REOPERATIVE
AESTHETIC & RECONSTRUCTIVE PLASTIC SURGERY

VOLUME II

REOPERATIVE AESTHETIC & RECONSTRUCTIVE PLASTIC SURGERY

EDITOR

JAMES C. GROTTING, M.D.

Professor

Division of Plastic Surgery, Department of Surgery

University of Alabama at Birmingham

Birmingham, Alabama

ILLUSTRATOR

BILL WINN

QMP

Quality Medical Publishing, Inc.

ST. LOUIS, MISSOURI

1995

Printed in the United States of America.

PUBLISHER *Karen Berger*
PROJECT MANAGER *Linda Kocher*
PRODUCTION *Susan Trail, Judy Bamert*
DESIGN *Diane M. Beasley*

Quality Medical Publishing, Inc.
11970 Borman Drive, Suite 222
St. Louis, Missouri 63146

LIBRARY OF CONGRESS CATALOGING-IN-PUBLICATION DATA

Reoperative aesthetic and reconstructive plastic surgery / editor, James C. Grotting ; illustrator, Bill Winn.
p. cm.
Includes bibliographical references and index.
ISBN 0-942219-25-2
1. Surgery, Plastic—Reoperation. I. Grotting, James C. II. Title: Reoperative aesthetic and reconstructive plastic surgery. III. Title: Aesthetic & reconstructive plastic surgery. IV. Title: Aesthetic and reconstructive plastic surgery.
[DNLM: 1. Surgery, Plastic—methods. 2. Reoperation—methods. WO 600 R424 1995]
RD118.7.R46 1995
617.9′5—dc20
DNLM/DLC
for Library of Congress 94-39605
CIP

VT/WW/WW
5 4 3 2 1

Contributors

Carl C. Askren, M.D.

Clinical Faculty, Department of Surgery, Plastic Surgery Section, University of California San Francisco–Fresno, Fresno, Calif.

Thomas J. Baker, M.D.

Assistant Clinical Professor of Surgery (Plastic), University of Miami School of Medicine, Miami, Fla.

Tracy M. Baker, M.D.

Attending Surgeon, Department of Plastic Surgery, Mercy Hospital, Miami, Fla.

Ricardo Baroudi, M.D.

Attendant Plastic Surgeon, Samaritan Hospital, Campinas City, São Paulo State, Brazil

John Bostwick III, M.D.

Professor and Chairman of Plastic, Reconstructive, and Maxillofacial Surgery, Department of Surgery, Emory University School of Medicine, Atlanta, Ga.

Gregory M. Buncke, M.D.

Clinical Assistant Professor of Surgery, Department of Surgery, Division of Plastic Surgery, University of California San Francisco, San Francisco, Calif.

Harry J. Buncke, M.D.

Clinical Professor, Department of Surgery, Division of Plastic Surgery, University of California San Francisco, San Francisco, Calif.

Dean E. Burget, Jr., M.D.

Director, West Grove Plastic Surgery Center, West Grove, Pa.

Gary C. Burget, M.D.

Clinical Assistant Professor, Section of Plastic and Reconstructive Surgery, The University of Chicago, Chicago, Ill.

H. Hollis Caffee, M.D.

Professor of Surgery, Department of Surgery, University of Florida College of Medicine, Gainesville, Fla.

James H. Carraway, M.D.

Professor of Plastic Surgery, Department of Plastic Surgery, Eastern Virginia Medical School, Norfolk, Va.

Grady B. Core, M.D.

Section Chief, Plastic and Reconstructive Surgery, Ochsner Medical Institutions; Assistant Clinical Professor of Surgery, Tulane University, New Orleans, La.

Paulo da Paula, M.D.

Visiting Fellow, Division of Plastic and Reconstructive Surgery, The Milton S. Hershey Medical Center, Pennsylvania State University, Hershey, Pa.

A. Lee Dellon, M.D.

Associate Professor of Plastic Surgery and Associate Professor of Neurosurgery, Johns Hopkins University School of Medicine, Baltimore, Md.

Loren H. Engrav, M.D.

Professor and Chief, Division of Plastic and Reconstructive Surgery, University of Washington/Harborview Medical Center, Seattle, Wash.

R. Jobe Fix, M.D.

Assistant Professor, Division of Plastic Surgery, Department of Surgery, The University of Alabama at Birmingham, Birmingham, Ala.

Leonard T. Furlow, Jr., M.D.

Clinical Professor, Department of Plastic Surgery, University of Florida College of Medicine, Gainesville, Fla.

Mabel Gamboa-Bobadilla, M.D.

Research Associate, Division of Plastic Surgery, Department of Surgery, University of Alabama at Birmingham, Birmingham, Ala.

PAUL M. GARDNER, M.D.

Fellow, Division of Plastic Surgery, Department of Surgery, University of Alabama at Birmingham, Birmingham, Ala.

ROBERT M. GOLDWYN, M.D.

Clinical Professor of Surgery, Harvard Medical School; Head, Division of Plastic Surgery, Beth Israel Hospital, Boston, Mass.

HOWARD L. GORDON, M.D.

Assistant Clinical Professor of Plastic Surgery, Department of Plastic Surgery, University of Miami School of Medicine, Miami, Fla.

JAMES C. GROTTING, M.D.

Professor, Division of Plastic Surgery, Department of Surgery, University of Alabama at Birmingham, Birmingham, Ala.

GABRIELA GUZMAN-STEIN, M.D.

Assistant Professor, Division of Plastic Surgery, Department of Surgery, University of Alabama at Birmingham, Birmingham, Ala.

JEFFREY M. HARTOG, D.M.D., M.D.

Former Fellow in Craniofacial Surgery, University of Miami School of Medicine, Miami, Fla.

CHARLES E. HORTON, M.D.

Professor of Plastic Surgery, Department of Plastic Surgery, Eastern Virginia Medical School, Norfolk, Va.

CHARLES E. HORTON, JR., M.D.

Assistant Professor of Clinical Urology, Department of Urology, Eastern Virginia Medical School, Norfolk, Va.

PAUL S. HOWARD, M.D.

Assistant Professor, Division of Plastic Surgery, Department of Surgery, University of Alabama at Birmingham, Birmingham, Ala.

IAN T. JACKSON, M.D., D.Sc. [Hon], F.R.C.S., F.A.C.S., F.R.A.C.S. [Hon]

Director, Institute for Craniofacial and Reconstructive Surgery; Director, Plastic Surgery Program; Section Chief, Plastic Surgery, Providence Hospital, Department of Plastic and Reconstructive Surgery, Institute for Craniofacial and Reconstructive Surgery, Southfield, Mich.

REBECCA L. JACKSON, M.D.
Private practice, Napa, Calif.

GARY S. KOPF, M.D.
Professor of Surgery, Department of Surgery, Yale University School of Medicine, New Haven, Conn.

BRADLEY K. LEWIS, M.D.
Resident, Department of General Surgery, Eastern Virginia Medical School, Norfolk, Va.

WILLIAM C. LINEAWEAVER, M.D.
Associate Professor, Division of Hand Surgery and Division of Plastic and Reconstructive Surgery, Stanford University Medical Center, Stanford, Calif.

ERNEST K. MANDERS, M.D.
Professor of Surgery and Pediatrics and Chief, Division of Plastic and Reconstructive Surgery, Department of Surgery, The Pennsylvania State University, Hershey, Pa.

PAUL N. MANSON, M.D.
Professor of Surgery, Department of Surgery, Johns Hopkins Hospital, Baltimore, Md.

VICTORIA R. MASEAR, M.D.
Associate Professor and Director of Orthopaedics, Department of Surgery, University of Alabama at Birmingham, Birmingham, Ala.

MARK W. MCCLUNG, M.D.
Assistant Professor, University of Missouri–Kansas City School of Medicine, Kansas City, Mo.

D. RALPH MILLARD, JR., M.D., Hon. F.R.C.S.Ed., Hon. F.R.C.S.Eng., O.D., Ja.
Light-Millard Professor of Plastic Surgery and Chief, Division of Plastic Surgery, Department of Surgery, University of Miami School of Medicine, Miami, Fla.

JAMES R. MILLER, M.D.
Chief Resident, Department of Plastic Surgery, Eastern Virginia Medical School, Norfolk, Va.

Alfonso Oliva, M.D.

Assistant Clinical Professor of Surgery, Department of Plastic and Reconstructive Surgery, University of California San Francisco, San Francisco, Calif.

F. Raymond Ortega, M.D.

Private practice, Bearwood Plastic and Reconstructive Surgery, Anderson, S.C.

Glenn E. Peters, M.D.

Associate Professor and Director, Division of Otolaryngology—Head and Neck Surgery, Department of Surgery, University of Alabama at Birmingham, Birmingham, Ala.

A. Esteban Reyes, M.D.

Research Fellow and Surgery Resident, Division of Plastic Surgery, Department of Surgery, University of Alabama at Birmingham, Birmingham, Ala.

Brunno Ristow, M.D.

Chief Emeritus, Division of Plastic Surgery, Pacific Presbyterian Medical Center, San Francisco, Calif.

Rod J. Rohrich, M.D.

Professor and Chairman, Division of Plastic Surgery, Department of Surgery, University of Texas Southwestern Medical Center at Dallas, Dallas, Tex.

Eva Rubin, M.D.

Professor, Chief of Mammography Section, Department of Radiology, University of Alabama at Birmingham, Birmingham, Ala.

Jack H. Sheen, M.D.

Clinical Professor of Surgery, Department of Surgery, Section of Plastic and Reconstructive Surgery, University of Southern California; Associate Clinical Professor, Department of Surgery, Division of Plastic Surgery, UCLA School of Medicine, Los Angeles, Calif.

Randy Sherman, M.D.

Associate Professor of Surgery, Orthopedic Surgery, and Neurologic Surgery; Chief, Division of Plastic and Reconstructive Surgery, University of Southern California, Los Angeles, Calif.

DAVID M. SION, M.D., F.R.C.S.(C)

Department of Plastic Surgery, Windsor Western Hospital, Windsor, Ontario, Canada

SUMNER A. SLAVIN, M.D.

Assistant Clinical Professor of Surgery (Plastic), Harvard Medical School; Associate in Plastic and Reconstructive Surgery, Beth Israel Hospital; Consultant in Surgical Oncology, Dana-Farber Cancer Institute, Boston, Mass.

RICHARD S. STAHL, M.D., M.B.A.

Associate Clinical Professor, Department of Surgery (Plastic), Yale University School of Medicine; Associate Chief, Department of Plastic Surgery, Yale–New Haven Hospital, New Haven, Conn.

DAVID R. STEPHENS, M.D.

Assistant Professor of Plastic Surgery and Director of Hand Surgery, Division of Plastic Surgery, Department of Surgery, University of Alabama at Birmingham, Birmingham, Ala.

JAMES M. STUZIN, M.D.

Clinical Instructor of Plastic Surgery, University of Miami School of Medicine, Miami, Fla.

MARSHALL M. URIST, M.D.

Professor and Director, Division of General Surgery, Department of Surgery, University of Alabama at Birmingham, Birmingham, Ala.

LUIS O. VASCONEZ, M.D.

Professor and Chief, Division of Plastic Surgery, Department of Surgery, University of Alabama at Birmingham, Birmingham, Ala.

S. ANTHONY WOLFE, M.D.

Clinical Professor of Plastic and Reconstructive Surgery, Department of Surgery, University of Miami School of Medicine, Miami, Fla.

To Ann, Jimmy, and Ben

and

To my mother, Shirley Bell Grotting,
and my father, John K. Grotting, M.D. (1915-1968),
who would have been awed by the tremendous advances in his beloved specialty of plastic surgery, yet reassured to know that kind and compassionate care of patients remains its foundation.

FOREWORD

All surgeons face reoperation as a routine part of their practices. We frequently find ourselves back in the operating room to refine results, manage complications, or complete the final stage in a sequenced procedure. The reoperative setting often tests even the most seasoned surgeon's skill and ingenuity.

Although the literature is filled with detailed accounts of primary operations, it is surprising how little attention has been devoted to secondary surgery. This excellent book edited by Dr. Grotting promises to fill that void. It is the first book devoted to this important subject and offers a wealth of information that will be of inestimable value to all plastic surgeons.

Dr. Grotting brings together an impressive group of contributors to share their personal experience in treating aesthetic and reconstructive patients undergoing difficult secondary or staged procedures. This book is filled with retrospective analyses by distinguished authors with extensive clinical experience who take a thoughtful look at some of their surgical conundrums.

Dr. Grotting has spent innumerable hours editing and collating the various contributions. In addition to this awesome responsibility he has also authored or co-authored many of the chapters himself. His skill as a surgeon and as an author and editor is evident throughout every page of this book. The final result represents a unique contribution that will benefit all plastic surgeons, both those just beginning their practice and the more experienced. Careful study of this remarkable two-volume work will not only permit us to face complications and the less than perfect result more confidently, but it will improve our primary results as well.

Luis O. Vasconez, M.D.

PREFACE

Reoperative plastic surgery assumes many guises in a plastic surgeon's practice. Although complications and salvage situations immediately come to mind when we think of reoperative surgery, the scope is far broader. It is the staged procedure carefully planned to preserve blood supply or the finishing touch that transforms a good result into a superlative one. Perhaps it represents a surgical intervention to treat the recurrence of disease or the continued biologic changes of aging. It may be the creative solution for improving an unsatisfactory result—the nemesis of all surgeons. Whatever the definition, much of our practice is reoperative in nature. The thread of commonality uniting all reoperative surgery is that the plastic surgeon finds himself confronting tissue planes biologically altered by the effects of wound healing. This challenge often demands more innovative solutions and greater skill than the initial surgical intervention; it is more right brained than left, more creative than analytic. Much like a chess game, strategic planning is the critical element defining a successful outcome.

When faced with any difficult problem, we typically turn to the literature and to the masters who have preceded us to guide our way. In secondary surgery the answers we seek are more elusive. Despite the complex nature of these procedures, their artful execution and pitfalls have received scant attention in the literature. Thus we often approach these secondary cases with surgical plans derived from our own personal and anecdotal experience only to find ourselves adrift without a nautical chart or compass.

This book is in response to the need for a source of information to which to turn when confronted with secondary problems—a synthesis if you will. Similar to the travel clubs so popular in plastic surgery that have long been a rich source of shared experience and verbal problem solving, this book culls the wisdom and clinical advice from a national and international group of expert contributors. It is an attempt to draw on the cumulative experience of master surgeons to increase our chances of obtaining a favorable result. It would serve us well to have a road map—to know in advance that a brilliantly conceived plan may already have been clinically applied with an unfortunate outcome because of unanticipated tissue failure and to know that an alternative surgical approach would provide a safer, more effective solution. We have focused on those clinical conditions in which previous surgery has resulted in significant tissue changes and in which secondary correction requires an approach that differs from the primary plan. By analyzing reoperative conditions, we seek to better understand the mechanisms by which they occur, thus developing a strategy for avoiding problems and promoting favorable outcomes. We also attempt to capture the surgical artistry and vision that enable experienced surgeons to produce unparalleled results.

The contributors to this book were carefully selected for their technical skill, their innovative approach to problem solving, and their extensive experience in a particular area. These chapters represent each author's personal approach to specific surgical conundrums. A virtual gold mine of untapped information is contained within these pages as these authors share personal insights, explain how they refine their results, and take the reader through the critical planning process essential to achieving superior results. The perspective of each chapter is dictated by its unique subject matter. Some chapters address primarily complications. Others discuss staged procedures, whereas others examine a mix of problems and planned revisions. Some chapters focus on one clinical case and use it as a springboard to discuss a wide range of problems, whereas others contain numerous case examples to highlight individual anatomic challenges.

The scope of this book is both aesthetic and reconstructive; the distinction becomes blurred in the reoperative setting. The 45 chapters are divided into seven sections starting with the reoperative environment and basic issues of scarring, tissue movement, and transplantation and then proceeding anatomically to investigate specific reoperative problems of the head and neck, breast, chest wall, trunk, and extremities. To make the reading process as smooth as possible, text and illustrations are in close proximity to each other. Hundreds of patient examples and operative sequences have been described and illustrated in color to assist the reader in understanding the nuances of various operative approaches.

One of the primary criticisms levied against any contributor work is the unevenness and overlapping of material from one chapter to another. A concentrated effort was made to obviate this problem by providing a basic format and structure to shape the authors' presentations and by investing enormous time and effort writing my own chapters and editing others to ensure a consistent approach. Notwithstanding these guiding principles, the contributors had the freedom to vary the format when the topic so dictated. In addition, to facilitate the learning process, some overlap still remains when the information is integral to the understanding of a problem or a clinical description. Every attempt was made, however, to retain the author's personality and distinctive style. The wit and individual style displayed by each contributor permit the reader a rare insight into the creative spirit that guides the scalpel.

As the writing process draws to a close, my initial enthusiasm and vitality begin to resurface. I trust that this legacy will be worth the sacrifices and the stolen moments from family and practice. My desire is that the reader and patients will be the beneficiaries of this first attempt to harvest the collective wisdom from those who have risen to the challenge of reoperative surgery.

James C. Grotting, M.D.

ACKNOWLEDGMENTS

No book of this type could possibly come to fruition without teamwork. Although I am privileged to have been the editor for these volumes, I am deeply indebted to my co-authors and contributors whose creative minds and vast experiences culminated in the breadth of information presented herein.

I have been very fortunate to have been associated with an outstanding team of publishing professionals. Karen Berger, president of QMP, deserves tremendous credit for her vision of the value of this type of resource to the specialty of plastic surgery. Her personal support during many weekends and late nights working together writing, rewriting, and editing manuscripts made my job tremendously easier, especially when spirits were low! During the writing of this book, many of the QMP staff became like family. Project manager, Linda Kocher, quarterbacked us inside the 20-yard line, and Carolita Deter, to whom I am especially grateful, took the ball into the end zone! To both of these exceptionally talented editors, I truly stand in awe and admiration. Once the pieces were in, Susan Trail produced the layout and Judy Bamert monitored the illustration program. They are responsible for making this book user friendly! Diane Beasley was able to sort through my ideas and old photographs and extract design elements to produce an attractive book. I am indebted to all of the other QMP professionals who have worked tirelessly to make this book happen.

Probably no one is happier to see this book completed than my administrative assistant, Judy Hunt. I am tremendously grateful to her for keeping me organized throughout the writing and editing process as well as serving as the point person for all communication with the contributors and publisher. Similarly, I want to express my sincere appreciation to my partners, our residents, and our nurses, who have offered suggestions for the book and participated in the care of many of the patients discussed in these pages. I also want to thank Dr. Mansoor Saleh for his review of the material related to coagulation.

We were extremely fortunate to be able to recruit Bill Winn for the artwork. He is one of the most gifted medical illustrators in the country. Bill has an exceptional talent for visualizing tissue movement and structure, and his illustrations have helped communicate ideas much more effectively than we could possibly have done with the written word alone.

Finally, I want to acknowledge the tremendous support of my wife, Ann. She has put up with my frequent absences during evenings and weekends while I pored over manuscripts and grew to accept this book as our constant companion. Similarly, my two boys, Jimmy and Ben, have been deprived of my attention and time during the many hours necessary to devote to this project. Without the understanding and support of my wife and children, I would not possibly have seen this book through to completion. I truly hope that all will be proud of the fruits of our labor.

CONTENTS

VOLUME I

III Reoperative Surgery of the Head and Neck

Volume II

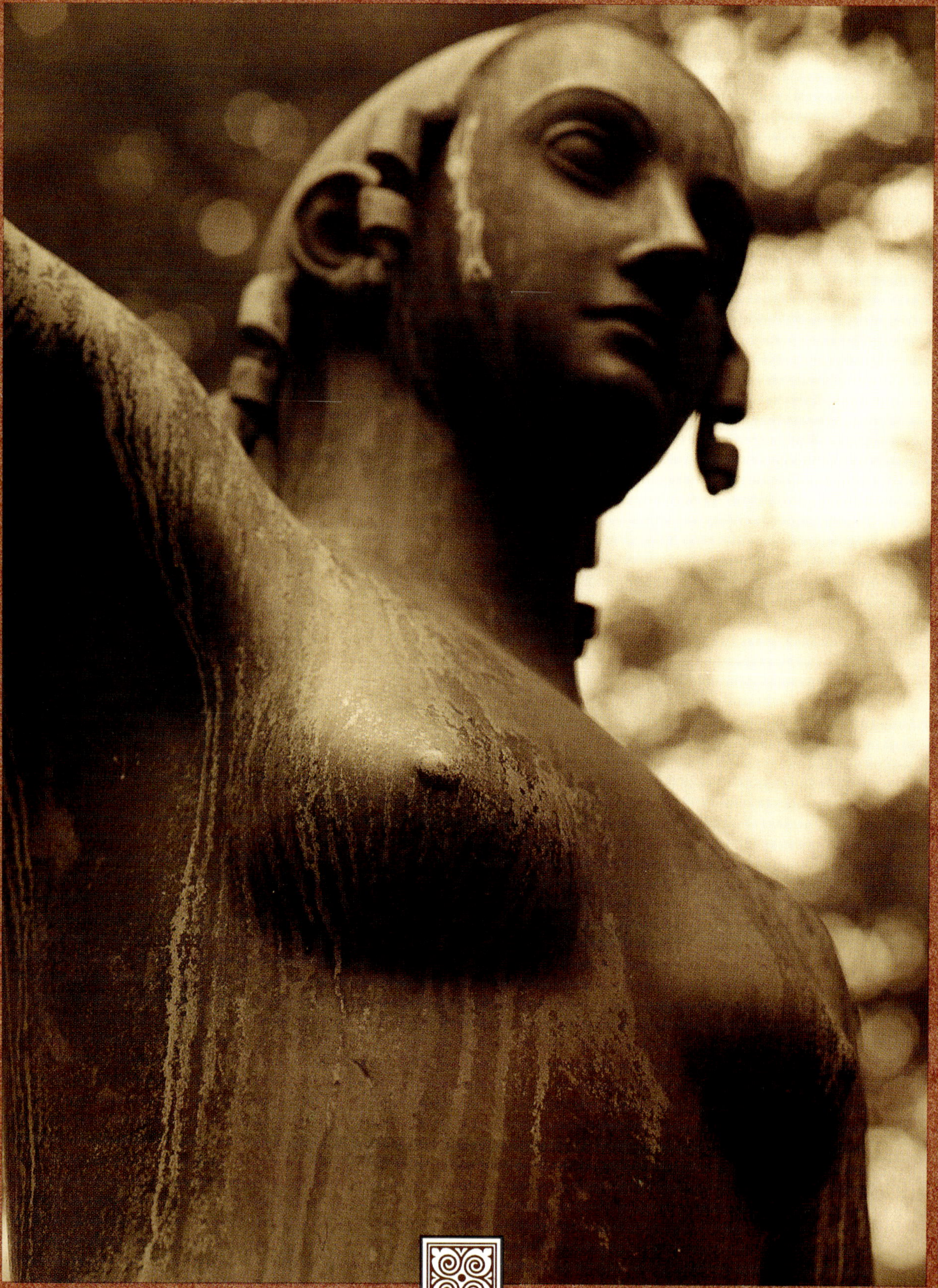

27

Reoperative Breast Surgery After Reduction Mammaplasty and Mastopexy

James C. Grotting, M.D., and Carl C. Askren, M.D.

Reoperative Problems

Complications
- Hematoma/seroma
- Fat necrosis
- Skin necrosis
- Wound dehiscence
- Infection
- Nipple-areola complex loss

Aesthetic problems
- Breast mound
  - Asymmetry
  - Contour deformity
  - Recurrent ptosis
  - Overreduction
  - Insufficient reduction
  - Scarring
- Nipple-areola complex
  - Malposition
  - Irregular size and shape
  - Depigmentation
  - Retraction or protrusion
  - Scarring

Other conditions
- Occult cancer
- Virginal hypertrophy

Every surgeon tries to obtain a perfect result in aesthetic breast surgery without resorting to revisional surgery. If a secondary surgery is needed following reduction mammaplasty or mastopexy, this situation implies that an unfavorable result developed and that the patient is somehow dissatisfied. The source of this dissatisfaction may range from inadequate counseling of the patient with unrealistic expectations (resulting in inadequate reduction) to a surgical mishap (resulting in massive fat necrosis).

In the past some surgeons advocated planned two-stage reductions in order to minimize the incidence of complications. As our understanding of the blood supply to the breasts has improved, these techniques have fallen by the wayside.[1] In an effort to maintain short scars, new approaches have also recommended staged reduction for large-volume breasts.[2]

The multitude of procedures available for breast reduction attest to the inability to find a universally applicable solution to the many different patient presentations. Most reduced breasts, no matter what technique is performed, change shape with time. The need for reoperation for aesthetic reasons depends on the original technique selected and the judgment used in applying that technique to a particular patient. This decision also depends on the ability of the patient and surgeon to cope with that imperfection.[3,4] Long-term follow-up is essential to fully assess the results of surgery. However, as these patients are among the most satisfied and gratifying to treat, they are also a mobile population and often may not return for follow-up once they are completely healed.

Reoperative surgery of the breast may be indicated for aesthetic problems or for complications of the primary surgery. Reoperation may also be necessary for miscellaneous conditions such as occult cancer or regrowth in cases of virginal hypertrophy.

The optimal timing for reoperation is determined by the clinical situation. For most secondary deformities reoperation is best carried out after the scars have fully matured (i.e., when the edema has resolved and the scars have become pale and soft). Complete healing may take up to 1 year or longer. Some situations such as impending nipple loss or wound dehiscence do require early intervention.

The goals of treatment echo those of the primary procedure: attractive breast shape, symmetry, minimal scars, round nipples with good sensibility, appropriate nipple-areola position, and long-lasting result.

ANATOMIC CONSIDERATIONS

The blood supply to the breast and the innervation of the nipple are two important anatomic considerations when planning reoperation of the breast. The incisions and parenchymal dissection performed in the previous surgery alter the vascular architecture, and these factors must be considered and integrated into the operative plan. For example, the inferior pedicle technique separates the nipple from the internal mammary perforators and the external mammary artery; the pedicle is based on the anterolateral and anteromedial intercostal perforators contained in the fat above the pectoralis fascia and in the subcutaneous plexus.

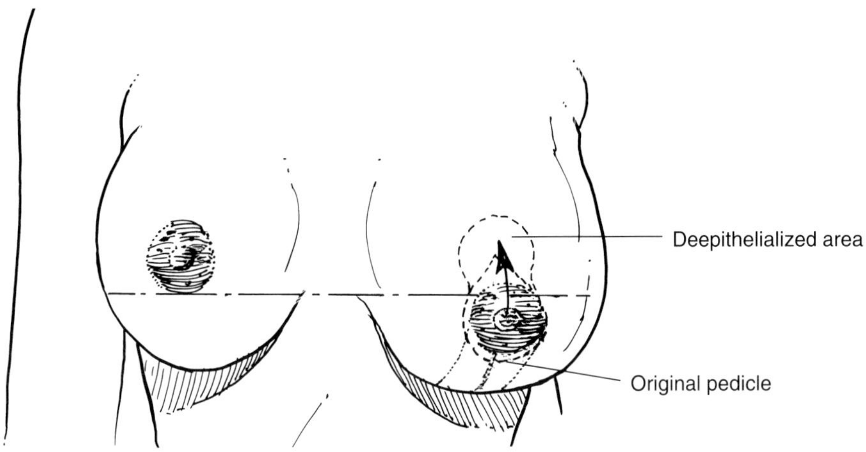

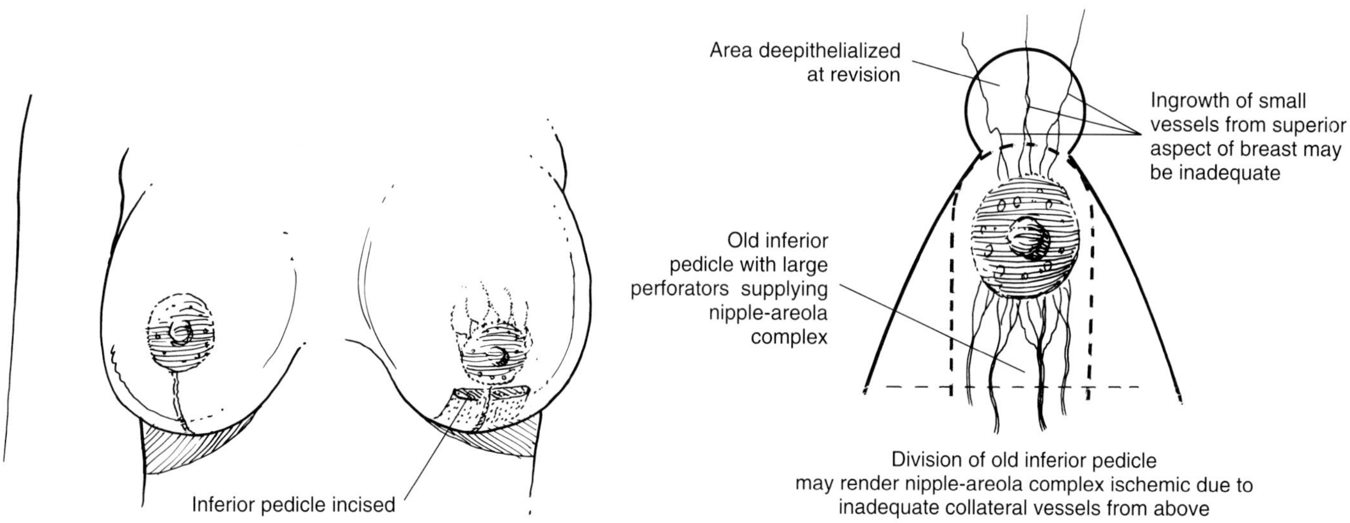

Secondary revisions based on a superior pedicle or other techniques that divides the inferior pole of the breast can risk causing necrosis of the nipple-areola complex. Fortunately most secondary surgeries do not require a large-volume reduction.

The risk of decreased sensibility in the nipple following secondary surgeries is increased with any procedure that involves resection of breast parenchyma. Since the course of the segmental nerves that supply the nipple follows that of the arteries, the same principles that hold true for the blood supply also apply to the nerves. The state of nipple-areola sensation should be documented before secondary revisions.

PATIENT EVALUATION

In general, patients who undergo reduction mammaplasty are among the most satisfied patients. However, no matter how much care is taken, complications occasionally occur. A discussion of complications is an integral part of the preoperative patient consultation. Complications involving the nipple-areola complex are particularly troublesome, and the possible need for intraoperative conversion to free nipple grafts must be discussed preoperatively. Preoperative consultations with the patient are essential for developing rapport, assessing whether the patient is a suitable candidate and does not have unreasonable expectations, and selecting the proper reoperative technique. Information learned from these sessions will aid in reducing the risk of postoperative complications or problems.

There are multiple reasons for patient dissatisfaction, not all of which can be remedied by additional surgery. Poor communication between the surgeon and patient may result in misunderstandings and unrealistic expectations. For example, in obese patients with true gigantomastia it is virtually impossible to reduce a breast to an aesthetically shaped B cup in a single stage; however, this scenario is often what patients request and expect.

The need for a secondary procedure may become obvious anytime from the first postoperative day to years later. However, aside from early complications, most deformities are well established by approximately 3 months postoperatively. Therefore the 3-month postoperative visit is an important turning point for the patient and surgeon. Does she like the result? Has her body image altered? Has her lifestyle changed? Has her ability to wear normal clothing improved? It is remarkable how many patients will be totally satisfied at this stage regardless of the small aesthetic deformities or asymmetries that the surgeon may notice! The surgeon must resist the urge to point out these minor imperfections to the patient. Why precipitate dissatisfaction in an otherwise “happy customer”?

On the other hand, there are a variety of secondary deformities that the patient may wish to have treated. If these problems become a source of concern for the patient, a clear plan must be laid out. The patient should be told what to expect and given a timetable for any secondary surgery that may be necessary.

COMPLICATIONS

Complications have a wide range of presentations: some minor, others major. Minor complications include nipple cyanosis (which may progress to necrosis), wound dehiscence, local infections, and inclusion cysts. Major complications include slough of the nipple-areola complex, large skin sloughs or hematomas, infection, and necrosis of large areas of fat or breast parenchyma.

Hematoma and Seroma

Hematomas are identified by an acute breast asymmetry with pain and ecchymosis. The patient usually complains of disproportionate unilateral pain. Hematomas may occur as late as 9 days postoperatively[5] and should be evacuated once detected. Exploration to rule out the presence of a hematoma is also indicated if there is impending necrosis of the nipple. We prefer to drain acute hematomas in the operating room with the patient under general anesthesia. To treat hematomas that are detected several days postoperatively, it may be possible to aspirate or drain the site by reopening only a small portion of the wound. We place a 1-inch Penrose drain, which seems to maintain an evacuated cavity better than a closed suction system.

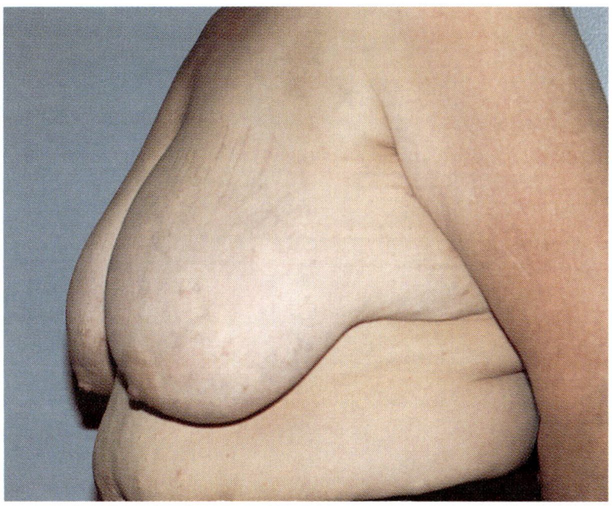

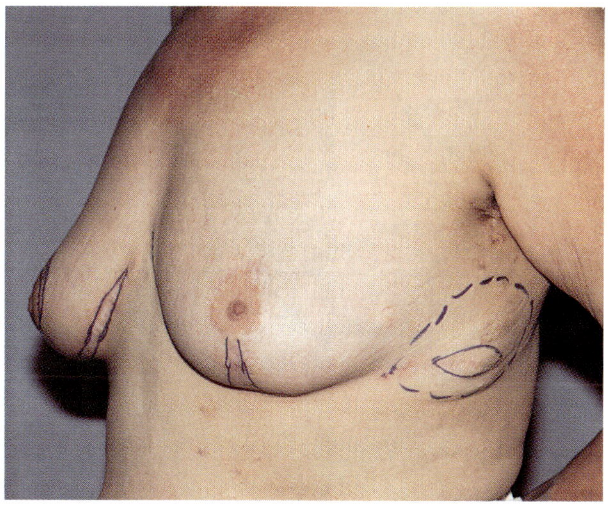

Hematomas can occur following secondary surgery as well as following primary surgery. After an inferior pedicled breast reduction, this patient had redundant fat and skin in the low area of the axilla, a common postoperative deformity in overweight patients. Because the lateral portion of the inframammary scar extended into this area, a direct excision was planned in addition to revision of the scars.

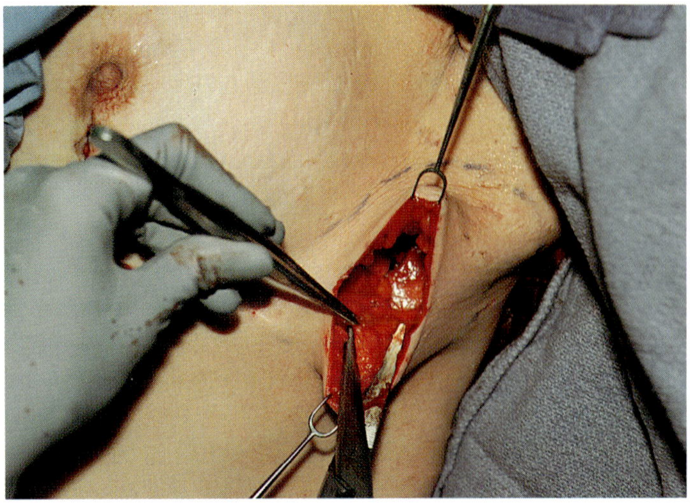

If no additional skin is to be resected, these deformities can be contoured using suction-assisted lipectomy. In this case direct defatting was performed. No drains were placed.

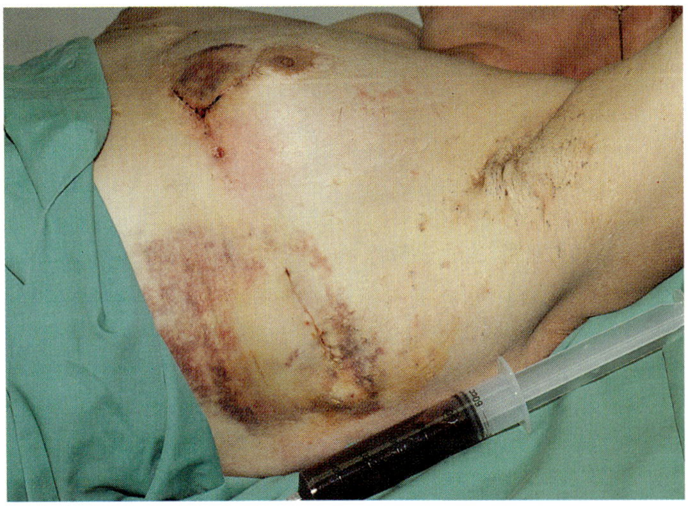

Five days postoperatively the patient returned to the office with an obvious hematoma at the operative site as well as early cellulitis, possibly related to chronic axillary hidradenitis.

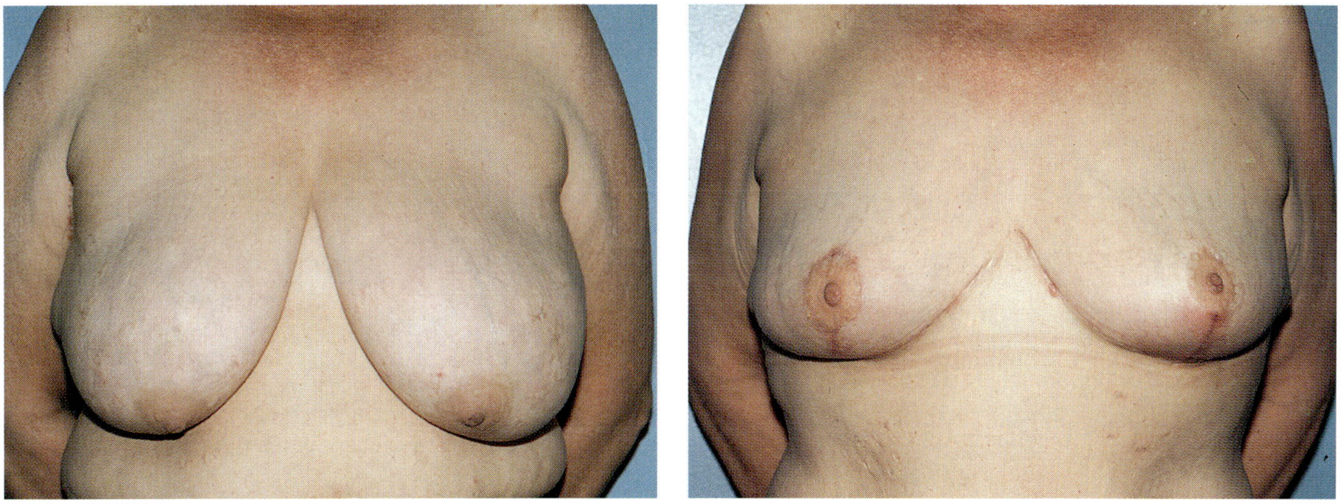

The hematoma was aspirated and the patient was prescribed an antibiotic regimen. She recovered uneventfully.

Seromas may have a more insidious onset. They usually occur laterally or even in the low area of the axilla. Treatment is similar to that for small late-onset hematomas. If small, seromas may be aspirated once or twice a week. However, a seroma of 50 cc or more will resolve most predictably by the placement of a Penrose drain for 1 week, which prevents reaccumulation.

Nipple Necrosis

Nipple necrosis results from vascular compromise. Vascular complications occur when the vasculature of the breast is disregarded, when technique selection is inappropriate, or in rare cases in association with certain conditions such as collagen vascular disease. Fortunately vascular complications diminish in frequency as a surgeon gains experience. The Biesenberger technique had a high percentage of these complications—up to one third of patients in some series experienced these problems.[6] Vascular compromise occurred as the result of the elevation of long, thin skin flaps with little regard for or understanding of the blood supply to the breast. With a better knowledge of the vascular anatomy of the breast, the rate of such complications has dropped significantly.

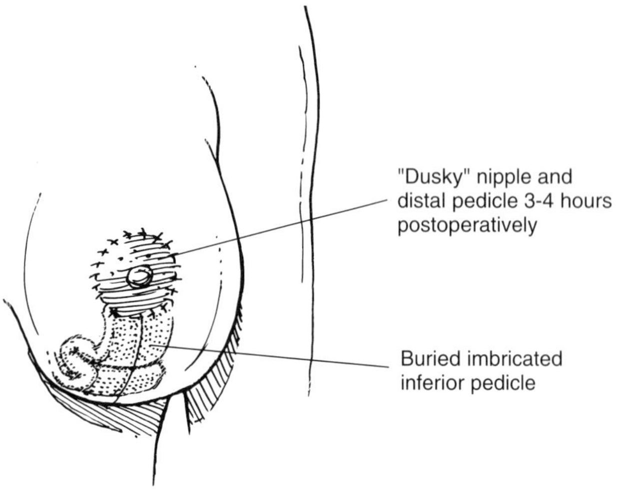

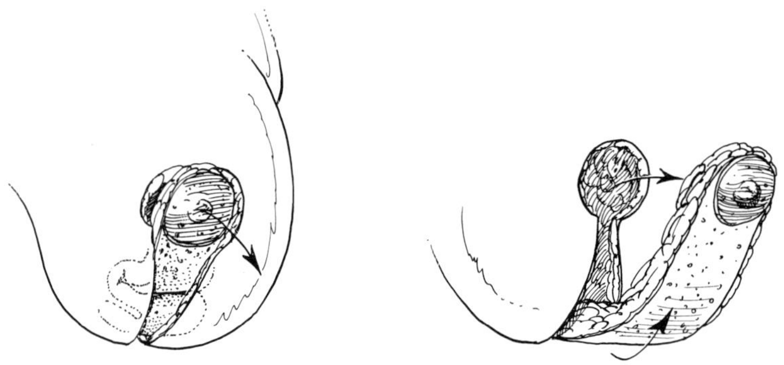

Wound is reopened, pedicle is unfolded, and pedicle is irrigated with warm saline solution

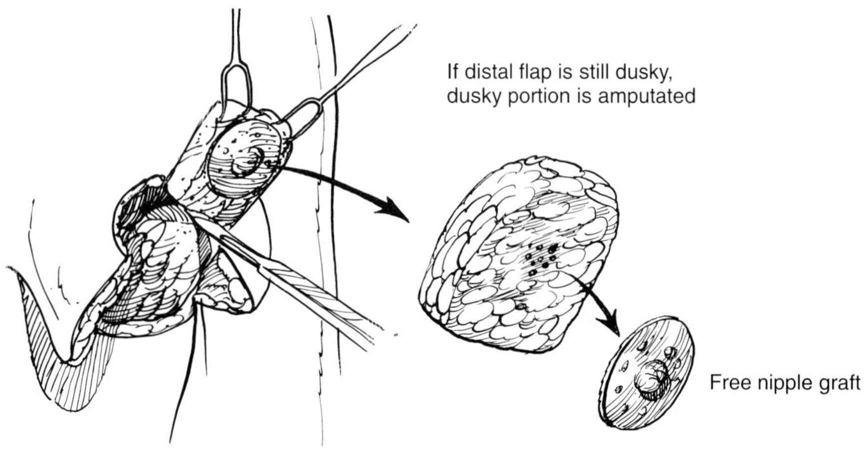

During the primary procedure the circulation of the nipple must be assessed at the final closure of the flaps. The vascularity of the pale, soft nipple can be expected to improve. The blue and engorged state of a nipple, however, may be the first signs of impending necrosis.[7] Fluorescein has been used to assess nipple viability.[8-10] If a viable nipple becomes congested as the keyhole window is closed, delayed primary closure with preplaced monofilament suture is an alternative.[9] If the closure is too tight, compromising the nipple or skin flap circulation, sutures may be released to improve circulation. The pedicle should be evaluated for kinking and/or excessive tension. Conversion of the pedicled nipple-areola complex to a free composite graft should be considered if no correctable cause can be identified.[7] Leeches have also been successfully employed to treat venous congestion when improvement cannot be obtained with any other mechanical manipulation.[11]

Free Composite Nipple Graft

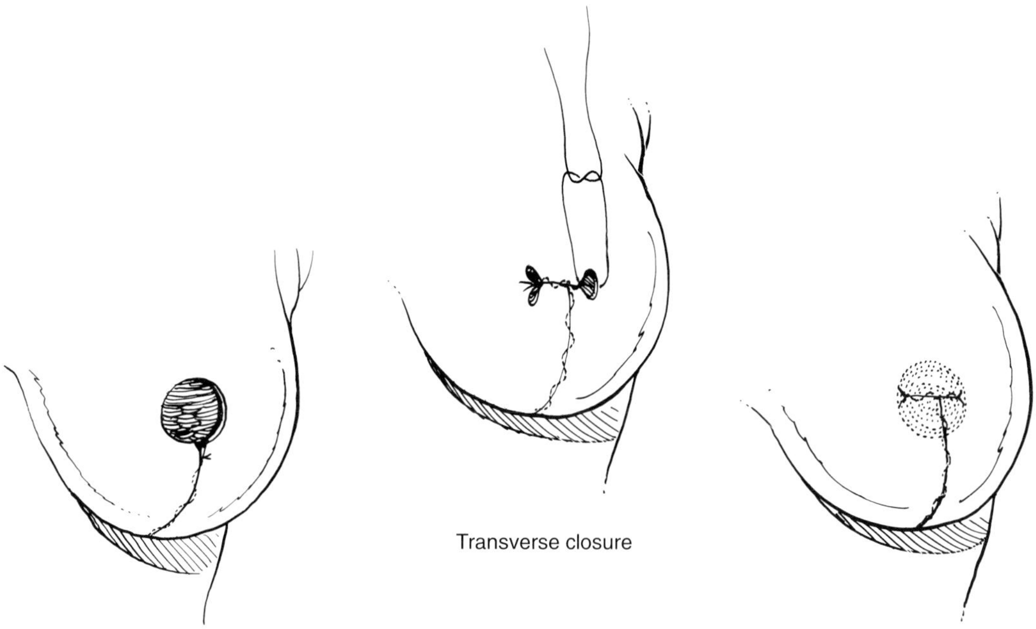

Once the decision has been made to convert the pedicled nipple-areola complex to a free composite nipple graft, the most important consideration is the vascularity of the recipient bed. Almost without exception if the nipple-areola complex is poorly perfused, then the pedicle from which it is excised will also have marginal vascularity for a variable distance. One has two choices—either to trim the pedicle back to healthy perfused tissue and advance the pedicle into the keyhole or to debride the pedicle as necessary and then close the keyhole with a pursestring suture or transversely. Since the pedicle often will not reach the keyhole, we prefer to graft directly to the breast skin. The keyhole can be closed either with a pursestring suture or transversely with medial advancement of the dog ears at either end of the closure. Regardless of how the keyhole is closed, one should attempt to limit the scar so that it does not extend beyond the perimeter of the graft.

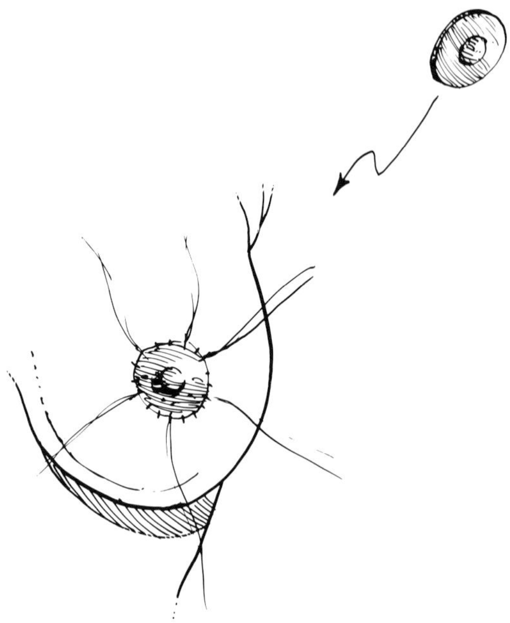

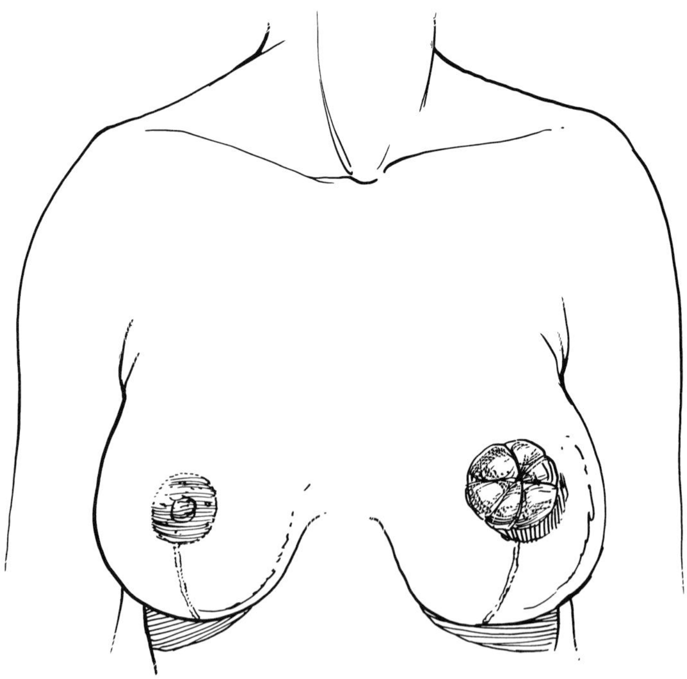

The nipple-areola complex is defatted, keeping in mind that this graft is intended to be a composite graft rather than a skin graft. As such, it should include at least some muscle fibers so that theoretically contractility of the complex is maintained. However, under these circumstances graft take with appropriate pigmentation is preferable to the inclusion of deep tissue components. Therefore one should err on the side of a thin composite graft. We prefer to stabilize the graft with a tie-over bolster dressing.

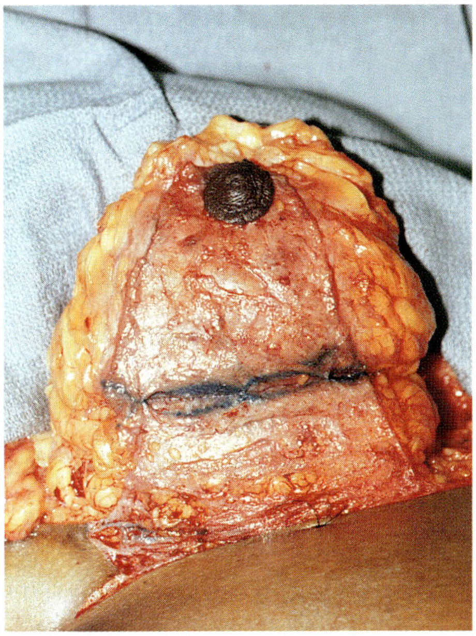

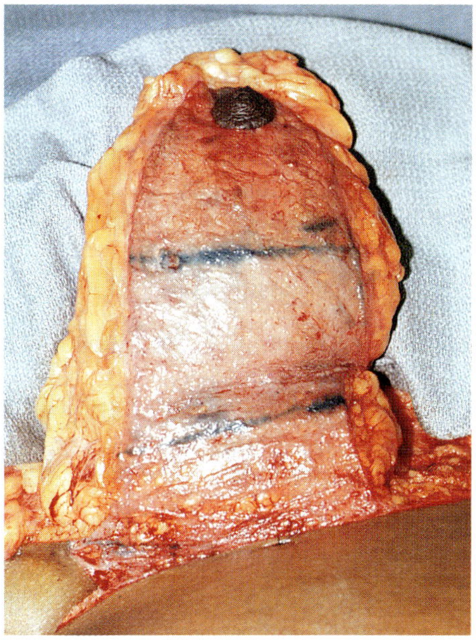

Intraoperatively the nipple-areola complex is noted to be soft and pale following the placement of dermal plication sutures to shorten the pedicle length. Therefore the sutures are immediately removed and the pedicle is irrigated with warm saline solution. No improvement in the perfusion occurs and the decision is made to convert to free nipple grafts.

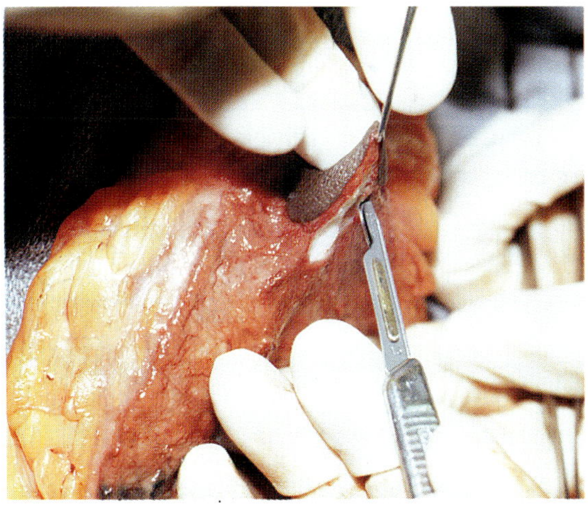

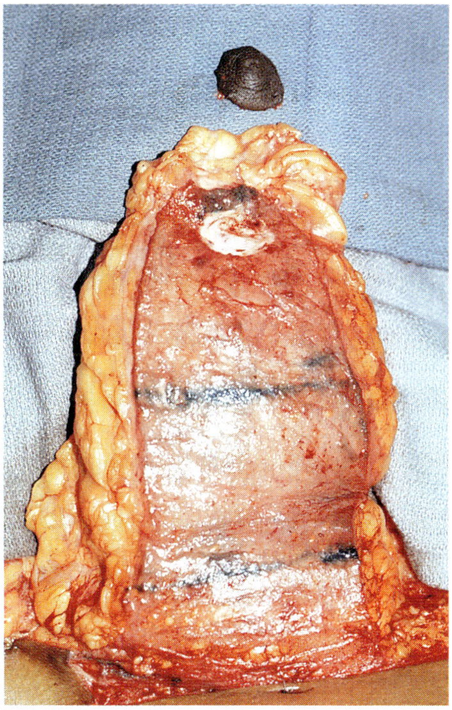

The nipple-areola complex is removed as a composite graft.

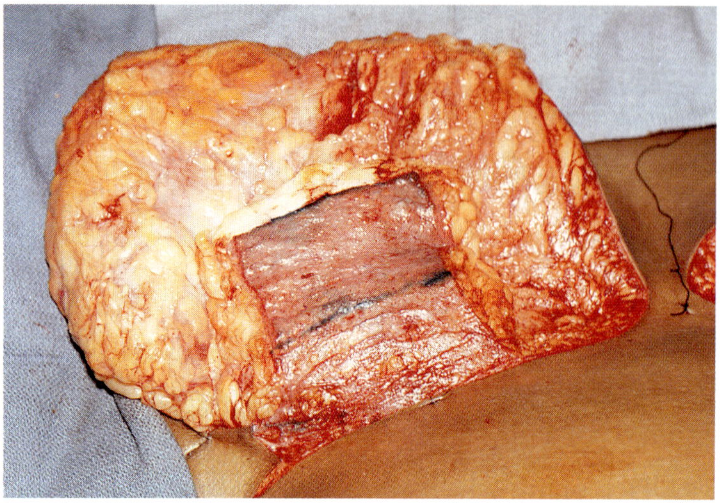

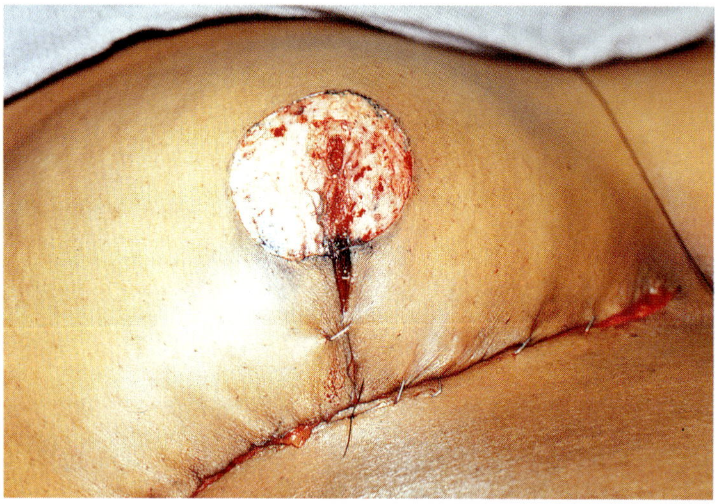

The inferior pedicle is trimmed back to the level at which satisfactory red bleeding is noted. This flap can then be simply tacked to the chest wall to improve projection and fill. The medial and lateral skin flaps are reapproximated, and a disk of skin is deepithelialized at the appropriate position to accept the composite graft.

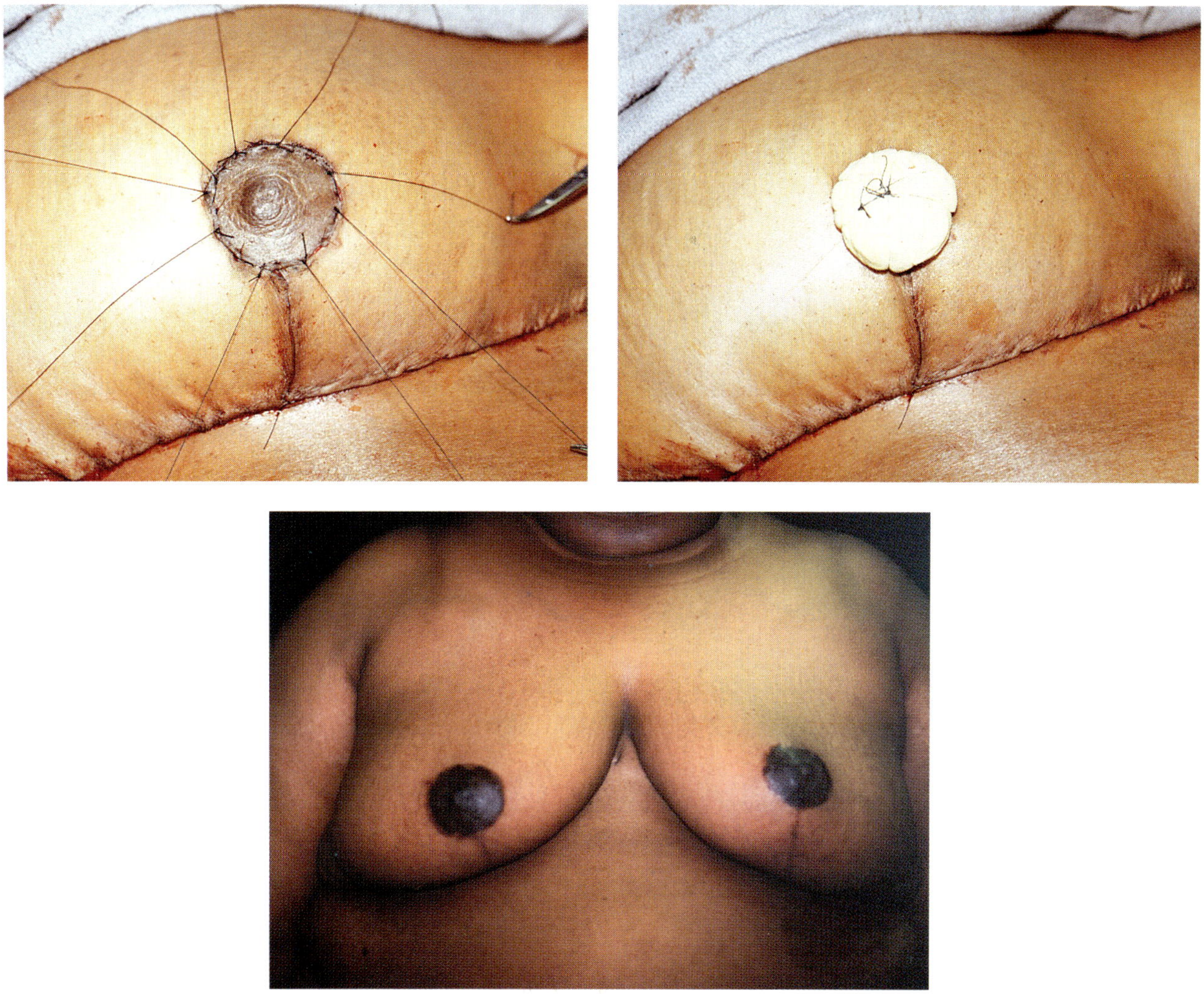

The composite graft is sutured into position and secured with a tie-over bolster dressing. The postoperative result is shown.

Postoperatively reoperation is indicated if the removal of a few stitches does not improve the situation. Hematoma or torsion of the pedicle may cause necrosis; these possibilities must be explored and addressed immediately. More breast tissue may need to be resected to decrease the tension of the closure. Areas for tissue resection are determined based on the blood supply of the nipple-areola. Again excision and free nipple grafting may be required.

Minor necrosis of the skin or areola will result in wound separation and can be treated conservatively with dressings. Major skin or nipple loss is best treated by surgical debridement. Delayed primary closure may be accomplished if the wound bed permits. Large sloughs should be treated with surgical debridement to reduce healing time. Loss of the nipple areola complex, either partial or complete, requires reconstruction by the same methods used for nipple-areola complex reconnection following mastectomy.

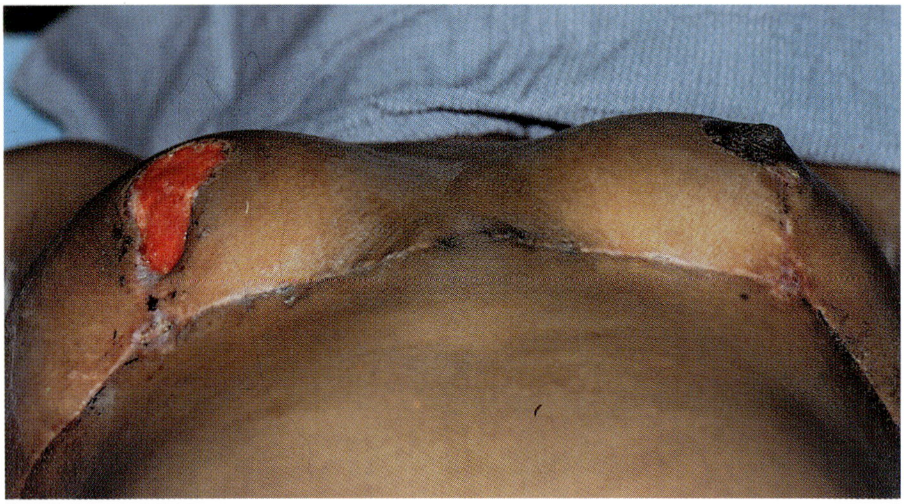

Despite pedicle reexploration and removal of tension sutures, this patient eventually suffered complete loss of the nipple-areola complex.

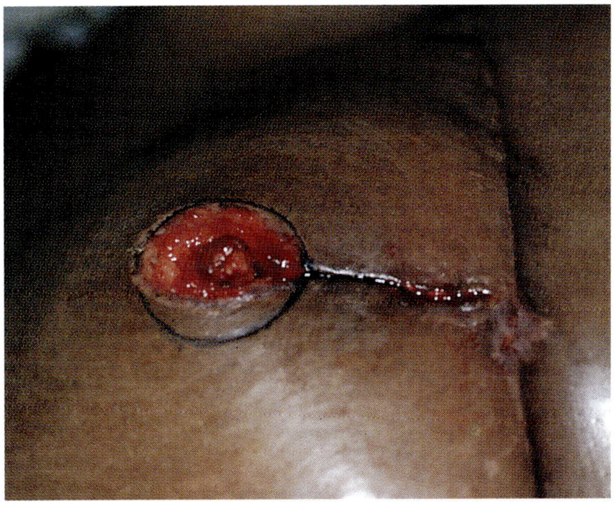
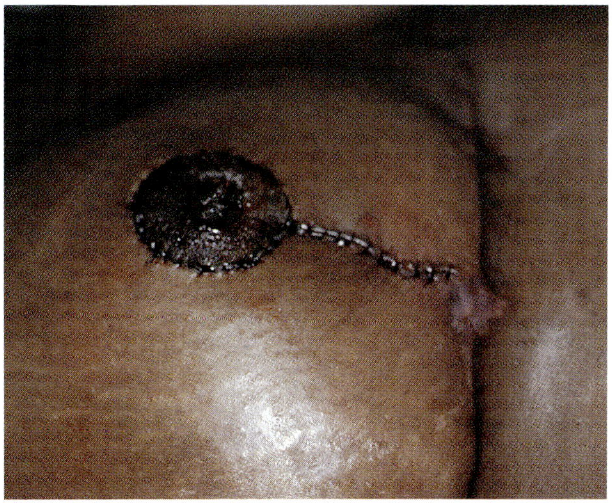

By 6 weeks postoperatively the wound had completely granulated. Under considerable pressure to correct the poor result, an attempt was made to secondarily close the vertical wound and reconstruct the nipple with a fat flap and full-thickness graft from the groin crease. Perhaps a more prudent course would have been simply to obtain a closed wound at this time and delay formal nipple reconstruction until the tissues were soft.

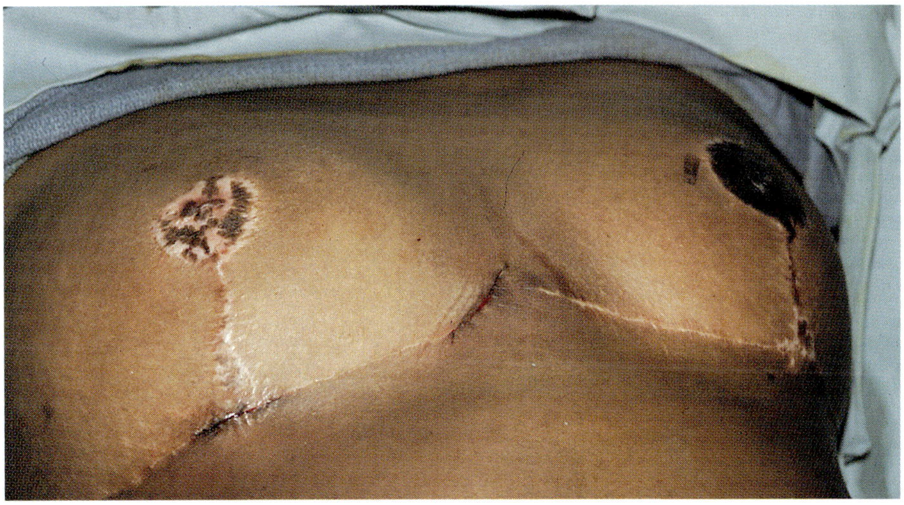

Ultimately, poor nipple shape and areolar depigmentation ensued. Although these problems could have been corrected with secondary nipple reconstruction and nipple-areola tattooing, the patient chose not to proceed with further surgery.

Fat Necrosis

Fat necrosis, if minor, manifests itself as localized drainage for days to weeks that ends with a wide scar or dimpling of the drainage tract. Secondary infection may develop. These problems may require a revisional procedure to improve the appearance. If fat necrosis is massive, there is associated glandular necrosis and the healing process is prolonged. Significant asymmetry can result because of volume loss. A major reconstructive effort may be needed, possibly requiring an implant, scar revision, and partial or total nipple reconstruction.

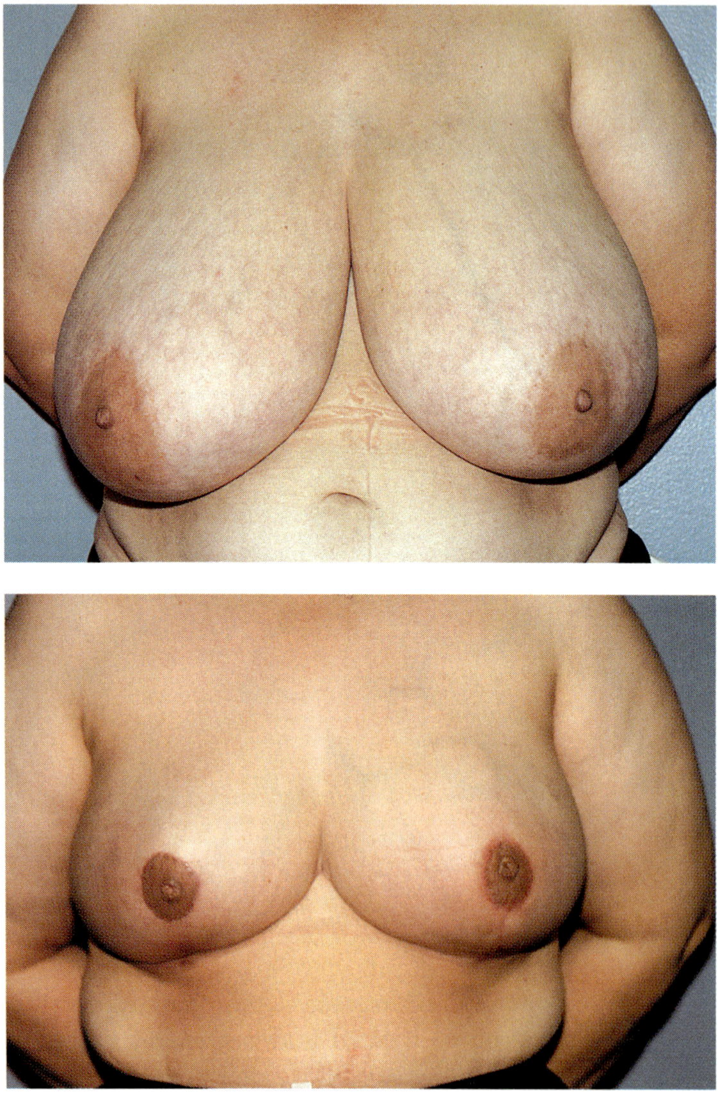

This patient underwent breast reduction via the inferior pedicle technique. Three months postoperatively an area of fat necrosis developed in the superior aspect of the left breast, which was manifested as a subtle fullness.

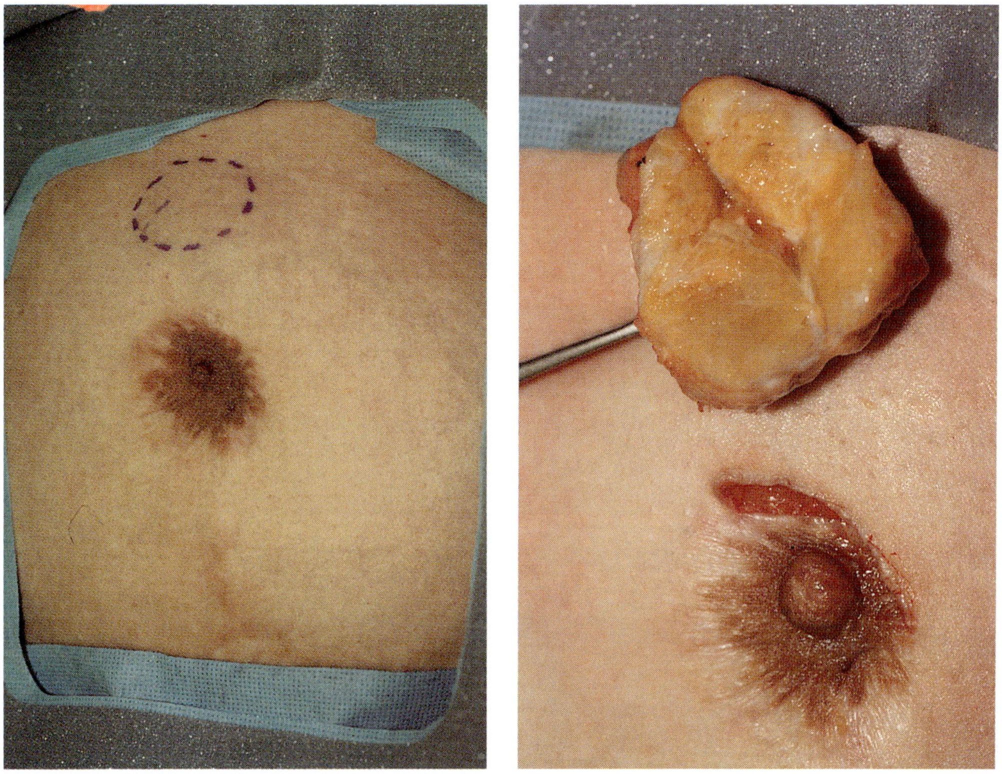

One year postoperatively the mass was smaller but persistent. For this reason the dense, calcified, necrotic tissue was excised through a periareolar incision. Healing was uneventful.

Wound Dehiscence

Wound dehiscence occurs most often after very large reductions. Breast weight is thought to be a major factor. It most commonly develops at the inverted T of the incision as a result of excessive tension. To prevent this complication, an adequate amount of breast tissue must be excised to allow closure with minimal tension. However, the breast flaps must not be thinned so much that circulation is impaired as this also will lead to wound breakdown.

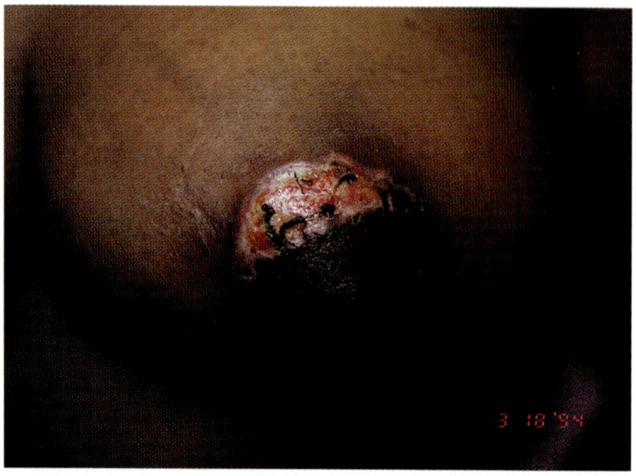

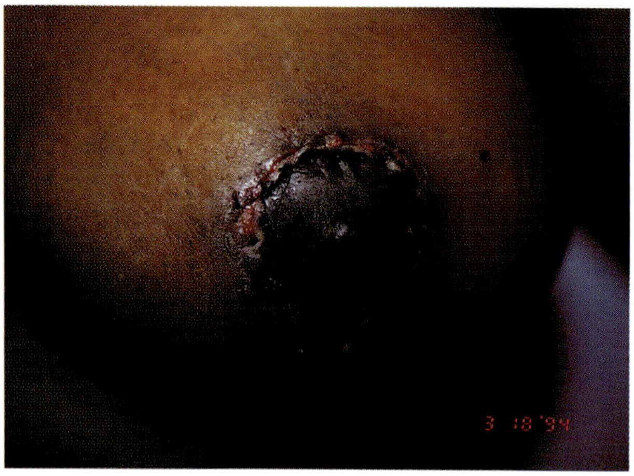

Early suture removal occasionally may account for wound disruption. In this event the skin should be immediately resutured, which was performed in this patient with areolar dehiscence following suture removal. However, if other factors such as excessive tension or marginal devascularization contribute to the dehiscence, resuturing will fail and the wound should be allowed to heal by secondary intention.

Local wound care is all that is required for the treatment of wound dehiscences that are not amenable to resuturing. Antibiotic therapy should be administered if there is associated infection. These patients must be examined frequently and reassured that in most cases conservative treatment yields the best results. A wide scar invariably results; scar revision can be performed secondarily.

AESTHETIC PROBLEMS

Aesthetic problems range from wide scars to nipple distortion to gland asymmetries. In general, breasts are asymmetric to varying degrees preoperatively. Pointing this fact out to the patient preoperatively will avoid a postoperative explanation by the surgeon that sounds like an excuse. Depending on the magnitude of the reduction, small degrees of asymmetry are common postoperatively. The smaller the breast, the more the asymmetry will be apparent.

BREAST MOUND PROBLEMS

Asymmetries

Correction of primary breast asymmetries can be a tremendous challenge to the plastic surgeon because the operated breast continues to change shape postoperatively, whereas the normal unoperated breast does not. Therefore one must try to preoperatively assess how these dynamic forces will eventually influence the final breast shape. Fortunately asymmetries that occur after primary reduction usually are not severe and the surgeon has a variety of surgical options from which to choose for revision. These asymmetries may be the result of differences in either volume or contour. With contour problems the patient will state usually that the problem is disguised by wearing a brassiere. With major volume discrepancies, one cup of the brassiere may fit normally, whereas she may "spill out" of the other side. Careful study of the postoperative photographs may assist the reoperative surgeon better than direct examination in diagnosing the problem.

Major asymmetries are largely preventable by careful preoperative assessment and removal of the correct amount of tissue. Sitting the patient up intraoperatively to assess symmetry before final closure is the best way to assess the volume of both breasts. In addition, palpating the thickness of the flaps on each side helps to judge whether excess tissue is being left behind. ***More attention should be paid to the volume of tissue left behind than to that which is removed.***

Correction of volume asymmetries is accomplished in much the same way that primary breast asymmetries are treated. It is usually best to reduce the large breast further rather than to augment the small side. The small breast is used as a model. Careful measurements are taken from the sternal notch to nipple, nipple to inframammary fold in the midline of the breast, and medial sternal line laterally to the nipple. These measurements are transferred to the large breast. The amount of additional volume resection necessary is sometimes difficult to determine. However, one must imagine how the final breast mound will look by pinching the marked lines together and comparing the appearance to that of the opposite side. Some settling of the breast mound will invariably occur in the first 3 postoperative months. Thus the nipple-areola complex will usually become elevated to some degree as the parenchyma settles into the lower pole of the breast, with resultant lengthening of the vertical limb of the closure.

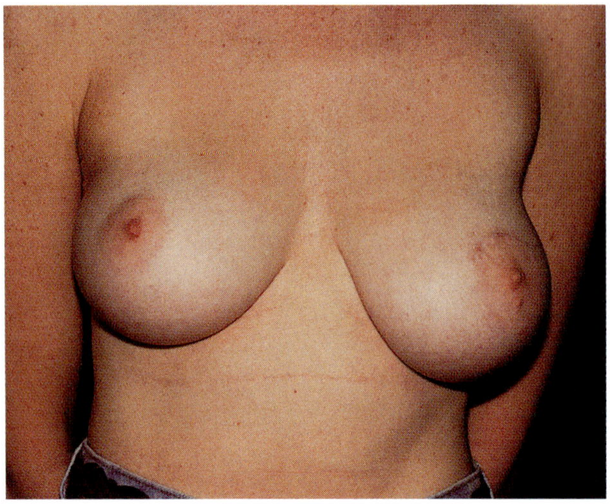

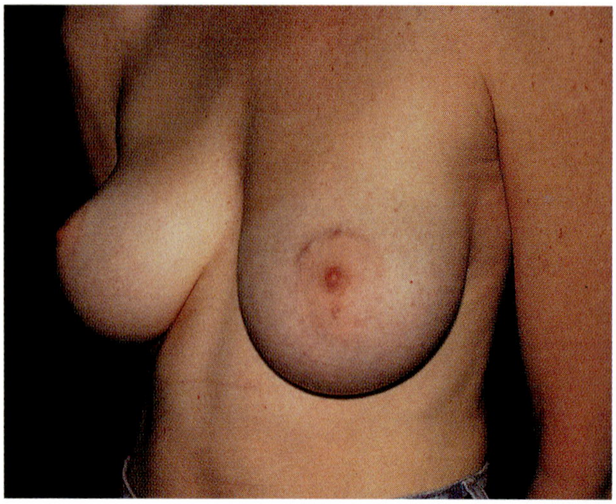

This 28-year-old patient sought correction of breast asymmetry. Since the right breast was to be matched, the initial operative plan was to attempt a periareolar reduction mammaplasty of the left breast.

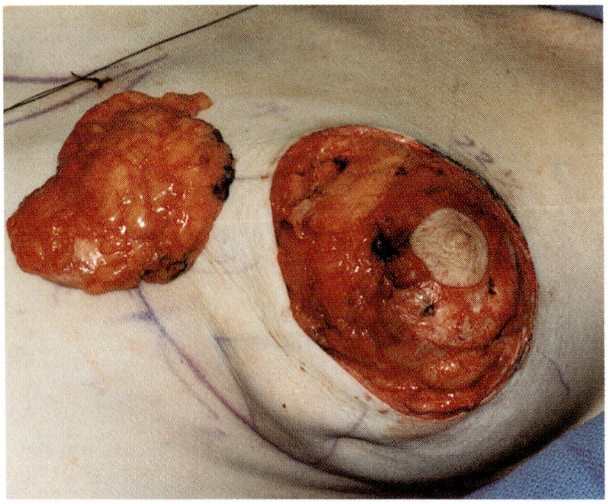

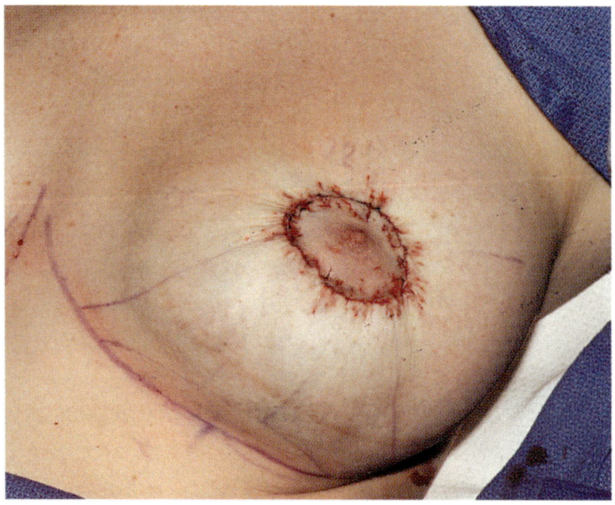

Following reduction of the periareolar skin, the skin of the lower pole of the breast was elevated from the parenchyma. The base of the breast was then elevated from the pectoral fascia. A radial wedge of breast tissue was removed from the inferior pole and the base was trimmed. The immediate postoperative result is shown.

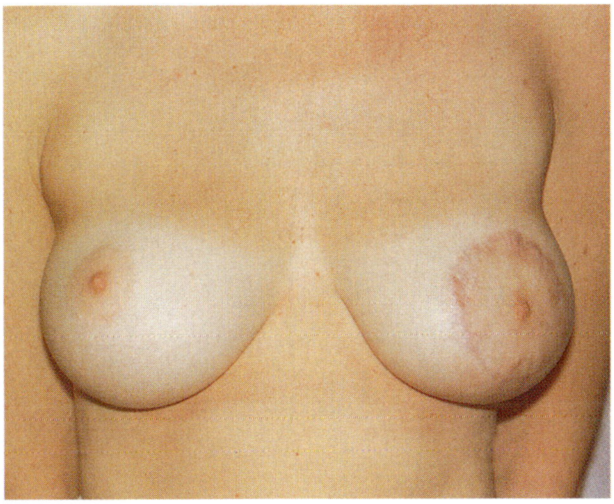

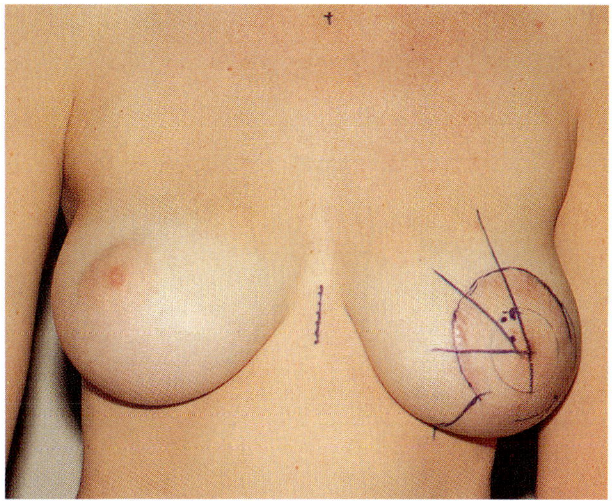

Unfortunately, the postoperative result was unacceptable to both the patient and surgeon, with excessive spreading of the areola and excess breast tissue inferiorly and laterally. We waited 1 full year before correction; the tissues were completely soft and stable by this time. The revision required a similar operative pattern of additional parenchymal resection. However, we did not believe that optimal shape could be achieved without resecting skin from the vertical midline of the breast. This resection would achieve a reduction in the base width, an important goal in obtaining symmetry.

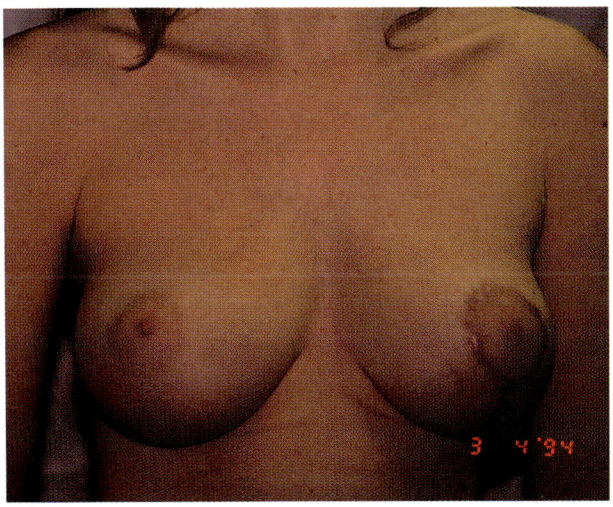

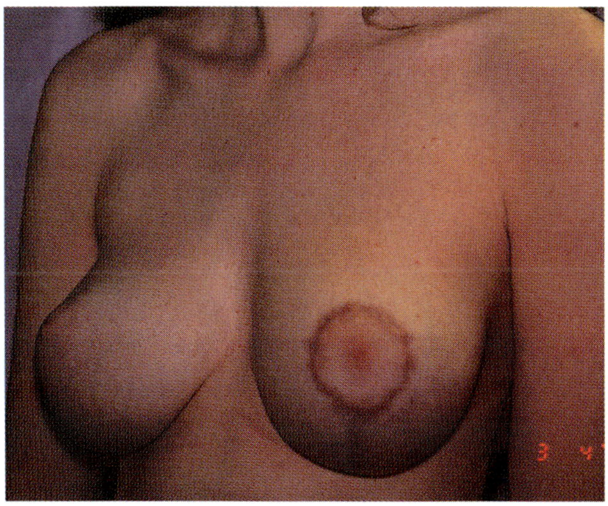

The final postoperative result is shown 1 year following final correction.

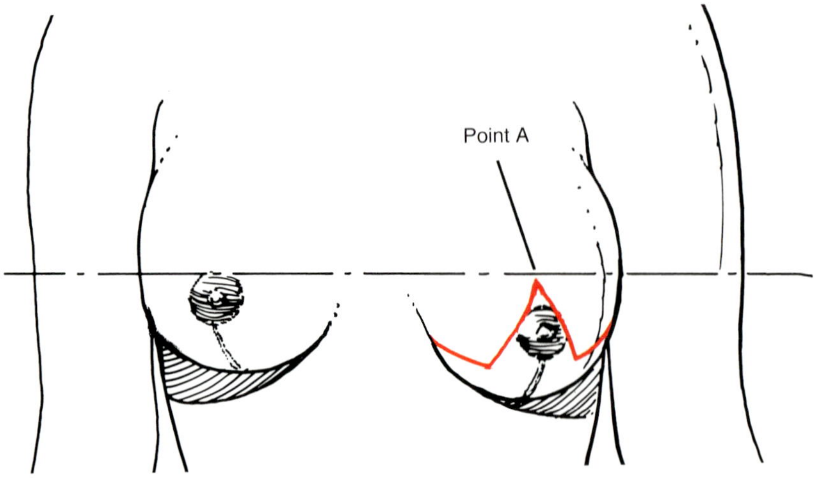

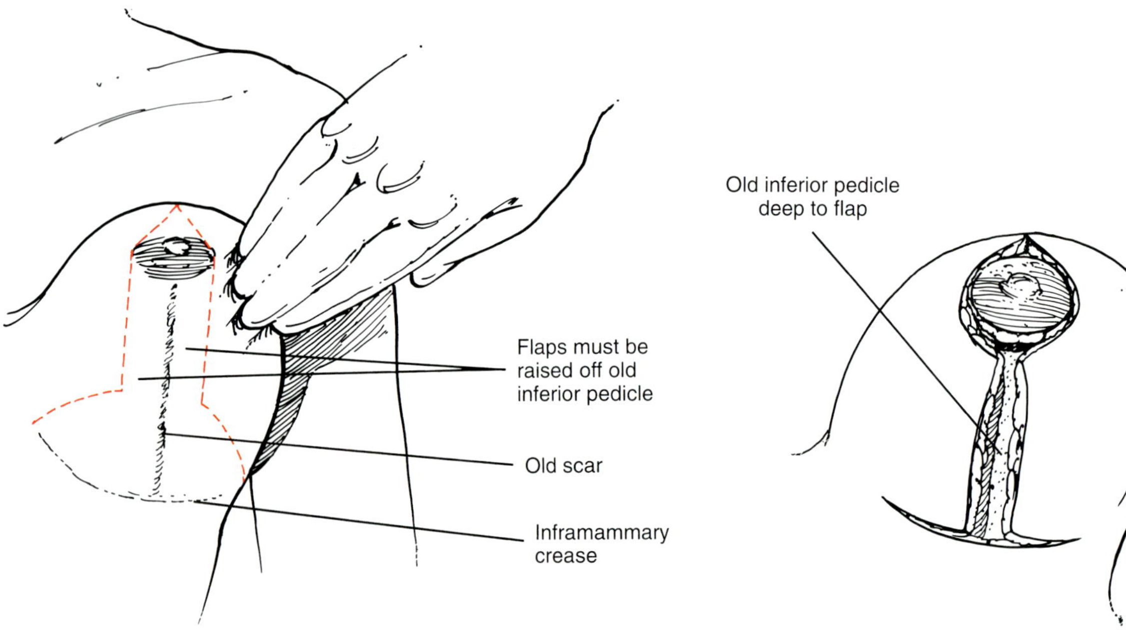

As for insufficient reduction, correction of asymmetry by further resection of a single breast should be accomplished using the same technique that was performed for the initial reduction. For instance, in the case of an inferior pedicle technique, since the skin overlying the previous inferior pedicle is probably not contributing to the circulation of the nipple-areola complex, the incisions can simply be reopened and the previous breast flaps dissected from the inferior pedicle.

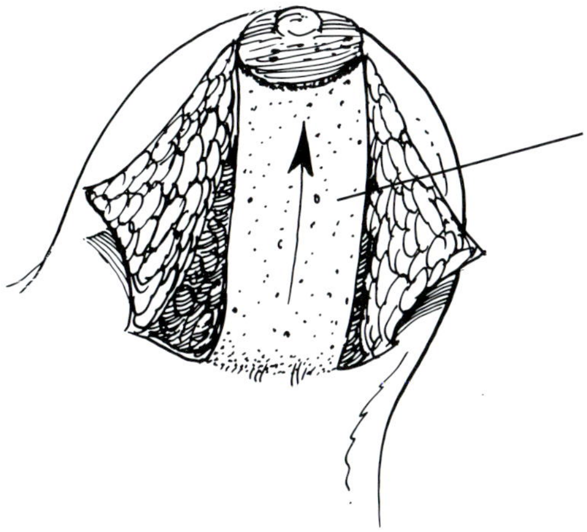

After the flaps are dissected from the previous pedicle to its lateral margin, the dissection plane is then continued deep around the lateral walls of the previous pedicle, thereby essentially redissecting the inferior pedicle in roughly the same shape and size as in the primary reduction procedure.

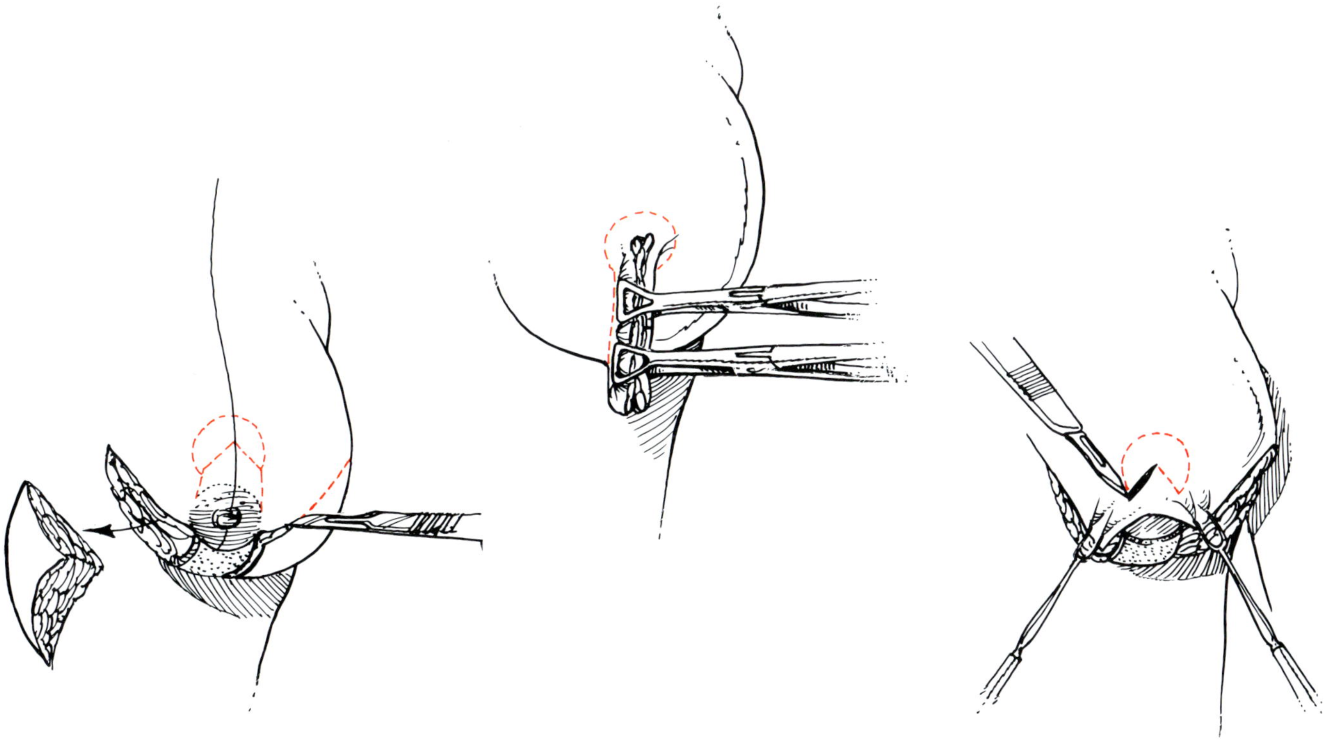

The resection can then be carried out after approximation of the breast shape using approximating clamps. The excess tissue is excised in both the vertical and horizontal directions depending on the amount of reduction necessary.

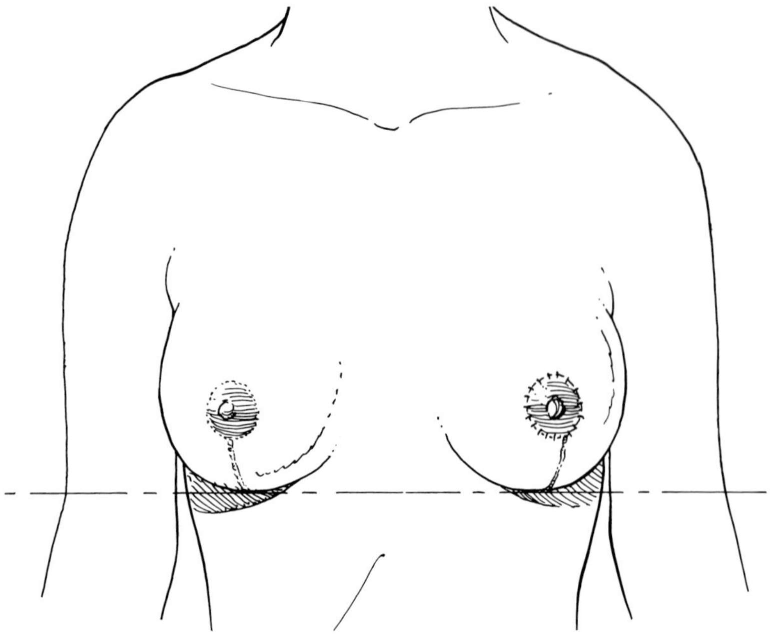

With the skin flaps temporarily closed, the patient should be placed in the upright sitting position so that volume and shape can be assessed. The lower pole of the breast should be kept somewhat flat and high in anticipation of the later dissent of the lower pole of the gland. One should anticipate the lengthening of this vertical limb by at least 1 to 2 cm, depending on the volume of remaining breast tissue. The incisions are closed in layers.

If one is unsure what type of technique was used initially and medical records cannot be obtained, the safest technique to equalize volume discrepancies is liposuction alone or in combination with skin envelope modification. This will work only in patients who have less dense, fatty breast parenchyma. However, it is simple and safe, and if the nipple-areola complexes are symmetric, no opening of old scars is necessary. Residual devascularized fat that is not aspirated may calcify and be visible mammographically, so liposuction patients should always inform mammographers that reduction mammaplasty and liposuction of the breast have been performed. Calcifications due to fat necrosis usually can be distinguished from those associated with neoplasms.

With contour asymmetries the problem is usually a result of excess skin left behind with roughly symmetric parenchymal volumes. These corrections can be performed in exactly the same manner, although often the inferior pedicle does not need to be completely dissected to make the correction. Rather the skin flaps are simply reelevated, approximation of the resection is performed, asymmetry is checked with the patient in the upright position, and excess skin is trimmed.

Minor discrepancies in breast volume are common after reduction and do not usually require correction. Final evaluation of symmetry must be deferred until postoperative edema has completely resolved because the size of the breasts will fluctuate for several months postoperatively. Such asymmetries are usually due to an asymmetric resection. If correction is desired by the patient, volume changes can be effected by suction lipectomy coupled with skin resection if necessary.

In secondary surgery to correct asymmetry it is better to reduce the large breast further rather than insert an implant.[12] The breast volume and the skin envelope are two components that must be addressed in secondary aesthetic breast surgeries. Skin tightening alone without resection of breast tissue does not seem to maintain the correction as well because of stretching.[13] Reduction of the skin envelope in the vertical direction will aid in projection and reduce the length of the lower scar.

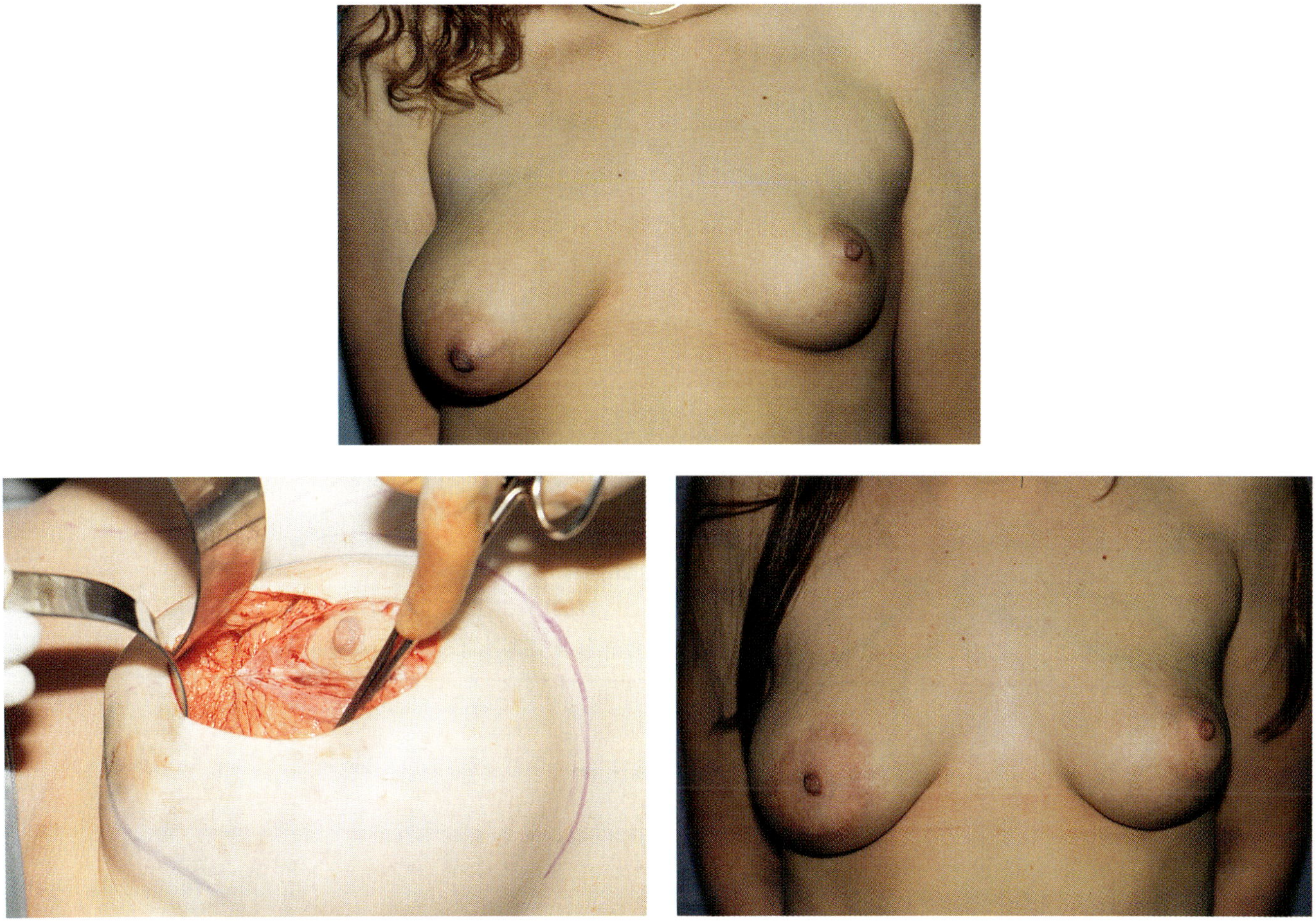

Periareolar mastopexy of the right breast and augmentation of the left breast were performed in an attempt to correct primary breast asymmetry in this 18-year-old woman. The postoperative result demonstrates the clear failure to achieve either the proper size or shape to match the left side. The parenchymal plication sutures were used to try to elevate the nipple-areola complex. These sutures, however, failed to produce permanent elevation of the nipple-areola complex.

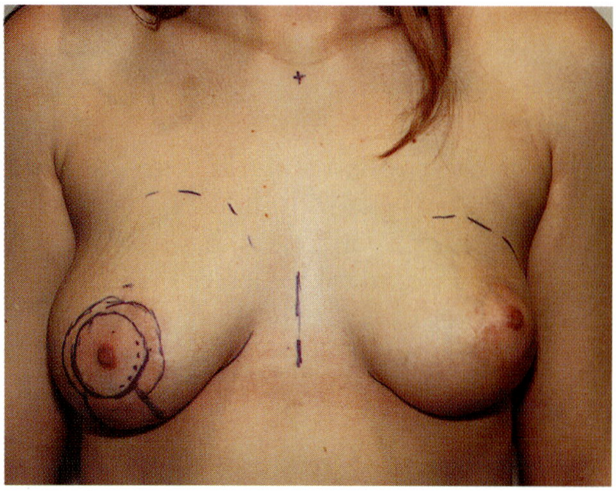

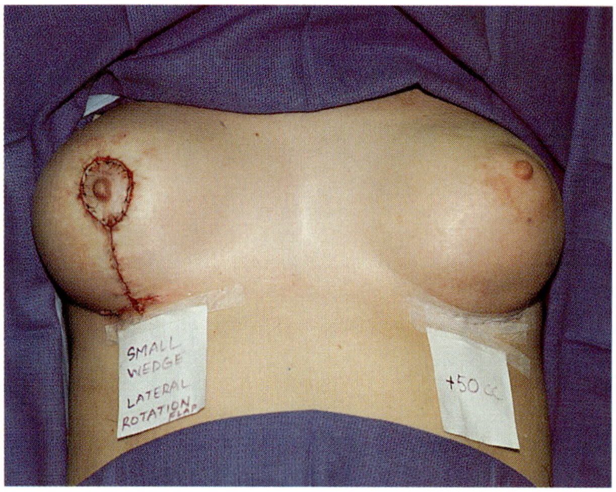

In the secondary correction vertical reduction with additional radial wedge excision in the inferior pole was performed in the right breast; a small lateral parenchymal flap was also pulled medially to produce the proper lateral contour. In addition, a larger implant was placed on the left side. The intraoperative result shows improved symmetry.

Contour Deformities

Many factors affect breast contour. The appearance of the breast is a function of the relationship between the breast volume and the skin envelope. With time, various influences have an effect on breast volume and the condition of the skin envelope. For example, with lactation, there is a temporary increase in breast volume that stretches the skin, at times to the point that the skin loses some of its elasticity. With involution, the breast volume decreases while the skin envelope remains disproportionately large, depending on its intrinsic residual elasticity. Of course, gravity exerts a constant effect. The result is breast ptosis.

Following reduction mammaplasty and mastopexy, some typical deformities may develop. Restoring an aesthetic appearance to the breast means correcting the relationship between parenchymal volume and skin envelope. Techniques that use a wedge excision of breast tissue[14] may produce a tubular deformity when performed on large-volume breasts. Vertical as well as horizontal skin excision is needed to correct the deformity.

Periareolar mammaplasty also may result in predictable patterns of deformity when inappropriately applied, particularly in the wrong type of patient. The amount of skin excess following large-volume reductions cannot be effectively removed with the maintenance of an appropriate breast contour. A flattened breast with stellate wrinkles in the surrounding skin often results when the technique is pushed to its limits. Recurrent ptosis and enlarged areolae are common. Correction requires excision of vertical excess.

Dog ears are common after the reduction of broad-based breasts. Exceedingly long scars will result if the dog ear is resected over the lateral chest wall. Aspirative lipoplasty,[15,16] a recent addition to aesthetic breast surgery, offers an excellent method of flattening dog ears without having to lengthen the scars.

Obese patients with true gigantomastia will invariably have residual folds of adipose tissue in the low area of the axilla that are not related to excess breast glandular tissue. These folds must be pointed out to the patient in advance of the reduction mammaplasty procedure because these folds often will appear more prominent once the breast has been reduced. The patient may actually see these rolls for the first time! She may think they are the residual effect of the surgery, but in actuality these folds are little changed from their preoperative contour unless vigorous fat reduction by liposuction or by direct excision is accomplished at the time of the reduction. Since vigorous fat removal by direct excision of this area can affect the sensation of the breast or even the vascularity of the lateral flap, I usually reduce these areas only minimally at the time of the initial surgery, but I wait 6 months to 1 year to perform a secondary revision.

Recurrent Ptosis

As the result of pregnancy, weight loss, menopause, or the constant force of gravity, recurrent ptosis is just about inevitable. Breasts that contain substantial amounts of fat may be prone to recurrent ptosis with weight reduction following aesthetic breast surgery. Suctioning the fat before breast reduction compacts the firm, glandular tissue and may reduce the likelihood of recurrent ptosis in patients with a significant fatty component to the breasts following weight loss.

"Bottoming out" represents a particular type of recurrent ptosis. This glandular descent is easily recognized as a lengthening of the vertical limb of the inverted T scar used for reduction mammaplasty. It results from a stretching of skin and scar. Attempts have been made to correct the problem using dermal strips, fascia lata tacking sutures, and autoaugmentation with deepithelialized segments. Because ptosis recurrence may not be evident in the early postoperative period, patients should be followed up long term in order to assess the results of surgery properly.

The surgical treatment of recurrent ptosis following reduction mammaplasty or mastopexy is best accomplished simply by additional skin or glandular excision using the same technique and incisions that were used for the primary procedure. Occasionally, if only a vertical incision was used, a horizontal resection may be necessary to shorten the vertical limb. Glandular plication may also be helpful. The gland can be undermined from the pectoralis major muscle and sutures placed between the parenchyma and the pectoralis fascia to draw the gland superiorly. In addition, glandular plication sutures can be placed in a vertical row between the areola and the inframammary fold to help to hold the gland in a higher position. The skin can then be tailored over the reshaped gland.

The long-term stability of ptosis correction alone may be improved with the use of a breast implant. However, if the patient does not want larger breasts, this is not an option.

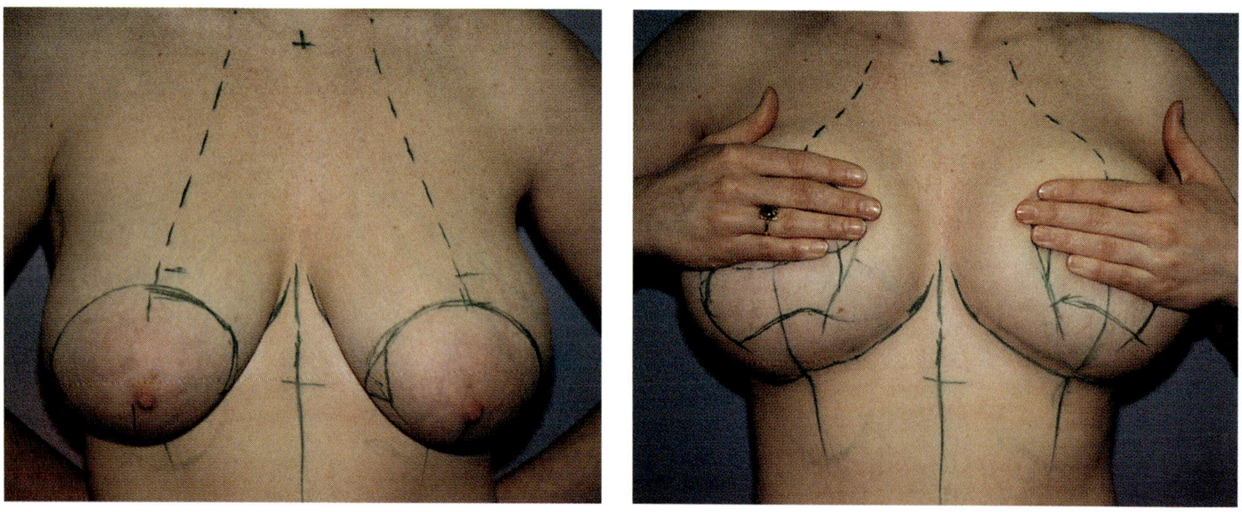

Recurrent ptosis can be unilateral as was evident in this 28-year-old patient. Reduction mammaplasty was performed using Marchac's technique.

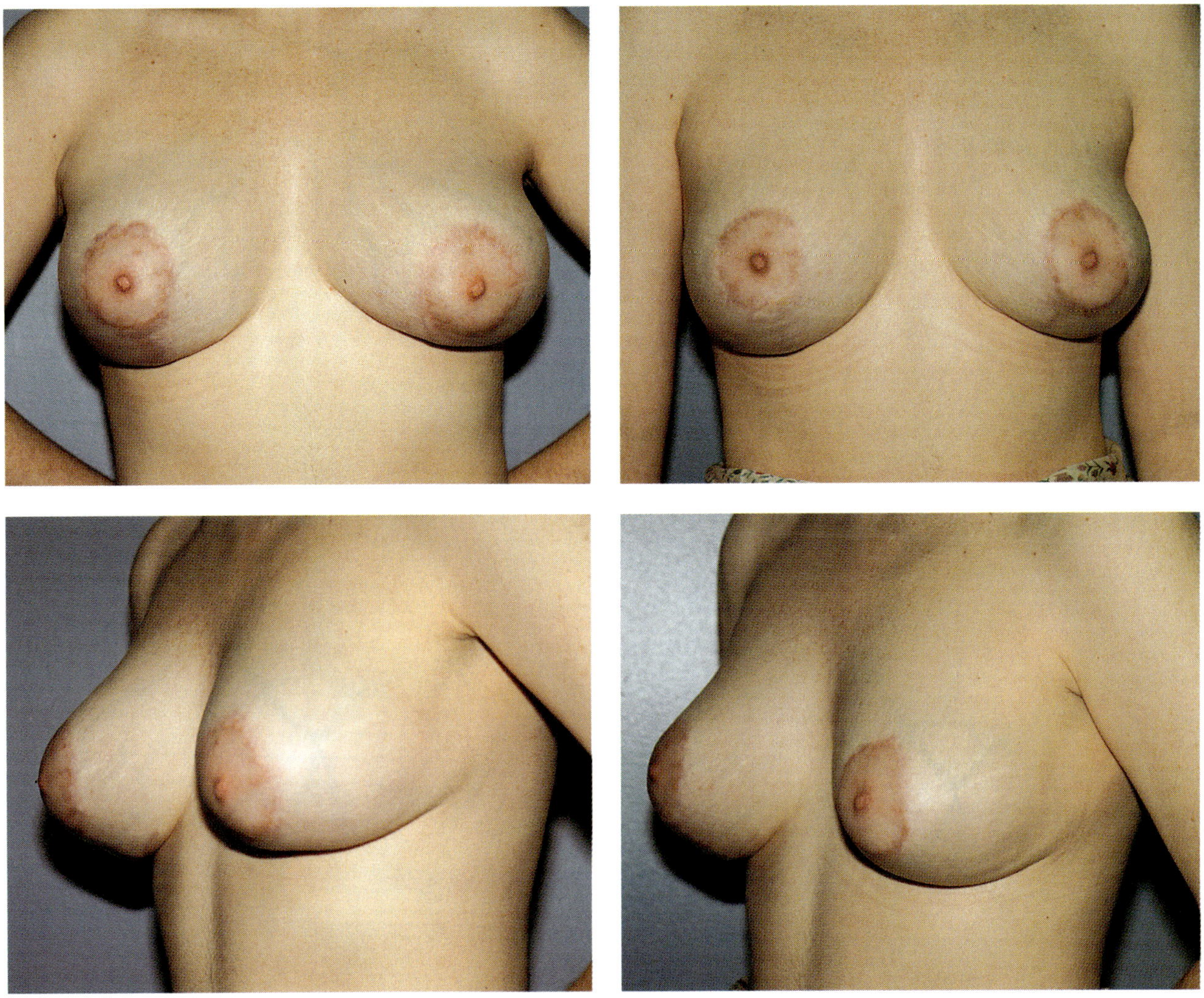

One year postoperatively the left breast was slightly larger than the right and had developed recurrent ptosis. A simple correction using the previous incisions was performed. A wedge of breast tissue in the inferior pole was resected, and the nipple-areola complex was raised approximately 2 cm.

Overreduction

Overreduction in specific quadrants of the breast may yield contour irregularities. These depressions may be quite visible to the patient and a considerable cause of concern. Yet treatment by parenchymal flaps requires reopening of the entire breast with the possibility of correcting one area of depression only to create another. One also risks further sensory changes when parenchymal flaps are used.

If the problem is a flat, nonprojecting breast, reopening the incisions and advancing the breast gland parenchyma toward the midline of the breast medially and laterally with parenchymal plication sutures may help to create a cone with the remaining parenchyma. Despite the small volume, this type of correction often satisfies the patient without the need for implants.

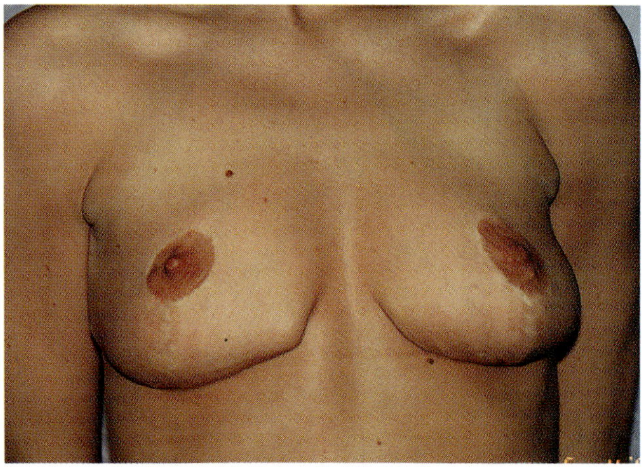

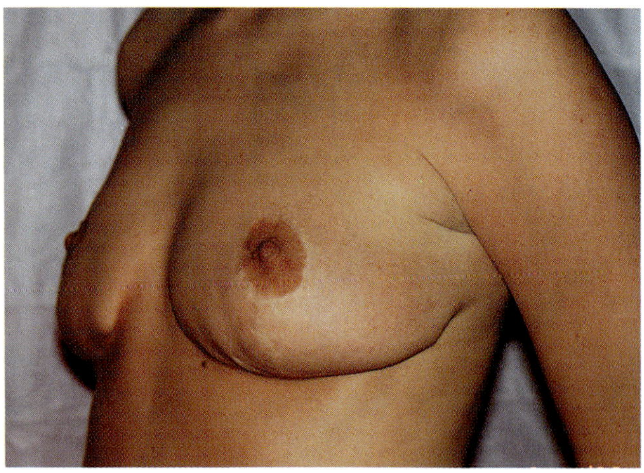

This 30-year-old woman was referred for secondary correction following an inferior pedicle reduction that had produced broad, flat, nonprojecting breasts that she believed had insufficient volume. Nevertheless, she did not desire to have an implant placed.

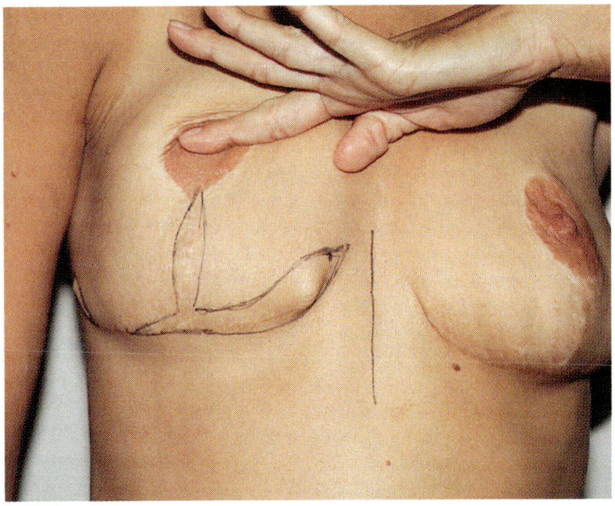

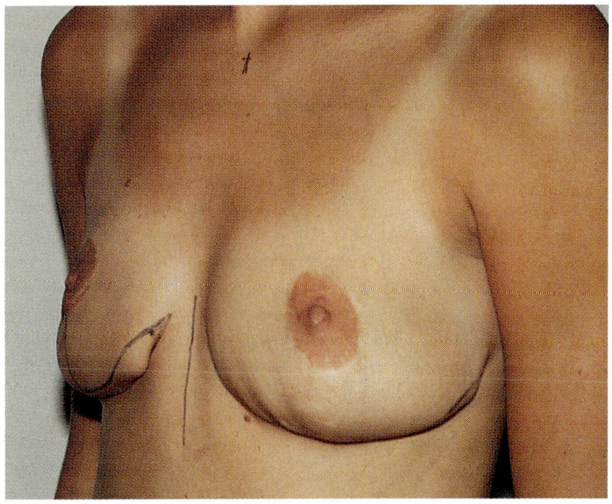

The previous incisions were reopened and further gland plication was performed. The lateral skin, particularly on the right breast, was tightened.

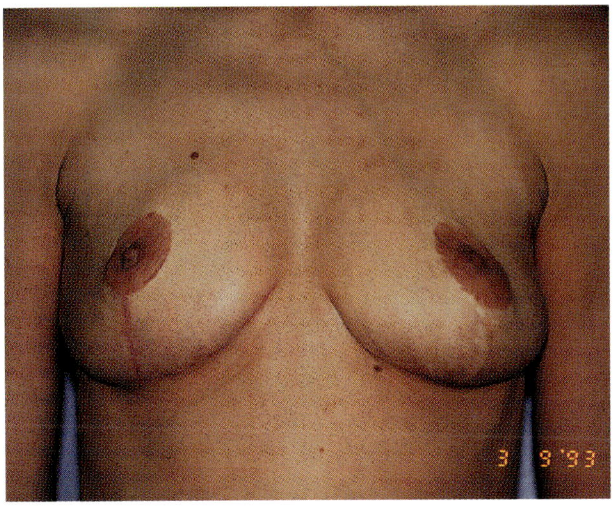

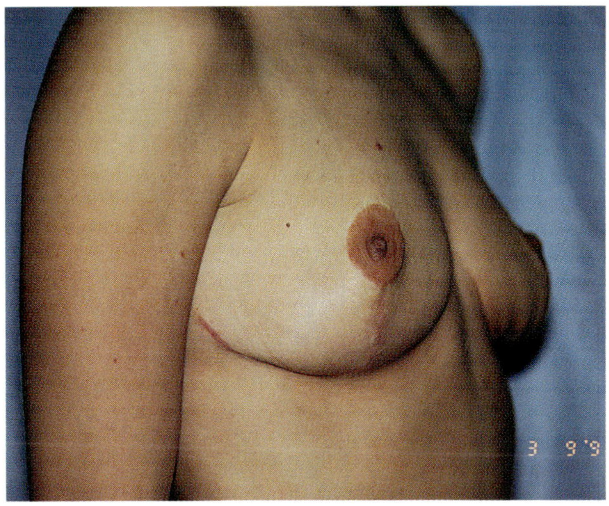

Although not an ideal result, the patient is pleased with this improvement.

Another possibility with small surface contour irregularities is cautious autogenous fat injection. This procedure is not advocated for breast enlargement in general, but it can be helpful to fill surface contour irregularities.

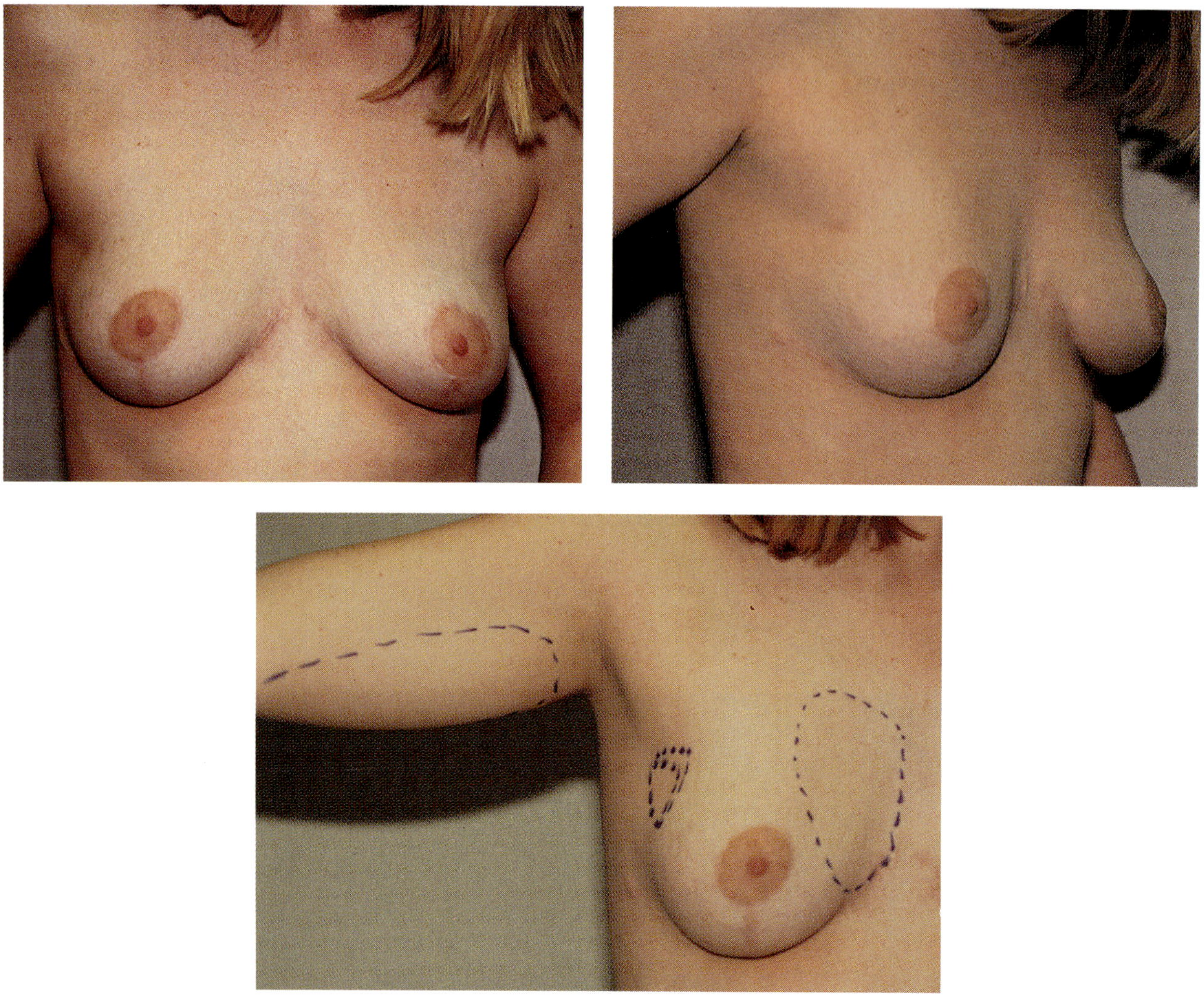

In this patient, a mediolateral hollow resulted from an inferior pedicle breast reduction. The patient was referred for correction. We did not consider redissection of the breast and correction with parenchymal flaps advisable. However, the patient was offered autogenous fat injection into the depressed areas as a treatment option. Donor sites were selected from the triceps area of the arm and the abdomen. The areas to be injected are outlined.

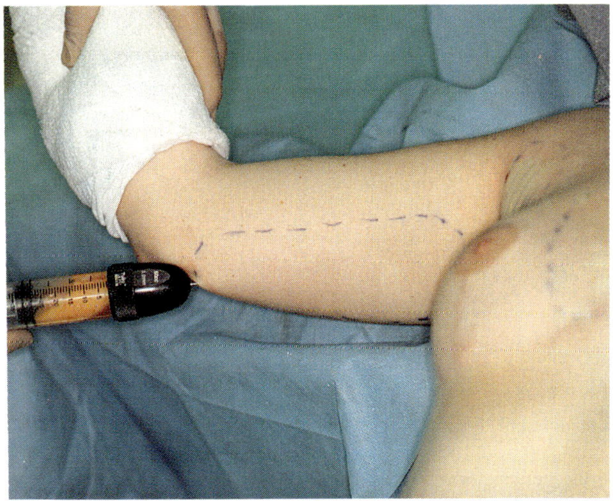

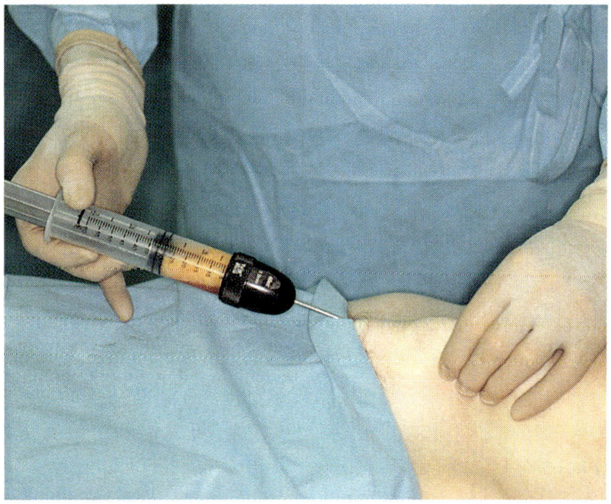

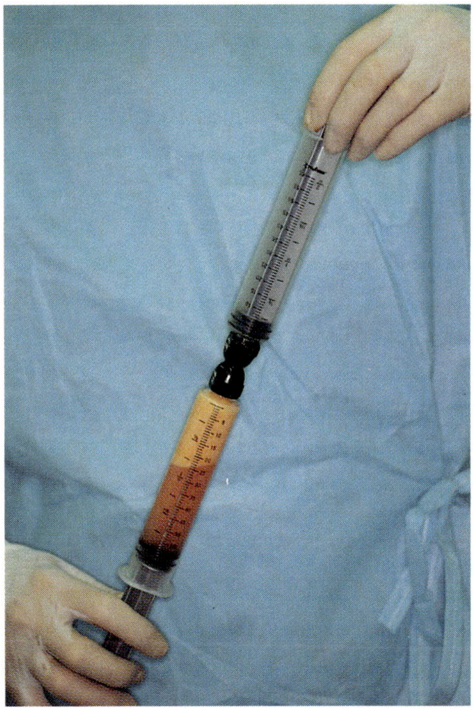

The fat was harvested using the tumescent technique. The harvested fat was washed with saline solution, and the pure fat component was separated for injection.

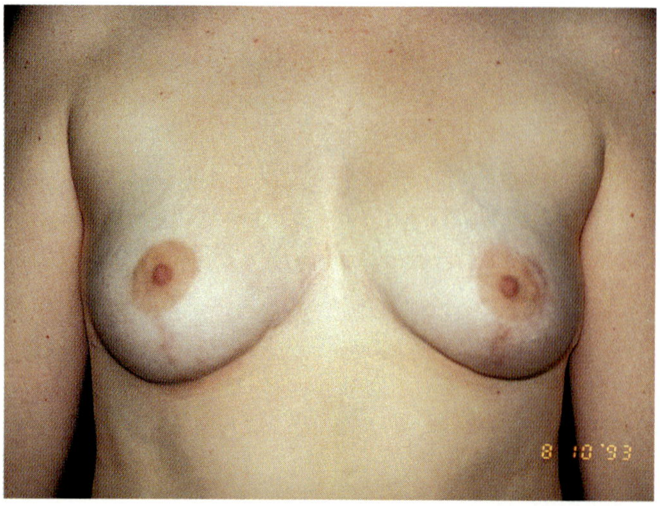

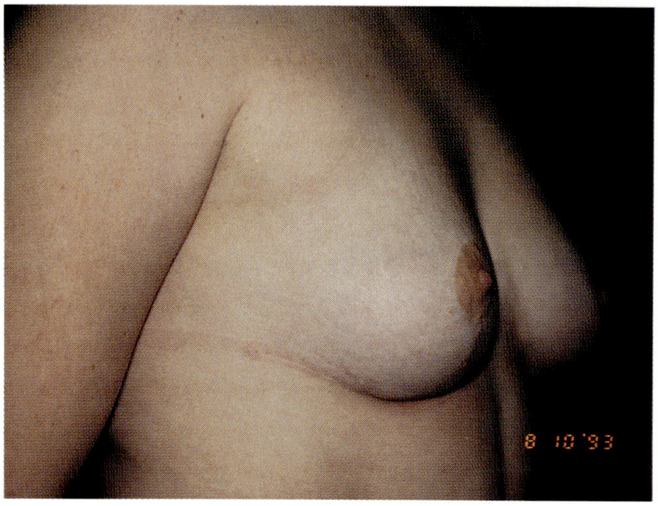

The postoperative result showed stable improvement at 1 year. Calcification and nodularity of the injected fat can be minimized by careful saline solution washing and removal of the impurities before injection. In the future the patient also must inform the mammographer that she has had autogenous fat injection into these limited areas so that a misinterpretation of calcifications by mammography is avoided.

Overreduction is a problem that is best avoided. Correction of severe overreduction requires augmentation either with a prosthetic implant or autogenous tissue, either of which may be unsatisfactory to the patient.

Insufficient Reduction

Whether a patient has been "sufficiently reduced" is a possible source of disagreement among patient, surgeon, and insurance company. This disagreement may result from poor communication between patient and surgeon preoperatively. Patient expectations may be unrealistic, or the surgeon may not have listened to or may disagree with the patient's expressed desires. The insurance company is interested only in the resolution of preoperative associated symptoms such as neck and back strain or skin problems. (Breast regrowth is discussed later in this chapter.)

In general, it is better to err on the side of a conservative reduction than to risk overreduction. However, if one attempts to reduce breast size so that it is in proportion with the remainder of the body, the patient will usually be satisfied as long as the result is symmetric. On occasion, however, insufficient reduction may occur. This problem is most common in young women who have only a slight hypertrophy in whom the result of an overcautious approach may not be in keeping with what the patient had expected.

Surgical correction of this problem is usually delayed at least 3 to 6 months until the breasts are soft and the shape has stabilized. The patient must be counseled that the scars may in fact be worse the second time around and sensibility may be reduced as the anatomy may now be distorted due to the previous surgery. In general, two approaches are available. One may use the same technique as the initial surgery to minimize risk of nipple-areola necrosis. The breast flaps are redissected as described for treatment of asymmetry. One can use either predetermined markings or a "cut as you go" approach in which the amount of resection is determined intraoperatively with the patient in the sitting position. Great care must be taken to ensure that the resections are symmetric and will result in correct breast proportion and nipple position.

Alternatively, liposuction may be useful for secondary reduction of breast fat in the underreduced patient. Clearly only breasts that contain a considerable amount of fat are amenable to this corrective method; breast parenchyma is not removed. When one is uncertain of the technique that was used primarily (e.g., as in the referred patient for whom medical records are unavailable), liposuction may afford the best margin of safety for the maintenance of circulation to the nipple-areola complex. If necessary, a skin reduction–type mastopexy may provide the necessary improvement in contour.

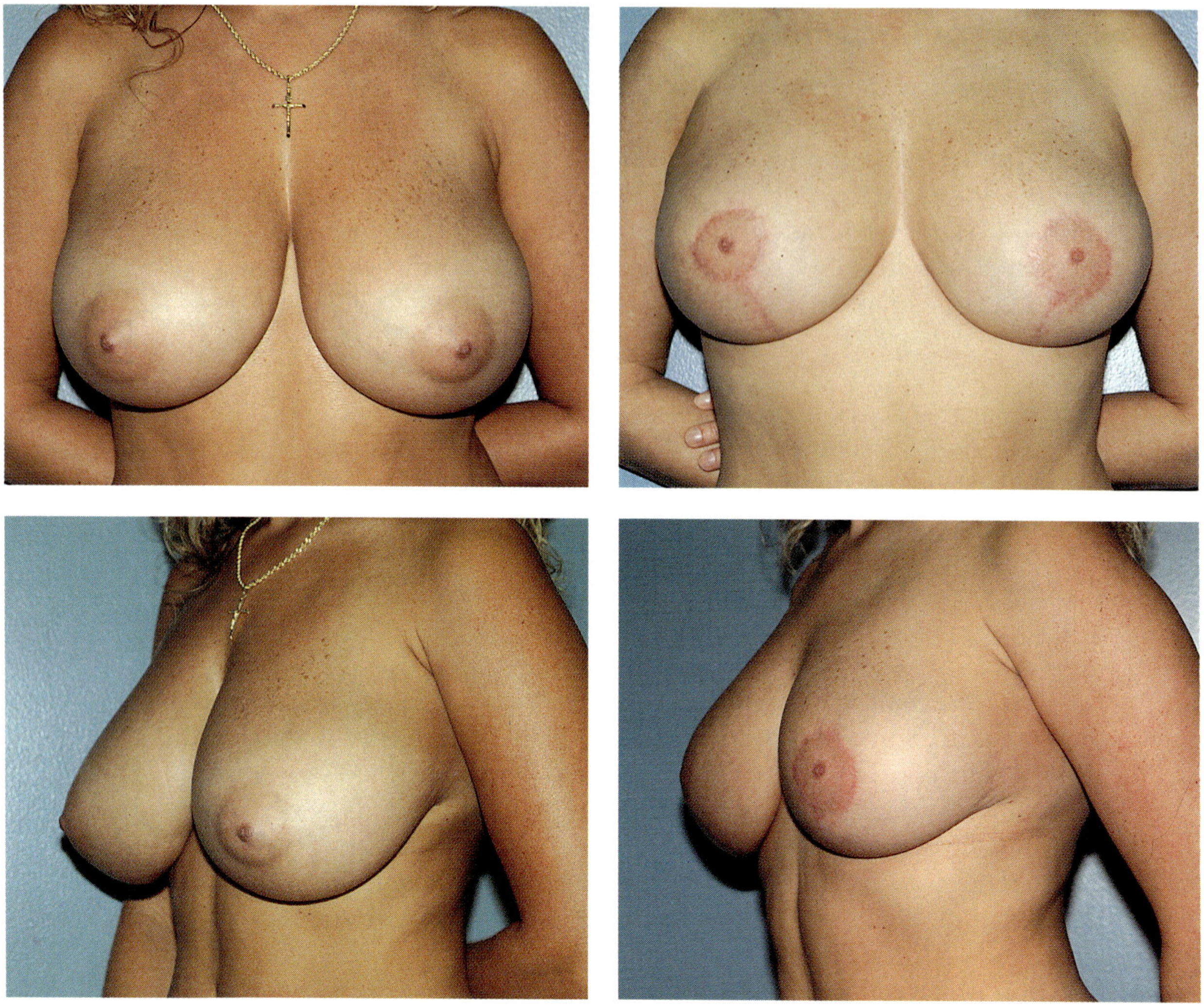

This young woman underwent reduction mammaplasty using the Marchac technique. A conservative reduction left her with fuller breasts than she desired. Rather than reopening all of the old incisions for additional direct parenchymal resection, liposuction is planned to help to reduce the fat content.

Insufficient reduction is a problem that occurs due to a miscommunication between the surgeon and the patient: her expectations do not match what the surgeon can deliver. With experience this outcome is less likely to occur.

NIPPLE-AREOLA COMPLEX

Although some authors attribute late postoperative changes to characteristics of an individual's body tissues, most believe them to be the result of incorrect planning or execution of the surgery. Smith and Gillen[17] have described some of these technical errors. Errors in planning can result from failure to keep the nipple-areola complex between 18 and 24 cm from the sternal notch. Similarly, for most standard reduction techniques, the distance from areola to inframammary fold should not exceed 4 to 5 cm. Flexibility is also required when pattern techniques (e.g., Wise, Strömbeck) are used.

Symmetry of the nipple-areola complexes must be checked before final suturing. We have found the pendulum suture technique with the patient in the sitting position to be of great help in verifying this symmetry. One full-length 2-0 silk suture is placed at the sternal notch and another one over the xiphoid. Triangulating these crossed sutures from one nipple to the other gives an accurate idea of the symmetry of the closure.

Malposition

In the preoperative plan, allowances must be made for skin elasticity, which may shorten the sternal notch to nipple distance after excess breast weight is removed. The nipples might otherwise be somewhat higher than desirable, and secondary repositioning may be requested by the patient. Lateral displacement can be accomplished by moving the nipple-areola complex medially on a central pedicle much like mastopexy.[18]

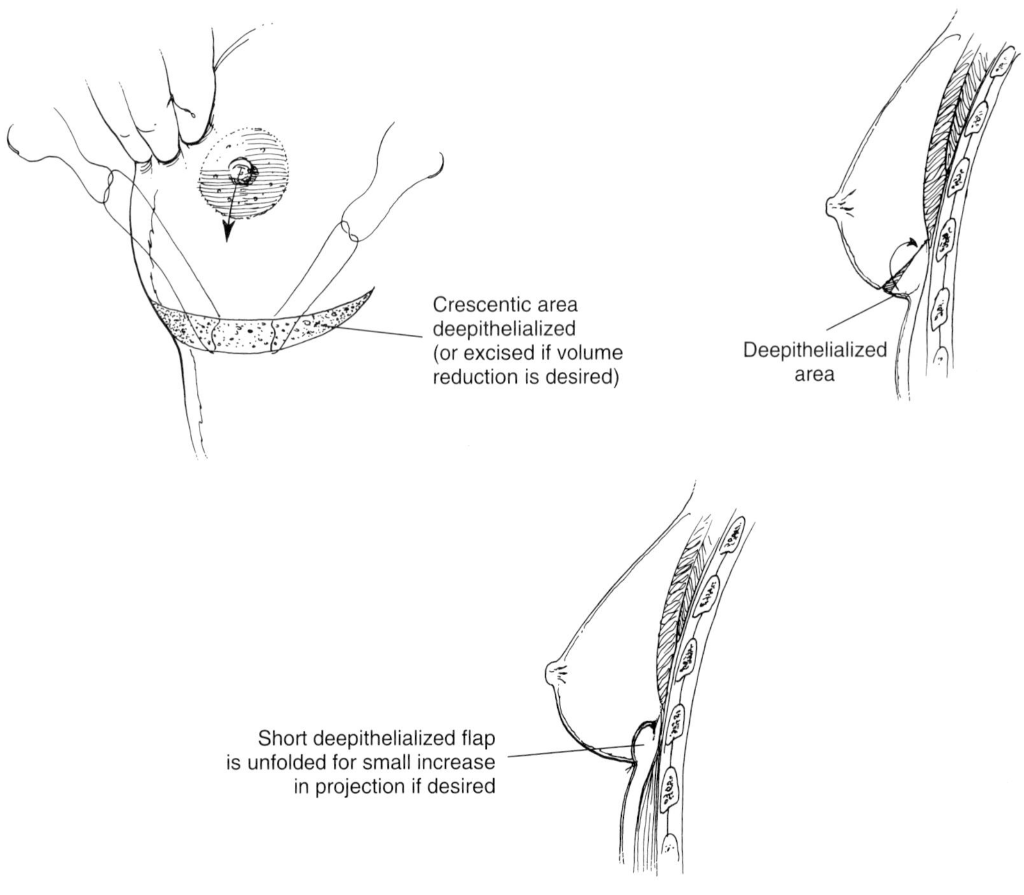

Superior displacement can be corrected using one of two methods: by repositioning the nipple-areola complex directly as a free nipple graft or by shortening the distance from the nipple to inframammary fold by direct excision of skin, tucking the lower pole up behind the breast.[19] This second method is preferred as no scars remain in the superior pole of the breast. Areolae that are displaced medially can be corrected by an inferior flap of dermis and fat[20,21] or by a crescent excision.

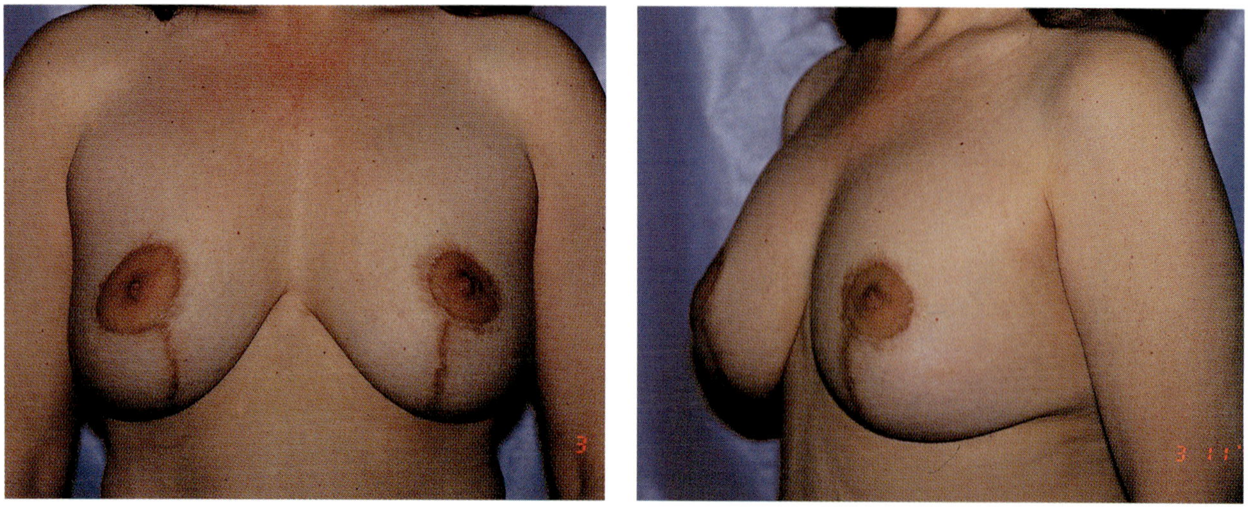

This patient was referred for correction 10 years following mastopexy and the placement of breast implants. She had never been happy with the result of the primary breast surgery and desired implant removal. Preoperative assessment revealed that the implants were positioned too high with respect to the breast mounds and that she had glandular ptosis and high nipple-areola complexes.

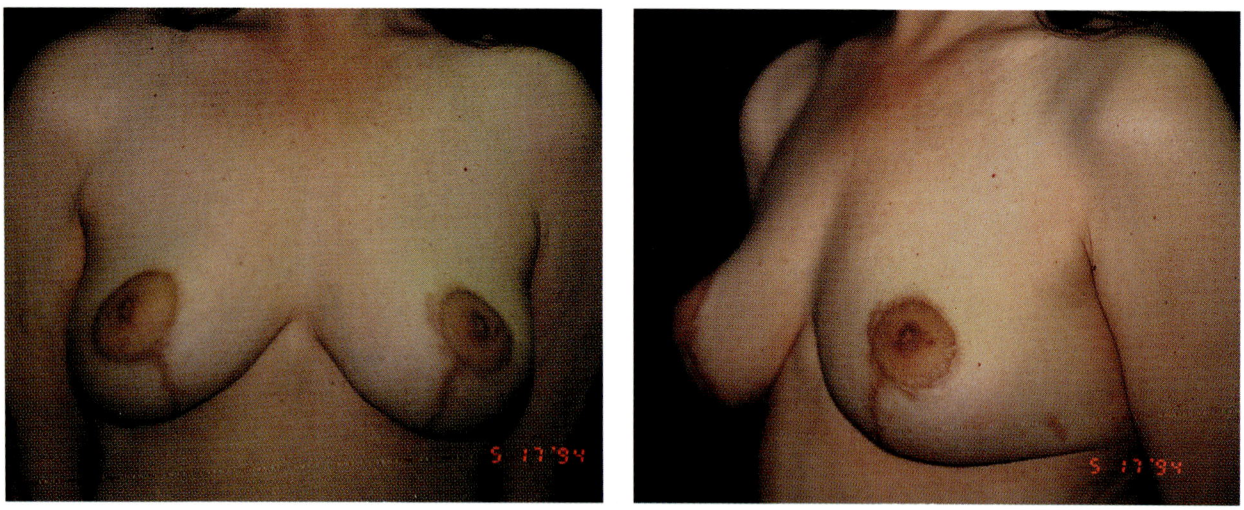

Correction was accomplished by shortening the distance between the nipple and inframammary fold, which had lengthened over time. The current inframammary fold was marked and incised, elevating the gland from the chest wall until the capsule of the implant was reached. The implants were removed, and a total capsulectomy was performed as the patient had requested. A deepithelialized flap was created from the excess gland in the inferior pole. This flap was turned up underneath for additional projection, creating an improved contour without implants.

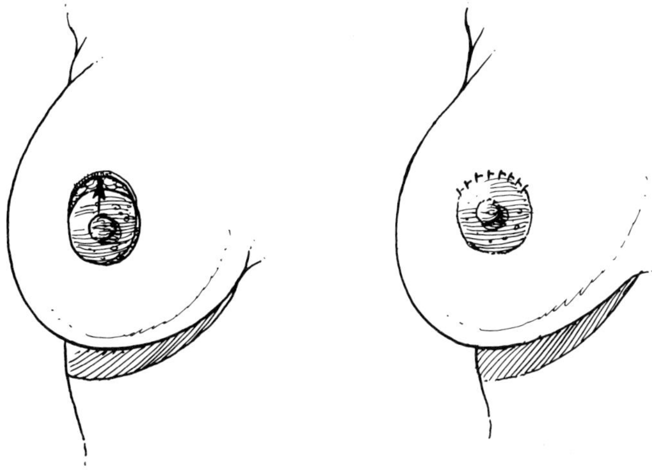

Nipples that are placed too low can similarly be repositioned with a crescentic excision. Only minimal elevations (2 to 3 cm) are advisable with crescentic excision alone because additional shape distortion may occur.

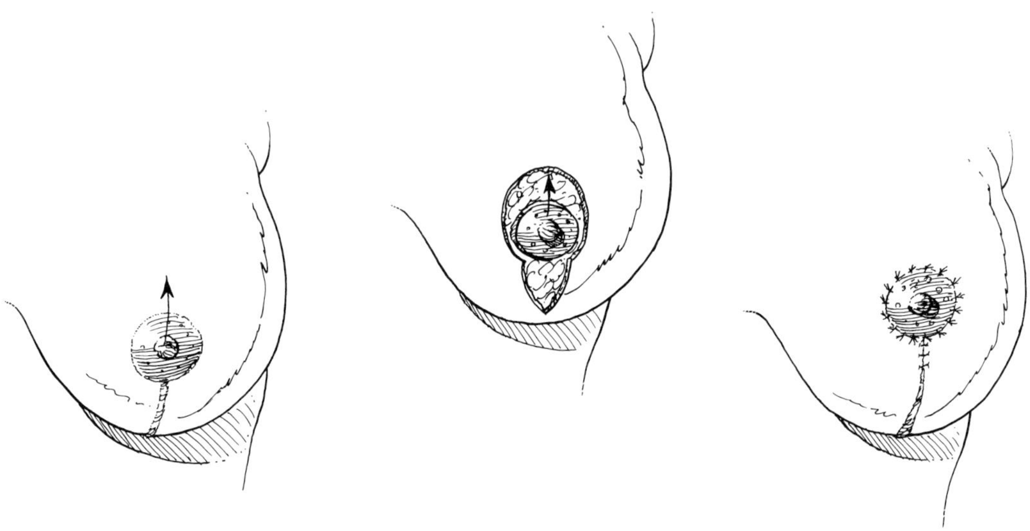

A vertical excision of skin may also need to be performed to avoid this problem.

Irregular Size and Shape and Depigmentation

The areola should be round, with the nipple centered precisely. Segmental contraction of the intrinsic musculature of the nipple or careless marking can account for an offset appearance. The oval nipple results when localized skin tension distorts the areolar window. Overresection of the breast parenchyma in relation to the skin envelope will result in an oval nipple as demonstrated by observing correction when the breast skin is placed under tension by medial and lateral compression. Also a tight vertical closure will cause medial and lateral bulging.[5] Spreading of the nipple-areola complex can result from motor denervation; more often it is simply the result of excessive circumferential tension created by periareolar skin excision.

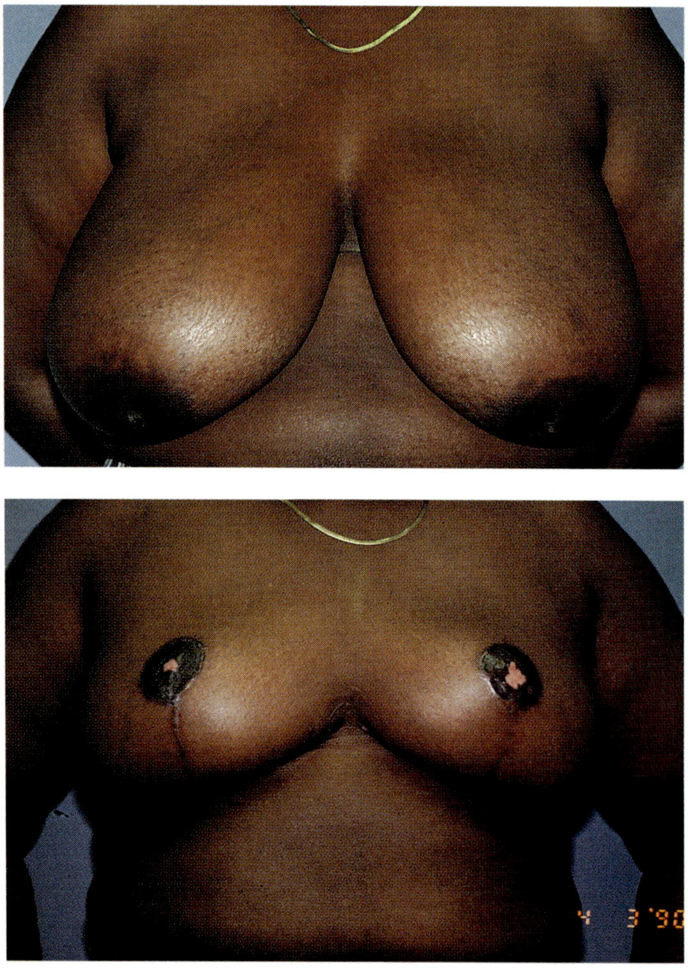

Depigmentation can be a source of dissatisfaction, particularly in the non-Caucasian patient. It is especially common with the free nipple graft technique if the pigment-producing basal layer is thinned from the composite graft. In this patient most of the pigmentation of the areola returned but the pigment in the nipple did not. If the pigmentation has not returned by 1 year, satisfactory correction can be obtained with nipple-areolar tattooing.

Retraction

Some breast reduction techniques such as Strömbeck's procedure are associated with nipple inversion. Certainly inversion will be present postoperatively if it was present preoperatively. If the overall bulk of the residual pedicle is insufficient to fill the skin envelope, the central pedicle will fall back from the areolar attachment. This situation may not necessarily require reoperation, but if needed, correction requires further reduction of the skin by widening the keyhole and reducing the medial and lateral inferior skin edges.[5] Support of the breast tissue underlying the nipple-areola complex by infolding the lower pole may be necessary.

Protrusion

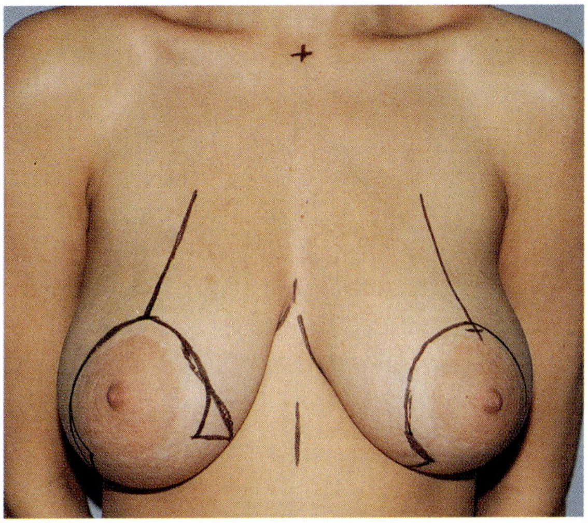

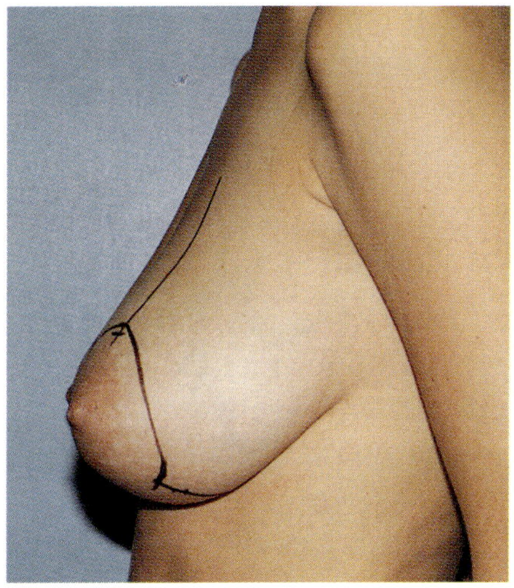

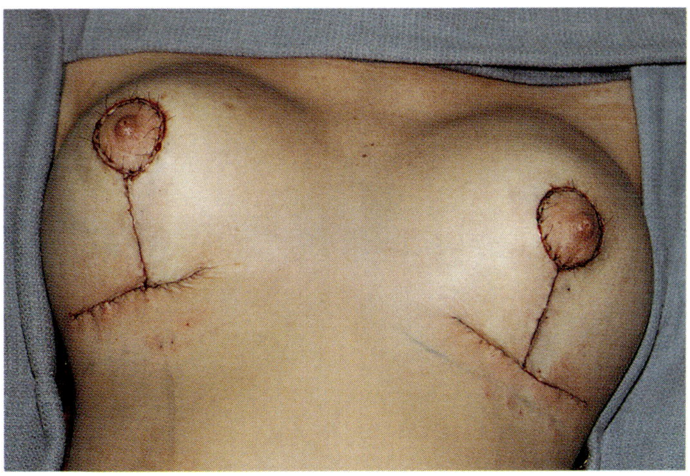

A redundant and pouting areola results from an excess of areolar tissue relative to the size of the keyhole. This 21-year-old patient had typical symptoms related to mammary hypertrophy. Reduction was carried out using the Marchac technique. The immediate postoperative result is shown.

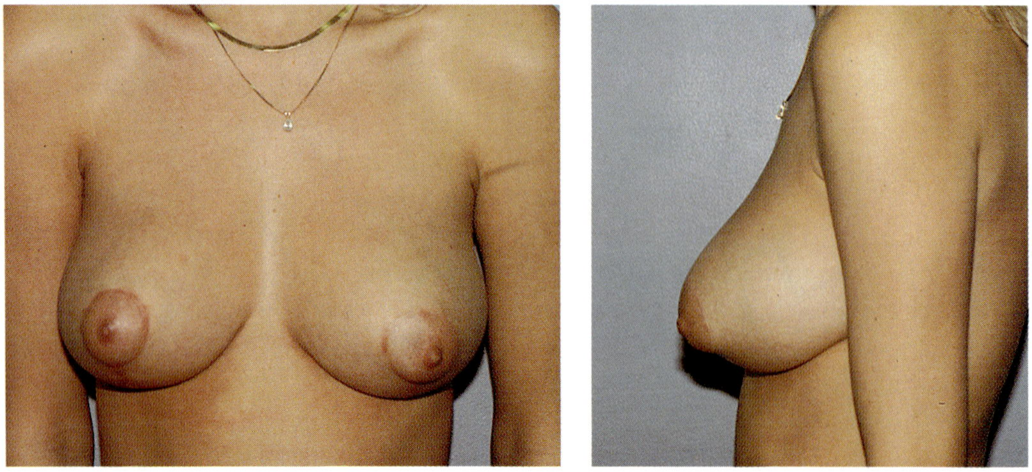

The pouting deformity of the left nipple-areola complex is clearly seen. Also, the left nipple-areola complex is slightly lower on the left side. This condition may be corrected by excising a circumferential strip of skin around the areola, including areolar tissue and/or surrounding skin.

SCARRING

Scarring is considered the biggest drawback of aesthetic breast surgery. Scars are generally unpredictable in appearance, and the patient should be made aware of this fact preoperatively. Keloid scars are an especially difficult problem. Excessive tension at the time of closure is thought to be a major contributing factor to poor scarring.

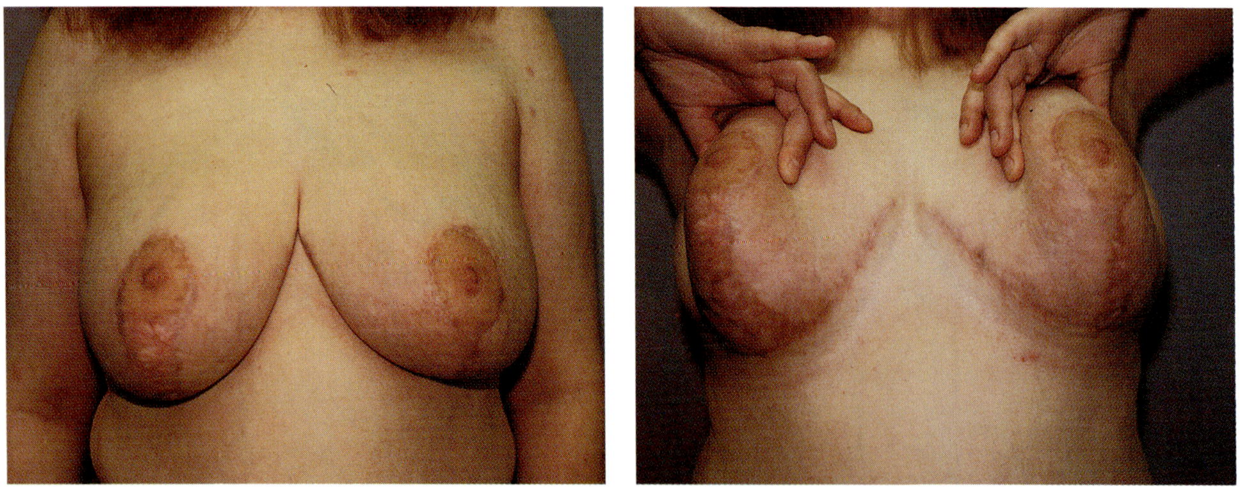

This patient underwent breast reduction using the inferior pedicle technique. Excessive tension on the skin flaps resulted in partial-thickness loss of breast skin along the vertical and horizontal lines of closure and caused excessive scarring.

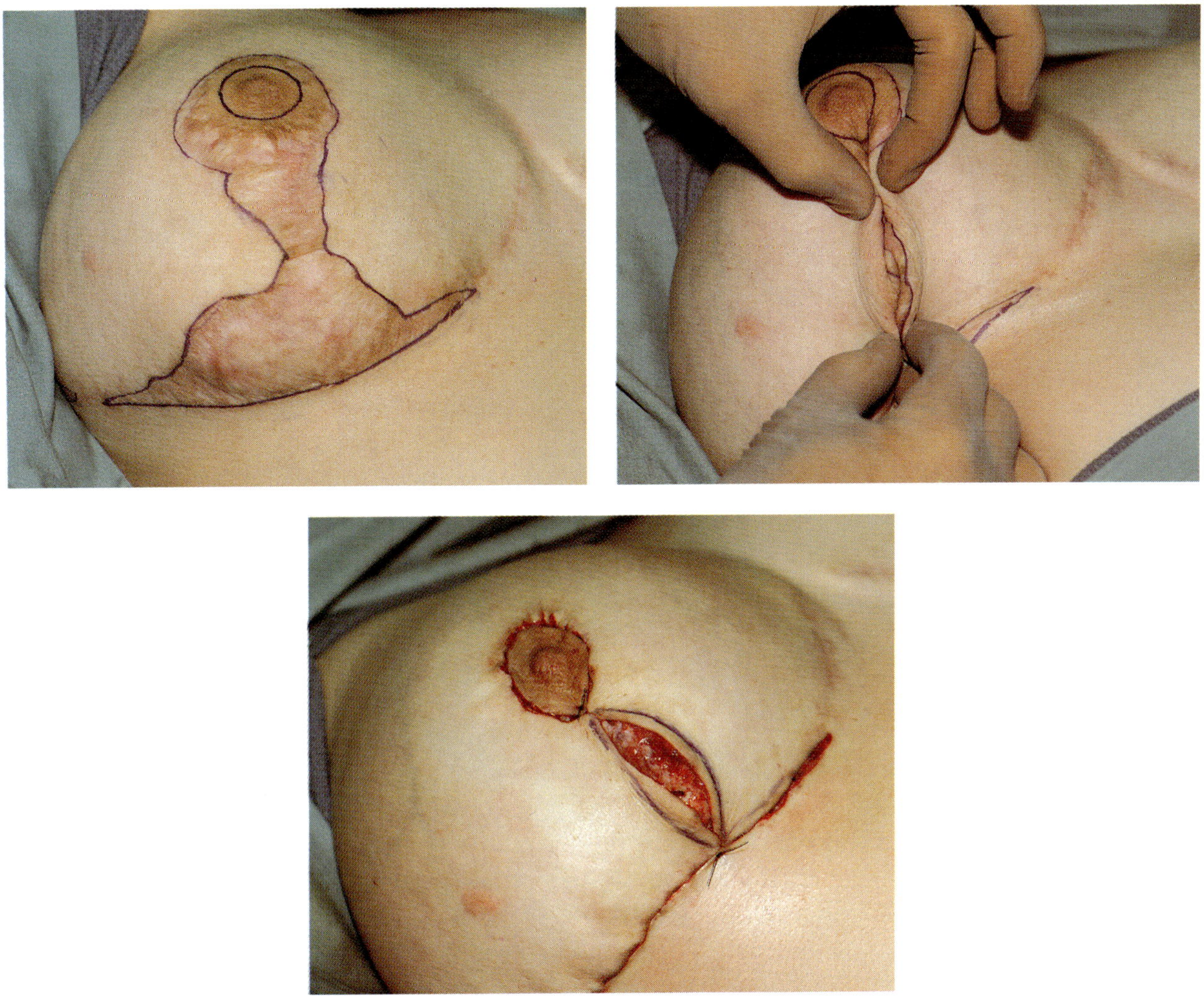

At the time of revision the area to be resected is marked. The bidigital pinch maneuver demonstrates that the scar can be easily resected and layered closure can be accomplished. Additional trimming of the vertical margin of the skin helps to create a straight-line closure.

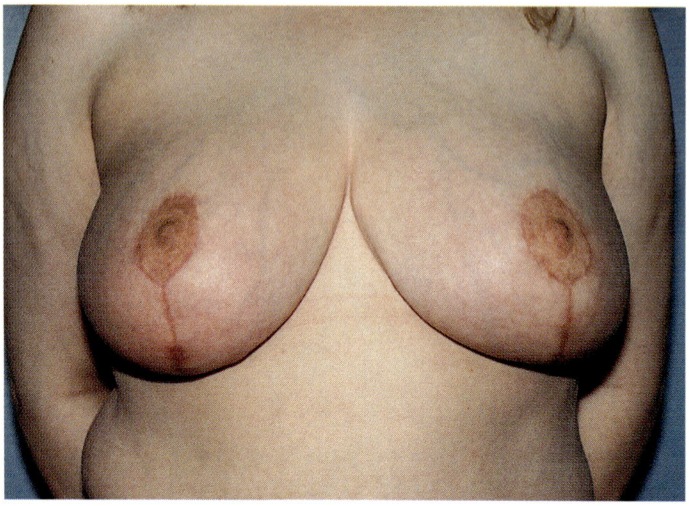

The postoperative result demonstrates improvement in the scar as well as the shape in the inferior pole of the breast.

Scar hypertrophy can be temporary and may subside with time. Revision is typically performed 6 months to 1 year following surgery. Even though late scar revision may allow closure with less tension, it still may not result in scar improvement. For this reason it is important to use the previous scars and not to add new ones. Silicone gel sheeting[22] offers an alternative therapy that shows some promise. Treatment with steroid injections may result in wide scars that inevitably require scar revision. Again, prevention is the ideal solution to scarring.

Newer techniques of breast reduction and mastopexy aim at reducing the length of the scars. L, J, or lateral scar techniques all seek to avoid creating a scar in the medial region, which is the area most vulnerable to hypertrophy.[2,23-27] Nevertheless, patients may still benefit from scar revision.

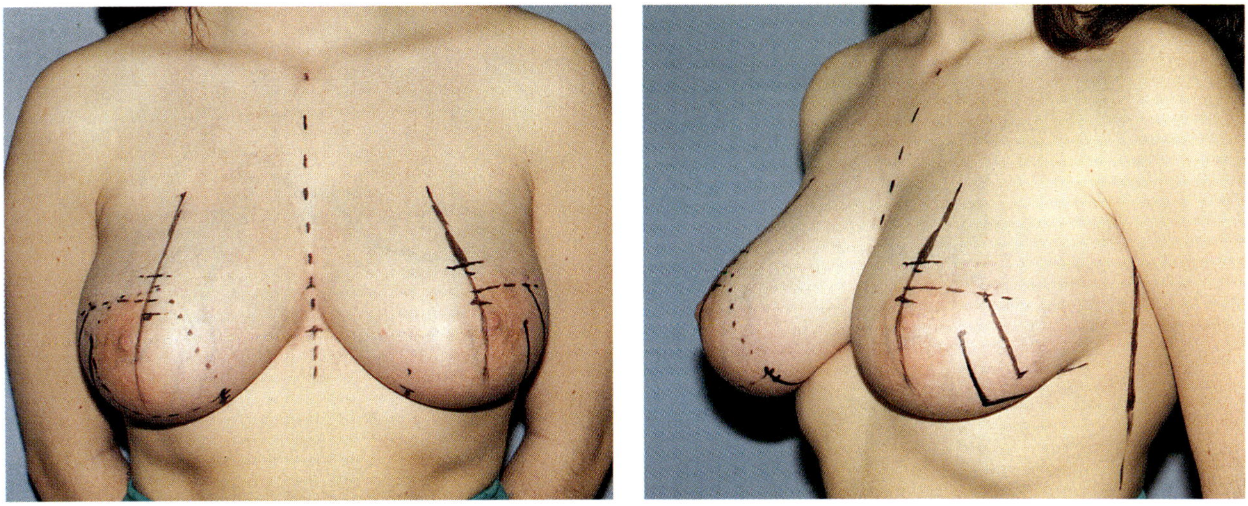

This 18-year-old patient underwent a 300 gm reduction mammaplasty using the L-shaped technique of Chiari.[2]

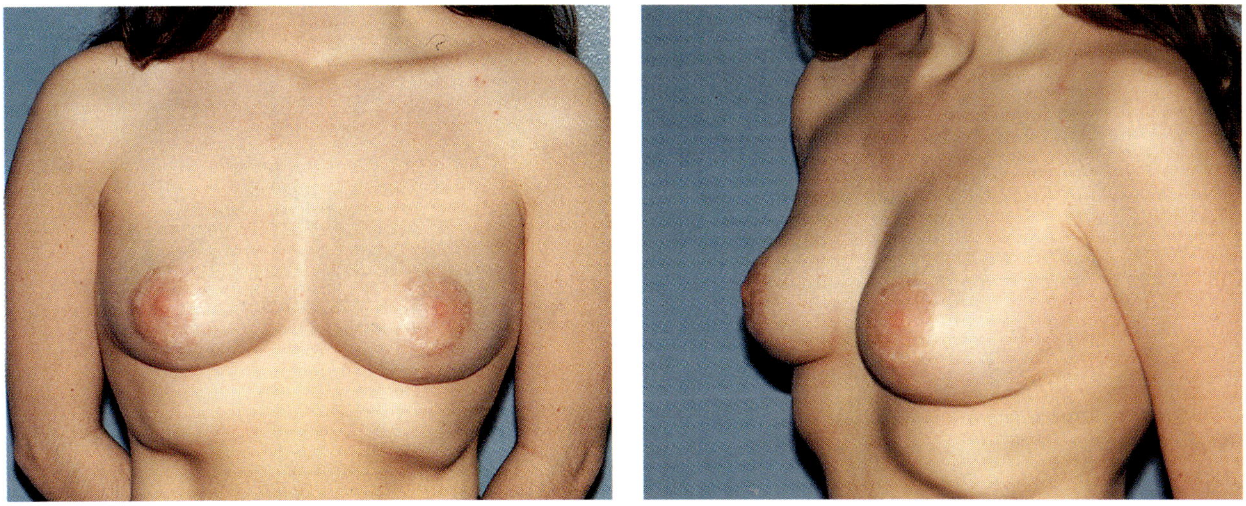

The postoperative result was satisfactory in terms of shape; however, at 1 year she was dissatisfied with the periareolar and vertical scars.

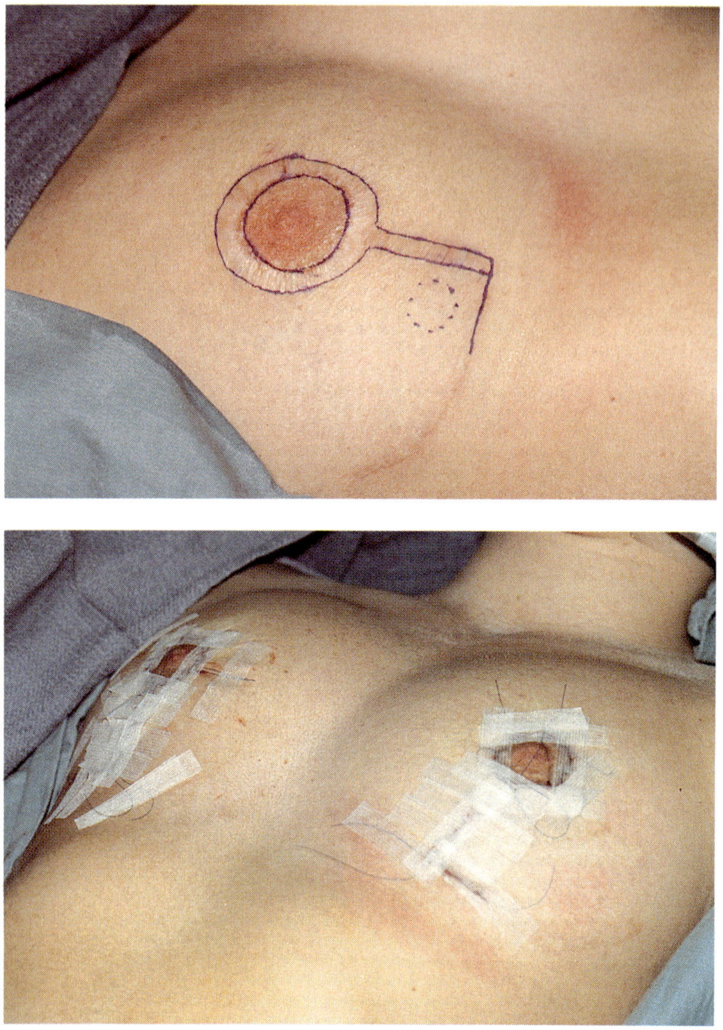

A simple revision was accomplished by full-thickness excision of the skin, layered closure with a periareolar pursestring suture, and taping.

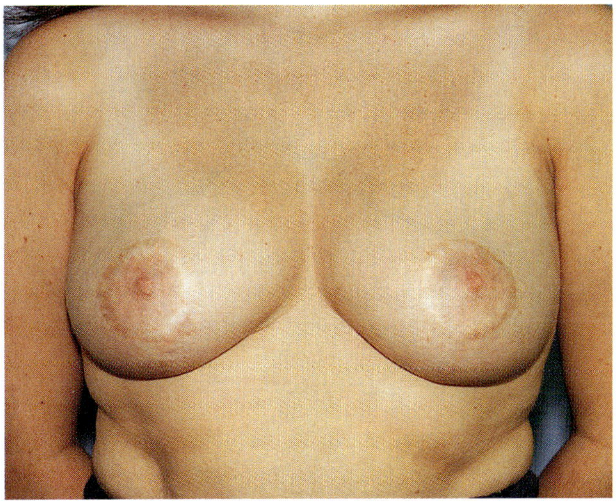

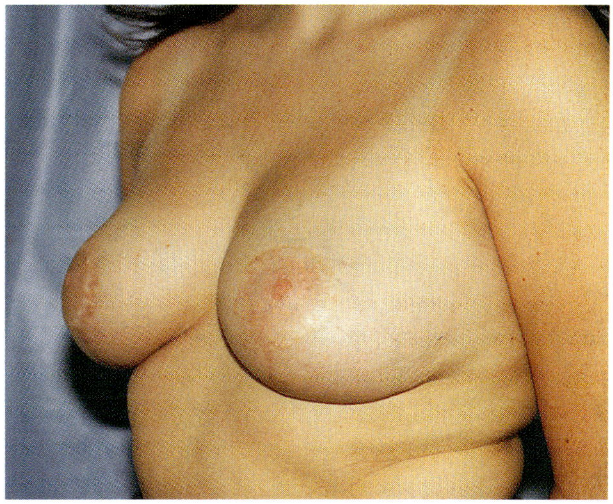

Three years postoperatively the scars are mature and satisfactory to the patient.

Periareolar techniques have a tendency to produce wide, radiating scars or enlarged areolae. The latter problem has been addressed by Benelli,[28] who uses a permanent pursestring stitch to prevent areolar enlargement. However, it is the large discrepancy between the areolar circumference and the skin excision that results in the stellate pattern of wrinkles, tension, and ultimate areolar spreading. This appearance does not always flatten with time. Other authors have used nonabsorbable[29] and absorbable[30] mesh to support the reshaped gland and to relieve tension from the periareolar closure. The best results are achieved with reductions of less than 400 gm or 40% of the breast volume.

OTHER CONDITIONS

Occult Cancer

Because breast cancer develops in one of every eight women, there is always a chance that a patient who has had a reduction mammaplasty or mastopexy may develop a mass, have an abnormal mammogram, or occasionally present for aesthetic surgery with an occult cancer.

Routine screening for breast cancer may reveal an indication for biopsy. In patients who have undergone aesthetic procedures, biopsies may be performed through old scars. Suspicious areas found during a reduction procedure should be examined with frozen section; definitive treatment may be performed later. A microscopic focus of in situ carcinoma might be adequately treated by the reduction procedure alone. For a large solitary tumor, radiotherapy and axillary dissection or mastectomy may be required.

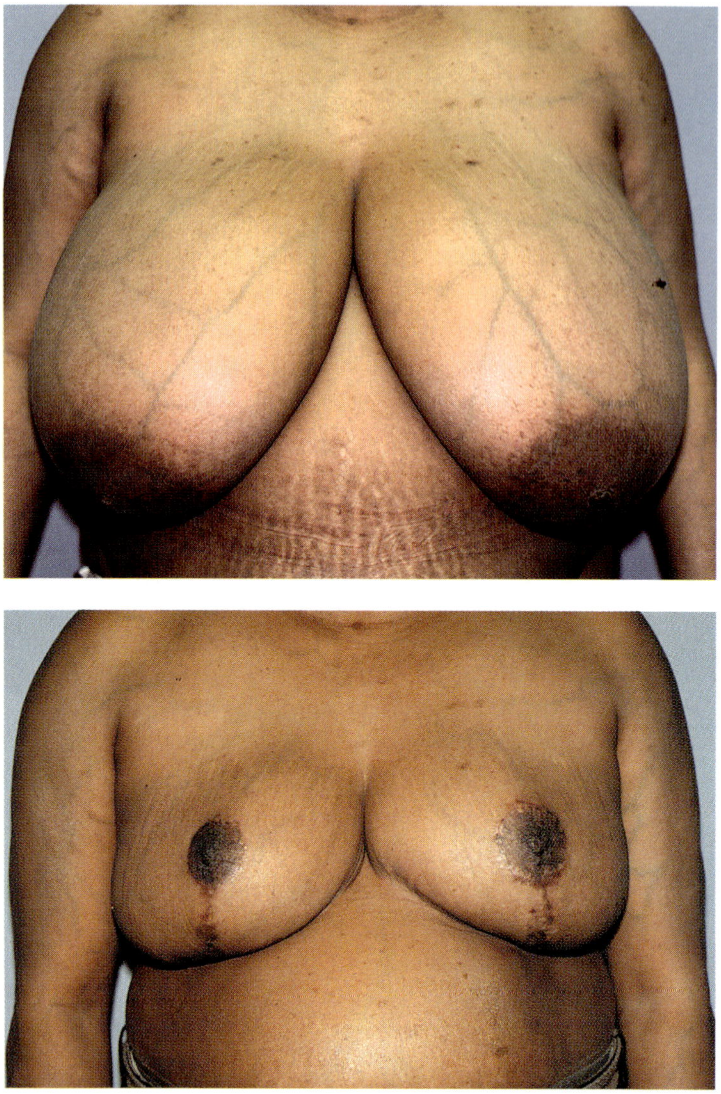

This 38-year-old woman presented for reduction mammaplasty using free nipple grafts. Histologic examination of the resected breast tissue revealed several small areas of both atypical lobular and intraductal hyperplasia and one focus of carcinoma in situ. Postoperative mammograms revealed no other suspicious areas. The patient has been followed up carefully. No further surgery has been necessary; it seems very likely that the cancer was adequately treated by the reduction procedure alone.

Radiographically breasts that have undergone reduction surgery exhibit a different appearance on mammography that the experienced mammographer can easily identify as postsurgical (see Chapter 32). When the mammographic appearance is difficult to differentiate from cancer, a biopsy is indicated. Should modified radical mastectomy be indicated, the same skin flaps designed for the reduction procedure may be used. The delay phenomenon should ensure a more robust skin flap and reduce the risk of flap necrosis. Hoffman[31] has described a mastectomy through an inverted T incision.

In patients with gigantomastia, a small mass may not be palpable preoperatively. Women 35 years of age and over should undergo screening mammography preoperatively to rule out the presence of these lesions.[32] If there is a family history of premenopausal breast cancer, then mammography at a younger age is indicated. If cancer is not detected preoperatively but is suspected intraoperatively, diagnosis may be based on histologic examination of the pathologic specimen.

Virginal Hypertrophy

Regrowth is more likely to occur in young patients (12 to 15 years of age) who have already manifested rapid breast development. One can anticipate a secondary reduction after several years in many of these patients. Lejour[33] has used staged liposuction in these patients followed by resection once breast growth ceases. Several reports appear in the literature in which antiestrogens were administered to prevent such regrowth,[34-38] but others have not found these drugs as useful. Mastectomy with reconstruction may need to be performed in unusually severe cases.[31]

UNSOLVED PROBLEMS

Scarring, contour irregularities, and durability of the postoperative result are persistent problems. Presently, wound healing research is aimed at unfolding the mystery of fetal wound repair. When this riddle is solved and scarring can be controlled, the length of scars may no longer be an issue. Until then, our efforts are focused on developing breast reduction techniques with short scars.

As noted in the introduction to this chapter, the diverse techniques available for breast reduction demonstrate our inability to find a universally applicable solution to the many different patient presentations. Each technique tends to have its own nuances and secondary aesthetic problems when applied to patients who are not ideal candidates. Until a universal technique is developed, the optimal aesthetic result will have to be attained with the best technique chosen based on the surgeon's judgment followed by secondary revisions, if needed.

Finally, durability of the result is a problem. If all of the variables affecting the volume and the skin envelope can be controlled, then we might expect a long-lasting result. Unfortunately this is not the case. The effects of hormones and gravity on tissue cannot be effectively controlled. Breasts change shape with time. Presently, the results achieved with breast-lift techniques must be regarded as temporary. Reduction techniques are successful in relieving patients of the discomforts of gigantomastia, but these patients are still subject to the same influences of gravity as seen in the mastopexy patient. Long-term follow-up remains an essential component in the evaluation of any procedure designed to reverse these influences, including secondary procedures.

References

1. Psillakis JM, deOliveira MC. History of reduction mammaplasty. In Goldwyn RM, ed. Reduction Mammaplasty, 2nd ed. Boston: Little, Brown, 1990, pp 1-15.
2. Chiari A. The short-scar mammaplasty: A new approach. Plast Reconstr Surg 90:233-246, 1992.
3. Goldwyn RM. The Unfavorable Result in Plastic Surgery: Avoidance and Treatment, 2nd ed. Boston: Little, Brown, 1984, pp 758-759.
4. Rees TD, Flagg SV. Reduction mammaplasty. In Goldwyn RM, ed. The Unfavorable Result in Plastic Surgery: Avoidance and Treatment, 2nd ed. Boston: Little, Brown, 1984, pp 371-385.
5. McKissock PK. Complications and undesirable results in reduction mammaplasty. In Goldwyn RM, ed. The Unfavorable Result in Plastic Surgery: Avoidance and Treatment, 2nd ed. Boston: Little, Brown, 1984, pp 739-759.
6. Biesenberger H. Eine neue Methode der Mammaplastik. Zentralbl Chir 55:2382, 1928.
7. Wray RC, Luce EA. Treatment of impending nipple necrosis following reduction mammaplasty. Plast Reconstr Surg 68:242-244, 1981.
8. Casanova R, Iribarren O, Grotting JC, Vasconez LO. Clinical evaluation of flap viability with a dermal surface fluorometer. Ann Plast Surg 20:112-116, 1988.
9. Hallock GG, Cusenz BJ. Salvage of the congested nipple during reduction mammaplasty. Aesthetic Plast Surg 10:143-145, 1986.
10. Singer R, Krant SM. Intravenous fluorescein for evaluating the dusky nipple-areola during reduction mammaplasty. Plast Reconstr Surg 67:534-550, 1981.
11. Gross MP, Apesos J. The use of leeches for treatment of venous congestion of the nipple following breast surgery. Aesthetic Plast Surg 16:343-348, 1992.
12. Hoffman S. Recurrent deformities following reduction mammaplasty and correction of breast asymmetry. Plast Reconstr Surg 77:55-60, 1986.
13. Goldwyn RM. Comments on Chapter 34. In Goldwyn RM, ed. The Unfavorable Result in Plastic Surgery: Avoidance and Treatment, 2nd ed. Boston: Little, Brown, 1984, p 716.
14. Dufourmentel CI, Mouly R. Chirurgie Plastique. Paris: Flammarion, 1959.
15. Lejour M, Abboud M. Vertical mammaplasty without inframammary scar and with liposuction. Perspect Plast Surg 4(2):67, 1990.
16. Matarasso A, Courtiss E. Suction mammaplasty: The use of suction lipectomy to reduce large breasts. Plast Reconstr Surg 87:709-717, 1991.
17. Smith JW, Gillen FJ. Repairing errors of nipple-areolar placement following reduction mammaplasty. Aesthetic Plast Surg 4:179-187, 1980.

18. Kroll SS, Doores S. Nipple centralization for the correction of breast deformity from segmental mastectomy. Ann Plast Surg 24:271-275, 1990.
19. Millard DR, Mullin WR, Lesavoy MA. Secondary correction of the too high areola and nipple after a mammaplasty. Plast Reconstr Surg 58:568-572, 1976.
20. Salema R, Abdoudib JH, DeCastro CC. Convergent nipple-areolar complexes corrected by inferior curve pedicle technique. Ann Plast Surg 19:555, 1987.
21. Elsahy NI. Correction of abnormally high nipples after reduction mammaplasty. Aesthetic Plast Surg 14:21-26, 1990.
22. Ahn ST, Monafo WW, Mustoe TA. Topical silicone gel: A new treatment for hypertrophic scars. Surgery 106:781-786, 1989.
23. Regnault P. Reduction mammaplasty by the "B" technique. Plast Reconstr Surg 53:19, 1974.
24. Peixoto G. Reduction mammaplasty: A personal technique. Plast Reconstr Surg 65:217-225, 1980.
25. Marchac D, de Olarte G. Reduction mammaplasty and correction of ptosis with a short inframammary scar. Plast Reconstr Surg 69:45-55, 1982.
26. Marchac D. Reduction mammaplasty with a short horizontal scar. In Goldwyn RM, ed. Reduction Mammaplasty. Boston: Little, Brown, 1990, pp 317-335.
27. Bozola AR. Reduction mammaplasty: Preferred techniques. In Goldwyn RM, ed. Reduction Mammaplasty. Boston: Little, Brown, 1990, pp 407-437.
28. Benelli L. A new periareolar mammaplasty: Round block technique. Aesthetic Plast Surg 14:93, 1990.
29. Bustos RA. Periareolar mammaplasty with silicone supporting lamina. Plast Reconstr Surg 89:646-659, 1992.
30. Sampaio Góes JC. Periareolar mammaplasty: Double skin technique with application of polyglactine 910 mesh. Rev Soc Bras Cir Plast 7:1-6, 1992.
31. Hoffman S. Mastectomy using a T-shaped incision. Breast Dis 1:135, 1988.
32. Brown FE, Sargent SK. Mammographic changes after reduction mammaplasty. In Goldwyn RM, ed. Reduction Mammaplasty, 2nd ed. Boston: Little, Brown, 1990, pp 35-43.
33. Lejour M. Vertical Mammaplasty and Liposuction. St. Louis: Quality Medical Publishing, 1993.
34. Gottlieb JR, McKinney P, Walkinshaw MD, Sperling RL. Occult breast carcinoma in patients undergoing reduction mammaplasty. Aesthetic Plast Surg 13:279-283, 1989.
35. Sperling RL, Gold JJ. Use of an antiestrogen after a reduction mammaplasty to prevent recurrence of virginal hypertrophy of breasts: Case report. Plast Reconstr Surg 52:439, 1973.
36. Mayl N, Vasconez LO, Jurkiewicz MJ. Treatment of macromastia in the actively enlarging breast. Plast Reconstr Surg 54:6, 1974.
37. Ryan RF, Pernoll ML. Virginal hypertrophy. Plast Reconstr Surg 75:737-742, 1985.
38. Kupfer D, Dingman D, Broadbent R. Juvenile breast hypertrophy: Report of a familial pattern and review of the literature. Plast Reconstr Surg 90:303-309, 1992.

28

Reoperative Surgery Following Breast Augmentation

James C. Grotting, M.D., Paul M. Gardner, M.D.,
and H. Hollis Caffee, M.D.

Reoperative Problems

Hypertrophic scarring	Malposition
Seroma	Capsular contracture
Hematoma	Device failure
Wound dehiscence	Silicone-associated problems

Following the introduction of silicone implants by Cronin in the 1960s, breast augmentation using implants became one of the most widely performed operations in plastic surgery. It is estimated over two million women in the United States have breast implants. Before 1992, over 150,000 augmentations were performed annually.[1] Since the Food and Drug Administration (FDA) hearings regarding the safety and efficacy of implant devices, many more women have sought the advice of plastic surgeons regarding reoperation.

Problems related to breast implants range from immediate postoperative complications such as hematoma and infection to the long-term problem of capsular contracture. For example, some patients may present with implant failure. Others may express dissatisfaction with the aesthetic results. The "breast implant crisis" has drawn attention to a whole new set of challenges for the plastic surgeon.

PATIENT EVALUATION

The decision to reoperate must be made with specific goals in mind. For problems such as infection and exposure, there is usually no other recourse but surgical intervention. However, when the patient presents for correction of unsatisfactory aesthetic results, the surgeon must be certain the patient has realistic expectations based on careful preoperative consultation.

In the past many breast augmentations were performed with relatively little preoperative counseling. The patient population was usually young, somewhat impulsive, and often focused only on short-term volume correction. Nevertheless, breast augmentation has had a very high success rate when measured in terms of patient satisfaction.[2]

The sources of dissatisfaction are often linked to aesthetic problems that can occur early or late in the postoperative period. The most common cause of early dissatisfaction among breast augmentation patients is volume undercorrection. Failure to preoperatively recognize significant breast ptosis, asymmetry, or a tight or high inframammary fold may also result in patient dissatisfaction, especially if these factors were not brought to the patient's attention before the initial augmentation. Subsequently various issues affecting both the doctor-patient relationship and finances come into play (see Chapters 2 and 3).

Breast augmentation enlarges the volume of the breast and can correct breast shape but rarely will improve significant ptosis. Failure to recognize the need for a concomitant mastopexy often will lead to a poor aesthetic outcome and a dissatisfied patient.

If the patient's breasts are asymmetric before augmentation and the asymmetry is unrecognized preoperatively, the breasts may become more noticeably asymmetric postoperatively. Careful study of preoperative photographs will generally reveal subtle volume differences that can be corrected at the time of surgery.

Any discussion of the goals of reoperation must include the possibility of recurrence of the problem addressed by the secondary surgery. For example, treatment of capsular contracture by either capsular alteration or implant exchange may well be complicated by ultimate recurrence of the contracture.

Similarly, mastopexy is often complicated by recurrent ptosis. Explantation surgery in the face of systemic symptoms may not produce any effective long-term relief. The patient must clearly understand all of these issues before consenting to reoperative surgery.

TIMING

The timing of reoperation is determined by the nature of the problem. Again, complications like infection often require surgery as soon as the problem is diagnosed. On the other hand, for problems such as malposition or asymmetry a certain period of time should elapse before a secondary procedure is attempted. This delay allows edema to resolve, scarring to mature, and the implant to settle.

Some conservative measures can obviate the need for reoperation. For example, Velcro strapping of the upper poles of the implants may help to lower them symmetrically, and implant displacement exercises and support bras may influence the development of capsular contracture and affect the shape of smooth-walled implants during the waiting period.

One special circumstance in which early surgical intervention is indicated can occur following the treatment of capsular contracture by implant site change. Most commonly an implant is removed from the subglandular space and reinserted in a subpectoral pocket. Occasionally, if the subglandular space is not sutured closed, the implant may slip over the inferior border of the pectoralis major muscle back into the original pocket.

Early implant displacement may also occur in patients who have undergone lateral capsulorrhaphy to try to revise a laterally displaced implant. If the suture repair fails early, the implant may again become displaced; implant positioning should be corrected by early reoperation.

APPLIED ANATOMY

Blood Supply

The arterial supply to the breast is derived from numerous sources, is closely related to the underlying pectoralis major and serratus anterior muscles, and is rich in collateralization. The major contributing arteries are the internal mammary, lateral thoracic, and intercostal arteries.[3] This extensive vascular network allows the plastic surgeon to use a number of different augmentation approaches with little concern of devascularization.

The main alterations in vascularity following augmentation result from the division of perforators as the pocket is made. With the subglandular approach, the pectoralis major perforators from the thoracoacromial artery, some internal mammary segmental perforators, and the intercostal perforators are divided. The breast can survive entirely on the lateral thoracic artery, which enters the breast through perforators lateral to and through the pectoralis major muscle as well as perforators that are not divided. Whether a poorly vascularized area created in the subglandular dissection is predisposed to infection and capsular contracture has not been substantiated.

During dissection of a subpectoral pocket, the lower internal mammary perforators and some of the more central intercostal perforators may be divided. Care should be taken to avoid injuring the second and third internal mammary perforators, the largest perforators. Injury to these vessels can be avoided by leaving the origin of the pectoralis major muscle attached to the second and third intercostal space.[4]

The nipple-areola complex receives its blood supply via numerous branches from the breast parenchyma as well as the subdermal periareolar plexus. Neither the subglandular or subpectoral approach risks injury to the nipple-areola complex as long as the underlying breast tissue is left intact.[5]

Vascular compromise of breast parenchyma is not usually an issue with implant exchange or removal. However, when mastopexy is performed concomitantly, certain combinations of operations could conceivably devascularize the parenchyma. For example, when a subglandular implant has been previously placed, any mastopexy procedure that requires wide undermining of the skin flaps could potentially result in devascularization of the parenchyma. Review of operative records might be helpful in planning reoperation to avoid this complication. Alternatively, avoiding any secondary mastopexy procedure that requires wide skin undermining when the integrity of pectoralis major muscle perforators is in question is a good practice.

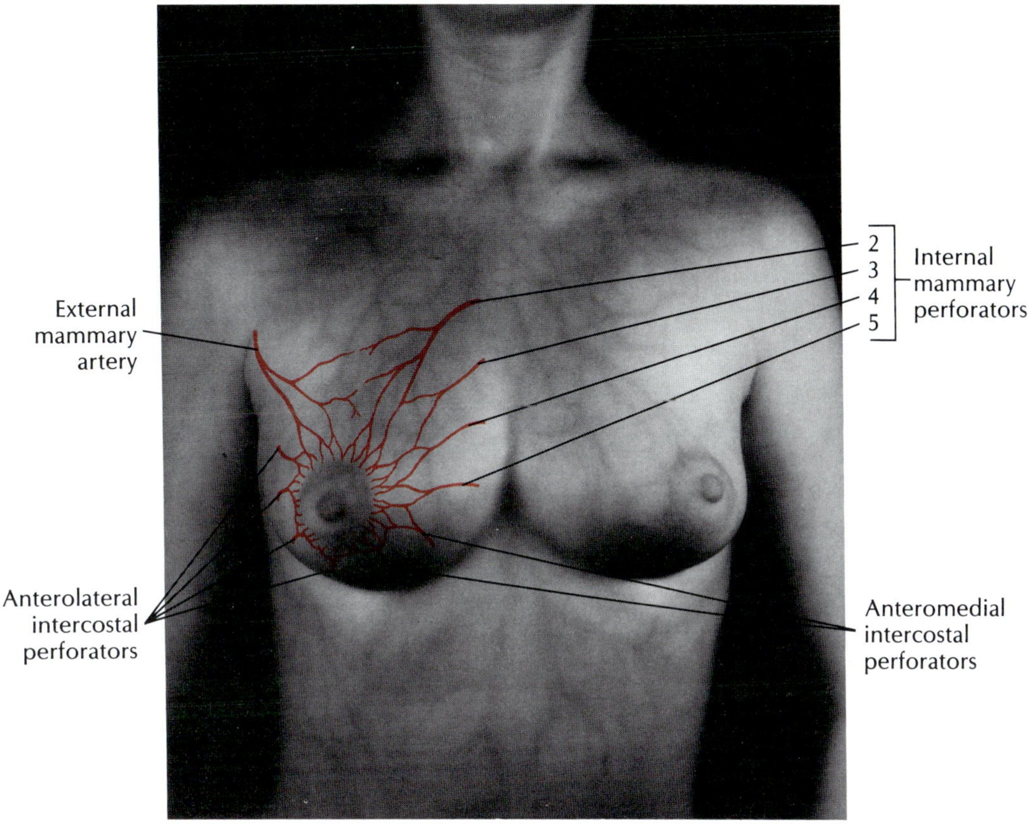

Illustration from Bostwick J III. Plastic and Reconstructive Breast Surgery. St. Louis: Quality Medical Publishing, 1990, p 63.

Nerves

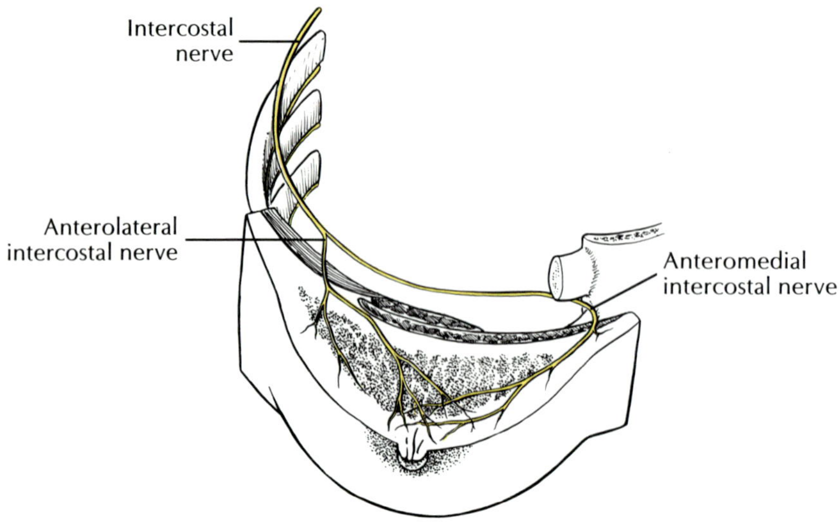

Sensation of the breast is provided by the intercostal segmental nerves as well as branches from the cervical plexus. The most disconcerting sensory change following breast augmentation is nipple hyposensitivity, which is reported to occur in between 15% and 49% of cases.[2,6] Postoperative anesthesia of the nipple is rare; when it occurs, it is usually the result of the division of the fourth anterolateral intercostal nerve.[7] This nerve penetrates the posterior aspect of the breast at the intersection of the lateral border of the pectoralis major muscle and the fourth intercostal space. This location is approximately the 4 o'clock position on the left breast and the 8 o'clock position on the right breast.[8]

With the axillary approach, injury to the second intercostal nerve (i.e., intercostobrachial cutaneous nerve) can occur if dissection is carried too deep into the axilla. The plane of dissection should be superficial to the lateral aspect of the pectoralis major muscle and then directly beneath it. Painful neuromas can occur if the lateral cutaneous nerves are divided or caught in the capsule.[4]

SPECIFIC PROBLEMS

The reoperative problems related to breast implants can be divided into complications resulting from the surgical procedure including malposition and capsular contracture and those associated with the device itself. The overall incidence of complications with breast augmentation is quite low if one excludes capsular contracture. Many of these complications, however, require reoperation.

Illustration from Bostwick J III. Plastic and Reconstructive Breast Surgery. St. Louis: Quality Medical Publishing, 1990, p 64.

Hypertrophic Scarring

Hypertrophic scarring occurs in approximately 2% to 5% of patients.[8] Keloid formation is rare. The best treatment is to make well-planned incisions that will camouflage the scar in the event it becomes hypertrophic. If the inframammary approach is used, the incision should be placed at the anticipated level of the new inframammary fold at or below the natural inframammary crease. If the incision is made in the axilla, a prominent crease should be chosen. The incision should never cross a crease[8] (see Chapter 5).

Seroma

Seroma formation is predictable and usually resolves without treatment. It usually becomes evident on the second or third postoperative day. Aspiration is performed only if the seroma is large and discrete enough to ensure that the needle will not be inadvertently introduced into the implant. Aspiration should not be performed through the incision but laterally while mechanically displacing the implant medially with fingertip pressure.[9] With sterile technique a 16-gauge intravenous catheter is slowly and carefully introduced. The needle is removed, leaving the flexible catheter within the fluid cavity. The fluid is aspirated and sent for the appropriate culture and sensitivity studies. This process is repeated on a serial basis until the seroma resolves or decreases to a negligible volume.

Hematoma

The incidence of hematoma following breast augmentation ranges from 1% to 6%.[10,11] Hematoma usually results from inadequate hemostasis at the time the pocket was dissected. However, some hematomas may appear up to 3 weeks following surgery. Most can be observed. Large hematomas should be evacuated in the operating room with the patient under general anesthesia. After the incision is opened, the implant is removed and placed in a dilute povidone-iodine (Betadine) solution. The hematoma is evacuated, and the source of bleeding is meticulously sought with the assistance of a fiberoptic retractor. Electrocautery is used to achieve hemostasis. After copious irrigation, the implant is replaced. Some studies link the incidence of hematoma with a higher rate of capsular contracture (see p. 974). In addition, a higher incidence of infection occurs when the hematoma is not drained.[12]

Infection

Infection with implants is rare. Some researchers report an incidence of approximately 2% to 4%.[13] *Staphylococcus aureus* and *Staphylococcus epidermidis* are the most commonly cultured organisms.[13] Patients with *Pseudomonas* infections typically present with pain out of proportion with the clinical findings; this type of infection must be suspected in patients with a low-grade fever and severe pain in the augmented breast.[8] *Mycobacterium* infections occur very rarely. The presence of this organism must be suspected when clinical signs of infection are present with negative "routine" culture results.[14]

LeRoy and Given[15] have reported that the prophylactic administration of antibiotics does not significantly decrease the incidence of infection. However, they irrigate the implant pockets with bacitracin or povidone-iodine. We prefer to prescribe a prophylactic antibiotic regimen. One gram of a first-generation cephalosporin is administered just before the skin incision is made. For patients with cardiac valve problems including mitral valve prolapse, intravenous or oral antibiotics are administered for 48 hours preoperatively.

If early cellulitis develops around the incision or involves the skin of the breast, this condition will frequently respond to aggressive intravenous antibiotic therapy. We admit our patients to the hospital and place them on a regimen of intravenous cephalosporin until the erythema resolves. The patient is then discharged from the hospital and prescribed oral antibiotics to be taken for at least 1 week with close follow-up. The standard treatment for infected implants is to remove them. The complications that can result from infected implants that are not removed include exposure with extrusion, capsular contracture, and even toxic shock syndrome.[16] Once gross purulence has formed around the implant, only open drainage with thorough irrigation can be expected to have any hope of salvaging the implant. There are reports of implants that have been saved in the face of infection. Courtiss, Goldwyn, and Anastasi[12] reported the salvage of 16 of 29 infected implants by draining the pocket and intravenous antibiotic treatment. Our preference is to remove the implant, thoroughly irrigate the pocket, and allow complete healing and softening of the breast to occur before implant replacement. This process usually requires several months. Occasionally a patient may wish to have both implants removed to avoid significant asymmetry during the waiting period. This approach also avoids the occasional situation in which an infection involving one breast may lead to subsequent infection of the contralateral breast.

Wound Dehiscence

Dehiscence and exposure may result from several technical problems including inadequate closure, hematoma, seroma, and infection. In addition, an inadequate pocket for the size of the implant may result in a tense closure that ultimately breaks down.[9] Implants inserted through an inframammary approach, especially when large, can exert considerable tension on the sutured wound. This tension is particularly accentuated when the patient is in the upright position. A separate layer of sutures in Scarpa's fascia will help to relieve tension from the skin closure and diminish the risk of dehiscence and exposure.

If dehiscence occurs within the first 2 or 3 days following implant placement, often the implant may be salvaged by returning the patient to the operating room, irrigating the wound carefully, and reclosing it in layers. However, when dehiscence occurs 1 week or more postoperatively, one must always suspect infection as the cause. An attempt might be made to salvage the implant by thorough irrigation of the pocket with an antibiotic solution, replacement of the implant, reclosure of the wound, and intravenous antibiotic therapy. ***However, the presence of frank purulence mandates removal.*** If the original placement was subglandular, replacement in the submuscular position may reduce the risk of recurrence.

When textured-surface implants are inserted, they are expected to adhere to the surrounding capsule. Lack of adherence may result from seroma formation or infection. When dehiscence occurs from seroma, pockets of nonadherence may contribute to further seroma collections and ultimately to infection. In this situation the wound pocket should be explored under sterile conditions and drains should be placed to try to prevent the development of further seroma collections. On exploration, if the entire implant is adherent to the surrounding capsule, then simple reclosure of the wound is likely to be successful.

Implant Malposition

Malposition can result in the implant being too high, too low, or too far laterally. Usually malposition is detected immediately postoperatively while the patient is still on the operating table. However, malposition may not become apparent until the pocket has had time to mature.

If the inferior dissection is too extensive, the implant will drop below the proposed inframammary line, creating a bulge or an unnatural elevation of the nipple-areola complex. If this problem is recognized intraoperatively, the subcutaneous tissue of the inferior flap can be sutured to the fascia. A compression garment is employed to maintain postoperative implant position.[17]

If the implant descends at some point after the initial operation, repositioning of the implant by the use of a compression garment may be attempted. However, this practice usually has little chance for success. Steroids placed in the pocket intraoperatively are known to cause gradual inferior displacement of the implant. Atrophy of the breast skin may also occur. Correction of the deformity usually requires reoperation. The adjusted fold is marked preoperatively. The stretched or thinned inframammary skin may need to be excised. However, it is usually better to redrape the skin than to create long scars. The capsule is dissected until it is exposed anteriorly and posteriorly. A crescent wedge of exposed capsule is excised. The implant is then removed. The subcutaneous tissue of the inferior flap is sutured to the underlying fascia. The implant is replaced with a textured-surface implant. The inferior capsule is reefed to maintain the superiorly repositioned implant. A compression garment is applied for at least 4 weeks.[18]

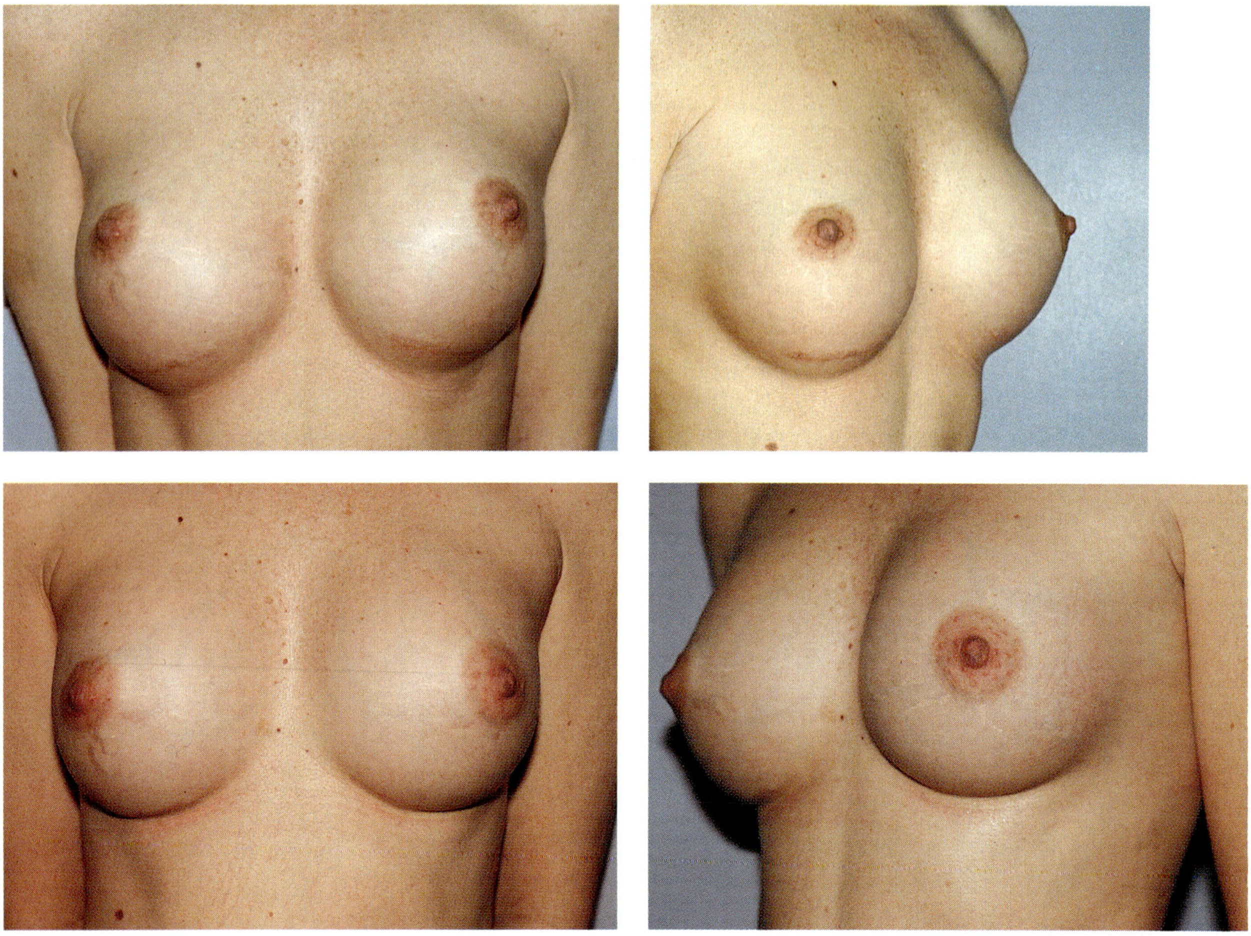

This patient demonstrates the effect of implant descent. Two years earlier steroids had been inserted into the implant pocket. The reoperative result is shown 1 year following correction using the technique described above.

An alternative way of correcting inferior descent is implant site change. If the primary pocket was subglandular, the implant is reinserted in the subpectoral position. Relocation of the implant prevents recurrence of malposition, which can occur if the inferior flap dehisces from the fascial plication.

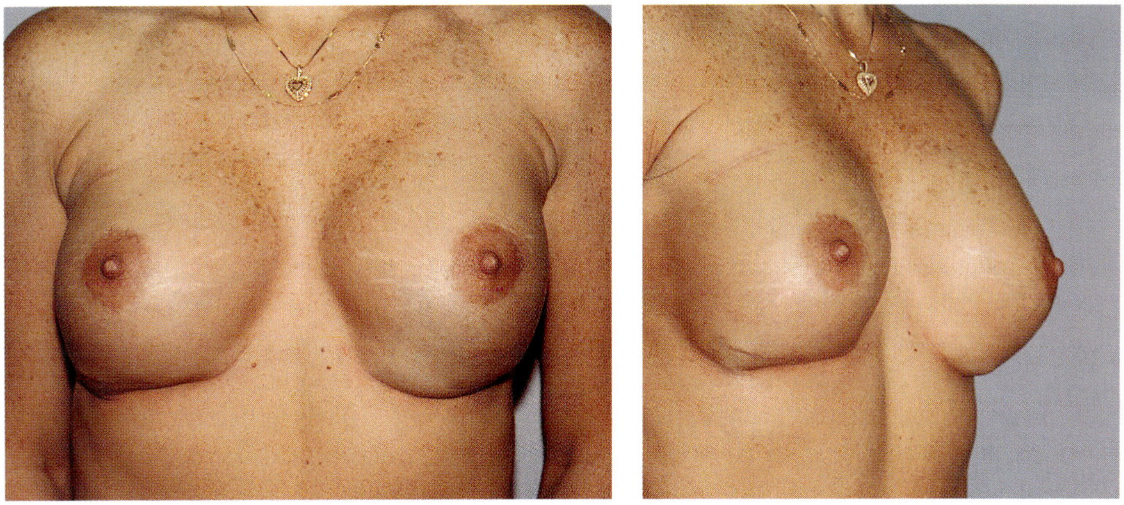

This 45-year-old woman underwent augmentation with subglandular bilumen silicone gel implants. She was referred for correction 1 year later following two additional procedures for implant malposition. The surgeon had attempted replacement of the implants with plication of the inframammary fold, but persistent herniation ensued with irregularities along the inframammary fold. Correction was accomplished by careful suturing inferiorly and laterally of the reopened capsule along the projected level of the inframammary fold. A textured-surface implant was placed in the subpectoral position.

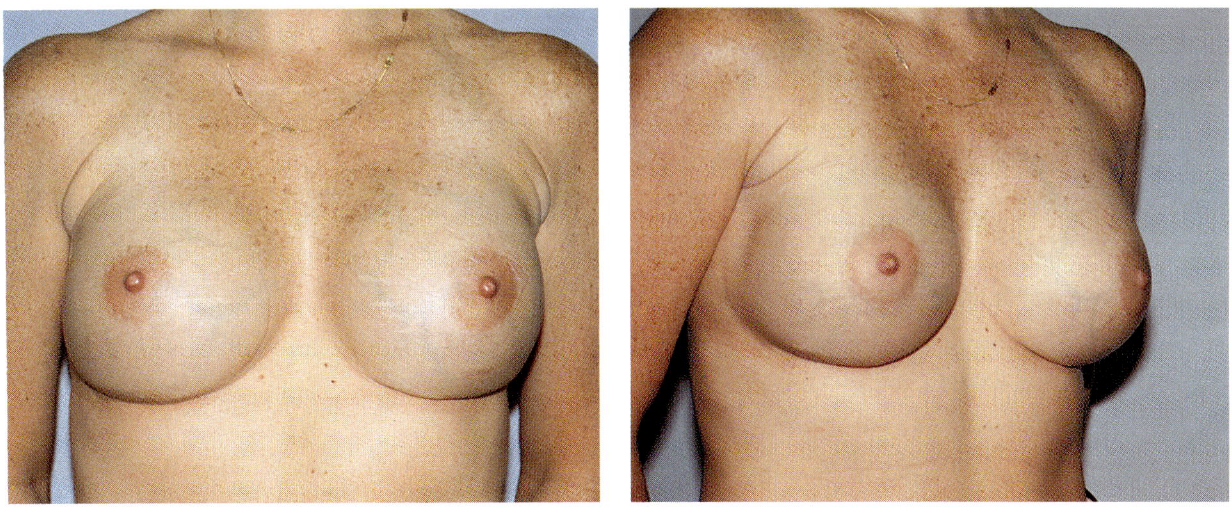

The postoperative result is shown at 1 year. The correction has been maintained.

When a large implant is placed in a small breast without adequately lowering the inframammary fold, a high-riding implant may result. This problem can often be treated with a superiorly placed compression strap. If this approach fails, surgical lowering of the implant is required. When implants are placed too far laterally or when an implant "drifts" postoperatively, the implants should be repositioned and the lateral pocket reinforced with several rows of sutures. We prefer to open the capsule anteriorly and posteriorly along the new anticipated lateral border to locate a part of the wound where solid fibrosis and healing can be expected to occur. If this location is not satisfactory, a new site is chosen.

For all malposition problems, we prefer to replace the primary implant with a textured-surface implant, which tends to remain where it is placed if it becomes adherent to the surrounding capsule. This attachment will diminish the gravitational forces that tend to allow inferior and lateral implant movement.

Capsular Contracture

The development of capsular contracture in the augmented breast is one of the most frustrating and difficult problems plastic surgeons face. Numerous etiologies have been proposed. Multiple strategies to prevent or reduce its incidence have been advocated. Despite intensive efforts, capsular contracture remains the most common complication of breast augmentation surgery.[19]

Causes

All foreign bodies implanted into the body incite an inflammatory response that results in the development of a fibrous capsule. This capsule consists largely of fibroblasts and an associated fibrous connective tissue matrix.[20] In some patients with breast implants this capsule contracts, resulting in varying degrees of contracture. A specialized fibroblast with smooth muscle characteristics, the myofibroblast, has been found in the capsules of patients with contractures and is considered by many to be responsible for contraction.[21] It is not understood what causes myofibroblasts to appear in the capsule and what regulates its contraction properties.

A single primary cause of capsular contracture has not been identified. Numerous associations have been proposed in the literature. Although none is conclusive, these hypotheses at least warrant consideration.

Hematoma has long been associated with increased rates of contracture. Hipps, Raju, and Straith[22] reported an 86% incidence of contracture in patients with hematoma vs. 32% incidence in patients without hematoma. Animal studies showed histologic evidence of a thicker capsule around the implants in baboons in which hematomas were allowed to develop.[23] The problem with this study is there is no correlation between the thickness of a capsule and the likelihood of significant contracture developing. Implants placed in rabbits in which a hematoma was allowed to develop on one side and not the other failed to show an increased incidence of contracture.[24] Finally, the low incidence of hematoma in breast implant patients (at the most, 6%) falls far below the observed incidence of contracture.

Infection has been linked to increased rates of contracture. Several authors have shown a causal relationship between bacterial contamination and capsular contracture in animals.[25,26] A number of experiments have been reported demonstrating a relationship between subclinical infection and contracture.[27,28] Burkhardt et al.[29] published a prospective, randomized, double-blind clinical study demonstrating a significant decrease in the incidence of contracture in patients who received local antibacterial agents at the time of implant placement. Again, the incidence of capsular contracture is far higher than the incidence of infection, defining infection as a contributing factor at best.

The discovery of silicone particles in breast implant capsules led some researchers to believe gel bleed was responsible for contracture.[30] This theory was indirectly supported clinically by a prospective randomized study in which the contracture rate of saline vs. that of gel-filled implants was lower.[31] Further evidence was provided by an animal study in which low-bleed implants had a lower rate of contracture than standard gel-filled implants in rabbits.[32] Despite these findings, contracture has continued to be observed in women with low-bleed implants.

Capsular contracture can be a considerable source of discomfort and dissatisfaction among patients. Any possible preventive measure should be used. The following considerations are theoretical and are based on percentages.

Implant type has a direct bearing on the incidence of contracture. Contracture developed with all of the early sponge implants.[33] The smooth-surface silicone gel implant fared much better but still had a high incidence of contracture ranging from 36% to 81% in the literature.[34] Saline implants have lower contracture rates ranging from 8% to 38%.[35] The type of surface on the implant also has a bearing on the rate of contracture. Textured-surface implants have been reported in several series to have a lower incidence of contracture than smooth-surface implants.[36] The foam-covered implant, particularly the polyurethane type, offers an even lower incidence of contracture. One series investigating this type of implant reported no contractures with up to 4½ years of follow-up.[37]

Based on these statistics, it is obvious that the choice of implant affects the risk of capsular contracture. At the time of this writing, silicone gel implants are under an FDA moratorium and can be used only in special circumstances under the silicone gel–implant clinical adjunct study protocol. Consequently saline implants are now used much more frequently than ever before. The drawbacks are the less natural "feel" and the increased incidence of deflation. The polyurethane-covered implant is no longer available in the United States. Therefore today the only choice in the United States is a textured-surface or a smooth-surface saline-filled implant.

Although not universally accepted,[38] many reports in the literature attribute a lower incidence of capsular contracture to the placement of implants in the submuscular vs. the subglandular position.[39,40] There are a variety of possible explanations. One is that the muscle repeatedly contracts over the implants, resulting in continuous stretching of the scar. Another possible explanation could relate to the different tissue characteristics of the submuscular space, which perhaps make this tissue less prone to scar contracture than glandular tissue. It is also possible that the submuscular space is less vulnerable to contamination by bacteria.[41] Naturally preoperative considerations such as breast size, degree of ptosis, and postpartum glandular involution must be considered when choosing the most appropriate implant site.

Reducing the incidence of infection has been shown to decrease the rate of contracture for 3 months postoperatively. Burkhardt et al.[10] demonstrated a statistically significant reduction in contracture rate when any of four antibacterial regimens was implemented. These protocols included intraluminal antibiotics alone and in combination with an irrigation solution, irrigation solution alone, and povidone-iodine antibiotic steroid foam instillation. The antibiotic used was 1 gm cephalothin in 100 cc of normal saline solution. The solution, 30 cc of 5% povidone-iodine solution, was distributed throughout the pocket. The antibiotic steroid foam consisted of a mixture of 50,000 U bacitracin, 250 mg of oxacillin, and 40 mg of triamcinolone.

A number of physicians advocate displacement exercises to decrease the incidence of contracture.[42,43] Patients are instructed to gently massage their breasts during dressing changes for the first postoperative week. Then more vigorous daily massage and even manual releases of fibrous tissue are performed on a weekly basis. It is thought that this manipulation preserves the implant pocket volume, thus decreasing contracture forces. None of the displacement exercise studies demonstrating favorable results was controlled for motion exercises alone. In fact, Marshall[44] reported better rates of contracture with motion restriction. Textured-surface implants that adhere to the surrounding capsule will not displace and are not intended to be moved.

The practice of steroid placement in the implant pocket to decrease the incidence of contracture is based on steroids' inhibitory effects on wound contraction.[45] Several early reports of success with steroids placed in the implant pocket and within the lumen of the implant were published.[46,47] Long-term follow-up, however, has demonstrated a significant incidence of associated complications including prosthesis ptosis, atrophy and thinning of overlying breast tissue, impending extrusion, and even capsular contracture.[48,49]

Treatment

H. Hollis Caffee, M.D.

Most contractures are minor and treatment is unnecessary. Some contractures are of moderate degree; in this case the patient may desire correction only if it can be achieved without the expense and inconvenience of a second operation. Occasionally contracture will cause symptoms problematic enough to justify aggressive treatment. Until recently it was only the rare patient who had severe enough symptoms that she was willing to have the implants removed.

In the past those women who desired treatment of contracture had three options: closed capsulotomy, open capsulotomy, and percutaneous capsulotomy. With the current controversy surrounding silicone and given the known risk of implant rupture with closed capsulotomy, closed capsulotomy is mentioned for historic interest only. Closed capsulotomy is no longer condoned by implant manufacturers. Most plastic surgeons avoid the procedure, especially for long-standing contractures around silicone gel implants.

Open capsulotomy has the distinct advantage of allowing greater control but involves the risks and expense of the original augmentation. The risk of recurrent contracture has not been well studied, but the logical conclusion would be that recurrence will occur in a similar manner as with closed capsulotomy. Recurrence with closed capsulotomy ranges from 30% to 67%.[2,50] The methods for reducing the risk of recurrent contracture are the same as those applicable for primary augmentation.

Our method of open capsulotomy is as follows. With the patient under general anesthesia, the previous incision is reused if possible. An inframammary approach is preferred, but endoscopy may allow this procedure to be performed via the transaxillary approach. The implant capsule is incised with cautery since the implant will not conduct electric current and will therefore not be cut by the instrument. However, the cautery will generate enough heat to melt the elastomer if there is prolonged contact in any one area. The capsule is usually incised around the entire circumference of the base. A variety of cuts in the dome can be created in an attempt to allow the implant to either drop or project inferiorly. Segmental or total capsulectomy, together with implant exchange and site change, is now more common.

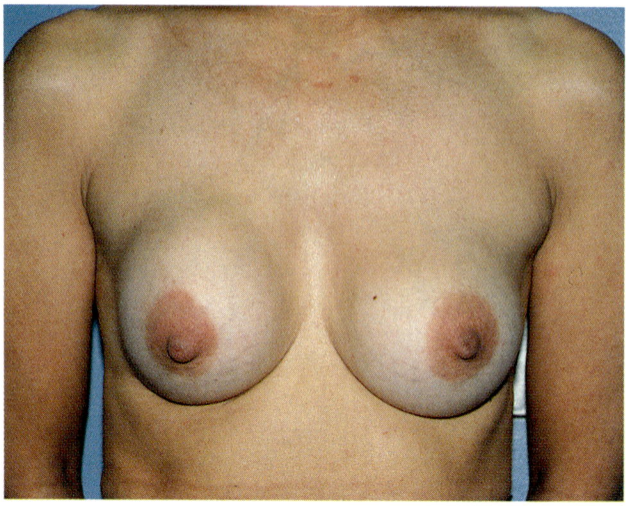

Twenty years earlier this 40-year-old patient underwent subglandular breast augmentation using smooth-surface silicone gel implants. Capsular contracture developed relatively soon after the primary augmentation, and closed capsulotomy had resulted in only temporary improvement. Because of continued discomfort around the implants, she sought correction.

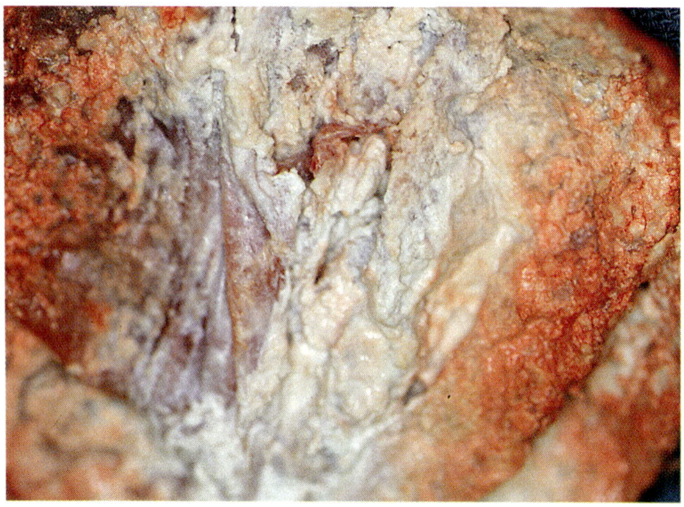

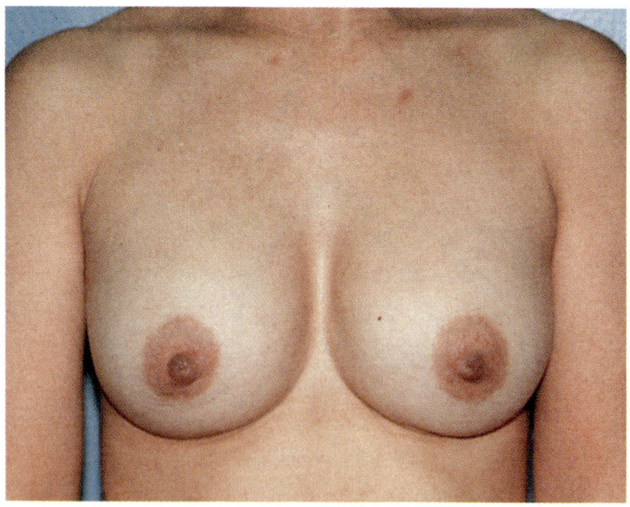

Intraoperatively the capsule was noted to be thick and heavily calcified. Free calcium deposits were present on and within the capsular wall. A total capsulectomy was performed along with implant removal. Conversion to saline implants in the subpectoral position was performed.

The postoperative result is shown at 3 months.

Deflation and Rupture of Implant

Deflation and rupture can occur early or late postoperatively. With saline implants deflation has been reported from 0 to 15%.[51] In the early postoperative period deflation can result from valve leakage or an inadvertent hole made in the implant shell. Over time, material fatigue occurs and deflation can result. Such material fatigue usually develops at the site of a fold and has been termed "fold flaw leak."[52]

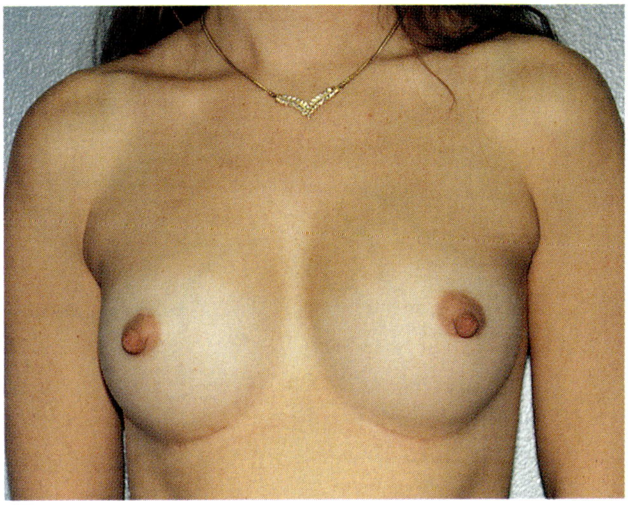

This patient is shown 4 months after undergoing subpectoral augmentation using smooth-walled inflatable saline breast implants.

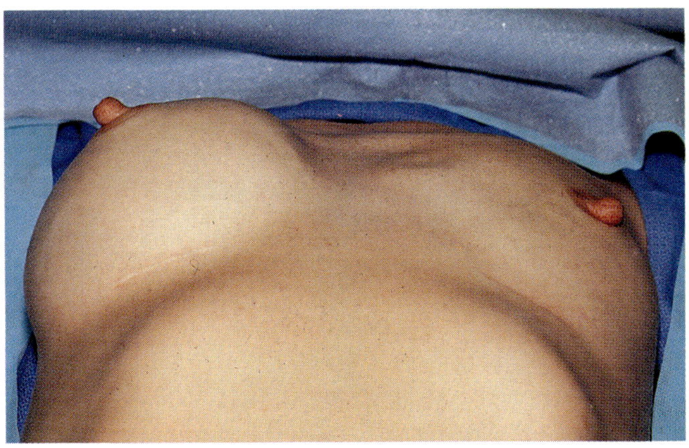

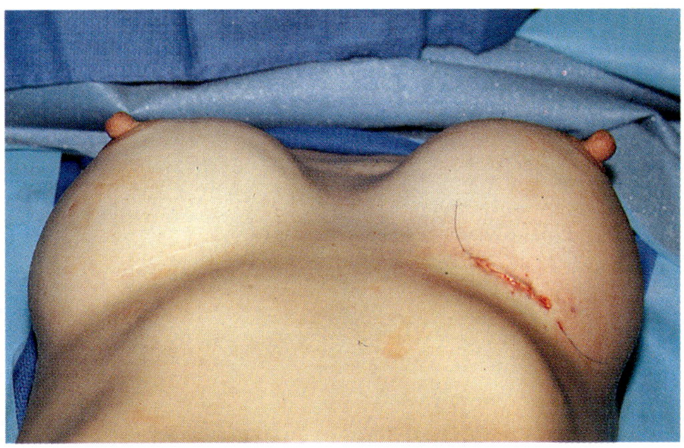

Two years following augmentation she returned, having noted a gradual diminished size of the left augmented breast over a period of several days. The deflated implant was removed through the previous inframammary fold incisions. An open capsulotomy around the entire base perimeter of the capsule was performed followed by replacement of another identical inflatable saline implant.

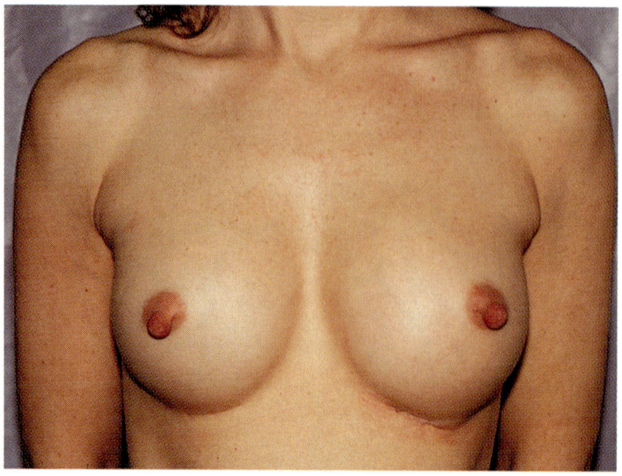

The postoperative result is shown 1 month following replacement.

Gel Leakage

As previously mentioned, one of the complications of closed capsulotomy is implant tear and gel extrusion. However, implants can also fail without a history of direct trauma or manipulation. The effect this free silicone gel has on women has become one of the most widely publicized and scrutinized aspects of current plastic surgery. In order to fully understand the significance, a brief review is necessary.

Implant rupture during closed compression capsulotomy was first reported in 1977.[53,54] The extent to which the silicone was extruded was anecdotally reported by several authors who described silicone at distant sites including the axilla, upper extremity, and groin.[55-57]

The first reports of gel leakage unrelated to closed capsulotomy date back to 1978 when it was noted that there was spontaneous diffusion of silicone from implants placed on cardboard.[58] To prove that the gel bleed phenomenon occurred in vivo, the capsule around implants was microscopically examined and found to have silicone-laden histiocytes.[59] A report from Austria introduced the next year made the association of leaking implants and lymphadenopathy.[60]

The Effects of Free Silicone Gel

At the time of the writing of this book, great concern exists in women with breast implants primarily due to the widely published reports of women having developed symptoms of connective tissue disease associated with their implants. Although no scientific study to this date has proved a causal relationship, the FDA has placed a moratorium on the use of silicone gel implants.

Before the history of this association is reviewed, a distinction must be made for clarification. The terms "connective tissue disease," "immune disease," "rheumatic disease," and "autoimmune disease" have all been used in association with breast implants. "Immune disease" refers to the broad category of disorders that are related to the immune system. A type of immune disease is "autoimmune disease," which refers to pathologic consequences of autoimmune responses (i.e., an immunologic reaction to an antigen of the host itself). "Rheumatic disease" refers to conditions that are of articular origin or are related to other elements of the musculoskeletal system.[61] The term "connective tissue disease" is an anatomic classification and does not necessarily result from immune disorders. For example, one can have connective tissue disease that is characterized by fibrous degeneration and inflammation. These sequelae can result from toxic, infectious, or immunologic reactions.[62] The point is, when reviewing the literature, one must be aware of how these terms are associated with breast implants to accurately interpret the data.

Silicone-Associated Problems

History

In 1964, Miyoshi et al.[63] described a condition exhibited in two patients with arthritis and hypergammaglobulinemia following breast augmentation with injected paraffin. His group called this condition "human adjuvant disease," a term that has been associated with silicone gel breast implants. They defined it with six characteristics: (1) autoimmune disease–like symptoms develop following foreign material injection, (2) silicone or other materials injected into the breast may have adjuvant effects, (3) foreign body granulomas occur in the injected area or the area of lymphocytic drainage, (4) serologic abnormalities become manifest, (5) symptoms may improve following removal of the foreign material (e.g., the patient's symptoms improved following mastectomy), and (6) infection or malignancy are not present.

The term "human adjuvant disease" is believed to be inaccurate by many and should be abandoned.[64] The term "adjuvant" refers to a vehicle used to enhance antigenicity.[61] No experimental evidence exists to label silicone as an adjuvant. In fact, the adjuvant disease evidenced in experimental animals does not resemble the autoimmune connective tissue disorder in humans.[64] In the April 10, 1991, *Federal Register,* the FDA even agreed that the term "human adjuvant disease" is "inappropriate" and should be abandoned.[65]

In 1973, Yoshida[66] described seven patients with autoimmune characteristics following the injection of paraffin or silicone for breast augmentation. Their symptoms included arthritis, local and regional adenopathy, fever, and breast induration. Improvement following mastectomy occurred in four of seven patients.

Kumagi et al.[67] first suggested the association of sclerodema and injection augmentation in 1984. They described a series of 46 patients in whom symptoms developed after being injected with paraffin, petroleum, or liquid silicone. The incidence was increased threefold over the population without injections.

The first report of immune disease following augmentation with silicone gel–filled prostheses was by Van Nunen, Gatenby, and Basten[68] in 1982. Systemic lupus erythematosus, mixed connective tissue disease, or rheumatoid arthritis with Sjögren's syndrome was diagnosed in three patients. Each experienced improvement with steroid therapy. The implants were not removed.

A case report of a patient with an immune syndrome that improved after implant removal was reported in 1983. Arthralgias, weakness, and lymphadenopathy developed in a woman 6 years following bilateral subcutaneous mastectomy with implant reconstruction. At the time of reoperation and removal, one of the implants was found to be ruptured.[69]

A number of patients with silicone gel–filled implants associated with symptoms of connective tissue disease have been reported in the literature. Patients report having a number of presentations. Some have been diagnosed by their physicians as having well-defined connective tissue diseases such as progressive systemic sclerosis, rheumatoid arthritis, polymyalgia rheumatica, eosinophilic fasciitis, and Sjögren's syndrome. Other patients have less well-defined diseases. Some reports in the literature give these patients the diagnosis of "human adjuvant disease," a term that has previously been discussed. One study examining the number of such patients since 1982 found the most common symptom to be arthralgia and the most commonly reported single diagnosis to be systemic sclerosis. Nearly half of the patients in that study had Raynaud's phenomenon.[70]

Despite the reported association between silicone gel–filled breast implants and immune disease, a causal relationship has not been scientifically established. In fact, the epidemiologic data are inconclusive as to whether there truly is an association. An excellent study performed by the Mayo group to examine the risk of a variety of connective tissue diseases and other disorders after breast implantation was performed in Olmstead County, Minnesota, between 1964 and 1991. They compared 749 women who had received a breast implant to 1498 controls to examine the risk of connective tissue disease and other specified disorders after breast implantation. They concluded that no association exists between breast implants and connective tissue diseases and other disorders in their study population.[71]

Another study was performed in which women who had undergone breast reconstruction with silicone gel were compared with those who had autogenous tissue breast reconstruction to see if there was a difference in the incidence of autoimmune disorders in patients with silicone gel implants. Reconstruction with autogenous tissue was performed on 353 patients, whereas 250 patients received silicone gel implants for reconstruction. One patient from each group had a documented autoimmune syndrome that required therapy. They concluded that the incidence of autoimmune disease in mastectomy patients who had autogenous tissue reconstruction was no different from that in patients who had breast reconstruction with silicone gel implants.[72]

A study evaluating the clinical and serologic features of 156 women with silicone gel–filled implants and symptoms of rheumatic disease was reported in 1993.[73] Three subgroups were defined based on clinical and laboratory findings: joint and muscle pain, joint swelling, and connective tissue diseases. Most of the women had no detectable serologic abnormalities. The conclusions of the study suggest that women with silicone implants are not at increased risk for rheumatoid arthritis and that serious connective tissue disease associated with silicone breast implants is uncommon. The researchers did, however, find a group of implant patients with clinical and serologic features of a scleroderma-like illness who differed from patients with idiopathic scleroderma reported in the literature. The significance of this finding has not been established, but the researchers concluded that atypical immunologic reactions may develop in some women with breast implants.[73]

The conclusion on the subject in the recent literature is that more research is needed. A breast implant registry has been established with particular emphasis on the follow-up of patients with symptoms of immune disease. The mode and results of treatment must be noted to develop management guidelines. Further work is necessary to determine the bioreactivity of silicone and its components.

Patient Evaluation

In view of the continued controversy regarding the safety of breast implants, plastic surgeons are facing a growing number of patients who are concerned about their implants. Many simply have questions regarding their implants and are confused about what they have heard. Others may have either local or systemic symptoms that they or their physicians relate to their implants. A careful methodical approach to each of these patients is warranted. A multidisciplinary team including the plastic surgeon, rheumatologist, radiologist, and psychiatrist may under certain circumstances be helpful. None of these patients should ever be dismissed without a complete consultation.

The majority of women who are currently returning for evaluation are primarily concerned with two issues: whether their implants are intact and whether any local or systemic symptoms they have been experiencing are related to their implants. One of the primary roles of the plastic surgeon is to educate each patient on what is currently known or unknown from a scientific standpoint. Each plastic surgeon caring for the postaugmentation mammaplasty patient must keep himself well informed regarding ongoing scientific studies and recommendations from industry and government. For the otherwise entirely asymptomatic patient, reassurance may be all that is necessary. Helping a woman sort out what is fact from what is fiction goes a long way toward this reassurance.

Although silicone gel implants may leak without producing any symptoms at all, some patients will experience changes that might be associated with a leak. As mentioned previously, the development of capsular contracture has been associated with gel bleed or implant failure. New onset of firmness, chest wall discomfort, or burning pain, which may radiate to the shoulder or around the chest wall, will sometimes develop in the presence of a failed or failing implant. Similarly, a change in the size or shape of an implant, particularly if unilateral, may be associated with rupture.

For the sake of this chapter, a "leak" refers to an implant that has a small amount of silicone gel on the outside of the silicone elastomer. This leak may be via either a small pinhole or by gel bleed. A "rupture" or "disrupted implant" refers to one with a larger tear in which a large amount or even the majority of gel is outside of a partially or completely collapsed silicone elastomer. If the gel is maintained within the capsule, this situation is referred to as an "intracapsular rupture." If the gel has migrated out of or has been forced through the capsule to appear in breast tissue or beyond, this problem is referred to as an "extracapsular rupture." Some patients may express a "feeling" that the implant has ruptured and may relate this suspicion to a history of localized trauma.

Implant failure is difficult to diagnose by simple physical examination. The edge of the capsule should be carefully palpated for areas of irregularity or possible masses within the capsule. Older, well-established capsules may be calcified, which may account for irregularities. However, distinct nodules within the capsule may also represent silicone granulomas or other benign masses. In addition, malignant disease can present as a nodule within the capsule.

The breast parenchyma must be carefully examined to rule out other breast pathologic conditions. Similarly, regional lymph nodes should be carefully palpated for evidence of lymphadenopathy, which has been associated with implant failure.

One sign occasionally present in patients who have a ruptured implant is a lateral bulge. It is most easily visualized with the patient in the supine position. The bulge can be felt along the lateral edge of the breast.

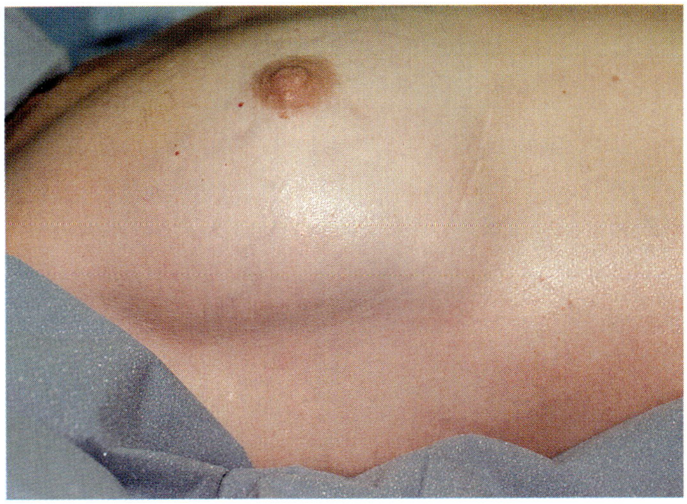

This patient experienced the new onset of a burning sensation around the right breast implant associated with a bulge created by free silicone gel within the capsule.

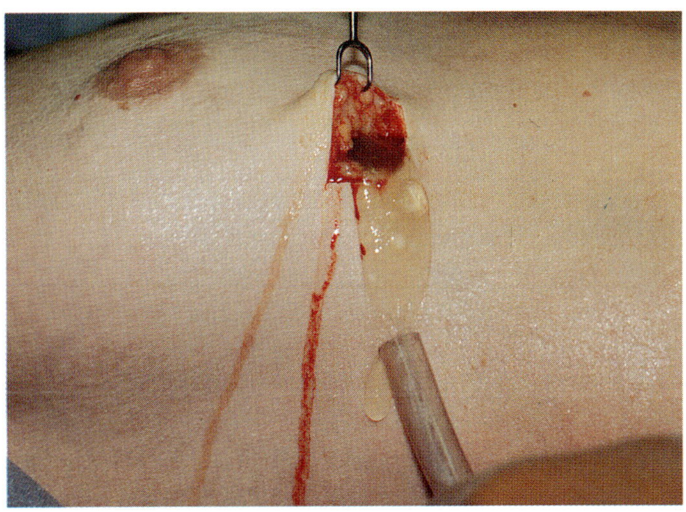

At the time of implant removal, the inframammary incision was opened. The capsule was quite thin and spontaneously tore, revealing the extruded gel. Large-bore suction tubing such as that used for suction lipectomy has been helpful in evacuating free gel in these circumstances. This method of gel removal helps to prevent the gel from contacting other dissected tissue planes.

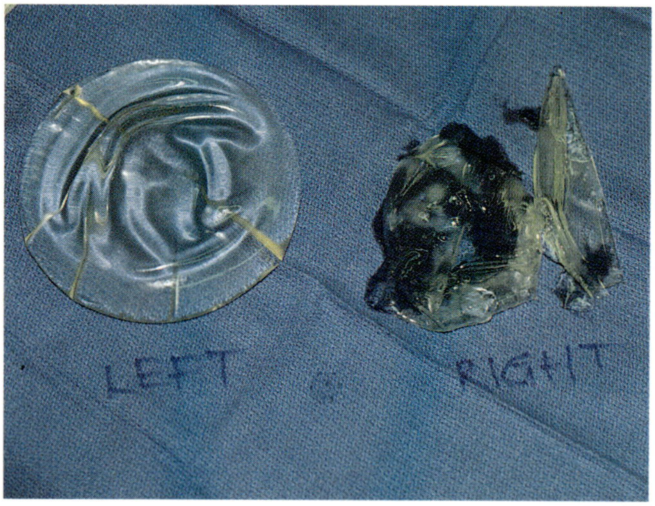

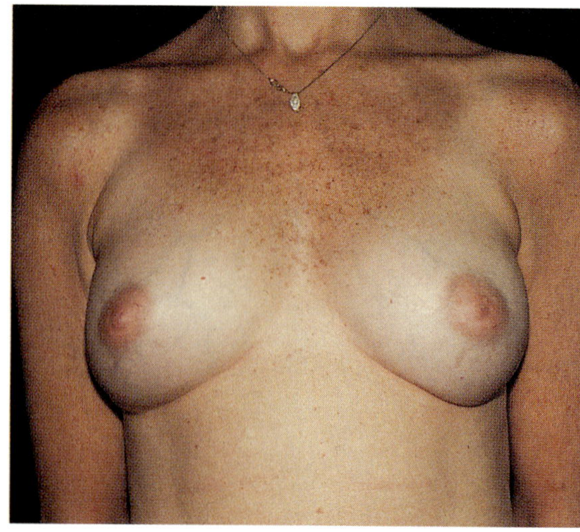

The left breast implant was also removed, but it was intact. Saline implants were placed into the same pockets.

Indications for Radiologic Workup

At present no single ideal radiologic method for diagnosing failed or leaking breast implants exists. Every patient does not need a radiologic workup because the results may have little bearing on management decisions. In addition, any view of the implant is only a "snapshot" in time. Therefore it is not practical or cost effective to routinely screen breast implant patients using radiologic methods.

Each radiologic method is described in detail in Chapter 32. If a plastic surgeon has access to good mammography, ultrasonography, and MRI, the decision as to which technique to use may be deferred to the radiologist. Mammography is satisfactory for detecting extracapsular rupture but is somewhat inaccurate for identifying leaking or failed implants in the intracapsular space. Ultrasonography has been quite effective for evaluating masses alongside the capsule or within the breast parenchyma. MRI has been the most helpful for the detection of intracapsular leak or rupture but only when used by experienced radiologists.

The starting point for a radiologic workup in women between 35 and 40 years of age should be a baseline mammogram if they have not already had one. Often the breast parenchyma can be screened and some information about the implant can be obtained. An MRI scan may be recommended to evaluate the intracapsular status of the implant.

The decision to perform any radiologic tests is determined on an individual basis. A patient who is otherwise asymptomatic and does not wish to have the implants removed needs no further workup. However, some patients will consider having their implants removed if radiologic workup indicates a possible leak or failure. In this case, because the results of an MRI scan will affect a patient's decision, proceeding with the examination is indicated. Women who have already decided to undergo explantation do not need further radiologic studies except under special circumstances. For example, radiologic evaluation of extracapsular masses might help the surgeon to plan whether the surgical removal of these masses should be performed at the time of explantation.

Patients With Local Symptoms

Pain or discomfort in the area surrounding a breast implant, particularly one that has been in place for many years, is common. Patients may describe a tightness that is often related to capsular contracture. Other times the pain is localized to a rib or a specific area of the capsule. The causes of pain around an implant include neuroma, capsular contracture, inflammatory response from a leaking implant, or mechanical pressure from a large or heavy implant. Some local pain syndromes simply cannot be accurately diagnosed.

If the patient is to be treated without surgery, utilization of certain types of brassiere support, massage, and administration of anti-inflammatory agents has been most helpful. Costochondritis, often due to mechanical shearing, will also often respond to these measures.

Chronic pain from capsular contracture or gel leak is often improved by reoperative surgery. In the case of contracture, capsulotomy or capsulectomy may offer relief. If gel leak is the cause, implant removal or replacement may be of benefit. However, improvement may be only temporary. For the patient who is debilitated by local pain, explantation with total capsulectomy may be necessary.

Patients With Systemic Symptoms

Many patients who now seek consultation with a plastic surgeon regarding their breast implants also complain of a variety of systemic symptoms. Whether or not these symptoms are related to the breast implants may be nearly impossible to confirm. Some patients seem to have been influenced by articles they have read or news stories they have watched on television. Others have experienced a variety of vague systemic complaints that they feel may be related to their implants. The most common symptoms are fatigue, muscle and joint aches and pain, weakness, memory loss, skin changes or rashes, and burning discomfort in the hands and feet.

It is important to document each symptom a patient mentions regardless of whether or not it can be logically attributed to the breast implant. We refer most patients with systemic symptoms to a rheumatologist for further testing. A rheumatologic workup includes a standardized questionnaire and laboratory evaluation consisting of rheumatoid factor and antinuclear antibody, thyroid function tests, and a cytokine profile. In our experience most women with such complaints have not had systemic rheumatologic disorders such as scleroderma or systemic lupus erythematosus. Some have had either fibromyalgia or a type of soft tissue rheumatism attributable to overuse syndromes. In some patients these symptoms have responded to local steroid injections.

TREATMENT

Removal of Breast Implants

Every patient who returns for evaluation of their implants, even if symptomatic, does not necessarily need an operation. However, explantation has now become a major part of breast implant surgery. Alarmed by the controversy surrounding the safety of breast implants, an increasing number of patients wish to have their implants removed. Many of these patients are women who underwent augmentation in earlier years but now have different motivations, priorities, and body habitus. Some have gained weight, have more breast tissue, and believe that the removal of their implants can be performed without making the residual breasts disproportionately small. Other women simply do not wish to "take a chance" that the implants might eventually be shown unsafe and therefore want to have them removed. In general, once a patient has been fully educated about what is known and what is not known regarding breast implants and has made a decision to have them removed, the role of the plastic surgeon should be to help to facilitate explantation.

Other than a patient's fear of her implants, there are other reasons to consider removal. Patients with known or suspected rupture should have implants removed or replaced. In addition, the development of painful capsular contracture is best treated by total capsulectomy and implant removal. Some patients have had poor surgical results as a result of poorly executed surgery. Others have capsular contracture, implant malposition, or continued glandular ptosis with aging. Once the aesthetic results have become poor, both patient and surgeon will usually agree to implant removal with possible subsequent reconstruction. Finally, breast cancer may develop in patients with implants although at a rate no greater than that for the general population.[74] Therefore the treatment of breast cancer may include removal of the implant.

The following options are offered to most augmentation patients who are experiencing problems: (1) observation only, (2) removal of the implant with or without capsulectomy, (3) removal of the implant with or without capsulectomy with saline implant replacement, (4) removal of the implant with or without capsulectomy with mastopexy.

■ ***Autogenous conversion using flaps such as the TRAM or latissimus dorsi flap is rarely indicated for patients who had their implants inserted for breast augmentation. These procedures have a prohibitive risk and medical cost, making them impractical options for implant replacement.*** Only under very rare circumstances in which the patient has undergone multiple failed implant procedures and is in a situation similar to that of a postoperative subcutaneous mastectomy patient are distant flap procedures a reasonable reconstructive alternative.

Capsulectomy

There are very few if any absolute indications for total capsulectomy. However, if one is trying to remove a ruptured implant, total capsulectomy is often an easy way to extract the device without leaving residual silicone. Certainly, established capsular contracture is well treated by capsulectomy, especially if one intends to replace the implant with a textured-surface implant in which an interface with native tissue may prevent future capsular contracture. However, total capsulectomy is not always a simple procedure and may result in additional morbidity, particularly if the capsule is beneath the pectoralis major muscle and is dense and adherent to the chest wall. Patients should be alerted to the fact that total capsulectomy may not be safe under all circumstances and that sometimes breast and muscle tissue must be sacrificed with this procedure, which can lead to additional bleeding and eventually to the thinning of the soft tissue coverage. If a patient specifically requests total capsulectomy, we discuss these factors and let her know we may decide intraoperatively to leave some intact capsule behind rather than create additional morbidity.

Whether or not to perform total capsulectomy at explantation remains a controversial issue among plastic surgeons at the present time. However, some patients have a great fear of silicone and may insist the entire capsule be removed. These patients must be carefully counseled that although most of the visible silicone can be removed, microscopic particles will be left behind. Although the impact of this residual silicone in the body is unknown as of this writing, it appears that MRI scanning will detect any significant amount of silicone left behind. The presence of residual silicone may serve as a possible source of confusion for patients concerned about the relationship between silicone and symptoms they might be experiencing. For example, a patient with systemic symptoms may want her implants removed because she believes that her symptoms might be caused by or related to her implants. If her symptoms fail to substantially improve following explantation, she may wonder whether silicone left behind in the capsule could be responsible for her lack of recovery, even in the absence of scientific data supporting such a contention. For this reason we believe a concerted effort should be made to remove as much of the capsule as possible in patients with systemic symptoms or ruptured implants.

Leaving the capsule behind, even parts of it, can also be a problem for screening mammography. Capsules containing calcium may cause confusion in future mammograms. In addition, residual capsules may result in persistent postoperative seromas. We prefer to place a drain any time significant surgery has been performed on a capsule.

Patients who undergo explantation of polyurethane-covered implants and capsulectomy are treated in a similar fashion. However, this type of implant has several features that require special attention. The polyurethane capsule may have become separated from the inner implant, which occasionally results in fluid accumulating within this space. In addition, the capsule may be slightly thicker than that which develops with silicone implants. By design the capsule grows within and among the open pore foam structure of the polyurethane coating. This intertwined growth makes capsulectomy more difficult. However, one can generally develop a plane of dissection just outside the capsule and accomplish capsule removal by sharp dissection.

Most explantation procedures are performed as an outpatient surgery. We prefer to have the patient under general anesthesia. If a total capsulectomy is performed, we prefer the inframammary approach. Usually the previous incision is satisfactory, although it may need to be extended to facilitate adequate visualization for dissection.

Handling of the Explanted Device and Specimens

Any removed implants or tissues must be handled according to hospital guidelines and federal regulations. These rules vary among institutions and states. Foremost the surgeon must carefully document the operative findings. This description should include whether or not the implant appeared to be intact, any defects of the integrity of the elastomer, whether gel was present on the surface of the implant or within the capsule, whether or not silicone was present elsewhere (i.e., within the capsule, breast tissue, or nodes), and any other abnormalities associated with the breast. The implants and capsules should be photographed and then delivered to the pathologist for gross and microscopic examination. Any removed tissues should likewise be sent for pathologic examination. Some patients request special tests suggested by consumer groups or legal counsel. It is important that the patient clearly understand in advance what guidelines a particular hospital and surgeon must heed regarding the handling and processing of the specimens.

Many patients request that implants be returned to them. Since explanted devices are considered biohazardous waste by most criteria, the patient must accept responsibility for the ultimate disposal if she is to be given the device. Patients are asked to sign a release that outlines the conditions under which they accept responsibility for the implant once pathologic examination has been completed.

Case Examples

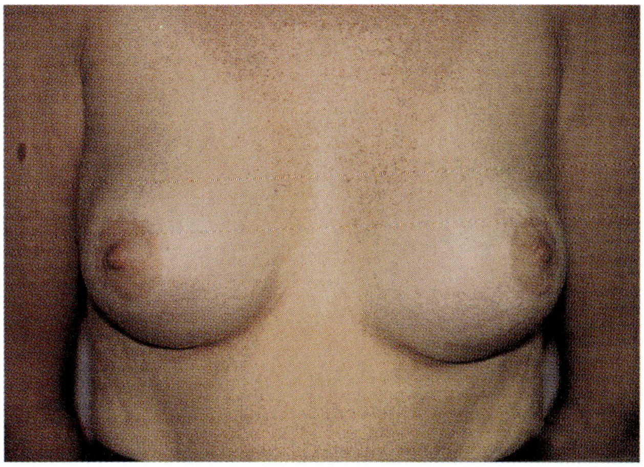

This 38-year-old patient had undergone breast augmentation using subpectoral smooth-surface silicone gel implants 8 years earlier. Although satisfied with the result, she developed intermittent muscular pain and weakness associated with fatigue. Rheumatologic evaluation was most consistent with fibromyalgia. The patient showed only moderate improvement with exercise and anti-inflammatory agents. She strongly desired that her implants be removed.

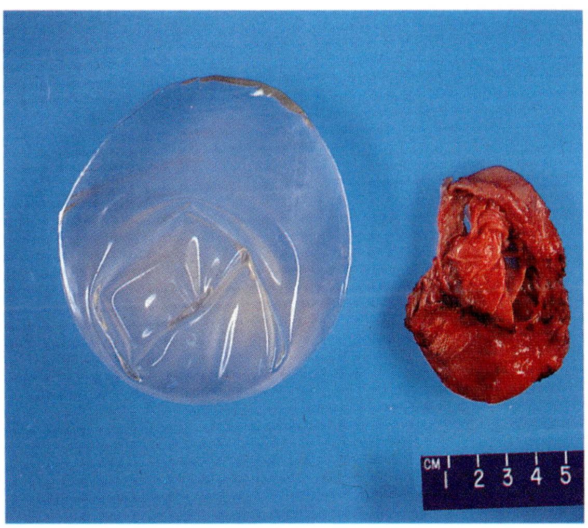

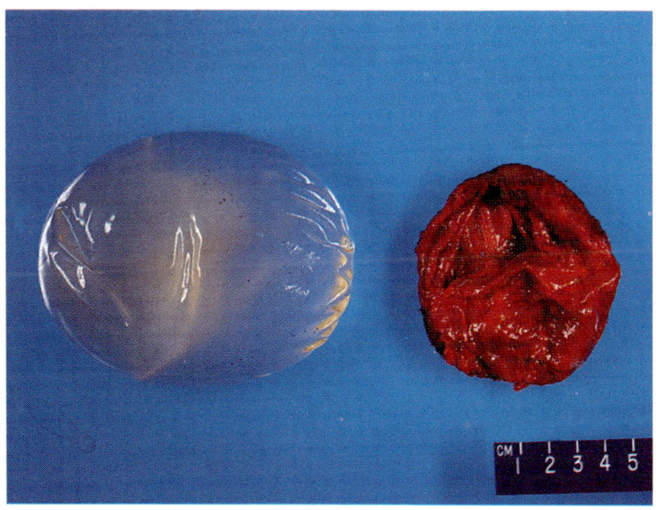

In view of the patient's concern about silicone and its relation to her symptoms, we believed that capsulectomy was indicated. On removal both the right and left implants appeared to be intact. The capsules were relatively thin. Histologically the capsules showed multinucleated giant cells and foreign body reaction.

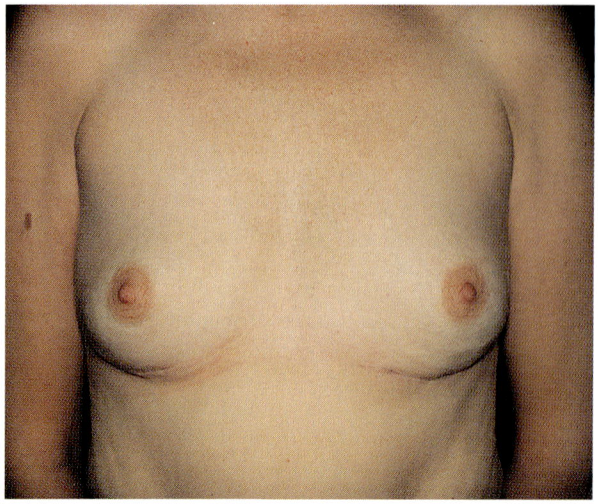

Postoperatively the aesthetic result is acceptable. The patient subjectively considered that her symptoms improved postoperatively. However, several months later they returned.

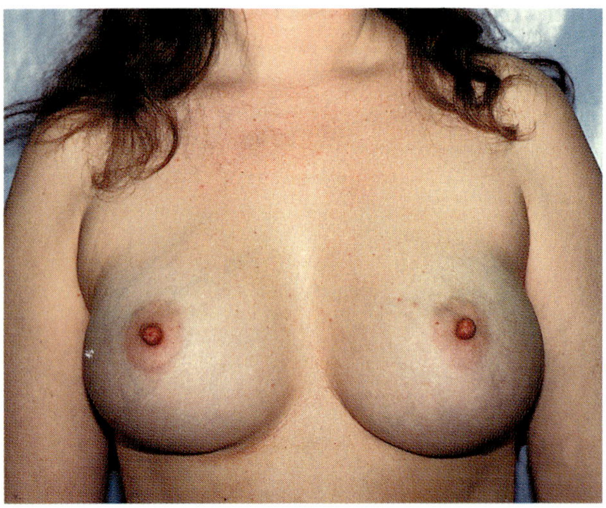

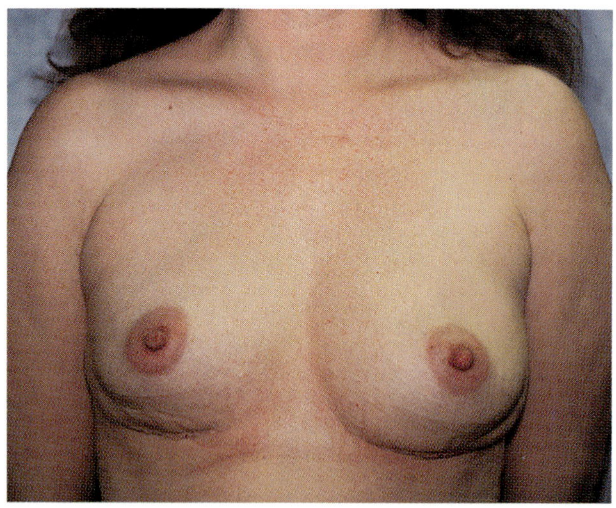

This 36-year-old woman underwent augmentation 8 years previously to correct breast asymmetry. She requested removal of her implants. Such patients must be carefully reminded that removal of the implants will again reveal the preexisting asymmetry, which may in fact be worsened by the intervening atrophy of the breast. The resultant asymmetry following explantation was acceptable to the patient. She did not desire replacement of the implants.

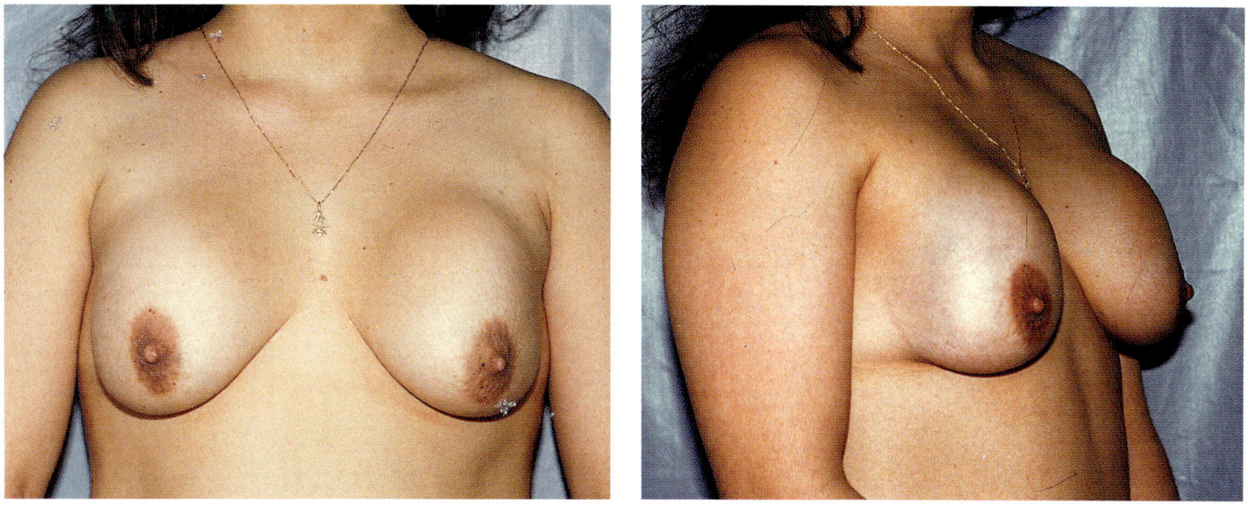

Established capsular contracture is best treated by total capsulectomy. Whether the patient wants to have the implants replaced is a matter of individual choice. This patient presented 12 years following subglandular augmentation using silicone gel breast implants. Firmness developed within the first year postoperatively, and she had undergone several previous attempts at closed capsulotomy many years before. Her main complaint was pain around the implants that extended into the shoulders. In addition, she complained of fatigue and generalized weakness. She strongly wanted her implants to be removed. Rheumatologic findings were consistent with fibromyalgia. She was offered mastopexy but declined because she did not wish to have additional scars.

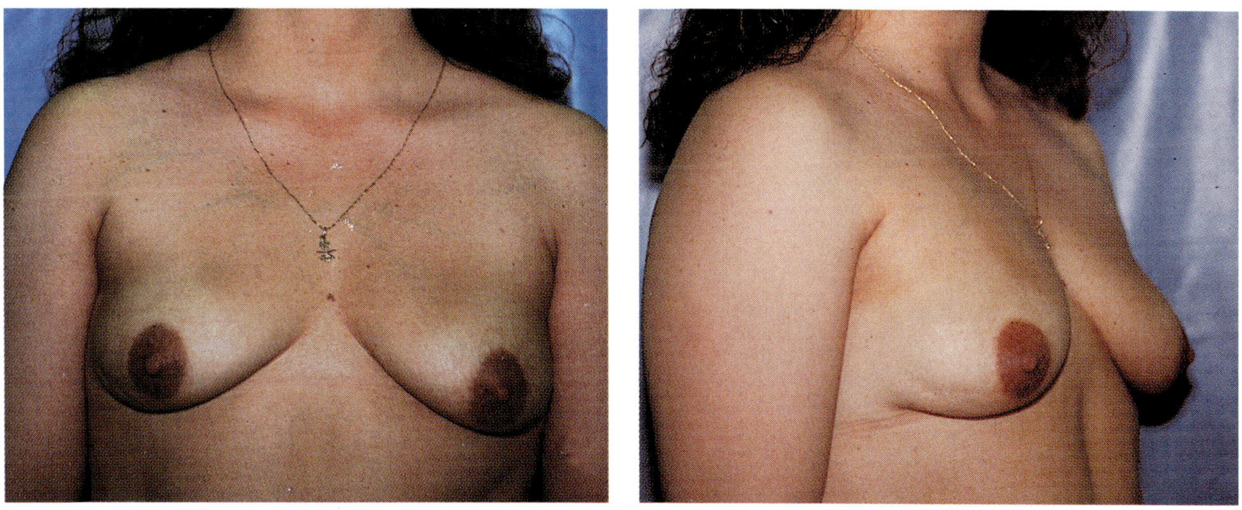

Postoperatively the patient had complete relief of breast pain and discomfort. However, the weakness and fatigue have persisted.

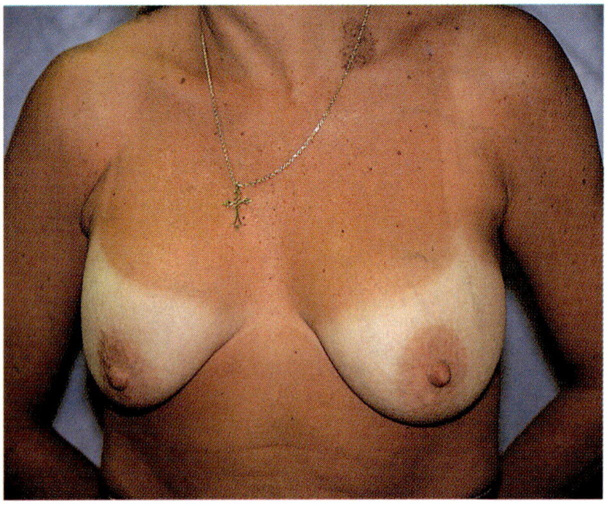

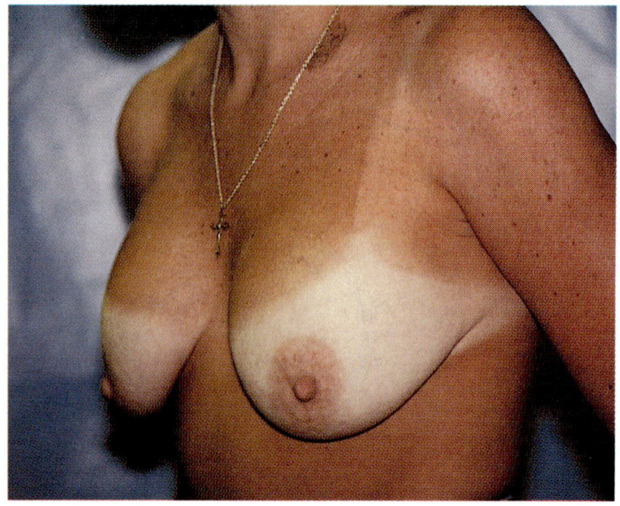

This 32-year-old flight attendant presented 10 years after augmentation mammaplasty and 2 years following pregnancy. She had become concerned about silicone gel and wanted the silicone gel implants to be removed. A mammogram suggested the possibility of implant rupture. MRI demonstrated that these were bilumen implants with possible collapse of the saline outer chamber.

Although preoperative breast aesthetics were poor and glandular ptosis was present, she wanted to maintain the breast size. She did not want additional scars from a mastopexy, which would have been required to improve the shape of the breasts. The silicone gel implants were removed. The bilumen implants were found to be intact. The capsule was quite thin and noninflamed. Therefore the implants were simply replaced with saline implants.

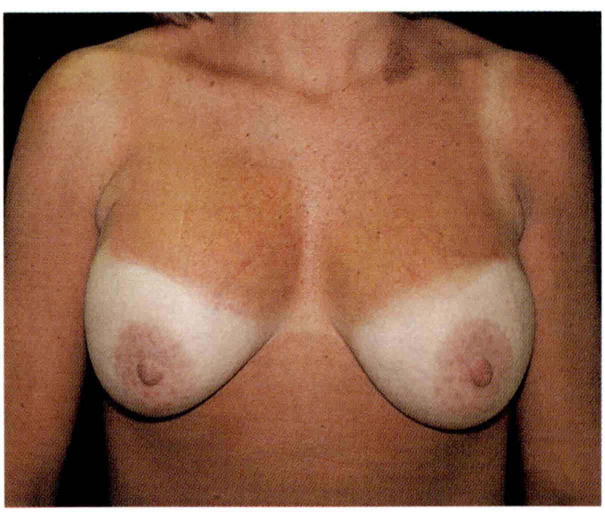

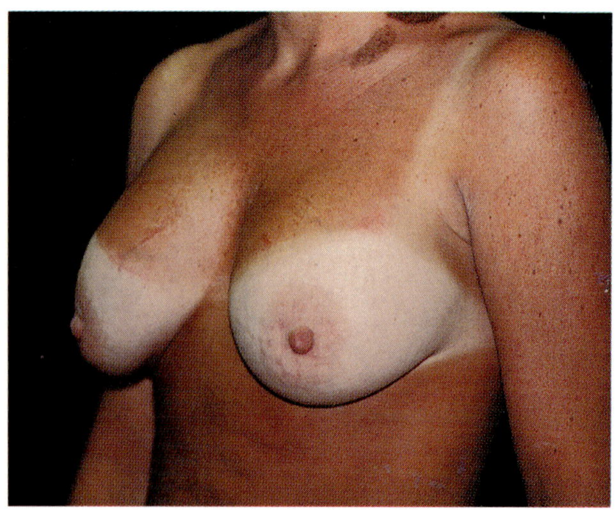

The postoperative result shows minimal change in breast aesthetics. However, the patient seemed relieved by this treatment.

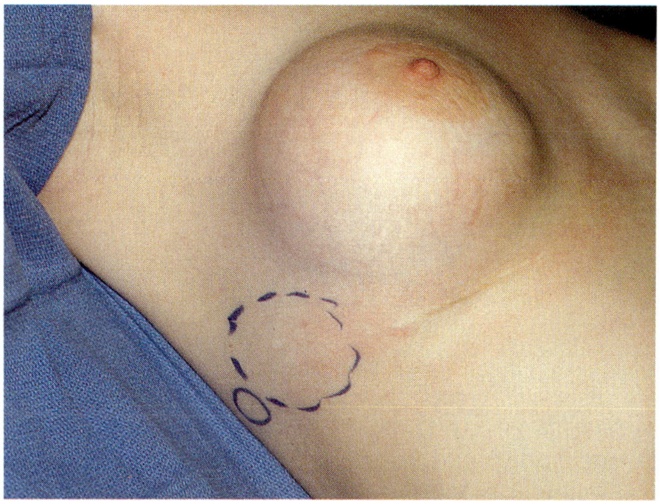

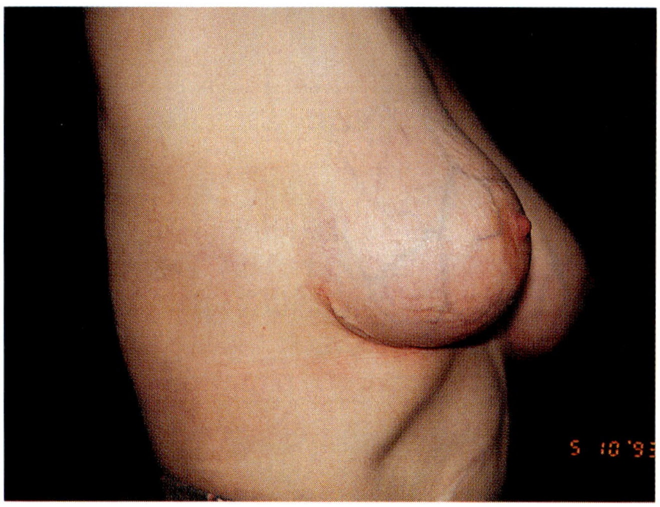

Tenderness surrounding palpable silicone granulomas is an indication for total capsulectomy and removal of the masses. This patient demonstrated established capsular contracture with silicone granulomas in the lateral chest wall as a result of implant rupture. Treatment consisted of total capsulectomy and excision of the silicone granulomas as marked. The postoperative result is shown. Unfortunately, local symptoms persisted. She ultimately elected to have the saline implants removed as well. Her symptoms have currently improved, but she is undergoing treatment in a pain clinic for chronic pain in the lateral chest wall, shoulder, and right arm.

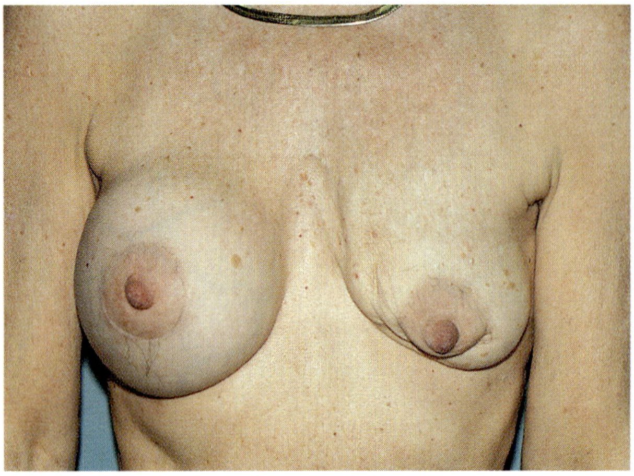

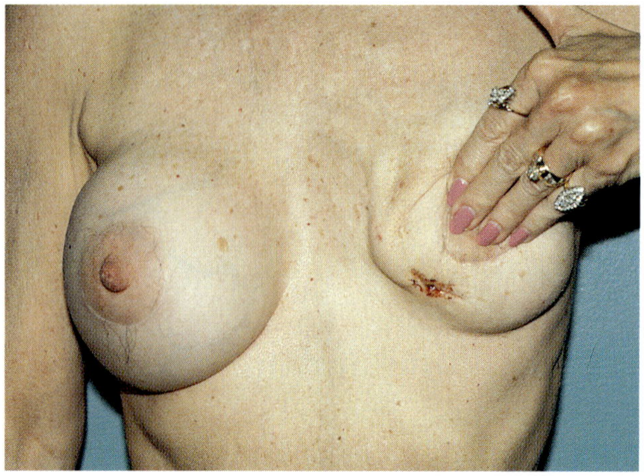

This unfortunate patient was referred after undergoing a series of procedures. In September 1990, she underwent transaxillary subglandular augmentation with smooth-surface silicone gel implants. Postoperatively a left-sided hematoma developed. In October 1990, the hematoma was drained. In February 1991, capsular contracture developed on both sides and was treated by exchanging the smooth-surface implants with subglandular polyurethane-covered implants. In March 1991, redness developed beneath the left implant. From June to August 1991, she was administered several regimens of antibiotics and she suffered recurrent bouts of cellulitis and drainage. Finally, in November 1991, the left polyurethane-covered implant was removed. From November to February 1992, she experienced multiple recurrent abscesses of the left breast. When first seen by us, the patient continued to have purulent drainage from the inframammary fold incision on the left side. She was presumed to have an infected retained polyurethane capsule. Open capsulectomy was recommended.

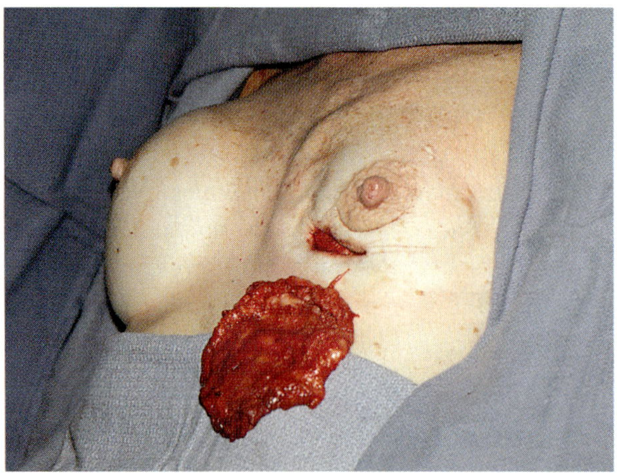

After removal of the residual polyurethane, the wound was simply allowed to heal. The plan was to wait for the breast to become soft, which ultimately occurred.

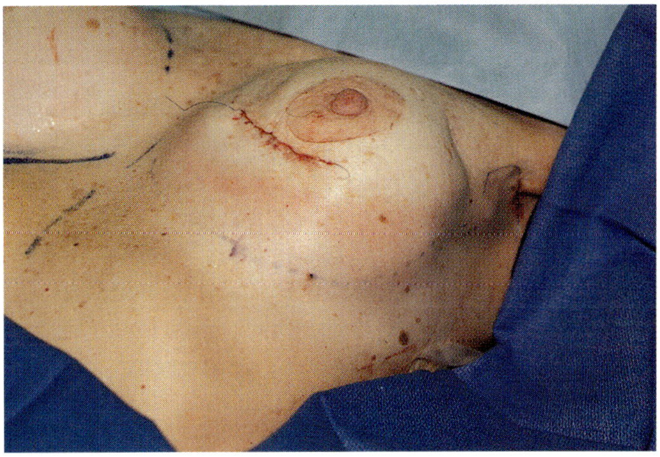

We elected to wait a full 9 months before placing a tissue expander. At that time the Becker expander-prosthesis was considered to be the best choice.

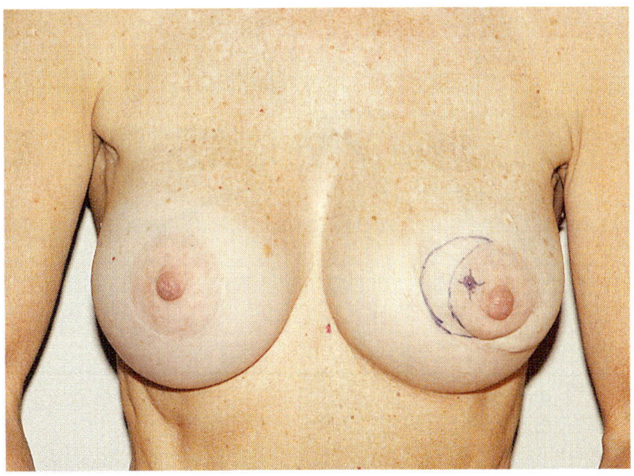

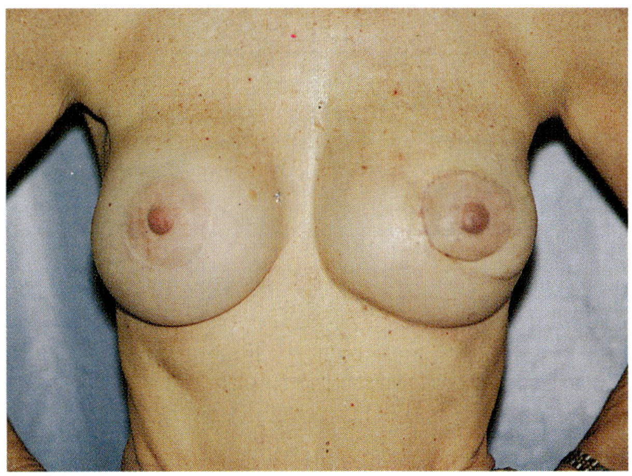

Gradual expansion was successful because the device was placed at the proper level. This placement allowed the inframammary fold to develop in the correct position. A small concentric periareolar mastopexy helped to improve the shape of the left breast. However, the postoperative result reflects the difference in the shape of the two implants. Replacement of the right polyurethane-covered implant with a Becker expander-prosthesis identical to that used on the left side was recently performed, resulting in improved symmetry.

This case demonstrates the importance of making certain that adequate debridement of the residual capsule is performed before another implant is inserted. Although these unfortunate patients may be frustrated and anxious to achieve the end result, the worst mistake one can make is to take shortcuts. It is imperative to ensure that infection has been adequately treated before a new implant is inserted. In retrospect, this patient would have been well served if the prosthesis and the infected capsule had been removed at the first sign of recurrent infection.

MASTOPEXY PROCEDURES FOLLOWING EXPLANTATION

Although some patients may benefit from small mastopexies following explantation, many refuse this surgery because they do not want additional scars on the breast. In general, those patients who have had only one previous procedure (e.g., augmentation) and had no significant ptosis to begin with will do well with explantation without mastopexy. If a patient is unsure how she might feel about the results of mastopexy, we believe it is best to delay mastopexy until the tissues have settled and contracted. It is sometimes surprising how good the result will be following explantation without mastopexy.

There are situations in which one can predict that some type of parenchymal reconstruction should be performed, particularly if the patient has elected not to have the implant replaced. In general, those patients who have a thin layer of atrophic soft tissue over the capsule on preoperative examination, particularly if large implants had previously been placed, are women who will benefit by immediate mastopexy.

Case Examples

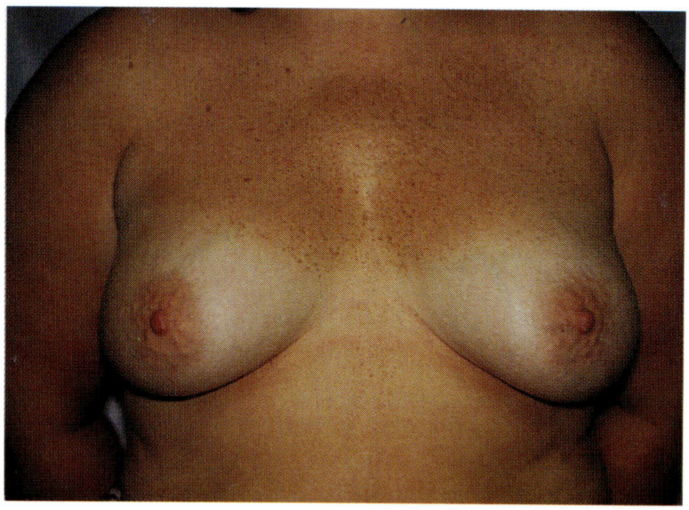

Twelve years earlier this 42-year-old patient had undergone augmentation using subglandular silicone gel implants. She presented with radiologically confirmed rupture on the right side. She desired that the implants be removed. With intervening weight gain and several pregnancies, ptosis had developed, and she wanted an aesthetic improvement to be performed at the time of explantation.

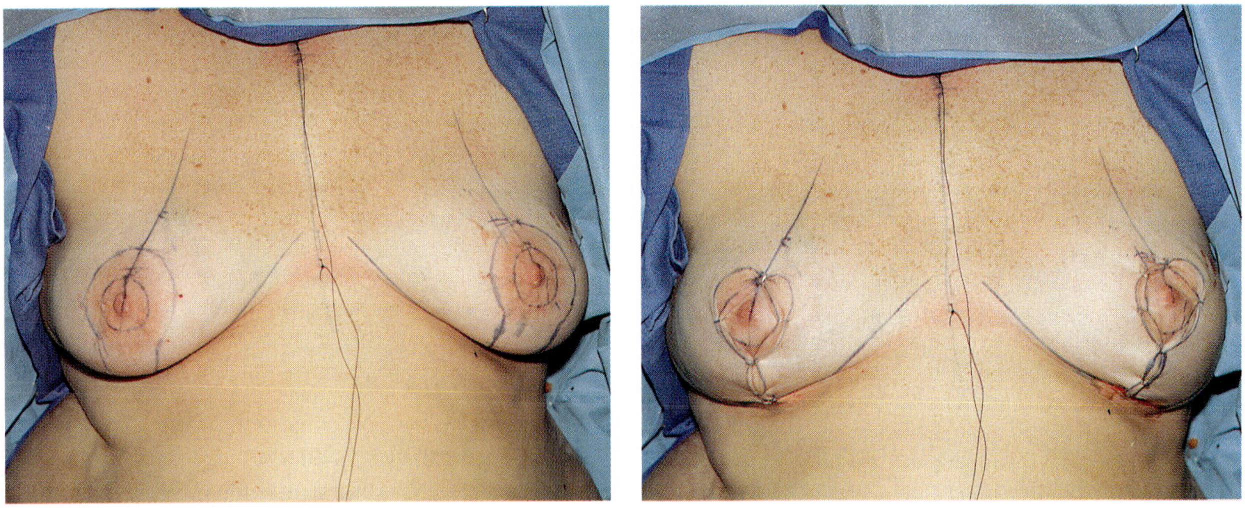

A simple skin-only mastopexy was outlined and the correction was assessed by a "stapled mastopexy" with the patient in the upright sitting position. The infolded areas were simply deepithelialized and sutured.

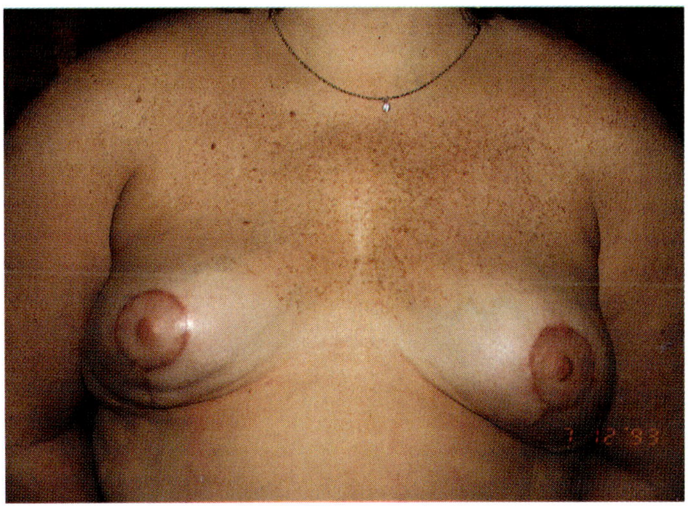

The postoperative result is shown at 3 months.

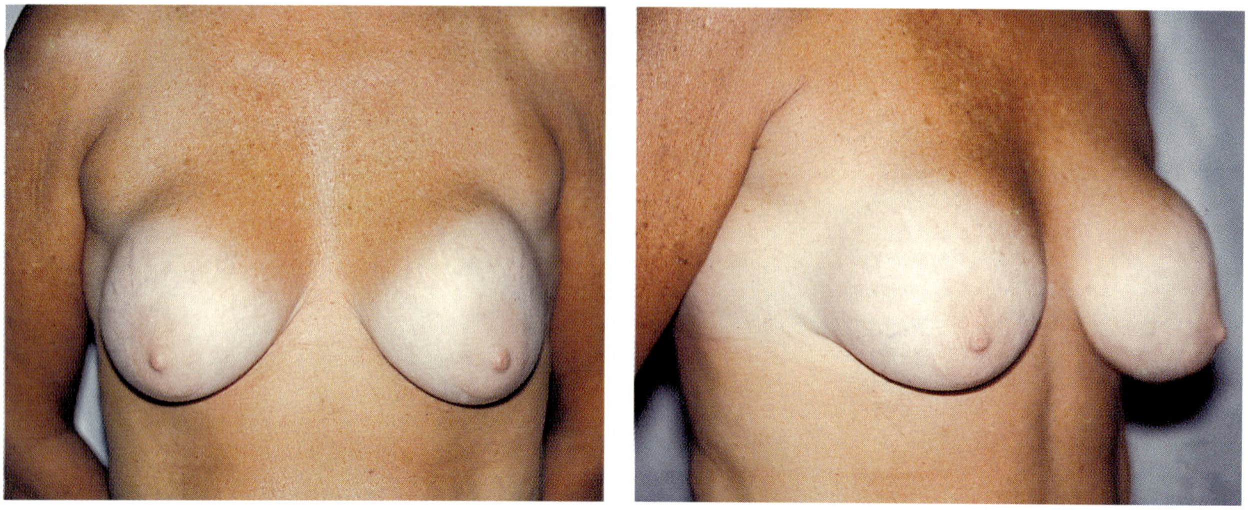

This 48-year-old patient presented 15 years following subglandular breast augmentation using silicone gel breast implants. Painful capsular contracture had developed, and she requested that the implants be exchanged for saline implants and that mastopexy be performed. Since the implants had originally been inserted through a periareolar incision, we planned the implant exchange via the same approach with a simultaneous periareolar mastopexy.

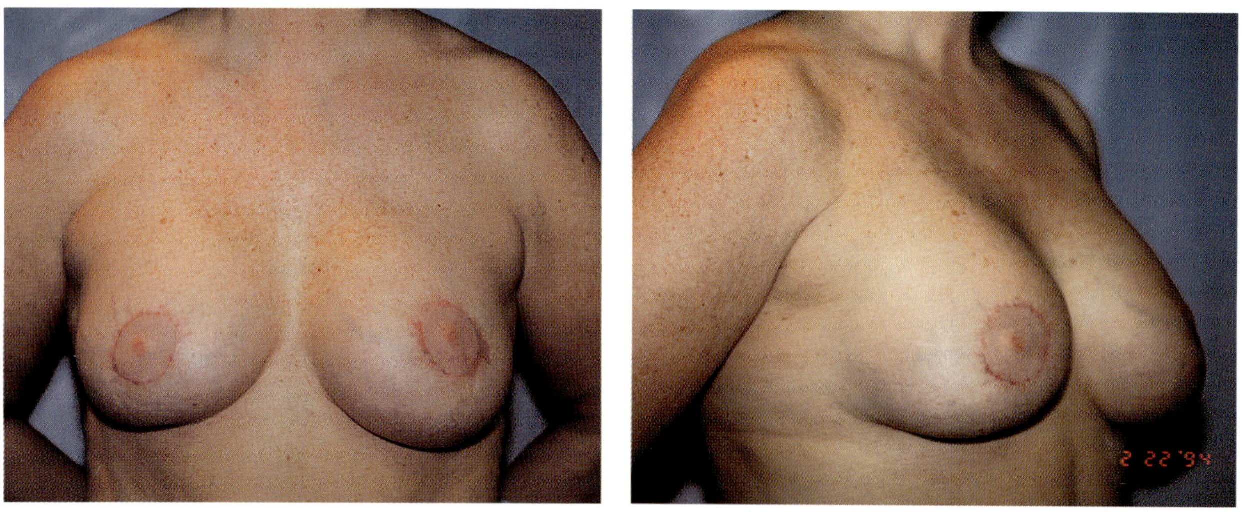

The postoperative result at 3 months is shown. The saline implants were inserted in the subpectoral position in an attempt to diminish subsequent capsular contracture and improve the effectiveness of mammographic surveillance.

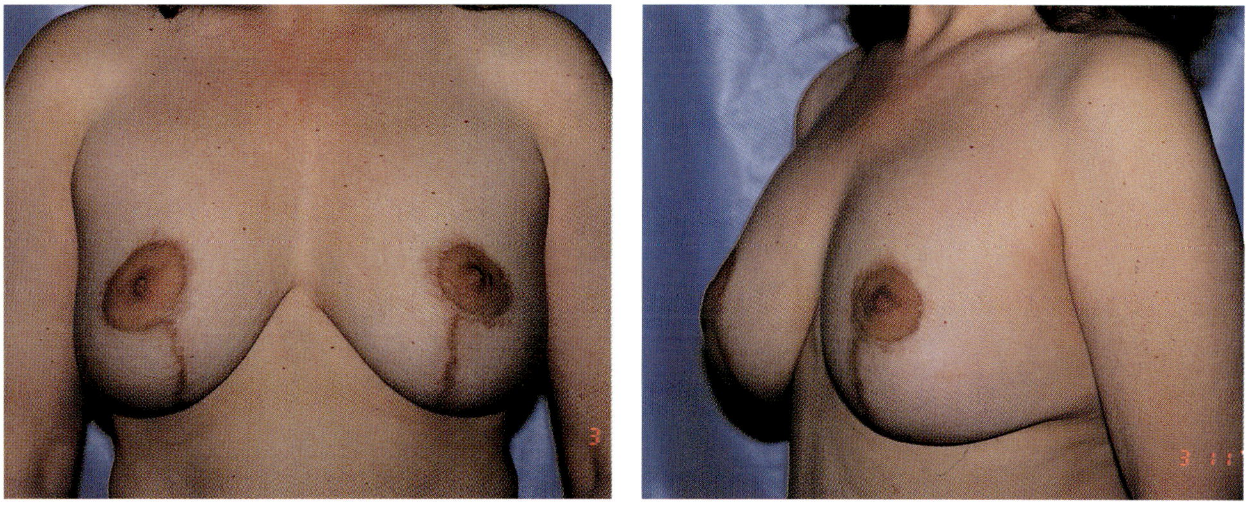

This patient presented for consultation 12 years following breast augmentation apparently to treat significant ptosis. Three years earlier the patient had returned to her original surgeon and requested correction of the ptosis. A Wise-pattern mastopexy was performed without an exchange of the implants. Six months later the patient developed systemic lupus erythematosus. She was under good medical control when she presented to us. However, she strongly desired that the implants be removed in hopes that her medical condition might resolve. In the preoperative photographs one can see that she still had glandular ptosis with high-riding submuscular implants. Radiologically these implants appeared to be leaking on both sides. The operative plan included explantation, total capsulectomy, and use of excess glandular tissue in the lower pole to try to improve ptosis. At operation, both implants were noted to have failed.

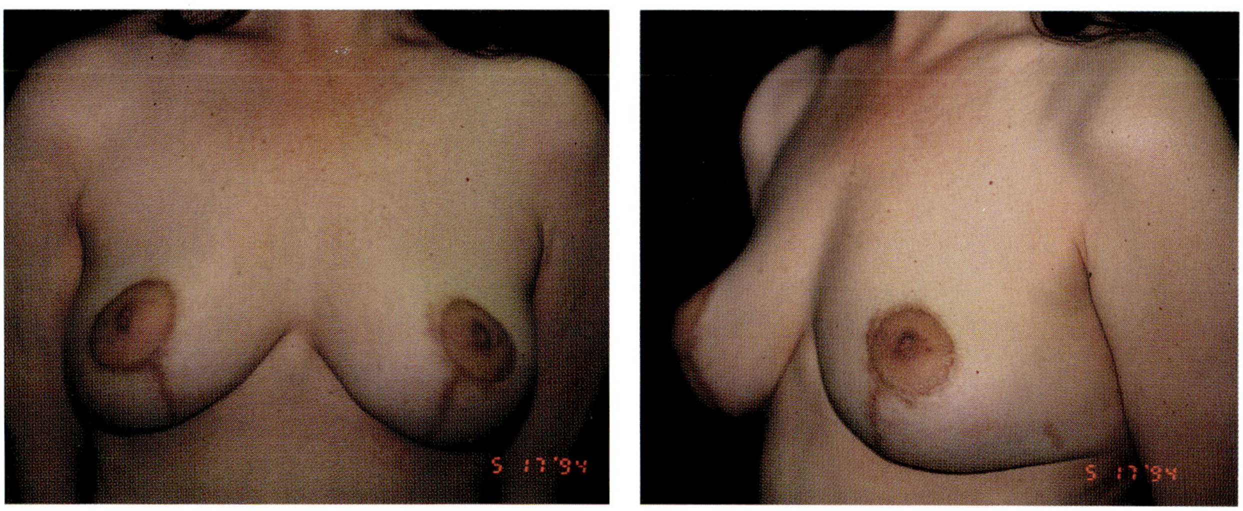

Postoperatively the shape of the breasts is modestly improved following de-epithelialization and inversion of the excess tissue along a secondary Wise pattern (see pp. 947 and 948).

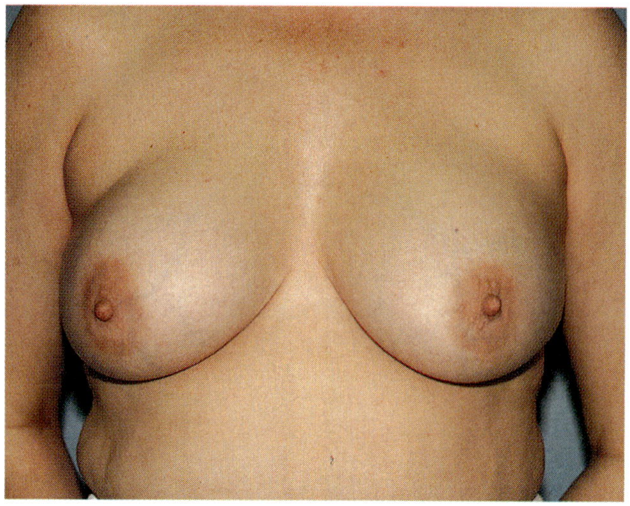

This 30-year-old patient presented for consultation regarding the removal of her breast implants. She and her referring physicians were convinced that multiple systemic symptoms she was experiencing were related to her implants. She strongly desired that the implants be removed. She also requested that simultaneous mastopexy be performed to improve the shape of the breasts since she did not want the implants to be replaced.

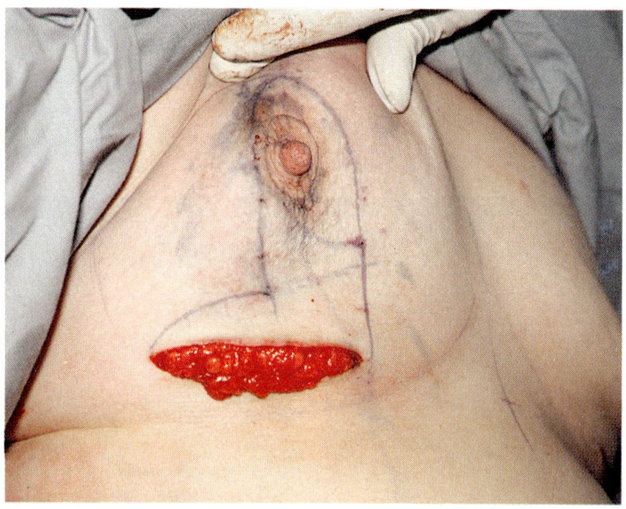

The implants were removed through the previous inframammary fold incision and total capsulectomy was performed. The remaining breast tissue was somewhat thin and atrophic. Therefore an L-shaped mastopexy was planned. With the patient in the sitting position, the markings for the mastopexy were drawn as shown.

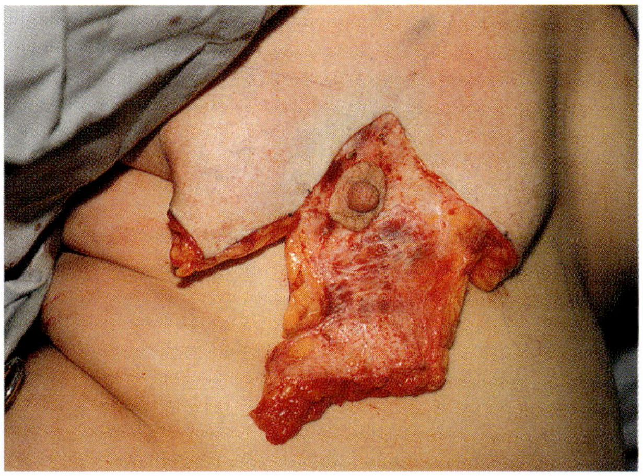

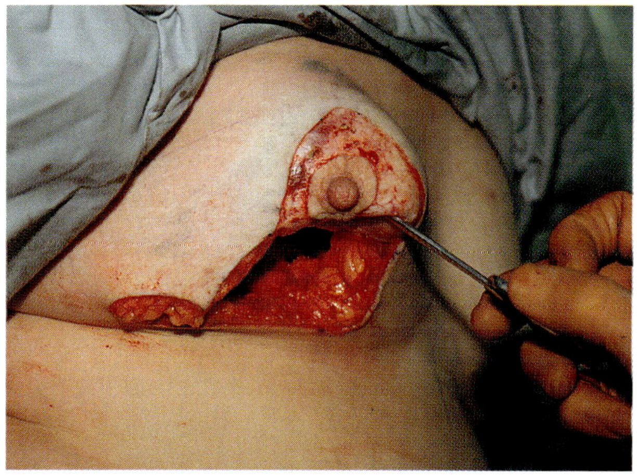

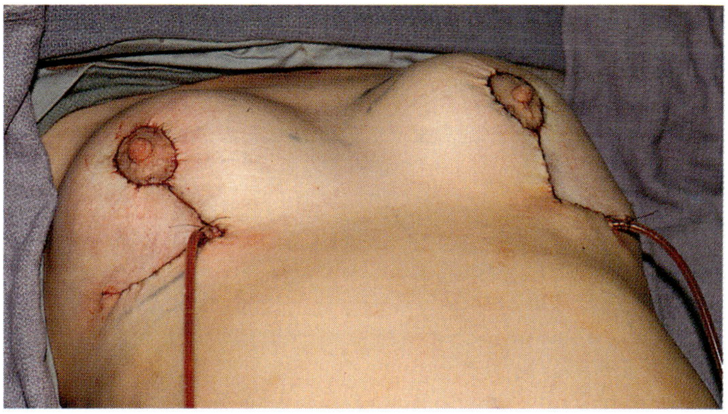

The superiorly based inferior flap was deepithelialized and turned inward to add fullness in the upper pole and projection of the nipple-areola complex. The remaining glandular tissue was rotated and the wound was closed in an L-shaped fashion.

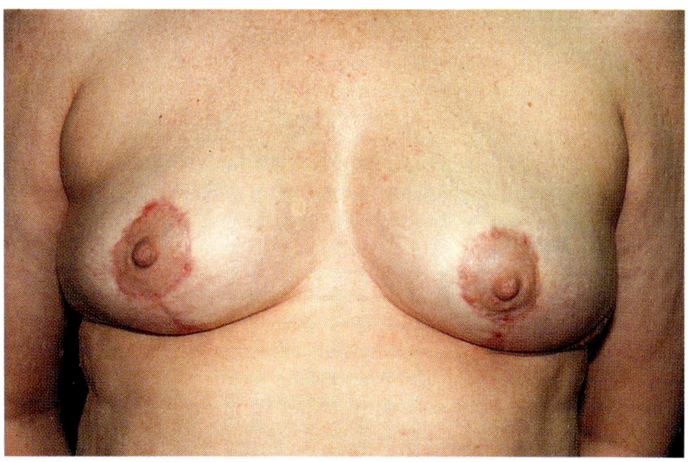

The postoperative result is shown at 6 weeks. The patient has not returned for further follow-up. However, we understand that her systemic symptoms remain unchanged following explantation.

CONCLUSION

Of all the reoperative conditions discussed in this book, none has undergone such a radical evolution in the past 2 years as those regarding patients with breast implants. The foregoing discussion represents our current approach to women with a variety of reoperative conditions. Research studies continue to establish the safety and efficacy of both silicone gel and saline breast implants. New product development is also under way. Certainly the results of these studies will impact the future surgical management of women with breast implants. It follows that reoperation for these types of problems will also change, particularly indications and techniques. Hopefully, with the improvement in devices, patient satisfaction will remain high and reoperative intervention can be kept to a minimum.

References

1. Estes EH Jr. Breast Implants (resolution 259, A-91). Report of the Council on Scientific Affairs, Report: M(I-91). December 1991.
2. Hetter GP. Satisfactions and dissatisfactions of patients with augmentation mammaplasty. Plast Reconstr Surg 64:151, 1979.
3. Maliniac JW. Arterial blood supply of the breast. Arch Surg 47:329, 1943.
4. Bostwick J III. Plastic and Reconstructive Surgery of the Breast. St. Louis: Quality Medical Publishing, 1990.
5. Shapiro MA. The nipple-areola and mammary blood supply. Plast Reconstr Surg 78:129, 1976.
6. Courtiss EH, Goldwyn RM. Breast sensation before and after plastic surgery. Plast Reconstr Surg 58:1-13, 1976.
7. Goldwyn RM. Plastic and Reconstructive Surgery of the Breast. Boston: Little, Brown, 1976.
8. Peck GC. Complications and Problems in Aesthetic Plastic Surgery. New York: Gower Medical Publishing, 1992.
9. Gurdin M. Complications of breast augmentation. Plast Reconstr Surg 40:530, 1967.
10. Burkhardt RB, Dempsey PD, Schnur PL, Tofield JJ. Capsular contracture: A prospective study of the effect of local antibacterial agents. Plast Reconstr Surg 77:919, 1986.
11. Brownstein ML, Owsley JQ Jr. Augmentation mammaplasty: A survey of major complications. In Owsley JQ, Peterson RA, eds. Symposium on Aesthetic Surgery of the Breast. St. Louis: Mosby, 1978, p 267.
12. Courtiss EH, Goldwyn RM, Anastasi GW. The fate of breast implants with infections around them. Plast Reconstr Surg 63:812, 1979.
13. McGrath MH, Burkhardt BR. The safety and efficacy of breast implants for augmentation mammaplasty. Plast Reconstr Surg 74:550, 1984.
14. Toranto IR, Malow JB. Atypical mycobacterial periprosthetic infections—Diagnosis and treatment. Plast Reconstr Surg 66:226, 1980.
15. LeRoy J, Given KS. Wound infection in breast augmentation: The role of prophylactic perioperative antibiotics. Aesthetic Plast Surg 15:303, 1991.

16. Barnett A, Lavey E, Peall RM, Vistnes LM. Toxic shock syndrome from an infected breast prosthesis. Ann Plast Surg 10:408, 1983.
17. Georgiade NG. Aesthetic Surgery of the Breast. Philadelphia: WB Saunders, 1990.
18. Clarendon CD. Implant descent: A complication of augmentation mammaplasty and its correction. Ann Plast Surg 21:452, 1988.
19. Biggs T, Cukier J, Worthing L. Augmentation mammaplasty: A review of eighteen years. Plast Reconstr Surg 69:445, 1982.
20. Gayou RM. A histologic comparison of contracted and noncontracted capsules around silicone breast implants. Plast Reconstr Surg 63:700, 1979.
21. Rudolph R, Abraham J, Vecchione T, et al. Myofibroblasts and free silicon around breast implants. Plast Reconstr Surg 62:185, 1978.
22. Hipps CJ, Raju DR, Straith RE. Influence of some operative and postoperative factors on capsular contracture around breast prostheses. Plast Reconstr Surg 61:384, 1978.
23. Williams C, Aston S, Rees TD. The effect of hematoma on the thicknesses of pseudosheaths around silicone implants. Plast Reconstr Surg 56:194, 1975.
24. Caffee HH. The effects of hematoma on implant capsules. Ann Plast Surg 16:102, 1986.
25. Shah Z, Lehman JA, Tan J. Does infection play a role in breast capsular contracture? Plast Reconstr Surg 68:34, 1981.
26. Kossovsky N, Heggers JP, Parsons RW, et al. Acceleration of capsule formation around silicone implants by infection in a guinea pig model. Plast Reconstr Surg 73:91, 1984.
27. Birnbaum LM, Hopp DD, Mertens BF. The role of iodine-releasing silicone implants in prevention of spherical contractures. Plast Reconstr Surg 69:956, 1982.
28. Dubin DB. The etiology, pathophysiology, predictability, and early detection of spherical scar contracture of the breast: A detailed explanation and protocol for prevention of spherical scar contracture of the breast. Presented at the 13th Annual Meeting of the American Society of Aesthetic Plastic Surgery. May 1980.
29. Burkhardt BR, Dempsey PD, Schnur TL, et al. A prospective study of the effect of local antibacterial agents. Plast Reconstr Surg 77:919, 1986.
30. Domanskis EJ, Owsley JQ. Histological investigation of the etiology of capsule contracture following augmentation mammaplasty. Plast Reconstr Surg 58:689, 1976.
31. Asplund O. Capsule contracture and silicone gel and saline filled breast implants after reconstruction. Plast Reconstr Surg 73:270, 1984.
32. Caffee HH. The influence of silicone bleed on capsule contracture. Ann Plast Surg 17:284, 1986.
33. Broadbent TR, Woolf RM. Augmentation mammaplasty. Plast Reconstr Surg 40:517, 1967.
34. Burkhardt BR. Comparing contracture rates: Probability theory and the unilateral contracture. Plast Reconstr Surg 74:527, 1984.
35. McKinney P, Treslie G. Long term comparison of patients with gel and saline mammary implants. Plast Reconstr Surg 72:27, 1983.
36. Caffee HH. Textured silicone and capsule contracture. Ann Plast Surg 24:197, 1990.
37. Eyssen JE, von Werssowetz AJ, Middleton GD. Reconstruction of the breast using polyurethane coated prostheses. Plast Reconstr Surg 73:415, 1984.
38. Rudolph R. Submuscular vs. submammary placement of breast prostheses. Presented at the 30th Annual Meeting of the Plastic Surgery Research Counsel. Portland, Ore.: 1985.
39. Mahler D, Hauben DJ. Retromammary vs. retropectoral breast augmentation: A comparative study. Ann Plast Surg 8:370, 1982.
40. Slade CL. Subcutaneous mastectomy: Acute complications and long-term follow-up. Plast Reconstr Surg 73:84, 1984.
41. Caffee HH. Breast implant capsule contracture. Unpublished data, 1987.
42. Terino E. Essential concepts in prosthetic plastic surgery. Aesthetic Plast Surg 626:25, 1982.
43. Finnick CA. Spherical contracture of fibrous contracture around breast implants. Plast Reconstr Surg 58:555, 1976.

44. Marshall WR. Amelioration of capsular contracture by motion restriction. Ann Plast Surg 16:211, 1986.
45. Stephens FO, Dunphy JE, Hunt KK. Effect of delayed administration of corticosteroids on wound contraction. Ann Surg 173:214, 1971.
46. Peterson HD, Burt GB Jr. The role of steroids in prevention of circumferential capsular scarring in augmentation mammaplasty. Plast Reconstr Surg 54:28, 1974.
47. Perrin ER. The use of soluble steroids within inflatable breast prosthesis. Plast Reconstr Surg 57:163, 1976.
48. Cohen IK, Carricco TJ. Capsular contracture and steroid-related complications in augmentation mammaplasty. Aesthetic Plast Surg 4:267, 1980.
49. Oneal RM, Argenta LC. Late side effects related to inflatable breast prosthesis containing soluble steroids. Plast Reconstr Surg 69:641, 1982.
50. Little G, Baker JL. Result of closed compression capsulotomy for treatment of contracted breast implant capsules. Plast Reconstr Surg 65:30, 1980.
51. McKinney P, Treslie G. Long-term comparison of patients with gel and saline mammary implants. Plast Reconstr Surg 72:27, 1983.
52. Derman GH, Argenta LC, Grabb WC. Delayed extrusion of inflatable breast prostheses. Ann Plast Surg 10:154, 1983.
53. Feliberti MD, Arrillage A, Colon GA. Rupture of inflated breast implants in closed compression capsulotomy. Plast Reconstr Surg 59:848, 1977.
54. Eisenberg HV, Bartels RJ. Rupture of a silicone bag–gel breast implant by closed compression capsulotomy. Plast Reconstr Surg 59:849, 1977.
55. Huang TT, Blackwell SJ, Louis SR. Migration of silicone gel after the capsule. Plast Reconstr Surg 61:277, 1978.
56. Capozzi A, Du Bou R, Pennisi VR. Distant migration of silicone gel from a ruptured breast implant. Plast Reconstr Surg 62:302, 1978.
57. Edmond J, Versaci A. Late complication of closed capsulotomy of the breast. Plast Reconstr Surg 66:478, 1980.
58. Bergman RB, Van Der Ende AE. Exudation of silicone through the envelope of gel-filled breast prostheses: An in-vitro study. Br J Plast Surg 32:31, 1979.
59. Barker DE, Ritsky MI, Schultz S. Bleeding of silicone from the bag-gel breast implants and its clinical relation to fibrous capsule reaction. Plast Reconstr Surg 61:836, 1978.
60. Whintsch W. Leaking Ashley prosthesis with lymphanopathy. Presented at the 5th Alpine Workshop on Plastic and Reconstructive Surgery. Austria: February 15, 1978.
61. Stedman's Medical Dictionary, 24th ed. Baltimore: Williams and Wilkins, 1982.
62. Rose NR. Invited commentary: Silicone breast implants and immune disease. Ann Plast Surg 28:499, 1992.
63. Miyoshi K, Miyramura T, Kobayashi Y, et al. Hypergammaglobulinemia by prolonged adjuvanticity in man. Disorders developed after augmentation mammaplasty. Jpn J Med 2122:9, 1964.
64. Shons AR, Schubert W. Silicone breast implants and immune disease. Ann Plast Surg 28:491, 1992.
65. Federal Register. 21 CFR Part 878, pp 14620-14627.
66. Yoshida K. Post mammaplasty disorder as an adjuvant disease of man. Shikoku Acta Med 29:318, 1973.
67. Kumagi Y, Shikowaka Y, Medsger TA Jr, et al. Clinical spectrum of connective tissue disease after cosmetic surgery. Arthritis Rheum 27:1, 1984.
68. Van Nunen SA, Gatenby PA, Basten A. Post mammaplasty connective tissue disease. Arthritis Rheum 25:694, 1982.
69. Baldwin CM Jr, Kaplan EN. Silicone-induced human adjuvant disease? Ann Plast Surg 10:270, 1983.
70. Elberg JJ, Kjoller KH, Krag C. Silicone mammary implants and connective tissue disease. Scand J Plast Reconstr Hand Surg 27:243, 1993.

71. Gabriel SE, O'Fallon WM, Kurland LT, Beard CM, Woods JE, Melton LJ III. Risk of connective tissue diseases and other disorders after breast implantation. New Engl J Med 330:1697, 1994.
72. Schusterman MA, Kroll SS, Reece GP, Miller MJ, Ainslie M, Halabi S, Balch CM. Incidence of autoimmune disease after breast reconstruction with silicone gel implants vs. autogenous tissue: A preliminary report. Ann Plast Surg 31:1, 1993.
73. Bridges AJ, Conley C, Wang G, Burns DE, Vasey FB. A clinical and immunologic evaluation with silicone breast implants and symptoms of rheumatic disease. Ann Intern Med 118:929, 1993.
74. Deapen DM, Pike FC, Casagrande JT, Brody GS. The relationship between breast cancer and augmentation mammaplasty: An epidemiologic study. Plast Reconstr Surg 77:361, 1986.

29

Reoperation Following Implant Breast Reconstruction

James C. Grotting, M.D.

Reoperative Problems

Inframammary fold displacement	Gel leakage
Lack of projection	Infection
Lateral displacement of implant	Hematoma
Chronic pain	Seroma
Capsular contracture	Skin loss
Flap failure	Valve leakage
Implant deflation	

The earliest attempts at breast reconstruction consisted of the simple placement of some type of filler material to construct a mound. Although today these early reconstructive efforts appear rudimentary at best, they laid the groundwork for the development of newer and better techniques for breast reconstruction, acceptance of breast reconstruction as an integral part of the breast cancer patient's rehabilitation, and inclusion of the plastic surgeon as a member of the breast cancer team. As a specialty, we are indebted to these surgeons and patients who embarked on this surgical adventure, paving the way for those of us who have followed.

However, the evolution of breast reconstruction is by no means concluded, and with the restriction of the availability of silicone gel–filled breast implants, which has been the mainstay of reconstruction over the past 30 years, there has been a corresponding increase in the use of saline breast implants and autogenous tissue for breast restoration as most plastic surgeons have altered their approach to primary breast reconstruction. Similarly, women who have previously undergone implant breast reconstruction and who return with new problems may require a change in reconstructive approach.

The goal of breast reconstruction is to produce a permanent, natural, and symmetric match to the opposite breast, if present. No surgeon can hope to always achieve perfect results in one operation. Staged procedures and secondary operations are often necessary, even commonplace, to perform refinements and to correct problems, particularly as more and more women with "state-of-the art" reconstructions from decades earlier return to discuss the possibility of improvement. We now have a variety of reliable techniques for treating patients with problems related to previous breast implant reconstructions.

STAGED BREAST RECONSTRUCTION

The majority of breast reconstructions remain staged procedures. Usually the second stage of an implant reconstruction can be accomplished in an outpatient facility. I prefer to perform such surgery with the patient under general anesthesia because I believe it is more comfortable for the patient and gives me the option of doing more extensive capsular surgery and adjustment of the fold area if necessary.

Secondary breast reconstruction requires a motivated patient and an experienced and careful surgeon. Realistic expectations are the key to eventual patient satisfaction. From the time of the first consultation the patient and her family should have a clear view of the sequence of the operations and the time required to complete the reconstruction.

Timing

Various factors affect timing in a staged breast reconstruction. In immediate reconstruction an expander is often placed at the initial procedure. The second-stage reconstruction, however, may need to be deferred until after the patient has completed chemotherapy. This variable must be carefully explained to the patient in advance of the reconstruction. Another factor that influences the timing of the second stage is the rate at which the skin envelope matures. Although maturity of the skin envelope predictably occurs between 2 and 3 months postoperatively, in some patients factors such as capsular contracture, persistent edema, or possibly even radiation will delay the return of pliability to the soft tissues overlying the expander. I prefer to wait until the skin envelope matures before I reoperate.

Planning

Whether an expander or an implant was placed at the initial stage in a staged implant reconstruction, the second stage of mound reconstruction usually will require removal and replacement of the device. At present, there is only one adjustable saline implant device available (Mentor Spectrum). Perfect reconstructed symmetry with implant devices in a single stage is usually possible only in bilateral mastectomies or in the case of a round nonptotic breast on the opposite side.

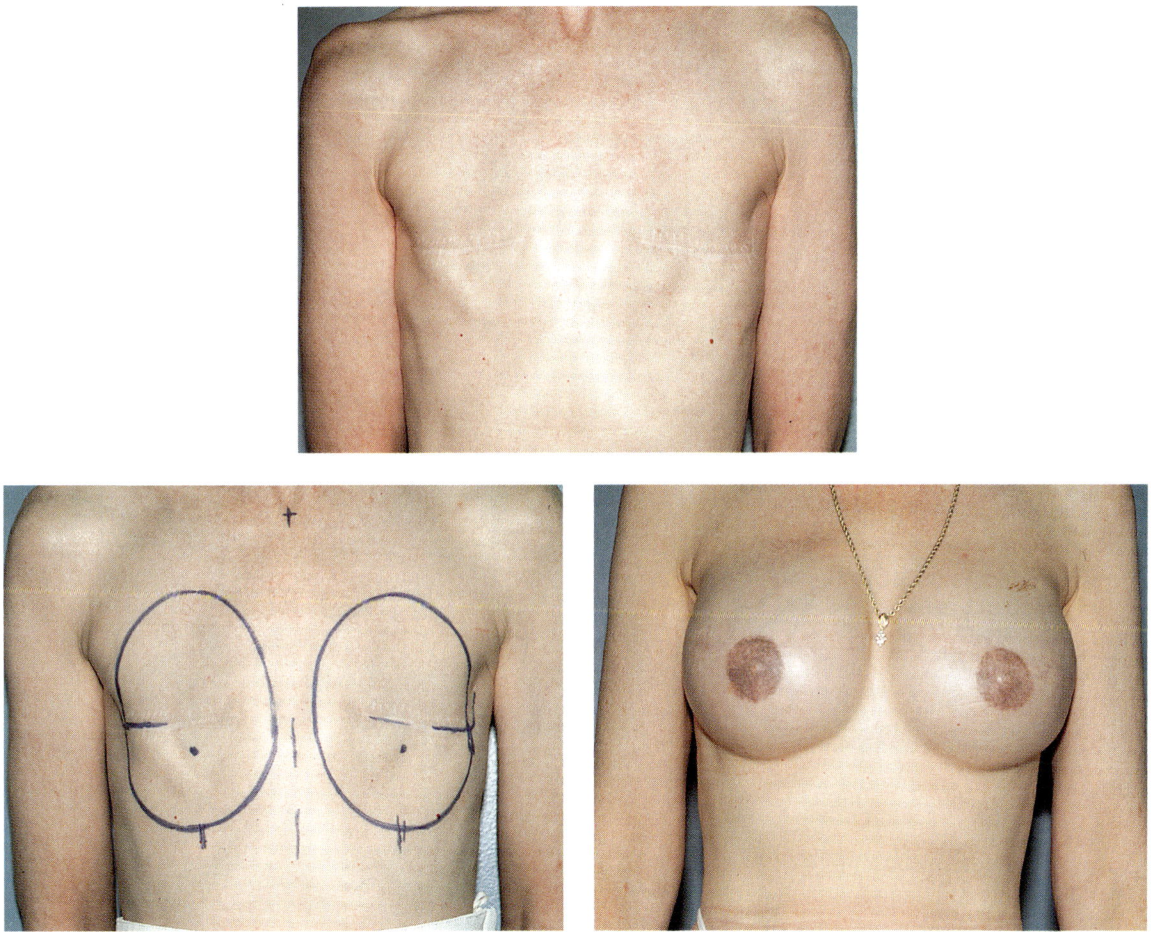

Mirror image expander placement in bilateral reconstruction virtually guarantees symmetry in patients in whom the quantity and quality of skin coverage is identical. This patient presented 2 years after undergoing bilateral modified radical mastectomies for carcinoma of the breast. Remote-valve adjustable implants were placed through short incisions in the lateral mastectomy scars. The pockets were submuscular in the upper portion and subcutaneous inferiorly and over the serratus anterior muscle. With the inframammary folds set at the proper position, symmetric expansion was accomplished, thereby simplifying the secondary procedure, which involved only nipple reconstruction and valve removal. The postoperative result is shown at 1 year.

Currently there is considerable pressure from insurance companies and other payors to minimize secondary surgeries or eliminate them as a patient benefit. Therefore proper planning becomes imperative to optimize results in as few procedures as possible. Care in selecting the proper expander and positioning it at the right level so that the inframammary fold develops symmetrically are key factors in minimizing the complexity of secondary revisions.

Planning errors, however, do occur. Although such errors are easy to recognize in retrospect, unfortunately they are not always easy to accept. One of the most difficult discussions to have with a patient is to honestly explain that things have not worked out according to plan and that a new tact must be taken. Remarkably the patient is often well aware of this situation even before the surgeon. With experience comes the judgment of how tissues will respond to an implanted device or a tissue transfer. Proper patient selection then becomes the key, thereby diminishing the requirement for reoperative adjustment or completely "changing gears."

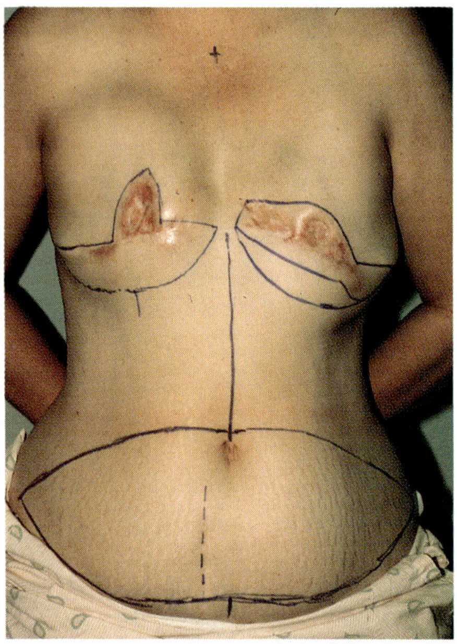

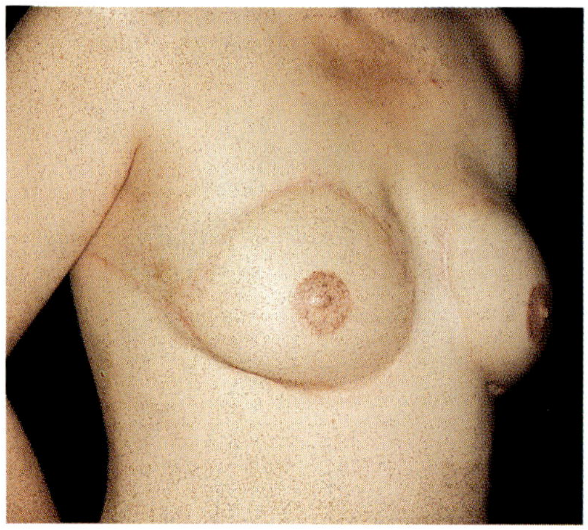

The need to completely "change course" is effectively demonstrated in this patient who sought consultation after having undergone several previous reconstructive procedures. Her past history included multiple silicone injections for breast enlargement, which resulted in painful, contracted, and nodular breasts. She underwent subcutaneous mastectomy and reconstruction using tissue expanders. Apparently these expanders became exposed due to skin loss and superficial infection. She is shown preoperatively with the expanders still in place. Clearly implant reconstruction did not produce the desired result. Therefore we elected to completely change plans and to proceed with autogenous reconstruction using bilateral free TRAM flaps. The final reconstruction was accomplished in two stages; despite the presence of a right lower paramedian incision, the perforators on the right side had not been completely disrupted. (The second operation is depicted in Chapter 31.)

The degree of tissue expansion will vary depending on the initial mode of expansion and how much overinflation may have been done. (I no longer greatly overfill an expander as I do not believe that this contributes to the creation of a ptotic breast.) The most important consideration, however, is the positioning of the reconstructed inframammary fold at the proper level and the development of a compliant soft tissue envelope that will be suspended from the inframammary fold. Textured-surface expander devices have been helpful in allowing the latter to occur.

In the situation in which the previously placed expander or implant has produced a reasonably good shape along the inframammary fold, then the most important considerations are the diameter of the base of the reconstructed breast and its projection. At the present time new saline devices are being designed to attempt to affect the shape in the upper pole. However, the key to implant selection is to choose the implant according to the optimal base diameter and projection, with the volume depending on the desired upper pole fill and firmness.

■ *The opposite breast will always serve as the model for symmetric reconstruction. It is the key to the operative plan for all stages of breast reconstruction.* For some surgeons careful study of the preoperative photographs is the most effective way to detect subtle differences in symmetry that occasionally escape the eye on direct examination. I find it helpful to compare the level of the lower pole overlying the costal margin on each side. Then I follow the fold laterally and study how much of the inferior lateral curve of the reconstructed breast projects beyond the lateral chest wall compared to the opposite side. Then examination of the symmetry of the medial curve of the breast and the plane of the upper pole as seen from the lateral view completes the reoperative evaluation of shape. The operative plan should address alterations in the shape and fill in all of these areas.

Operative Options

The operative options available for breast mound correction during the second stage include:

Alteration or replacement of saline device

- Alteration of volume, base diameter, or projection
- Use of a textured-surface or smooth-surface device
- Use of a postoperatively adjustable or permanent-volume device
- Use of a custom device

Alteration of the soft tissue envelope capsule
- Total capsulectomy
- Partial capsulectomy
- Segmental capsulotomy
- Capsular plication

Opposite breast adjustments
- Prophylactic simple or subcutaneous mastectomy
- Augmentation
- Reduction
- Mastopexy

All of these techniques can be used singly or in combination to produce a symmetric reconstructed breast. Although stacking of multiple polyurethane-covered implants was an effective way to alter shape and projection, no data are currently available as to whether textured-surface silicone saline-filled implants can be handled in the same way.

Correction of Problems Associated With Saline Implant

Inflatable saline implants are currently the only type of widely available implants used by plastic surgeons. Although these devices have been satisfactory for breast augmentation, they have not produced the same degree of success in reconstruction. Deflation rates have been reported as low as 1%/year, but this rate may actually be considerably higher. The incidence of capsular contracture may be somewhat less than that for silicone gel implants; however, the wrinkling phenomenon seems to be more common with saline implants. Wrinkling or rippling is related to underfilling and will occur in all underfilled implants in the upright position. With textured-surface silicone inflatable implants in which the surrounding capsule is adherent to the outer surface of the implant, wrinkling can be a source of dissatisfaction. Textured-surface implants are not freely mobile within the capsule and therefore wrinkling may be more visible. Sometimes these corrugations are simply palpable, but other times they are visible through the skin. As the capsule adheres into the surface folds in the implant, the overlying subcutaneous tissue and skin will deform into this corrugated pattern. It is difficult to either prevent or treat this problem. Overinflation of implants is effective at reducing wrinkling but not at completely eliminating it. Overinflation may also void the manufacturer's warranty on the implant in the same way that using any medications other than saline inside the implant can affect the warranty. Use of a smooth-surface implant rather than a textured-surface implant increases implant mobility within the pocket but does not necessarily diminish upper pole wrinkling. However, the wrinkling may not be as visible with the smooth-surface implants.

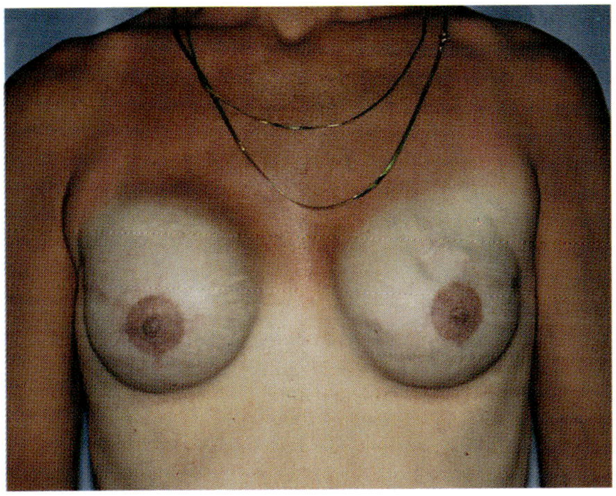

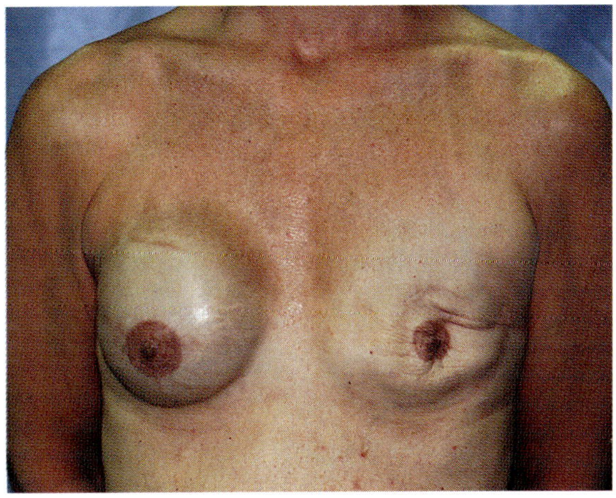

This 41-year-old patient underwent bilateral breast reconstruction using saline inflatable implants. She had an infiltrating ductal carcinoma of the right breast and premalignant changes of the left breast. Simple mastectomies were performed on successive occasions with saline implant insertion. Notice the rippling in the upper pole of the reconstructed left breast. Six months after completion of the reconstruction she presented with the deflation of the left-sided implant. At surgery a small perforation was found on the base of the implant away from the valve area. The implant was removed through the lateral mastectomy scar, a perimeter capsulotomy was performed, and an identical implant was replaced into the same pocket. She has experienced no further problems.

Correction of the base diameter of the reconstructed breast can be accomplished simply by measuring the base diameter of the opposite breast. The expander or previous implant is then replaced by a saline implant of appropriate base diameter. In actuality the base diameter is a much more important factor than the ultimate volume in terms of achieving symmetry. Capsular alterations may also be necessary.

Occasionally it is helpful to place an adjustable implant rather than a fixed-volume implant in the second stage. When treating recurrent capsular contracture, some surgeons have advocated maintaining slight overcorrection for a period of 3 to 6 months while the new capsule is forming; then saline solution is withdrawn from the implant to achieve the appropriate volume. However, one must be aware of the possibility of "uncovering" upper pole wrinkling as the saline solution is withdrawn.

A variety of new saline devices is being introduced at the time of this writing that can purportedly affect breast shape based on the variable thickness of the silicone elastomer envelope. In this way one might be able to create a more mature-looking breast using an implant that is flatter in the upper pole.

Inframammary Fold Alterations

■ ***The inframammary fold is the key to achieving a good result no matter what kind of breast reconstruction is being performed. Unless this fold is set at the proper level, all other natural curves of the breast will be difficult to simulate.***

Inframammary Fold Too High

A high inframammary fold is a common problem after breast reconstruction; fortunately it is also the easiest to correct during reoperative breast implant surgery. An inframammary fold that is too high may result from the initial implant or expander being placed too high or from the natural elevation that occurs with encapsulation.

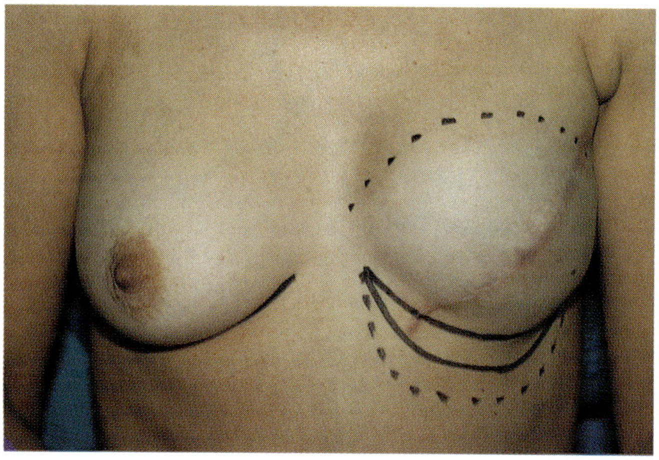

With the patient standing preoperatively, the proper inframammary fold level is marked on the chest wall. Usually the fold can be lowered by simply incising the perimeter of the capsule in the lower pole of the breast and dissecting the subcutaneous tissue off the muscle fascia to the marked level. However, it is possible to lower the fold too much by dissecting too low. In addition, in patients who have thick subcutaneous tissues, the fold is easily blunted so that there is not a distinct emergence of the lower pole of the breast from the chest wall. This appearance is unaesthetic and difficult to correct. Therefore in these patients I prefer to thin the fat slightly and place internal plication sutures between Scarpa's fascia and the chest wall. If this maneuver does not give the distinct, crisp inframammary fold that I am trying to achieve, it may be necessary to actually plicate the dermis to the chest wall using 2-0 Prolene sutures. These sutures may need to be placed from the medialmost extent of the inframammary fold all the way to the anterior axillary line. More commonly, however, only a portion of the inframammary fold will need to be plicated in this way. This determination is best made in the operating room with the patient in the upright position. It must be kept in mind that the fold will often elevate 1 to 2 cm postoperatively as the capsule develops, especially with smooth-surface implants. Therefore this correction is taken into account when the fold level is chosen preoperatively.

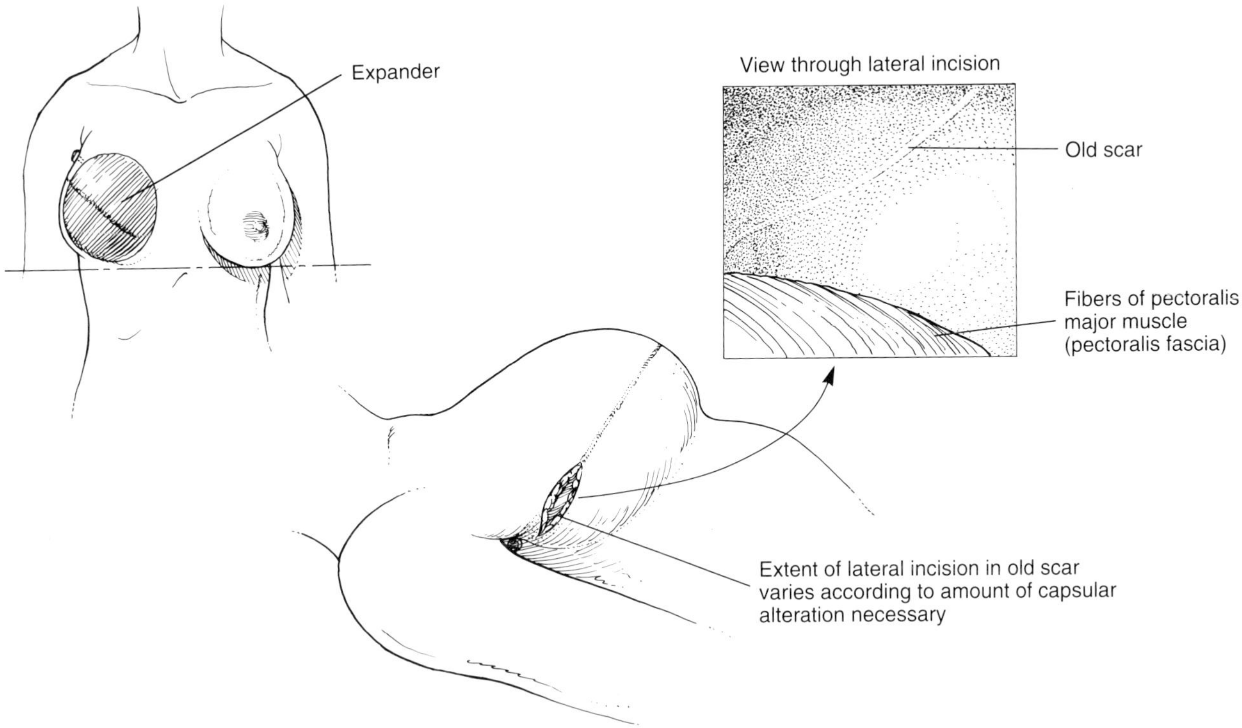
Expander
View through lateral incision
Old scar
Fibers of pectoralis major muscle (pectoralis fascia)
Extent of lateral incision in old scar varies according to amount of capsular alteration necessary

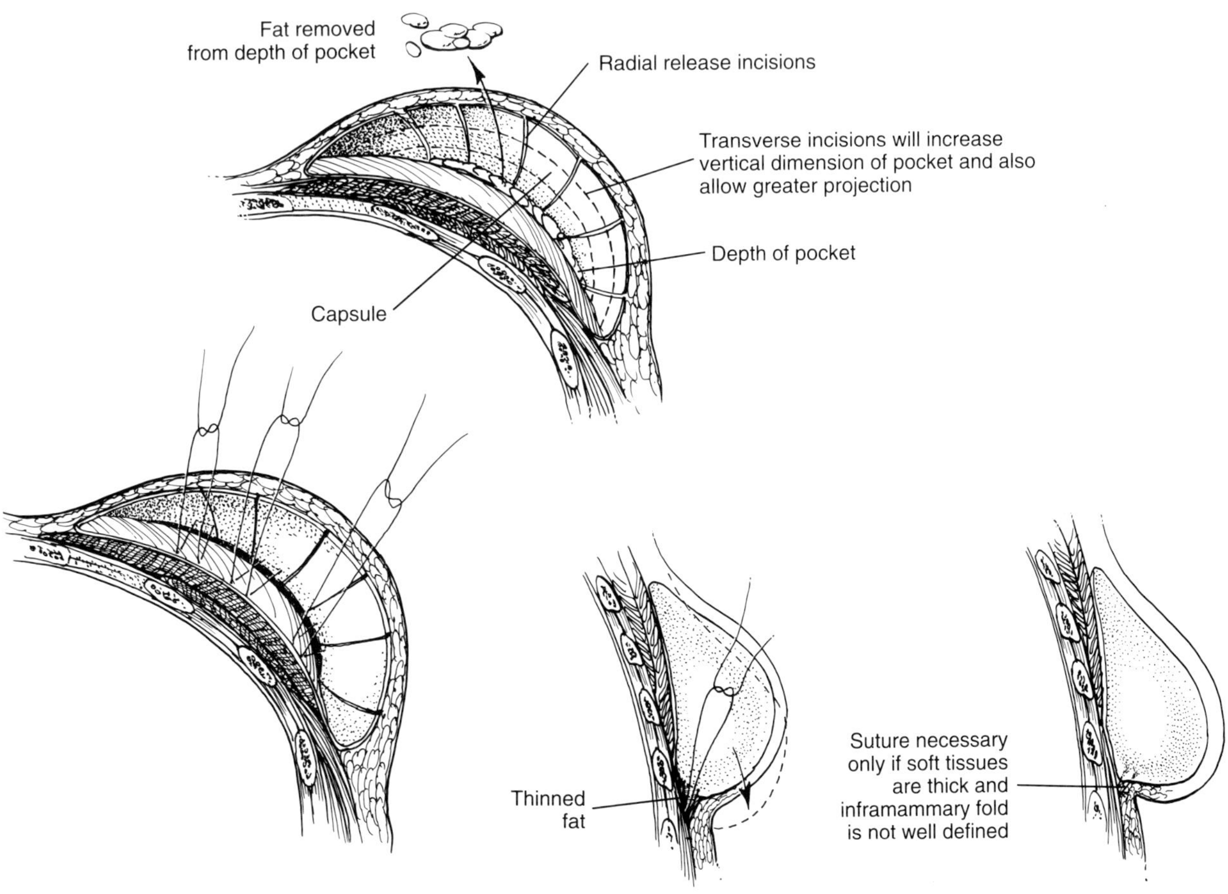
Fat removed from depth of pocket
Radial release incisions
Transverse incisions will increase vertical dimension of pocket and also allow greater projection
Depth of pocket
Capsule
Thinned fat
Suture necessary only if soft tissues are thick and inframammary fold is not well defined

Inframammary Fold Too Low

Purposely constructing a low inframammary fold has been suggested as a way of simulating a ptotic opposite breast. Although this technique can give the visual impression of ptosis on anterior view, particularly in a photograph, the patient finds it difficult to wear a brassiere or other fitted clothing when the inframammary folds are at different levels. Therefore I prefer not to use this technique for creating ptosis. If, however, the fold is too low from a low expansion or a descended implant, this problem can be corrected in the second stage of a planned staged reconstruction. I prefer to use the internal plication technique rather than external dermal flap procedures as proposed by Ryan.

The lateral portion of the previous skin incision is reopened, and a short subcutaneous flap is developed so that the muscle pocket can be entered at a different level. This approach is taken so that if one of the incisions opens postoperatively, implant exposure or extrusion is less likely to result. The pectoralis major muscle is divided along its fibers to expose the capsule.

The capsule is then entered and opened widely enough so that the entire lower portion of the capsule can be visualized following the removal of the expander or previous implant. If the skin and subcutaneous tissue overlying the capsule in the lower pole are quite thin, the inframammary fold can sometimes be re-created by capsular plication sutures alone that extend from the medialmost aspect to the anterior axillary line. Heavy sutures of 2-0 Prolene are most effective. If the subcutaneous tissues are thick or if capsular plication sutures do not create a crisp inframammary fold when the patient is in the sitting position, then the capsule must be opened and a capsular flap dissected from the level of the old inframammary fold up to the level of the new one.

The subcutaneous tissues beneath the capsule are then thinned because this tissue is being converted to abdominal wall skin rather than breast skin. The capsular flap is then advanced superiorly and plicated to the posterior capsule on the chest wall. In addition, I find it helpful to place heavy sutures through either the Scarpa's fascia or the dermis to the chest wall in a manner similar to that described for lowering the inframammary fold. A double row of sutures will help to secure the new inframammary fold and prevent descent of the new implant. A textured-surface implant is a good choice under these circumstances as it is more likely than a smooth-surface implant to stay fixed in position.

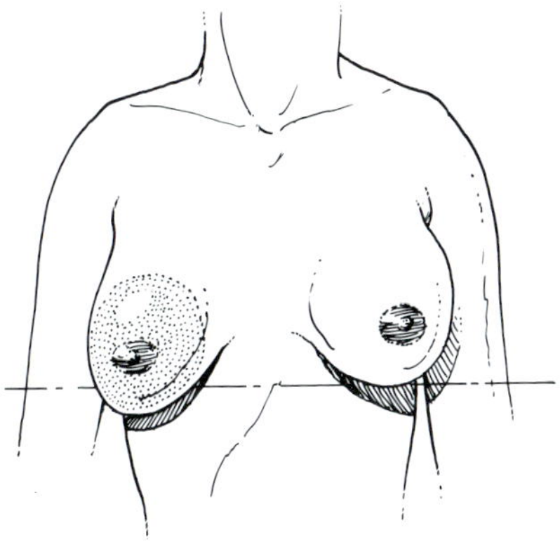

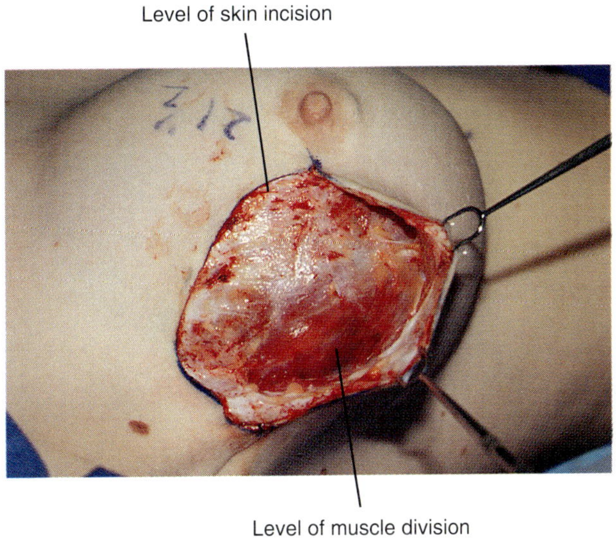
Level of skin incision
Level of muscle division

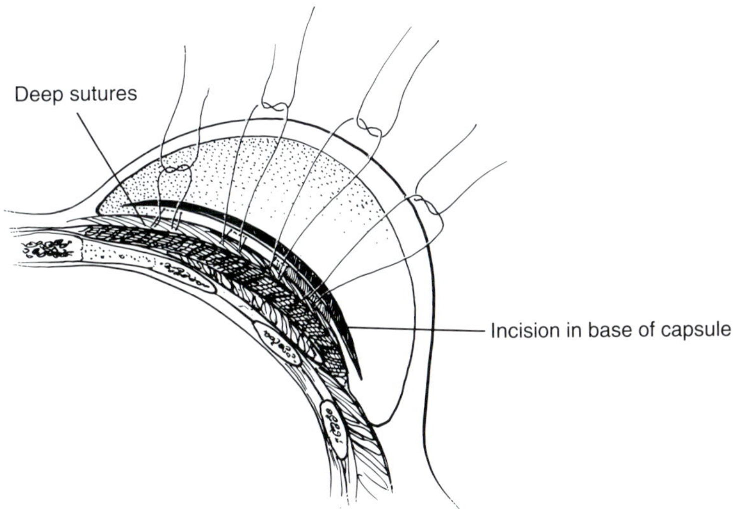
Deep sutures
Incision in base of capsule

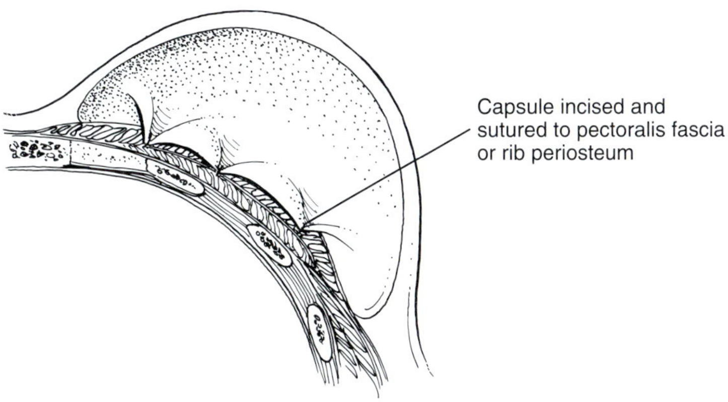
Capsule incised and
sutured to pectoralis fascia
or rib periosteum

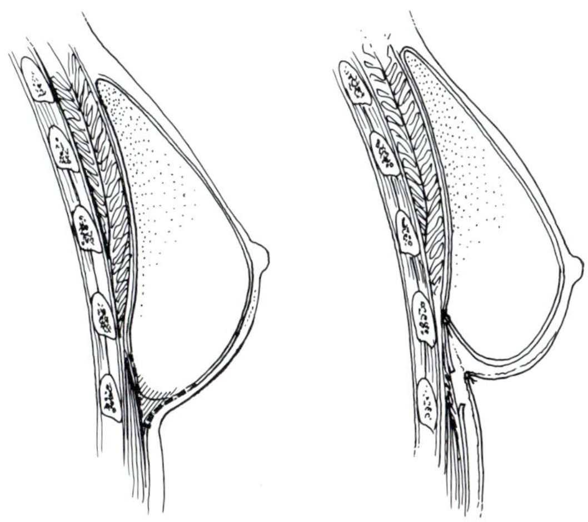

Alteration of Projection

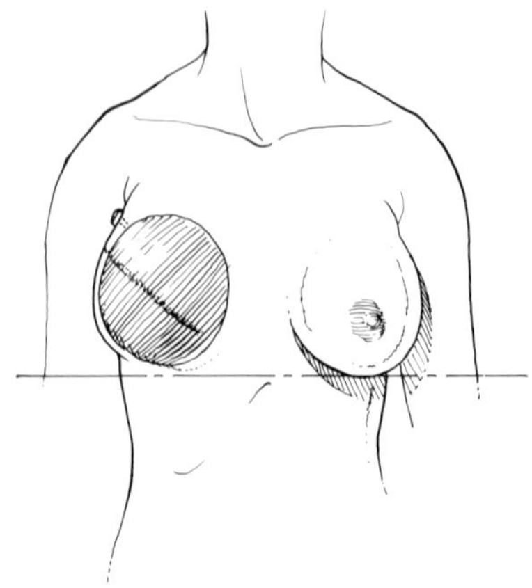

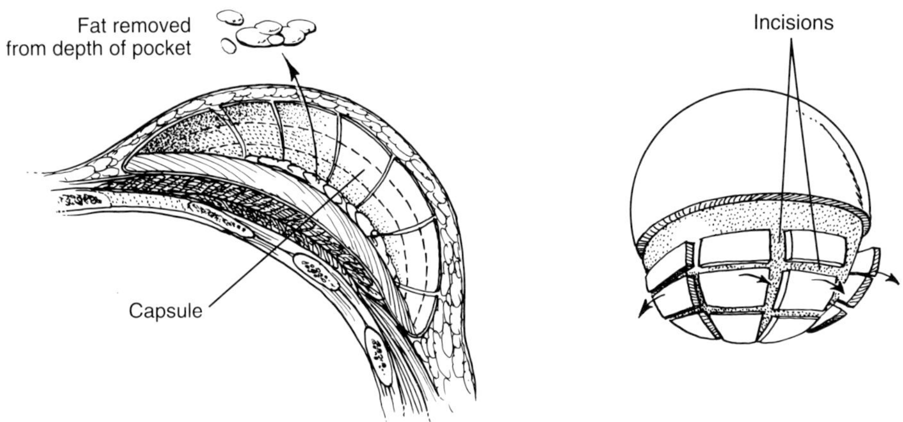

Altering the projection of a saline implant reconstruction is difficult because if one simply adds volume, the shape may be adversely affected and an unnatural fullness may result, particularly in the upper pole. If breast flattening is caused by capsular contracture in the lower pole, this problem can be improved in the second stage. Preoperatively the horizontal level that corresponds with the point of maximum projection on the opposite breast is marked. This marking is continued over the reconstructed breast. Below this level the capsule must be either removed or incised. The capsule is entered as before; the level of the skin incision and the capsular incision laterally can vary.

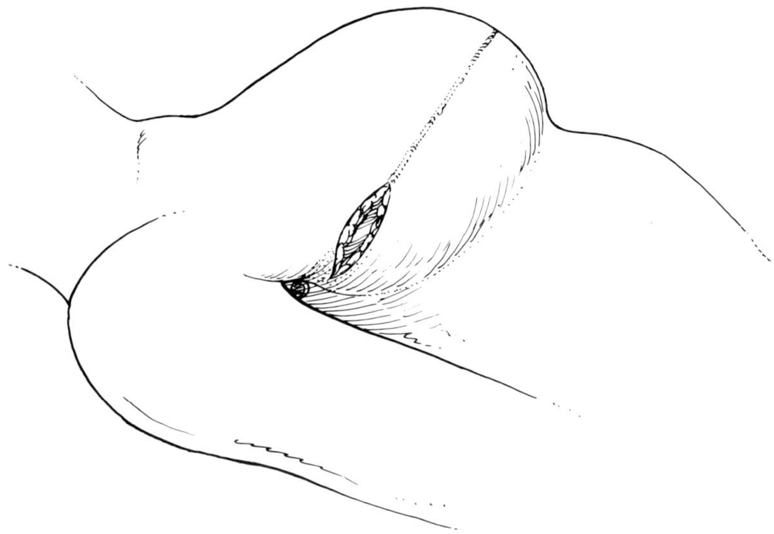

The implant or expander is removed. The initial horizontal capsular incision demarcates the upper from the lower pole. Perpendicular radial incisions are then made to expand the capsule and the lower pole soft tissue envelope in the anterior and horizontal direction. "Dicing" the capsule or removing it entirely in the lower pole allows the soft tissue envelope to expand in all directions. These incisions are really the only way to change the shape in the lower pole of the breast reconstructed with saline implants at the present time.

Correction of Lateral Implant Displacement

The youthful breast is full medially, is nonptotic, and does not extend beyond the anterior axillary line. However, due to the effects of gravity, implants or expanders inserted for immediate reconstruction that develop soft capsules may shift laterally or descend into the inferior part of the axillary dissection. This problem is bothersome to patients and is a frequent source of asymmetry and dissatisfaction.

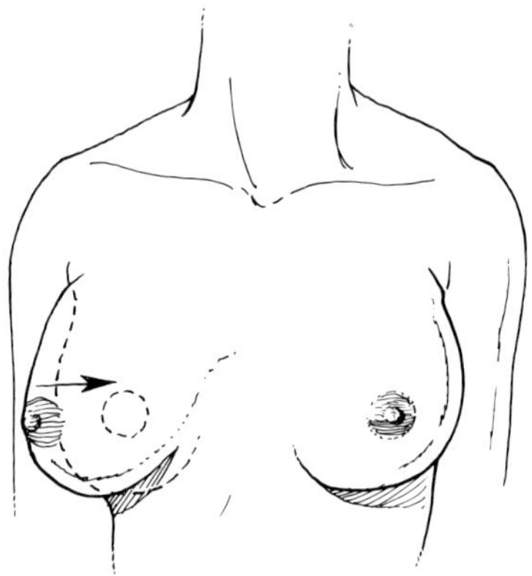

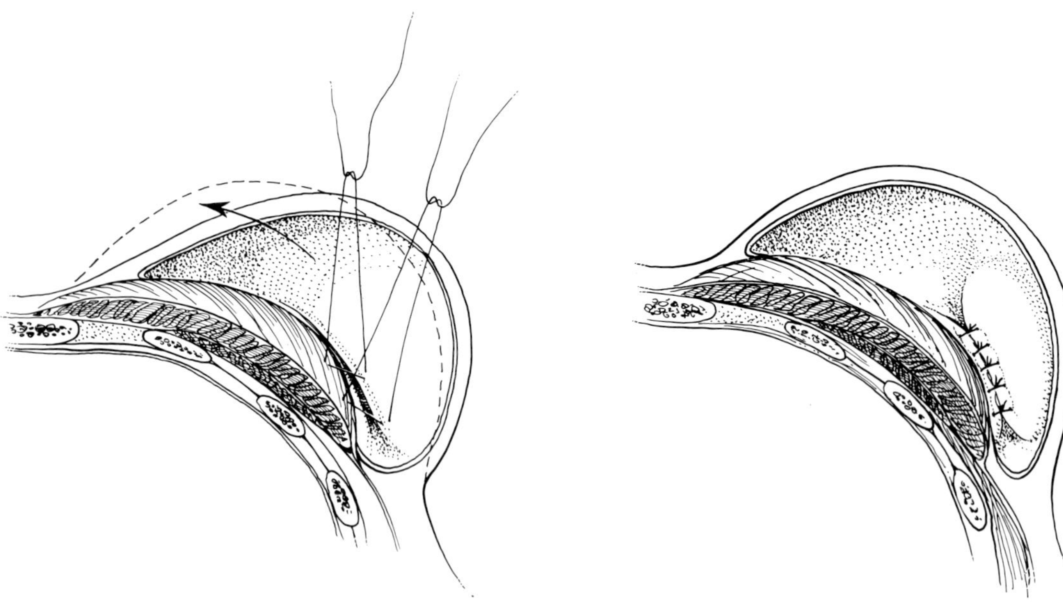

Lateral implant displacement is best corrected internally. Preoperatively with the patient in the standing position, the implant is manually compressed into the proper position and a line is drawn on the skin extending from the inframammary fold laterally to mark the lateral limit of the base of the breast. This line will be translated to the capsule and chest wall for the plication.

With the patient under general anesthesia, the mastectomy scar is reopened laterally and the capsule is entered at a separate level. The implant can sometimes simply be distracted medially while these sutures are placed. Other times it is best to temporarily remove the implant, particularly if any other capsular surgery is to be performed. The capsule and chest wall are then marked internally according to the preoperative skin markings. The marking is scored with electrocautery to create a fresh tissue plane to promote healing. A double row of running 2-0 Prolene sutures is used to plicate the lateral capsule to the chest wall. After the plication is completed, the implant can be reinserted, and the patient is placed in a sitting position to check the correction.

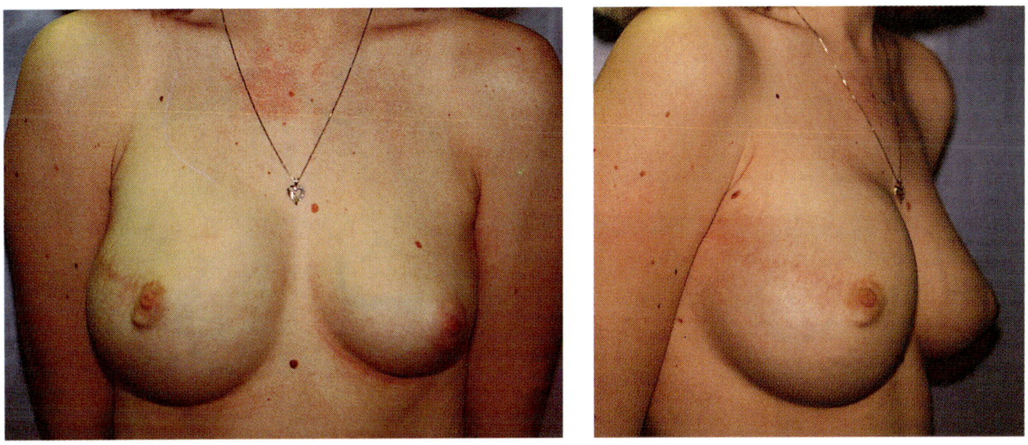

This patient underwent a right simple mastectomy for recurrent cystosarcoma phylloides. An integrated valve textured-surface expander was placed at the time of mastectomy. Overexpansion has created an ample soft tissue envelope. However, the inframammary fold is at least 2 cm too low and laterally displaced.

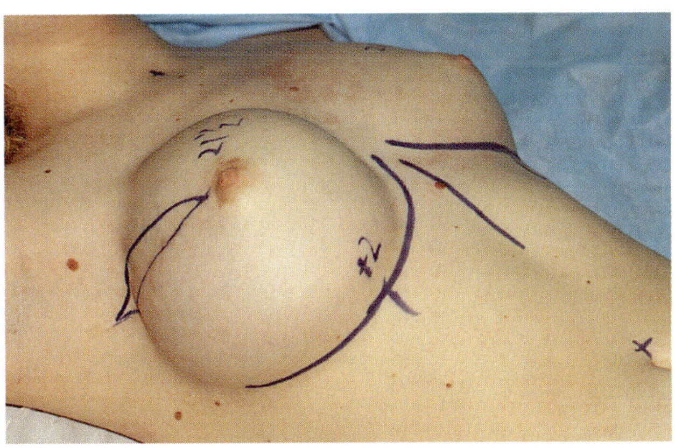

The second stage requires both a change of the device and the alteration of the soft tissue envelope. The inframammary fold needed to be raised 2 cm, and the lateral portion of the capsule had to be plicated. A scar revision of the lateral mastectomy scar was accomplished at the same time.

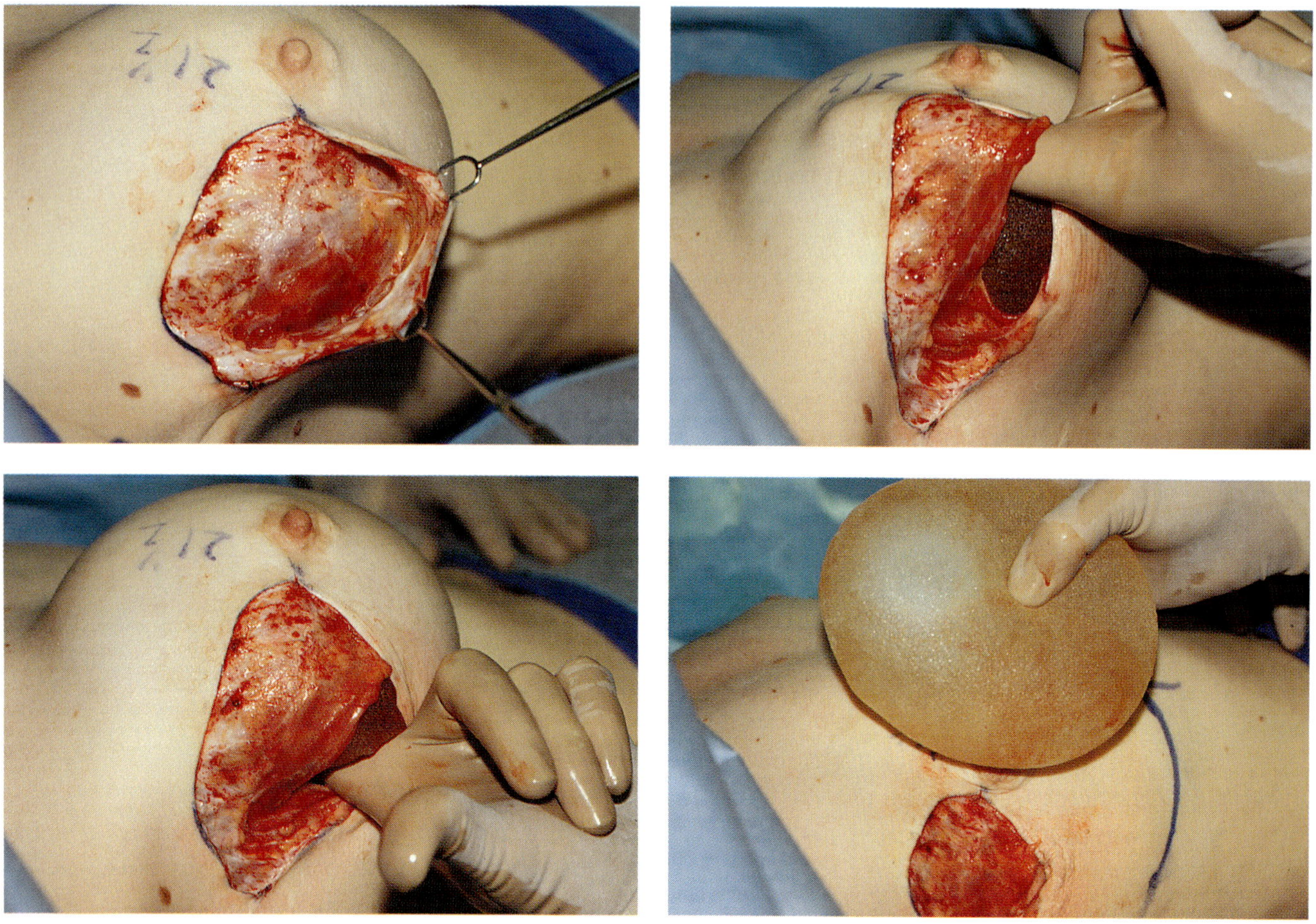

Following the resection of the mastectomy scar, the inferior mastectomy flap was elevated from the muscle cover so that the muscle could be entered at a separate level from the skin incision. This approach ensures that if either the skin incision or the muscular closure were to dehisce postoperatively, neither would necessarily result in implant exposure. The textured-surface implant was separated bluntly from the capsule first over the dome of the implant and then at its base. The expander was then removed.

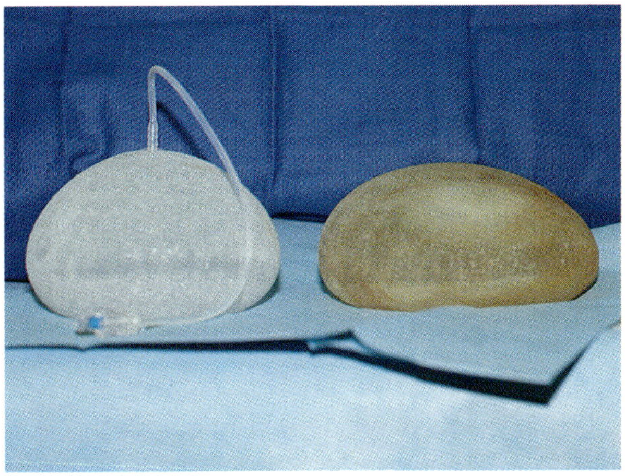

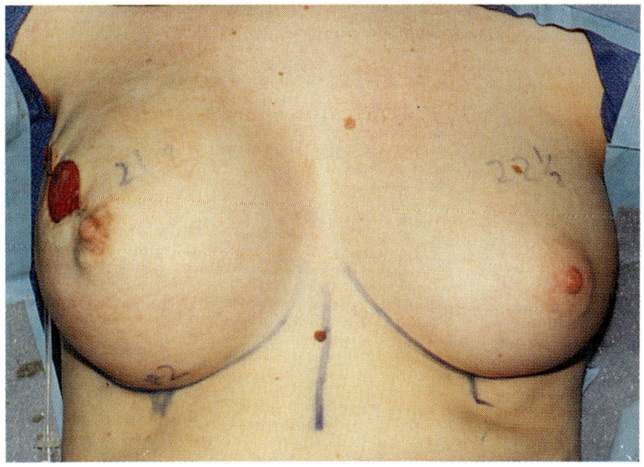

In this case a custom-designed textured-surface saline implant was designed based on measurements taken from the opposite normal breast. One can see the increased projection and decreased base diameter of the custom implant compared to those of the expander. Intraoperatively the patient was placed in a sitting position to make final adjustments. The capsule was scored over its inferior half as well as plicated inferiorly and laterally to raise the position of the reconstructed breast on the chest wall.

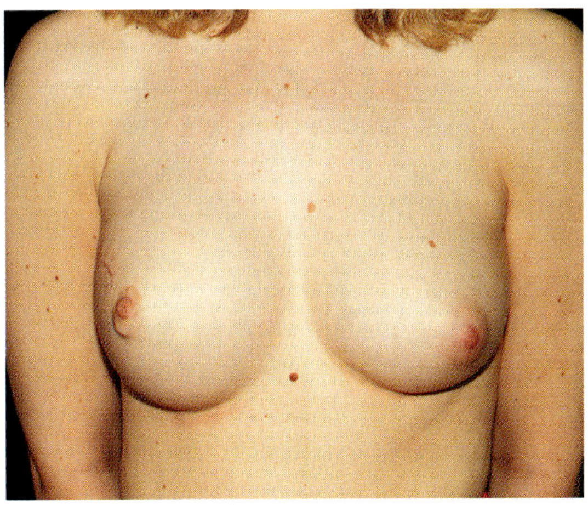

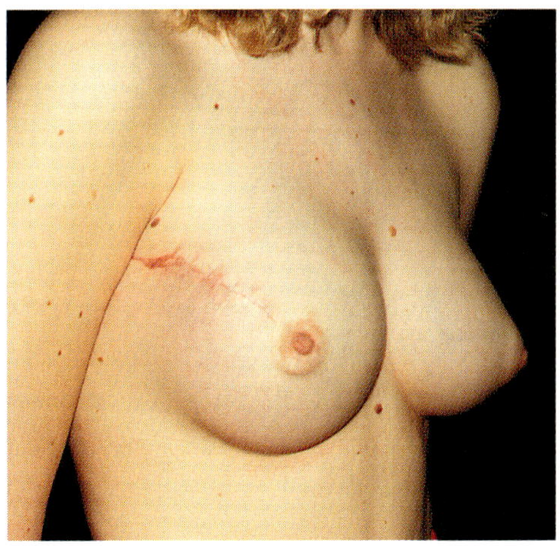

The early postoperative result is shown.

Opposite Breast Adjustments

Although we should strive to match the opposite breast without altering it, this is not always possible, particularly when breast implants are used. ***My philosophy is to keep opposite breast alterations to a minimum. The surgeon should never do anything to the opposite breast that would significantly impact the patient's ability to do breast self-examination or to be followed up for the development of breast cancer.***

It is difficult to match a very small opposite breast without augmenting it. If augmentation is acceptable to the patient, I prefer a saline implant in the submuscular position in order to optimize mammographic screening.

If a reduction mammaplasty is to be performed, I try to select a technique that will minimize the chances of fat necrosis and subsequent parenchymal calcification. In a very large breast this might mean employing a free nipple graft technique. In a moderate-sized breast a superior pedicle or short scar technique might be selected. If an inferior pedicle technique is used, the blood supply to the pedicle must be maximized by keeping the base wide and chest wall attachments liberal. In any event preoperative screening mammography should be performed before reduction.

In circumstances in which I am quite certain that an opposite side correction will be required, my preference has been to proceed with opposite breast corrections at the time of the initial mastectomy and implant or expander placement. I then have the opportunity to adjust the opposite side correction at the time of expander replacement or nipple-areola reconstruction. It is often difficult to perform a primary opposite breast correction at the second stage and achieve perfect symmetry because recurrent settling of the breast following reduction or mastopexy can lead to persistent asymmetry. However, by 3 months postoperatively, at the time most expanders are exchanged for permanent implants, this anticipated settling will have occurred and a small adjustment of the previously altered normal breast can be completed at that time to optimize symmetry.

Women who have a small nonptotic breast on the opposite side are difficult to match with use of expansion and a saline implant alone. Most often symmetry is achieved only by altering the opposite breast by the placement of a submuscular saline implant. Or, if the patient is a candidate for prophylactic mastectomy of the opposite breast, then bilateral expander breast reconstruction can be accomplished.

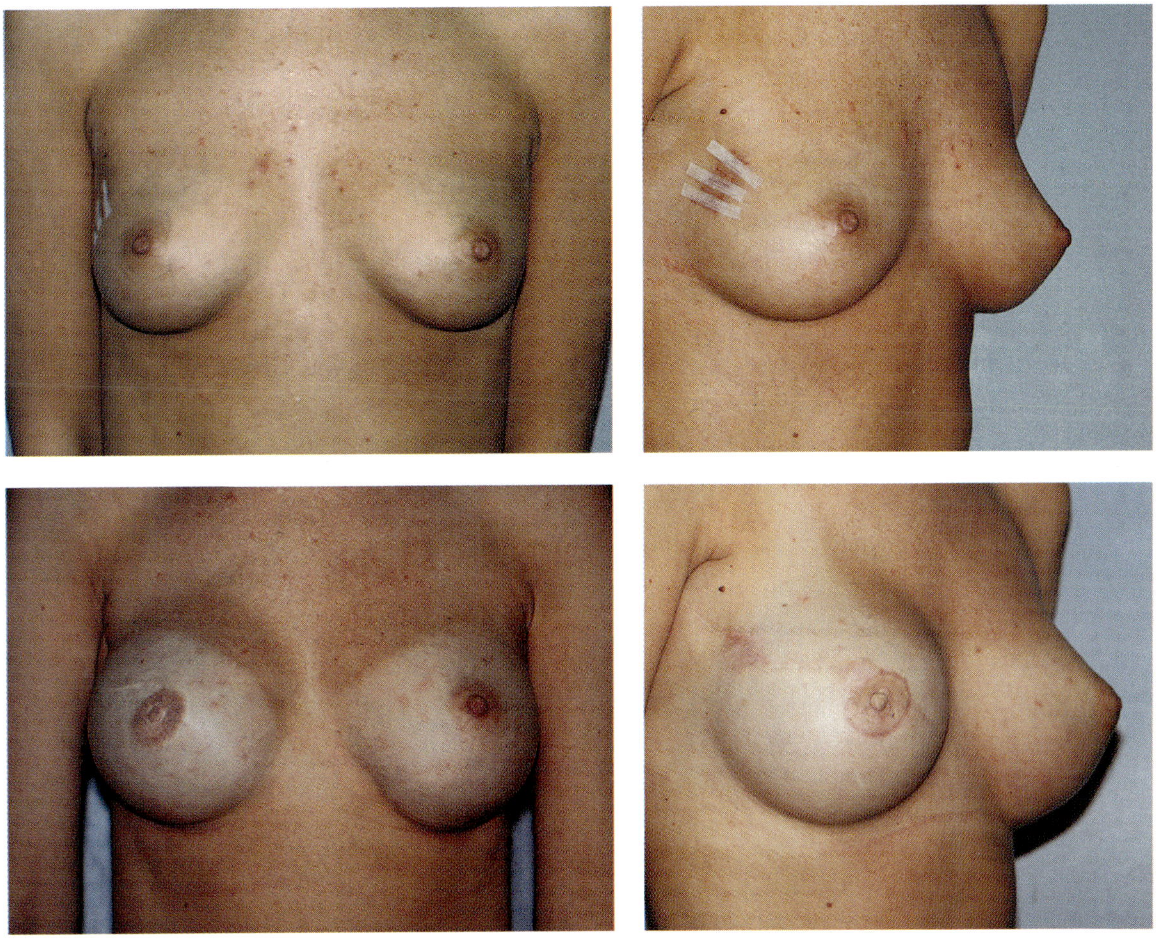

In this patient the second stage included removal of the right expander and placement of a permanent implant along with augmentation of the left breast. Nipple-areola reconstruction was performed simultaneously. She is shown 3 years postoperatively.

Nipple-Areola Reconstruction

With implant reconstructions the technique of nipple-areola reconstruction depends most on the thickness of the subcutaneous tissue overlying the pectoralis major muscle. I prefer the modified fish tail flap (see Chapter 31) unless the opposite nipple is large and therefore available for a composite graft-sharing technique. The pectoralis major fascia if present should be included in the "wings" of the fish tail, particularly if the subcutaneous tissue is thin.

Nipple-areola reconstruction can usually be performed at the planned second stage following an implant reconstruction. However, there are situations in which it is difficult to ascertain whether the ultimate breast mound will be satisfactory to both the surgeon and the patient. If I am still unsure intraoperatively as to whether acceptable symmetry has been achieved in the second stage, I will defer nipple-areola reconstruction until healing has occurred and this determination can be accurately made. Otherwise nipple-areola reconstruction is accomplished at the same time as mound correction during the second stage. I usually try to preselect the location for the nipple-areola reconstruction while manually adjusting the expander or implant to simulate what the corrected mound will look like. This maneuver gives me at least some idea as to the general location for the ultimate reconstruction once the patient is in the operating room and again supine. Following mound correction, pendulum sutures at the sternal notch and xiphoid can be used to determine the proper position of the nipple-areola based on that of the opposite breast (see Chapter 31). Usually if the nipple-areola complex is less than 1 cm off in terms of perfect symmetry, the eye will not detect this minor difference. Therefore, if there is slight persistent mound asymmetry, I will offset the nipple by less than 1 cm so that it appears in the proper location relative to the size and shape of the reconstructed breast rather than exactly symmetric with the opposite side.

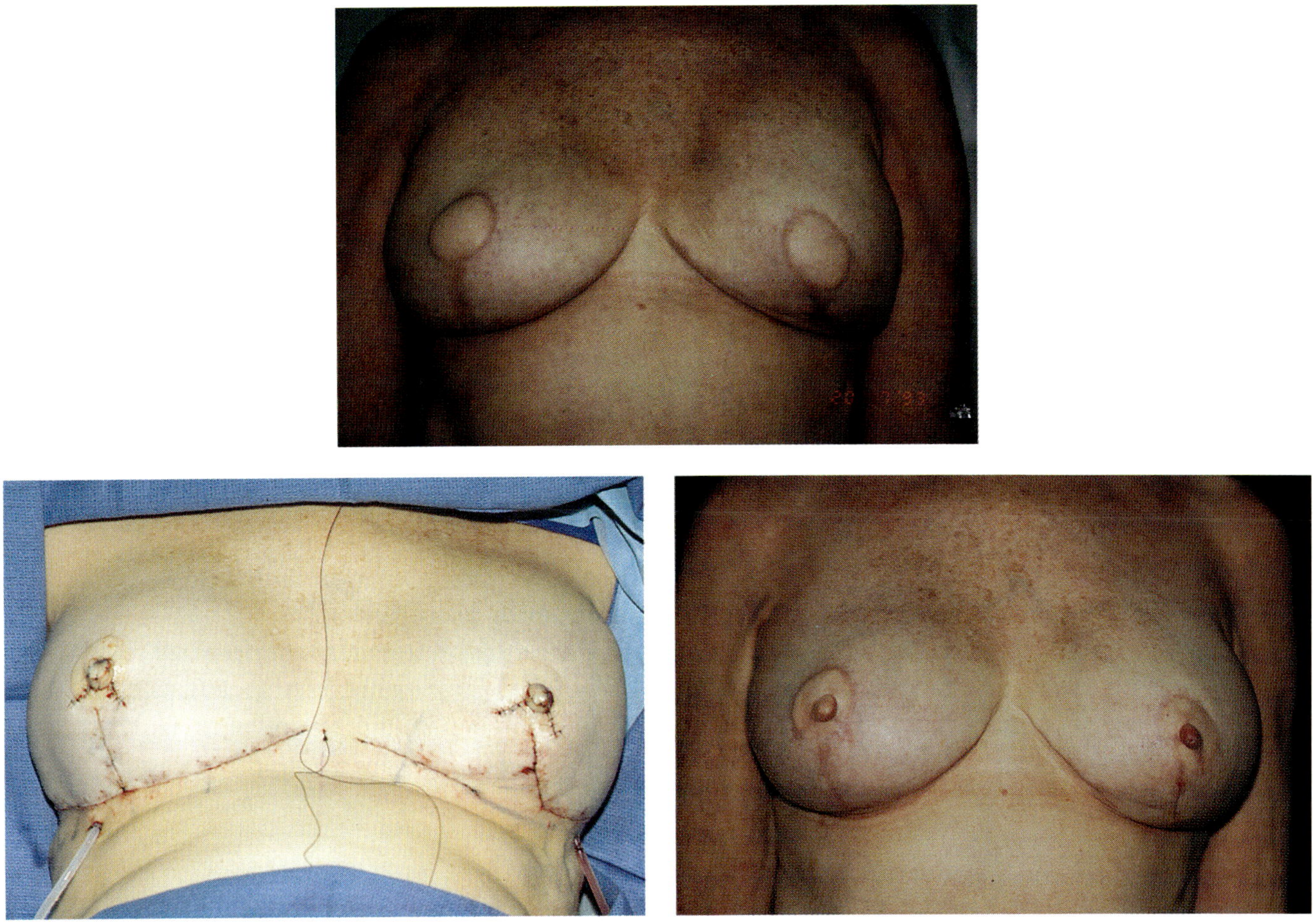

Excellent execution of the first stage in breast reconstruction simplifies the requirements for the second stage. This patient had a small infiltrating ductal carcinoma of the right breast with premalignant changes of the left breast. Bilateral simple mastectomies and immediate reconstruction using bilateral latissimus dorsi musculocutaneous flaps and tissue expanders were performed for the initial reconstruction. Expansion proceeded only to the desired volume. The use of a flap in this case improved coverage in the lower pole and provided tissue for a more natural, ptotic appearance. The second stage required skin envelope modification and elevation of the nipple-areola complex location on the left side. Although there is still slight asymmetry between the nipples, each is placed accurately with respect to breast contour. Nipple-areolar tattooing will complete the reconstruction.

EARLY PROBLEMS FOLLOWING BREAST IMPLANT RECONSTRUCTION

Although implants remain the mainstay of most breast reconstructions, they cannot match all opposite breast shapes. Recognition of this fact before embarking on an implant reconstruction may influence the surgeon to select an alternate technique or to alter the opposite breast.

Problems Associated With Flaps Used in Conjunction With Implants

Some of the best results in breast reconstruction can be achieved using flaps and implants in combination. Flaps used in this context are generally among the most reliable in any type of reconstructive plastic surgery. However, total or partial flap failure continues to occur and leads to the need for secondary breast surgery. More commonly, however, choosing the wrong flap, placing or shaping it poorly, or giving inadequate attention to technique leads to less than satisfactory results. When an implant has been used in combination with a flap, capsular contracture is less common but deflation or leak may still occur. Accordingly, reoperative procedures may range from small adjustments performed with the patient under local anesthesia in the clinic to complex microsurgical flap transfers when primary reconstruction has resulted in flap failure. (Flap failure is discussed in greater detail in Chapters 30 and 31.)

Complications

Immediate breast reconstruction using implants or expanders has a higher complication rate than that associated with delayed reconstruction. This is understandable when one considers the wider field of dissection, thin mastectomy flaps, axillary dissection, and wider field of exposure that is open for a longer period of time. Most surgeons find that in time their own success with immediate reconstruction using implants increases and the complications diminish. Nevertheless, a certain number of immediate reconstructions can be expected to fail.

Infection is probably the most common cause of total failure both in immediate and delayed reconstruction using implants. Infection is heralded by cellulitis that if treated early and vigorously with antibiotics may occasionally resolve without the need for immediate implant removal. Some surgeons have reported success in salvaging an infected implant by open irrigation and drainage with reclosure over a suction irrigation system. Capsulectomy and replacement of the implant are also possible methods of treating minor chronic recurrent infection. However, most often in the face of significant infection, the implant will need to be removed and the wound drained and allowed to heal. Although one might be tempted to reinsert the implant within 2 months after the infection has resolved, this move is usually a mistake. It is best to wait at least 3 months, or in the case of immediate reconstruction until the patient has completed chemotherapy, before considering replacement of the expander or implant.

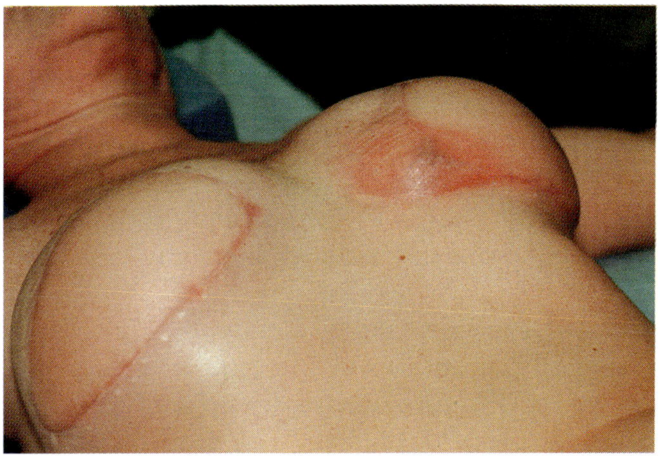

This patient presented 8 weeks following reconstruction of both breasts using latissimus dorsi musculocutaneous flaps and tissue expanders. She had cellulitis with impending expander extrusion. Interestingly these problems developed approximately 10 days following a severe dental infection and may have been related. Management required removal of the implant and drainage of the purulence with irrigation and the placement of Penrose drains. Four months later the expander was replaced.

Hematoma is also more common following immediate reconstruction with implants than delayed reconstruction probably due to the increased amount of sharp dissection. Hematoma becomes apparent in the first 24 hours postoperatively with pain, swelling, and bluish discoloration beneath the mastectomy flaps. The mastectomy flaps might even become compromised because of the pressure exerted from the hematoma beneath them. Under these circumstances immediate evacuation of the hematoma is indicated. The implant or expander can usually be left in place unless the viability of the mastectomy flaps is in question. In this case saline solution may need to be removed from an expander or an implant might need to be removed. Hematoma has been implicated as a cause of capsular contracture, and therefore operative evacuation is almost always preferred to conservative management.

Seromas most commonly occur in the axilla and usually can be treated by serial syringe evacuation or the placement of a dependent Penrose drain.

Skin loss is an early complication almost entirely limited to immediate reconstruction. The use of tissue expanders has diminished the incidence of this complication but has not entirely eliminated it. The viability of mastectomy skin flaps during immediate reconstruction should be assessed by observing the quality of skin edge bleeding or the use of intravenous fluorescein and Wood's lamp evaluation. Any portion of the mastectomy skin flaps that is in question should be debrided. When areas of partial-thickness or full-thickness loss appear to be developing in skin flaps in the early postoperative period, operative debridement and reclosure should be performed. Areas of skin that become progressively more cyanotic will virtually always progress to full-thickness loss and possible late implant or expander exposure. At that point the expander or implant may need to be removed. Certainly early expansion will not be possible. Therefore it is best to return the patient directly to the operating room for excision of these areas and closure of unquestionably viable skin edges.

Remote valves on tissue expanders can be a cause of early complications as well. Valve leakage is a possibility and is sometimes related to the use of large-bore filling needles. Valves can also turn over or flip up on their sides, making filling difficult or impossible. Occasionally they can retract into the pocket of the expander itself so that they are no longer palpable and filling cannot be accomplished. If this happens, a minor operation performed with the patient under local anesthesia to reposition the valve is necessary.

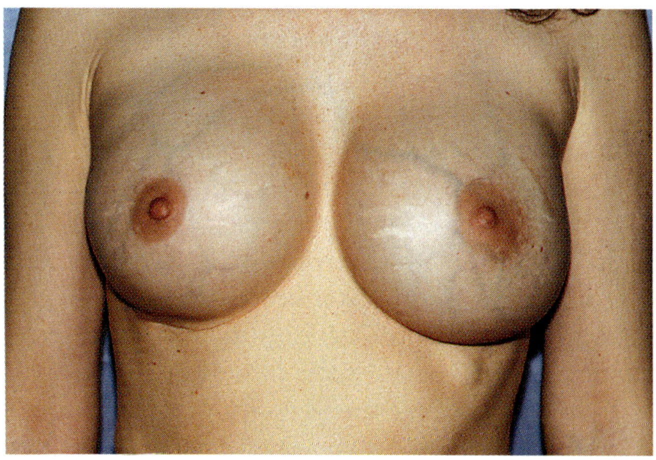

This patient underwent bilateral subcutaneous mastectomy and expander reconstruction for premalignant mastopathy. The remote valve is visible beneath the inframammary fold on the left side. However, the valve on the right side retracted under the expander, making any further volume adjustments impossible. Fortunately expansion was nearly complete by this time, and we were able to make final adjustments and remove the valves as an outpatient procedure performed with the patient under local anesthesia.

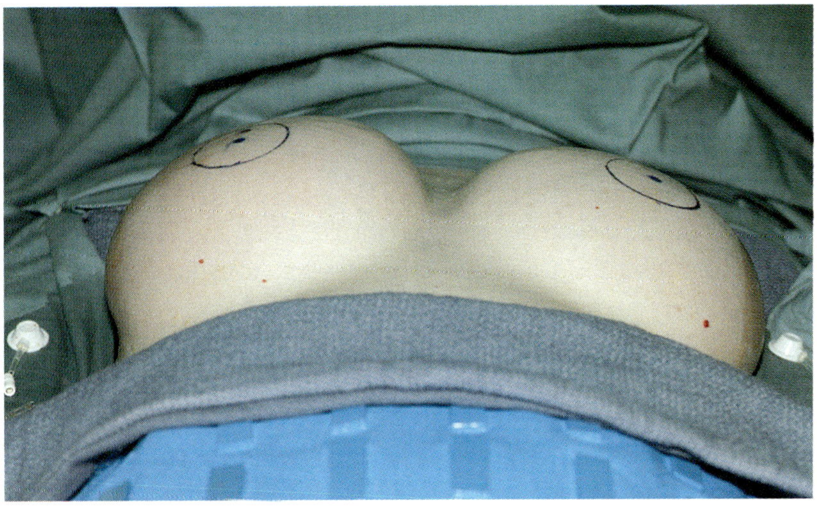

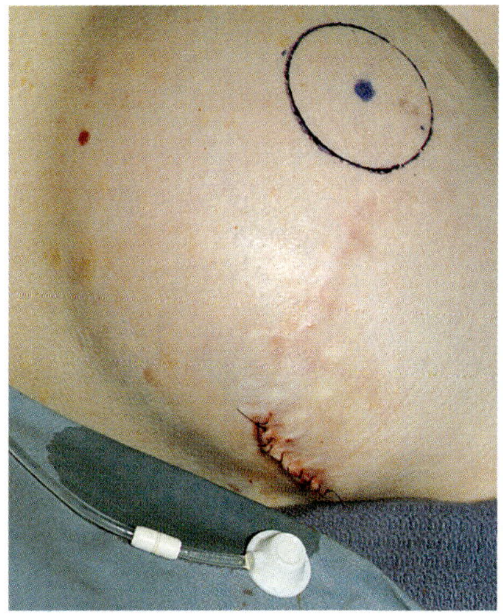

This patient demonstrates two additional minor problems associated with tissue expander valves. With the type of sleeve connector shown, encapsulation around the connector may occur to the point at which removal is difficult and the tubing can be pulled apart. In addition, the fluid on the drapes represents a small seroma that formed around the valve itself.

LATE PROBLEMS FOLLOWING BREAST IMPLANT RECONSTRUCTION

Capsular Contracture

The most common late problem following breast implant reconstruction is capsular contracture. Capsular contracture may present in a variety of ways. Usually the patient notices progressive hardening of the reconstructed breast. Pain may develop in specific portions of the reconstructed breast. This pain may be intermittent, occurring more commonly with certain activities or positions. The patient may not be able to sleep on the reconstructed breast any longer without discomfort. Sometimes the pain may radiate into the axilla or around to the back. The source of this discomfort is often difficult to pinpoint; sometimes it is attributable to the capsule pulling on rib periosteum.

At the present time we no longer perform closed capsulotomy for the release of capsular contracture. The maneuver may be associated with implant rupture or even injury to the surgeon's hands! However, some plastic surgeons continue to perform this maneuver within the first 3 months following implant placement for cases of early capsular contracture. Late capsular contracture cannot be effectively released by closed capsulotomy and is not recommended. Open capsulotomy and percutaneous endoscopic capsular release are alternatives for treatment of this condition (see Chapter 28).

Chronic Pain

Costochondritis

This condition is more common with submuscular implants, which most breast reconstruction patients have, than with subglandular implants. Costochondritis has a waxing and waning course. It usually can be easily localized by physical examination; the affected site can be quite tender and the disease can be debilitating. It will usually respond to local measures such as moist heat and anti-inflammatory agents. I prefer to prescribe a 2-week course of a nonsteroidal anti-inflammatory agent.

Neuroma

Neuromas usually do not become apparent until at least 6 months to 1 year following implant reconstruction. The patient can usually localize the affected site quite specifically and avoids any type of brassiere or clothing that rubs on this region. Tinel's sign may be present. Relief can be achieved by the injection of local anesthesia into the specific area. Although this information is anecdotal, I have had two patients with neuromas who have required reoperation for other reasons. In both cases the symptoms improved after the lateral capsular area was redissected. In one patient I was able to find what appeared to be two subcutaneous nerve branches in this area. I trimmed these branches back and allowed them to retract into a thicker pad of subcutaneous fat; ultimate relief of symptoms was achieved.

Possible Loss of Implant Integrity and Associated Conditions

Many patients at the present time are concerned about the condition of their silicone gel breast implants and the possibility of alleged associated health risks. The Food and Drug Administration (FDA) investigation into the safety and efficacy of the silicone gel breast implant and the subsequent media attention have generated considerable concern and confusion among women with breast implants. Consequently many women with breast implants that were placed years earlier are now coming to plastic surgeons for reevaluation.

Implants are manmade devices and as such have a limited life expectancy. Rupture, leak, and recurrent capsular contracture are possible modes of failure among implant reconstruction patients. Reoperation may be necessary for women with these types of problems as well as for women who simply wish to have the implants removed. Those women who are currently returning for reevaluation are primarily concerned about whether these devices are "intact" and if it is safe to leave the implants in place. Many are patients who previously underwent subcutaneous mastectomy and implant reconstruction and have not been evaluated in several years. Plastic surgeons are also seeing patients who were reconstructed elsewhere many years before. Asymmetry and capsular contracture are common in this patient population. Some patients will have their records available and others may not. Some may know the model of implant; most do not.

Some silicone gel implants appear to undergo some degree of gel bleed in which gel material is able to pass through the silicone elastomer and appear outside the implant. Whether this is a true physical phenomenon or the result of a microperforation is unknown at this time. The low-bleed models of implants that have been produced in recent years seem to reduce but not completely eliminate this phenomenon. It is probably safe to assume that of women with a silicone gel implant in place, at least some may have a very small amount of silicone gel outside the silicone elastomer. The impact of free silicone on the patient's overall health is unknown at this time.

In an unknown number of patients the elastomer has developed either a small leak or total disruption, allowing the gel material to escape. When this occurs, the majority of the gel material virtually always remains inside the implant capsule unless it is mechanically forced through a tear in the capsule. Gel within breast parenchyma or axillary lymph nodes has been noted following closed capsulotomy or traumatic injury in which the gel material is mechanically forced into new planes of dissection outside the capsule.

Occasionally patients will describe specific events after which localized symptoms apparently related to implant disruption have developed. An automobile accident, a forceful hug, or occasionally a mammogram may precipitate implant failure. Many patients who experience implant failure will note the sudden onset of a burning discomfort around the disrupted implant. They may describe an aching pain that radiates into the axilla, shoulder, or back. Patients may also note a sudden change in the size or shape of the implant. As the gel material escapes into the pocket, it may begin to dissect into the low axillary area or toward the apex of the axilla simply from capsular distention. In some patients an inflammatory response to the silicone gel also apparently develops and may cause symptoms. The pooled gel laterally or in the apex of the capsule may be visible as a new "bulge" or may even be palpable as an irregularity along the edge of the implant. Gel material that has escaped into or through the capsule may also solidify into a nodule or silicone granuloma.

Silent leakage may also occur. In fact mammographers will intermittently detect disrupted implants in patients who are otherwise totally asymptomatic.

At this point in time the clinical significance of a leaking breast implant is unknown. Many patients seem to tolerate this situation with no clinically detectable abnormalities. On the other hand, in other patients symptoms do appear to develop and these patients benefit by reoperative treatment. Most plastic surgeons would agree that once an implant has been shown to have disrupted in some way, it should be removed or replaced. Manufacturers also recommend removal or replacement of any implant that is known to have failed.

Evaluation of Patients With Implant-Associated Problems

Currently, new patients with possible problems associated with their breast implants require thorough evaluation and counseling regarding their treatment options. Some are simply scared by what they have read or heard. Others have experienced new symptoms and wonder whether they are related to their breast implants. Still others are referred by attorneys or consumer groups for evaluation. All are seeking information and recommendations as to whether secondary surgery or other treatments might be indicated.

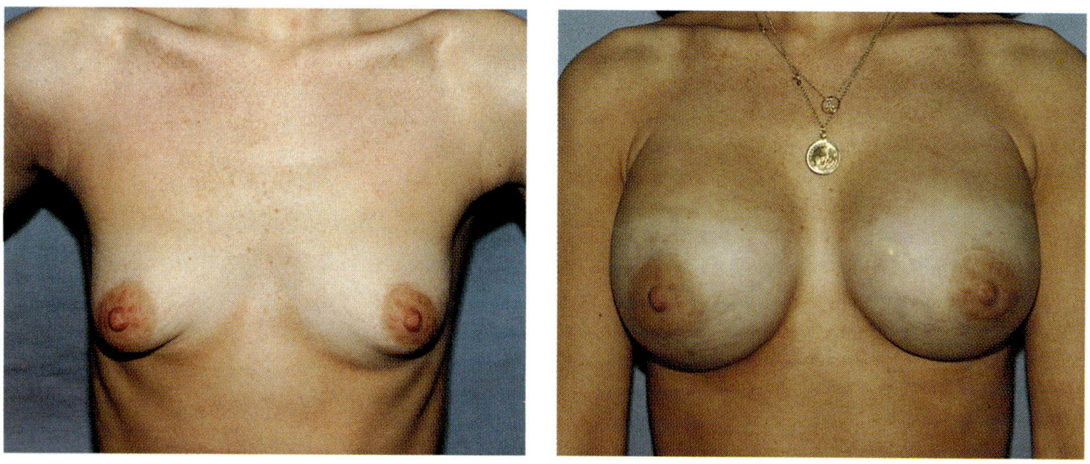

This 36-year-old patient contacted me 8 years after undergoing bilateral subcutaneous mastectomies and adjustable implant reconstruction. She had become pregnant and following delivery noticed that her breasts were swollen and she was able to express fluid. She was concerned that this condition might represent ruptured silicone gel implants. In actuality, the small amount of breast tissue remaining beneath the nipple-areola complexes and within the subcutaneous fat had begun to lactate. She was not aware that this was possible following mastectomy. She was reassured that her implants were intact and her fears were resolved.

A careful history should be obtained that notes exactly why mastectomy was performed and whether reconstruction was accomplished immediately or in a delayed fashion. Knowledge of the type of reconstruction including the model of implant is helpful. The approximate date of onset of the symptoms if any should be noted. The symptoms should be described in detail, including the exact anatomic location of any change that has occurred. In general, patients fall into three categories: (1) those with essentially no symptoms, (2) those with local symptoms related to the breast and chest wall, and (3) those with systemic complaints. A patient may relate any or all of her symptoms to the breast implants. For most plastic surgeons it is difficult to be certain which symptoms if any are caused by the breast implants. The pathophysiologic mechanisms of such associations are simply unknown at this time. If the patient is consulting with other specialists and has been evaluated for other problems, the results of these tests and evaluations should be obtained. In addition, if the patient has preexisting medical problems, these conditions as well as any medications or allergies should be noted.

A full physical examination should be performed, and any abnormal findings associated with the skin, joints, lymph nodes, or palpable organs should be noted. Since many of these patients may be at risk for a local recurrence of breast cancer or a second primary cancer in the opposite breast or any remaining breast tissue, the examination must be carefully performed to rule out these possibilities.

Examination of the reconstructed breast or breasts should focus on the degree of firmness or any abnormalities palpable at the edge of the implant in the skin, subcutaneous tissue, scar, or regional nodes. Evidence of leakage demonstrated by the presence of siliconomas or visible bulges from pooled gel must be sought.

If the patient has undergone previous subcutaneous mastectomy and implant reconstruction, there may be other reasons for localized symptoms. Many such patients appear to have considerable amounts of residual breast tissue. A degree of the localized pain that some of these women experience may be attributable to residual fibrocystic disease. On careful questioning, some will state that the symptoms that they are now experiencing are similar to those that they were having before the subcutaneous mastectomy procedures.

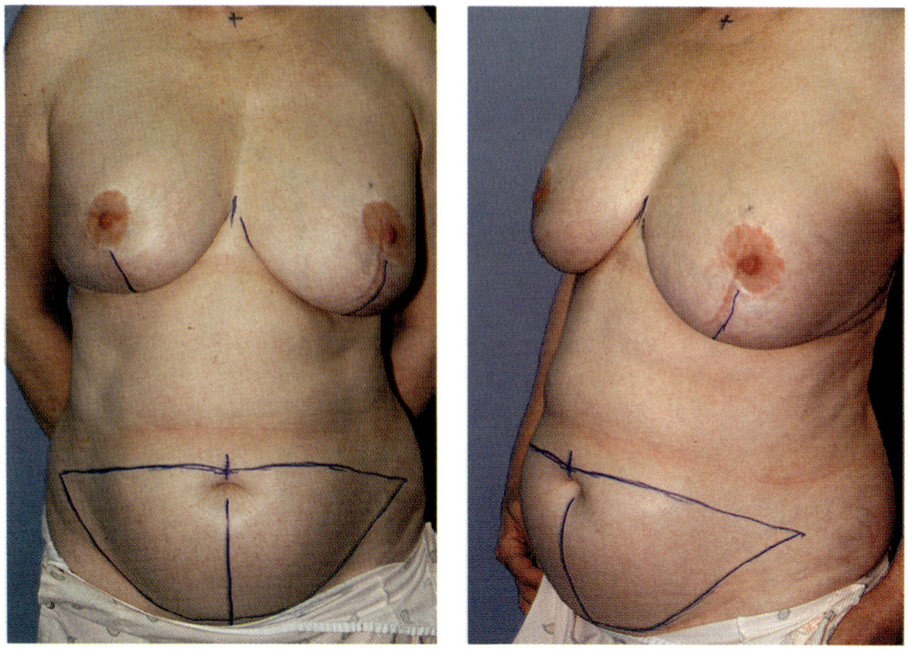

This 48-year-old patient presented 6 years following bilateral subcutaneous mastectomies and implant reconstruction. She was referred for the evaluation of continued cyclic discomfort in the breasts and pain around the implants. She had become quite concerned about the silicone gel implants and wanted to have them removed. On examination she was noted to have a considerable amount of residual breast tissue underlying the contracted implant capsules. Reoperation was planned including implant removal with total capsulectomy, complete subcutaneous mastectomy, replacement of the pectoralis major muscles against the chest wall, and bilateral reconstruction using bilateral microvascular free TRAM flaps.

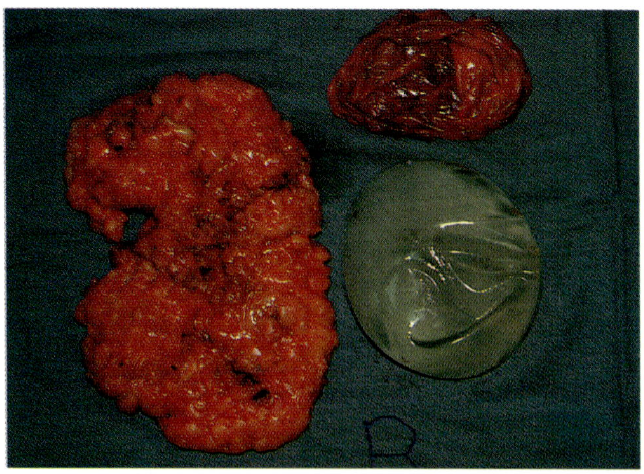

At operation a considerable amount of residual fibrocystic breast tissue was removed. There was evidence of gel bleed but no frank rupture. The residual breast tissue, implant capsule, and implant are shown.

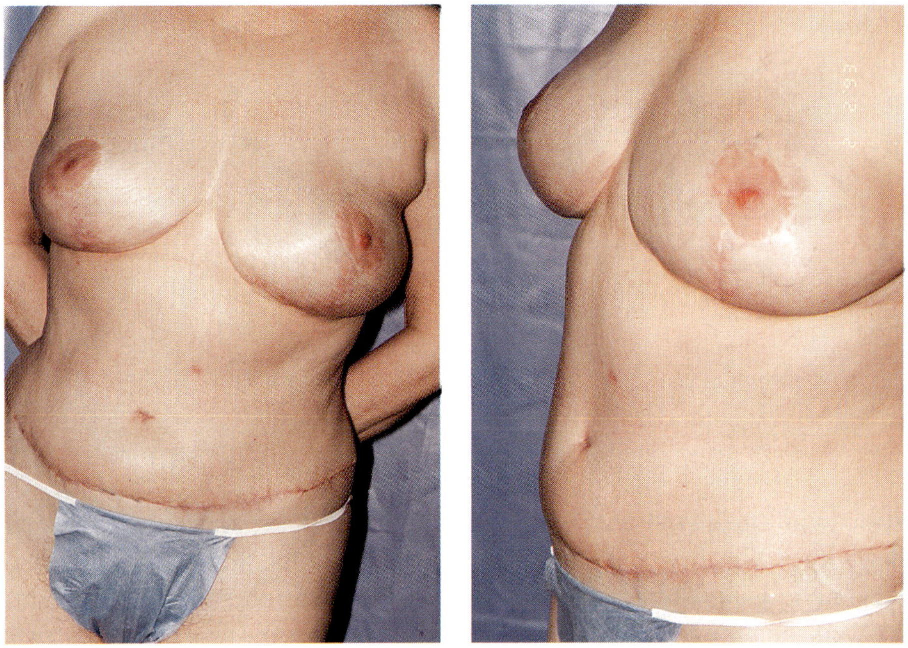

The postoperative result is shown. The patient is free of symptoms and is quite pleased with the appearance and feel of her reconstructed breasts. It is likely in this patient's case that most of the local symptoms were due to residual fibrocystic breast tissue rather than the implants themselves.

Some patients will have considerable distortion of the reconstruction with poor aesthetic results. This residual deformity may be the source of dissatisfaction by the patient and the reason she seeks additional consultation. Although she may state that her main concern is whether the implants are intact, she may really be asking whether an aesthetic improvement might be possible. Some of these patients operated on years ago may have profound capsular contracture around their implants with associated distortion. Considerable asymmetry may be present. The patient may also have had recurrent capsular contracture treated by closed capsulotomy or other procedures. She may have had multiple attempts at correction by implant replacement or readjustment.

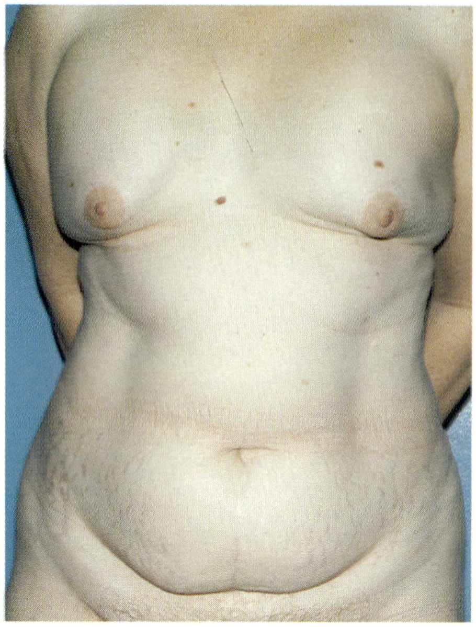

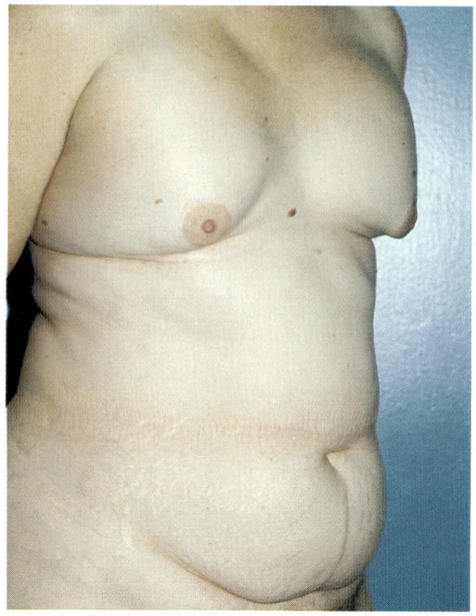

Distortion and capsular contracture following implant reconstruction can be treated by capsulotomy and replacement of implants. However, increasingly patients are choosing to have their implants removed and replaced with autogenous tissue if they are otherwise good candidates. This patient primarily suffered from local chest wall symptoms as a result of long-standing capsular contracture.

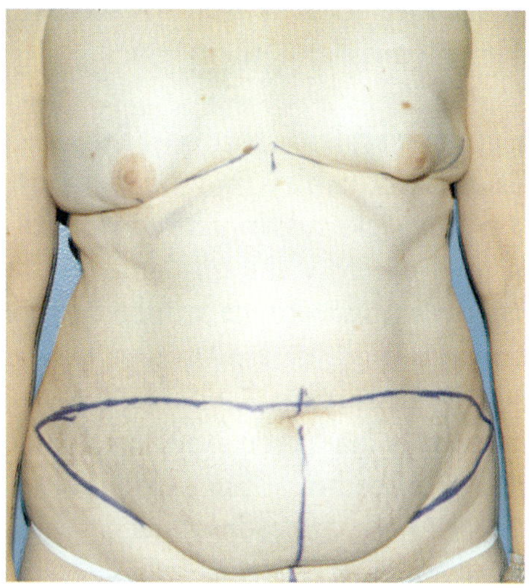

After a careful discussion of the options of implant readjustment vs. conversion to autogenous tissue reconstruction, she preferred the latter. Bilateral free TRAM flaps were designed to be inserted through the inframammary fold incisions. An important part of this procedure is to replace the pectoralis major muscles against the chest wall as I believe some of the pain associated with implant reconstructions is due to capsular contracture beneath the muscle.

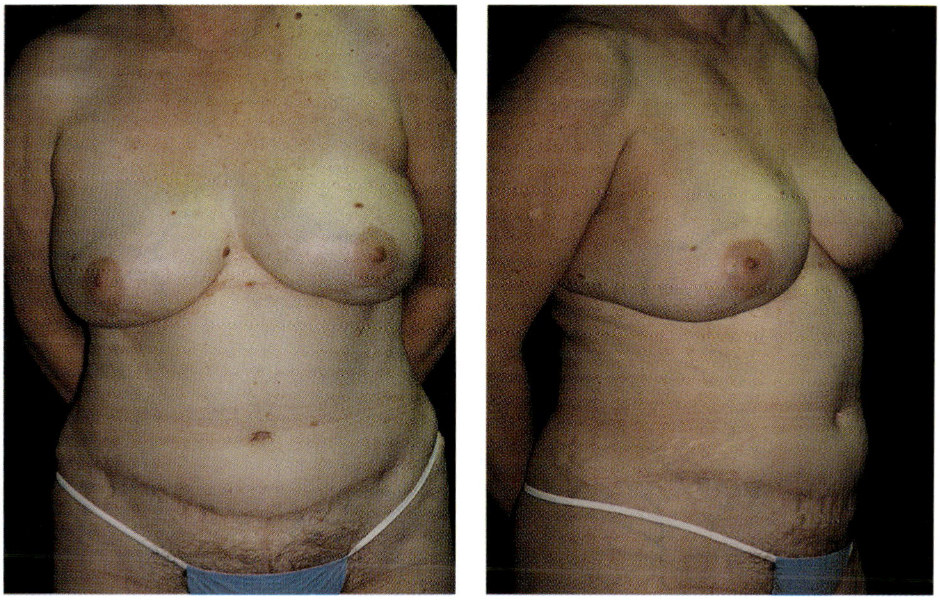

The postoperative result is shown. She had complete resolution of her symptoms in one procedure with considerable improvement in breast shape and body proportion.

Imaging Studies

I do not submit every breast implant reconstruction patient who is experiencing problems to a full radiologic workup. This decision depends on why the patient is seeking consultation. If the patient has already decided that she does not want to continue with an implant reconstruction, I see little reason to attempt to make a preoperative diagnosis of implant rupture by sophisticated x-ray studies. On the other hand, if the patient is reasonably happy with her reconstruction and would consider additional surgery only if the implant were shown to be not intact, then I believe that x-ray studies are indicated. These studies are described in greater detail in Chapter 32. However, I can summarize my own algorithm as follows. I start out with a mammogram for screening of the normal breast if present and to examine the status of the implants. If any suspicious findings are noted, an ultrasound scan may be performed. If the radiologist is reluctant to perform a mammogram or if the examination is inadequate, I believe that obtaining an MRI scan is indicated. MRI has emerged as the most sensitive and specific method for determining whether a breast implant is intact.

Evaluation by Other Consultants

In patients with systemic symptoms it is often difficult to diagnose their condition. I suggest that these women be fully evaluated by a rheumatologist or other specialist depending on the symptoms. The rheumatologist will generally order a battery of laboratory tests to screen for systemic rheumatologic disorders. Patients with breast implants who are found to have systemic rheumatologic disorders may wish to have the implants removed. Again sufficient evidence for whether the symptoms of these patients will be improved by breast implant removal is lacking at the time of this writing. However, many such patients do not wish to "take a chance" and wait for the publication of scientific studies; they will request that the implants be removed or replaced or that some other type of reconstruction be performed.

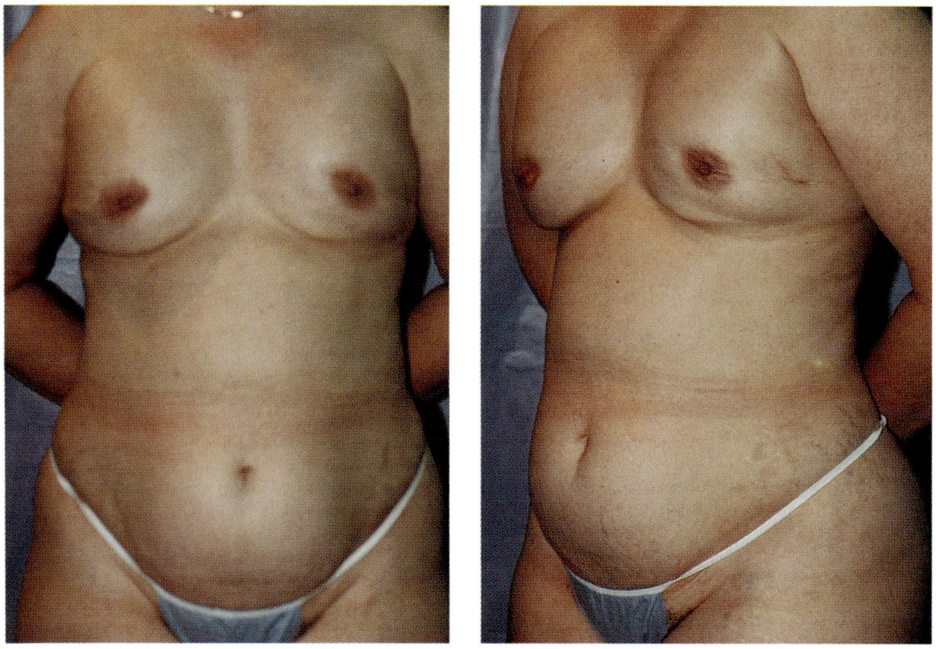

This 46-year-old patient presented 10 years following subcutaneous mastectomy and implant reconstruction. She had recently noticed a change in the shape of as well as an increased burning discomfort in her left breast. In addition, she had been diagnosed with fibromyalgia and was concerned that some of her systemic symptoms might be related to her breast implants. Clinically she was considered to have a ruptured left breast implant. Saline replacement and autogenous conversion were offered to her as reconstruction options. She felt strongly that she would prefer not to have further implant reconstruction.

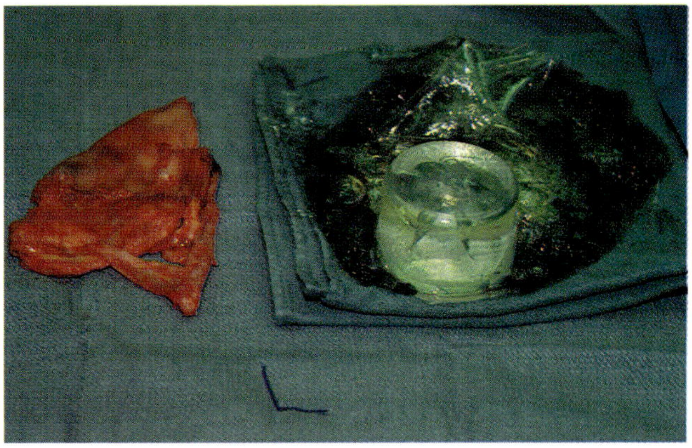

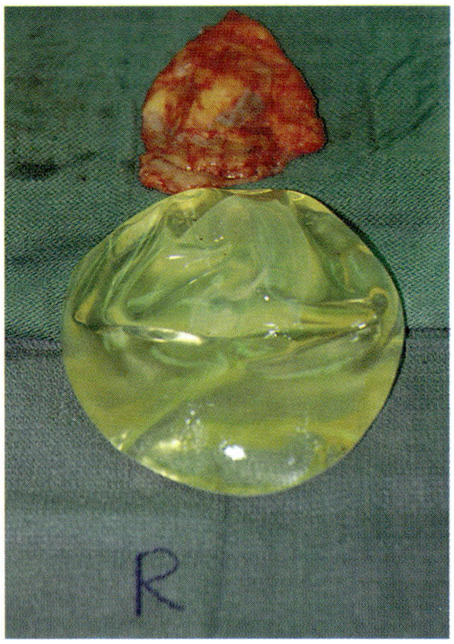

At the time of operation she was found to have a ruptured left breast implant and an intact right breast implant. Total capsulectomies were performed on both sides at her request and to facilitate removal of the ruptured left implant.

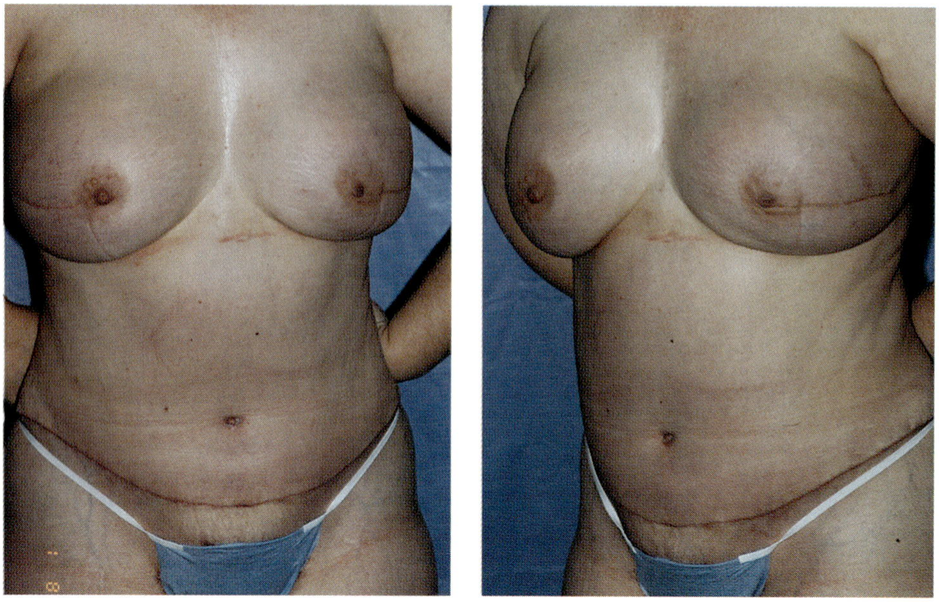

The postoperative result is shown following one operation for implant removal, bilateral capsulectomy, replacement of the pectoralis major muscles, and bilateral microvascular free TRAM flap reconstruction.

Weighing Treatment Alternatives

Patients who are concerned about their silicone gel breast implant reconstructions are in a difficult situation. They may have been quite happy with their reconstruction but are simply anxious based on what they have read and heard in the media. Many of these women can simply be reassured that they, like vast numbers of other women, do not appear to be at significant risk for developing health problems as a result of their implant breast reconstructions. Some women, however, are unable to accept this additional risk no matter how small and will wish to have their silicone gel–filled implant reconstruction be converted to some other type of reconstruction.

Explantation and Replacement

For women who have a satisfactory aesthetic result with good symmetry and who will accept a saline breast implant, then certainly the most satisfactory alternative is to replace a gel implant with a saline implant. If the gel implant is intact, then this is a relatively simple procedure whereby the gel implant is replaced with a saline implant of similar volume. Usually in a breast reconstruction patient we would place the saline implant directly back into the same pocket as before. If the integrity of the gel implant has been disrupted and if the patient has local or systemic symptoms, then total or subtotal capsulectomy is performed simply as an efficient way to control the free silicone and reduce the amount of silicone gel left behind. However, I should quickly point out that there is little evidence to support the use of total capsulectomy other than anecdotal case reports. Whether this additional procedure has any bearing on reducing the recurrence of symptoms is unknown, but it does have the advantage of allowing a smooth redraping of the soft tissues over the new implant. Probably some additional microscopic amounts of silicone are removed with the capsule, but any relationship between capsular silicone to local or systemic symptoms is unproven at this time. However, if the posterior capsule is densely adherent to the chest wall, I do not believe that the additional morbidity associated with this dissection and the risk of hemorrhage or penetration into the intrapleural space are worth the trade-off of a small amount of additional silicone removal. I therefore would leave the posterior capsule under these circumstances. Similarly, if the anterior subcutaneous tissue is thin, removal of the anterior capsule might leave insufficient coverage over the implant and a more unnatural-appearing result.

Any patient undergoing explantation and replacement must be carefully counseled as to the possible clinical sequelae of this procedure (see box). Although most of these sequelae are uncommon, educating the patient as to these possibilities is part of informed consent for the explantation procedure. In addition, patients who desire to have their silicone gel–filled implants replaced with saline breast implants should be shown a saline implant and counseled regarding the differences in the feel and appearance of a saline reconstruction vs. those of the previous reconstruction with gel implants.

Possible Sequelae of Breast Explantation

Bleeding or hematoma
Infection
Seroma or edema
Additional incisions
Excessive scarring
Asymmetry
Breast indentation
Unaesthetic appearance (breast may look worse than prior to augmentation or reconstruction)
Loss of sensation in nipple-areola complex or breast itself
Chronic pain
Implant damage on removal
General disappointment or depression
Anesthetic-related complications including death

Autogenous Conversion

Patients who are candidates for conversion to autogenous tissue reconstruction generally fall into two categories. First, there are the women who have had previous implant reconstructions who for one reason or another no longer wish to have breast implants but still desire breast reconstruction.

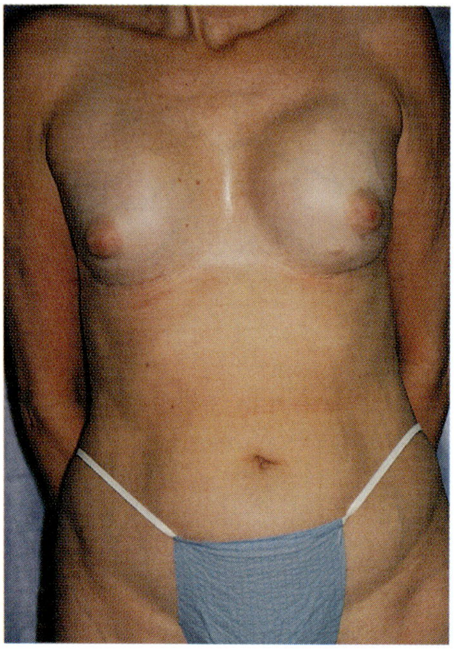

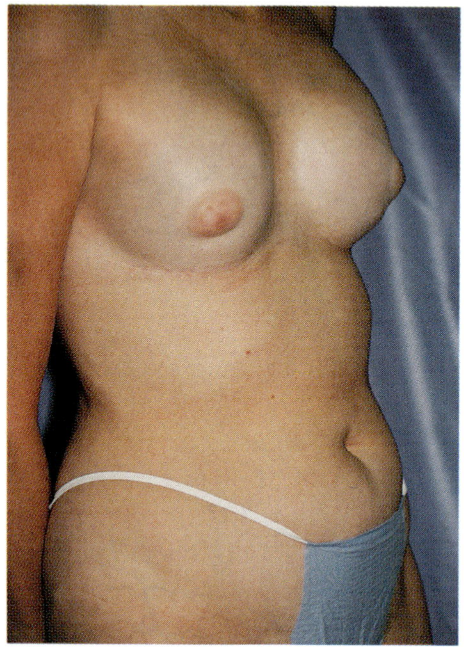

This patient is an example of a woman with a reasonably good implant reconstruction following subcutaneous mastectomy for premalignant disease. However, her main problem was pain surrounding the left implant. The reconstructed breasts were quite firm as a result of capsular contracture. Although the patient tolerated this pain for a period of time, once she became concerned about the safety of silicone gel, she could no longer accept the implant reconstruction and wanted the implants removed.

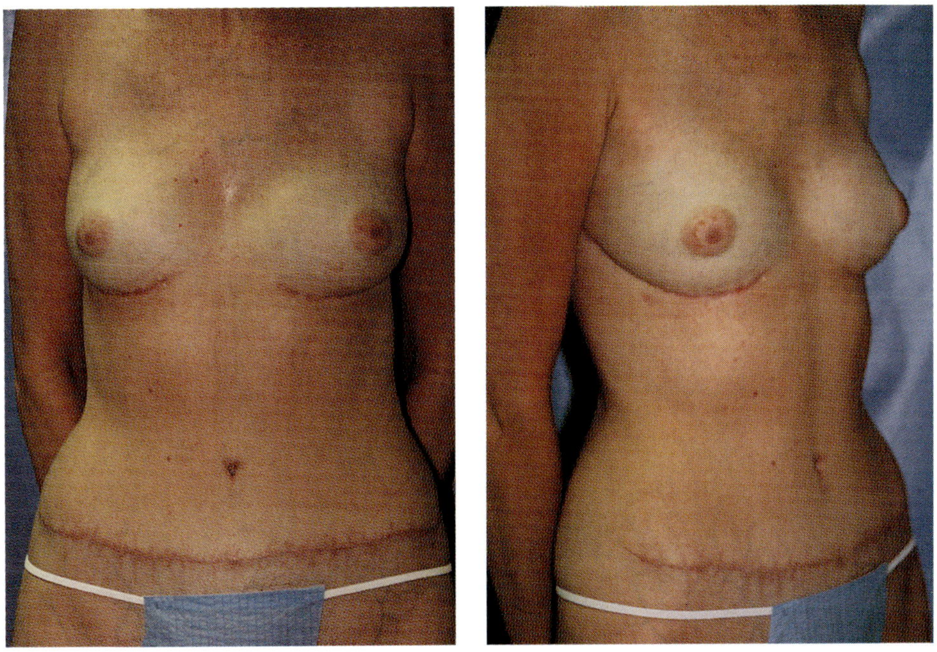

TRAM flap reconstruction ultimately produced a softer and more natural result. Replacing the pectoralis major muscles against the chest wall seems to provide relief in a number of women with painful implant reconstructions. The postoperative result is shown.

The second group of women who may benefit by autogenous conversion are those who have had one or more previous implant reconstructions but have continued to experience asymmetry, distortion, recurrent implant failure, or recurrent capsular contracture. This group of women seems to have the most satisfactory outcome following autogenous conversion.

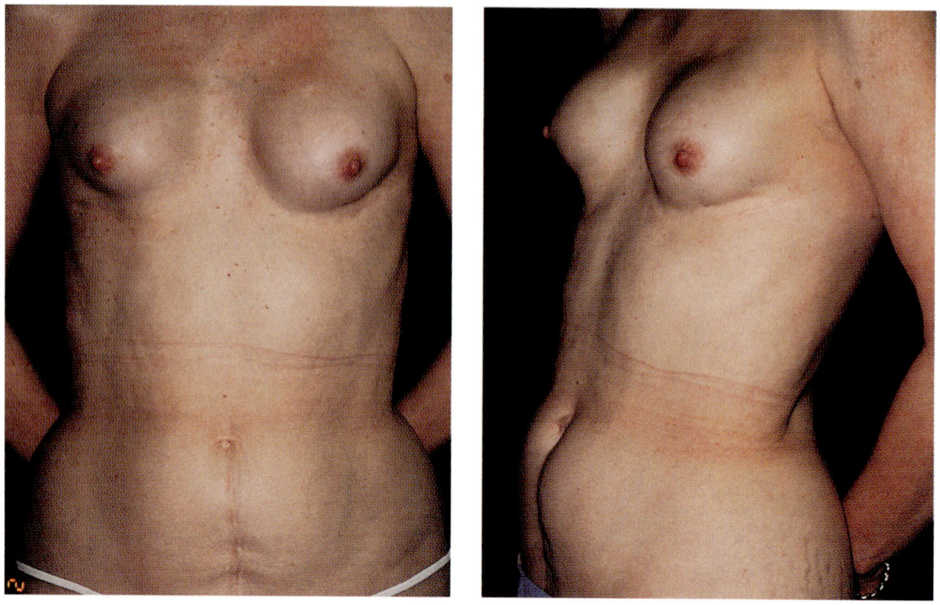

This 46-year-old patient is shown 12 years following bilateral subcutaneous mastectomies and implant reconstruction. Her postoperative course was complicated by hematoma, implant rupture, and implant replacement. She has undergone several attempts at closed capsulotomy for capsular contracture that subsequently developed. Her preoperative condition demonstrated distortion, asymmetry, and contracture.

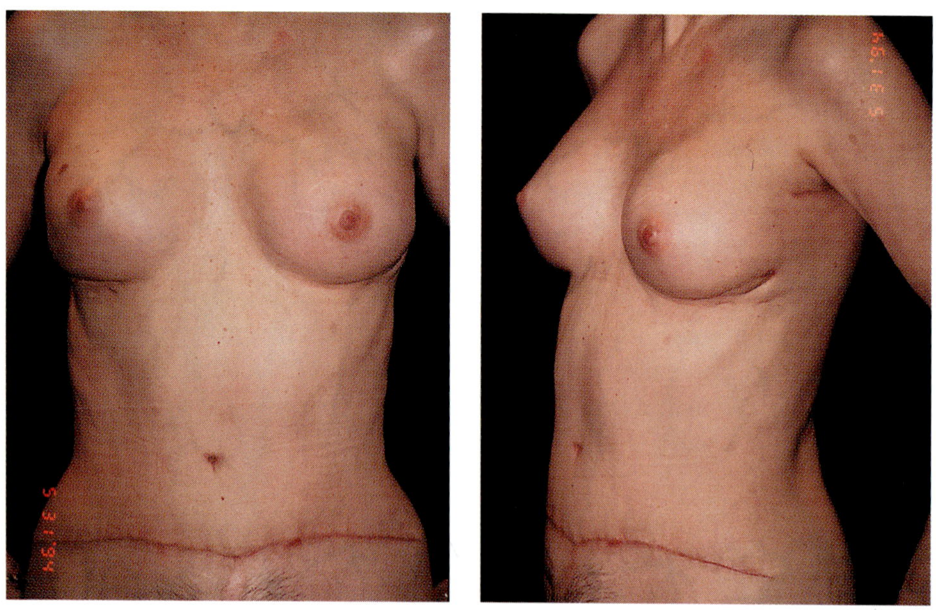

This group of patients benefits greatly by autogenous conversion. The surgical approach consists of implant removal with total or subtotal capsulectomy, replacement of the pectoralis major muscles against the chest wall, and autogenous reconstruction using bilateral free TRAM flaps in the subcutaneous position.

Although this approach is one that carries significant risks, the postoperative results are unparalleled in my opinion.

Patients who have been through breast reconstruction using implants may not be prepared for the commitment and the magnitude of autogenous reconstruction. They must be very carefully counseled regarding the commitment, risks, and complications associated with this major operation. Nevertheless, our ability to use autogenous tissue for breast reconstruction has allowed us to greatly improve the results of patients who did not have aesthetic reconstructions using implants. This type of reoperative breast reconstruction demands excellent patient rapport and cooperation, careful patient education, and precise technical execution to minimize further complications. Most patients who desire or require autogenous conversion do not wish to have any other implants used for reconstruction. Therefore the TRAM flap and the latissimus dorsi flap are the mainstays of autogenous conversion. Other microsurgical flaps can be considered. If the patient has sufficient tissue available in the lower abdomen, the TRAM flap is my preference. It is also my personal preference to transfer the TRAM flap as a microsurgical free flap, particularly in the case of bilateral reconstruction in which more rectus abdominis muscle can be left in the abdominal wall. Nevertheless, the conventional TRAM flap is a perfectly satisfactory solution for autogenous conversion of implant patients.

CONCLUSION

Despite the advances in breast implant reconstruction over the past 20 years, breast reconstruction essentially remains a staged procedure. In addition, with recent restrictions in the use of breast implants, plastic surgeons are relearning how to effectively use inflatable saline implants for primary and secondary breast reconstruction. This type of implant clearly has its limitations, and secondary surgery with inflatable saline implants is common to achieve the desired result.

In addition, women who have previously been reconstructed with silicone gel implants are returning for reevaluation. In some of these patients implant-related problems have developed that can be improved by reoperation. Such sequelae as capsular contracture, implant failure, and distortion can often be improved by either capsular surgery and implant replacement or in some cases conversion to autogenous tissue reconstruction. Although the implant choices are now restricted, the flap choices are more numerous and safer than a decade ago.

The role of implant removal for the treatment of systemic symptoms remains controversial. In my experience few systemic symptoms are predictably improved by the removal of breast implants. On the other hand, local symptoms are reliably treated by reoperative surgery. Patients who desire that their breast implants be removed out of concern that their symptoms may be related to systemic complaints often request capsulectomy. Although it is likely that only microscopic amounts of silicone are removed by this procedure, it does avoid the unpleasant circumstance in which the patient's symptoms do not improve and she fears that residual silicone could be the continued cause of these symptoms. The choice of reoperative procedure following breast implant reconstruction is best left to the judgment of the operating surgeon. All procedures must be weighed carefully in terms of the risks and benefits in the context of a well-informed patient.

Bibliography

Apfelberg DB, Laub DR, Maser MR, Lash H. Submuscular breast reconstruction—Indications and techniques. Ann Plast Surg 7:213, 1981.

Argenta LC. Reconstruction of the breast by tissue expansion. Clin Plast Surg 11:257, 1984.

Argenta LC, Marks MW, Grabb WC. Selective use of serial expansion in breast reconstruction. Ann Plast Surg 11:188, 1983.

Asplund O. Capsular contracture in silicone gel and saline-filled breast implants after reconstruction. Plast Reconstr Surg 73:270, 1984.

Asplund O. Breast reconstruction with submuscular prosthesis after modified radical or simple mastectomy. Surgical technique and early complications. Scand J Plast Reconstr Surg 17:141, 1983.

Bailey MH, Smith JW, Casas L, Johnson P, Serra E, de la Fuente R, Sullivan M, Scanlon EF. Immediate breast reconstruction: Reducing the risks. Plast Reconstr Surg 83:845, 1989.

Becker H. Expansion augmentation. Clin Plast Surg 15:587, 1988.

Becker H. The expandable mammary implant. Plast Reconstr Surg 79:631, 1987.

Becker H. Breast reconstruction using an inflatable breast implant with detachable reservoir. Plast Reconstr Surg 73:678, 1984.

Bostwick J III. Breast reconstruction using modified tissue expansion for matching a small opposite breast. Perspect Plast Surg 1(1):79, 1987.

Bostwick J. Breast reconstruction: A comprehensive approach. Clin Plast Surg 6:143, 1979.

Chisholm EM, Marr S, Macfie J, Broughton AC, Brennan TG. Postmastectomy breast reconstruction using the inflatable tissue expander. Br J Surg 73:817, 1986.

Copeland M, Kressel A, Spiera H, Herman G, Bleiweiss I. Systemic inflammatory disorders related to fibrous breast capsules after silicone implant removal. Plast Reconstr Surg 92:1179, 1993.

Cronin TD, Upton J, McDonough JM. Reconstruction of the breast after mastectomy. Plast Reconstr Surg 59:1, 1977.

Darnell EK, Demars RV. Ultrasonographic localization of breast tissue expander valves. J Ultrasound Med 6:531, 1987.

Dickson MG, Sharpe DT. The complications of tissue expansion in breast reconstruction: A review of 75 cases. Br J Plast Surg 40:629, 1987.

Dowden RV. Achieving a natural inframammary fold and ptotic effect in the reconstructed breast. Ann Plast Surg 19:524, 1987.

Gibney J. The long-term results of tissue expansion for breast reconstruction. Clin Plast Surg 14:509, 1987.

Gruber RP, Kahn RA, Lash H, Maser MR, Apfelberg DB, Laub DR. Breast reconstruction following mastectomy: A comparison of submuscular and subcutaneous techniques. Plast Reconstr Surg 67:312, 1981.

Hartrampf CR, Scheflan M, Black PW. Breast reconstruction following mastectomy with a transverse abdominal island flap: Anatomical and clinical observations. Plast Reconstr Surg 69:216, 1982.

Hester TR Jr, Nahai F, Bostwick J, Cukic J. A 5-year experience with polyurethane-covered mammary prostheses for treatment of capsular contracture, primary augmentation mammoplasty, and breast reconstruction. Clin Plast Surg 15:569, 1988.

Lemperle G. Unfavorable results after breast reconstruction with silicone breast implants. Acta Chir Belg 79(2):159, 1980.

Little JW III, Golembe EV, Fisher JB. The "living bra" in immediate and delayed reconstruction of the breast following mastectomy for malignant and nonmalignant disease. Plast Reconstr Surg 68:392, 1981.

Maxwell GP. Latissimus dorsi breast reconstruction: An aesthetic assessment. Clin Plast Surg 8:373, 1981.

May JW Jr, Attwood J, Bartlett S. Staged use of soft-tissue expansion and lower thoracic advancement flap in breast reconstruction. Plast Reconstr Surg 79:272, 1987.

McKinney P, Edelson R, Terrasse A, Zukowski M. Chest-wall deformity following soft-tissue expansion for breast reconstruction. Plast Reconstr Surg 80:442, 1987.

McShane RH, Omotunde O, Weatherly-White RC. Individualized muscle coverage of implants in breast reconstruction. Plast Reconstr Surg 67:318, 1981.

Olbrisch RR, Miericke B. Tissue expander in breast reconstruction. Experiences and results with more than 300 expanders. Chirurg 58:553, 1987.

Pakiam AI, Young CS. Submuscular breast reconstruction: A one-stage method of tissue expansion. Ann Plast Surg 19:312, 1987.

Rosato FE, Horton EE, Maxwell GP. Postmastectomy breast reconstruction. Curr Probl Surg 17:585, 1980.

Ryan JJ. A lower thoracic advancement flap in breast reconstruction after mastectomy. Plast Reconstr Surg 70:153, 1982.

Versaci AD. A method of reconstructing a pendulous breast utilizing the tissue expander. Plast Reconstr Surg 80:387, 1987.

Versaci AD. Reconstruction of a pendulous breast utilizing a tissue expander. Clin Plast Surg 14:499, 1987.

Ward J, Cohen IK, Knaysi GA, Brown PW. Immediate breast reconstruction with tissue expansion. Plast Reconstr Surg 80:559, 1987.

Woods JE. Unusual complication of submuscular placement of implants in breast surgery. Plast Reconstr Surg 73:972, 1984.

Woods JE, Irons GB Jr, Arnold PG. The case for submuscular implantation of prostheses in reconstructive breast surgery. Ann Plast Surg 5:115, 1980.

30

Finishing Touches After Breast Reconstruction With Pedicled Flaps

John Bostwick III, M.D.

Reoperative Problems

- Tissue deficiency
- Asymmetry
- Tissue loss
- Excess fullness
- Seroma
- Inadequate central breast projection
- Capsular contracture
- Donor site contracture
- Missing anterior axillary fold
- Axillary hollowness
- Malpositioned nipple-areola reconstruction
- Excess tissue in abdominal wall
- Hernia
- Incorrect placement of inframammary fold

Before the introduction of the silicone breast implant in the early 1960s, pedicled flaps were the only viable method for breast reconstruction. These were random flaps from the lateral and inferior abdominal wall that were transferred as tubed pedicles; they required multiple staged procedures and were characteristically fraught with problems of tissue loss and aesthetic shortcomings. Even after the development of silicone breast implants, pedicled flaps were still the method of choice because most mastectomies were radical. Current breast reconstruction techniques have evolved considerably since the time when pedicled tube flaps were the standard. Modern pedicled flap operations require far fewer stages with the promise of superior results. With the advent of the latissimus dorsi flap and the TRAM flap, the two most popular and effective sources of autogenous tissue for these operations, a woman can now expect to have a natural, well-contoured breast reconstruction with her own tissues and without many of the problems that plagued earlier flap operations. Interestingly, the abdomen, which offers the most abundant source of tissue, has once again become the primary source of donor tissue for women seeking breast reconstruction with autogenous tissue; thus it appears we have come full circle in our reconstructive efforts.

Although the results of the TRAM flap and the latissimus dorsi flap are far superior to those possible with earlier techniques and most women today have less significant deformities to reconstruct, these operations are not simple or trouble free. These procedures are artistically and technically demanding and like their predecessors may require secondary procedures to attain the desired result. Careful patient selection, detailed preoperative planning, knowledge of the pertinent anatomy, and excellent and diligent care postoperatively all contribute to the ultimate quality of the result expected after a pedicled TRAM or latissimus dorsi flap breast reconstruction. These operations should be performed by a reconstructive surgeon experienced in these procedures who has an excellent aesthetic eye and can properly position and shape the musculocutaneous back or lower abdominal flap into a breast symmetric with the opposite breast. Ideally the flap should be positioned and shaped for optimal breast appearance, size, form, and symmetry during the first operation. Secondary operations can then focus on nipple-areola placement and minor corrections. In reality, however, additional modifications may be needed to improve breast contour, volume, or shape after breast reconstruction with the TRAM or latissimus dorsi flap. Fine adjustments of the volume and position of the autogenous tissue or tissue expander and adjustments of the donor site may be necessary. Suction-assisted lipectomy and scar revision may also be required. Nipple-areola reconstruction should be delayed until good symmetry is obtained.

This chapter addresses the most common problems that require reoperation or revisional surgery after pedicled TRAM or latissimus dorsi flap breast reconstruction. These secondary procedures may be necessary revisions as a part of a staged procedure, aesthetic improvements to refine the results of the primary operation, or maneuvers to treat complications or to improve on aesthetic shortfalls.

PATIENT EVALUATION

A woman seeking breast reconstruction desires a return to wholeness; this desire is clearly voiced by most patients during consultation. The reconstructive surgeon is ill-advised, however, if he believes that mere restoration of breast form is sufficient to satisfy the patient. Most expect the same artistry as would be demanded from an aesthetic operation. Patient expectations for breast reconstruction must be accurately determined before the primary breast reconstruction and again before any reoperative procedures. Although some patients say that they would be satisfied if their breasts were to appear symmetric in a brassiere without the need for an external prosthesis, usually this is not the case. Most breast reconstruction patients desire a reconstructed breast that is symmetric with the opposite breast when they are naked and a donor site that is unobtrusive and enhances the overall appearance. These patients are highly motivated to have their breasts symmetric and are often willing to undergo additional procedures to achieve this goal. They want to have this part of their life resolved, and an acceptable breast reconstruction is needed for them to be satisfied. Because pedicled flap reconstructions are more complex, I always advise my patients that a minimum of two procedures are needed to achieve the expected result. That way there are no surprises and the need for reoperation is considered part of the operative plan.

When a patient is evaluated for secondary breast reconstruction or for finishing touches, the reconstructive surgeon should take the time to listen to the patient and to consider her requests. Patient communication and understanding are most important before a secondary operation. The patient who is adequately informed can best understand the procedure and its limitations and approach it with realistic expectations.

When a complication occurs, whether severe as in total flap loss or minor, honesty and careful explanation are essential. The patient needs to understand why this problem has occurred and that there is a solution. I find it helpful to outline the operative plan to the patient to relieve her anxiety and to let her feel that the problem is under control.

When the patient is referred from another reconstructive surgeon, then the referring physician should be contacted to obtain important information about the patient. If the patient has a relatively satisfactory result yet voices intense displeasure with the result or with previous surgeons, then she may have unrealistic expectations or other concerns or psychologic conditions that cannot be resolved within the limits of improving the breast reconstruction. The wisest course for some of these patients is not to perpetuate their dissatisfaction with another operation.

Some patients have a long history of cigarette smoking and have significant complications related to previous pedicled flaps or breast reconstruction with available tissue or tissue expanders. The TRAM flap is susceptible to complications related to cigarette smoking; the latissimus dorsi flap is prone to a lesser degree. Patients with previous breast reconstruction complications who are heavy cigarette smokers should be instructed to refrain from cigarette smoking for approximately 2 weeks before these secondary procedures. The use of the lower vascular delay of the TRAM flap is a means of enhancing the upper flow into the flap as well as the venous drainage. A delay, or even better, a free flap is considered when the patient has risk factors such as cigarette smoking, radiation to the mediastinum, and obesity.

It is important to remember that most patients who have breast reconstruction have had breast cancer and that breast cancer is generally a chronic disease. The surgeon must always consider the oncologic aspects of the patient's treatment and be alert to the possibility of a local or systemic recurrence. Before modification of the opposite breast, this breast should be evaluated oncologically and aesthetically. Treatment needs to be coordinated with the other members of the breast management team in order to provide adequate surveillance and follow-up.

A complete medical history is necessary to identify any psychologic or medical conditions that would mean an increased risk of complications or contraindicate plans for reoperation. Systemic conditions such as diabetes mellitus and autoimmune conditions such as lupus erythematosus and scleroderma are associated with problems with flap microcirculation and survival and may be contraindications to flap surgery. These patients also may not be candidates for breast implants. The presence of a hypercoagulable state such as polycythemia or a history of deep vein thrombosis will also affect the success of a pedicled flap reconstruction, especially with a TRAM flap with which there is a fine line between satisfactory microcirculation and inadequate perfusion.

The patient's weight and general medical condition are important considerations in planning reoperation. Breast reconstruction with flaps has physical limitations. I have found that patients who are significantly overweight (i.e., more than 50 pounds over their ideal body weight) often have unsatisfactory breast reconstructions because of physical limitations of the procedure, possible complications of moving large pedicled flaps, or psychologic dynamics of the patient who can develop serious complaints related to the appearance of the breast reconstruction or the donor site. The significantly overweight patient experiences an increased incidence of complications from pedicled flap procedures and is more likely than a patient of normal weight not to be satisfied with the result despite additional operations.

PLANNING

After a pedicled TRAM flap or latissimus dorsi flap breast reconstruction, the reconstructive surgeon should determine whether the reconstructed breast has adequate volume and is shaped properly before proceeding with a nipple-areola reconstruction. The opposite breast is the model for the breast reconstruction and for any secondary procedures that may be necessary to improve breast form. If a match with the opposite breast is not possible, then the corrected opposite breast is the model for the finishing touches. The reconstructive surgeon should consult with the patient to determine whether the opposite breast is to be changed to match the reconstructed breast, the reconstructed breast should be modified, or both.

When either the opposite breast or the patient are so large that the breast reconstruction cannot be done safely, then the opposite breast may need to be reduced to achieve an adequate breast reconstruction. After a TRAM flap or latissimus dorsi flap breast reconstruction when the opposite breast is somewhat ptotic and a mastopexy is planned, periareolar purse-string mastopexy is a good choice. This technique produces a breast with some central flattening, which matches the profile produced by a TRAM flap breast reconstruction; therefore the opposite breast can be modified to more closely resemble a breast reconstructed with a TRAM flap. When a breast implant has been used under the TRAM or latissimus dorsi flap, then to achieve symmetry the placement of a textured-surface breast implant on the side of the mastopexy can be considered. When a small breast reduction is also needed, this can be performed through the periareolar approach with the breast maintained as a central parenchymal pedicle.

Breast implants can be used to supplement the breast reconstruction and thus provide additional breast volume, which is sometimes lacking with pedicled flaps. In this case the patient will need to decide whether she wants a silicone breast implant or whether she prefers only autogenous tissue. When the flap reconstruction is too small to match the opposite breast and implant or expander placement is planned, consideration must be given as to whether there is sufficient tissue cover in the primary reconstruction.

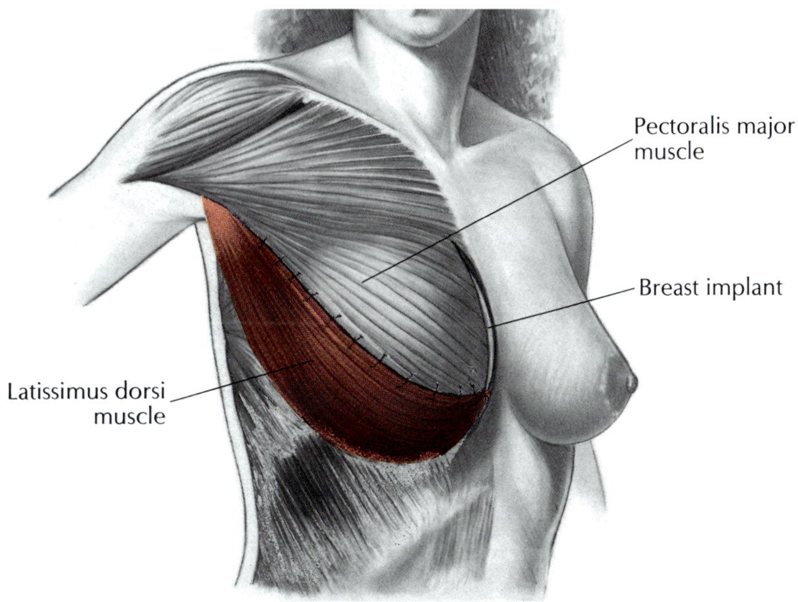

When there is not sufficient tissue cover, the latissimus dorsi muscle can be transferred to cover and protect the lower portion of the breast implant. This muscle transfer also serves to provide an additional source of blood and oxygen supply to the region.

Alternatively, when autogenous tissue is insufficient resulting in a volume deficit, and a silicone breast implant is not desired, then the transfer of a second pedicled flap should be considered. The latissimus dorsi musculocutaneous flap often can be used to enhance the upper breast reconstruction after a TRAM flap restores the lower breast contour. For example, for a radical mastectomy defect, the TRAM flap can be used for the lower breast reconstruction and the latissimus dorsi flap used for replacement of the upper breast and axillary region.

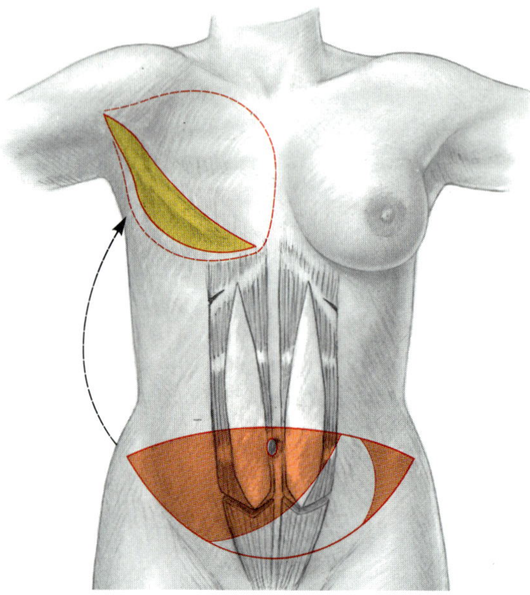

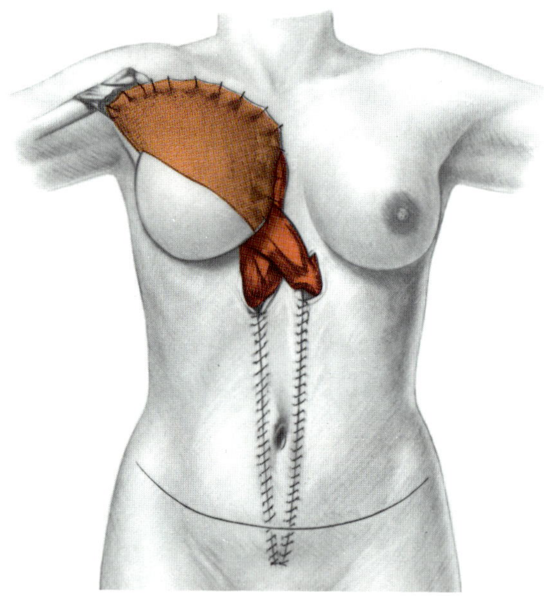

In this situation breast reconstruction is carried out in two stages. At the first operation a bilateral lower TRAM flap procedure is performed. The ipsilateral flap is deepithelialized and positioned to provide upper chest fill and some axillary fill. The contralateral flap is used for the right breast reconstruction.

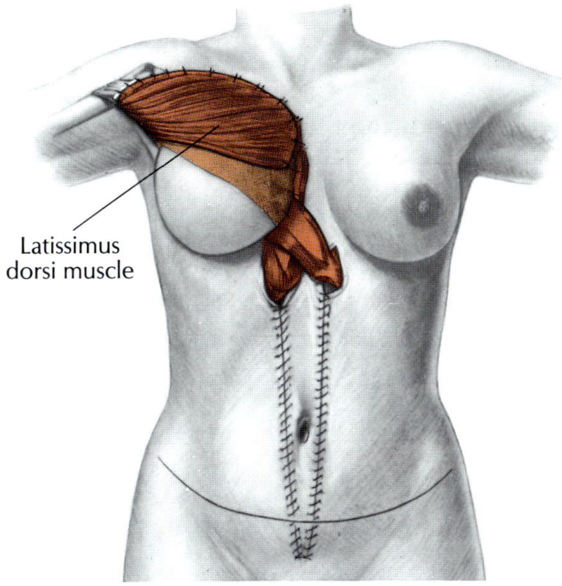

During a second stage a right latissimus dorsi muscle flap with a small deepithelialized skin island is transferred to the divided insertion of the pectoralis major muscle to further define the anterior axillary fold.

After disappointing results, especially capsular contracture with a silicone breast implant under a latissimus dorsi flap, a TRAM flap can be used to provide a soft breast reconstruction. If the volume of tissue required for reoperation is not available from pedicled flaps, then reconstruction with either implants or free flaps is needed to obtain the proper volume.

Anatomic Considerations

When reoperative surgery is performed after a pedicled flap reconstruction, the primary concern is to avoid harming the remaining breast reconstruction or worsening the deformity. Familiarity with the surgical anatomy of the TRAM flap and the latissimus dorsi flap and with the position of the vascular pedicles after transfer for breast reconstruction is a requirement. The source of the blood supply of the flap should always be considered because any interventions that compromise the vasculature can result in an even larger problem. I know of several instances of partial TRAM flap loss that occurred because the muscle pedicle was thinned or divided to reduce fullness in the epigastrium. The proximal muscle and pedicle of the latissimus dorsi flap can produce a similar fullness or even a mass in the axilla. Care should be taken not to confuse this anatomic appearance with an axillary recurrence, which might lead to involved and unnecessary workups.

TRAM Flap

The TRAM flap is unforgiving of technical shortfalls. Its blood supply is less reliable when patient selection, operative technique, and perioperative management are extended beyond recognized limits. For instance, if the pedicle of a TRAM flap is divided while an implant is placed to enlarge the reconstructed breast, the blood supply to the TRAM flap can be compromised and portions of the flap lost.

Knowledge of the blood flow in the TRAM flap is particularly important when reoperative surgery involves the use of this transferred tissue with another technique, such as an implant reconstruction or a latissimus dorsi flap reconstruction.

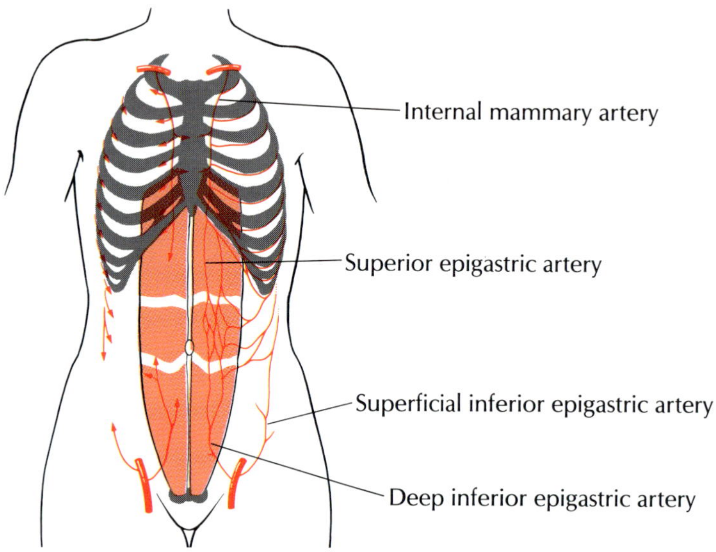

The vertical epigastric vascular system provides the major source of blood supply to the rectus abdominis muscle and the overlying musculocutaneous territories of the anterior abdominal wall.

The superior epigastric artery, a terminal branch of the internal mammary artery, nourishes the superiorly based TRAM flap. Musculocutaneous arterial perforators extend from the vertical epigastric system within the rectus abdominis muscle and pass through the anterior rectus sheath, providing nourishment to the skin and subcutaneous tissue of the anterior abdominal wall.

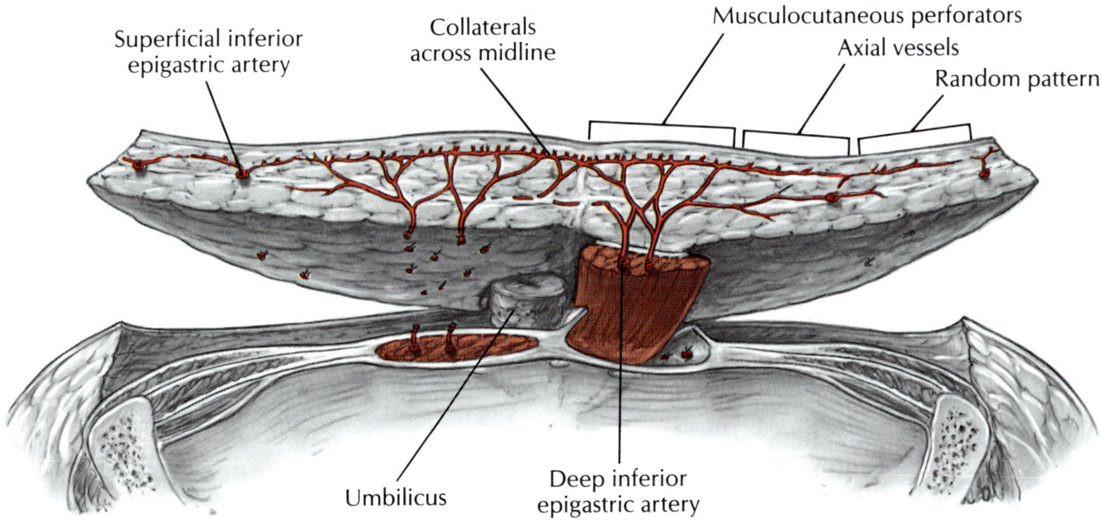

These perforating vessels branch into axially coursing vessels that are primarily located above the superficial layer of the abdominal wall fascia and are especially concentrated in the subdermal plexus. In the upper abdomen these vessels supply the primary flow into the thoracoepigastric flap, with the subdermal plexus providing significant collateral flow.

Axial vessels branching from the direct periumbilical rectus abdominis muscular perforators nourish the lateral extensions of the TRAM flap that are not directly over the rectus abdominis muscle. A rich vascular network and interconnected vessels branch in the subcutaneous tissues across the midline of the abdomen. The vascular network is present primarily at the level of the subdermal plexus. It communicates with the axial vascular system and subdermal plexus of the contralateral anterior abdominal wall, providing flow to the skin on the contralateral side. TRAM flap elevation across the entire anterior abdominal wall laterally to the anterior axillary line is dependent on this collateral flow and that of the subdermal plexus across the midline into the opposite sides of the abdominal wall subcutaneous vascular network.

Radiation, atherosclerosis, age-associated problems, anatomic variations, previous operations, and vasoconstrictors can affect normal flow in this vascular network. A midline incision effectively destroys this midline vascular connection. After an abdominoplasty, the perforators that supply the TRAM flap are divided; therefore in patients who have had a previous abdominoplasty, a reoperative plan that relies on the elevation of a TRAM flap risks total flap loss. Decreased vascularity to the TRAM flap and a small skin island may be a problem in patients who smoke. Division of the lower deep inferior epigastric artery allows greater flow into the system from the superior deep epigastric artery. For this reason vascular delay of a TRAM flap is advantageous.

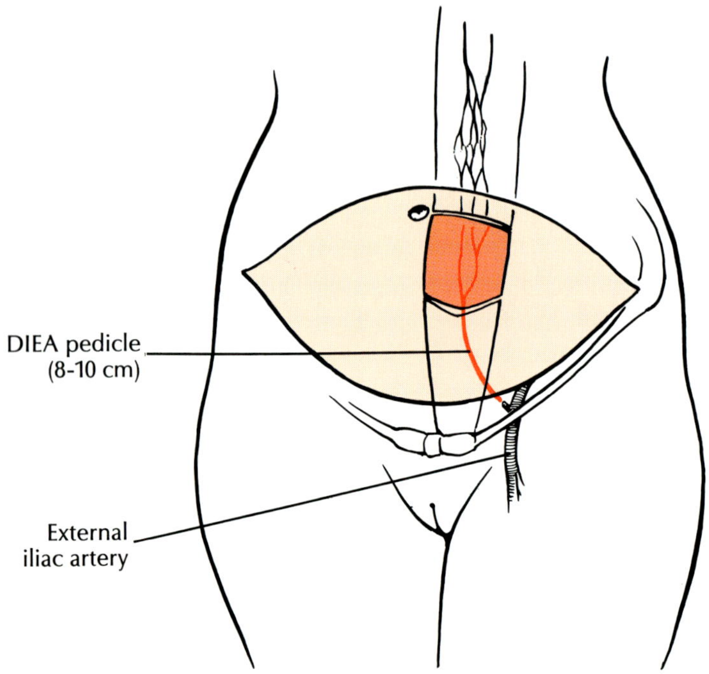

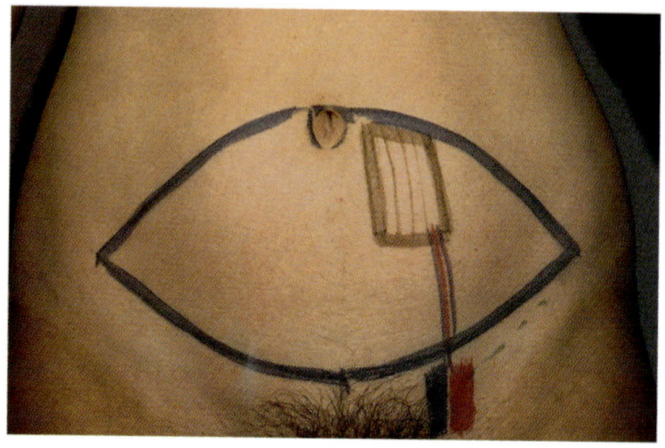

For patients with risk factors, a free TRAM flap may be a better option than a pedicled TRAM flap because it offers an alternative pattern of blood flow. The dominant blood supply to this area is the musculocutaneous perforating branches of the deep inferior epigastric artery (DIEA) through the rectus abdominis muscle and the superficial inferior epigastric artery (SIEA). The entire lower abdominal ellipse of skin and subcutaneous tissues may be elevated as a free flap based on either of these vessels (see Chapter 31).

Latissimus Dorsi Flap

The anatomy of the latissimus dorsi musculocutaneous flap is more forgiving than that of the TRAM flap. The latissimus dorsi flap is based on the thoracodorsal pedicle, a branch of the subscapular artery arising from the axillary artery, which is usually spared with today's method of axillary lymph node dissection. In the past this was not the case with a radical mastectomy.

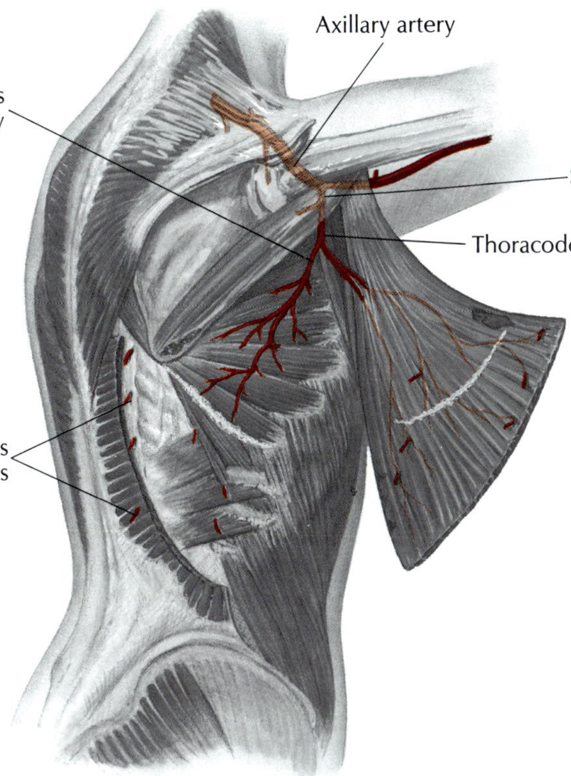

The thoracodorsal artery has a relatively large diameter of 1 to 2.5 mm. An intramuscular pattern of vasculature radiates from the thoracodorsal pedicle to nourish the latissimus dorsi flap. Successful latissimus dorsi flap reconstruction, both primary and secondary, depends on the reconstructive surgeon's knowledge of this intramuscular branching of the thoracodorsal artery. The primary intramuscular vessel courses vertically in the same direction as the pedicle, approximately 3 cm inside the lateral edge of the latissimus dorsi muscle. The intramuscular network, radiating from the entrance of the thoracodorsal pedicle into the latissimus dorsi muscle 10 cm below the axilla, permits the splitting of the latissimus dorsi muscle into two or three muscle strips that can support several skin islands if necessary for specialized secondary procedures. The largest perforators branch from this primary vessel; therefore a vertical lateral orientation of a latissimus dorsi flap provides the safest skin island. Several other major branches extend in a radial manner from the primary pedicle. The intramuscular branching pattern permits division of the latissimus dorsi muscle while preserving the proximal blood supply and the integrity of the musculocutaneous unit. A collateral pedicle from the serratus anterior fascia is also usually preserved and is a constant vessel in this region. The latissimus dorsi flap can survive on this vessel when the thoracodorsal pedicle has been injured or divided.

The flap can be harvested either laterally or transversely for a variety of flap designs that can be customized to replace the tissue needed for the reconstructed breast. When there has been a previous axillary lymph node dissection, the reconstructive surgeon should always assume that the thoracodorsal pedicle has been injured. He should check with the original surgeon and the operative report to determine if the pedicle has been divided. He can also check for function in the latissimus dorsi muscle by palpating the muscle while the patient's arm is abducted and the patient pushes down. Absence of latissimus dorsi muscle function indicates pedicle division. There is still some flow into the muscle via the serratus collateral artery, but flap reliability in our experience is usually about 75%. With these findings, it may be best to select another flap or to use a free flap. Patient selection also plays a role in the use of the latissimus dorsi flap; when there is heavy radiation damage in the axilla, there may be some concern for the thoracodorsal pedicle and for the ultimate vascular nourishment of the flap.

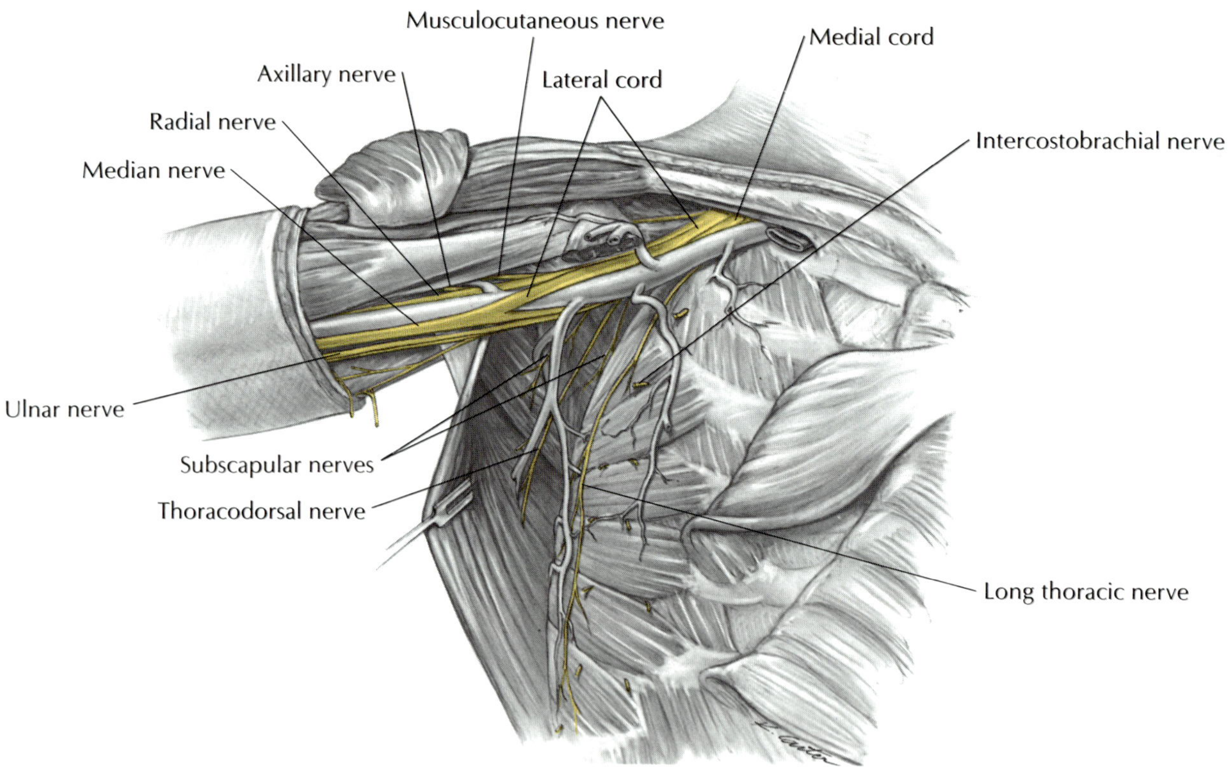

The thoracodorsal nerve, arising from the C6-8 roots of the posterior cord of the brachial plexus, is the motor nerve to the latissimus dorsi muscle. This nerve, along with the thoracodorsal vessels, passes downward through the axilla and enters the muscle with the thoracodorsal vascular pedicle. The thoracodorsal nerve is responsible for muscular contraction of the latissimus dorsi muscle. If muscle contraction is a problem to the patient after a latissimus dorsi flap reconstruction, the nerve can be divided during a secondary procedure. This division paralyzes the muscle and induces denervation atrophy of the latissimus dorsi muscle without compromising the blood flow to the flap through the muscle and skin island as long as the collateral arteries from the serratus anterior muscle are preserved.

The surgeon should also be familiar with the anatomy of the insertion of the latissimus dorsi muscle. The insertion is through a 3 cm broad tendon attached to the bottom of the intertubercular groove of the humerus. The tendon and proximal latissimus dorsi muscle actually encircle the teres major muscle, which is the muscle that primarily contributes to the form of the posterior axillary fold. In many reoperative situations the result can be enhanced by dividing and transferring the proximal latissimus dorsi muscle and its tendon around to the pectoralis major muscle insertion or to the axilla and the upper outer chest wall.

Reoperation After a TRAM Flap

Reduction of flap excess, augmentation of a deficient flap (from either tissue loss or inadequate tissue transfer), and contouring of the abdominal donor site are three reasons for reoperation after a TRAM flap reconstruction. Flap deficiency can be caused by tissue loss because of improper patient selection (e.g., a cigarette smoker, a massively overweight patient, or a patient with unrecognized or improperly considered abdominal wall scars), improper flap planning (e.g., placing the skin island too low below the periumbilical perforators), a technical shortcoming during the procedure (e.g., injury to the deep superior epigastric artery), or an unrecognized and untreated postoperative situation (e.g., compression of the pedicle from a hematoma or a low hematocrit level with reduced oxygen delivery to the flap, which may result in tissue loss). Tissue deficiency with lack of fullness in the upper breast region after TRAM flap reconstruction can result from inadequate preoperative planning such that the length of the pedicle limits the surgeon's ability to place the tissue in the upper breast or axillary region. Although reduction of a large flap can be corrected with liposuction or excision of the excess, insufficient tissue is more difficult to correct. In this situation either a breast implant, tissue expander, or another flap is required.

Flap Deficiency

Asymmetry

When a breast reconstructed with a TRAM flap is too small, exhibiting a tissue deficit of the breast mound or the upper chest wall, a textured-surface implant or a textured-surface permanent expander-implant can be used to provide additional volume. When an expander is used, a small subcutaneous fill valve can be retained to permit fine adjustments of the volume of the reconstructed breast. Smooth implants are not recommended; when positioned under a TRAM flap, they have a high incidence of capsular contracture.

Alternatively a pedicled flap, most often a latissimus dorsi muscle flap with or without a skin island, can be used to supplement the TRAM flap. The choice of technique depends on the patient's feelings about the use of implants and her physical condition. A latissimus dorsi flap provides the best solution for obtaining additional autogenous tissue to supplement a deficient TRAM flap reconstruction.

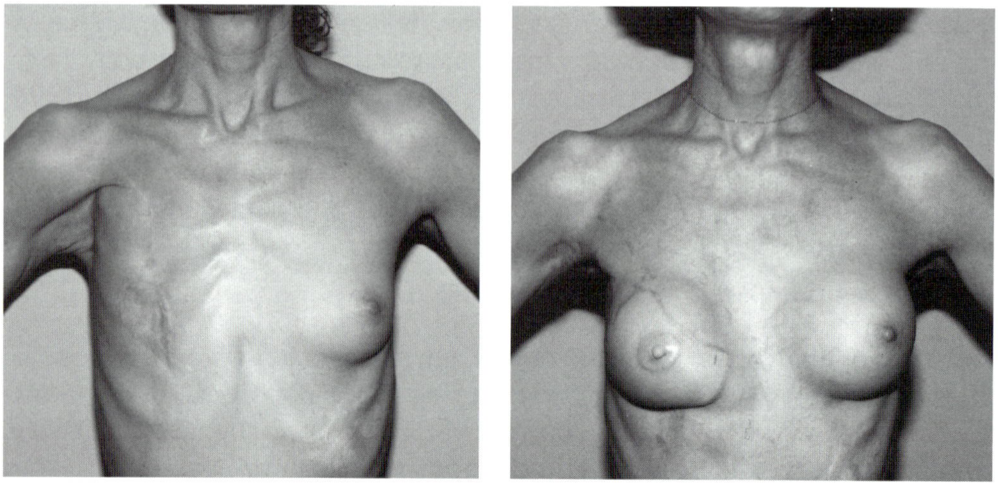

This 43-year-old woman had a radical mastectomy and breast reconstruction with a TRAM flap. Because there was not enough lower abdominal tissue available for reconstruction of the axilla and anterior axillary fold, a latissimus dorsi flap was rotated to provide this additional tissue. Because the patient also wanted to have larger breasts, breast implants were placed for both breasts.

Small Area of Flap Loss

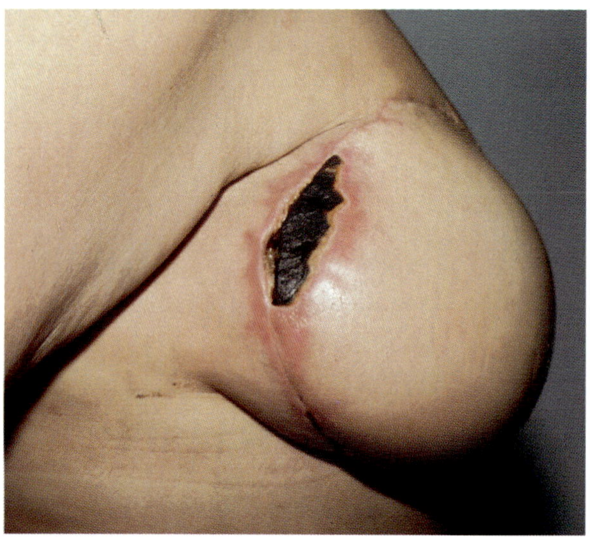

When a small area of the TRAM flap is lost, the area is allowed to become defined, and debridement is performed with secondary closure. Revision is then undertaken at a secondary reconstruction.

Partial Tissue Loss

After partial loss of a TRAM flap, the preferred method of handling the problem is to excise the nonviable tissue and reapproximate the tissues of the TRAM flap in the local area to achieve a satisfactory breast reconstruction. Sometimes a breast implant can be used for the reconstruction.

When the patient desires only autogenous tissue for reconstruction or when there is a more substantial tissue loss following TRAM flap reconstruction (25% or more) and autogenous tissue is needed, particularly when the defect is in the upper lateral chest wall, then the latissimus dorsi flap is the first and safest choice. An approach should be planned to maximize flap survival. I generally administer additional steroids, maintain the patient's hematocrit level so it is at least 30%, and use systemic supplemental oxygen. I prefer delayed rather than early flap debridement because it is difficult to ascertain the exact amount of flap compromise, especially in fat, for the first few days. I believe that extension of fat necrosis can occur from early debridement, desiccation, spreading infection, and additional trauma, leading to additional tissue loss. I prefer to wait until a distinct skin margin develops with better delineation of the necrotic tissue, which usually takes 1 to 2 weeks. The TRAM flap is positioned so that the least vascular portion is lateral. When this flap is positioned horizontally, the ipsilateral pedicle should be considered.

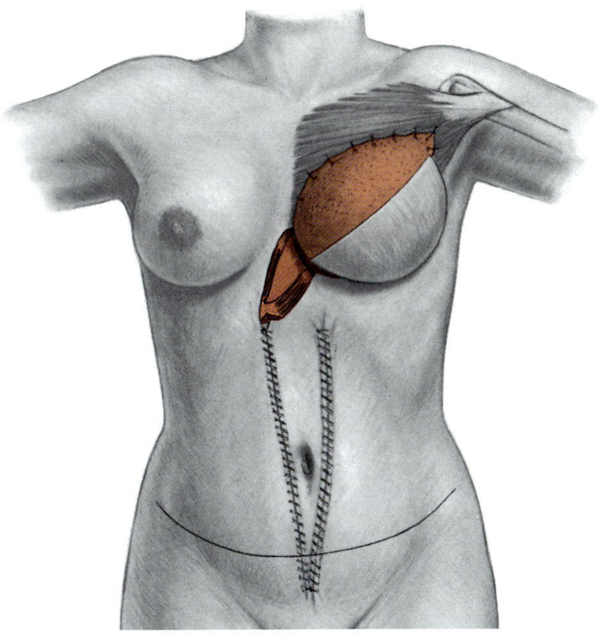

When the TRAM flap is used for breast reconstruction, the best blood supply in the pedicled tissue should be in the medial portion of the flap. With this strategy, if there is partial loss of the flap, it occurs laterally. A lateral defect is not as critical as a large central or medial defect. A latissimus dorsi flap can easily fill the lateral deficit. A small area of flap nonviability can be directly excised in the early postoperative period or, if the area of loss is large, a latissimus dorsi flap can be used to salvage the breast reconstruction.

The anatomic details and standard technique of elevation of the latissimus dorsi flap are described in detail in other texts.[1] When the latissimus dorsi flap is used in a secondary operation to improve the result after a TRAM flap complication, I prefer not to make an additional back scar.

If the patient has excess lateral tissue at the site of the mastectomy and the mastectomy scar extends under the arm, I usually use this excess tissue for the reconstruction or use the mastectomy scar as access to the latissimus dorsi muscle. A considerable volume of autogenous tissue often can be obtained from the latissimus dorsi muscle without the need for a major skin island and large back scar.

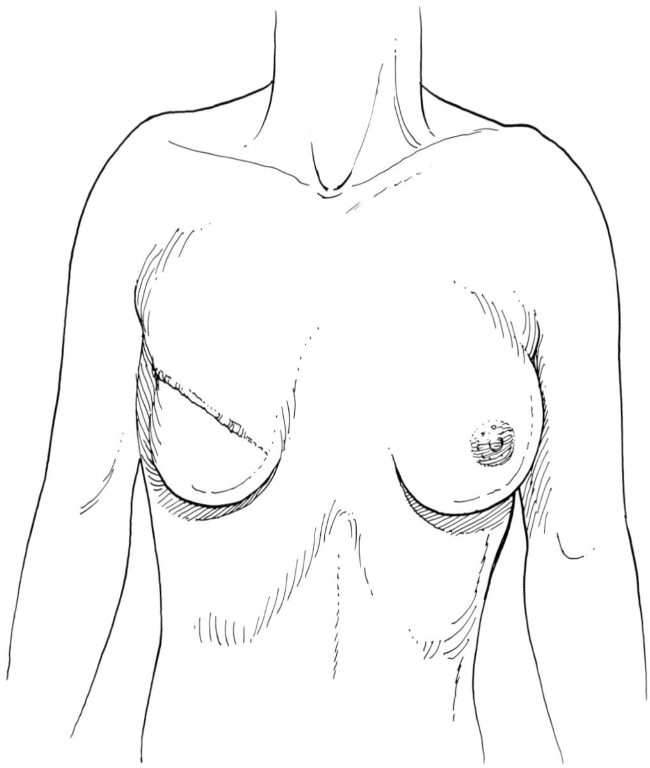

When a lateral deformity results from tissue loss after a TRAM flap, a latissimus dorsi flap can be used to fill this deficit.

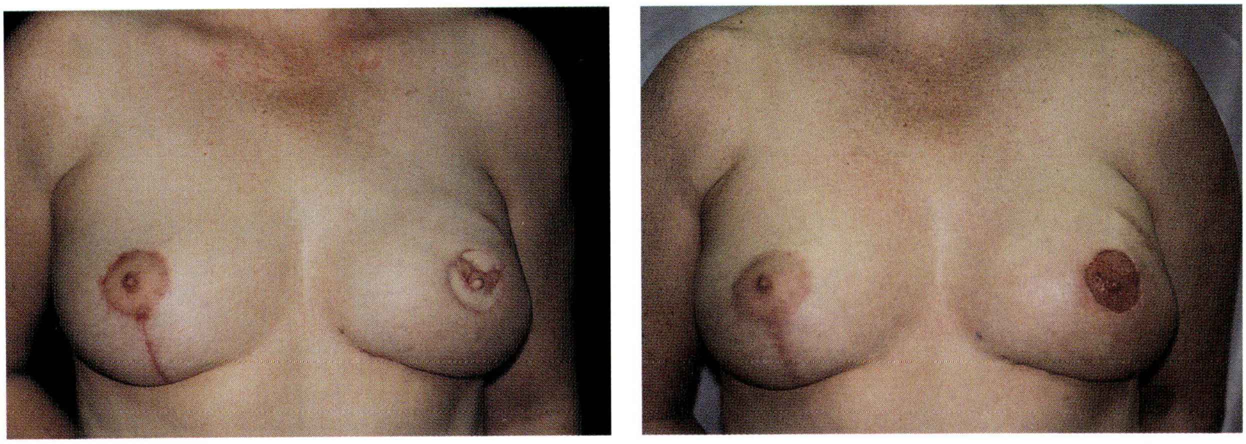

The immediate postoperative result shows the improved contours of the breast mound. Eight weeks later nipple-areolar tattooing was performed.

If the inframammary fold is too high, it must be released and dropped down. Usually the flap can be mobilized slightly to drop into the new fold area; however, occasionally the insertion of an implant will give more distinct contour in this area.

Smaller Contour Defects

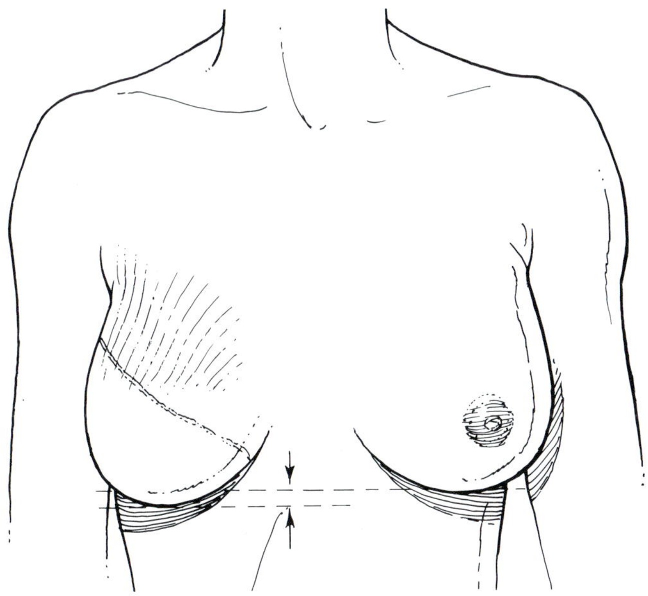

No matter what type of free flap is used, it is often difficult to construct a breast mound that has both satisfactory infraclavicular fill and ptosis. If ptosis is created, tissue may be lacking in the infraclavicular hollow as well as tail of breast area. Small asymmetries in these areas are usually accepted by the patient. However, larger depressions cannot be well disguised in swimming suits or low-cut dresses. For this reason, patients may request secondary correction. To correct an infraclavicular depression, I usually try to mobilize the free flap in a direct superior direction.

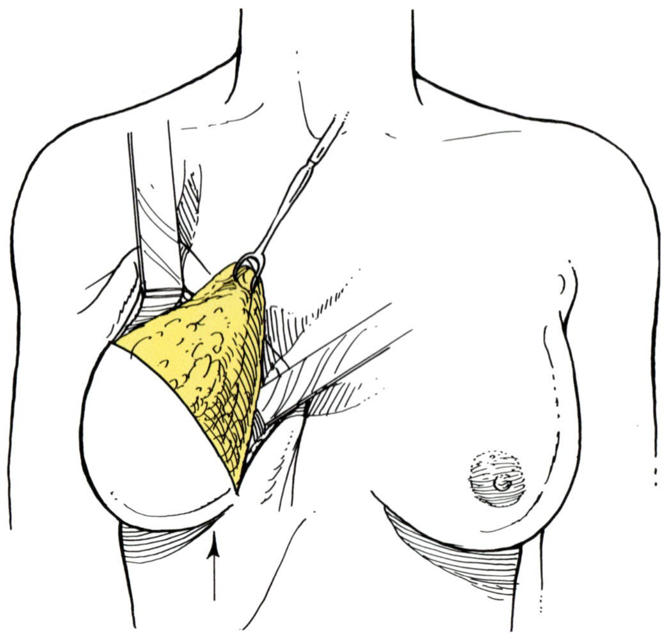

The mastectomy flap is elevated and the superior pole of the reconstructed breast is mobilized to the level of the muscular pedicle but usually not beyond this point.

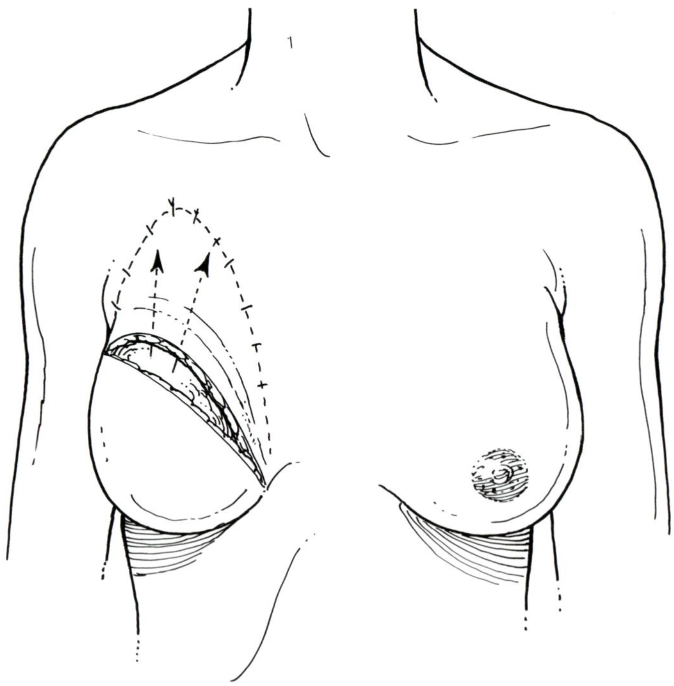

The free flap can then be elevated superiorly and plicated to the pectoralis major muscle in the infraclavicular fold with large permanent sutures.

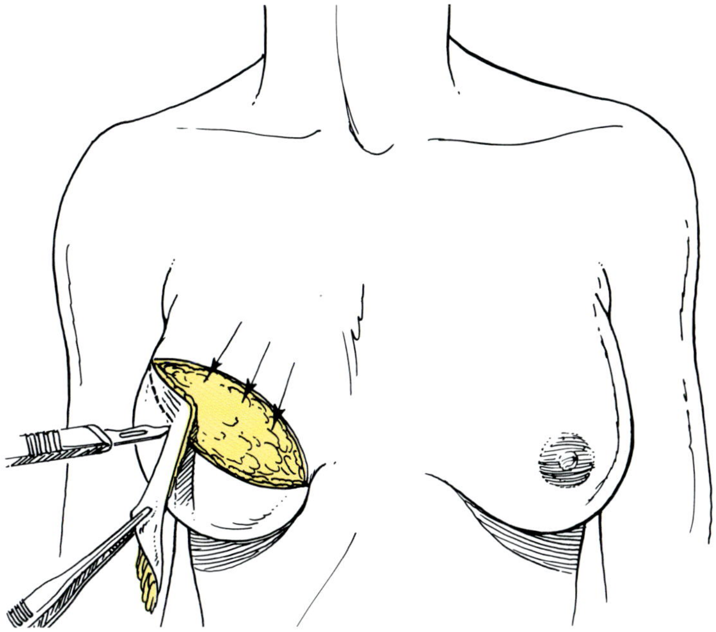

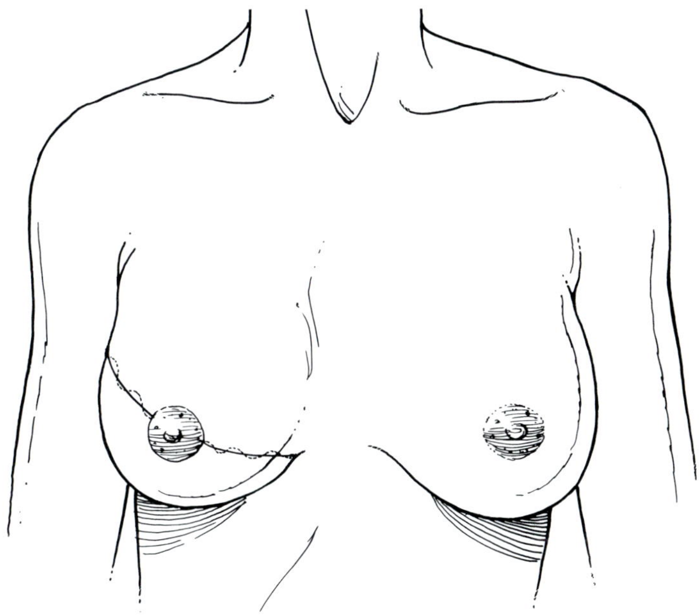

To minimize tension on the plication, the mastectomy flap is sutured more inferiorly over the free flap skin island. ***The TRAM skin island, not the mastectomy flap, is trimmed before closure in order to create a lower scar and preserve normal breast skin.*** This technique will usually provide adequate fill in this area as long as slight ptosis existed preoperatively. If there was no ptosis and superior mobilization of the flap would create asymmetry inferiorly and inferolaterally, then an alternative method must be sought. Occasionally, the lateral portion of the flap can be mobilized and rotated into the tail of the breast area. However, this method cannot correct more medial defects.

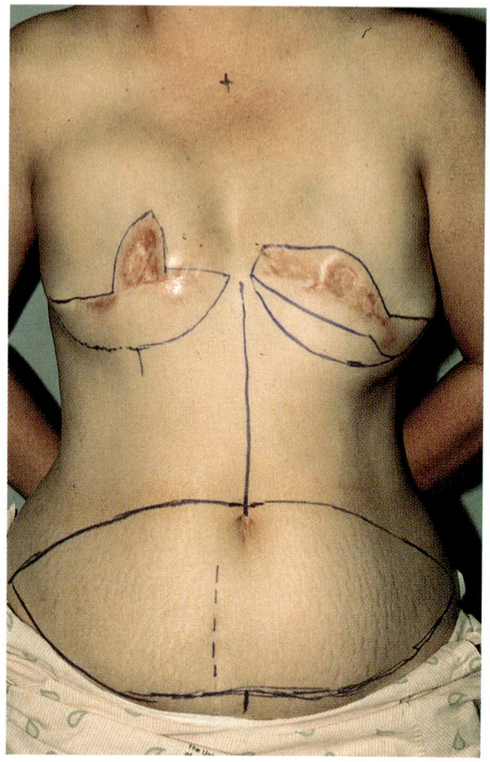

This unfortunate patient was referred for salvage breast reconstruction following simple bilateral mastectomies and failed expander reconstruction. Mastectomies had been performed because of a history of free silicone injection and premalignant mastopathy. Bilateral free TRAM flap breast reconstruction was planned.

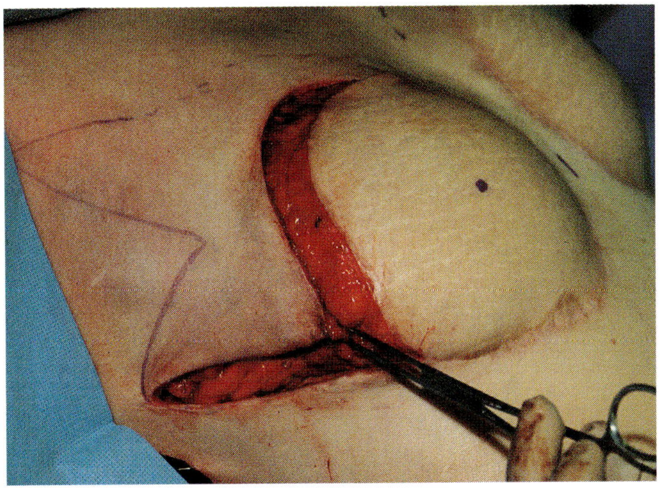

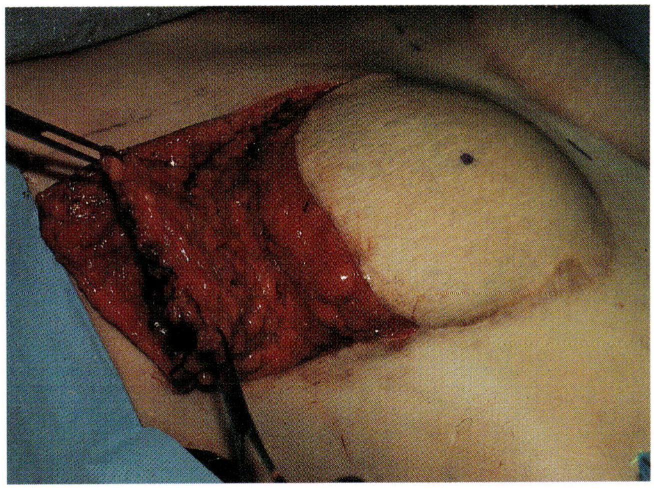

Three months following the flap transfer, a small deficiency in the tail of the reconstructed right breast was evident. No other flap excesses were available to rotate into this area. Therefore a medially based fat flap was mobilized from the lateral portion of the reconstructed breast mound and transposed into the deficiency in the tail of the breast.

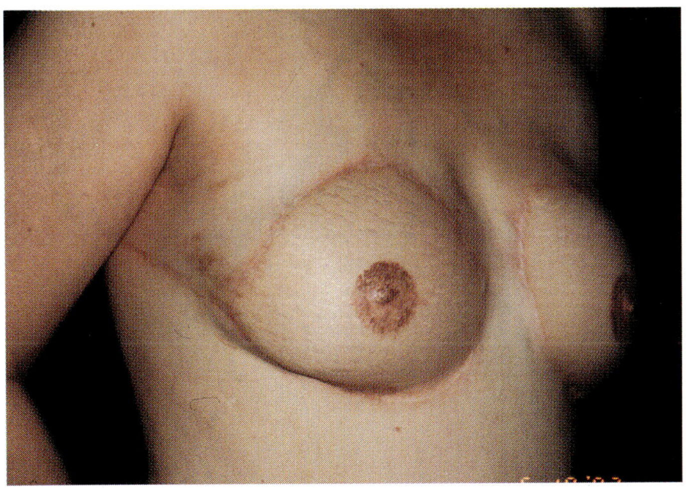

The postoperative result was satisfactory.

To correct very severe contour deformities, the insertion of a custom implant or the transfer of a second flap such as the latissimus dorsi could be considered.

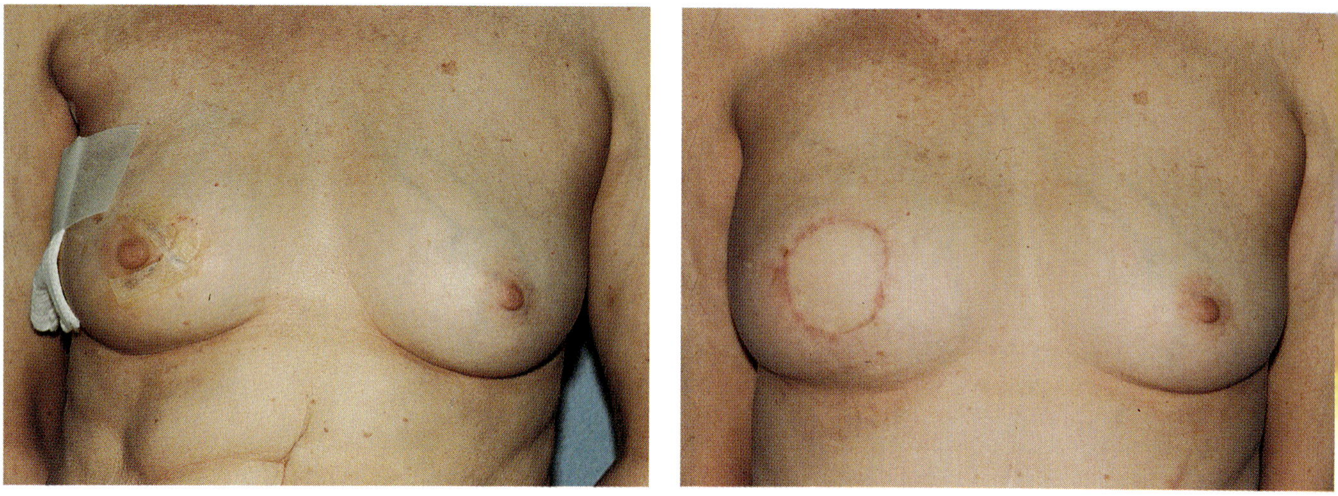

Following immediate free TRAM reconstruction of the right breast, this patient had a breast mound that was somewhat large and full laterally.

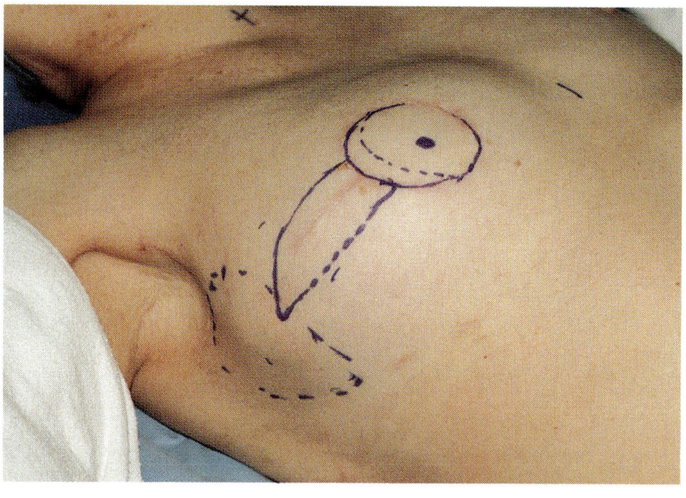

In the first correction, the breast was elevated slightly by excision along the scar, the lateral aspect was contoured, and the nipple-areola was reconstructed.

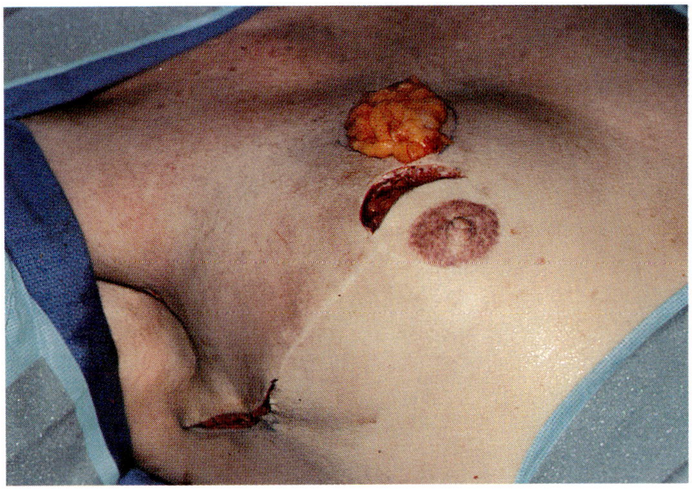

Postoperatively, she continued to complain of a small medial contour defect. Therefore in a second revisional procedure a small fat graft was harvested from the axillary area and transplanted into the medial aspect of the reconstructed right breast.

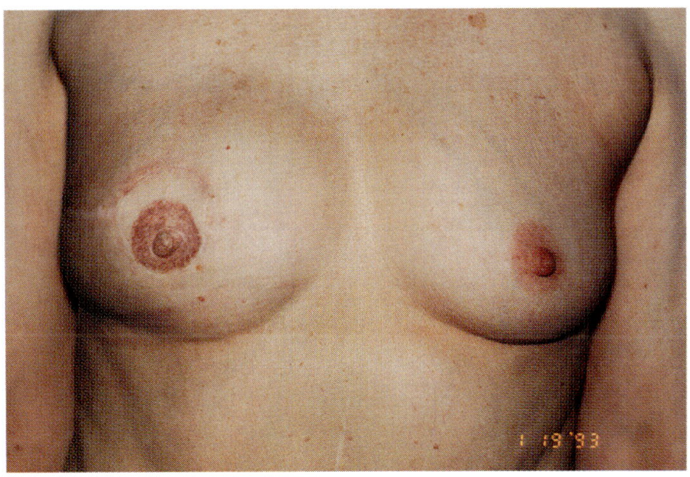

These fat grafts become firm initially but seem to hold up well over time. Fat injection can also be used.

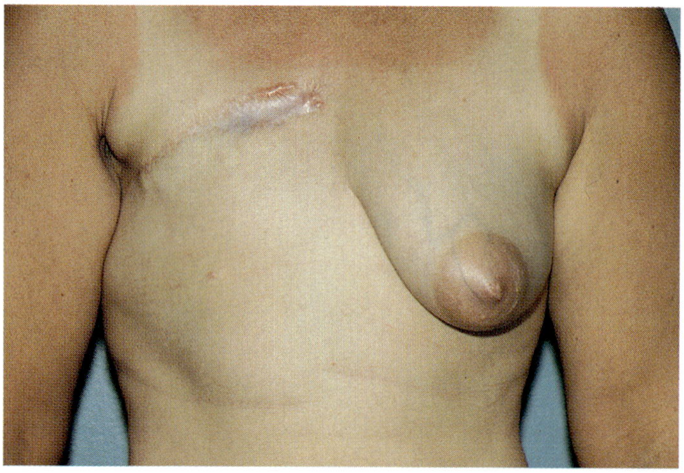

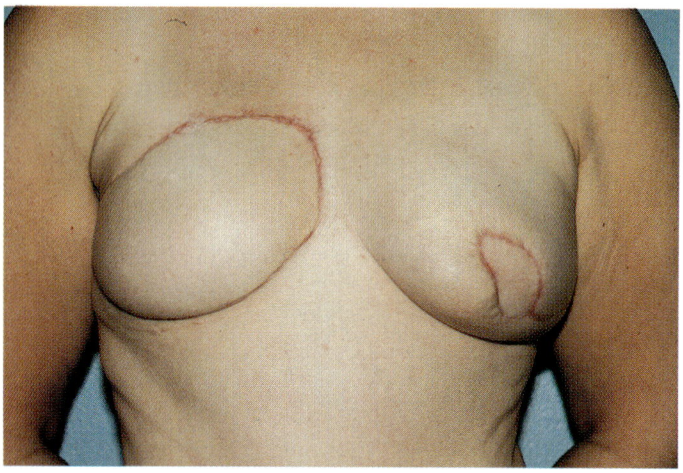

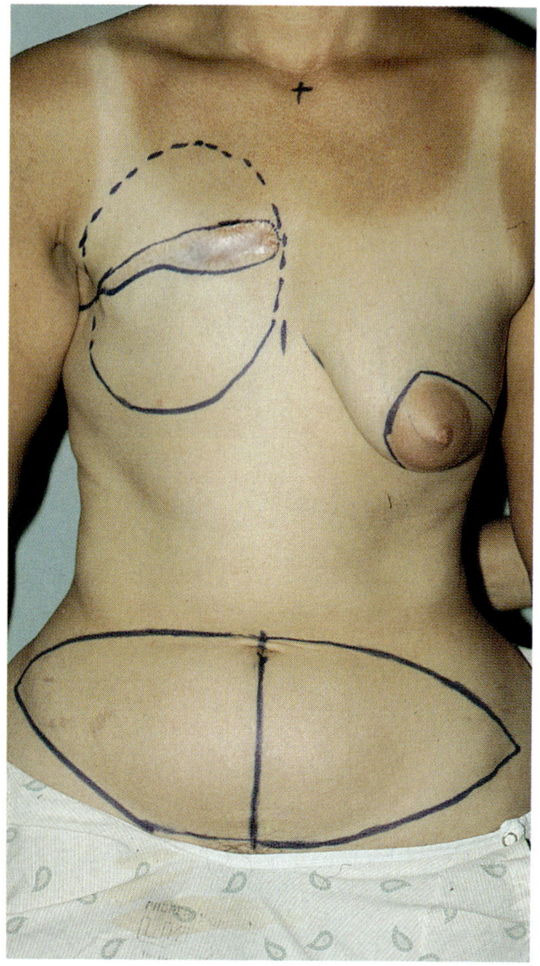

This patient provides a good example of the difference between the anticipated aesthetic result achievable with immediate reconstruction vs. that possible with delayed reconstruction. The patient had had a previous modified radical mastectomy on the right side; a new cancer subsequently developed in the left breast. She desired bilateral breast reconstruction, which was performed using bilateral free TRAM flaps. Following the initial reconstructive procedure, symmetry was close in terms of volume but there was an obvious difference in the skin color and texture between the two sides. The high right mastectomy scar will always limit the type and style of clothing that she can wear.

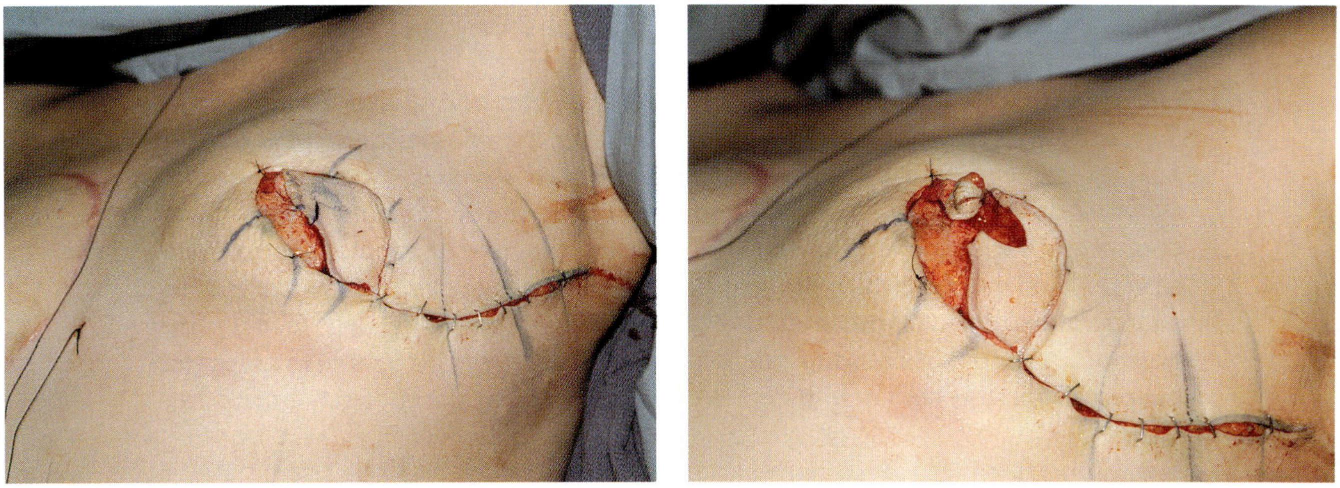

During the revision, the monitoring skin island, which had been left exposed on the left breast, was excised. The superior mastectomy flap was rotated inferiorly, closing the monitoring skin island area much like a diaphragm.

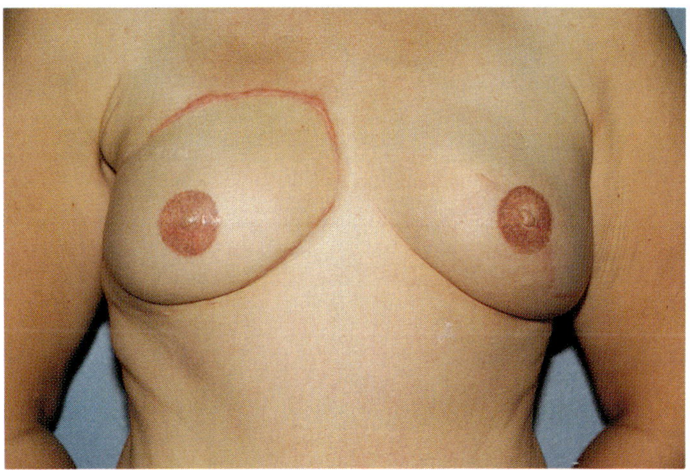

Following tattooing, the TRAM skin island is no longer visible on the left but is readily apparent on the right breast. The skin island itself was elevated as a fish tail flap and fashioned into a nipple.

Scars

As a matter of routine, during secondary surgery I try to improve any scar on the breast that I think will respond to the usual techniques of scar revision. When asked, patients will always point out which scars they find most difficult to conceal with clothing. With delayed reconstruction, a transverse scar usually extends across the middle or upper portion of the breast. ***Any time the mastectomy flap can be brought lower during mound revision, the scar will subsequently be easier to hide beneath clothing.*** With skin-sparing mastectomy we often leave a monitoring skin island at the future site of the nipple-areola complex. The intent is to try to completely excise the monitoring skin island at the time of nipple-areola reconstruction and areolar tattoo. However, complete excision is not always possible, and occasionally a segment of the periareolar scar must be left in a visible position. Although these scars fade with time, it is always preferable to complete the reconstruction with only native breast skin covering a completely buried free flap.

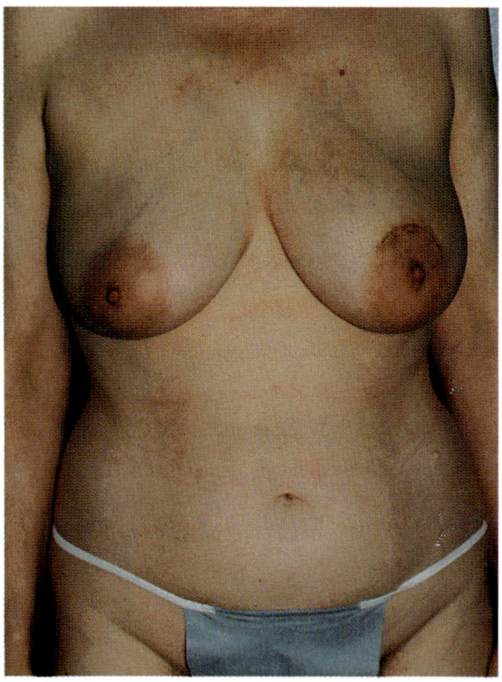

This 45-year-old patient underwent a modified radical mastectomy for intraductal carcinoma of the left breast.

Photograph from Grotting JC. Immediate breast reconstruction using free TRAM flap. Clin Plast Surg 21:207-221, 1994.

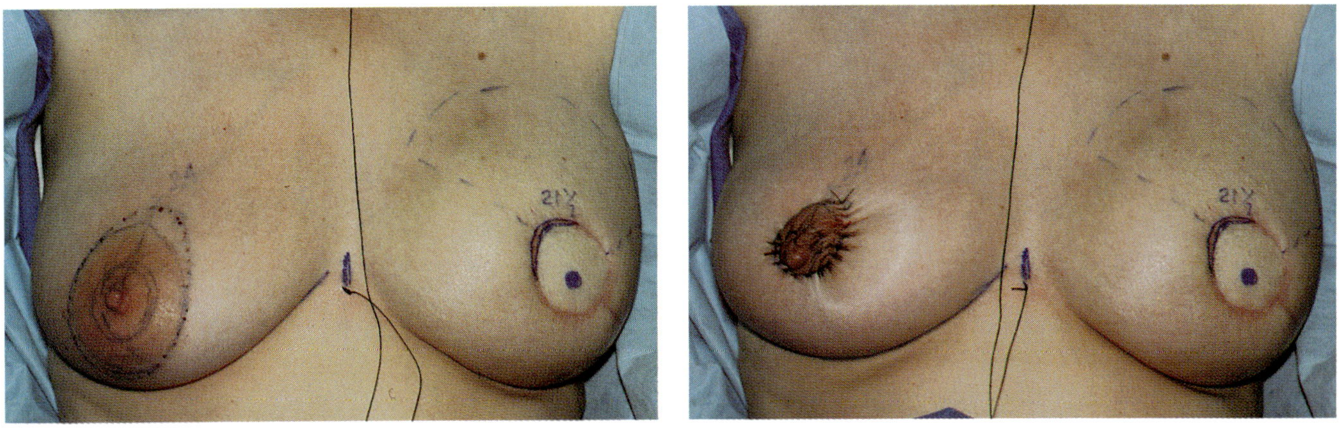

Immediate reconstruction was performed using a free TRAM flap. Postoperatively the reconstructed left breast was slightly higher than the ptotic right breast. She desired a modest mastopexy of the right breast for symmetry. Periareolar mastopexy of the right breast, mound correction via liposuction of the left breast, and then nipple-areola reconstruction were performed.

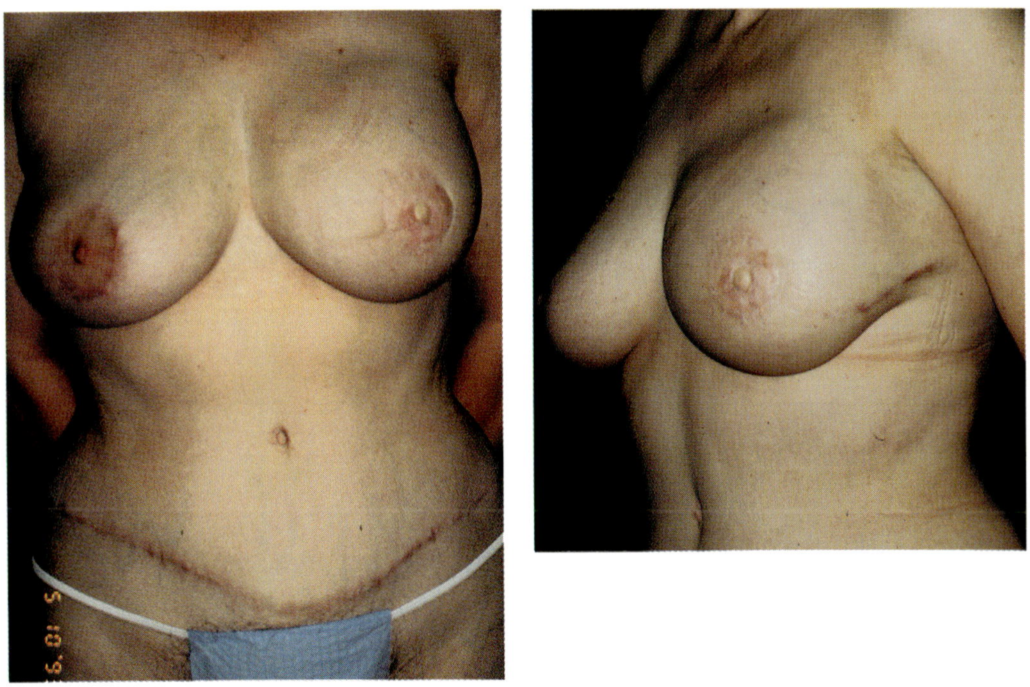

The postoperative result before nipple-areolar tattooing demonstrates good positioning of scars, which will allow the patient to wear a variety of clothing styles.

Photographs from Grotting JC. Immediate breast reconstruction using free TRAM flap. Clin Plast Surg 21:207-221, 1994.

NIPPLE-AREOLA RECONSTRUCTION

I prefer to delay nipple-areola reconstruction until all revisions of the breast mound have been completed and the patient and I are satisfied with the symmetry. If a major mound revision was required, I sometimes even perform nipple-areola reconstruction as a separate procedure to allow settling and softening of the breast mound to occur. However nipple-areola reconstruction can usually be easily performed at the same time as mound revision.

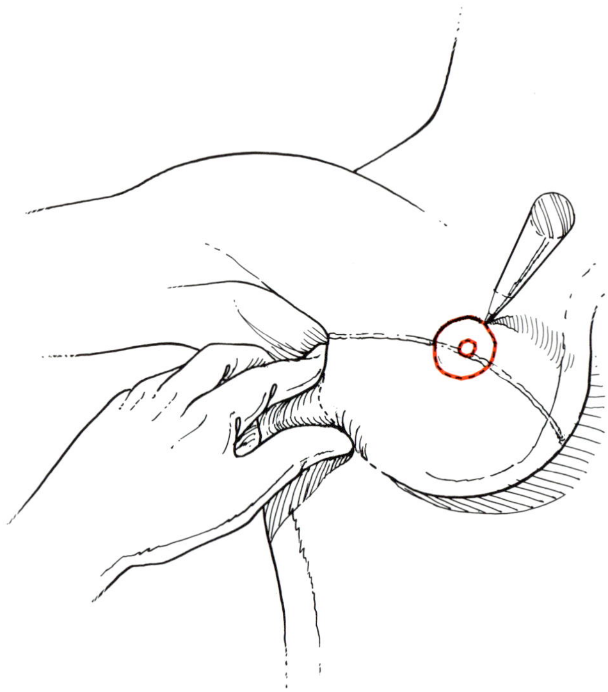

Even when the mound is to be revised in the same operation, it is possible to determine the position of the reconstructed nipple by manually holding the breast mound in its corrected position as the patient is viewed from the front and marking the nipple position according to how it will look best on the reconstructed breast mound and in relation to the opposite nipple-areola complex. I also ask the patient to place a small circular adhesive bandage the day before surgery at the position where she believes the reconstructed nipple-areola would look best.

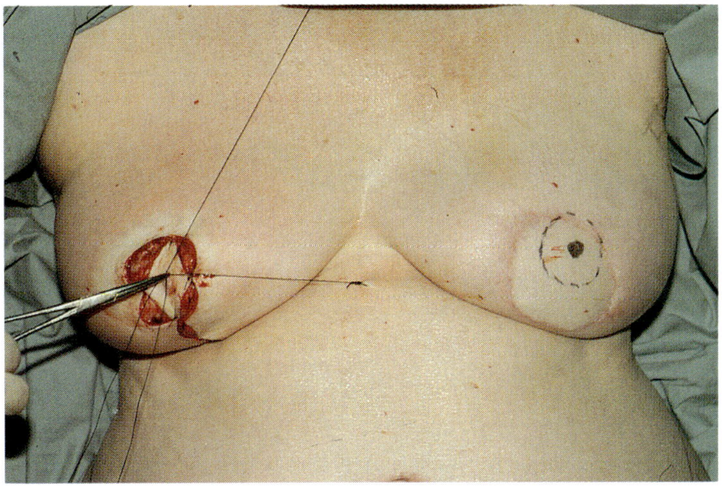

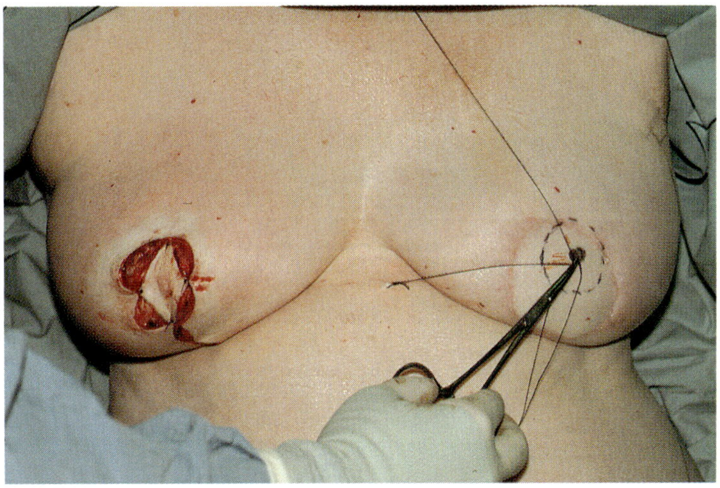

At the time of operation, one 2-0 silk suture can be placed at the manubrium and a second suture placed at the xiphoid in the midline. Based on the use of these two sutures in pendulum fashion, nipple position can be symmetrically placed after mound revision with the patient in the sitting position.

If the opposite nipple is large or broad, my procedure of choice is a nipple-sharing composite graft if the patient concurs. Otherwise, my preferred technique of nipple reconstruction is either the star flap[29] or a modification of the fish tail flap.[30] The latter technique utilizes two small skin fat flaps from the breast mound itself and allows primary closure of donor sites without skin grafts.

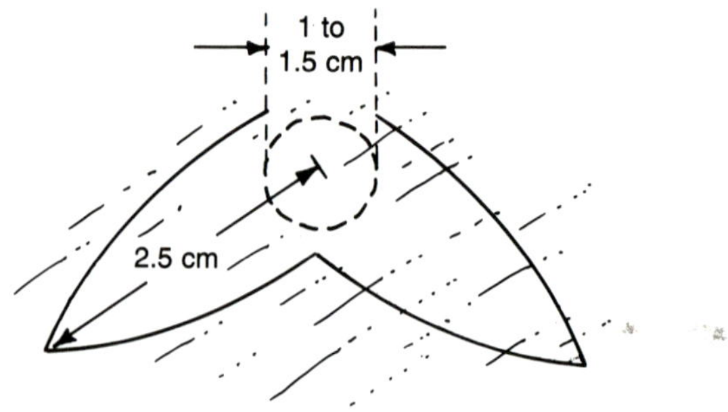

The modified fish tail flap is designed as shown, although the angle between the two flaps and their orientation can vary. The design of these flaps occasionally must be altered depending on the periareolar scars. However, they can be oriented in virtually any direction by simply designing the flaps where skin and fat are most available.

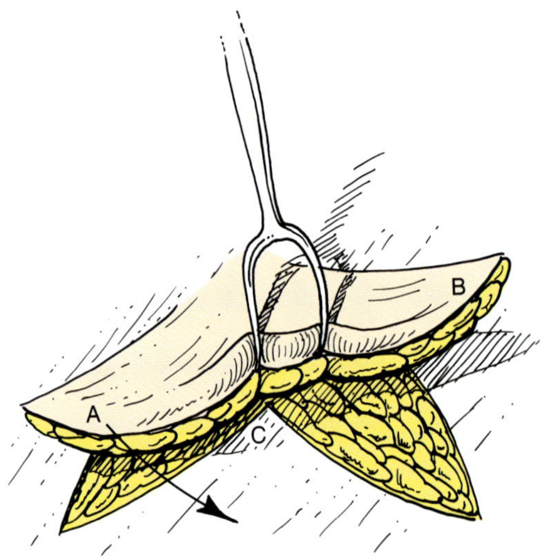

The wings of the flap are elevated from the apex toward the central pedicle. As the edge of the proposed nipple is reached, the dissection is deepened into the subcutaneous fat without further undermining beneath the center of the nipple. The superior aspect of the nipple is left intact. The inferior portion is incised and the two flaps are tilted up.

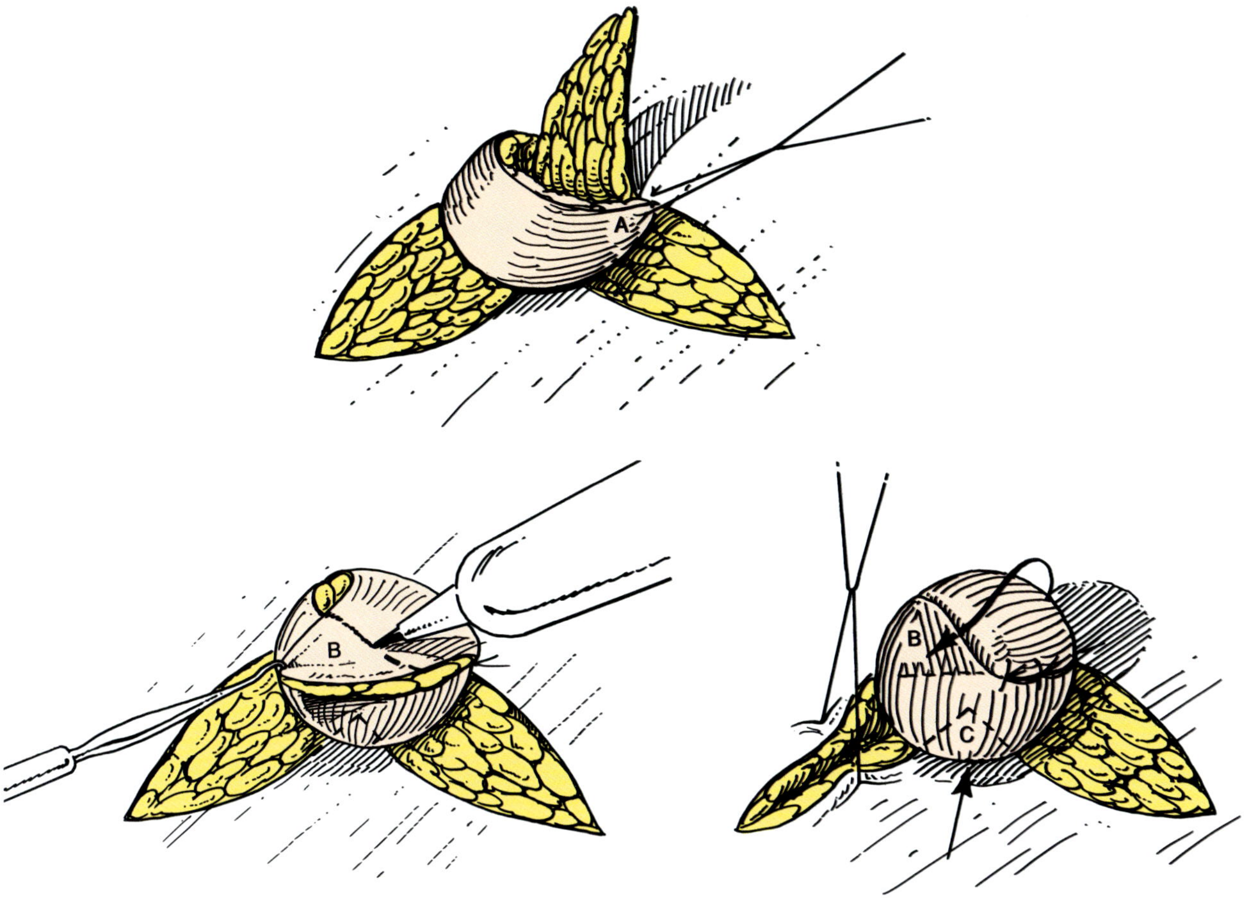

Flap A is then rotated around the base. Flap B is folded over to form the top of the nipple. The tip of flap B can be deepithelialized and tucked into the central part of the nipple to increase bulk. The donor sites can be closed primarily. The apex of flap C, which slides underneath the nipple, is deepithelialized to serve as a supporting platform and to prevent retrusion of the reconstructed nipple.

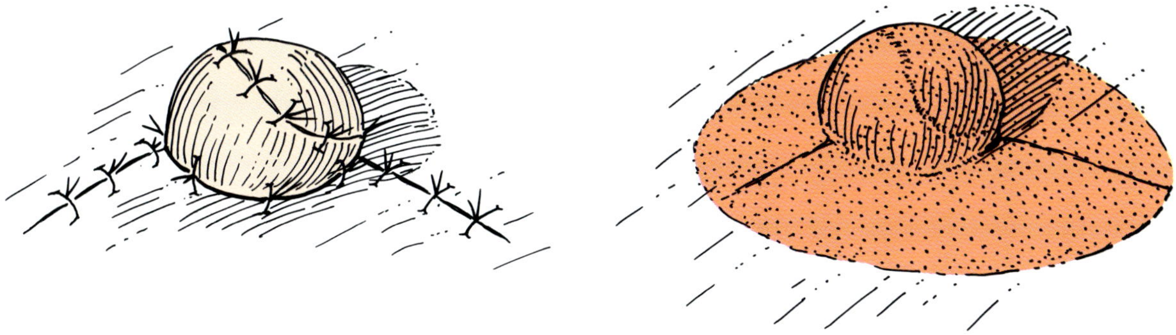

Nipple-areolar tattooing is usually delayed 6 weeks to allow stabilization of the tissues. Alternatively, tattooing can be performed first, followed by flap elevation and nipple-areola reconstruction.[31]

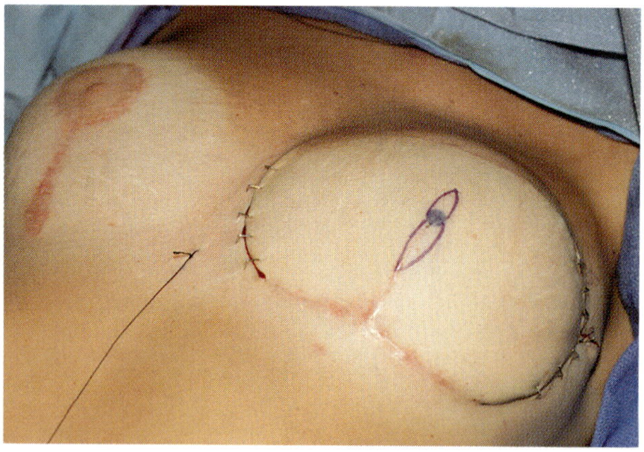

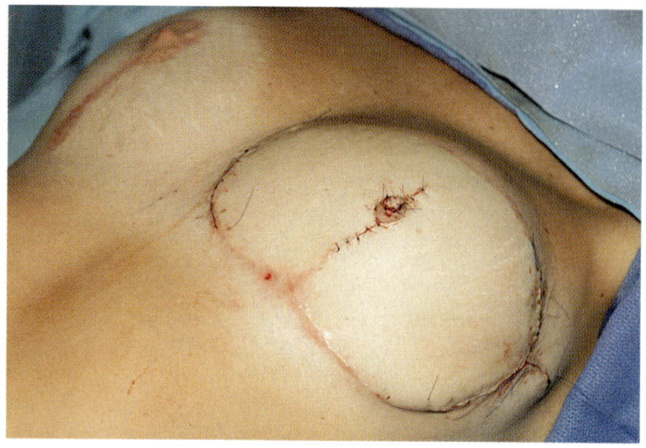

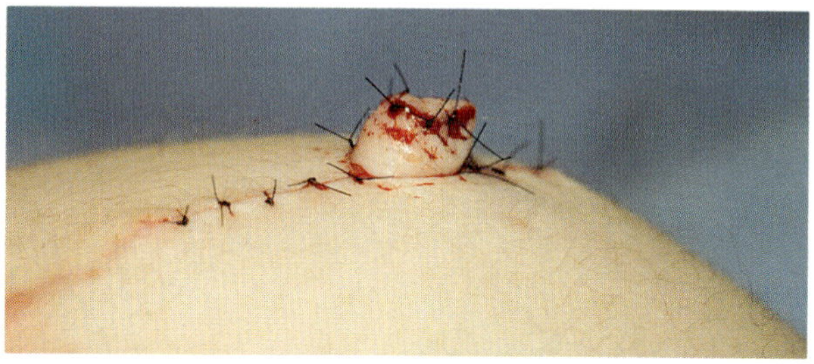

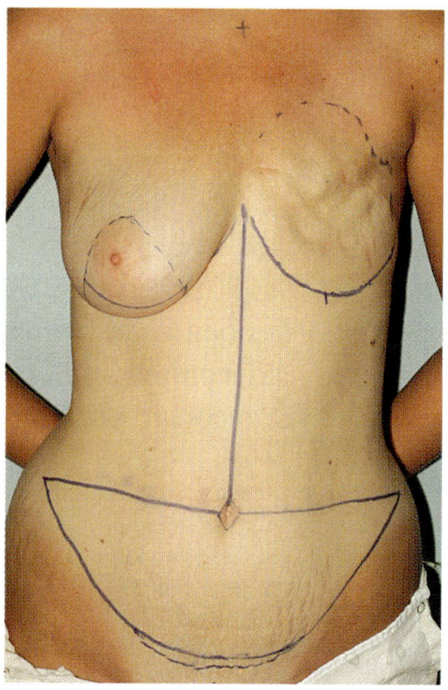

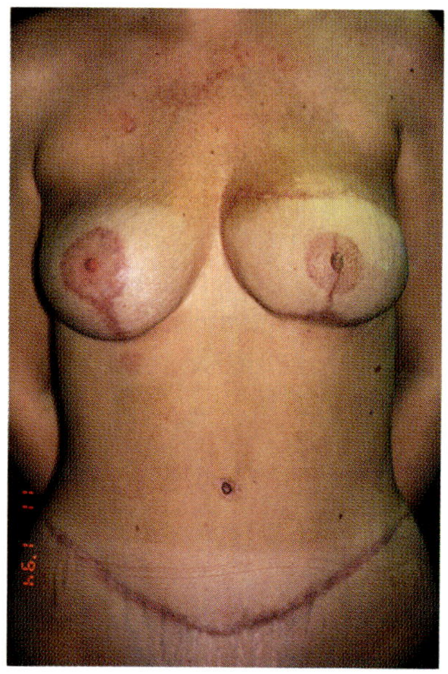

In this patient, the flaps were oriented vertically; this position seemed to result in less constriction of the cone of the reconstructed breast. The flaps were dissected, elevated, and transposed. The postoperative result is shown 1 month following tattooing of the areola.

As we have gained more experience with permanent pigmentation techniques, I now prefer to create the illusion of an areola by tattooing as opposed to skin grafting. The native skin of the breast or the flap will accept the pigments much more readily than a skin graft and therefore the color appears more stable long term.

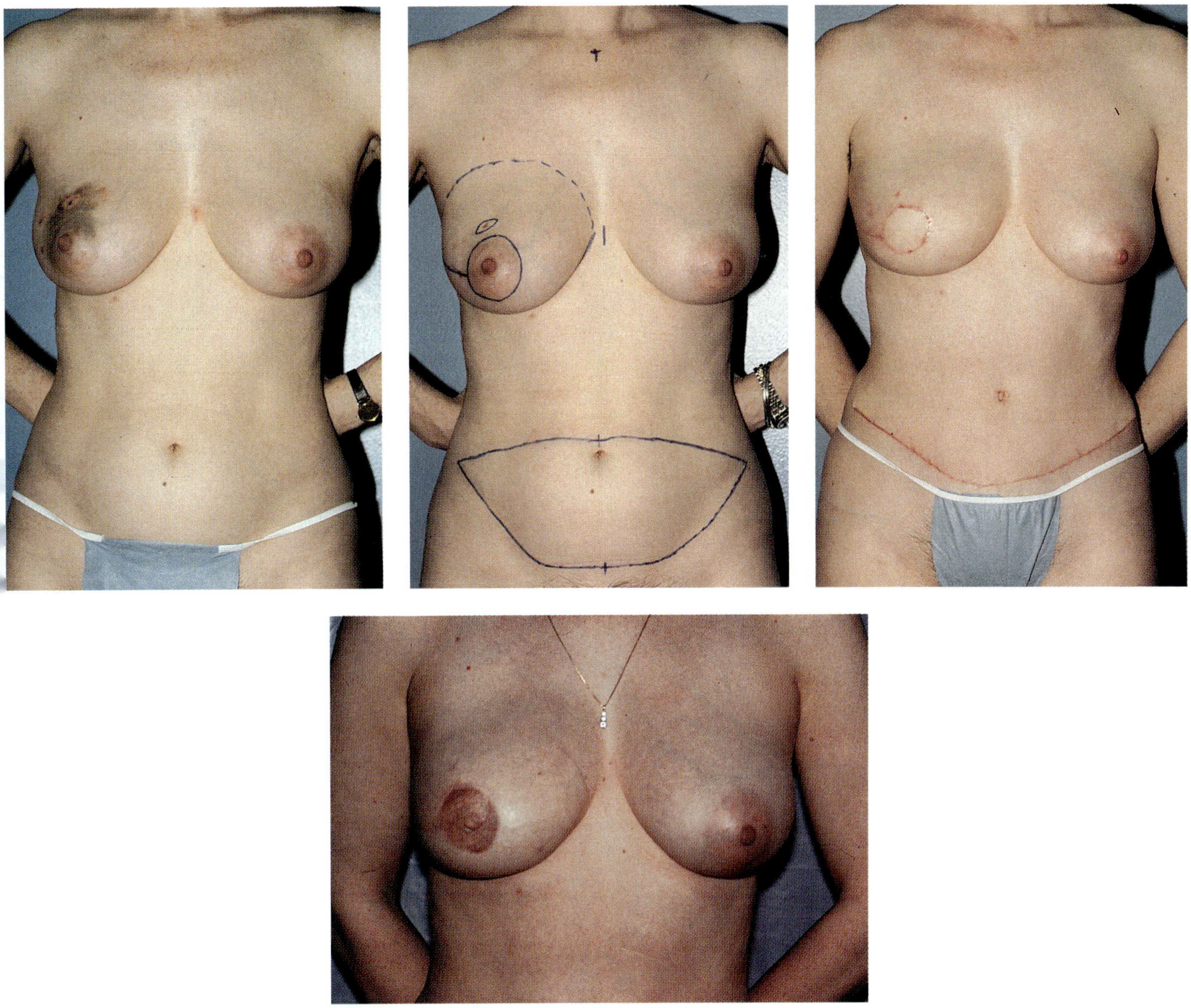

This 40-year-old woman presented with a small infiltrating ductal carcinoma of the right breast. Autogenous reconstruction using the free TRAM flap was performed. Following the initial procedure, the breast was slightly full in the lateral axillary area. Small corrections in this area as well as in the flanks were made using liposuction. Nipple reconstruction further reduced the size of the monitoring skin island from the TRAM flap. Postoperative tattooing completed the reconstruction, resulting in a completely buried flap and a good symmetric match.

Photographs from Grotting JC. Immediate breast reconstruction using free TRAM flap. Clin Plast Surg 21:207-221, 1994.

REVISIONS OF THE RECONSTRUCTED NIPPLE-AREOLA COMPLEX

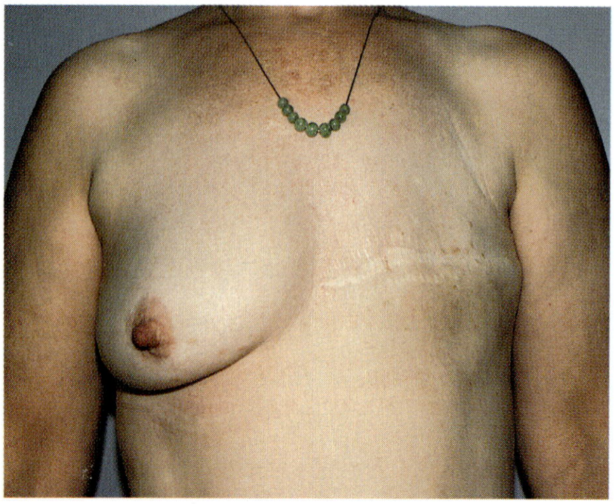

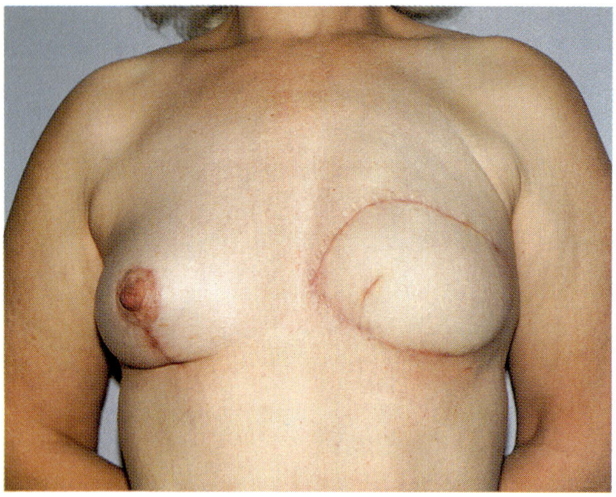

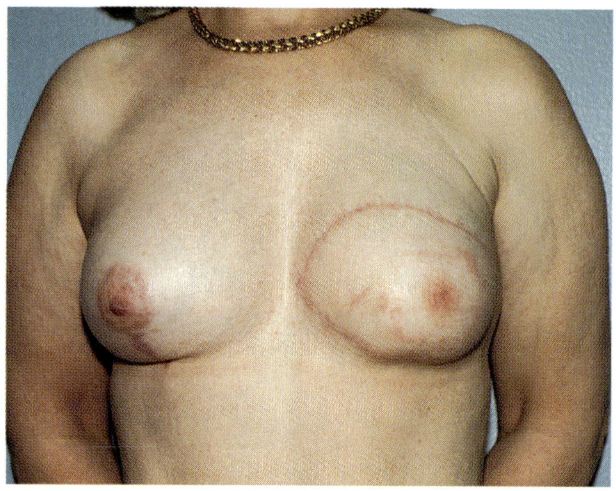

Complete loss of a reconstructed nipple is unusual, but composite grafts are particularly at risk for this complication. This patient suffered complete loss of a composite graft. I believe this was due to the fact that when the breast mound, created with a free TRAM flap, was revised, the pedicle to the flap was divided. The flap immediately became pale but appeared to have bleeding at the skin edges. We elected to proceed with nipple reconstruction using a composite graft. However, when the recipient site was deepithelialized, dermal bleeding was minimal. Although the breast flap survived in its entirety, the nipple reconstruction was lost.

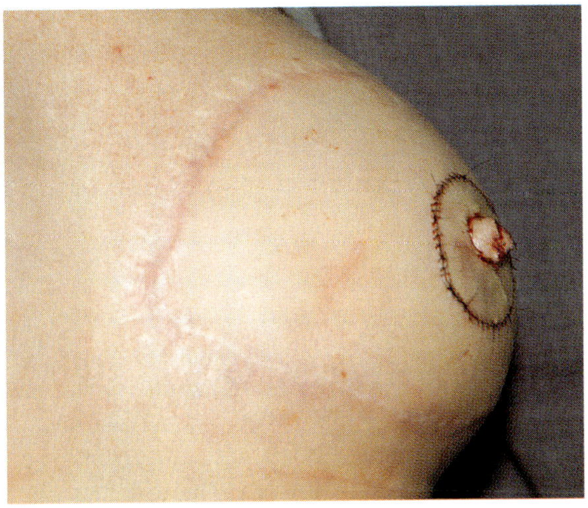 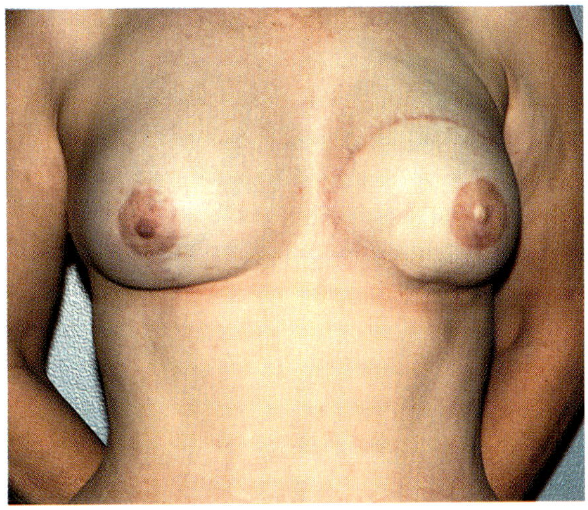

Secondary reconstruction using a skate flap was required.

Minor revisions of the reconstructed nipple are occasionally indicated. For example, the reconstructed nipple may heal with a small overhang of tissue or be tilted to one side. These problems are usually easily corrected on an outpatient basis at the time of tattooing. Some patients experience more atrophy of a reconstructed nipple than is desirable and request secondary correction. I have improved several such nipples by simply performing a second star flap reconstruction at the same location designed to include the original atrophied nipple. Another method of correction is to transfer a composite graft from the opposite nipple as an "on top–plasty." The previous inadequate nipple is simply bivalved and the composite graft is sutured into position on top.

In every case the tattooed areolar pigmentation will fade. It usually stabilizes 6 months to 1 year following initial application. Touch-ups are sometimes requested by the patient or suggested by our office nurse who now does most of these finishing touches. If the nurse believes that the color can be improved, this procedure is easily accomplished in the office. If the tattoo is too dark, lightening is more problematic: either a lighter color needs to be added on top of the darker pigment or a partial-thickness excision or dermabrasion must be performed to lighten the area before tattooing the area again.

DONOR SITE PROBLEMS

Some of the problems affecting donor sites from free flap breast reconstruction are discussed in Chapter 6. Specific problems that may need to be addressed at the time of revisional surgery for breast reconstruction are presented here.

TRAM Flap

Abdominal deformities following free TRAM flap transfer fall into the following categories: (1) hernia, (2) contour irregularities, (3) umbilical malposition or necrosis, and (4) scarring.

Hernia

To date, the incidence of hernia formation following free TRAM flap transfer has not dramatically lessened compared to that following conventional TRAM reconstructions. The reason is that both techniques violate the fascia in the most susceptible region of the abdominal wall: the interior rectus sheath at the level of the arcuate line and below. The internal oblique muscle and fascia play an important role in maintaining the integrity of the abdominal wall and must be carefully resutured following the harvest of the TRAM flap. Without innervated muscular support in this region, the fascia can attenuate, resulting in the characteristic bulge between the umbilicus and the pubis at the site of the muscle harvest. This hernia may be entirely asymptomatic except for a contour deformity. Other times, the patient may complain of general discomfort or a sharp pain in this area. A distinct fascial ring is usually not palpable. The patient may or may not request surgical correction. I have never seen an intestinal incarceration or other surgical emergency precipitated by this type of hernia.

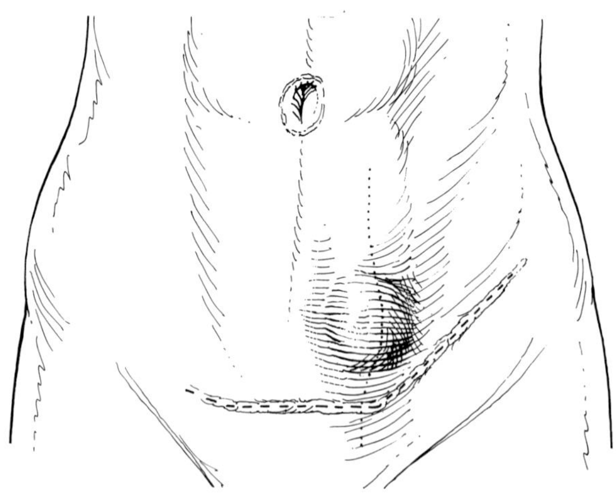

A bulge of this type can be corrected by reelevating, advancing, and reclosing the abdominal skin flap on the symptomatic side. Depending on the size and location of the defect, the umbilicus usually does not need to be released. In most cases it is not necessary to enter the abdominal cavity.

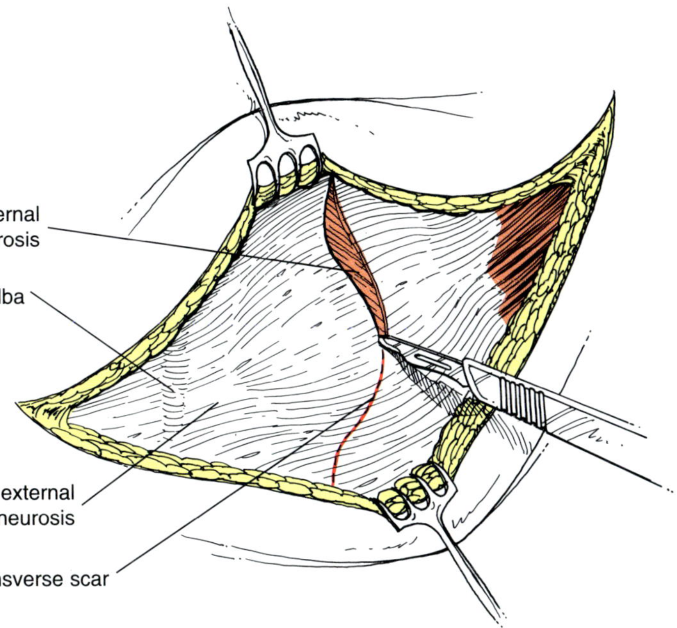

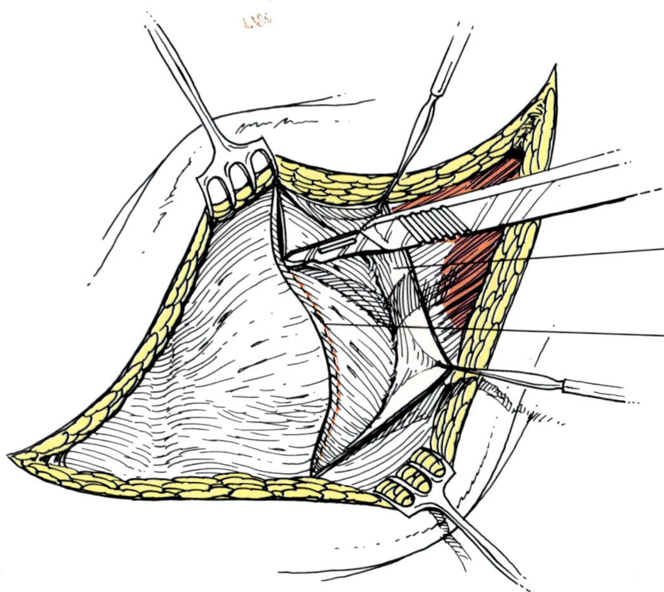

The external oblique fascia and internal oblique muscle are located laterally by palpation and the scarred edge is trimmed. Immediately and inferiorly, the linea alba and fascia above the pubis are incised sharply.

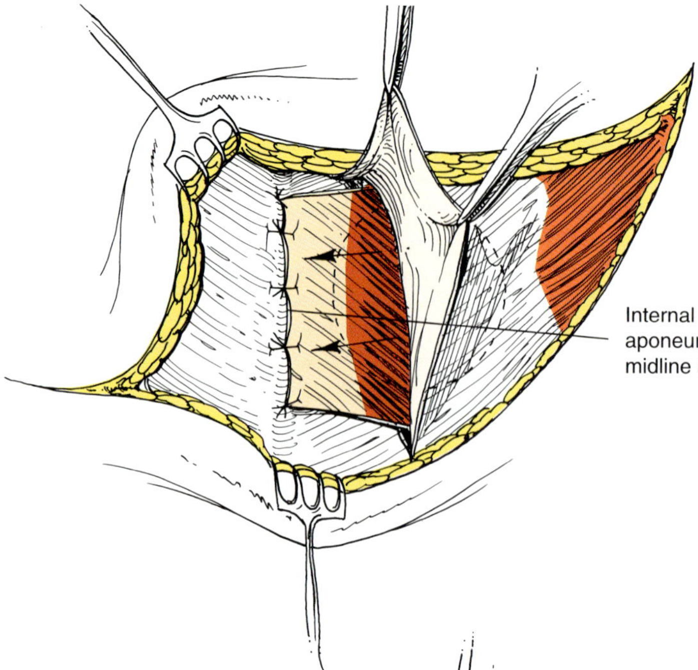

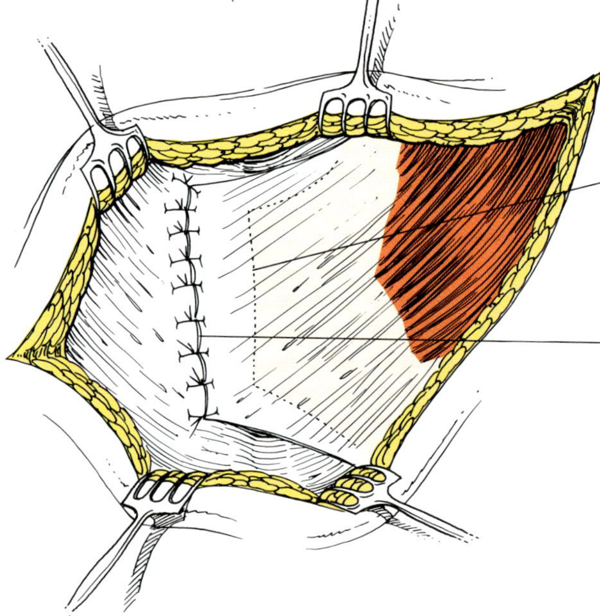

■ If the internal oblique and external oblique aponeuroses can be advanced medially and inferiorly for primary repair, this method of correction is preferred. ***For strong, long-term support, special care must be taken to achieve secure and accurate closure of the internal oblique aponeurosis.***

It is often not possible to primarily close the defect in larger hernias. Therefore a sheet of polypropylene mesh must be inserted. The mesh is stretched taut to maintain long-term support in the area and is sutured circumferentially inside the fascial rim circumference using mattress sutures. Drains are placed and the wounds are closed.

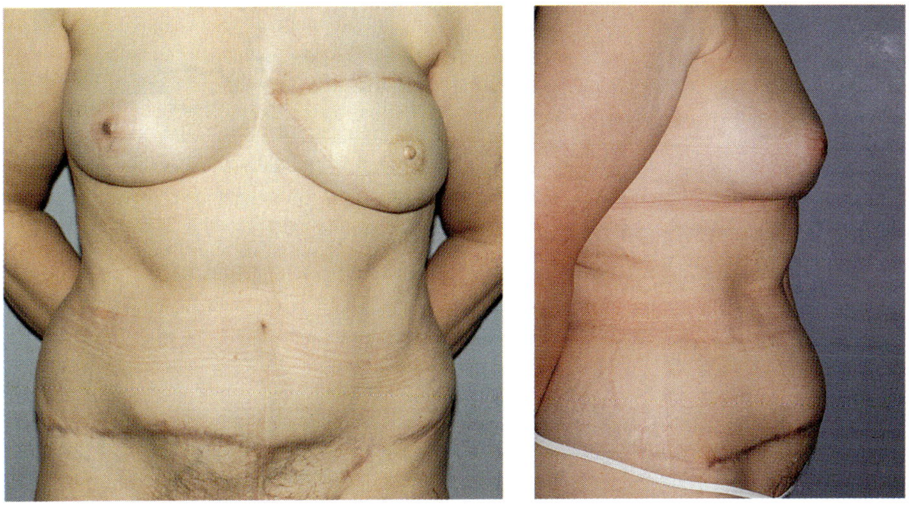

This 50-year-old patient underwent delayed reconstruction of the left breast using a contralateral microvascular free TRAM flap. Four months postoperatively, she noted the sudden onset of pain in the right inferior portion of the hypogastrium associated with the appearance of a visible bulge.

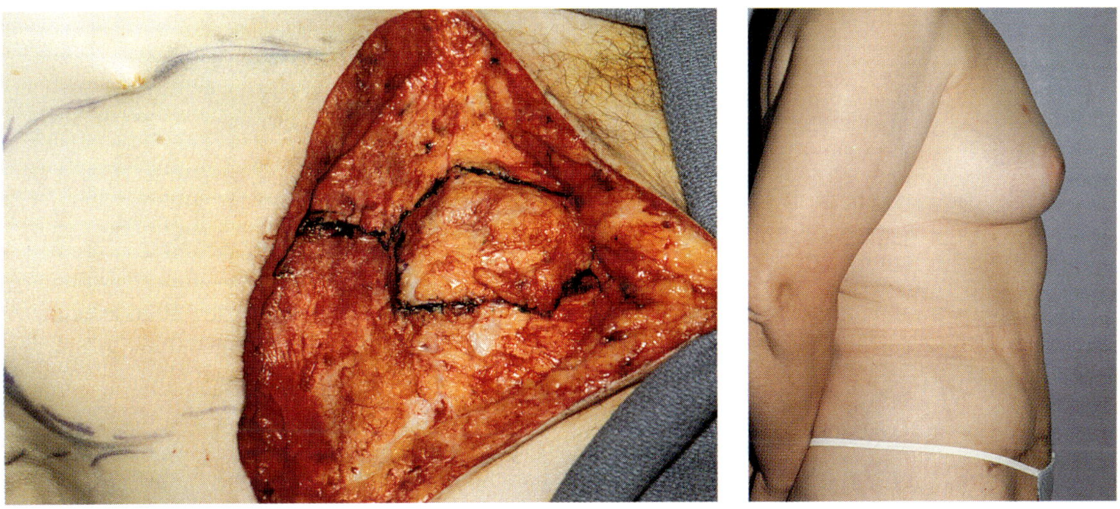

Exploration of this bulge revealed that the internal oblique and external oblique muscles had retracted well beyond the semilunar line. It was not possible to readvance these muscles; therefore a sheet of Marlex mesh was used to close the defect. Long-term correction has been maintained.

Photographs from Grotting JC. The TRAM flap. In Hartrampf CR Jr, ed. Hartrampf's Breast Reconstruction With Living Tissue. New York: Raven, 1991.

Contour Irregularities

Removal of an ellipse of skin and fat from the lower abdomen coupled with tightening of the epigastrium results in bulging of the flank fat and a change in the dimensions of the waistline. The abdominal closure can accentuate the bulging appearance. This deformity can be aggravating to some patients, particularly those who had excess fat in that area preoperatively. These contour irregularities are easily corrected at the time of nipple-areola reconstruction.

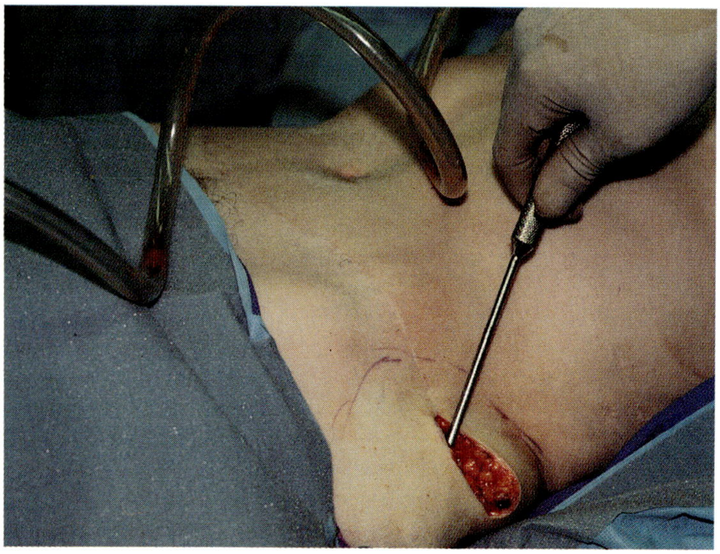

While the patient is in a standing position, the areas of excess fat are marked. These sites usually include the flank and occasionally a thick epigastric area as well. A small dog ear correction in the flank is often carried out at this time; liposuction of this area is performed through this incision. I prefer to use the syringe liposculpture technique for contouring. These regions may also be accessed through small stab wounds in the previous lateral abdominal scar.

Umbilical Malposition and Necrosis

If following the harvest of one or both rectus abdominis muscles the umbilicus is not brought back to the midline before fascial closure, it will heal off-center. This defect, which patients often find disturbing, can be difficult to correct. Occasionally slight malposition will result from the disruption of the tacking sutures placed between the dermis of the umbilical stalk and the rectus sheath. If this appears to be the cause of the deformity, a small incision is made at the border of the umbilicus, the dissection is carried down to the rectus sheath, and plication sutures are placed to draw the umbilicus into the midline. Only a small correction is possible via this local approach.

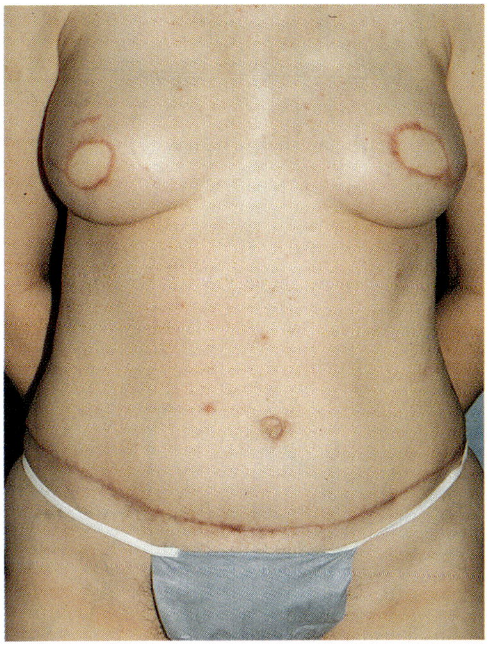

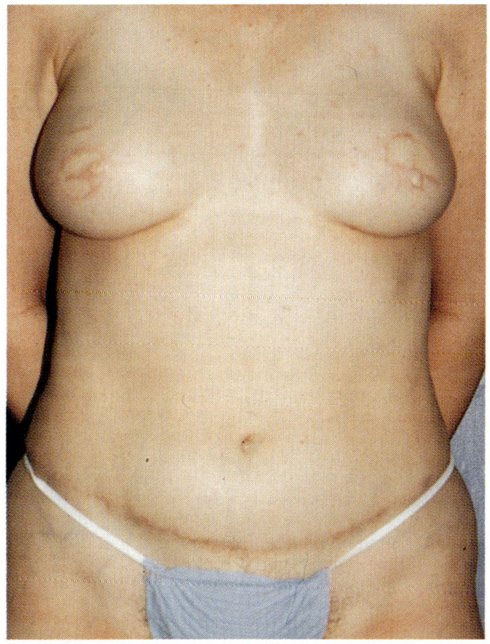

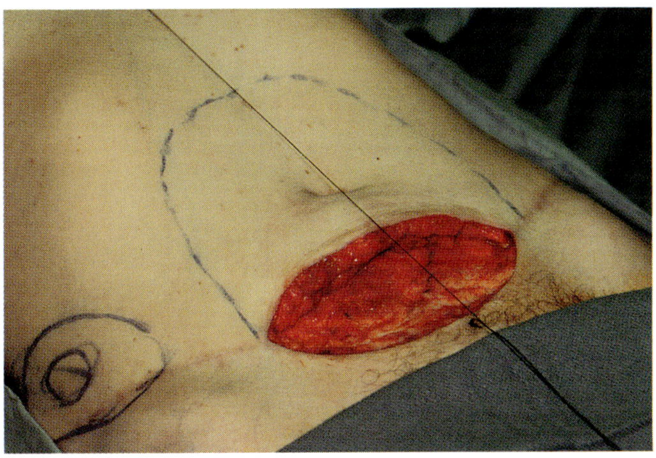

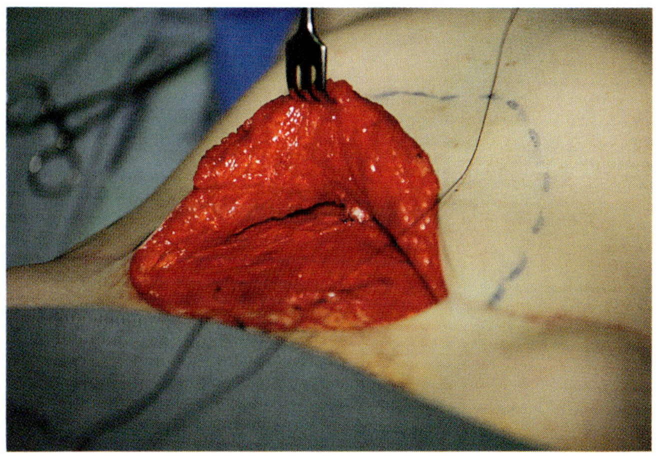

If the malposition is significantly more off-center, as it was in this patient, a more involved surgical repair is necessary.

The abdominal incision is reopened, the lower abdominal skin flap is reelevated, and the umbilical stalk is transected. The abdominal fascial defect is oversewn and the stalk is then drawn back into the midline and sutured with a heavy Prolene permanent suture. Drains are placed and the wound is reclosed.

Umbilical necrosis is an unfortunate complication that results from either the critical disruption of the circulation to the umbilicus or the suturing of the umbilicus under excess tension. Both result in death of the umbilical stalk, slough, and healing by secondary intention. A superficial depression and discolored scar occur but with none of the aesthetic features of the native umbilicus. Also, if the abdominal skin dehisces from the umbilical stalk, overhealing will result. The umbilical stalk may still be alive but healed underneath the abdominal skin. Cyst formation or local infection may ensue. Neoumbilicoplasty is recommended for both of these situations.

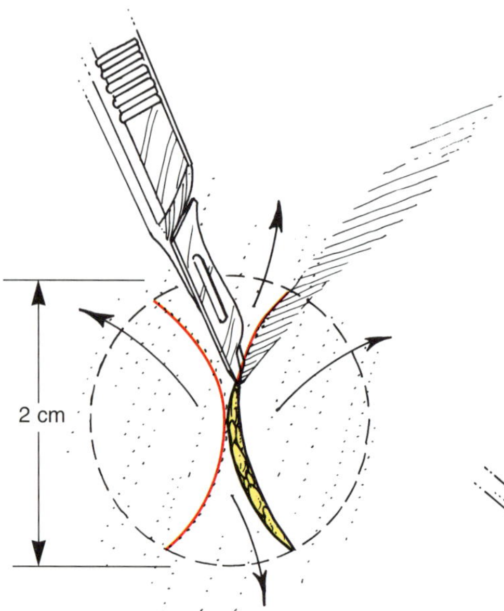

After Illouz

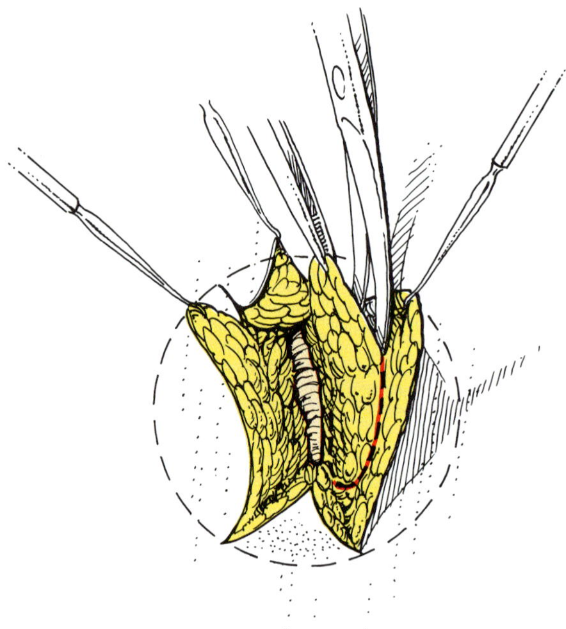

The umbilical position is determined and marked. Usually this site is at the location of the umbilical necrosis. The technique of Illouz[32] gives the best results.

Two semicircular flaps are incised and thinned. Small superior and inferior triangular flaps are also developed. The dissection is carried down to the anterior rectus sheath. Ideally the umbilical stalk is located and resutured to the abdominal skin flaps.

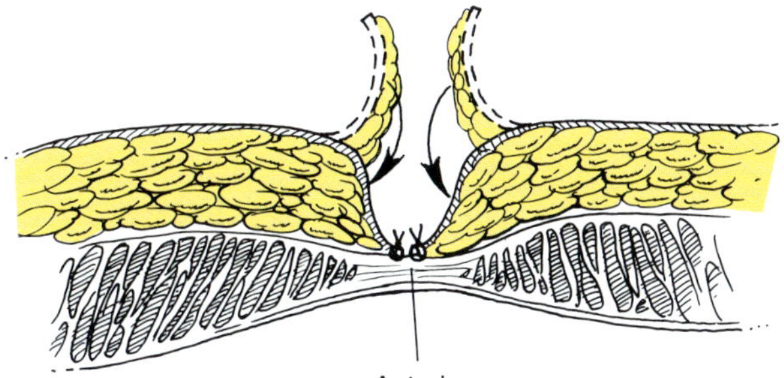

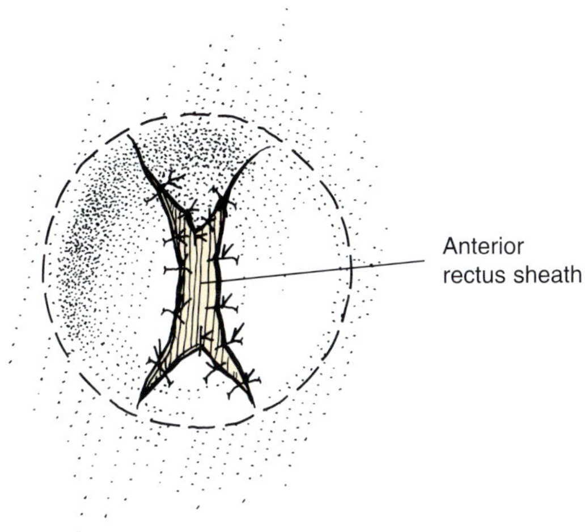

If the umbilical stalk is completely necrosed, then the skin flaps are sutured with permanent sutures to the linea alba or anterior rectus sheath. A skin graft in the depths of the wound can be used but is usually unnecessary.

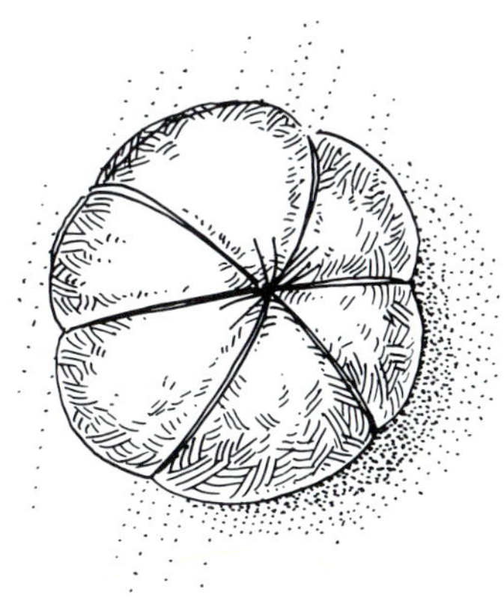

The umbilicus is then filled with a greasy gauze tie-over bolster dressing. This dressing is left in place for 5 days. Complete healing usually occurs in 10 to 14 days.

Scarring

Another minor problem following TRAM free flap harvest involves the abdominal scar. The scar may be widened or hypertrophic and require simple excision and layered closure. Occasionally, painful sutures may benefit by excision. In addition, not infrequently a small dog ear is present at either end of the abdominal scar. These dog ears can be elliptically excised and the wounds closed, creating a smoother contour to the abdominal scar.

Thigh Flap

Unilateral harvest of a lateral transverse thigh flap virtually always results in asymmetry of the trochanteric areas. Bilateral harvest is most frequently complicated by over-resection of fat and resultant depressions.

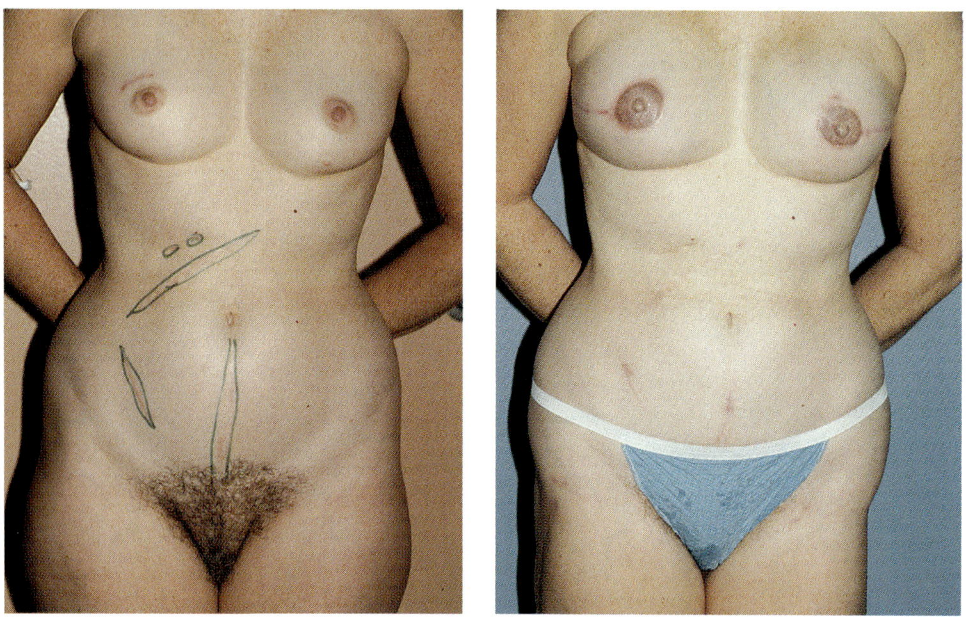

This 53-year-old patient required bilateral mastectomy and desired breast reconstruction using autogenous tissue. She was not a candidate for TRAM flap reconstruction because of multiple abdominal scars. On subsequent days during the same hospitalization she underwent bilateral mastectomy and reconstruction using lateral transverse thigh flaps. Although the shape and symmetry of the

Photographs from Grotting JC. Breast reconstruction with free tissue transfer. In Cohen M, ed. Mastery of Plastic and Reconstructive Surgery. Boston: Little, Brown, 1994.

breast reconstruction are satisfactory, the depressions left by overzealous harvesting of the thigh fat are quite apparent. This deformity is almost impossible to fully correct. Some additional liposculpturing could smooth out the surrounding area. Fat injection would be insufficient to fill the defects in this case.

The lateral vertical thigh flap causes the same problem if only a unilateral flap is harvested. However, the bilateral harvest of this flap improves the contour of the lateral thighs. The trade-off is a visible vertical scar similar to that which occurs with femoral osteotomies. However, the patients we have treated seem to accept this scar better than the resultant scar following harvest of the lateral transverse thigh flap. Contour deformities that occur following the harvest of the lateral vertical thigh flap can sometimes be treated with the transfer of local flaps. A small flap of subcutaneous fat designed in an area of excess fat is simply transposed into the area of deficit.

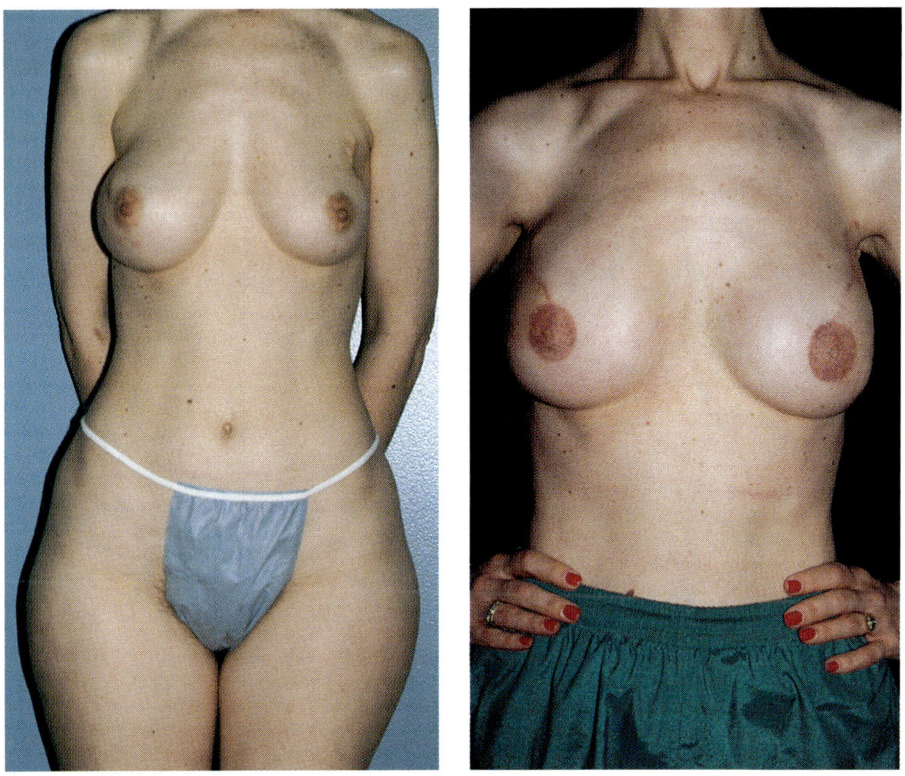

This 40-year-old patient required bilateral mastectomy and bilateral reconstruction. Due to insufficient abdominal tissue and her desire for autogenous reconstruction, lateral vertical thigh flaps were used.

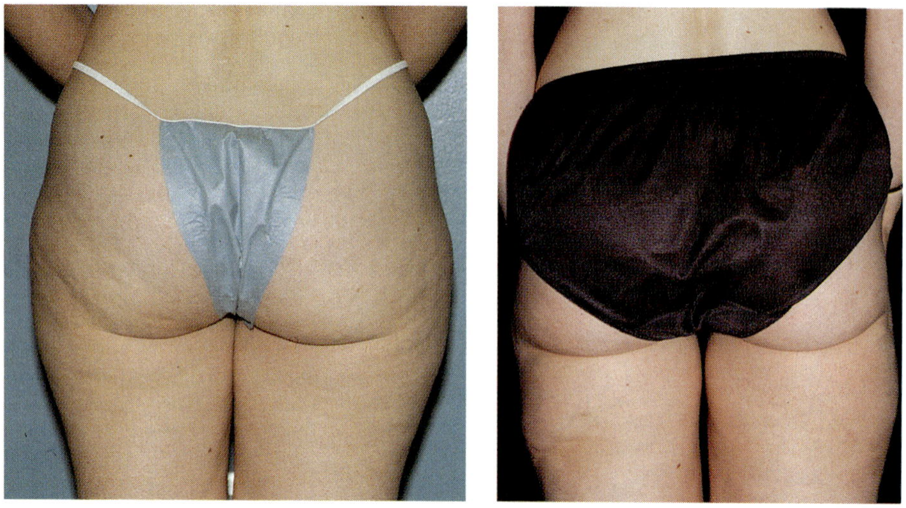

Comparison of the preoperative and postoperative contour of the donor site demonstrates a more acceptable appearance than that following the harvest of the lateral transverse thigh flap. Nevertheless, a minor revision was required using a small flap of subcutaneous fat transposed into a surface contour depression.

Gluteal Flap

Planning errors with the gluteal flap can result in wide, visible scars. Misplaced scars are not easily treated by any scar revision technique. Widened scars can be excised and reclosed in layers. When the superior gluteal flap is designed to be more transverse and in a lower position, the scar is more easily concealed. Similarly, the harvest of the inferior gluteal flap ideally should leave the scar in the infragluteal fold, where it is well hidden.

Unilateral flap harvest will always result in some degree of asymmetry. The lesser the amount of tissue harvested, the more symmetric the final result will be. If the asymmetry is marked, opposite buttock liposuction will help to balance it. Direct excision of the opposite buttock is a less preferable option; the patient must be willing to accept a contralateral scar.

NERVE INJURY

Peripheral nerve injuries can occur in free flap breast reconstruction. In the upper extremity these may be noted during the early postoperative period as a result of intraoperative positioning. For TRAM flap harvest and transfer the arms are usually positioned on arm boards at approximately 90 degrees.

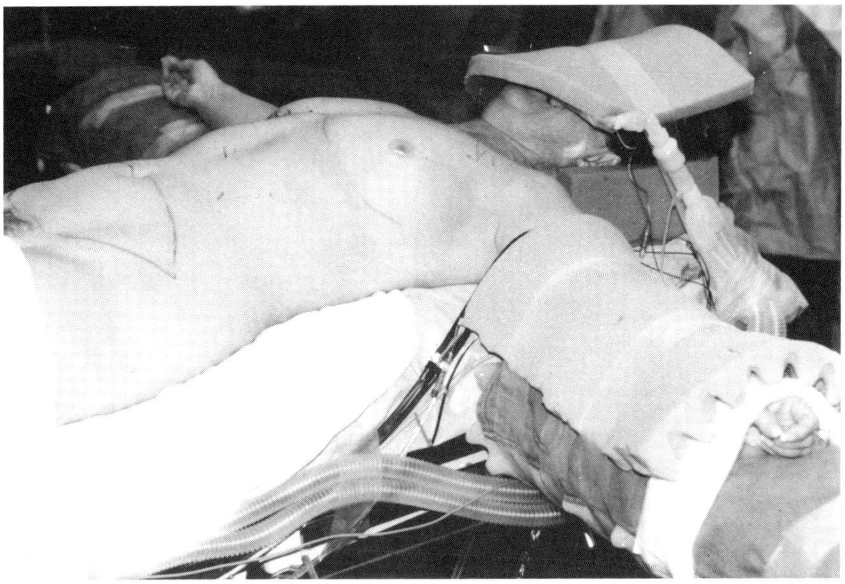

■ ***Careful padding and positioning of the arms is essential to prevent compression or stretch of the brachial plexus.*** The arms must not be abducted more than 90 degrees. The elbows should be slightly flexed and the forearms should be in the neutral position, neither supinated nor pronated.

Prevention of nerve injuries is the key. If neurapraxia occurs, conservative treatment is usually indicated. Patients with preexisting but possibly asymptomatic compression neuropathies are at risk for this problem. With diminished axonal flow due to pressure on the brachial plexus, patients may become symptomatic at the distal site of preexisting compression due to a "double crush injury." Most minor neurapraxias resolve within 30 days. If they persist, a baseline electromyogram and a nerve conduction study are indicated. Usually, however, even recalcitrant neurapraxias will completely resolve. If the patient does remain symptomatic and unimproved at 3 months, nerve release at the specific point of compression is indicated.[33]

In the lower extremity, sciatic nerve neurapraxia may be noted following inferior gluteal flap harvesting. Again, this is generally caused by intraoperative positioning and will virtually always resolve with conservative treatment.

Photograph from Core GB, Grotting JC. Peripheral nerve injury in the free TRAM procedure. Perspect Plast Surg 7(2):49–57, 1993.

CONCLUSION

Although free flap breast reconstruction has greatly increased in popularity among microsurgeons, the initial flap transfer represents only the first step on the path to a satisfying result. Most often, a planned second-stage breast mound revision coupled with skillful nipple-areola reconstruction will provide excellent symmetry, particularly in the context of immediate breast reconstruction. The reconstruction of a sensate breast remains investigational at the present time. Similarly, various surgeons are working toward a one-stage total breast reconstruction, including reconstruction of the nipple-areola complex. In the meantime, mere mortals need to be prepared for reoperations in the quest for perfect results.

References

1. Holmstrom H. The free abdominoplasty flap and its use in breast reconstruction. Scand J Plast Reconstr Surg 13:423, 1979.
2. Pennington DG. The rectus abdominis myocutaneous free flap. Br J Plast Surg 33:277, 1980.
3. Arnez ZM, Smith RW, Eder E, Solinc M, Kersnic M. Breast reconstruction by the free lower transverse rectus abdominis musculocutaneous flap. Br J Plast Surg 41:500, 1988.
4. Grotting JC, Urist MM, Maddox WA, Vasconez LO. Conventional TRAM flap versus free microsurgical TRAM flap for immediate breast reconstruction. Plast Reconstr Surg 83:828, 1989.
5. Nahai F, Bostwick J III. Microsurgical techniques. In Bostwick J III. Plastic and Reconstructive Breast Surgery. St. Louis: Quality Medical Publishing, 1991.
6. Friedman RJ, Argenta LC, Anderson R. Deep inferior epigastric free flap for breast reconstruction after radical mastectomy. Plast Reconstr Surg 76:455, 1985.
7. Grotting JC. Breast reconstruction with free tissue transfer. In Cohen M, ed. Mastery of Plastic and Reconstructive Surgery. Boston: Little, Brown, 1994.
8. Elliott LF. The lateral transverse thigh free flap for autologous tissue breast reconstruction. Perspect Plast Surg 3(2):80, 1989.
9. Fujino T, Harashina T, Aoyagi F. Reconstruction for aplasia of the breast and pectoral region by microvascular transfer of a free flap from the buttock. Plast Reconstr Surg 56:178, 1975.
10. Fujino T, Harashina T, Enomoto K. Primary breast reconstruction after a standard radical mastectomy by a free flap transfer. Plast Reconstr Surg 58:372, 1976.
11. Shaw WW. Breast reconstruction by superior gluteal microvascular free flaps without silicone implants. Plast Reconstr Surg 72:490, 1983.
12. Harashina T, Imai T, Nakajima H, Fujino T. Breast reconstruction with microsurgical free composite tissue transplantation. Br J Plast Surg 33:30, 1980.
13. Le Quang C. Two new free flaps developed from aesthetic surgery. II. The inferior gluteal flap. Aesthetic Plast Surg 4:159, 1980.
14. Paletta CE, Bostwick J III, Nahai F. The inferior gluteal free flap in breast reconstruction. Plast Reconstr Surg 84:875, 1989.
15. Jones GT, Cramer A, Cohen LB, McCraw B. The inferior gluteal-posterior thigh flap (the trefoil flap) for autologous reconstruction of the breast. Presented at the annual meeting of the American Society for Reconstructive Microsurgery. Kansas City, Mo.: September 1993.
16. Volpe AG, Rothkopf DM, Walton RL. The versatile superficial inferior epigastric flap for breast reconstruction. Ann Plast Surg 32:113-117, 1994.

17. Grotting JC. The free abdominoplasty flap for immediate breast reconstruction. Ann Plast Surg 27:351-354, 1991.
18. Allen RJ, Treece P. Deep inferior epigastric perforator flap for breast reconstruction. Ann Plast Surg 32:32-38, 1994.
19. Koshima I, Soeda S. Inferior epigastric artery skin flaps without rectus abdominis muscle. Br J Plast Surg 42:645-648, 1989.
20. Serafin D, Georgiade NG, Given KS. Transfer of free flaps to provide well-vascularized thick cover for breast reconstruction after radical mastectomy. Plast Reconstr Surg 62:527, 1978.
21. Serafin D, Voci V, Georgiade N. Microsurgical composite tissue transplantation: Indications and technical considerations in breast reconstruction following mastectomy. Plast Reconstr Surg 70:24, 1982.
22. Elliott LF, Hartrampf CR Jr. The "Rubens" flap for breast reconstruction. Presented at the annual meeting of the Southeastern Society of Plastic and Reconstructive Surgeons. Amelia Island, Fla.: June 1993.
23. Hartrampf CR Jr, Noel RT, Drazan L, Elliott LF, Bennett GK, Beegle PH. Rubens's fat pad for breast reconstruction: A peri-iliac soft-tissue free flap. Plast Reconstr Surg 93:402-407, 1994.
24. Yousif JN, Kolachalam RB, Matloub HS, Sanger JR. The axial orientation of perforators in the upper medial thigh: Anatomic basis of the transverse upper gracilis musculocutaneous flap. Presented at the Thirty-fourth Annual Meeting of the Plastic Surgery Research Council. Atlanta, Ga.: April 1989.
25. Vila R, Guinot A. Post-mastectomy breast reconstruction in an irradiated field using a contralateral latissimus dorsi free flap. Br J Plast Surg 35:371, 1982.
26. Le Quang C. Microvascular tissue transfer in plastic surgery. In Lie TS, ed. Microsurgery: Proceedings of the International Conference of the International Microscopical Society. Amsterdam: Excerpta Medica, 1979.
27. Le Quang C. Two new free flaps developed from aesthetic surgery. I. The lateral mammary flap. Aesthetic Plast Surg 4:147-157, 1980.
28. Schusterman M, Kroll SS, Weldon ME. Immediate breast reconstruction: Why the free TRAM over the conventional TRAM flap? Plast Reconstr Surg 90:255-262, 1992.
29. Anton MA, Eskenazi LB, Hartrampf CR Jr. Nipple reconstruction with local flaps: Star and wrap flaps. Perspect Plast Surg 5(1):67-78, 1991.
30. McCraw JB. Fish tail flap [poster session]. Presented at the annual meeting of the American Society of Plastic and Reconstructive Surgeons. Washington, D.C.: September 1992.
31. Wong RKM, Feldman S, Banducci DR. A modification of the Anton-Hartrampf star flap using pre-reconstruction tattooing. Perspect Plast Surg 7(1):137-140, 1993.
32. Illouz Y-G. How to create a new umbilicus. Aesthetic Surgery Newsletter, Summer 1992, p 16.
33. Core GB, Grotting JC. Peripheral nerve injury in the free TRAM procedure. Perspect Plast Surg 7(2):49-57, 1993.

32

Imaging Considerations in Plastic Surgery of the Breast

Eva Rubin, M.D.

Imaging Challenges

- Detection of silicone leakage
- Verification of implant integrity
- Breast tissue partially obscured by implant
- Difficulty differentiating abnormalities
- Recognition of postsurgical parenchymal alterations after breast surgery

For many years plastic surgical procedures of the breast, particularly augmentations with breast implants, were of relatively little interest to imagers. Screening mammography was in its infancy and implants had not been in place long enough to raise questions about the durability of these devices. When the occasion to perform mammography on women with breast implants presented itself, the mammographer was usually able to see very little breast tissue. The imaging procedure was effective in defining the contour of the implant but yielded little useful information about overlying breast tissue.

With the aging of these implanted devices and the recent FDA inquiry into their safety and their potential for masking the diagnosis of breast cancer on x-ray mammography, a tremendous interest has been generated in observing this patient population, with a corresponding increase in the number of related publications. Recent publications in the radiology literature focus on two major areas: the efficacy of mammography in the detection of significant breast disease in the patient with augmented breasts and the ability of various imaging procedures (including x-ray mammography, ultrasonography, CT, and MRI) to determine implant leakage or rupture.

In the energized setting created by the adverse publicity regarding implants, it is important not to lose sight of the fact that over 1 million women with implants will choose to keep them and that the potential risk from the implants themselves is likely to be substantially less than the natural lifetime risk of developing breast cancer, now estimated to be one in eight for American women.

The indications for screening mammography in women with implants should thus be the same as those in women without implants. A *diagnostic* x-ray mammogram may be indicated in a woman of any age for evaluation of a localized breast mass or other significant breast symptom (e.g., bloody discharge, nipple or skin retraction). *Screening* mammograms are currently recommended annually for women 50 years of age and older and every 1 to 2 years for women aged 40 to 49 years.[1] Some[2,3] believe that if screening is to be effective in women under 50 years of age that annual examinations are required. Others believe that routine mammographic screening of women under the age of 50 is not indicated.[4]

The recent massive media attention and questions raised by the FDA inquiry have caused some asymptomatic women under 40 years of age to request mammograms to determine if their implants are intact. Mammography at this age should not be encouraged unless there are indications to suggest rupture. The guidelines restricting the use of screening mammography in women under the age of 35 are based on sensible considerations of the risk-benefit ratio for this population. There are no data to suggest that these guidelines should be altered for women with implants. Optimal imaging of the patient with augmented breasts requires modifications in both radiographic technique and positioning.[5] Ultrasonography is extremely useful as an adjunct to the x-ray mammogram in some cases. CT and MRI may also be helpful in selected patients. The American Society of Plastic and Reconstructive Surgeons has issued guidelines to suggest that the imaging of patients with breast implants should be performed only at centers with demonstrated expertise in the handling of these patients.[6] The following discussion focuses on the use of radiographic methods for diagnosis and screening of women after aesthetic breast surgery.

PREOPERATIVE IMAGING EVALUATION

There are no data to suggest that women who undergo cosmetic breast surgery are at higher risk for development of breast cancer at an early age than other women. Thus there is little sense in performing routine preoperative x-ray mammography on women in their 20s before cosmetic breast surgery. The probability that a 20-year-old American woman will develop breast cancer in her third decade is less than 0.07%.[7] Sadowsky[8] has recommended that routine preoperative mammograms before cosmetic breast surgery be performed beginning at the age of 30 years. The rationale for the use of an earlier age for the initiation of screening in this patient population is unclear. We believe baseline mammograms before the age of 35 years should be reserved for the small subset of the population with a family history of premenopausal breast cancer.

If an abnormality is suspected on preoperative physical examination of the breasts, this should be investigated regardless of the patient's age. In women in their 20s and early 30s, ultrasonography may be the initial diagnostic imaging method for a palpable breast mass.[9,10] If a simple cyst is found, an x-ray mammogram may be unnecessary. Ultrasonography is capable of identifying breast cysts with nearly 100% accuracy[11]; unless the cyst is symptomatic, further intervention is also unnecessary. In young women with a dominant breast mass, fibroadenoma is more likely to be the cause than cystic disease. Since the ultrasonographic appearance of fibroadenoma may mimic a well-circumscribed carcinoma,[12,13] opinion is divided as to whether all such lesions require biopsy. This decision may be less problematic in the case of women undergoing cosmetic breast surgery in that excisional biopsy of a palpable solid mass can usually be performed at the time of the scheduled cosmetic procedure. Alternatively, fine-needle aspiration cytology[14] or core biopsy[15] may provide a definitive diagnosis if excisional biopsy is deemed undesirable. In cases in which a palpable abnormality is not depicted on ultrasonography or the ultrasonographic findings are suspicious for malignancy, an x-ray mammogram should be performed regardless of the patient's age.

THE AUGMENTED BREAST

The earliest attempts at breast augmentation involved the insertion or injection of a variety of foreign substances into the breast ranging from autogenous fat to ping-pong balls.[16] Direct injections of paraffin or silicone into breast tissue were popular in the early 1960s. These substances produce an intense foreign body reaction in the breast, resulting in the formation of numerous nodules (paraffinomas, siliconomas). The nodules typically range in size from several millimeters to 2 cm and most will calcify. Peripheral "eggshell" calcifications are perhaps the most common pattern, but extensive fine punctate or ring-shaped calcification may also occur.[17] Diagnostic breast imaging in these women using any presently known method is severely compromised. Fortunately, direct injection of silicone into breast tissue was banned by the FDA, and such augmentations are now rarely performed in the United States.

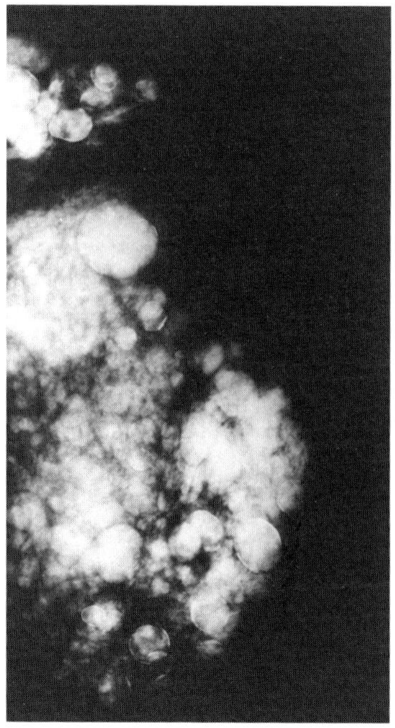

This detail from an x-ray mammogram of a woman who underwent augmentation with the injection of liquid silicone shows multiple, rounded, dense nodules of varying size throughout the breast. Many are surrounded by rim ("eggshell") calcification. The high kilovoltage required to depict the siliconomas results in overpenetration of the surrounding fatty breast tissue and skin.

Since the introduction of silicone gel–filled implants in 1963,[18] it is estimated that at least 1 million American women have undergone augmentation mammaplasty. The vast majority of implants used have contained either saline or silicone gel encased in a silicone elastomer envelope. Saline-filled silicone implants have advantages in breast imaging due to their relative radiolucency; however, fold-flaw fractures and valve leakage with these implants have resulted in higher reported leakage rates than silicone gel–filled implants. The spontaneous deflation rate of saline-filled implants is estimated to be about 1% per year.[19] Due to the current restrictions on the availability of silicone gel–filled implants, utilization rates of saline-filled implants have increased and will probably continue to do so until better alternatives are found. Experimental research using peanut oil– or radiolucent gel–filled implants[20-23] suggests that it is possible to modify implant construction to facilitate breast imaging.

In addition to the relative radiolucency of a breast implant, its position in the breast significantly affects the diagnostic quality of the image obtained. Implants may be placed in either the subglandular or subpectoral position. Ease of placement, more natural breast contour, and freedom from displacement due to contraction of the pectoralis major muscle have led some surgeons to favor subglandular insertion. However, it is possible to image a larger volume of breast tissue when the implant is placed subpectorally. Subpectoral placement also has the advantages of lower rates of capsular contracture and of loss of nipple sensation than subglandular insertion.[24]

There have been a number of publications regarding the volume of breast tissue obscured by a breast implant. In 1978, Wolfe[25] estimated that only 25% of breast tissue capable of generating a breast cancer was visible on xerograms in the presence of a gel-filled implant. The method by which this estimate was derived is unclear. More recently, Hayes, Vandergrift, and Diner[26] using planimetric measurements, calculated that 22% to 83% of breast glandular tissue was obscured on lateral and craniocaudal film screen mammograms. These statistics have been widely quoted in the literature to indicate that mammography is of limited usefulness after augmentation mammaplasty. However, the assumptions used in the calculation of obscured volume by Hayes and associates are questionable (e.g., the assumption that implant volume corresponds to that of a sphere), and measurements were performed on very few patients. There is no available study comparing the volume of breast tissue visible on a preoperative mammogram to that of breast tissue visible in the same patient after placement of an implant. Since the typical implant candidate is a woman with very small, usually dense-appearing breasts, preaugmentation x-ray mammography is usually not optimal in any case.

There is no doubt that some breast tissue is obscured by implants. The relatively rigid nature of implants limits the amount of compression that can be applied to breast tissue, and compression of the breast tissue produced by the implant itself compacts the tissue into a thin layer between implant and skin, resulting in apparent increased density of breast tissue. Both of these factors impair the quality of the diagnostic image; for this reason methods have been sought to rectify this problem.

In 1988, Eklund[27] published an article describing modified positioning for women with breast implants. In the Eklund technique the implant is displaced posteriorly against the chest wall and the breast tissue is pulled over and in front of the implant. The compression device is then lowered, in effect treating the implant as if it were the chest wall; the imaged area includes mainly breast tissue with little or no implant projected in the imaged field. This technique has resulted in a remarkable improvement in both the quality of the image and the volume of breast tissue imaged. Silverstein et al.[28] calculated the reduction in breast area imaged with standard nondisplacement mammography to be 49% in women with subglandular implants and 28% in women with subpectoral implants. Displacement mammography improved this reduction to 39% and 9%, respectively.

Although the optimal number of views for imaging patients with breast implants has yet to be firmly established, in many centers the examination of the implant patient consists of the four standard views (mediolateral oblique and craniocaudal views with the implant imaged on the film) and the four modified displacement or pushback views (mediolateral oblique and craniocaudal views with the implant off the film) or double the number of films required for a patient without implants. In patients with firm encapsulation of the implants, a supplemental true lateral view in the pushback position is often helpful.

The standard views obtained with the implant included are most helpful in depicting abnormalities related to the implant itself, whereas the modified views optimize the imaging of the breast tissue. Abnormalities of the implant include displacement, deformity of contour, rounding, puckers, protrusions, diverticula, and collapse. In women with abnormalities of the breast identified on the modified views, additional projections such as coned compression spots or magnification views can also be obtained using the pushback technique. Needle localization of nonpalpable lesions is also readily accomplished with the pushback technique.[29]

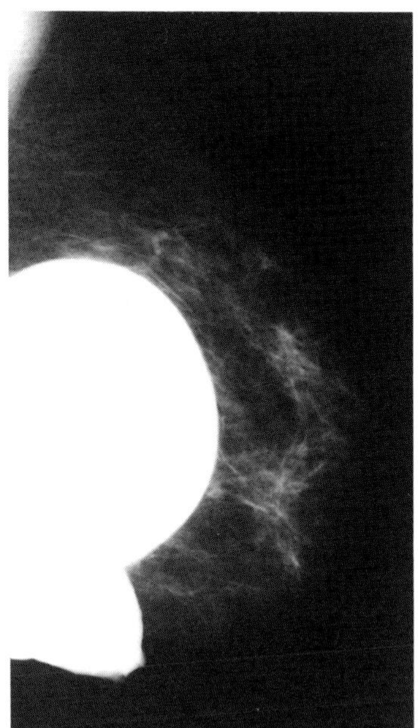

Courtesy Barbara Bear, M.D.

This mediolateral oblique mammogram shows a subglandular implant with a large triangular outpouching of the inferior portion of the implant. Films of the same breast earlier in the examination showed no evidence of this outpouching, which suggested that this deformity was produced or exaggerated by the mammographic compression. A small amount of leakage is visible and was unchanged from the year before.

Implant-Related Abnormalities

The issue of greatest concern currently is whether imaging is able to reliably detect leakage of silicone from the implant. The silicone elastomer envelope of an implant is not entirely impermeable to the silicone gel contained within it.[30] Although there is no scientific evidence that silicone is carcinogenic other than the induction of soft tissue sarcomas in rodents,[31] recent reports suggesting an association between silicone gel–filled implants and autoimmune or connective tissue disorders, particularly scleroderma,[32–38] have made detection of small amounts of leakage a major concern. Permeation of microscopic particles through the envelope is thought to be responsible for the fibrous capsule that forms around many implants.[39,40] The transudation of microscopic amounts of silicone gel through an intact implant envelope is called "bleed" and is contained within the fibrous capsule. The incidence of silicone bleed is unknown, but this phenomenon may occur normally with all silicone gel implants. By definition, it should be undetectable by imaging.

Microscopic amounts of silicone extruded through a detectable small hole in the implant envelope produce a thin (usually less than 0.5 mm thick) coating of silicone gel on the external surface of the implant and are best designated as "leaks." Frank "rupture" of the implant is best defined as those instances in which a major tear in the implant shell results in a large amount of silicone gel located between the implant shell and the capsule, whereas "extrusion" defines the situation in which the displaced silicone gel is present external to the capsule and in direct contact with mammary or extramammary tissue.[41] "Intracapsular rupture" and "extracapsular rupture" are also commonly used terms to describe "rupture" and "extrusion," respectively.

Silicone gel extrusion into breast tissue may occur due to puncture at the time of insertion, manufacturing defects in the implant device, spontaneous failure, and trauma. The most common cause of rupture in published series[42] has been closed capsulotomy, a forceful manual procedure performed to relax capsular contracture. Unusual causes of rupture include depressurization during airplane flight[43] possibly due to air inadvertently injected into an expandable implant at the time of surgery. There is at least one reported case of implant rupture occurring at the time of mammography.[44] It is considered that the compressive force applied during mammography is insufficient to rupture an intact implant. However, two studies have shown an inverse relationship between the pressure resistance[45] and integrity[46] of implants and the duration of implantation.

The incidence of rupture and extrusion is unknown but is likely more common than previously recognized. In one study of 51 silicone gel implants removed between 1987 and 1990, all 22 implants inserted more than 10 years previously were leaking or ruptured.[46] The age of a silicone-containing implant device should probably be kept in mind when applying mammographic compression or performing closed capsulotomy.

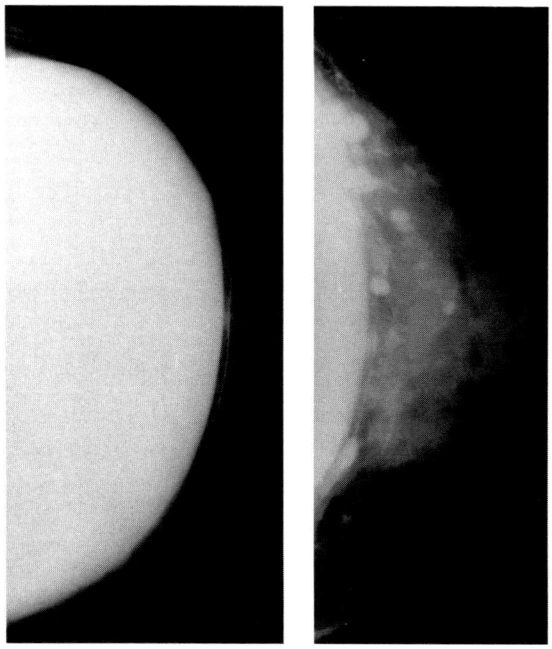

Extracapsular rupture is usually readily diagnosed on x-ray mammograms performed with the displacement technique. Such rupture may be diagnosed when globules of silicone are visible in the breast tissue on the x-ray mammogram. The standard nondisplacement view of a breast with a subglandular implant (left) shows a few rounded, dense nodules in the subareolar area. However, the displacement view of the same breast (right) shows multiple dense globules of silicone in breast parenchyma, confirming extracapsular rupture. Note the significantly improved visualization of the breast parenchyma with the displacement view.

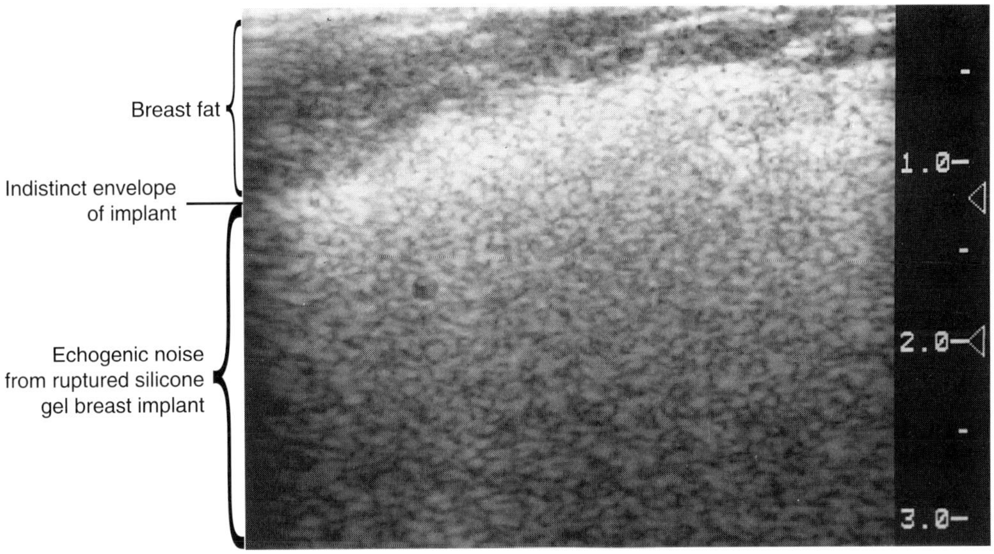

Extracapsular rupture can also be detected with ultrasonographic examination, which discloses abnormal echoes within the implant, showing disruption of normal breast-implant interface, or "echogenic noise" arising at the outer surface of the implant.[47,48]

Diagnosis of extracapsular rupture is facilitated by the detection of the migration of the silicone along tissue planes such as the fibers of the pectoralis major muscle. Silicone may be absorbed by lymph nodes in the axilla and rarely may migrate out of the breast into the infraclavicular area, arm, lower chest, abdomen, or groin. These latter findings may be best demonstrated by CT[49] or MRI.[50] In most cases of major extracapsular rupture, collapse or deformity of the implant will be identified on the imaging studies. There has been one case report of intraductal extension of silicone from ruptured breast implants[51] and several anecdotal reports of this phenomenon.[52]

Intracapsular ruptures are usually imperceptible on standard x-ray mammography since the intact fibrous capsule results in maintenance of the implant contour. Such ruptures may be recognizable on ultrasonography[53] but are probably best demonstrated by MRI.[54] MRI allows demonstration of the collapsed implant shell floating within the silicone gel, which remains contained within the fibrous capsule. The visible fragments of floating shell produce what has been called the "linguine sign" by Gorcyzca et al.[54]

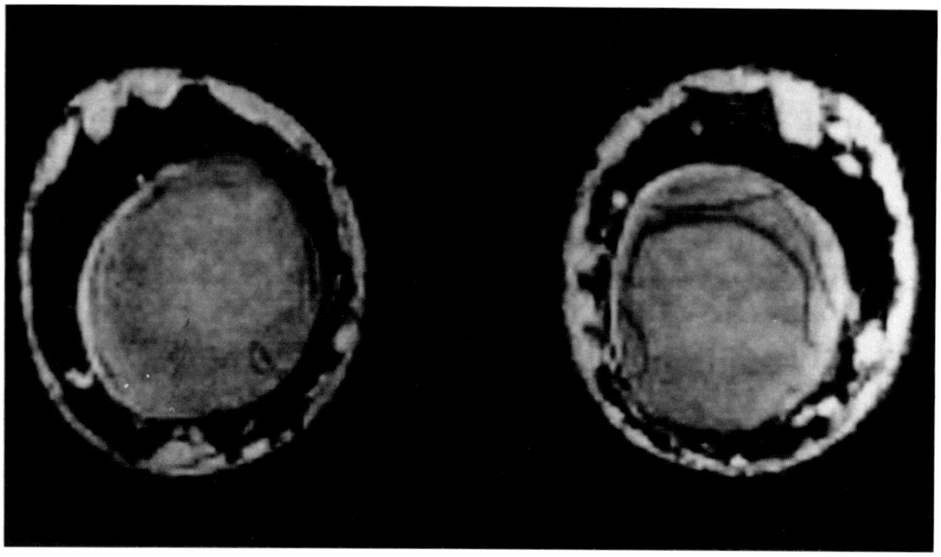

This MRI in axial projection shows intracapsular rupture manifest by serpiginous strands of low-signal intensity (linguine) in high-signal intensity silicone gel contained within the fibrous capsule. No abnormality was appreciable on the corresponding x-ray mammogram.

Fat-suppression sequences appear to be best for demonstrating the location of extruded silicone globules. These globules are usually manifest as round or curvilinear areas of decreased signal. Contour abnormalities are readily depicted on MRI as is fluid surrounding the implant. Neither of these findings is a reliable indicator of implant rupture. Both MRI and ultrasonography may yield false positive interpretations due to infoldings of the implant and pericapsular calcifications.

Periprosthetic calcification occurs in some implant patients. This complication was described as extremely rare in one reported study,[55] but in our experience, as well as in the more recent literature,[56] it is not uncommon if actively sought. The calcification is presumed to be dystrophic calcification and may simply be a foreign body reaction to the implant or may be the result of silicone "bleed" or "leakage." In any case it is the fibrous capsule that calcifies and not the implant itself.

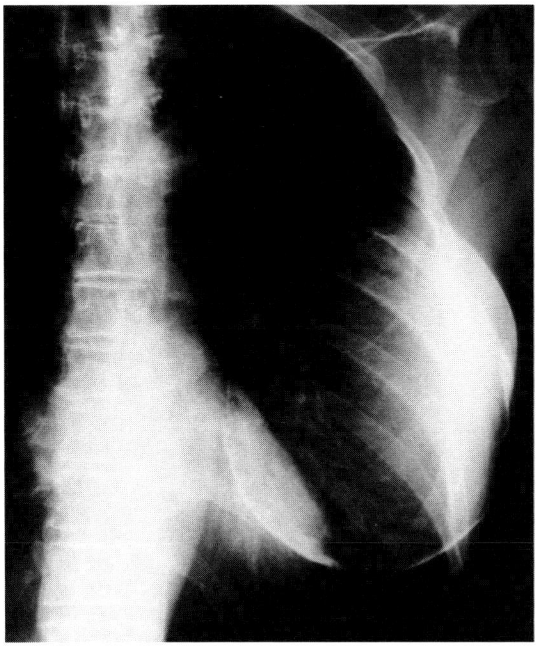

This detail from a rib film of a patient demonstrates extensive calcification of implant capsule.

If calcification adjacent to the implant is extensive and the implant is in subglandular position, abnormalities arising close to the implant may be obscured. In most cases pericapsular calcification is readily recognized as benign on the x-ray mammogram. Thin plaques of calcification or bulky curvilinear calcifications as well as the distinctive coarse calcifications of fat necrosis are most common. However, when the calcifications are fine and localized as may occur in the early stages of fat necrosis, distinction from malignant calcification may not be possible and biopsy will be required.[57]

Occasionally, deformities of contour of the implant may mimic breast masses. These are usually readily visible on the standard mammographic projections. Ultrasonography may also help to verify that a palpable abnormality represents the implant itself.[58,59] One must be cautious, however, not to mistake infoldings and wrinkles of the silicone envelope for tears.

Breast-Related Abnormalities

The fibrous capsule that forms around many implants is radiographically visible and should not be confused with leakage or rupture of the implant. Irregularity, distortion, or indentation of the capsule may be an indirect sign of a breast mass on the standard views. Most often, however, breast lesions are best identified on the modified Eklund views. Breast abnormalities include soft tissue nodules or masses, areas of architectural distortion, and calcifications. The criteria used for identifying the possible presence of malignancy are the same as for nonimplant patients: irregularity or spiculation of the margins of a dominant mass, parenchymal distortion in the absence of a history of biopsy in the distorted area, and clustered microcalcifications. All of these characteristics may be seen in the implant patient with or without a clinically detectable mass.

In 1988, Silverstein et al.[60] reported that breast cancers in implant patients were detected at a later stage than in patients without implants due to the obscuring effect of the implant on x-ray mammography. Although this report was not substantiated by others[61] and in fact was not supported by further accumulation of the data by the same authors,[62] many women continue to be fearful that mammography will not be effective in the presence of implants.

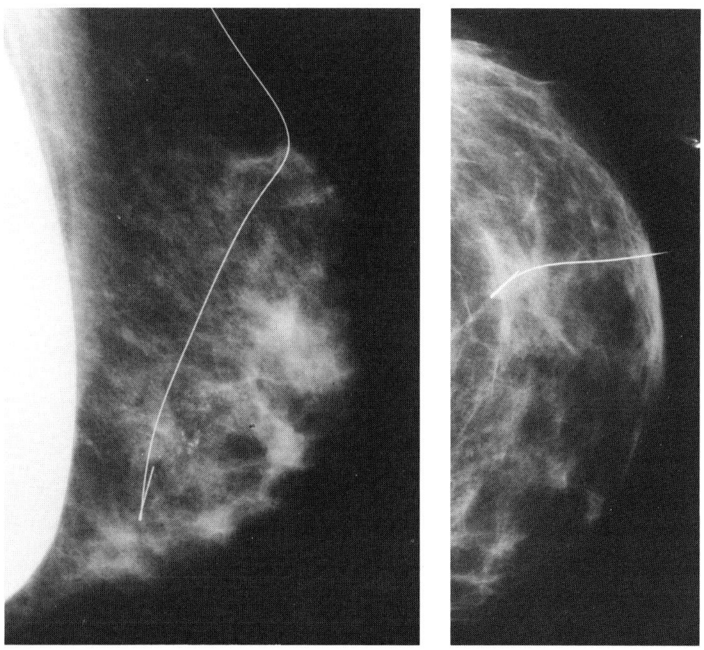

With careful attention to technique and positioning,[27,63-67] the diagnosis of early breast cancer should not be seriously impeded in women with breast implants. This mediolateral oblique pushback view of a breast with a subpectoral implant shows the needle localization wire in an area of pleomorphic malignant-appearing calcification. Histologic examination revealed ductal carcinoma in situ with microinvasion.

In this pushback craniocaudal view of another patient the needle localization wire is in a small, spiculated mass. Histologic study detected a 1 cm invasive ductal cancer. No abnormality was visible on the nonpushback projections.

There are relatively few cases of breast cancer reported to date in women who have had augmentation mammaplasty. However, most women who had implants placed 20 or 30 years ago are only now entering the age of major breast cancer risk. As the population of women with implants ages, one can anticipate a significant increase in the number of cancers found in women who have had augmentation.

Women with implants do not appear to be at increased risk for breast cancer[68]; their risk is similar to that of the general population. Thus it can be estimated that at least 100,000 to 200,000 cases of breast cancer will occur in the 2 million women who have undergone augmentation. Breast cancer screening should be encouraged in this population just as it is in other women.

Just as in nonimplant patients, if breast tissue is dense in the breast implant patient, masses may be obscured, especially if there is no associated distortion or calcification. If a palpable abnormality is present and is not identified on the x-ray mammogram because of dense tissue, ultrasonography may provide helpful diagnostic information. As mentioned earlier, cysts can be diagnosed with virtually 100% accuracy on ultrasonographic examination of the breasts. Since aspiration in the implant patient entails some risk of implant puncture, ultrasonographic evaluation may be preferable. If necessary, aspiration can be performed with ultrasonographic guidance, thereby minimizing the risk of entering the implant with the aspiration needle.

If a solid mass is detected on ultrasonography of a patient with a palpable abnormality, it may underscore the fact that biopsy is indicated. This is particularly true when the clinical findings are not definitive and the x-ray mammogram is unrevealing. There is as yet no proven use of ultrasonography in the absence of clinical or mammographic abnormality; its use simply for screening purposes in women with dense breast tissue is unproven.

Reduction Mammaplasty

Although surgical techniques for breast reduction vary, most involve a combination of three incisions: a vertical incision from nipple to inframammary fold along the 6-o'clock axis of the breast, an incision along the inframammary fold, and a circumareolar incision. The scars produced by these incisions are quite distinctive, and recognition by the experienced mammographer of the previous surgery is not a problem in the majority of cases.[69,70] Redistribution of the breast parenchymal tissue is usually clearly evident on the x-ray mammogram.

The alterations of parenchymal distribution occur in nonanatomic fashion but are usually bilaterally symmetric. Residual fibroglandular tissue often is transposed from its normal upper outer quadrant position toward the lower half of the breast. Bandlike configurations of parenchyma, long linear strands, and a whorled pattern of the residual parenchyma are common. Skin thickening is usually evident in the infra-areolar area. The bilateral symmetry of the findings and nonanatomic alterations in the parenchymal pattern are clues that the parenchymal distortion is postsurgical rather than neoplastic.

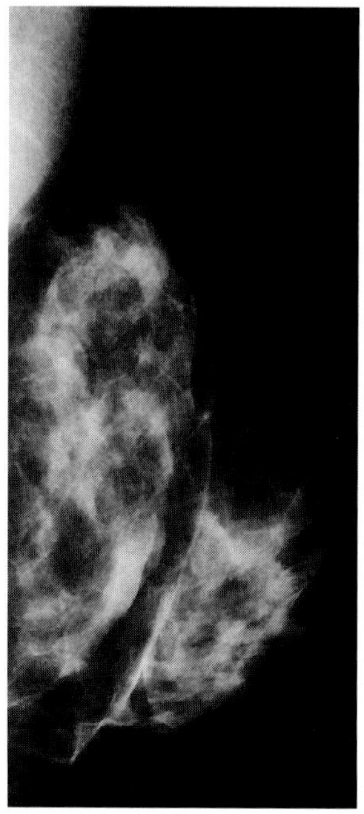

This mediolateral oblique mammogram of a patient following reduction mammaplasty shows separation of residual fibroglandular tissue into two distinct clumps, with nonanatomic transposition of parenchyma into the anterior region of the breast.

Dystrophic calcifications along scars or elsewhere in breast parenchyma commonly occur after reduction mammaplasty as do other manifestations of fat necrosis: lucent areas (oil cysts) with or without calcification and spiculated soft tissue densities that are usually of low density. In the early stages, when calcifications are still fine or when spiculation is not accompanied by distinctive coarse calcifications, differentiation from carcinoma may not be possible and biopsy may be indicated.

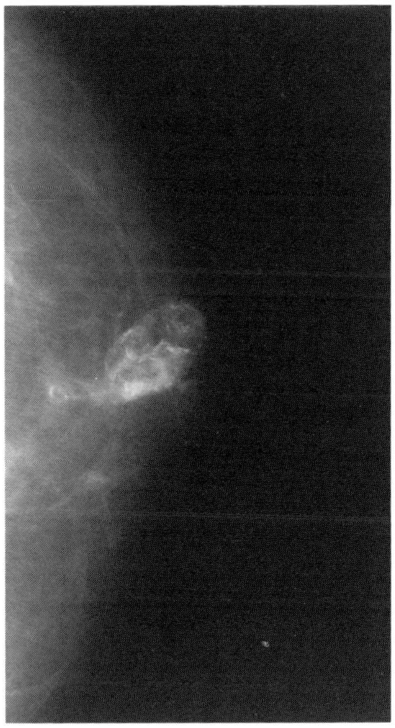

This craniocaudal x-ray mammogram of a patient 5 years after reduction mammaplasty shows a large area of calcified fat necrosis in the subareolar area.

Epidermal inclusion cysts are also found in breasts that have undergone reduction mammaplasty.[71] These cysts occur when infolding of the dermis during repositioning of the nipple-areola complex results in inclusion of some epidermal elements. Such cysts commonly develop along the inframammary incision or the vertical infra-areolar incision. They are usually nonpalpable and radiographically are depicted as well-defined noncalcified nodules. They often contain internal echoes on ultrasonography, mimicking solid masses. Rupture of an epidermal inclusion cyst may produce a pericystic inflammatory reaction, simulating the appearance of carcinoma on x-ray mammography. Knowledge of the usual location and appearance of these cysts may be sufficient for diagnosis.

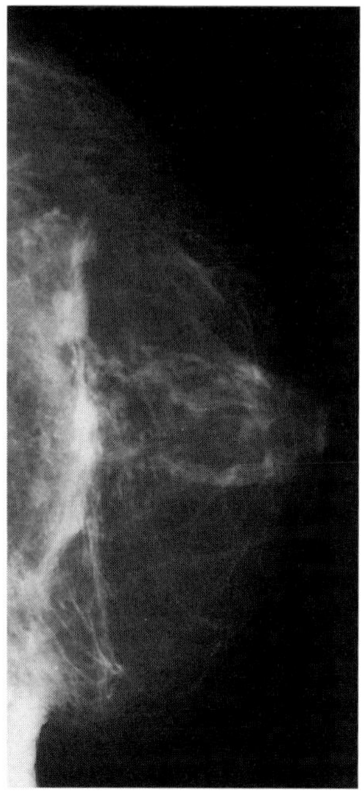

This mediolateral oblique mammogram shows numerous dense ovoid nodules—epidermal inclusion cysts—projected along the line of a reduction mammaplasty scar.

Stereotaxic or ultrasonographic guided fine-needle aspiration or core biopsy may be used if a more definitive diagnosis is deemed necessary.

Unlike the usual patient presenting for augmentation, the patient requesting reduction often has fatty breast tissue and on average is somewhat older. Reduction is also commonly performed after reconstruction of the contralateral breast after mastectomy. The benefits of preoperative mammography in the patient population in whom reduction mammaplasty is indicated are clear both because physical examination is hampered in breasts of large volume and because most of these patients are in a high-risk age group. Diagnosis of breast cancer in these patients at the time of or following surgery is clearly not ideal.[72]

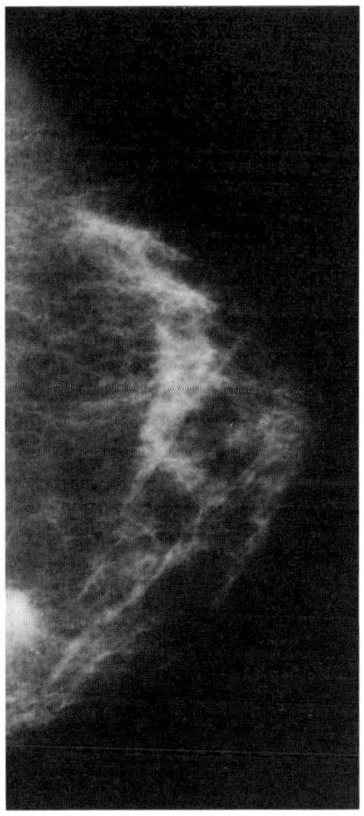

This craniocaudal mammogram of the left breast was obtained from a 45-year-old woman who 2 years previously had undergone contralateral mastectomy and reconstruction. Reduction mammaplasty of the left breast had been performed for symmetry. The irregularly marginated nodule in the medial area of the breast was new and in an atypical location for an epidermal inclusion cyst.

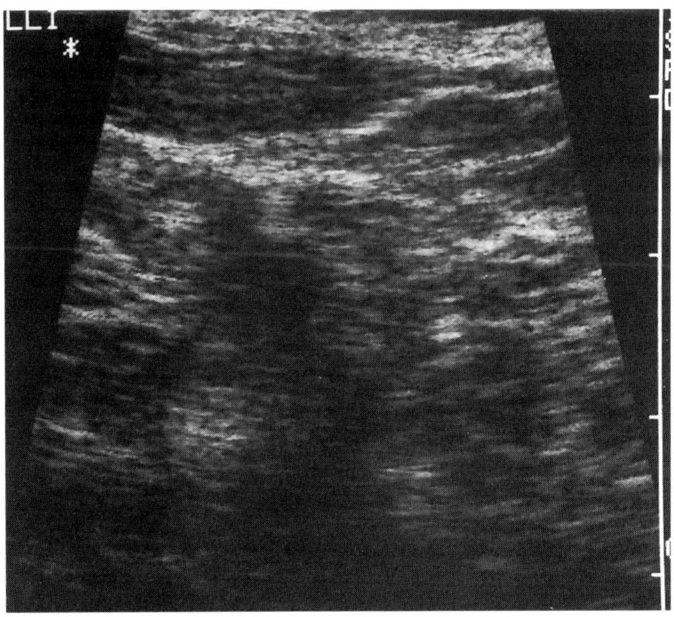

Ultrasonography revealed an irregularly shaped, solid nodule with acoustic shadowing that was highly suspicious for malignancy.

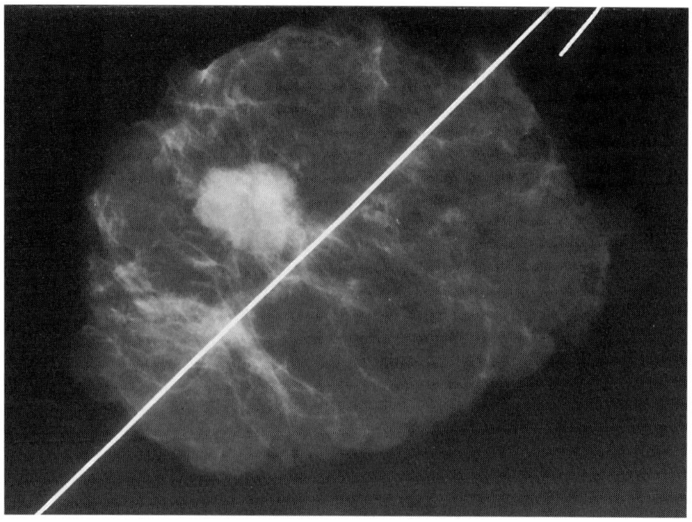

The specimen radiograph shows the excised nodule—an 8 mm invasive ductal cancer.

RECONSTRUCTIVE BREAST SURGERY

To date there has been relatively little published regarding imaging of the reconstructed breast. Reconstruction may be performed with a tissue expander (implant) or by transfer of a musculocutaneous flap, most often from the rectus abdominis muscle. With more and more women taking advantage of this procedure following surgery for breast cancer, studies are needed to determine the utility of imaging the reconstructed breast.

Masses in the reconstructed breast may occur due to fat necrosis, epidermal inclusion cysts, or chest wall recurrence. In cases in which breast tissue has not been completely excised, a true local breast recurrence is possible. Mammography is an excellent way of depicting the changes of fat necrosis in the reconstructed breast and may have some utility in the investigation of postoperative breast pain or other complications in these patients. Whether it also has utility in the detection of breast cancer recurrence has yet to be established. Unfortunately chest wall recurrence is virtually always an indicator of disseminated metastasis when it occurs and is not presently curable.[73] Even if mammography or chest wall CT[74] were able to detect recurrence earlier, one can question whether the asymptomatic patient needs to know this at an earlier time than when the disease would become clinically apparent.

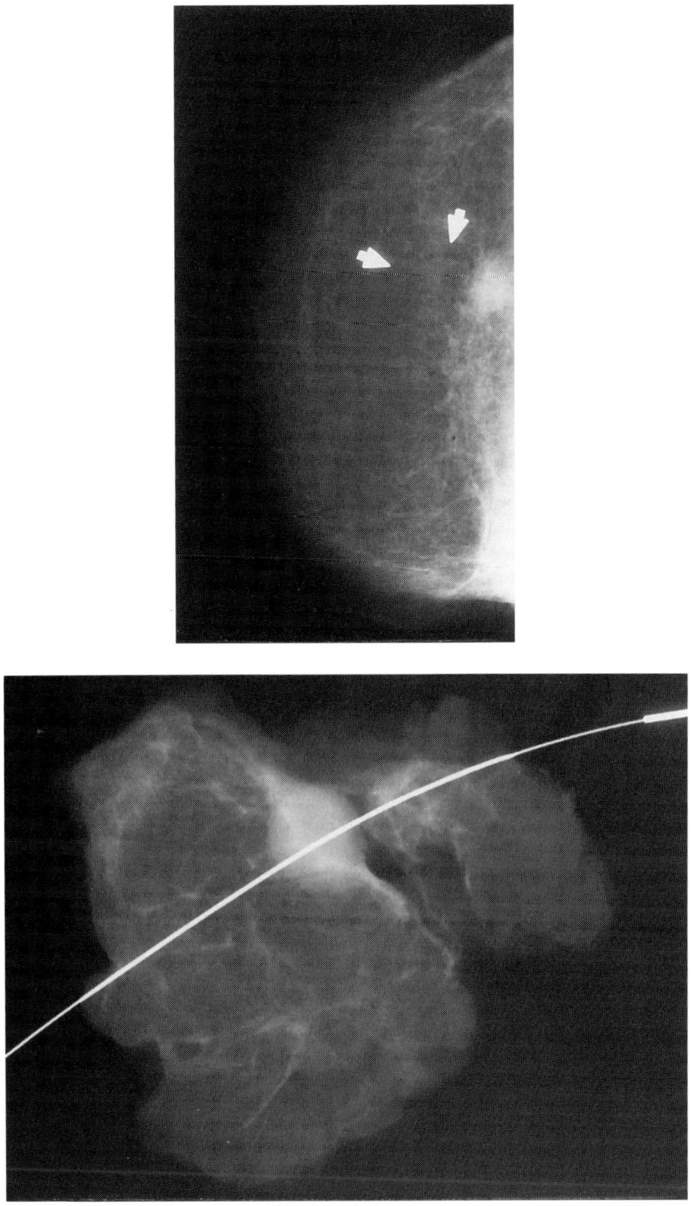

On craniocaudal view (top) of this TRAM flap–reconstructed breast, an irregularly marginated nodule (arrows) was thought to be suspicious for recurrence. However, the specimen radiograph of the excised nodule (bottom) proved the nodule to be an epidermal inclusion cyst. Note the sharp margins of the nodule compared to those of the lesion depicted on the opposite page.

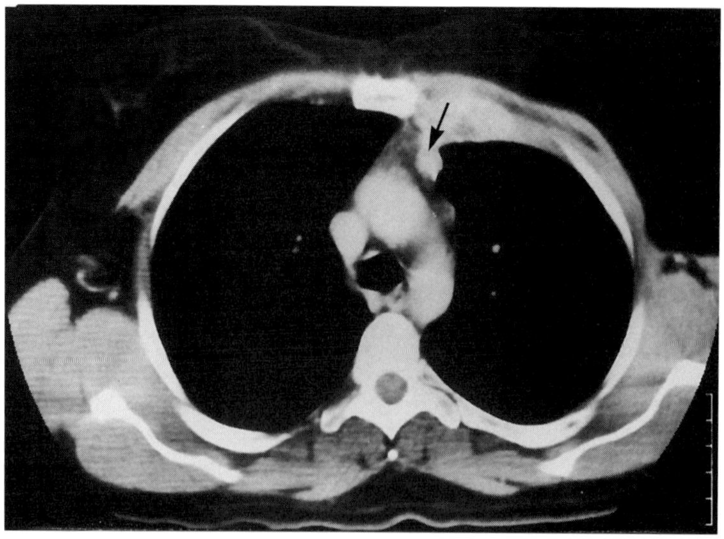

This axial CT of the chest of a 35-year-old woman following mastectomy of the left breast with free TRAM flap breast reconstruction shows a large internal mammary recurrence extending into the pectoralis major muscle.

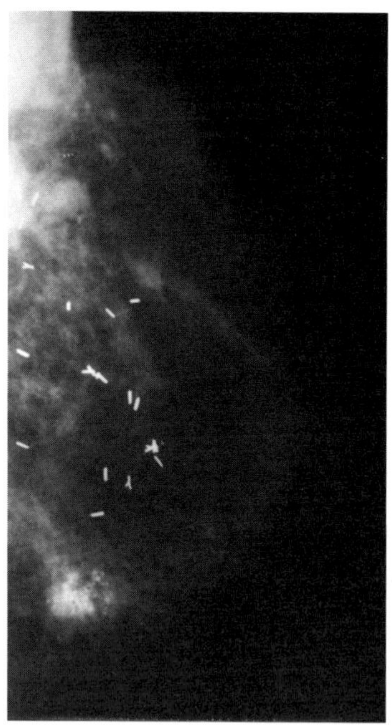

On this mediolateral oblique view of a TRAM flap breast reconstruction, an area of calcified fat necrosis is visible in the lower region of the breast. In the upper region of the breast, extending from the chest wall, is an irregular, dense, nodular area, which was found to be invasive ductal cancer on fine-needle aspiration biopsy performed under ultrasonographic guidance.

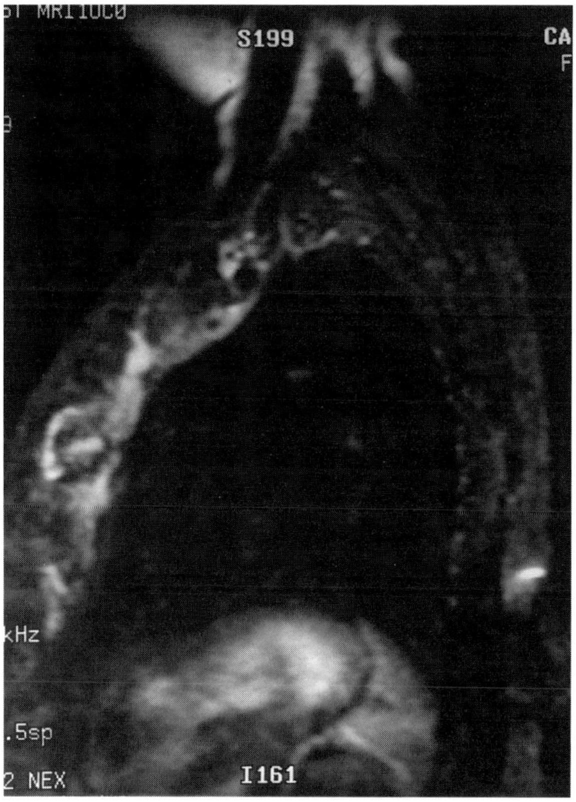

The gadolinium-enhanced MRI in lateral projection depicts a high-intensity signal, which represents an extensive breast cancer recurrence that extends along the upper posterior portion of the TRAM flap reconstruction toward the infraclavicular area.

Routine imaging of the reconstructed breast is probably not justified outside a clinical trial. However, since development of masses (usually due to fat necrosis) in the reconstructed breast is not uncommon and is certainly worrisome to the patient and her physicians when it occurs, a baseline postoperative x-ray mammogram of the reconstructed breast is suggested 1 year after surgery. Whether such mammograms should be repeated annually or only at the onset of symptoms remains to be established.

CONCLUSION

Currently there is no diagnostic imaging method that surpasses the x-ray mammogram for evaluation of diseases of the breast. Mammography provides helpful information both in symptomatic (diagnosis) and asymptomatic (screening) women. Women whose breasts have been altered by plastic surgery provide special problems in diagnostic imaging. Modified imaging techniques are now available to maximize the amount of breast tissue visible in the presence of a breast implant.

The verification of implant integrity is a problem unique to the woman who has undergone augmentation with a silicone gel prosthesis. Initial imaging of women with suspicion of this complication should consist of an x-ray mammogram with standard and displacement techniques. If extracapsular rupture is demonstrated, further imaging is unnecessary. If findings suspicious for carcinoma are found, additional mammographic views and/or ultrasonography should be performed. If x-ray mammography is negative or indeterminate and there is clinical suspicion of rupture, ultrasonography is the examination of choice. Ultrasonography may confirm rupture or identify a mass not visible on x-ray mammogram and is considerably less costly than other alternatives. If ultrasonography fails to elucidate the situation, MRI should be considered because it is the best available method for the detection of intracapsular rupture and anatomic depiction of the location of extruded silicone relative to vital structures.

Women who have had cosmetic breast surgery and who are of an appropriate age should undergo screening mammograms according to currently accepted guidelines. Preoperative mammograms should be performed no earlier than baseline mammograms recommended for women in general unless there is clinical suspicion of a localized breast lesion.

Some of the changes that occur in the postoperative breast mimic those of breast carcinoma. Recognition of the expected changes following augmentation, reduction, and reconstruction mammaplasty should avoid the need for biopsy for most benign postsurgical abnormalities. The use of additional views, spot compression, and magnification can and should be performed in the postsurgical breast when indicated for evaluation of breast lesions detected clinically or by mammography. Ultrasonography is particularly useful in the evaluation of palpable masses in patients with breast implants but should be used as an adjunct and not as a substitute for x-ray mammography. With careful attention to detail and knowledge of the alterations that may occur due to the various surgical procedures, the diagnosis of disease (both clinical and occult) in the cosmetically altered breast should not be compromised.

References

1. American Cancer Society. Mammography guidelines 1983: Background statement and update of cancer-related checkup guidelines for breast cancer detection in asymptomatic women age 40 to 49. CA 33:25, 1983.
2. Tabar L, Fagerberg G, Day ME, et al. What is the optimum interval between mammography screening examinations? Br J Cancer 55:547, 1987.
3. Moskowitz M. Guidelines for screening for breast cancer. Is a revision in order? Radiol Clin North Am 30:221, 1992.
4. Smigel K. NCI's proposed breast cancer screening guidelines. J Natl Cancer Inst 85:1627, 1993.
5. Bassett LW, Brenner RJ. Considerations when imaging women with breast implants. Am J Roentgenol 159:979, 1992.
6. Position Statement: Detection of Breast Pathology in Women With Breast Implants. Arlington Heights, Ill.: American Society of Plastic and Reconstructive Surgeons, 1987.
7. Seidman H, Mushinski MH, Gelb SK, et al. Probabilities of eventually developing or dying of breast cancer: United States, 1985. CA 33:25, 1985.
8. Sadowsky NL. Discussion of Hayes H, Vandergrift J, Diner WC. Mammography and breast implants. Plast Reconstr Surg 82:7, 1988.
9. Rubin E, Miller VE, Berland LL, et al. Hand-held real-time breast sonography. Am J Roentgenol 144:623, 1985.
10. Hilton SVW, Leopold G, Olson LK, et al. Real-time breast sonography: Application in 300 consecutive patients. Am J Roentgenol 147:479, 1986.
11. Sickles EA, Filly RA, Calley PW. Benign breast lesions: Ultrasound detection and diagnosis. Radiology 151:467, 1984.
12. Cole-Beuglet C, Soriano RZ, Kurtz AB, et al. Fibroadenoma of the breast: Sonomammography correlated with pathology in 122 patients. Am J Roentgenol 140:369, 1983.
13. Fornage BD, Lorigan JG, Audry E. Fibroadenomas of the breast: Sonographic appearance. Radiology 172:671, 1989.
14. Fornage BD, Faroux MJ, Simatos A. Breast masses: US-guided fine-needle aspiration-biopsy. Radiology 162:409, 1987.
15. Parker SH, Lovin JD, Jobe WE, et al. Nonpalpable breast lesions: Stereotactic automated large-core biopsies. Radiology 180:403, 1991.
16. Bostwick J III. Aesthetic breast surgery. In Plastic and Reconstructive Breast Surgery. St. Louis: Quality Medical Publishing, 1990, p 195.
17. Jensen SR, Mackey JK. Xeromammography after augmentation mammoplasty. Am J Roentgenol 144:629, 1985.
18. Safety of silicone breast prostheses. FDA Drug Bull 19:2, 1989.
19. Worton FW, Seifert LN, Sherwood R. Late leakage of inflatable silicone breast prostheses. Plast Reconstr Surg 65:302, 1980.
20. Gumicio CA, Pin P, Young VL, et al. The effect of breast implants on the radiographic detection of microcalcification and soft-tissue masses. Plast Reconstr Surg 84:772, 1989.
21. Beisang AA III, Geise RA, Ersek RA. Radiolucent prosthetic gel. Plast Reconstr Surg 87:885, 1991.
22. Handel N, Silverstein MJ, Gamagami P, et al. An in vivo study of the effect of various breast implant filler materials on mammography. Plast Reconstr Surg 91:1057, 1993.
23. Steinbach BG, Hiskes SK, Fitzsimmons JR, et al. Phantom evaluation of imaging modalities for silicone breast implants. Invest Radiol 27:841, 1992.
24. Mahler D, Hauben DJ. Retromammary versus retropectoral breast augmentation—A comparative study. Ann Plast Surg 8:370, 1982.

25. Wolfe JN. On mammography in the presence of breast implants. Plast Reconstr Surg 62:286, 1978.
26. Hayes H, Vandergrift J, Diner WC. Mammography and breast implants. Plast Reconstr Surg 82:1, 1988.
27. Eklund GW, Busby RC, Miller SH, et al. Improved imaging of the augmented breast. Am J Roentgenol 151:469, 1988.
28. Silverstein MJ, Handel N, Gamagami P, et al. Mammographic measurements before and after augmentation mammoplasty. Plast Reconstr Surg 86:1126, 1990.
29. Robertson CL, Kopans DB, McCarthy KA, et al. Nonpalpable lesions in the augmented breast: Preoperative localization. Radiology 173:873, 1989.
30. Barker D, Retsky M, Schultz S. "Bleeding" of silicone from bag-gel breast implants and its clinical relation to fibrous capsule reaction. Plast Reconstr Surg 61:836, 1978.
31. Oppenheimer BS, Oppenheimer ET, Stout AP. Sarcomas induced in rodents by imbedding various plastic films. Proc Soc Exp Biol Med 79:366-369, 1952.
32. Spiera H. Scleroderma after silicone augmentation mammoplasty. JAMA 260:236, 1988.
33. Brozena SJ, Fenske NA, Cruse W, et al. Human adjuvant disease following augmentation mammoplasty. Arch Dermatol 124:1383, 1988.
34. Varga J, Schumacher R, Jimenez SA. Systemic sclerosis after augmentation mammoplasty with silicone implants. Ann Intern Med 111:377, 1989.
35. Jennings DA, Morykwas MJ, DeFranzo AJ, et al. Analysis of silicon in human breast and capsular tissue surrounding prostheses and expanders. Ann Plast Surg 27:553, 1991.
36. Silver RM, Sahn EE, Allen JA, et al. Demonstration of silicon in sites of connective-tissue disease in patients with silicone-gel breast implants. Arch Dermatol 129:63, 1993.
37. Fenske NA, Vasey FB. Silicone-associated connective-tissue disease. The debate rages. Arch Dermatol 129:97-98, 1993.
38. Bridges AJ, Conley C, Wang G, et al. A clinical and immunologic evaluation of women with silicone breast implants and symptoms of rheumatic disease. Ann Intern Med 129: 97, 1993.
39. Rees TD, Platt J, Ballantyne DL. An investigation of cutaneous response to dimethyl polysilicone (silicone liquid) in animals and humans—A preliminary report. Plast Reconstr Surg 35:131, 1965.
40. Wickham MG, Rudolph R. Silicone identification in prosthesis-associated fibrous capsules. Science 199:432, 1978.
41. Dowden RV. Definition of terms for describing loss of gel from breast implants. Am J Roentgenol 160:1360, 1993.
42. Anderson B, Hawtof D, Alani H. The diagnosis of ruptured breast implants. Plast Reconstr Surg 84:903, 1989.
43. Lovich SF. Breast implants and air flight. Plast Reconstr Surg 85:172, 1990.
44. Hawes DR. Collapse of a breast implant after mammography. Am J Roentgenol 154:1345, 1990.
45. van Rappard JHA, Sonneveld GJ, van Twisk, et al. Pressure resistance of breast implants as a function of implantation time. Ann Plast Surg 21:566, 1988.
46. deCamara DL, Sheridan JM, Kammer BA. Rupture and aging of silicone implants. Plast Reconstr Surg 91:1828, 1993.
47. Levine RA, Collins TL. Definitive diagnosis of breast implant rupture on ultrasonography. Plast Reconstr Surg 87:1126, 1991.
48. Harris KM, Ganott MA, Shestak K, et al. Detection of silicone leaks: A new sonographic sign. Radiology 183:145, 1992.
49. Scott IR, Miller NL, Fitzpatrick DG, et al. Ruptured breast implant: Computed tomographic and mammographic findings. Can Assoc Radiol J 39:152, 1988.
50. Bilbey JH, Connell DG. MRI diagnosis of a ruptured breast implant presenting as an infraclavicular mass. Can Assoc Radiol J 44:224-226, 1993.
51. Leibman AJ, Korsoff MB, Kruse BD. Intraductal extension of silicone from a ruptured breast implant. Plast Reconstr Surg 89:546, 1992.

52. Robinson G. Personal communication, 1992.
53. DeBruhl ND, Gorczyca DP, Ahn C, et al. Silicone breast implants: Ultrasound evaluation. Radiology 189:95, 1993.
54. Gorczyca DP, Sinha S, Ahn C, et al. Silicone breast implants in vivo: MR imaging. Radiology 185:407, 1992.
55. Young VL, Bartell T, Destouet JM, et al. Calcification of breast implant capsule. South Med J 82:1171, 1989.
56. Ganott MA, Harris KM, Ilkhanipour ZS, et al. Augmentation mammoplasty: Normal and abnormal findings with mammography and US. Radiographics 12:281, 1992.
57. Mendelson EB. Evaluation of the postoperative breast. Radiol Clin North Am 30:107, 1992.
58. Mendelson EB. Imaging the post-surgical breast. Semin Ultrasound CT MR 10:154, 1989.
59. Shestak KC, Ganott MA, Harris KM, et al. Breast masses in the augmentation mammaplasty patient: The role of ultrasound. Plast Reconstr Surg 92:209, 1993.
60. Silverstein MJ, Handel N, Gamagami P, et al. Breast cancer in women after augmentation mammoplasty. Arch Surg 123:681, 1988.
61. Brody GS. Breast implants and cancer detection [letter]. Plast Reconstr Surg 85:204, 1990.
62. Silverstein MJ, Gierson ED, Gamagami P, et al. Breast cancer diagnosis and prognosis in women augmented with silicone gel-filled implants. Cancer 66:97, 1990.
63. Dershaw DD, Chaglassian TA. Mammography after prosthesis placement for augmentation or reconstructive mammoplasty. Radiology 170:69, 1989.
64. Leibman AJ, Kruse B. Breast cancer: Mammographic and sonographic findings after augmentation mammoplasty. Radiology 174:195, 1990.
65. Grace GT, Roberts C, Kelman Cohen I. The role of mammography in detecting breast cancer in augmented breasts. Ann Plast Surg 25:119, 1990.
66. Carlson GW, Curley SA, Martin JE, et al. The detection of breast cancer after augmentation mammoplasty. Plast Reconstr Surg 91:337, 1993.
67. Leibman AJ, Kruse BD. Imaging of breast cancer after augmentation mammoplasty. Ann Plast Surg 30:111, 1993.
68. Berkel H, Birdsell DC, Jenkins H, et al. Breast augmentation: A risk factor for breast cancer? New Engl J Med 326:1649, 1992.
69. Miller CL, Feig SA, Fox JW IV. Mammographic change after reduction mammoplasty. Am J Roentgenol 149:35, 1987.
70. Buhtz C, Freitag J, Berge G, et al. Mammographische Befunde nach Mammareduktionsplastik. Zentralbl Chir 114:36, 1989.
71. Fajardo LL, Bessen SC. Epidermal inclusion cyst after reduction mammoplasty. Radiology 186:103, 1993.
72. Gottlieb JR, McKinney P, Walkinshaw MD, et al. Occult breast carcinoma in patients undergoing reduction mammaplasty. Aesthetic Plast Surg 13:279, 1989.
73. Gilliland MD, Barton RM, Copeland EM III. The implication of local recurrence of breast cancer as the first site of therapeutic failure. Ann Surg 197:284, 1983.
74. Loyer EM, Krott S, David CL, et al. Mammographic and CT findings after breast reconstruction with a rectus abdominis musculocutaneous flap. Am J Roentgenol 156:1159, 1991.

33

Local Recurrence After Mastectomy and Breast Reconstruction

Sumner A. Slavin, M.D.

Reoperative Problems

- Metastasis
- Carcinoma-en-cuirasse
- Incomplete resection of tumor at mastectomy
- Irradiated chest wall

Local recurrence, a term often used interchangeably with locoregional recurrence, is defined as any reappearance of breast cancer on the ipsilateral chest wall or its skin or in adjacent node-bearing areas. Current concepts of tumor immunology consider a local recurrence to be a sign of systemic disease. As such, the recurrence is related to the prognosis of the particular breast cancer and is not related to the patient's breast reconstruction.[1] According to this theory, neither the type of reconstruction nor the timing of the surgery has any effect on the patient's ultimate course of illness or survival.

The factors that increase the risk of developing a local recurrence, such as a large primary tumor, skin and nodal involvement, absence of estrogen receptors, and dermal lymphatic infiltration, also correlate with an adverse outcome. Reducing the risk of local recurrence begins with using the most effective mastectomy technique. Controversy still exists as to which technique most thoroughly eradicates breast cancer.[2] The slightly reduced rate of local recurrence after total (radical) mastectomy has uncertain clinical significance[3] and must be weighed against the lower complication rate seen with the modified radical mastectomy.[4]

Although the extent of the incisional margins does not appear to influence the likelihood of a recurrence,[5] questions remain regarding the thoroughness of any mastectomy technique at removing all of the glandular tissue of the breast.[3,6] Total mastectomy and modified radical mastectomy achieve an equally effective excision of breast parenchyma, but they also leave microscopically identifiable residual foci of mammary tissue seen in 5% of all biopsy specimens performed after either technique.[6a] It has not been determined whether these foci are important and whether improving the completeness of glandular tissue excision would reduce the rate of local recurrence. Since most local recurrences do not contain breast tissue, it is unlikely that a recurrence would originate from these residual glandular cells. Nevertheless, the possibility that the tumor has completely replaced the breast tissue cells cannot be completely ruled out.

BREAST RECONSTRUCTION AND LOCAL RECURRENCE

The growing popularity of breast reconstruction following mastectomy,[7,8] as well as the increased availability and variety of reconstructive techniques, has raised questions regarding the safety of these procedures.[9,10] The primary focus of concern has been on oncologic issues,[11-13] such as (1) whether reconstruction compromises the effectiveness of the tumor ablation (either by restricting its extent or by inhibiting the body's immune response), (2) whether the opening of new tissue planes disseminates tumor cells, and (3) whether a breast reconstruction may impede detection of a recurrent tumor, delay its diagnosis, interfere with subsequent treatment, or diminish the patient's disease-free interval or survival.

The optimal timing of treatment has been a particularly perplexing issue; some clinicians favor deferred rather than immediate treatment of local disease. Traditionally patients were advised to delay breast reconstruction for 2 years after mastectomy out of concern that the tissue or prosthesis used to reconstruct the breast might mask a local recurrence.[14,15] The concept of delayed reconstruction became obsolete as a new understanding of the clinical significance of recurrence emerged. The 2-year disease-free interval for patients with stage I disease has been reported at 100%, and patients with stage II disease have an 80% rate for the same period.[14] Since none of the patients with stage I disease developed a recurrence within 2 years of mastectomy and patients with stage II disease had an average disease-free interval of over 4 years, delaying reconstruction would appear to be unreasonable. Moreover, since most local recurrences (up to 66%) occur in or about the area of the mastectomy scar, it is extremely unlikely that a subpectoral breast reconstruction would obstruct the detection of a recurrent tumor.[14]

Other potential objections to immediate reconstruction were based on the size of the primary lesion and the number of positive axillary nodes.[15a] Although some studies have reported no correlation between the size of the initial tumor and the length of the disease-free interval, lymph node metastasis, more than any other single factor, is linked to an increased rate of relapse. Research by Fowble et al.[16] showed that the local recurrence rate rose as high as 11% within 3 years after mastectomy in patients with more than four positive lymph nodes. Therefore the possibility of lymph node metastasis is a major consideration of many surgeons when evaluating a patient for reconstruction.

A newer approach to the timing of reconstruction examines the quality of life of the patient with a poor prognosis. If the treatment of a local recurrence is considered as primarily palliative rather than curative, then the emotional value of breast reconstruction might be considered as beneficial as the palliative benefits of chemotherapy or radiation therapy. ***The past decade of increasing patient demand for reconstruction has led to a gradual consensus by oncologists, surgeons, and plastic surgeons that breast reconstruction is an appropriate option for all breast cancer patients undergoing mastectomy, regardless of the size of the tumor, stage of the disease, or status of the lymph nodes.***

ORIGINS OF LOCAL RECURRENCE

Recurrent lesions are treatable and sometimes can be eradicated[17]; thus it is important to understand their pathogenesis, clinical manifestations, and mechanisms of spread. Most local recurrences are probably generated by the following three mechanisms:

1. The surgical technique directly implants tumor cells into the wound or inadequate excision leaves residual cells at the mastectomy site (this is more likely to occur when a thicker but more viable skin flap is used).
2. The intrinsic lymphatic system of the native skin and chest wall soft tissue either harbors persistent tumor cells, or the system communicates with other tumor-bearing areas.
3. Cancer cells spread systemically through the bloodstream.

Since nearly 90% of patients with local recurrence have concomitant systemic disease, circulating cancer cells would appear to be the most likely source of recurrent cancer.[1] However, lymphatic channels also can disseminate tumor cells by either reconnecting with tumor-infested lymphatic vessels or regenerating with adjacent normal tissues. For example, when musculocutaneous flaps are transposed as part of breast reconstruction, lymphatic channels become reestablished between the flap and the native chest wall. These new pathways can provide access for tumor cells into the previously uninvolved flap.

Local recurrence has been associated with efforts to preserve part or all of the nipple-areola complex.[18-23] The size and location of the tumor are not accurate predictors as to whether nipple-areolar structures are involved. Involvement of the nipple-areola complex with tumor has been demonstrated in 31% to 37.5% of breast cancer patients.[19,23] In another series tumor cells were found as close as 6 mm from the nipple in 39% of specimens. Heterotopically transplanted nipples can contribute to breast cancer metastases at the recipient site. Recent findings of ductal epithelium in the areolar tissues of mastectomy specimens[23a] should discourage attempts to save the areola after sacrifice of the nipple or nipple core. ***Salvage of any portion of the nipple-areola complex, including the areola without the nipple, is potentially dangerous and could lead to an increased incidence of local recurrence.***

SIGNS AND SYMPTOMS

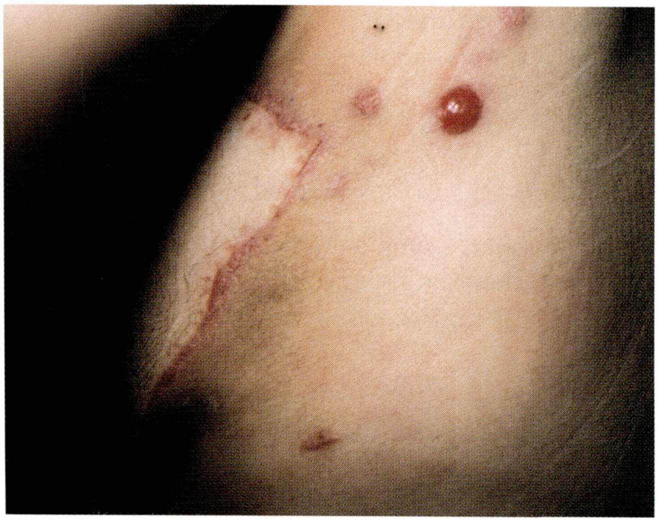

A local recurrence usually begins as a painless, erythematous rash or a solitary nodular lesion in the native skin or subcutaneous tissues adjacent to the mastectomy scar.[1] The growths have a cobblestone appearance caused by aggregates of tumor cells in the lymphatic spaces of the dermis. As the tumor grows, the malignant cells spread rapidly through the soft tissues, often forming a confluent firmness and thickening of the skin. When a recurrence occurs in a patient with a subpectoral implant, the lesions are usually superficially located and are easily visible and palpable. A physical examination unaided by sophisticated scanning and imaging techniques can typically yield an accurate diagnosis. Although deep, submuscular chest wall recurrences are extremely rare and it is unlikely that a subpectoral prosthesis would impede detection, this remote possibility must be considered.[24] Other known sites of chest wall recurrence include axillary lymph nodes, supraclavicular nodes, and parasternal skin.[25] In half of all local recurrences, only the native skin of the chest wall is involved.[17]

ROLE OF BIOPSY FOR SUSPECTED LOCAL RECURRENCE

Since other conditions may mimic the recurrence of a tumor, any suspicious physical finding on the chest wall following mastectomy (with or without breast reconstruction) requires prompt biopsy confirmation of its histologic makeup. Benign conditions that need to be differentiated from recurrent malignancy include cysts,[26] lipoma, fat necrosis (with and without calcification), scar tissue, and suture granuloma. Malignant conditions, such as sarcomas of bone or cartilage, can develop after surgical trauma or radiation therapy and may be totally unrelated to the original breast cancer. ***Although most local recurrences are clinically detectable skin lesions, biopsy is always mandated to avoid confusion with other conditions.*** For the more superficial types of lesions the biopsy often can be performed in a surgeon's office with the patient under local anesthesia. Conditions that are subcutaneous or deeper or those that involve large and sometimes vascular structures should be biopsied in an operating room with the patient anesthetized. The fresh specimen should be properly assayed for appropriate hormonal receptors.

Other examinations such as CT scanning, ultrasonographic scanning, or mammography are helpful in determining the nature or extent of a potential recurrent lesion in the subcutaneous tissues of the native chest wall or the musculocutaneous flap after breast reconstruction. Patients who have had a musculocutaneous flap reconstruction may have palpable areas of firmness in the subcutaneous tissues of the flap that are suggestive of recurrent cancer. In such situations it is important to explain to a patient that mammography can be used as a diagnostic tool despite the removal of all mammary tissues. Although benign calcifications in fat are particularly well visualized by this type of examination, imaging techniques can never provide the complete certainty of a tissue diagnosis.

Case Examples

A 44-year-old woman with lobular carcinoma of the breast had a right modified radical mastectomy performed in conjunction with immediate breast reconstruction using a TRAM flap. The initial postoperative course was uneventful. All drains were removed on the fifth postoperative day when drainage from the abdominal donor site was <30 ml/day.

Six months later, an epigastric mass was noted when the patient complained of abdominal discomfort and a sense of fullness. No weakness or hernia was identified, but a mass measuring 8 × 10 cm was palpated.

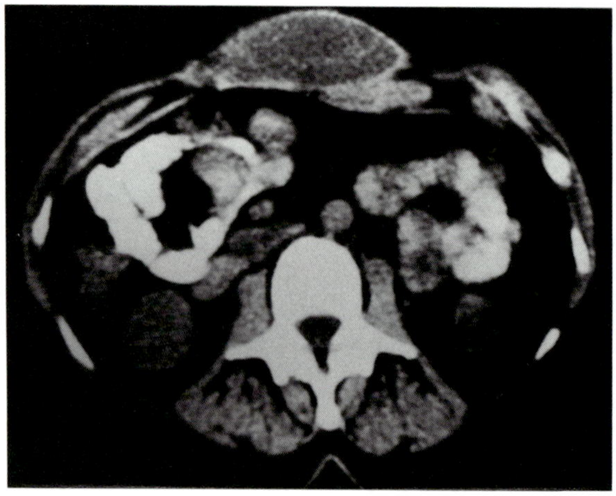

A CT scan of the abdomen revealed a large, subcutaneous mass adherent to the posterior sheath of the ipsilateral rectus abdominis muscle below the xiphoid process.

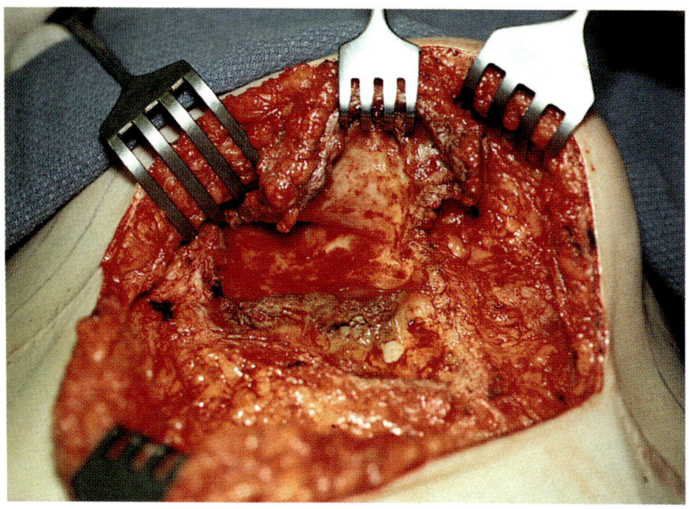

An 8 × 10 cm epigastric cyst filled with straw-colored fluid was surgically removed. Histologic examination revealed a benign cyst containing fibrinous material. No further abnormalities have appeared since the cyst was excised.

In this patient the epigastric mass was presumed to be a local recurrence, possibly resulting from dissemination of tumor cells from the mastectomy site to the extensive abdominal donor tissues at the time of the immediate breast reconstruction. Such spread of tumor has rarely, if ever, been reported. Nevertheless, the presence of a large mass raised the possibility of a local recurrence of breast cancer in an area adjacent to the mastectomy site. Although the CT image indicated a benign-appearing cyst, a similar lesion in another patient was explored and found to harbor a recurrence of adenocarcinoma of the breast in the cyst wall. This clinical example underscores the importance of confirming the precise histologic state with a biopsy rather than relying solely on imaging techniques.

A large cystic mass may occur at or near the donor site of a musculocutaneous flap. The exact mechanism of how these cysts form is not well understood, but it appears that either undrained or clinically undetected collections of serous fluid organize into a mass of fibrin, then the outer layers of fibrin solidify as the liquid is sequestered within. Despite the absence of a true histologic layer of secretory epithelium, the mass can increase in size, presumably by attracting serous fluid osmotically from the surrounding tissues. Ultimately these pseudocysts become large enough to be detected clinically. The diagnosis is established by biopsy of the cyst wall, and the anterior wall of the cyst must be excised to ensure eradication. When these lesions develop after the transposition of a TRAM flap, it is common to find the posterior wall of the mass firmly adherent to the posterior rectus sheath, rendering its removal risky. In such situations a hernia or entry into the peritoneal cavity could result in surgical complications. The liquid contents of a pseudocyst can be aspirated to temporarily alleviate the swelling; however, the aspirated fluid should not be used for tissue diagnosis.

▪ ▪ ▪

A 39-year-old woman with inflammatory breast cancer underwent mastectomy of the right breast and immediate breast reconstruction with a latissimus dorsi musculocutaneous flap. She received a course of chemotherapy followed by irradiation of the right breast and chest wall. Eleven months after the surgery, a solitary nodular mass was palpated in the subcutaneous tissues of the latissimus dorsi flap. The lesion was moderately firm and distinguishable from both the flap and chest wall soft tissues. Ultrasonographic examination showed a solid mass without any cystic component. An excisional biopsy was performed, and a 4×5 cm encapsulated yellow mass was dissected from the soft tissues of the latissimus dorsi flap. Subsequent examination of the mass revealed that it was a lipoma arising from the subcutaneous fatty layer of the flap. Four years after the surgery, there has been no recurrence of the lipoma.

This case demonstrates how a benign mass such as a lipoma can be confused with recurrent breast cancer, especially in a high-risk patient with inflammatory cancer of the breast. The mass was identified within the flap soft tissues, initially suggesting a local recurrence. However, the latissimus dorsi flap encompasses subcutaneous tissues harvested from the back and has a recognized potential for generating mature encapsulated lipomas from its lipocytes. In this instance, the ultrasonographic examination accurately predicted the solid nature of the mass, but only an excisional biopsy could provide the certainty of a tissue diagnosis.

▪ ▪ ▪

A 47-year-old woman with breast cancer had a mastectomy of the right breast and immediate breast reconstruction with a latissimus dorsi musculocutaneous flap. The drains were removed on the fifth postoperative day of an uncomplicated recovery.

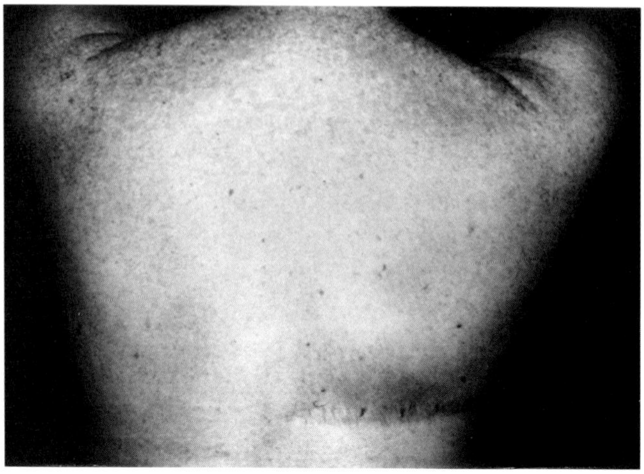

Two years later, the patient became aware of a firm mass growing within the donor site of the latissimus dorsi flap. As the mass gradually enlarged, it became more painful. When alerted to the presence of the mass, the oncologist became concerned about the possibility of a recurrence of cancer. CT imaging, however, revealed a solid mass in the donor site scar without any deformity of the adjacent ribs. An 8 cm fibroma was surgically removed, and the mass has not recurred in the 2 years since the procedure.

Unlike the two previous case histories, in this patient the development of a suspicious mass on the posterior chest wall was the first clinical manifestation of presumed recurrent breast cancer. Because of the location of the mass, a possible metastasis to the ribs was suspected, but CT imaging accurately demonstrated no involvement of adjacent ribs. Nevertheless, a local recurrence within the dermis and underlying fat could not be definitively ruled out until the mass was excised and examination confirmed it to be an aggregate of fibrous (scar) tissue.

DISCUSSING BIOPSY RESULTS: A POTENTIAL PITFALL

The initial detection of a local recurrence can become an emotionally charged event for both the patient and the plastic surgeon. To many patients, mastectomy, radiation therapy, and chemotherapy create a false sense of security, causing some patients to react defensively to the possibility of disease recurrence. Given the physical and emotional exhaustion that inevitably accompany a prolonged course of treatment for cancer, the patient may be poorly prepared to tolerate the prospect of any further disease. Unlike distant metastases to liver, lungs, or bone (which are not immediately apparent to the patient), local recurrence is especially disturbing to the breast cancer patient because it is a visible reminder of the disease. The predilection of locally recurrent lesions for growth on native chest wall skin abutting the skin flaps or musculocutaneous flaps of a breast reconstruction[27] means that the plastic surgeon may be the first member of a team of treating specialists to discover and biopsy the lesion. Ironically the earlier restorative role of the plastic surgeon is quickly subverted as the positive aspects of breast reconstruction give way to the negative implications of a biopsy-proven local recurrence. The tendency of any patient to reject distressing information can be increased when the tidings come from an unexpected source: the plastic surgeon. The surgeon must be extremely sensitive to the patient's feelings when discussing this disturbing finding. Sometimes it may be best for the oncologist to inform the patient of the biopsy results, but each physician should decide these important issues on an individual basis. ***Patients always appreciate a physician's considerate handling of this frightening situation.***

Local Recurrence After Mastectomy and Breast Reconstruction With Musculocutaneous Flaps

Breast reconstruction techniques that use flaps of musculocutaneous tissue (e.g., latissimus dorsi or rectus abdominis) bring extensive amounts of soft tissue to the mastectomy site. A patient with a tissue flap reconstruction may require a different method of monitoring for recurrent cancer than a patient with a breast reconstructed with an implant. Unfortunately, the influence, if any, of a musculocutaneous flap breast reconstruction on the diagnosis or treatment of a local recurrence has not been widely addressed by reviews of reconstructions using implants.

A study by Webster, Mansel, and Hughes[9] reviewed the results of immediate breast reconstruction in 85 patients, 68 of whom had reconstruction with musculocutaneous flaps: 35 patients with a rectus abdominis flap and 33 patients with a latissimus dorsi flap. The incidence of local recurrence was less than 5% for patients with either stage I or stage II disease. Local recurrence (located in the skin adjacent to the mastectomy site) was identified in two patients. There was no delay or difficulty in making an accurate diagnosis or in commencing treatment of the recurrent tumor. The authors concluded that local disease (1) usually develops in the skin adjacent to the flap, (2) is accompanied by simultaneous distant disease, and (3) is more easily recognized than a local recurrence following conservative surgery (lumpectomy) and radiation therapy. Unfortunately the period of follow-up covered by the study was quite brief, lasting approximately 2 years.

In a larger review by Slavin, Love, and Goldwyn,[27] the specific problem of local recurrence following immediate breast reconstruction with a musculocutaneous flap was examined in 161 patients with breast cancer.* All patients had either a rectus abdominis (65) or latissimus dorsi (97) musculocutaneous flap breast reconstruction performed immediately after mastectomy. Of the 161 patients reviewed, 120 had primary mastectomy and reconstruction; the remaining 41 patients underwent salvage mastectomy and immediate reconstruction after failed conservative surgery and radiation therapy. All patients requesting immediate breast reconstruction were included in the review, regardless of tumor size, nodal involvement, or estrogen receptor status. Locoregional recurrence was observed in 17 of the 161 patients (10.6%). Most of the recurrences developed in patients with stage II and III disease.

In this study[27] all of the local recurrences developed in the native skin and subcutaneous tissues of the chest wall adjacent to the mastectomy site regardless of the type of breast reconstruction technique used, including those with subpectoral implants. Typically the local recurrence was heralded by the appearance of an erythematous rash with a cobblestone appearance. Biopsy confirmation obtained in all of the patients demonstrated tumor-filled lymphatic spaces in the dermal tissues. A predictable pattern of tumor growth was observed in all patients with local recurrence, manifested initially by involvement of the skin next to the flap borders and followed by gradual encroachment on the flap. Late invasion of the musculocutaneous flap occurred as the disease became clinically apparent in the contralateral breast and continued to spread by carcinoma-en-cuirasse, reaching as far posteriorly as the latissimus dorsi donor site. Diagnosis of a local recurrence was performed by physical examination without the need for imaging techniques.

Local recurrences in this series[27] were detected as early as 1 month and as late as 3.8 years after mastectomy and reconstruction. In this series the 5-year survival rate for patients with a local recurrence of cancer (25%) reflects the known severe prognosis for patients having recurrent cancer after mastectomy. The authors assert that the diagnosis and treatment of a local recurrence were not delayed by the breast reconstruction in any patient, but they question whether early detection had any positive effect on the patient's survival.

Patients who had salvage mastectomy after failed conservative surgery and radiation therapy had a lower incidence of locoregional recurrence (7.3%) than patients who underwent primary mastectomy (11.7%).[27] Despite the metastases, the salvage mastectomy patients also survived longer. Although the reasons for improved survival in patients having salvage mastectomy are not well understood, the locally recurrent lesions in these patients tended to be smaller and confined to the breast.

*One patient had bilateral flaps.

This review[27] also addressed whether there was any correlation between the type of flap reconstruction performed and the incidence of local recurrence. Patients with early stage breast cancer tended to choose a latissimus dorsi flap; among patients with more advanced breast cancer (stage III), 66% had a TRAM flap and 34% had a latissimus dorsi flap. Since more extensive resections were anticipated for patients with stage III disease, the surgeons preferred the more expansive TRAM flap over the latissimus dorsi flap. Thus the increased incidence of local recurrence among TRAM flap recipients most likely reflected the surgeon's preference for that flap in patients who were at greatest risk for recurrence. The authors concluded that reconstruction with musculocutaneous flaps after mastectomy is oncologically safe. Furthermore, the presence of a musculocutaneous flap did not conceal tumor growth or hinder its treatment.

Case Presentation

A 42-year-old woman had a history of in situ carcinoma of the left breast that was treated by partial mastectomy and radiation therapy. Two years later she was diagnosed with inflammatory carcinoma of the right breast and was referred for mastectomy of the right breast and immediate reconstruction with a TRAM flap. She was treated initially with chemotherapy and a course of 5000 rads to the left breast, but the tumor persisted. It was determined that mastectomy would offer her the best opportunity for local control.

The right breast and extensive portions of the cutaneous surface of the right hemithorax were resected. Tumor cells were present in the dermal lymphatic system and in five of the six lymph nodes. The breast was reconstructed with a large TRAM flap measuring 16 × 35 cm.

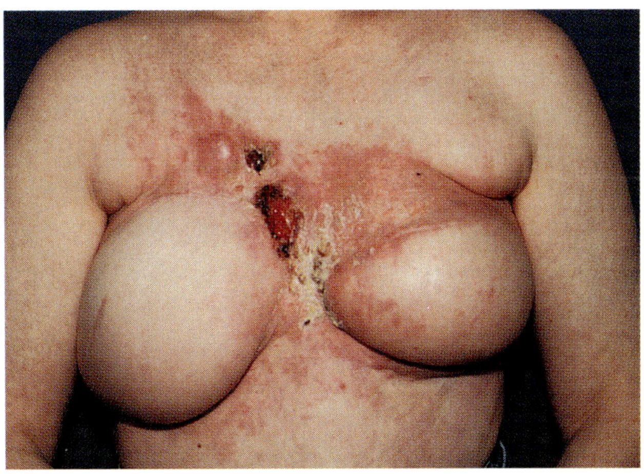

Seven months later an erythematous rash and multiple nodular lesions in the native skin of the chest wall adjacent to the mastectomy scar and musculocutaneous flap reconstruction developed. Biopsy of these lesions demonstrated cancer within the dermal lymphatic spaces, but clinical staging, including CT imaging of the chest and abdomen, did not show any evidence of distant metastasis.

A new mass that developed in the left breast was found to be intraductal carcinoma, necessitating a left salvage mastectomy and reconstruction with a left latissimus dorsi musculocutaneous flap. Eighteen months after the diagnosis of inflammatory cancer of the right breast, metastases to the lung and spine were found. After undergoing additional chemotherapy regimens, she lived 3 more years until finally succumbing to metastatic carcinoma.

This case history illustrates the usual clinical presentation of recurrent breast carcinoma after mastectomy and immediate reconstruction with a musculocutaneous flap. ***Although tumor nodules may involve extensive areas of the native skin of the chest wall, distant metastases may not be detectable at the time the skin lesions are diagnosed. However, distant disease can develop quickly thereafter.*** Most of these patients will be diagnosed with distant metastases within months to 1 or 2 years after the appearance of the local recurrence.

LOCAL SPREAD OF RECURRENT BREAST CANCER

When tumor cells reach an advanced stage of growth, major complications can occur, such as bleeding, ulceration, sepsis, and death.[28] Carcinoma-en-cuirasse, a rare form of tumor growth, can originate in the skin and subcutaneous tissues and infiltrate the lateral and posterior aspects of the chest wall in a bandlike manner, severely restricting chest wall mechanics. Often characterized by nodular lesions and areas of ulceration, carcinoma-en-cuirasse tends to be a late manifestation of a local recurrence that is particularly resistant to local or systemic treatment. The following case history underscores the severity of locally recurrent lesions and the difficulty in treating them.

Case Presentation

A 33-year-old woman had mastectomy of the left breast for infiltrating ductal carcinoma; axillary sampling demonstrated tumor cells in four of eight lymph nodes. Immediate breast reconstruction was performed with a latissimus dorsi flap. Despite a course of chemotherapy, nodular lesions rapidly developed over the native skin of the chest wall, which became progressively ulcerated and necrotic. Additional chemotherapy was administered in an unsuccessful attempt to control the spread of the tumor.

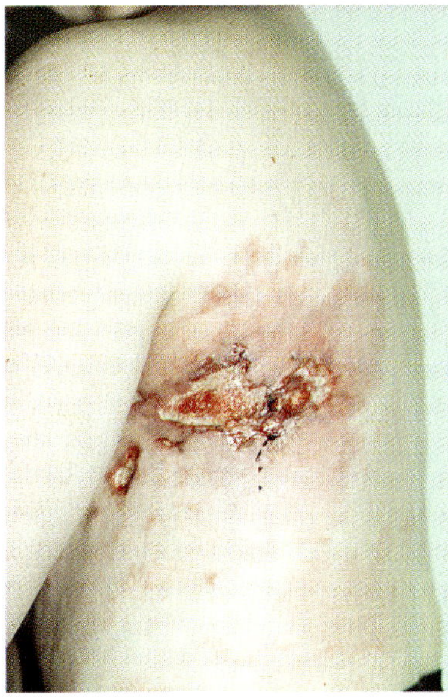

As tumor growth progressed through the skin and subcutaneous tissues of the chest wall, it not only invaded the latissimus dorsi flap tissue but also advanced to the latissimus dorsi donor site by the process of carcinoma-en-cuirasse. The patient was treated with local radiation therapy and thermotherapy followed by another course of aggressive chemotherapy, but she showed no clinical evidence of improvement. She died 1 year after the mastectomy and reconstruction.

This case history illustrates complications of ulceration, necrosis, and carcinoma-en-cuirasse occurring in association with a local recurrence. Even the posteriorly located donor site was vulnerable to the spread of the tumor along the chest wall. In addition, this case history demonstrates the refractory nature of such lesions to any type of treatment, including chemotherapy, radiation, and thermotherapy.

Local Recurrence After Microvascular Free Flap Breast Reconstruction

During the past decade advances in free tissue transfer have made possible the use of microvascular techniques for both immediate and delayed breast reconstruction.[29-31] Although a number of different donor sites have been described, gluteus maximus and TRAM free flaps have been the most widely used. Unfortunately there is little information available regarding local recurrence after mastectomy and free flap breast reconstruction. In a study by Grotting et al.[29] of ten patients undergoing TRAM free flap breast reconstruction, no instances of local recurrence were observed during a 3-year follow-up.

Because microvascular free flaps and pedicled grafts provide comparable amounts and types of soft tissue for breast reconstruction, the findings related to the detection and treatment of a local recurrence might be assumed to be similar, but studies are not available to substantiate this conclusion.

LOCAL RECURRENCE AFTER MASTECTOMY AND BREAST RECONSTRUCTION WITH IMPLANTS

The use of implants in breast reconstruction originated before the development of musculocutaneous and microvascular free flap tissue transfers, and prostheses continue to be more commonly used for reconstruction than the more complex and risky flap procedures. Because of the popularity of implants for reconstruction, there is more information available concerning local recurrence of breast cancer after reconstruction with a prosthesis. Most of these reports are concerned with oncologic safety, especially in regard to detection, treatment, and survival after local recurrence.[32-39] It is generally agreed that placement of a subpectoral prosthesis will not conceal a recurrent breast cancer lesion or inhibit its detection. ***Reconstruction with implants does not compromise the ablative procedure, open new tissue planes for dissemination of cancer cells, or inhibit the body's immune response.*** Georgiade et al.[12] studied the long-term clinical outcome in 147 patients followed up for 3 years after mastectomy and immediate reconstruction with a prosthesis; the disease-free interval of patients who had breast reconstruction was comparable to that of patients who did not undergo breast reconstruction.

Noone et al.[13] conducted a similar study of a 6-year experience with 185 patients who had immediate reconstruction after mastectomy for cancer, including patients with either large primary tumors or gross axillary disease. The rates of recurrence were consistent with the expected range reported in earlier published research.[40,41] All recurrences were easily diagnosed by physical examination while the recurrent lesions were still small. Some early bone scans after submuscular placement of the implant yielded false positive findings caused by subperiosteal reaction in the ribs after detachment of pectoralis major and serratus anterior muscle segments. All false positive findings reverted to normal within 6 to 12 months. The authors concluded that recurrence rates after mastectomy and immediate reconstruction were the same as those after mastectomy alone.

The study by Noone et al.[13] also noted that the mastectomy technique usually was not compromised by a need for musculocutaneous flap coverage of the prosthesis. In situations in which complete coverage of the prosthesis was not feasible, inflatable expanders were usually inserted. Only rarely was a musculocutaneous flap substituted for the usual closure with skin flaps.

Johnson et al.[11] reported on 118 patients who had immediate reconstruction with implants after mastectomy, fourteen (12%) of whom had recurrent lesions. Seven local recurrences (6%) were detected early enough that they could be treated without requiring the removal of the prosthesis. Again, the disease-free interval and survival rate for patients with reconstructed breasts was comparable with the rate for patients who underwent mastectomy alone; recurrence of disease was associated with larger primary tumors, increased number of positive axillary nodes, and absence of tumor estrogen receptors. The mastectomy technique was never altered or compromised to accommodate the reconstruction.

Several small studies[10,42-47] examining possible silicone gel implant inhibition of antitumor immunity found no evidence that tumor growth is abetted by a silicone gel prosthesis. ***Local recurrences arising adjacent to a silicone gel prosthesis apparently resulted from incomplete resection of tumor at the time of mastectomy.*** Since patients referred for delayed breast reconstruction may harbor recurrent tumor cells,[48-50] these recurrences should not be automatically attributed to a silicone-induced diminution of host immunity. In one report,[51] six of 26 patients referred for reconstruction had either local recurrence or distant metastases discovered at the time of the breast reconstruction. The patient should be informed that the presence of a silicone gel implant will not interfere with the administration of radiation therapy.[43,52-54] However, the development of fibrous scar tissue or increased encapsulation may adversely affect the aesthetic result.

TREATMENT OF LOCAL RECURRENCE

The controversy regarding treatment of the patient with local recurrence[17] includes areas of disagreement concerning the selection of modality and the condition for treatment. Most local recurrences can be treated with various combinations of local excision, radical excision, radiation therapy, and systemic therapy. The myriad clinical manifestations of locally recurrent cancer have made it difficult to assess the efficacy of any single approach. Occasionally, local excision may control a recurrence in a patient with a small lesion, but the extent of local disease on the chest wall can severely restrict the use of a surgical procedure. A study by Aberizk et al.[55] showed that radiation therapy is a useful option for palliation but that it does not necessarily result in improved survival. Systemic therapy would seem to be an appropriate treatment for patients with locoregional recurrence after mastectomy since they are more likely to have distant metastases as well, but clinical trials of this treatment regimen have shown no clear benefit for the patient in these circumstances. Combining chemotherapy with radiation therapy to treat a local recurrence might seem appealing, but Janjan et al.[56] have found no evidence of improved survival with this combination of treatments.

Although treatment of a local recurrence can prevent or reduce the local morbidity of wound complications, it is not known if it can affect favorably the disease-free interval or overall survival time. Patients free of concomitant distant disease are likely to benefit the most.

Surgical Treatment

Whether palliative or curative, surgical management is possible for most recurrent breast cancer lesions. Most of these lesions tend to occur on the chest wall adjacent to the mastectomy scar or the breast reconstruction site. Lesions in a nonirradiated area can be managed by wide excision and closure with local rotation or advancement flaps. Extensive lesions that involve large cutaneous surface areas or those that invade deep chest wall structures including the ribs should be widely excised and the wound closed with a musculocutaneous flap to ensure satisfactory healing. ***Use of a musculocutaneous flap is particularly suitable when necrosis of the bone following radiation therapy is present since this type of flap will provide the necessary vascularity and soft tissue elements.***

If a TRAM flap has already been used for breast reconstruction, an alternative flap donor site must be selected for closure of the repair wound. The latissimus dorsi musculocutaneous unit is an excellent choice as either a microvascular free flap or a pedicled graft (if the size of the wound is large or if the patient has a history of irradiation). Excision of locally recurrent breast cancer can create a defect whose dimensions exceed the availability of donor site skin. Recently, I have tried tissue expansion of the latissimus dorsi musculocutaneous unit in a small study of patients requiring breast and chest wall reconstruction and found that the axial dimensions of the flap increased by a factor of approximately 1.5.

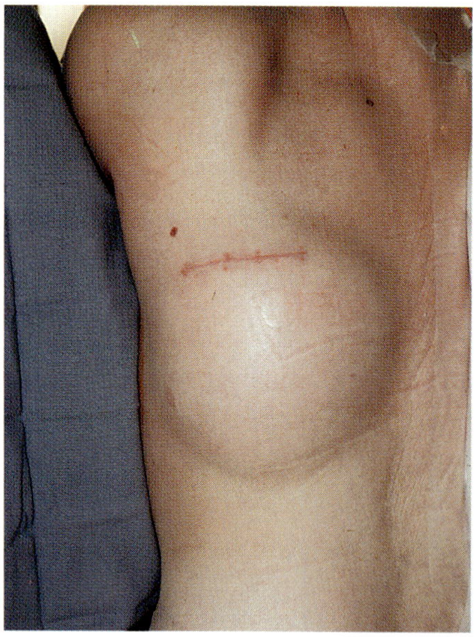

The proposed muscle flap is expanded at the donor site before it is transposed to cover a large sternal osteonecrotic wound. The latissimus dorsi muscle is particularly suitable for this application because it provides a broad, flat surface that is readily expanded. The tissue expander is inserted through an incision along the superior border of the muscle and then is intraoperatively expanded to a volume of approximately 300 ml. Two or three outpatient percutaneous injections continue the process, which creates a thinned, pliable latissimus dorsi musculocutaneous flap of augmented dimensions.

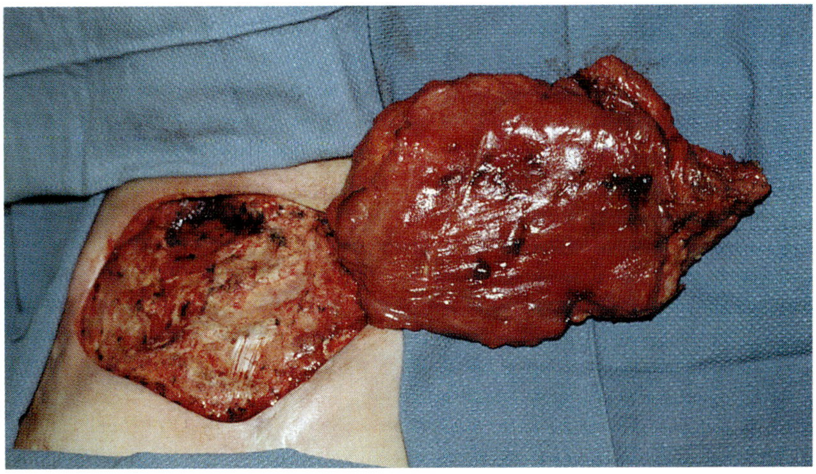

After the local recurrence is resected, the expanded latissimus dorsi flap is reflected back and then transposed into the wound. ***The expanded flaps are ideal for covering wounds on irradiated chest walls in patients with or without locally recurrent breast cancer.***

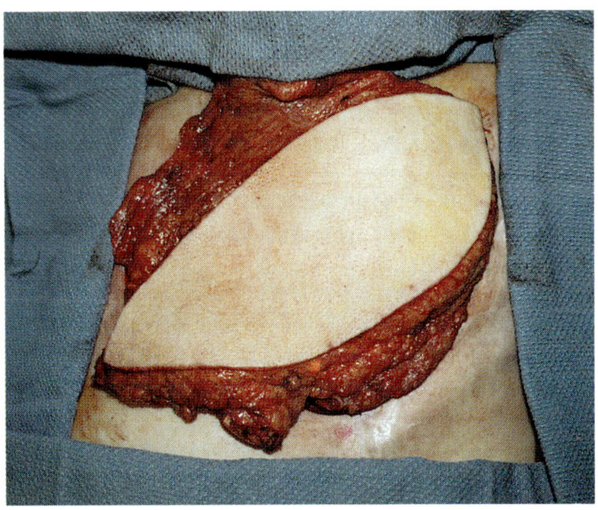

When cancer is present, wide excisions can be performed since the unusually large size of the expanded flap will provide the needed skin and soft tissues to cover the large defect. Mustoe, Bartell, and Garner[58] have collected experimental data showing that hyperplasia occurs in the vascular and microvascular components of the flap, along with thinning of dermal, subcutaneous, and muscular tissues. These findings explain the clinical success experienced with expanded musculocutaneous flaps.

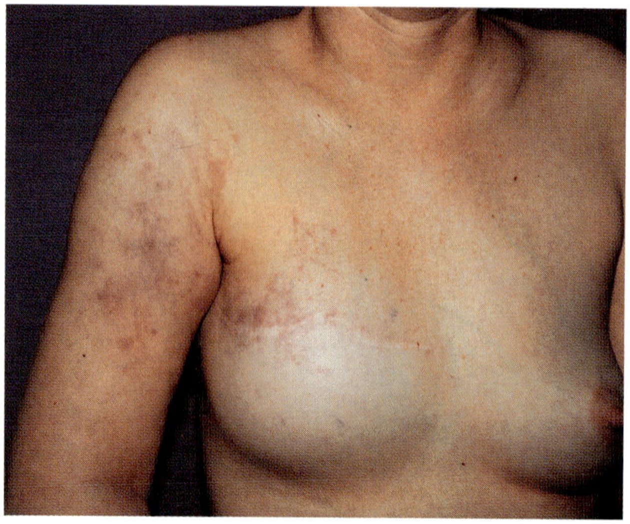

Sometimes recurrent breast cancer can manifest itself as a locoregional rather than a strictly local recurrence, and lesions may develop in the ipsilateral axilla or upper extremity. This patient has lymphedema with tumor nodules studding the skin. ***Locoregional recurrent breast cancer lesions are often the result of lymphatic rather than hematogenous dissemination; they are particularly refractory to treatment because of their diffuse mode of spread.*** Well-localized recurrent lesions of the axilla can be treated in the manner described for chest wall and breast lesions (i.e., with either local or musculocutaneous flaps), but multiple nodular tumor masses in the dermis of the upper extremity are too widespread for this approach. Short of combined chemotherapy and radiation therapy, no effective treatment appears to exist for these difficult locoregional metastases.

PROGNOSIS OF A LOCAL RECURRENCE

Most of the information regarding prognosis has been obtained from reviews of patients with local recurrence after mastectomy alone, but breast reconstruction has not been shown to adversely affect the disease-free interval or patient survival. Most patients are unaware of the poor prognosis associated with a local recurrence of breast cancer after mastectomy. The most difficult fact to communicate to the patient is the proven correlation between the onset of local recurrence and the probability of distant metastases since in more than 90% of patients with local recurrence, a distant metastasis develops within 5 years. What is even more emotionally stressful for the patient (and the physician) is the 5-year survival rate, which ranges from 0% to 50%.[1,17,55,59] The 10-year survival rate drops to a range of 0% to 33%. However, those patients who do survive 10 years are not necessarily disease free. In a review of 90 patients undergoing radiation therapy for the control of local recurrence of breast cancer after mastectomy, only 7% of the patients were free of distant disease at 10 years. The overall survival rate for the group at 10 years was 26%. Survival rates were found to be greatest in patients whose disease-free interval was at least 2 years.[55]

In a review from M.D. Anderson Hospital,[1] when local recurrence of breast cancer is the first site of therapeutic failure, only three of 60 patients (5%) survived for 10 years. The mean time interval between treatment of the local recurrence and death for patients with stage I, II, and III disease was 7.2, 6, and 2.5 years, respectively. All patients in the series eventually died of cancer, one patient as late as 27 years after the local recurrence. Although local recurrence was observed to be a major cause of chest wall morbidity in terms of uncontrolled infection and necrosis, these lesions are rarely the direct cause of death. ■ ***Rather, local recurrence means the patient will most likely die of metastatic disease within 10 years.*** More pessimistically, local recurrence may imply a 100% mortality rate, with a small fraction of patients with distant disease alive longer than 10 years. These findings of reduced survival strongly support the thesis that a local recurrence is an earlier manifestation of systemic disease, sometimes appearing concomitant with or only weeks or months before distant metastases are discovered.

■ ■ ■

Patients undergoing breast reconstruction are extremely fearful that the growth of occult or dormant tumor cells can be activated by the surgery itself. The finding of a local recurrence near the breast reconstruction site can evoke strong feelings of guilt and regret. Some will voice their concerns that the breast reconstruction might have caused the recurrence. It becomes especially important to communicate to the breast reconstruction candidate the shared concerns of the reconstructive surgeon regarding the diagnosis and treatment of recurrent lesions. The proven oncologic safety of a breast reconstruction should be emphasized during the preoperative consultation.

In summary, the incidence of local recurrence is not increased in patients having either immediate or delayed reconstruction with implants. Detection, treatment, and survival after local recurrence are unchanged as a result of the breast reconstruction. However, local recurrence is an early sign of probable metastatic disease that is notoriously refractory to treatment.

References

1. Gilliland MD, Barton RM, Copeland EM. The implications of local recurrence of breast cancer as the first site of therapeutic failure. Ann Surg 197:284, 1983.
2. Maddox WA, Carpenter JT, Laws HH, et al. Does radical mastectomy still have a place in the treatment of primary, operable breast cancer? Arch Surg 122:1317, 1987.
3. Barton FE, English JM, Kingsley WB, et al. Glandular excision in total glandular mastectomy: A comparison. Plast Reconstr Surg 88:389, 1992.
4. Martin JK Jr, van Heerden JA, Taylor WF, et al. Is modified radical mastectomy really equivalent to radical mastectomy in treatment of carcinoma of the breast? Cancer 57:510, 1986.
5. Donegan WL, Perez-Mesa CM, Watson FR. A biostatistical study of locally recurrent breast carcinoma. Surg Gynecol Obstet 122:529, 1966.
6. Goldman L, Goldwyn RM. Glandular excision in total glandular mastectomy and modified radical mastectomy: A comparison. Plast Reconstr Surg 88:393, 1991.

6a. Barton FE, English JM, Kingsley W, et al. Glandular excision in total glandular mastectomy and modified radical mastectomy: A comparison. Plast Reconstr Surg 88:389, 1991.

7. Noone RB, Frazier TG, Hayward CZ, et al. Patient acceptance of immediate reconstruction following mastectomy. Plast Reconstr Surg 69:632, 1982.
8. Frazier TG, Noone RB. An objective analysis of immediate simultaneous reconstruction in the treatment of primary carcinoma of the breast. Cancer 55:1202, 1985.
9. Webster TJT, Mansel RC, Hughes LE. Immediate reconstruction of the breast after mastectomy: Is it safe? Cancer 53:1418, 1984.
10. Dowden RV, Blanchard JM, Greenstreet RL. Breast reconstruction: Selection, timing, and local recurrence. Ann Plast Surg 10:265, 1983.
11. Johnson CH, van Heerden JA, Donahue JH, et al. Oncological aspects of immediate breast reconstruction following mastectomy for malignancy. Arch Surg 124:819, 1989.
12. Georgiade GS, Riefkohl R, Cox E, et al. Long-term clinical outcome of immediate reconstruction after mastectomy. Plast Reconstr Surg 76:417, 1985.
13. Noone RB, Murphy JB, Spear SL, et al. A 6-year experience with immediate reconstruction after mastectomy for cancer. Plast Reconstr Surg 76:258, 1985.
14. Gilliland MD, Larson DL, Copeland EM. Appropriate timing for breast reconstruction. Plast Reconstr Surg 72:335, 1983.
15. Henderson IC. Appropriate timing for breast reconstruction. Plast Reconstr Surg 72:338, 1983.

15a. Chen KKY, Montague ED, Oswald MJ. Results of irradiation in the treatment of locoregional breast cancer recurrence. Cancer 56:1269, 1985.

16. Fowble B, Gray R, Gilchrist K, et al. Identification of a sub-group of patients with breast cancer and histologically positive axillary nodes receiving adjuvant chemotherapy who may benefit from post-operative radiotherapy. J Clin Oncol 6:1107, 1988.
17. Recht A, Hayes DF. Local recurrence following mastectomy. In Harris JR, Hellman S, Henderson IC, Kinne DW, eds. Breast Diseases. Philadelphia: JB Lippincott, 1991, p 527.
18. McCarty KS Jr, Kesterson GH, Barton TK, et al. Selection of patients for heterotopic implantation of the areola and nipple. Surg Gynecol Obstet 150:545, 1980.
19. Anderson JA, Rallensen RM. Spread to the nipple and areola in carcinoma of breast. Ann Surg 189:367, 1979.
20. Rose JH. Carcinoma in a transplanted nipple. Arch Surg 115:1131, 1980.
21. Smith I, Payne WS, Carney JA. Involvement of the nipple and areola in carcinoma of the breast. Surg Gynecol Obstet 143:546, 1976.
22. Parry RG, Cochran TC Jr, Wolfort FG. When is there nipple involvement in carcinoma of the breast? Plast Reconstr Surg 59:539, 1977.

23. Lagios MD, Gates EA, Westdahl PR, et al. A guide to the frequency of nipple involvement in breast cancer: A study of 149 consecutive mastectomies using a serial subgross and correlated radiographic techniques. Am J Surg 138:135, 1979.
23a. Schnitt SJ, Goldwyn RM, Slavin SA. Mammary ducts in the areola: Implications for patients undergoing reconstructive surgery of the breast. Plast Reconstr Surg 92:1290, 1993.
24. Scanlon EF. Local recurrence in the pectoralis muscles following modified radical mastectomy for carcinoma. J Surg Oncol 30:149, 1985.
25. Kwai AH, Stomper PC, Kaplan WD. Clinical significance of isolated scintigraphic sternal lesions in patients with breast cancer. J Nucl Med 29:324, 1988.
26. Slavin SA, Howrigan PJ, Goldwyn PM. Pseudocyst formation after rectus flap breast reconstruction: Diagnosis and treatment. Plast Reconstr Surg 83:670, 1989.
27. Slavin SA, Love SM, Goldwyn RM. Recurrent breast cancer following immediate reconstruction with myocutaneous flaps. Plast Reconstr Surg 93:1191, 1994.
28. Bedwinek JM, Fineberg B, Lee J, et al. Analysis of failures following local treatment of isolated local-regional recurrence of breast cancer. Int J Radiat Oncol Biol Phys 7:581, 1981.
29. Grotting JC, Urist MM, Maddox WA, et al. Conventional TRAM flap versus free microsurgical TRAM flap for immediate breast reconstruction. Plast Reconstr Surg 83:828, 1989.
30. Arnez ZM, Bajee J, Bardsley AF, et al. Experience with 50 free TRAM flap breast reconstructions. Plast Reconstr Surg 87:470, 1991.
31. Shaw WW, Ahn CY. Breast reconstruction with free flaps. In Noone RB, ed. Plastic and Reconstructive Surgery of the Breast. Philadelphia: BC Decker, 1991, p 437.
32. Georgiade GS, Georgiade NG, McCarty KS Jr, et al. Rationale for immediate reconstruction of the breast following modified radical mastectomy. Ann Plast Surg 8:20, 1982.
33. Georgiade GS, Georgiade NG, McCarty KS Jr, et al. Modified radical mastectomy with immediate reconstruction for carcinoma of the breast. Ann Surg 193:565, 1981.
34. Georgiade GS. Immediate reconstruction of the breast following modified radical mastectomy for carcinoma of the breast. Clin Plast Surg 6:37, 1979.
35. Hueston JT, McKenzie G. Breast reconstruction after radical mastectomy. Aust N Z J Surg 39:367, 1970.
36. Woods JE, Irons GB, Arnold PG. The case for submuscular implantation of prostheses in reconstructive surgery. Ann Plast Surg 5:115, 1980.
37. McCraw J, Bostwick J, Horton CE. Methods of soft tissue coverage for the mastectomy defect. Clin Plast Surg 6:57, 1979.
38. Frazier TG, Noone RB. Immediate reconstruction in the treatment of primary carcinoma of the breast. Surg Gynecol Obstet 157:413, 1983.
39. Horton CE, Rosato RA, McCraw JB, et al. Immediate reconstruction following mastectomy for cancer. Clin Plast Surg 6:37, 1979.
40. Rosen PP, Saigo PE, Braun DW, et al. Predictors of recurrence in Stage I (T1 N0 M0) breast carcinoma. Ann Surg 193:15, 1981.
41. Rosen PP, Saigo PE, Braun DW, et al. Prognosis in Stage II (T1 N0 M0) breast cancer. Ann Surg 194:576, 1981.
42. de Cholnocky T. Augmentation mammoplasty: Survey of complications in 10,941 patients by 265 surgeons. Plast Reconstr Surg 45:573, 1970.
43. Krishnan L, St. George FJ, Mansfield CM, et al. Effect of silicone gel prosthesis on electron and photon dose distributions. Med Phys 10:96, 1983.
44. Leis HP Jr. Selective and reconstructive surgical procedures for carcinoma of the breast. Surg Gynecol Obstet 148:17, 1979.
45. Albo RJ, Gruber R, Kahn R. Immediate breast reconstruction after modified mastectomy for carcinoma of the breast. Am J Surg 140:141, 1980.
46. Harris HI. Surgery of breast implants from the point of view of carcinogenesis. Plast Reconstr Surg 28:81, 1961.
47. Schuler FA, Rosato F, Horton CE. Silicone prosthesis and anti-tumor immunity. Plast Reconstr Surg 61:762, 1978.

48. Lejour M, DeMey A, Mattheiem W. Local recurrences and metastases of breast cancer after 194 reconstructions. Acta Chir Plast 7:131, 1983.
49. Lejour M, Eder H, DeMey A, et al. Breast reconstruction at the Tumor Centre of the University of Brussels: A three-year report. Acta Chir Belg 79:135, 1980.
50. Der Hagopian RP, Zaworski PC, Sugarbaker EV, et al. Management of locally recurrent breast cancer adjacent to prosthetic implants. Am J Surg 141:590, 1981.
51. Montandon D. Incidental discovery of recurrent breast carcinoma in patients seeking breast reconstruction. Br J Plast Surg 32:318, 1979.
52. Shedbaker AR, Devata A, Padamilam T. A study of efforts of radiation on silicone prosthesis. Radiology 135:223, 1980.
53. McGinley PH, Powell WR, Bostwick J III. Dosimetry of a silicone breast prosthesis. Radiology 135:223, 1980.
54. Jacobson GM, Sause WT, Thomson JW, et al. Breast irradiation following silicone gel implants. Int J Radiat Oncol Biol Phys 12:835, 1986.
55. Aberizk WJ, Silver B, Henderson IC, et al. The use of radiotherapy for treatment of isolated locoregional recurrence of breast carcinoma after mastectomy. Cancer 58:1214, 1986.
56. Janjan NA, McNeese MD, Buzdar AV, et al. Management of locoregional recurrent breast cancer. Cancer 58:1552, 1986.
57. Slavin SA. Improving the latissimus dorsi myocutaneous flap with tissue expansion. Plast Reconstr Surg 93:811, 1994.
58. Mustoe TA, Bartell TH, Garner WL. Physical, biomechanical, histologic, and biochemical effects of rapid versus conventional tissue expansion. Plast Reconstr Surg 83:687, 1989.
59. Fentiman IS, Mathews PN, Davison OW, et al. Survival following local skin recurrence after mastectomy. Br J Surg 72:14, 1985.

34

Reoperative Surgery of the Chest Wall

Richard S. Stahl, M.D., M.B.A., and Gary S. Kopf, M.D.

Reoperative Problems

Sternal wounds	Infection
Empyema	Depression deformities
Bronchopleural fistula	Protrusion deformities
Tumor	Poland's syndrome

The thorax is a complex array of vital organs and great vessels housed by a special multilaminate musculoskeleton overlain by skin, subcutaneous tissue, and breasts. Processes within this body region are essential for normal bodily function.

Modern chest reconstruction is usually performed for defects resulting from cardiothoracic surgical complications or extirpative resections. As such, the majority of plastic surgery of the chest wall—strictly speaking—follows a primary intervention and is reoperative surgery. Notable exceptions include the reconstruction of traumatic defects or procedures for the primary treatment of congenital chest wall deformities. Heart failure, ischemia, or anomaly can, singly or in combination, necessitate further reoperation.

Sometimes the indications for secondary surgery are those for which the primary procedure itself was originally performed. Examples include repeat coronary bypass and redo thoracotomy in the setting of prior chest wall reconstruction.

Not all recurrent wounds, fluid collections, and dehiscences require intervention. Indications for reoperation may be clear-cut and absolute or relative and subject to debate. If support or protection of vital organs is inadequate to maintain acceptable homeostasis, surgery may be virtually mandatory. In some cases a patient's general condition or risk factors can be so adverse that a more conservative approach is advised. For example, a nutritionally depleted, catabolic patient with multiple organ failure makes an unfavorable, if not unacceptable, operative candidate. Such a patient can virtually always be managed safely during a period of preoperative preparation.

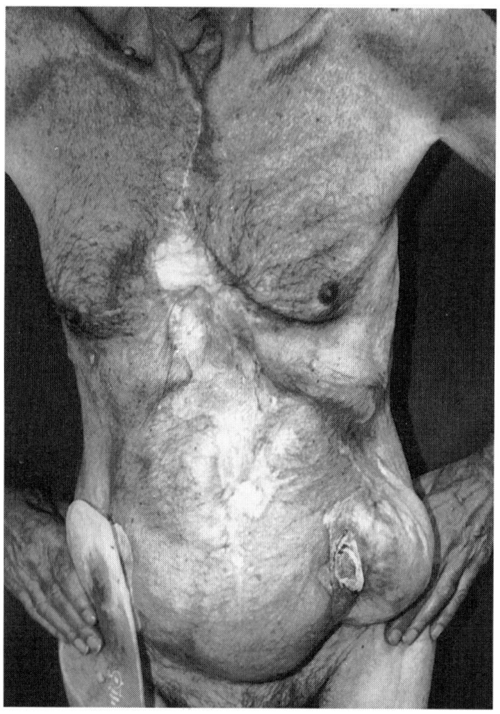

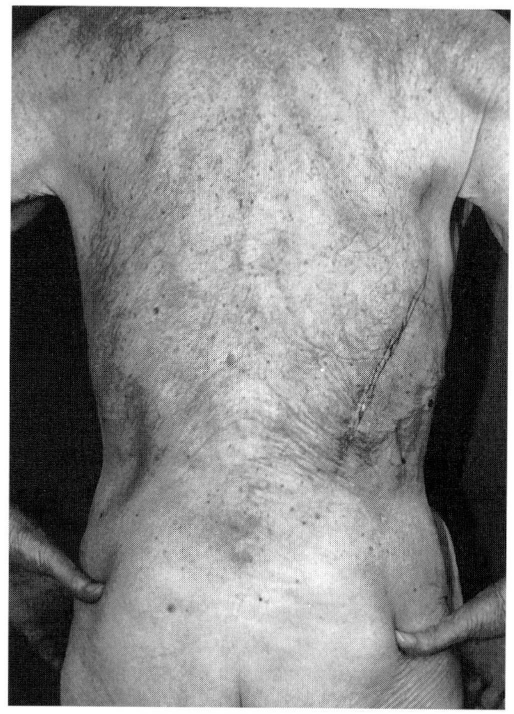

Not all patients are reasonable operative candidates. This elderly gentleman, referred for reoperative chest and abdominal reconstruction, had experienced numerous complications following coronary artery bypass surgery. After reconstruction with multiple flaps, he continued to have a healed but unstable sternal wound and abdominal hernias. The patient was ambulatory but severely depressed and in poor nutritional condition. This patient was discharged for a period of aggressive outpatient nutritional and psychiatric care. Had reoperative thoracic or abdominal wall reconstruction been performed, this patient would almost certainly have tolerated the procedure poorly.

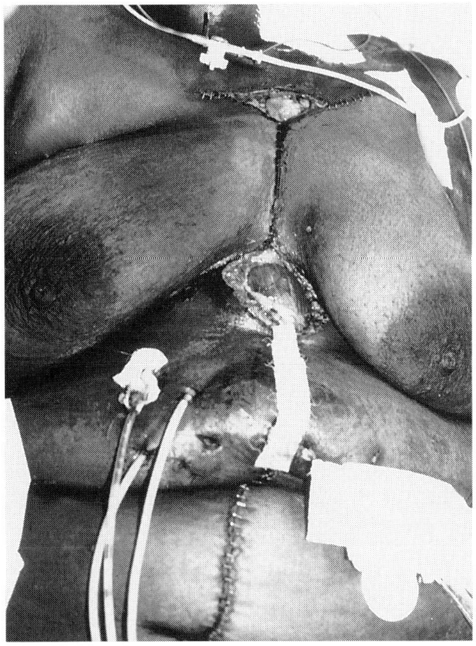

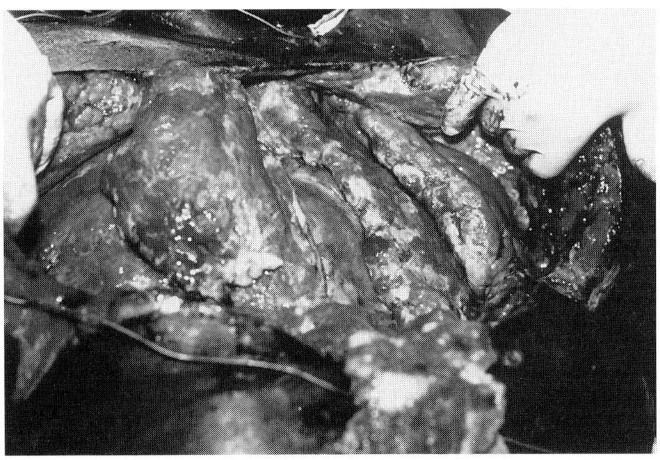

This 350-pound woman with marked macromastia had also been a poor candidate for reoperative surgery. She refused a transfusion for religious reasons despite a hematocrit of 16 following a coronary artery bypass. She was also in poor nutritional balance with greatly depleted protein stores.

A sternal wound reconstruction had been performed nonetheless using bilateral pectoralis major and unilateral rectus abdominis muscle flaps with pectoral cutaneous advancement flaps. Not surprisingly she manifested poor wound healing postoperatively. Despite all attempts to avoid the inevitable dehiscence of the central intermammary segment of the incision, the widely undermined submammary-pectoral cutaneous advancement flaps ultimately dehisced, resulting in a massive, extensively undermined wound that never healed. Without adequate nutritional support, transfusion, and avoidance of the traction effects of widely undermined mammary-pectoral flaps, this patient was unlikely to recover under any circumstances.

Restraint is also advised when planning treatment for the patient with advanced systemic malignancy who will not derive significant palliation from repeated attempts at advanced tumor resection or prolonged treatment of complications resulting from these procedures. The decision of when to operate vs. "when to say no" depends on a comprehensive analysis of the clinical situation.

This chapter discusses the major problems encountered in reoperative thoracic surgery and the decision-making process crucial to planning and executing that surgery. It reviews the treatment of chest wall defects in the setting of multiple failed debridements and/or failed prior flap reconstructions. Secondary chest wall reconstructions for multiply recurrent malignancy and problems of unsuccessful prior treatment of congenital chest wall anomalies are also addressed.

ANATOMIC AND PHYSIOLOGIC CONSIDERATIONS

Reconstructive surgery of the thorax requires a thorough knowledge of three-dimensional thoracic anatomy and cardiopulmonary physiology and careful attention to the special problems of that body region. Assessing the risk to and preserving the function of the underlying organs are important considerations. In thoracic reoperation it is particularly dangerous to assume that the anatomy and the physiologic processes contained within the thorax remain as they were at the time of the previous intervention—even when interoperative intervals are short. The potential for changes in these vital functions from the time of primary intervention *must* be considered. Life-threatening manifestations of cardiopulmonary abnormalities often develop due to the stress of reoperation when they might otherwise remain subclinical or compensated.

Specifically the patient's cardiac status must have adequate reserve for any major operation. Patients undergoing thoracic operations can have a myriad of congenital or acquired cardiopulmonary problems. In most cases, however—especially after successful coronary revascularization or other cardiac reconstruction—the heart's function or vulnerability to dysfunction may be significantly improved over the preoperative state. Consultation with colleagues in cardiology and the performance of studies suggested by them to assess these potential problems can now be frequently performed noninvasively (see p. 1212).

At times the planned reoperation may be expected to further restrict or otherwise interfere with cardiopulmonary function. Ventricular aneurysm, recurrent or persistent tumor or infection, or refractory pulmonary air leak can each require further resectional compromise of the heart, lungs, or supporting structures. Wound closure can occasionally add a small but critical degree of cardiovascular restriction in patients with low output or cyanotic states.

The reoperative thoracic reconstructive surgeon must be concerned with locating and exposing these troubled vital organs and effecting the desired remedies in a fibrotic, opaque, yet intricate encasement of scar. Overzealous resection or debridement can lead to intraoperative calamities or short- or long-term morbidity and mortality from hemorrhage or cardiac or pulmonary insufficiency. Overly conservative debridement, resection, and reconstruction, however, will inevitably subject the patient to yet another recurrent or persistent problem with its own inherent morbidity and mortality. Surgical therapy is thus executed, striking a balance between a number of competing factors.

TIMING

If performed at the wrong time, even the best operation can be doomed to failure. This is especially true in patients requiring cardiothoracic interventions. As a group these patients have limited reserve and cannot tolerate poorly timed interventions. Taking the extra time to aliment such a patient, reduce the bacterial burden within the wound, improve fluid balance or pulmonary toilet, or evaluate and optimize other general medical problems can make the critical difference in preventing complications and achieving a satisfactory result. Since thoracic reoperation is performed for chronic, persistent, or multiply recurrent wounds or problems, there is no excuse for proceeding before all such issues are addressed. A thorough investigation and understanding of prior interventions are also required before an appropriate plan can be executed.

Occasionally emergency situations, such as when exposed vascular or prosthetic suture lines threaten hemorrhage, precipitate the need for prompt intervention or definitive reconstruction. Although such hemorrhagic complications occasionally occur, this circumstance is actually less common than many think since proper debridement, reduction of contamination, and prevention of desiccation usually preclude such complications. In our experience such hemorrhage occurs more commonly as a result of preventable mechanical erosion of the heart by irregular bony margins. Earlier intervention may also be mandated by the presence of exposed, irradiated vital organs, which granulate and tolerate desiccation or contamination poorly.

Consideration of the patient's psychosocial situation is often neglected in the timing of intervention. In select cases definitive resection and/or reconstruction can be performed semielectively, if not electively. In this situation the interval before surgery can be used to enlist the patient's full cooperation. Thus improved efforts at pulmonary toilet, ambulation, and general mobilization can be more easily achieved.

PATIENT EVALUATION

The assessment and planning phases are crucial in all of reconstructive surgery, especially in reoperation for chest wall reconstruction. Many questions must be answered to ensure satisfactory results. The most crucial questions to be answered are: What operations and treatments have been performed and by whom? Why have previous treatments failed? Why has the problem recurred or persisted?

Reviewing prior operative and radiotherapy summaries, discussing operative findings and previous surgery with the primary surgeons, and carefully examining the patient to document previous incisions and operations are invaluable for addressing these questions. It is important to inventory even previously violated or used flaps since they or their remnants may be of use when properly re-elevated and readvanced or transposed. In addition, a list of unviolated reconstructive donor units can be generated in this manner for use in reoperation. A careful patient examination and records analysis will pinpoint the likely causes of recurrence or persistence of the patient's problem or at least guide the way for reoperation in the previously operated field.

Recurrent wound complications, sinuses, or fistulae most commonly result from inadequate identification and resection of involved bone, cartilage, soft tissues, foreign body, or tumor. The second likely cause of local failure is inadequate soft tissue reconstruction in terms of donor bulk, vascularity, inset, or drainage. These potential causes and sites of recurrence must be sought first in the records and patient review so they can be detected at operation. The causes and sites of recurrent wound problems are most successfully determined intraoperatively when they have been first studied and anticipated in the preoperative analysis and planning stages.

The patient's general health status must also be assessed so that other disease processes such as diabetes mellitus, conditions requiring immunosuppressive therapy, and nutritional deficits can be adequately managed. A complete evaluation of the patient's pulmonary and cardiac function must be made before thoracic intervention. It cannot be taken for granted that coronary artery bypass grafts, for example, remain patent. A number of noninvasive studies are now available to ascertain the adequacy of cardiopulmonary function. Occasionally, cardiac catheterization can be of help in verifying graft patency and/or proximity of the graft to the wound that requires debridement. Although most patients can be treated without cardiac catheterization, sometimes biplane arteriographic views of bypass grafts, especially of the internal mammary artery, will help to avoid injury to this structure if it remains patent. Arteriography can also confirm the integrity of the internal mammary–superior epigastric axis supplying the rectus abdominis or pectoralis major turnover flap.

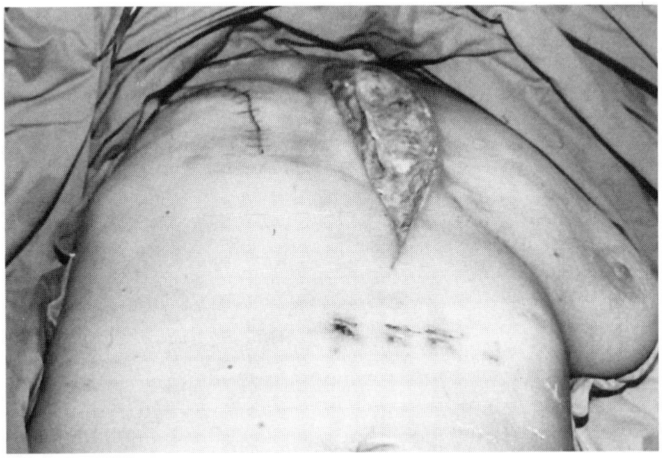

This 64-year-old woman was referred for treatment 6 weeks after a coronary artery bypass graft with left internal mammary artery and multiple saphenous vein grafts. She had previously undergone classic right radical mastectomy for carcinoma of the breast followed by right thoracic radiation therapy.

One month postoperatively she developed signs of an acute staphylococcal infection; the wound was subsequently drained and debrided surgically. The pectoralis major muscle was absent because of the mastectomy, and it was unlikely that either rectus abdominis muscle could be used in its entirety because of the harvest of the left internal mammary artery for the coronary artery bypass and the possible injury to the right internal mammary artery secondary to radiation therapy. The significant size of the left breast was also of concern due to the weight it placed on the presternal region. The stress caused by the weight of the breast was considered to be a risk for further wound healing problems with the unstable, irradiated skin.

Extensive bony and cartilaginous involvement with copious purulent drainage emanating from the wound and multiple sternal fractures were evident. Erythematous and indurated skin margins were also visible. Given the intense fibrosis that had occurred in the 6 weeks since the surgery, the cardiac surgeon believed it would be helpful to obtain an arteriogram before sternal wound reconstruction to assess the internal mammary artery–left anterior descending coronary artery bypass with regard to patency and proximity to the wound.

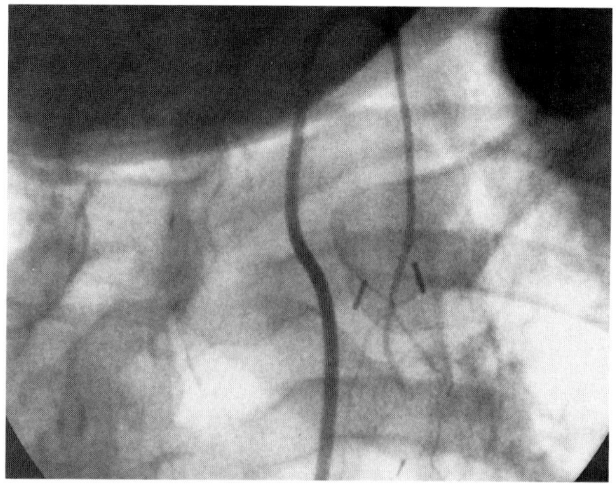

Right and left internal mammary artery: Anteroposterior view

Coronary angiograms were obtained before sternal wound reconstruction. Selective injections of the left internal mammary artery, which had been used to revascularize the left anterior descending coronary artery, were performed. The anteroposterior view as well as the sequential lateral views demonstrate an abrupt cutoff of flow in the internal mammary–left anterior descending coronary artery revascularization. It was consequently believed that this particular coronary artery revascularization had not been successful and that intraoperative injury to the left internal mammary artery would not be as dangerous as if the bypass had been successful. The left internal mammary artery is in close proximity to the sternum as seen on lateral view and would be at risk to injury when resection of a densely fibrotic mediastinum was performed for sternal debridement. Coincidentally, injection of the right internal mammary artery demonstrated robust flow, with patency all the way down to the superior epigastric artery.

The operative plan was thus to avoid mobilizing the left pectoralis major muscle because it was considered to have insufficient bulk and because of concerns about the effect that elevation and mobilization of the totally undermined, heavy left breast would have on the wound. An extremely long, vertically oriented, right rectus abdominis musculocutaneous flap was planned, realizing that the venous or arterial circulation might require supplementation. The right rectus abdominis musculocutaneous flap was elevated, preserving a long inferior epigastric arteriovenous pedicle for anastomosis to recipient vessels in the neck if necessary.

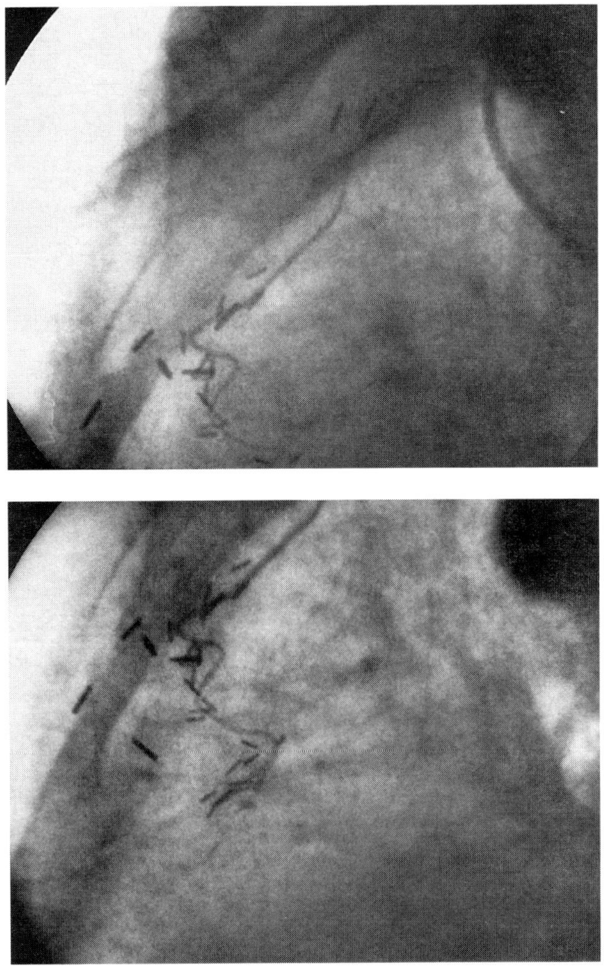

Left internal mammary artery: Sequential lateral views

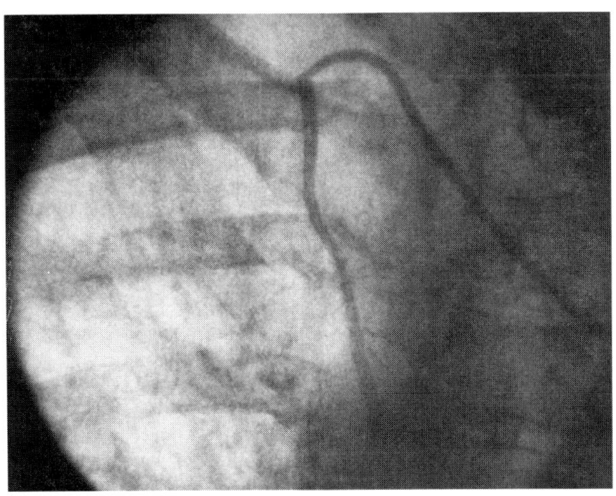

Right internal mammary artery: Selective injection

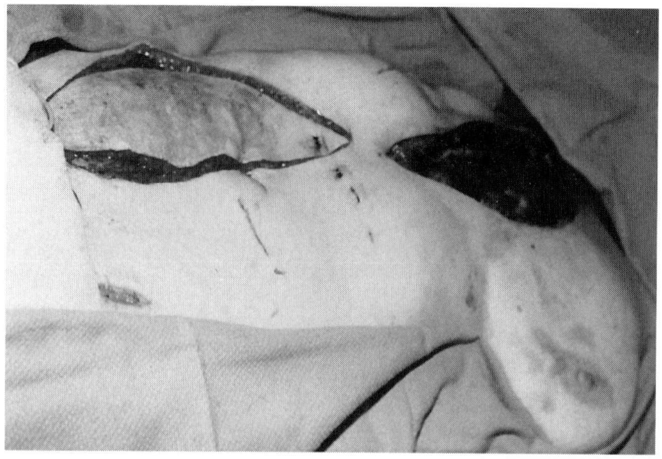

Elevation of the flap was performed, and the flap appeared quite healthy except for equivocal venous congestion at the inferior-most suprapubic rectus territory. Accordingly, the flap was inset without microvascular hookups. The equivocal venous congestion was treated with leeches for 2 to 3 days. Their use did not appear necessary beyond this point. The flap survived in its entirety.

Use of a rectus musculocutaneous flap is not often necessary in sternal wound reconstruction, but in this case it provided the advantage of allowing for further resection of the compromised right presternal cutaneous margin and avoided the tension that elevation and mobilization of the heavy left breast and pectoral region would have placed on the wound.

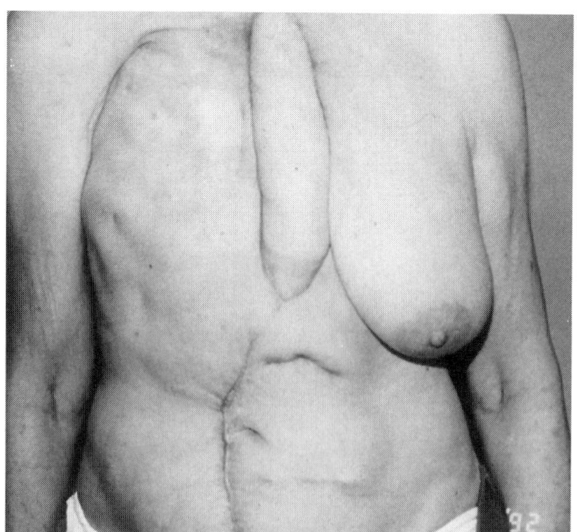

The postoperative result is demonstrated 3 months later, with the patient having healed *per primum* without complications.

Preoperative pulmonary evaluation and therapy can minimize systemic and local wound complications that might result from pulmonary-related wound complications. An assessment of the likely reasons for failure must be made. Postero-anterior and lateral chest x-ray films can help in the search for certain foreign bodies such as retained pacemaker wire remnants or sternal wires that may be infected. Although it is usually not necessary, it should be remembered that other radiographic and nuclear medicine studies such as bone, indium, or gallium scans, CT scan or MRI, and sonograms can help with the preoperative determination of the extent of infection or exploration and debridement that might be necessary.

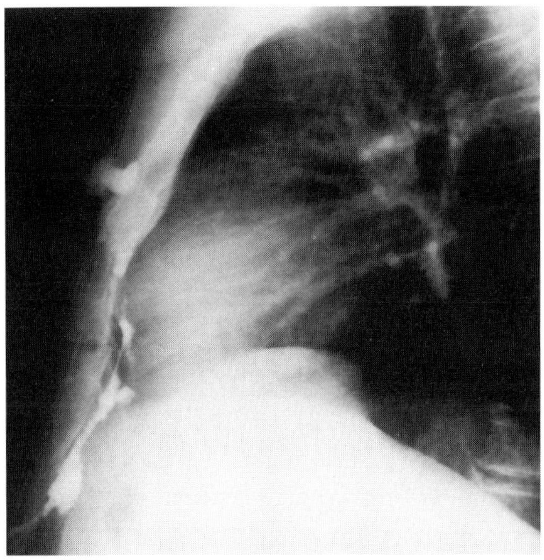

Radiographic contrast injection studies proved beneficial in evaluating this 58-year-old man who was plagued with multiple recurrent infections and sinus tract infection after an urgent coronary artery bypass graft. The midsternal sinus demonstrated apparent extension directly to underlying bone, where a smoldering sequestrum, infected sternal wire segment, or other foreign body was presumed to account for the wound. Injection of a less prominent but recurrent left epigastric sinus opacified a tract extending beneath the xiphoid to an inferior cardiac–diaphragmatic collection and a more superior retrosternal-precardiac collection. Preoperative cultures were also obtained so that the use of sensitivity-directed antibiotic therapy could be ensured.

In recurrent benign processes of the chest wall a determination must be made as to whether the problem or wound is probably going to be self-limited or to heal spontaneously in a reasonable time frame. Factors or conditions that would make spontaneous wound healing more protracted, if not unlikely, include exposed foreign body, exposed rib cartilage or bone, radiation therapy itself, persistent significant air leak in the presence of obstructive pulmonary disease, poor nutrition, high levels of contamination, a large residual dead space or cavity, and a persistent inflammatory or malignant condition.

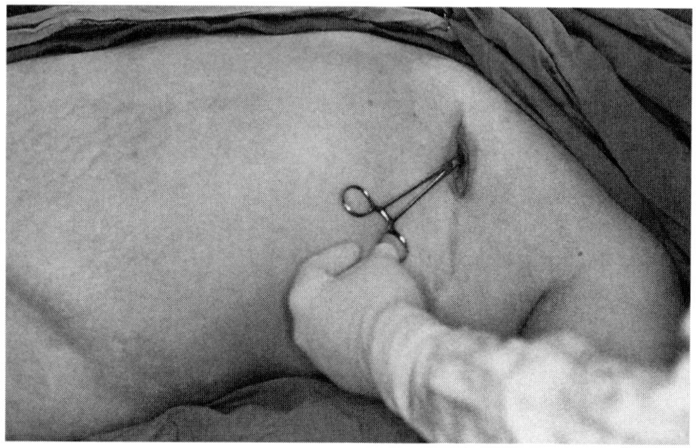

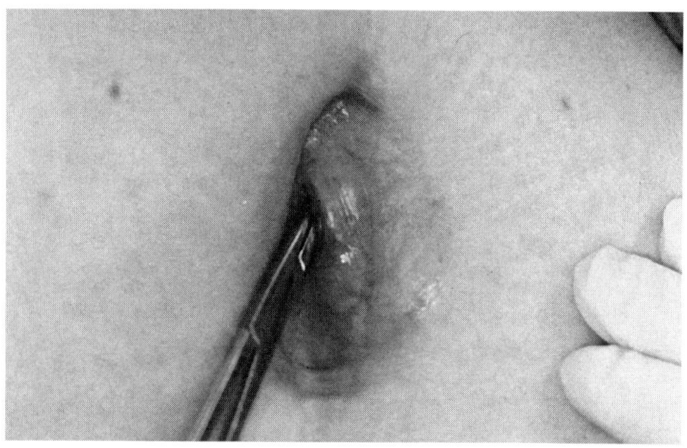

This 42-year-old woman presented with a nonhealing wound of the left anterolateral chest wall secondary to recurrent infection of 4 years' duration. She had undergone multiple procedures for the infection, including ultimately a mastectomy in an unsuccessful attempt at cure. Her past medical history was also significant for inflammatory bowel disease treated with steroids and other immunosuppressive agents.

The wound tracked down to underlying rib. The bone scan was positive for osteomyelitis in this area as well. Given the multiple previous drainage procedures, resections, and soft tissue manipulations, it was decided to attempt chest wall resection and reconstruction to cure this wound.

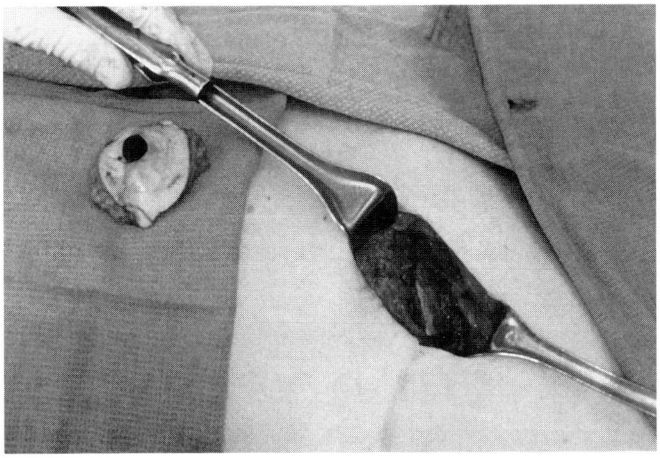

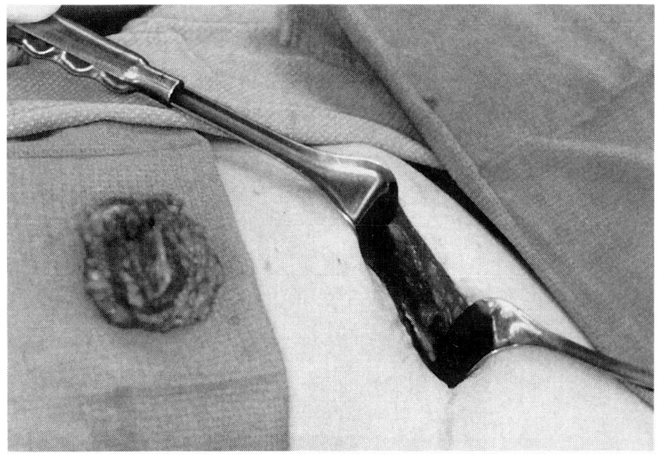

The resection included segmental resection of the underlying rib and a 4 cm soft tissue margin. The wound cavity was stained with methylene blue before the initiation of the procedure to facilitate its resection. The wound was obturated with a pectoralis major muscle flap, and closure was completed with cutaneous advancement flaps.

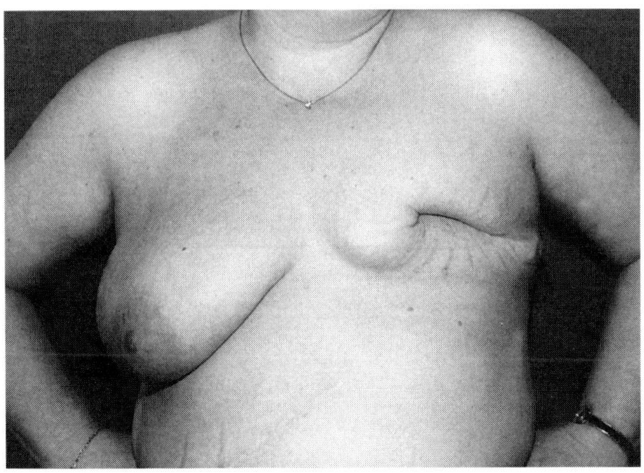

Because of the chronic nature of the infection, she was treated with a 6-week postoperative course of intravenous antibiotics. The healed wound is demonstrated 6 months postoperatively.

With recurrent or persistent malignancy the possibility of distant disease might affect the indications or extent of planned resection. In this situation, before a major reoperative reconstruction is attempted, a full metastatic workup, usually consisting of an MRI or CT scan of appropriate body cavities, should be obtained.

A problem-oriented workup should also be performed as indicated to fully assess the extent and course of bronchopleural fistula, empyema, or sinus tracts. If there is any question as to these parameters after reviewing suitable posteroanterior and lateral chest radiographs, CT scan, MRI, injection studies with both posteroanterior and lateral views, or injection studies in conjunction with a CT scan can be of great help. Such injection studies aid in assessing the three-dimensional anatomy of the wound, planning the execution of the reoperative procedure, and ascertaining the arcs of flap rotation. Occasionally a three-dimensional CT scan or MRI can give an even more descriptive illustration of the anatomy of these entities. In addition, a three-dimensional CT scan or MRI can be helpful in the preoperative evaluation of depression and protrusion deformities.

When injection studies are performed, the most appropriate contrast medium must be selected by the radiologist for each study, particularly in cases in which the contrast material is likely to enter the tracheobronchial tree. In these cases, for example, fat-soluble contrast material is best tolerated by the tracheobronchial tree and least likely to cause aspiration pneumonia. When recurrent tumor occurs in proximity to major vessels (usually the subclavian vessels), vascular examination and angiography are indicated to detail the underlying vascular anatomy, ascertain the degree of vascular disease, and make any necessary contingency plans for localizing, resecting, or bypassing involved vessels. In irradiated or multiply operated patients, these issues can be especially complicated and require special care.

PLANNING

When reoperative thoracic surgery is necessary, careful forethought and contingency planning are important for maximizing the margin of safety. A multitude of life-threatening contingencies may arise rapidly and without warning in the thorax. Effective surgical planning requires that any operation and all imaginable consequences and subsequent actions be envisioned in advance in a step-by-step manner to ensure the success of the intervention. In this way intraoperative problems as well as short- and long-term sequelae can be anticipated and management planned accordingly.

A three-dimensional analysis of the wound, structures to be resected, flaps available for reconstruction and their arcs of rotation, and vital organs that need to be covered is important in this planning process. In postsurgical empyema or bronchopleural fistula, for example, the hilum and the diaphragm may typically shift superiorly and laterally. This movement effectively elevates the pleural defect or bronchial stump to a more superior (and usually more favorable) territory for coverage. The diaphragm elevation effectively decreases the volume of the pleural cavity and thus its demand for vascularized fill. Failure to appreciate the mediastinal hilar shift makes injury during debridement more likely. The three-dimensional appreciation of the intrathoracic wound is also invaluable in making counterincisions or creating transcostal or transdiaphragmatic windows or tunnels to optimize flap use or inset.

Resection of the soft tissue margins of the wound must also be planned. These must be resected as best possible. Although true resection of the surfaces of the heart and great vessels is impractical, the bacterial burden at these sites is greatly reduced by curettage of these surfaces, gentle stripping of exudates and peels, and jet lavage. When infection of synthetic-pledgeted sutures, overly prominent sternal wires, or vascular patches or conduits occurs, however, the intimidating task of their resection, removal, or replacement must be pursued if cure is to be achieved. Grafts of biologic origin are more likely to tolerate infection than synthetic ones. Such homografts or heterografts typically respond favorably to adequate cleansing or debridement of the wound and flap coverage *without* replacement.

Three-dimensional planning also comes into play when the effects of bony-cartilaginous debridement for sternal wound reconstruction are considered. The antibacterial benefits of ridding the wound of contaminated or desiccated bone and cartilage have been well described. No cartilage should be left exposed in the wound as it is a frequent source of smoldering chondritis. A less frequently recognized favorable effect of this debridement is its creation of a less acutely concave, more shallow mediastinal wound. This effect also decreases the volume of wound requiring vascularized fill. With the reduction of the anteroposterior height of the lateral wound margins, the reach of the pectoralis major or latissimus dorsi muscle is increased as it is advanced medially into the wound. Similarly there is no bowstringing of taut muscle flaps draped across the potential space of a steeply concave wound.

The short- and long-term cardiorespiratory effects of any required skeletal, cardiac, pulmonary, or prosthetic resection must also be anticipated. How likely is the proposed operation to make the patient a cardiac or respiratory cripple? Will any resultant vital organ compromise likely be transient or permanent? Will the procedure interfere with subsequent growth? To what other problems will the patient be prone as a result of the operation? An assessment of such problems in advance allows the surgeon to minimize risks.

The amount of bony resection required must be analyzed relative to the maximum amount that can be tolerated. Risk factors that increase the chances of infection, exposure, or nontake of bone grafts or prosthetic materials include the presence of contamination, prior or planned radiation, and questionable soft tissue coverage. Exposure of the skeletal reconstruction or prosthetic mesh at the site of thoracic skeletal resection to a pulmonary air leak—especially in the presence of anticipated continued positive pressure ventilation—also renders bony reconstruction susceptible to postoperative complications or failure. At times the location of rib grafts may be such that they compress flap circulation or the flap pedicle.

When bony reconstruction is planned, it must be remembered that harvesting multiple rib grafts—especially if split rib grafts are not used to stabilize the donor site—can result in paradoxical motion at the donor site, an effect that may outweigh the benefits of stabilizing the area of resection.

Most patients can tolerate segments of two to three rib resections without replacement if necessary. Taut prosthetic mesh helps to stabilize such segments without bone graft replacement. If flaps are not adequately mechanically supported without the presence of mesh and if support is the only indication for the placement of mesh, absorbable mesh (e.g., Vicryl) may be used if contamination is a concern. Defects larger than two to three ribs can be tolerated in some patients, especially in certain areas such as beneath the scapula. Most adult patients also can tolerate the total absence of a sternum, if necessary. Adults with pulmonary compromise and children, whose thoracic musculoskeletons are virtually all cartilaginous, tend to have greater difficulty with respiratory recuperation when larger skeletal defects are created.

When bony reconstruction is elected, bone stabilization is crucial in establishing an adequate union. Maximizing contact at the junction of the bone graft to the margins of bony resection and the use of rigid stabilization can help. This is often a cause of failure of primary reconstructions in situations such as pectus deformities.

Chest wall reconstruction in the pediatric population requires other special general considerations. Some patients with congenital heart disease may have persistent low output or cyanotic disease that may not have been corrected at the time of chest wall reconstruction. These patients require highly specialized perioperative critical care. They often will require future cardiothoracic surgical interventions. Consideration and analysis of future operative interventions, the possible surgical incisions required for these future procedures, and the need to reenter any reconstructed site must be performed in the planning of such procedures.

The analysis must include verifying that all tissues to be used in the current reconstruction and as many as possible that might be used in possible future corrective procedures or reconstructions have an adequate vascular supply. Foresight is mandatory in considering the issue of future growth in the pediatric population. Primary thoracic musculoskeletal deformities are often present in this population. Reconstructive procedures can additionally adversely affect the growth of the musculoskeleton as well as the breast. Minimizing bony debridement, restoring the musculoskeleton as anatomically as practical, and avoiding dissection beyond the minimum required can help to minimize subsequent secondary growth deformities. Special care should be taken in the prepectoral or subcutaneous plane, especially in young women, since disturbance of breast growth can be severe, dramatic, and disfiguring, even with minimal interventions in the early years of life.

GOALS OF TREATMENT

The goal of treatment in reoperative chest wall reconstruction, as with all of reconstructive surgery, is the restoration of function and form. Since the function of this body region is to facilitate and protect a multitude of vital processes, returning the chest wall to a functional state is the highest priority. Although the goal of such procedures should be to anatomically restore normal form as well, this cannot practicably be obtained in all cases yet.

In the pediatric age group subsequent operations, especially breast reconstructive procedures, or correction of progressive thoracic skeletal deformities may become necessary in the future, and long-term follow-up must be performed for surveillance of such problems. In certain secondary deformities, early intervention can facilitate the ease of their treatment.

STERNAL WOUNDS

Sternal wound reconstructions may fail in the early or late postoperative phase. Early complications typically present as a wound separation, dehiscence, or early septic complications. Late problems arise from recurrent infection, often manifesting themselves as one or more sinus tracts.

Early wound separations following sternal wound reconstruction may be multifactorial but usually are caused by inadequate debridement leading to infection or persistent chondritis, unevenly debrided bony or cartilaginous margins causing mechanical trauma to the suture line, poor soft tissue coverage of the bony and cartilaginous margins, or inadequate attention to the details of achieving an adequate, meticulous, layered soft tissue coverage. Inadequate hemostasis, suction drainage, or pulmonary toilet with resultant excessive coughing can contribute to local factors and wound separations.

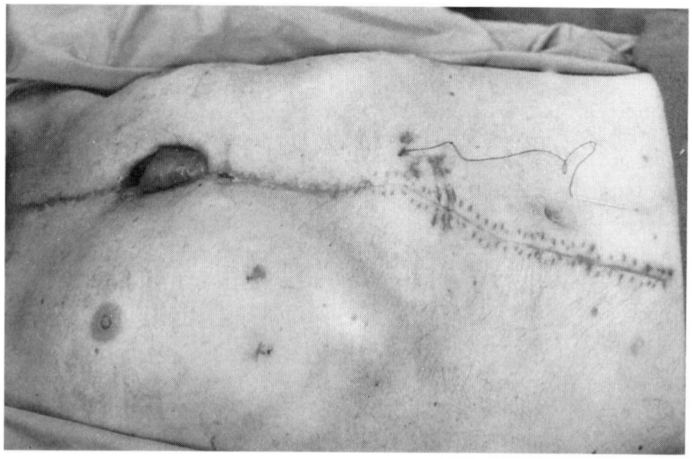

This 68-year-old man with a prior history of chronic obstructive pulmonary disease experienced episodes of severe coughing postoperatively after coronary artery bypass graft, which resulted in the dehiscence and fragmentation of the sternum by the sternal wires. He was returned to the operating room at that time for debridement of the involved bony-cartilaginous margins and reconstruction of the wound with bilateral pectoralis major and unilateral rectus abdominis muscle flaps and cutaneous advancement flaps. Two to 3 weeks postoperatively, during recurrent fits of coughing, a segment of the left sternal margin and associated costal prominences disrupted the incision as seen above.

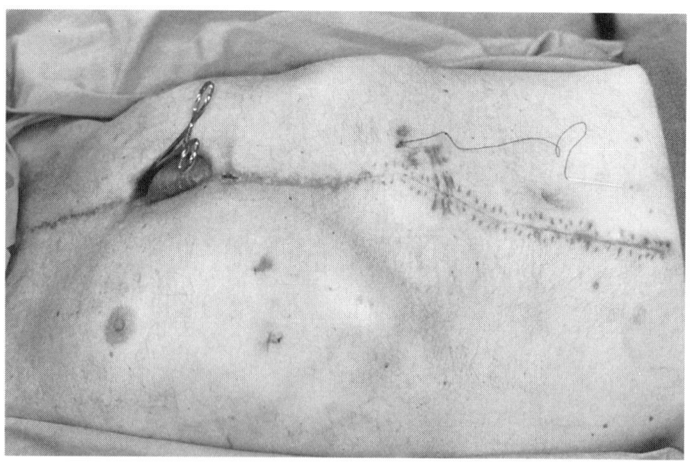

The entire undermined subcutaneous space communicated with this wound. This wound would not close in a stable fashion in any reasonable time interval. He was returned to the operating room for complete debridement-resection of the residual sternal and costal margins and salvage reconstruction with a greater omental flap and skin grafts. At the time of surgery the undermined spaces were vigorously curetted and jet lavaged. The omental flap was secured to the dermal margins, and multiple suction catheters were used to adequately evacuate the subcutaneous space.

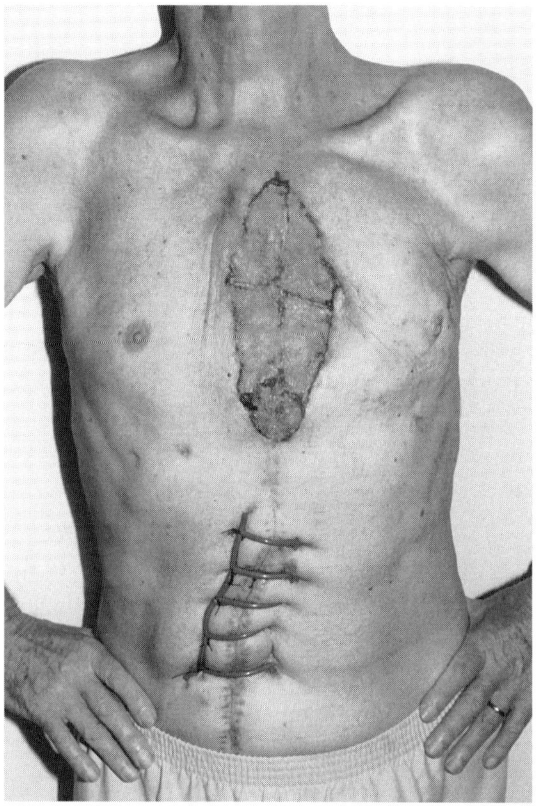

At the 3-week postoperative visit, the healing omental flap and skin graft were in place. There were no complications from this salvage procedure.

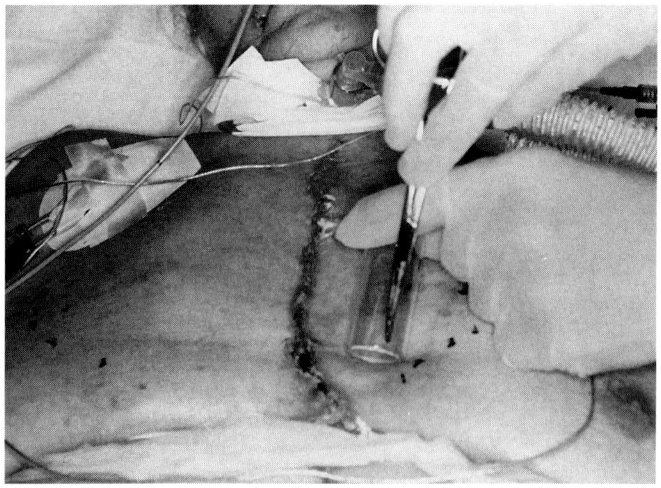

Occasionally, tracheostomy placement in a patient who has had sternal wound reconstruction can lead to a recurrent wound secondary to disruption of the layered closure by subcutaneous emphysema. This elderly obese diabetic woman had undergone sternal wound reconstruction with bilateral pectoralis major flaps and a rectus abdominis flap for mediastinitis, which had developed after coronary artery bypass surgery. She also suffered from acute systemic herpes and systemic candidiasis. She required tracheostomy for refractory pulmonary failure. Despite waiting 1 month after sternal wound reconstruction to perform the tracheostomy and taking precautions to place the tracheostomy as high as possible, massive subcutaneous emphysema developed in the entire pectoral region on both sides. Ultimately the wound had to be reopened and packed, thus representing a late cause for failure of the sternal wound reconstruction. The patient did not survive.

The soft tissue planes can take a great deal of time to heal in a secure manner, especially in debilitated, immunosuppressed, or malnourished patients. The operating surgeon thus must continue to carefully supervise all treatments rendered to the patient for a long interval postoperatively.

Preoperative Preparation

The following precautions should be taken when performing mediastinal reoperation. First, antiembolic intermittent compression garments are placed on at least one if not two extremities. Even if the lower extremities must remain draped into the operative field for other purposes, placement of such a garment on one of the upper extremities can help to reduce the incidence of pulmonary embolism. Cleansing and draping large areas of the body will help to prepare for any number of contingencies. An adequate lower extremity donor site should be available for harvesting vein grafts should replacement of a coronary artery bypass graft be necessary. Similarly access to the groin should be available for cannulation of the femoral vessels should emergency extracorporeal circulatory support need to be instituted. This is important in the reoperative situation because dense mediastinal fibrosis from prior procedures makes inadvertent injury to the heart or great vessels more likely.

The thigh can also be used to obtain fascia lata or deepithelialized full-thickness skin grafts for use as an outflow tract patch or autologous pledget material if an indwelling infected synthetic patch is to be replaced or a cardiac suture line is to be reinforced. A skin graft may also be needed from the thigh if cutaneous advancement flaps are not used for the completion of closure. This is especially true when the greater omentum is used. The entire abdomen is included in the operative field and prepared, giving access to both rectus abdominis muscles as well as the greater omentum.

When all of the pectoralis major and rectus abdominis muscles have been violated or rendered unusable and the omentum is not suitable, the latissimus dorsi muscles are available for coverage of the sternal region. If it seems likely that this contingency will arise, it is advisable to prepare the back, staple or suture sterile drapes along the posterior midline, and then place the patient in the supine position on sterile sheets placed over a beanbag before preparing and draping the anterior thorax for debridement or resection. This will obviate the need to turn the patient in the midst of a prolonged and complex operation for redraping and will also facilitate the stable positioning of the patient in the appropriate lateral decubitus position.

At this point the appropriate body regions are prepared and draped, and culture-directed antibiotic doses are given intravenously before the initiation of the operation. Suitable anesthesia is achieved with the appropriate monitoring lines and devices.

The degree of anticipated resection is assessed, and the desired incisions are outlined with methylene blue. Furthermore, if feasible, any sinus tracts are injected with methylene blue via a syringe and small catheter. Often infiltration with dilute epinephrine-containing solutions into the region of the incisions can help to minimize bleeding in the superficial planes and help with precise visualization of the location of the sinus tracts or other areas of abnormal anatomy.

Technique

The dissection proceeds first with the elevation of any previously used cutaneous flaps to allow for wide exposure. Next, any previously used muscles are re-elevated anatomically to preserve their maximal bulk so that they may be reused if possible. Previously used pectoralis major flaps may have been advanced and sutured in the midline. It is often difficult to anatomically dissect them from each other where they overlap or are secured. If both flaps have been advanced, it works well to divide them in the midline and reflect the soft tissues to their respective lateral direction. Review of prior operative notes or discussions with the previous surgeons should determine the pedicle on which each previously elevated flap was raised.

If reexploration is performed for a staged cardiac procedure in the setting of prior chest wall reconstruction, reelevation or dissection of the flaps from the heart and great vessels does not have a prohibitive risk. In some cases it is much more straightforward than expected, even when extensive cardiac procedures or the placement of large amounts of synthetic material is necessary. Alternatively the procedure may be performed via a previously unoperated alternative route (Table 34-1).

Table 34-1 Alternate Surgical Approaches for Cardiothoracic Procedures

Surgical Incision	*Procedures Feasible Via Given Incision*
Sternotomy	All cardiac procedures Select systemic-pulmonary shunts Pericardial window Pericardiectomy Pulmonary band Right pneumonectomy Left pneumonectomy Left upper lobectomy Right upper lobectomy Right middle lobectomy
Right anterior/anterolateral thoracotomy	Atrial septal defect repair Mitral valve replacement Tricuspid valve replacement Anomalous pulmonary venous return repair Select systemic-pulmonary venous return Select esophageal procedures Right upper lobectomy Right middle lobectomy Right lower lobectomy
Right lateral/posterolateral thoracotomy	Any pulmonary procedure Select esophageal procedures
Left anterior/anterolateral thoracotomy	Redo coronary artery bypass graft Select systemic-pulmonary shunts Pulmonary band Pericardial window Left upper lobectomy Left lower lobectomy
Left posterior/posterolateral thoracotomy	Redo coronary artery bypass graft Patent ductus arteriosus ligation Aortic coarctation Vascular rings Left upper lobectomy Left lower lobectomy
Combined bilateral thoracotomy	Any cardiac procedure Any pulmonary procedure

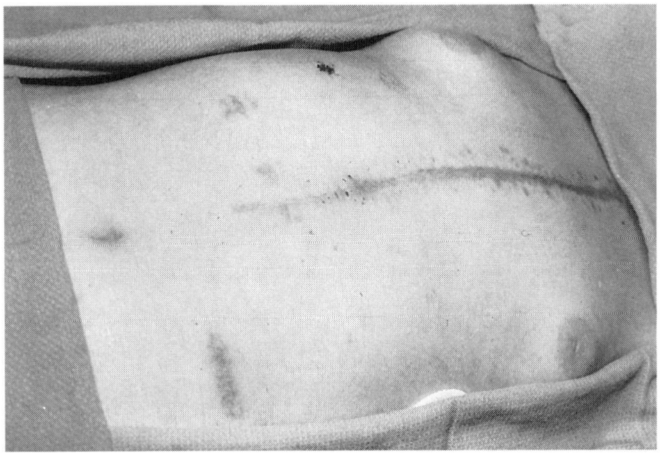

This 12-year-old girl is seen 4 months following omental obturation of a retrosternal abscess cavity that had occurred as a complication of right ventricular outflow tract patch repair with a biologic patch. Her cardiac condition required that she be returned to the operating room for reexploration and revision of the cardiac reconstruction.

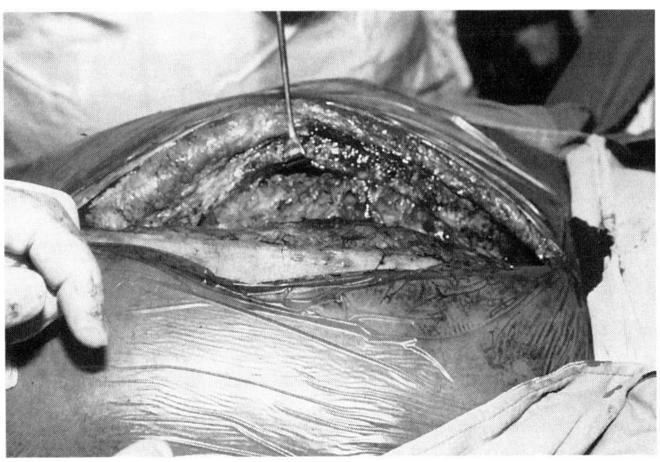

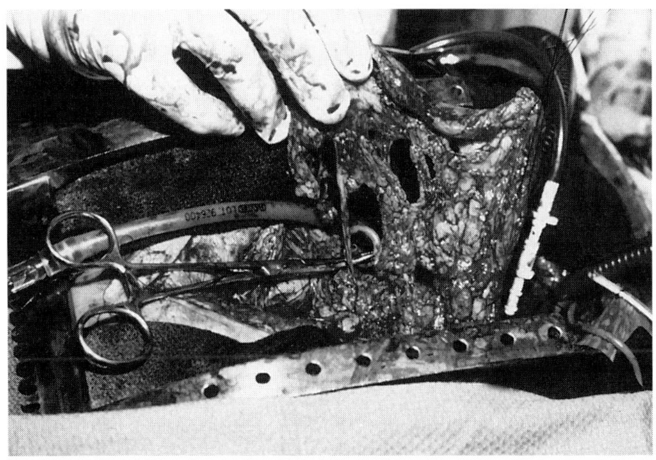

The well-healed sternotomy was reopened without difficulty and demonstrated the lack of dense adhesions to the posterior sternum. The omentum remained pliable and was easily manipulated within the former abscess cavity. The omentum was partially elevated and reflected to allow cannulation for cardiopulmonary bypass. The procedure was completed without incident and the omentum was returned to the cavity for closure.

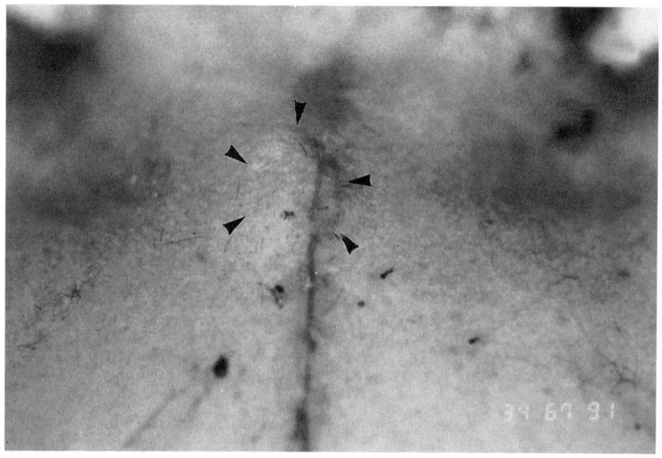

Another example of reexploration for a staged cardiac procedure is illustrated by this 30-year-old man who presented with high fever and a suprasternal abscess 2 weeks following the replacement of a prosthetic pulmonary valve and the placement of a right ventricular outflow tract patch for complex congenital anomalies. He had undergone multiple previous surgical procedures since infancy.

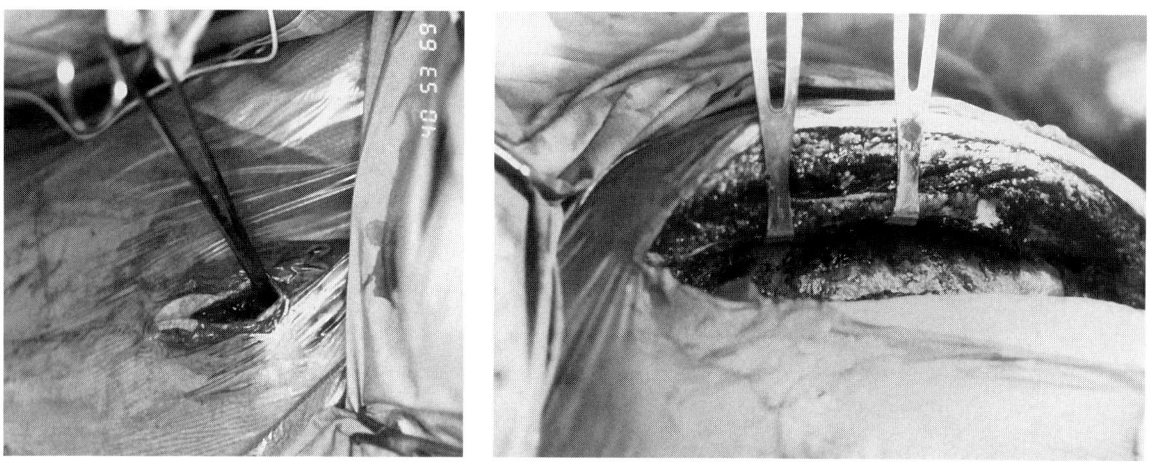

The upper sternotomy incision was incised and the abscess was drained. It tracked around the sternal notch superiorly and seemed to track further beneath the sternum. The entire sternotomy incision was reopened, and the sternal wires were removed to allow inspection of the retrosternal space. The suprasternal cavity was found to communicate with a large abscess cavity on the surface of the right ventricular outflow tract bioprosthetic patch behind the left hemisternum, which is seen being lifted by the retractors.

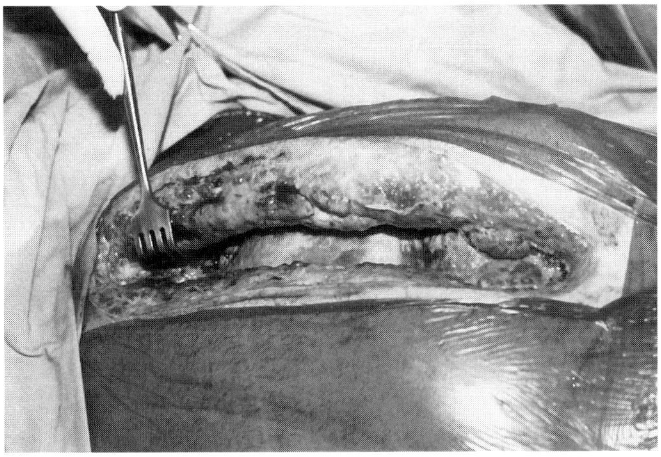

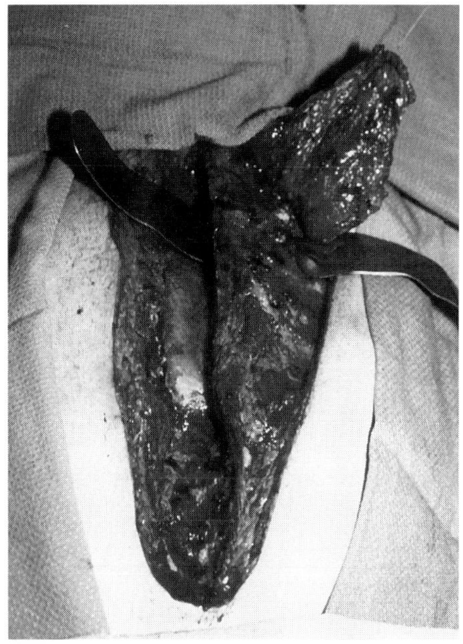

Because of the patient's systemic toxicity and extensive suppuration found locally, he was treated with several days of topical wound care and culture-specific antibiotics. He was returned to the operating room for further debridement and flap reconstruction. The rake is seen retracting the portion of the sternum behind which the fixed, uncollapsed abscess cavity was located. After limited debridement of the sternal margins involved by the process and debridement and curettage of the abscess cavity, heart, and great vessels, the wound was extensively jet lavaged with a dilute hypochlorite solution.

To obturate the unyielding abscess cavity with well-vascularized tissue, the left pectoralis major muscle was elevated on its dominant thoracoacromial pedicle (shown retracted by suture). The insertion was divided to achieve greater mobility. To deliver the muscle to the mediastinal abscess cavity and still allow reapproximation of the uninvolved sternum, a costal window or tunnel was created by resecting three costal cartilages on the left (malleable retractor traverses costal window). With cautious dissection, violation of the left pleura and the left internal mammary artery was avoided.

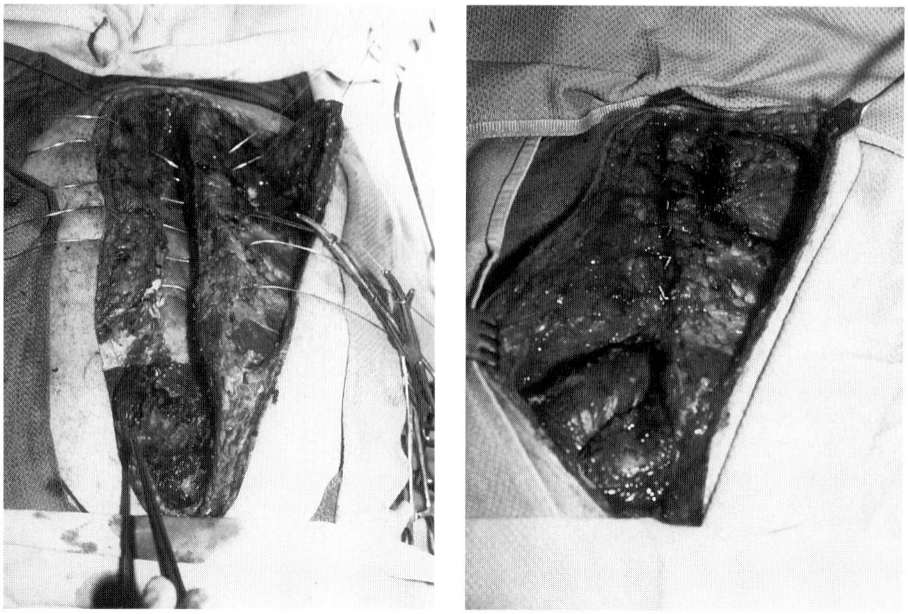

The muscle was secured to the costal window margins, placing the sutures in such a way as to advance the muscle into the defect and hold it in place in the cavity. The sternal wires were then placed and tied. Note the pectoralis major muscle entering the costal window in the patient's upper left thorax.

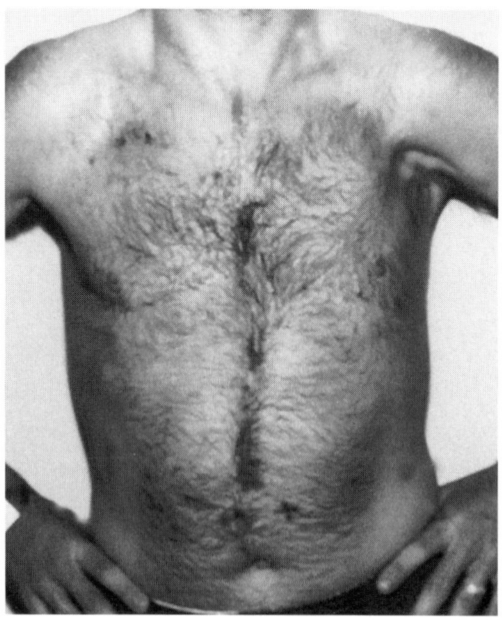

Four months later he returned with a healed wound ready to undergo the next cardiac procedure.

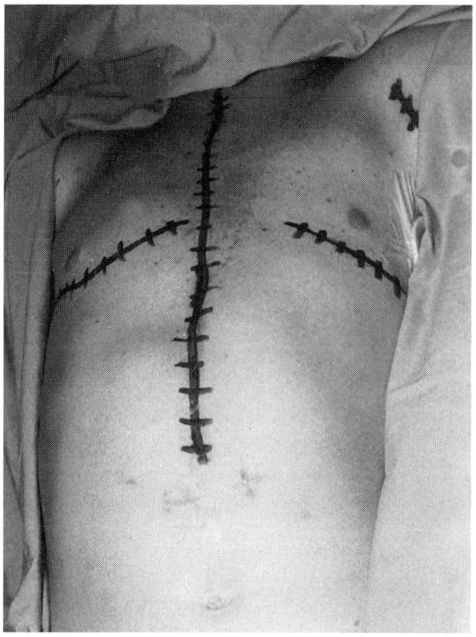

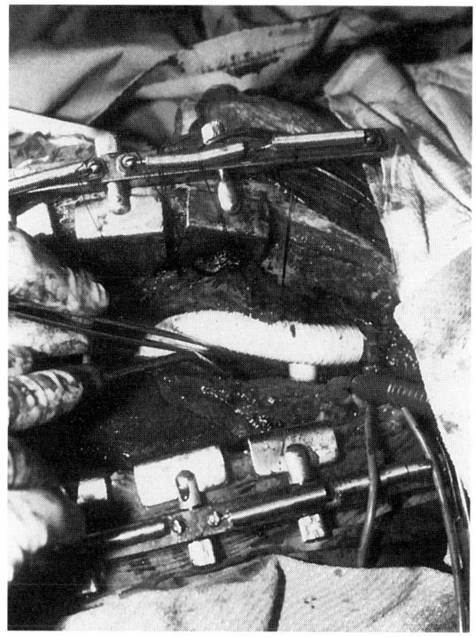

He was returned to the operating room, where the previous bilateral thoracotomy, sternotomy, and left pectoral flap tendon (axillary) release incisions are outlined. The sternotomy was opened and the muscle flap was taken down uneventfully. A large Dacron superior vena cava–right atrial shunt and, behind it, a main pulmonary artery–left pulmonary artery shunt were placed, and the muscle and sternum were closed over them without difficulty. There was no evidence of persistent fluid collection or cavity found at this reexploration. Healing proceeded without difficulty despite the complex nature of this reconstructive effort.

▪ ▪ ▪

If sinus tracts exist, they are circumscribed with separate counterincisions if they are not in proximity to the primary incision. Otherwise excisional extensions of the primary incision will include these in the original incision.

After reflection of previously used flaps from the problem site, the recurrent wound or sinus is traced, with the help of the methylene blue–stained tissues, to its origin. This origin is most commonly a smoldering, infected, or desiccated costal cartilage or sternocostal remnant or a foreign body such as sternal wires, pledgeted sutures or patches, or other synthetic prostheses or materials. The involved materials or tissues are then resected in a methodical, thorough, and safe manner.

This eradication of the offending materials typically requires several techniques. Progressing from "known" to "unknown" tissues is a safe principle of dissection and usually is achieved by exposing an adjacent uninvolved segment of bone or cartilage and proceeding with subperiosteal or subperichondrial dissection along it. In this manner the involved bone and cartilage can be fully removed from the underlying vital structures without violating the healthy tissue.

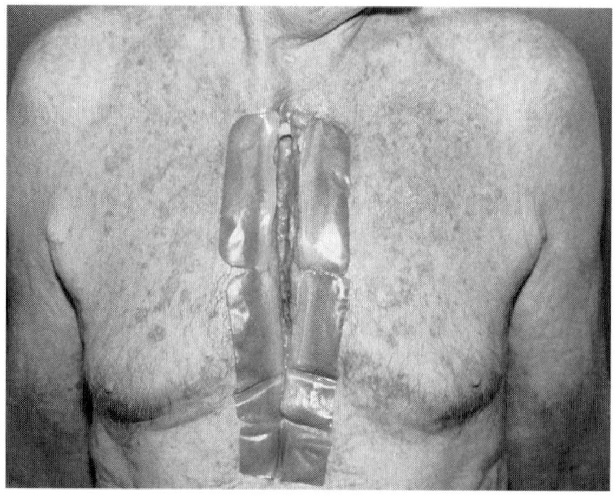

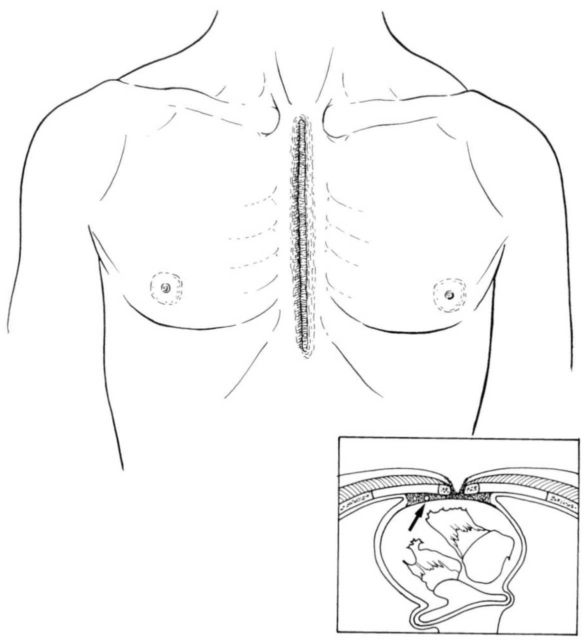

The use of various techniques to eliminate offending materials is effectively demonstrated in the treatment of this 65-year-old man who was referred 14 months after a coronary artery bypass operation. He had been returned to the operating room 2 hours postoperatively for retrieval of a surgical sponge. He was then readmitted 2 to 3 weeks postoperatively with signs of what proved to be a staphylococcal infection. He had undergone multiple surgical debridements and many months of intravenous and oral antibiotic therapy.

In the setting of multiple previous surgical procedures in this area, the wound was densely fibrotic, with the heart quite adherent to the anterior mediastinal structures. There was evidence of continuing smoldering infection of the margins of the sternum, and it was believed that sternal resection carried significant morbidity because of cardiac adhesions. A faded, long, right subcostal incision was evidence of a gastrectomy performed 20 years earlier. His past medical history was also significant for psoriasis. Because of multiple prior operations and the uncertain nature of the multiple previous episodes of sternal debridement, it was decided to widely resect the sternocostal region to give the best possible chance of completely removing the smoldering bony and cartilaginous tissues and give the greatest chance of recovery in this chronic multiply operated patient.

A chronic, nonhealing wound was evident at the site of the patient's previous median sternotomy with signs of peripheral skin involvement with psoriasis. The heart was adherent to the posterior sternum and costal cartilages. The underlying nearby internal mammary artery conduit was used for bypass of the left anterior descending coronary artery (arrow).

At this operation the soft tissue wound was first incised through skin, subcutaneous tissues, and muscle over areas where the presence of bone and cartilage could be confirmed by palpation.

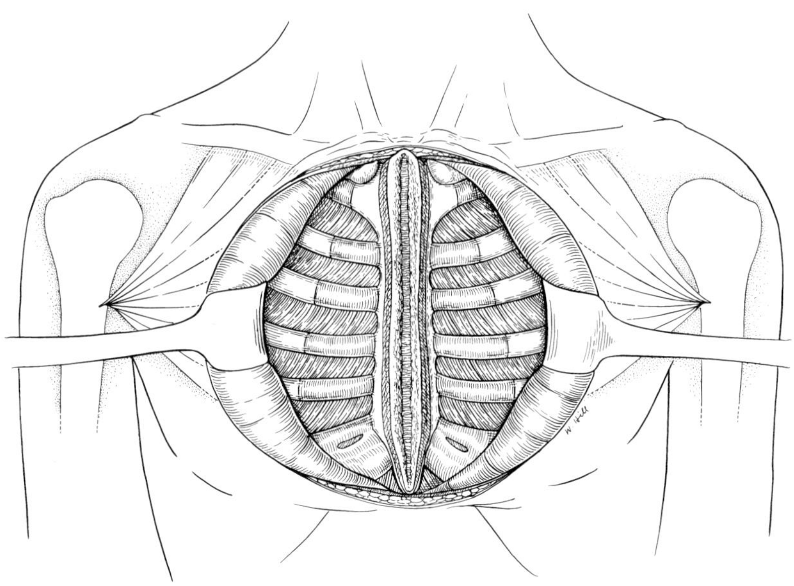

Composite musculocutaneous flaps were then elevated from the rib surfaces so that these units were widely undermined and elevated from the underlying structures to be further dissected and resected. The residual central full-thickness wound is shown with the adjacent/continuous unroofed costal cartilages and sternum. The retractors are holding the composite flaps laterally to expose the costal cartilages for piecemeal resection.

Sequential subperichondrial dissection of the costal cartilages was performed, with care taken to closely adhere to the cartilage surface to maintain a safe plane of dissection and thus avoid cardiac injury. In this manner all costal cartilages were removed and the lateral sternocostal junctions and lateral sternum were safely delineated so that the dissection could proceed most safely centripetally toward the area of greatest fibrosis and danger. Once the costal cartilages on both sides have all been resected, sternal dissection and resection can take place in a methodical manner from each sternal margin until the entire sternum is progressively elevated and resected on a piecemeal basis if necessary.

Use of a fine elevator such as the Freer with rongeurs is invaluable in this tedious, cautious subperiosteal sternal elevation. Once all the costal cartilages have been resected subperichondrially and the bone has been removed subperiosteally, a clean wound with fresh tissues, devoid of sequestra and any other nidus for infection, has been exposed without injury to the heart. At this point no bridges have been burned with regard to preservation of all flap units except for the additional division of internal mammary perforators (which are often injured by previous debridements or pectoralis major elevation), precluding the use of pectoral turnover flaps. The left internal mammary artery had already been used as a vascular conduit for coronary bypass.

During the debridement several fragments of bone and cartilage not contiguous with the body of the sternum were detected. These fragments resulted from the prior surgeon's failure to sequentially debride the sternal margins. In reoperative situations it is critical to detect and remove all questionable bone and cartilage fragments. It is easy to not appreciate certain of these free-floating incompletely debrided fragments when multiple previous debridements by other surgeons have been performed. Bony landmarks are also lost in these situations and make the debridement more dangerous with regard to cardiac injury.

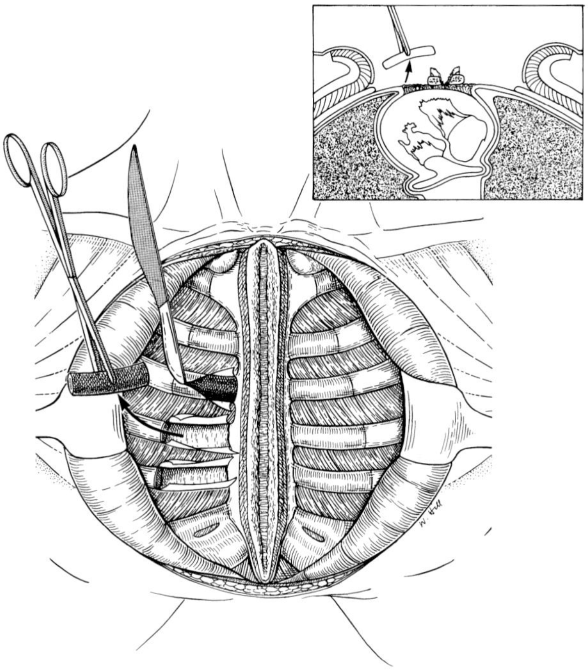

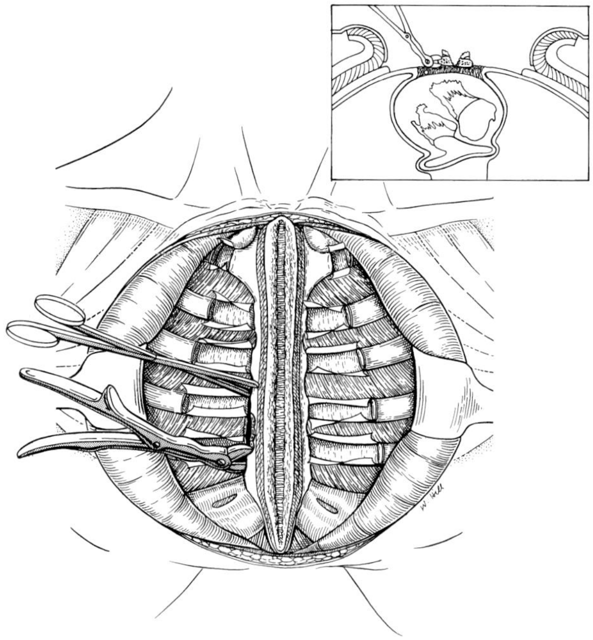

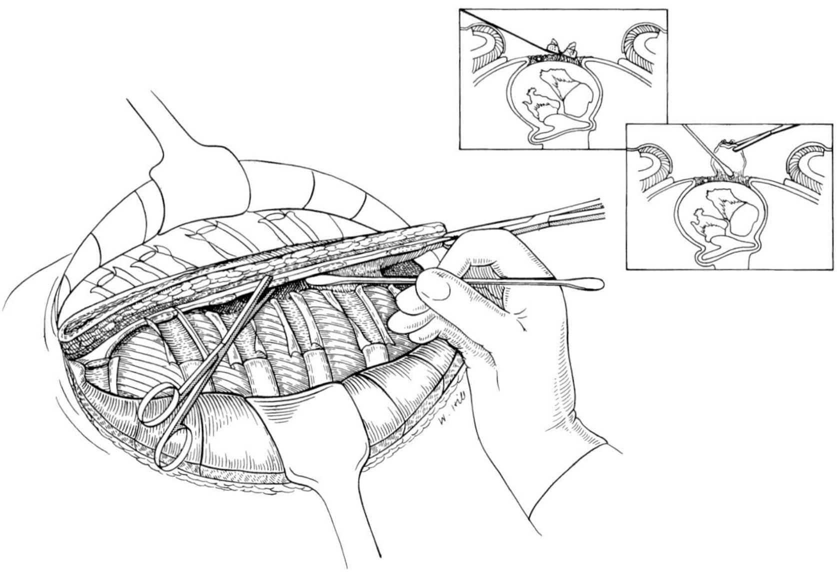

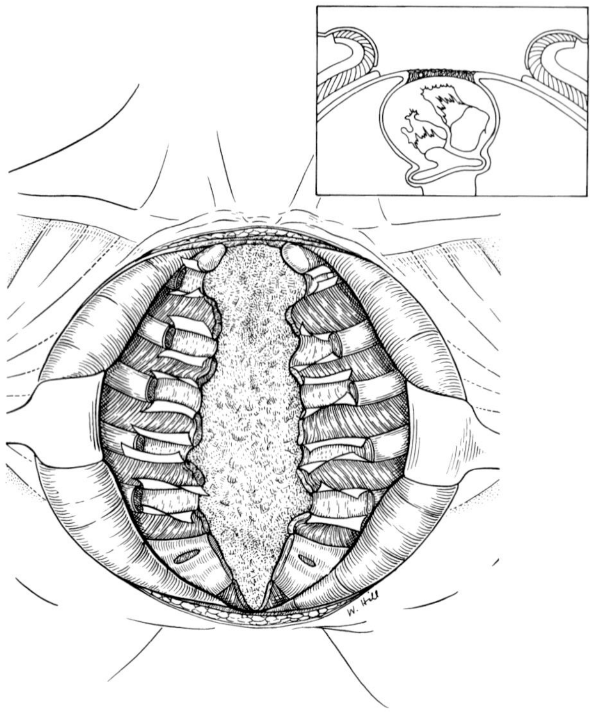

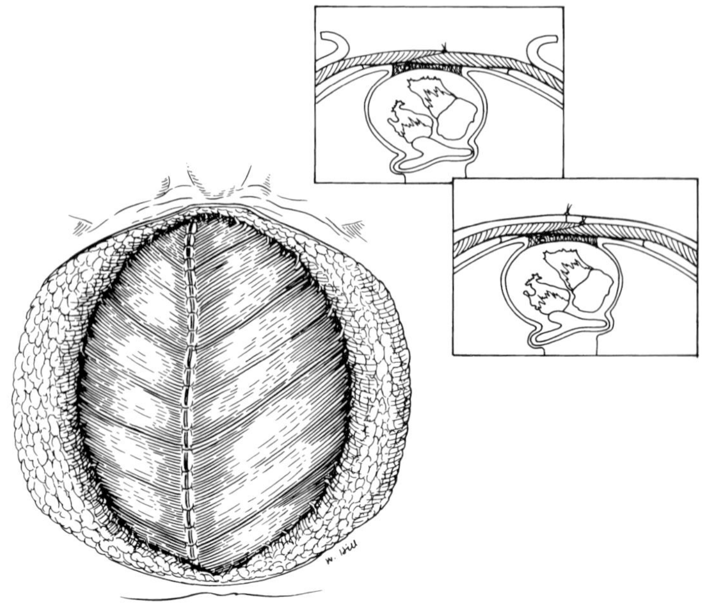

After curettage of the surfaces of the wound overlying the heart and jet lavage irrigation, the pectoralis major muscles were remobilized and the tendinous insertions were released bilaterally. They were approximated to each other, and closure was completed with mobilization and approximation of bilateral cutaneous advancement flaps over multiple suction catheters.

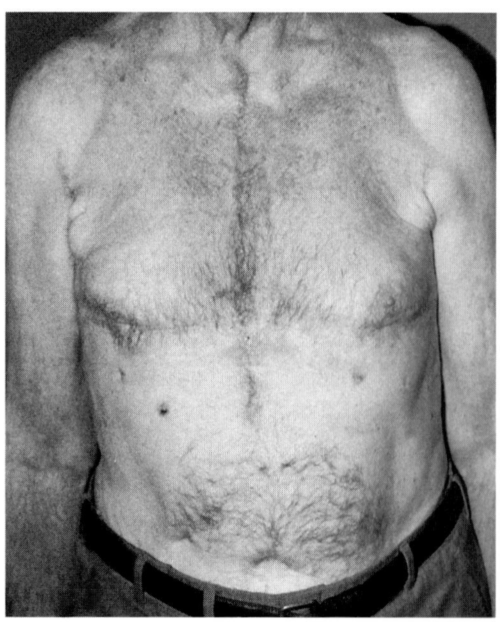

At 2-year follow-up the wound remained healed.

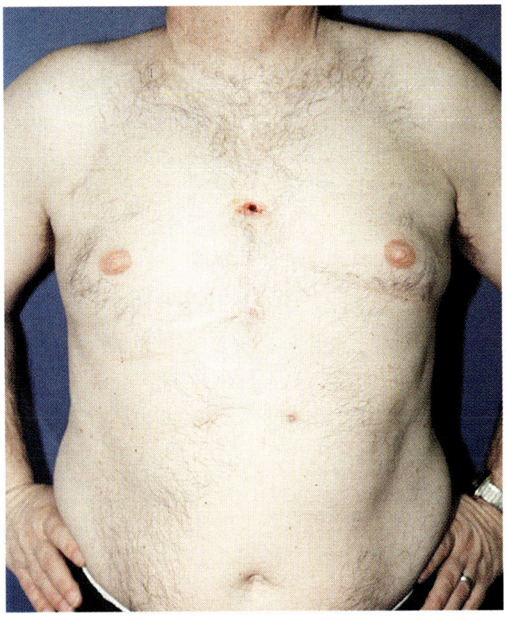

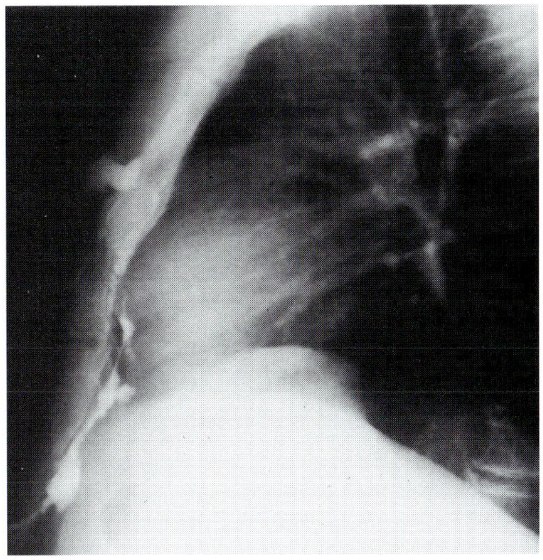

Another technique that can be useful in achieving the goal of successful healing is to approach the involved tissues via internal or external counterincisions to facilitate safe exposure as was performed in this 58-year-old man. Seven years earlier he had undergone an urgent coronary artery bypass graft, which had been complicated by multiply recurrent infections and sinus tract formation. He had been treated with multiple surgical debridements and flap reconstruction at another hospital. The most recent procedure included reconstruction with bilateral pectoralis major muscles and bilateral pectoral cutaneous advancement flaps. He had also been treated with many long-term courses of parenteral and oral antibiotics. At several of the prior surgical debridements, temporary pacing wire fragments were removed.

Radiographic contrast injection studies of the midsternal sinus demonstrated extension of the wound directly to underlying bone where a smoldering sequestrum and infected foreign body were thought to be the cause. A recurrent left epigastric sinus was injected in order to opacify a tract extending beneath the xiphoid to an inferior cardiac–diaphragmatic collection and a more superior retrosternal-precardiac collection.

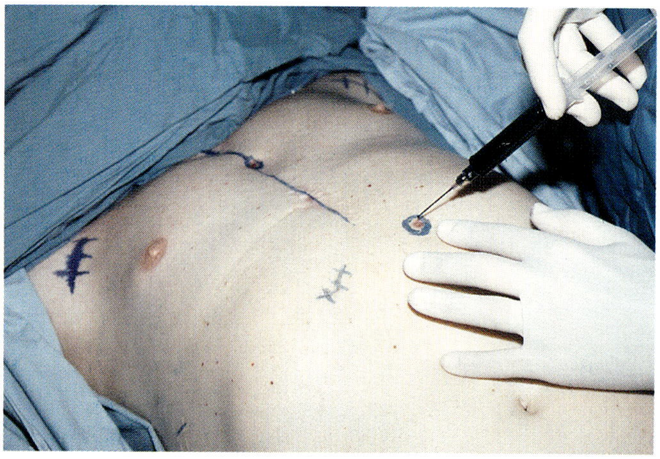

At reoperation for chest wall reconstruction, incisional scars were noted at the original median sternotomy site, pectoral humeral tenotomy counterincision sites, and multiple former chest tube sites. The left epigastric and the midsternal sinus tracts were forcefully injected with methylene blue before surgery.

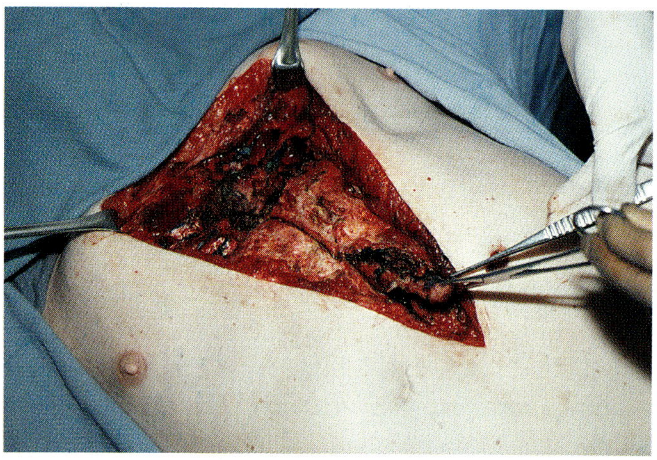

The entire sternotomy incision was opened through the underlying, previously advanced pectoralis major muscle flaps to the periosteum. An excisional incision (behind the forceps and clamp) was made around the orifice of the left epigastric sinus tract. The well-formed sinus tract was dissected until it could be drawn into the main wound cavity. Dissection continued around this well-formed tract, following it through the bone itself into fibrotic, treacherous planes between the heart and the diaphragm and between the sternum and the heart. Segments of the xiphisternum were resected piecemeal to unroof the extension between the heart and the sternum. Staining of the tract and cavities with methylene blue helped to verify the adequacy of the resection of the involved tissue. This long tract is shown held under traction at the inferior aspect of the wound by the surgeon's two forceps and clamp.

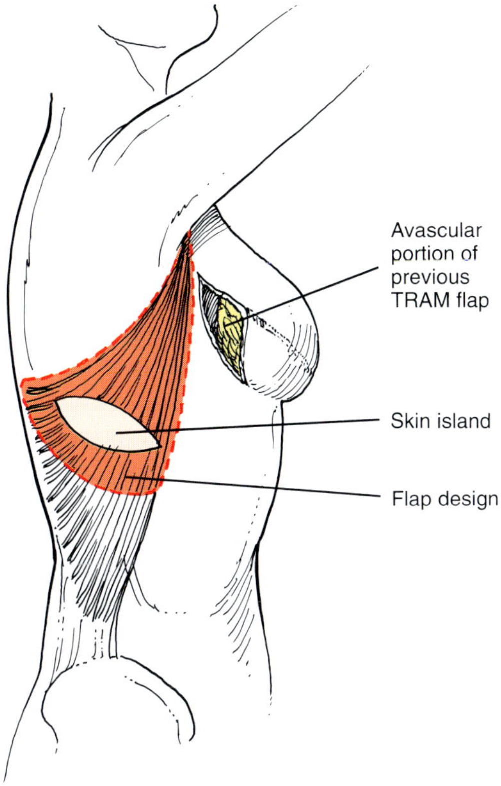

The latissimus dorsi flap may be designed transversely to include some excess tissue in the subaxillary region or vertically along the lateral muscle border.

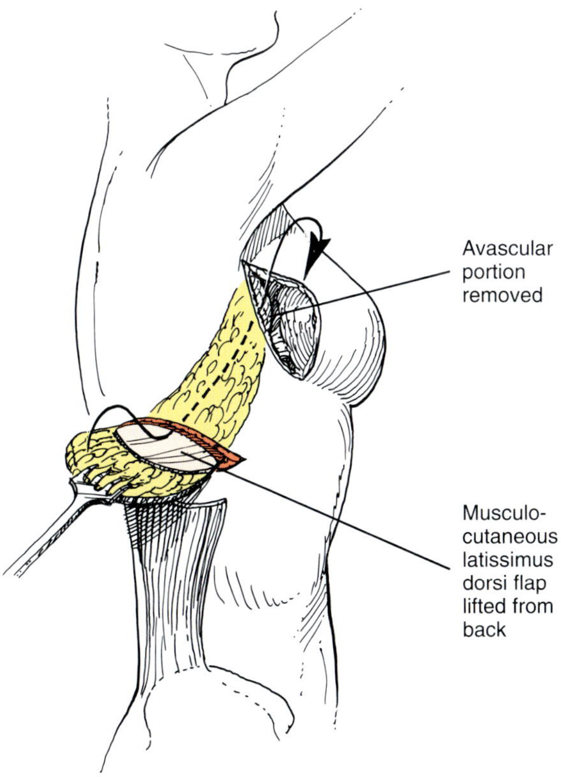

The latissimus dorsi flap is elevated laterally, and the skin island is designed to provide sufficient fill.

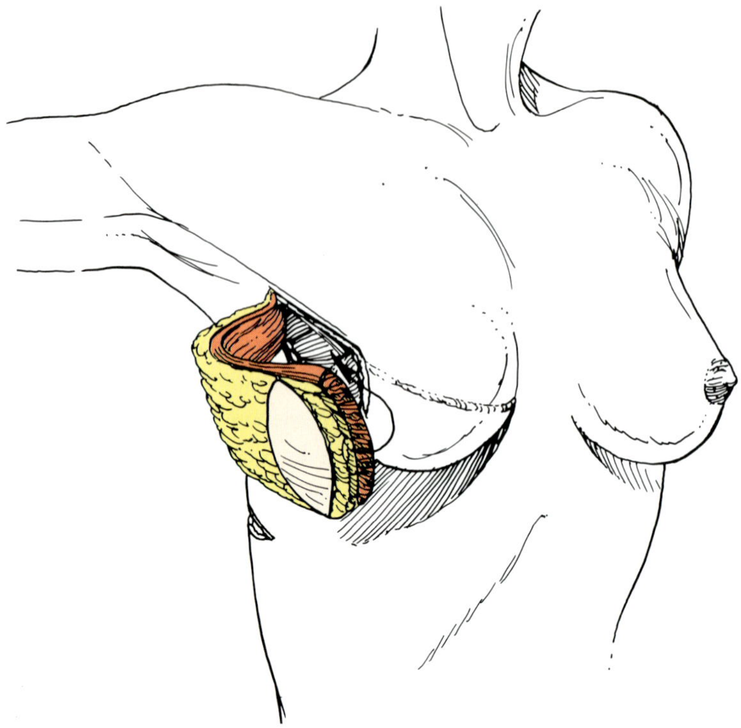

The flap is transferred to supplement the deficient lateral area of the breast.

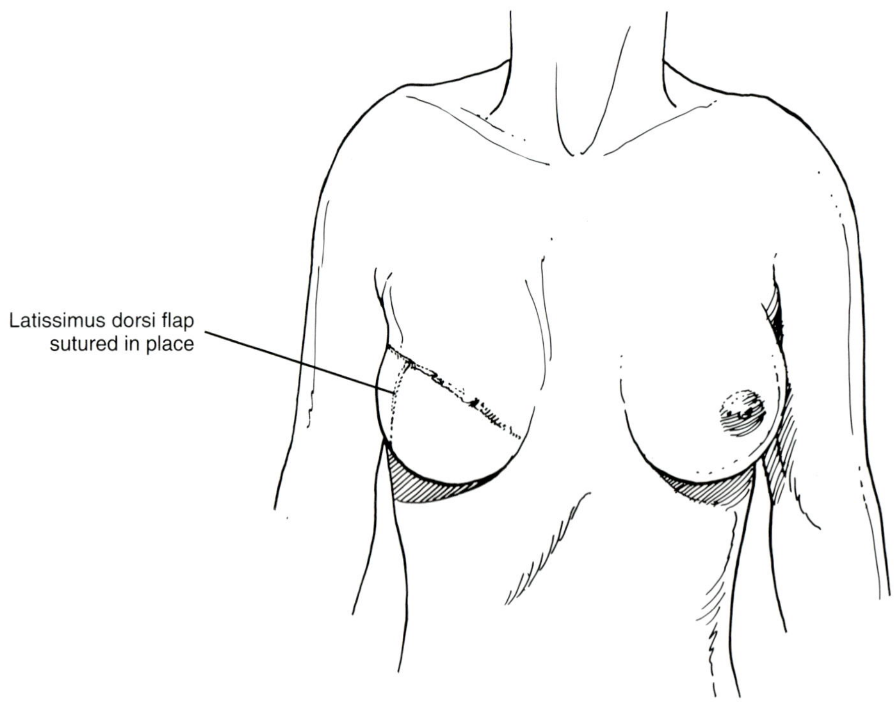

The latissimus dorsi flap restores breast symmetry without the need for a breast implant.

Total Flap Loss

When there is total loss of a TRAM flap, it is important that the secondary breast reconstruction be successful with special consideration given to safety. Usually there is insufficient tissue for tissue expansion and the transfer of a second flap is needed.

The latissimus dorsi flap is the safest, most reliable alternative and can be a source of autogenous tissue with additional subcutaneous harvest. A fleur-de-lis flap may be used when there is available back tissue. When the TRAM flap has been completely lost, a major latissimus dorsi flap is needed, usually supplemented by a textured-surface permanent expander-implant to provide sufficient volume. A gluteus free flap is considered when the latissimus dorsi flap is not available or when the patient wants autogenous tissue breast reconstruction and not enough tissue is available with the latissimus dorsi flap. Before attempting microsurgical breast reconstruction, the surgeon should be experienced with microsurgery technique and should have an excellent success rate with microsurgery.

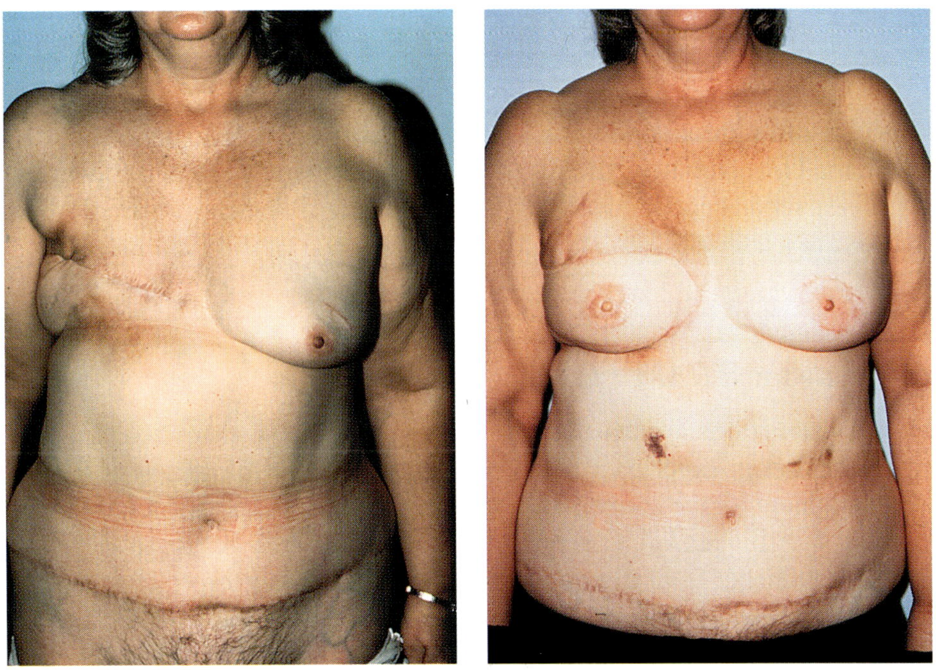

This 45-year-old woman experienced total flap loss after breast reconstruction with a TRAM flap. Because she wanted only autogenous tissue used for the reconstructive surgery, reoperation with a latissimus dorsi flap was planned. A mastopexy was performed on the remaining breast for symmetry.

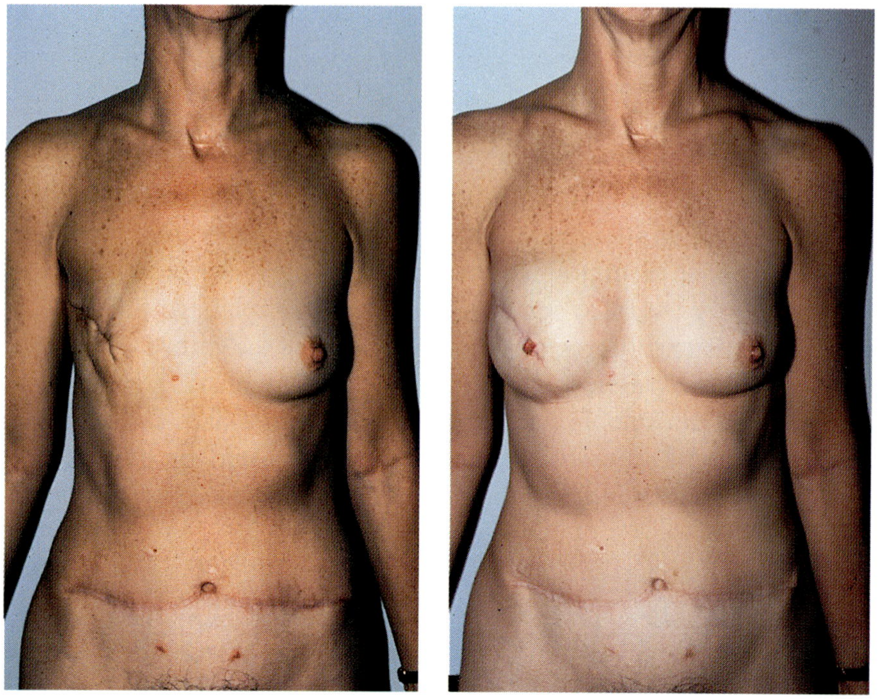

This 43-year-old woman underwent immediate breast reconstruction with a free TRAM flap. Unfortunately the flap was lost. Reoperation was performed as a staged breast reconstruction with a tissue expander. The nipple-areola was reconstructed in a later operation with a tattoo planned as the final procedure.

Tissue Excess
Recontouring the TRAM Flap

Breast reconstructions are usually too big or too little; seldom are they exactly the right size. In my experience it is generally better psychologically and aesthetically for patients to have a reconstructed breast that is a little too big rather than the reverse; for this reason I prefer for the reconstructed breast to be the same size or slightly larger than the opposite breast. Then no correction is needed or only suction-assisted lipectomy or tissue excision is required to obtain the desired symmetry. Suction-assisted lipectomy reduces flap bulk, softens the breast, and improves symmetry. I usually wait at least 3 months after the TRAM flap procedure to perform this correction.

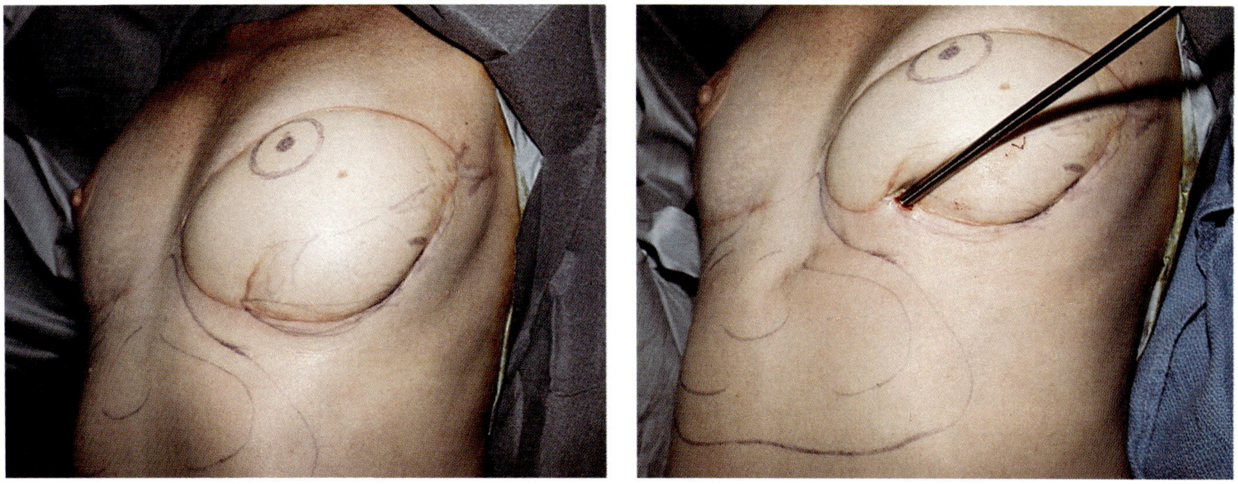

To avoid the possibility of flap or fat necrosis and atrophy of the TRAM flap, a musculovascular pedicle should not be excised after the primary breast reconstruction. The existence of this pedicle, however, causes the medial inferior breast to lack definition where it meets the juncture of the pedicle. Liposuction or tissue excision during a secondary procedure can help to define the crease.

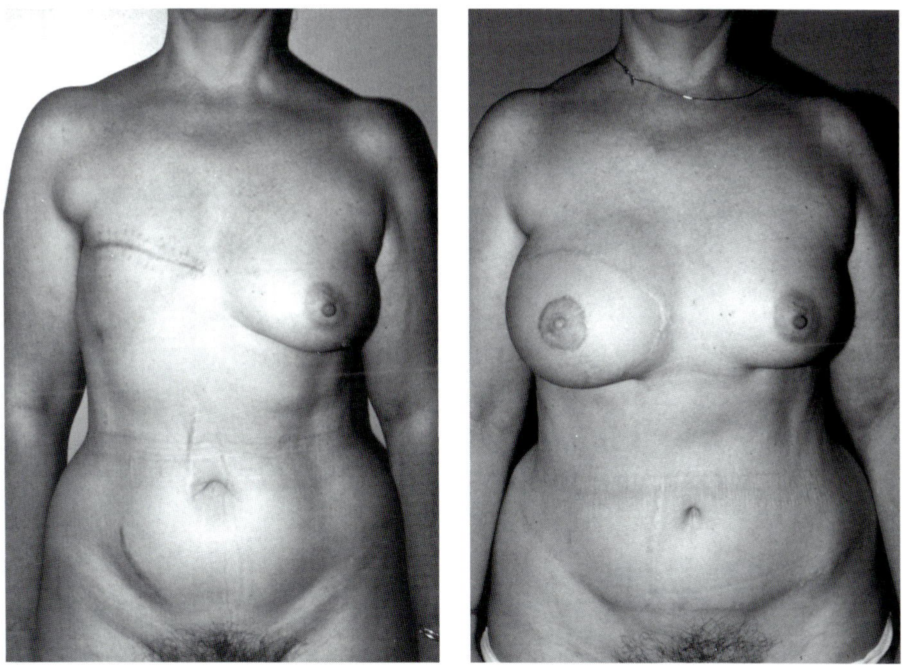

In this 52-year-old woman the right breast was reconstructed with a TRAM flap. After several years she gained 15 pounds and the reconstructed breast became larger than the opposite breast. Suction-assisted lipectomy of the TRAM flap would be a good solution for improving breast symmetry and contour.

Abdominal Wall Contouring and Scar Revision

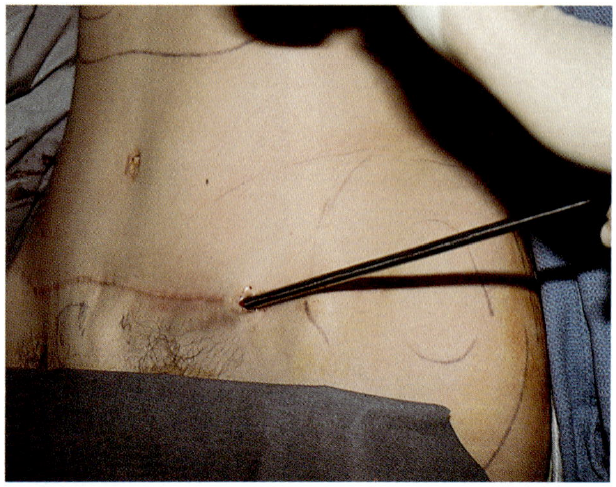

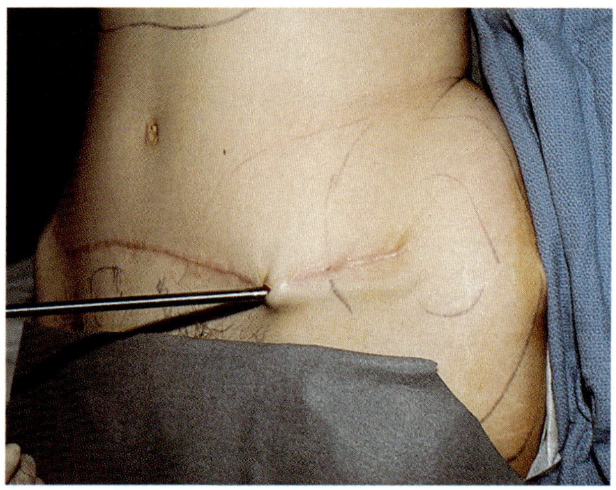

The abdominal wall may require secondary correction to contour and reduce areas of excess. Usually the lower abdominal area is flattened after a TRAM flap has been harvested; however, the overall abdomen may still have excess tissue, especially at the site of the pedicle in the upper, lateral, and mons pubis regions and in the lateral hip area. If the nerves to the upper rectus abdominis muscle are not divided, especially the eighth intercostal nerve, additional upper abdominal wall fullness may be present. Although some of these areas can be contoured at the time of the TRAM flap surgery, they may also require suction-assisted lipectomy at the time of the finishing touches or during secondary procedures. Suction-assisted lipectomy in this region can improve contour; however, it cannot be expected to flatten a protruding upper abdominal wall if the closure of the upper abdomen was not tight and secure. Sometimes the abdominoplasty scar can also be improved with scar revision.

Seroma

Because of the large dead space created by the harvest of abdominal flaps, a seroma can form. The blood supply to the abdominal wall fat below Scarpa's fascia comes mostly from the superficial tissues. When a seroma develops after a TRAM flap, excision of this layer beneath the Scarpa's fascia along with the seroma capsule is the best opportunity for correction.

Hernia Repair

An abdominal wall bulge or hernia can develop in the postoperative period after TRAM flap harvest. This condition usually develops within the first year. Analysis of our TRAM flap patients reveals that postoperative development of this condition is most commonly related to the failure of the primary direct approximation of well-vascularized healthy, strong fascia. An accurate knowledge of the position of the periumbilical perforators permits a selective fascial inclusion and muscle harvest in this region and allows for primary suture of the fascial margins even when a bipedicled TRAM flap is elevated. Choice of anesthetic technique also influences the risk of postoperative hernia. When nitrous oxide is avoided, the gas is not deposited intraluminally and the bowel is not distended, thereby facilitating primary closure.

When a hernia of the abdominal wall is being repaired after TRAM flap harvest, consideration should be given to the intra-abdominal contents. Care must be taken to avoid injury to the bowel; when in doubt concerning this area, the reconstructive surgeon should consult with a general surgeon. It is necessary to obtain wide exposure of the defect by elevating the abdominal wall flap.

The margins of the defect are identified. With good muscular relaxation and with a prepared bowel without intraluminal gas (no nitrous oxide), a primary closure is sometimes possible. Whether primary closure is possible or not, a double sheet of Prolene mesh is placed over the defect to prevent further protrusion (see Chapter 6).

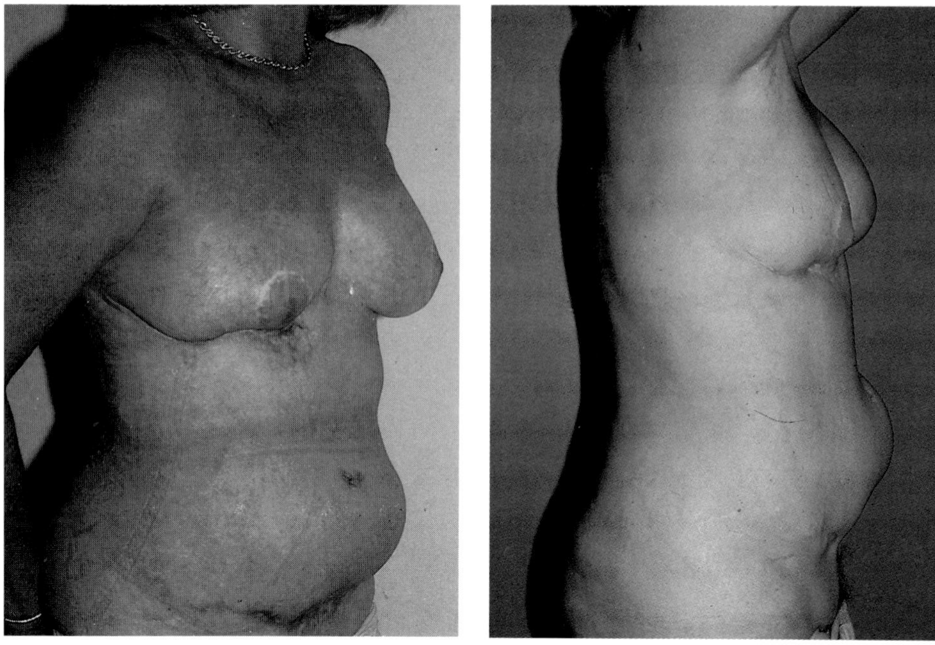

Two years before referral, a ventral hernia developed in this 45-year-old woman after a right unilateral TRAM flap breast reconstruction.

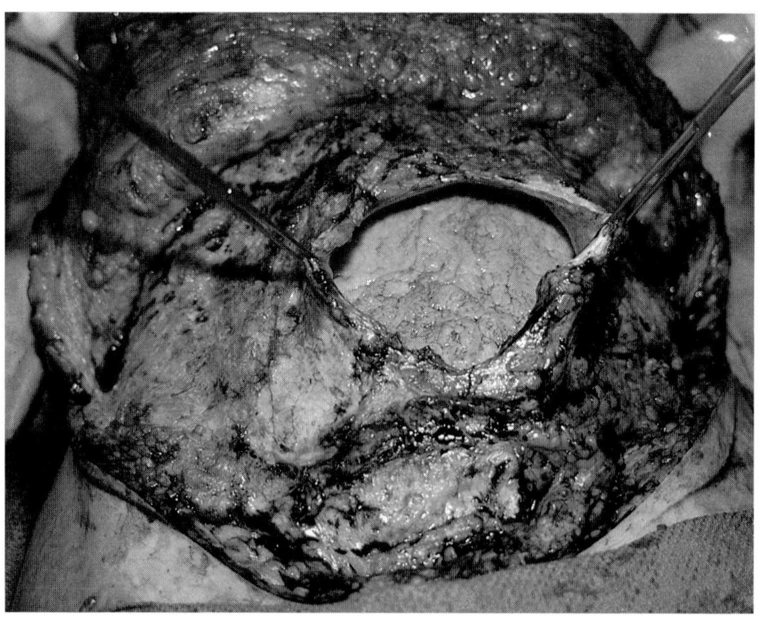

Repair was accomplished by reelevation of the abdominal skin flap. The ventral hernia was defined, the attenuated margins of the fascia were approximated, and additional plications were made laterally and centrally.

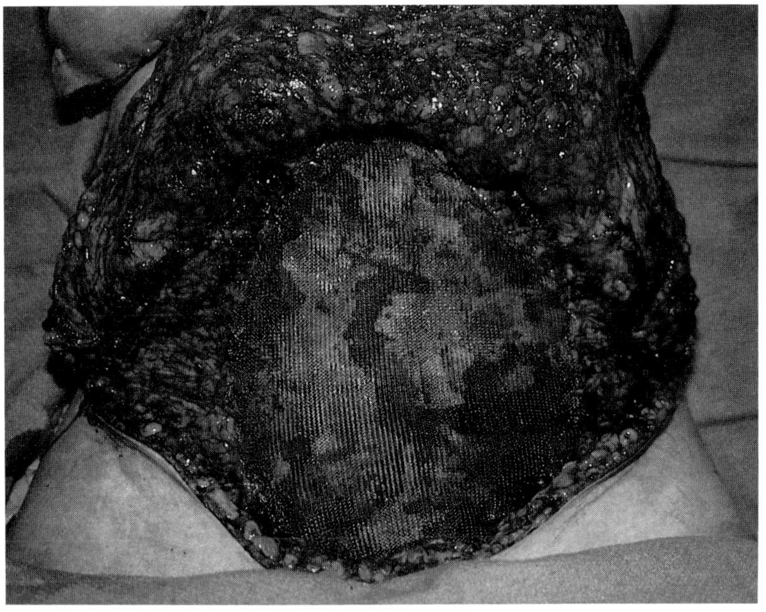

A double-thickness layer of Prolene mesh was sutured over the abdominal wall to reinforce the repair.

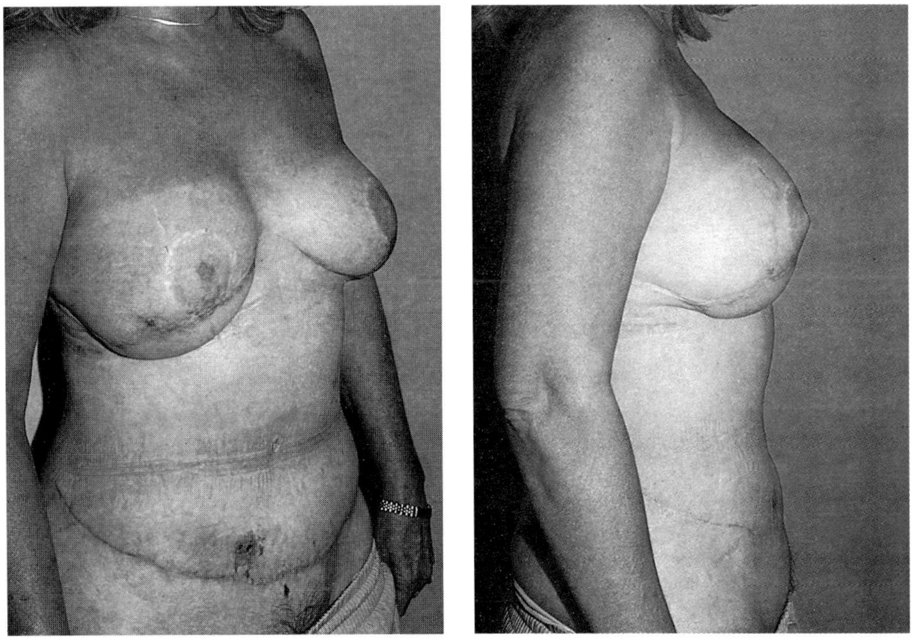

Interestingly, this former heavy smoker, despite the previous elevation of the abdominal skin flap, developed an area of delayed skin healing in the lower abdomen. This site healed with conservative care and the hernia repair remained intact. The patient is shown 2 months after hernia repair.

Inframammary Fold Correction

Incorrect placement of the inframammary fold can be a problem with autogenous tissue breast reconstruction because the tendency is to place the inframammary fold too low. Several factors account for incorrect positioning. If the inframammary fold is marked and cut symmetric with the opposite breast, the abdominal wall closure will release skin and allow it to settle lower. When the incision is made at the inframammary fold, the tension on the tissues from the mastectomy wound closure will lessen with time, and the inframammary fold will again assume a low position. When breast definition is combined with lower pole enhancement using an abdominal wall advancement flap, the inframammary fold tends to drift downward. During the second operation the inframammary crease must be defined or redefined, the flap may need to be repositioned, or an abdominal wall advancement flap may be necessary to correctly position the inframammary fold. Suction-assisted lipectomy of the upper abdomen can further define the fold.

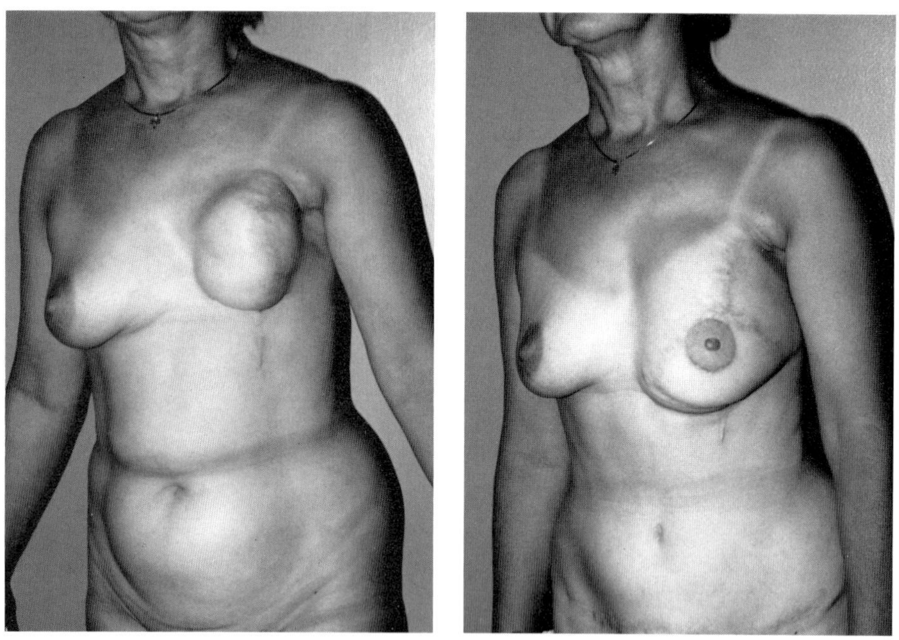

This woman had a modified radical mastectomy and implant breast reconstruction. She was disappointed with the resulting symmetry and requested a staged autogenous breast reconstruction. A TRAM flap breast reconstruction was performed after the removal of the breast implant. Unfortunately the reconstructed breast was larger and fuller than the opposite breast. Correction of this problem required resection and liposuction of the excess lower fullness of the TRAM flap and elevation and advancement of the inframammary fold to position the fold symmetric with that on the opposite side.

Inadequate Central Breast Projection

The normal breast, although it may be flat when the patient is in the supine position, has distinct central projection when the patient is upright. One of the problems with breast reconstruction, particularly with TRAM flap and with implant breast reconstruction, has been the difficulty in obtaining central mound projection that is symmetric with that of the opposite breast. In this situation an implant may be needed to restore projection.

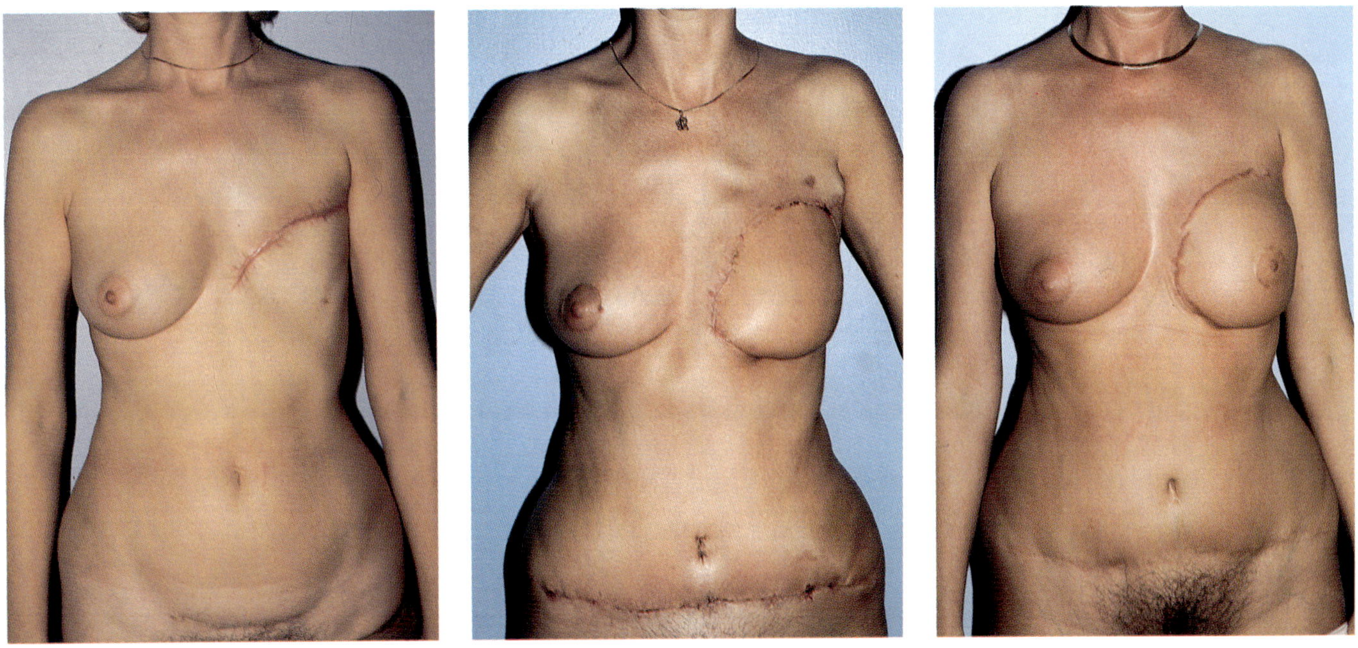

This woman had a TRAM flap breast reconstruction after modified radical mastectomy. Postoperatively she believed that she did not have sufficient central breast fullness. She also wished to have more breast volume, both in the reconstructed breast and in the opposite breast, which she wanted augmented. To improve this situation, breast implants were placed bilaterally. To reduce the probability of capsular contracture, a textured-surface breast implant should be used behind the TRAM flap.

REOPERATION AFTER A LATISSIMUS DORSI FLAP

The latissimus dorsi flap is one of the most reliable pedicled flaps; the incidence of tissue loss with this flap is usually less than 1%.[1] Most secondary procedures after latissimus dorsi flap breast reconstruction are needed because of improper planning (e.g., failure to transfer enough autogenous tissue to the chest wall to provide symmetry with the opposite breast), aesthetic shortcomings related to unaesthetic positioning of the flap high on the reconstructed breast in the mastectomy scar, and implant problems such as capsular contracture or incorrect implant size. Volume or position discrepancies may also necessitate reoperation. The donor site may require attention because of seroma or tightness.

Flap Deficiency

Asymmetry

When there is breast asymmetry, the decision is made to modify the reconstructed breast, the opposite breast, or both. ***As a principle, it is usually preferable to reshape the reconstructed breast with the latissimus dorsi flap.*** The tissue expander or breast implant can be repositioned or the shape or volume of the reconstructed breast can be changed. Some atrophy of the latissimus dorsi muscle is to be expected after the initial procedure. The placement of a saline-filled adjustable implant behind the flap provides the best opportunity to plan for this occurrence and to keep the volume of the reconstructed breast symmetric with that of the opposite breast. If a fixed-volume implant has been used in the initial reconstruction, then it may need to be exchanged for an adjustable implant. Alternatively, implants can be avoided altogether and a TRAM flap could be used to provide additional volume.

Partial and Total Flap Loss

After partial latissimus dorsi flap loss, the preferred correction is to modify the reconstructed breast with a tissue expander or breast implant. After complete loss of the latissimus dorsi flap, which is a rare occurrence, another autogenous tissue breast reconstruction is usually needed; a TRAM flap or free TRAM flap is usually the first choice.

Capsular Contracture and Breast Asymmetry

Experience with the latissimus dorsi flap for breast reconstruction following radical mastectomy has demonstrated that the muscle flap atrophies over time, with resulting deterioration of the shape of the reconstructed breast. Frequently this flap does not provide adequate tissue to fill substantial upper chest wall tissue defects, particularly for patients with a full opposite breast and thick subcutaneous tissues. In addition, capsular contracture can develop, especially when a smooth-surface breast implant has been placed under the latissimus dorsi flap. This problem is the most common complication after a latissimus dorsi flap breast reconstruction. Contracture along with the muscle atrophy can cause asymmetry and breast distortion.

When a latissimus dorsi flap reconstruction has deteriorated and contracture occurs, strategies for correction include the replacement of the implant with autogenous tissue (usually the TRAM flap) or capsulectomy with placement of a textured-surface saline-filled implant or expander. My current approach to this problem is to perform a total capsulectomy and replace the smooth-surface silicone breast implant with a textured-surface implant or textured-surface permanent expander-implant. A small subcutaneous fill valve can be retained to allow fine adjustments to the volume of the reconstructed breast. To remove the silicone breast implant, it is exposed through a scar that does not require division of the latissimus dorsi muscle; division could devitalize the distal flap. If a supplemental TRAM flap is used, it may be bisected, with one flap used for additional upper breast fill and the second flap employed for breast reconstruction. The latissimus dorsi flap is then used for upper breast reconstruction and anterior axillary fold reconstruction (if a radical mastectomy defect was reconstructed). A large skin island is deepithelialized to supplement breast fill, and the latissimus dorsi muscle is transposed to the pectoralis major insertion to satisfactorily restore the missing anterior axillary fold.

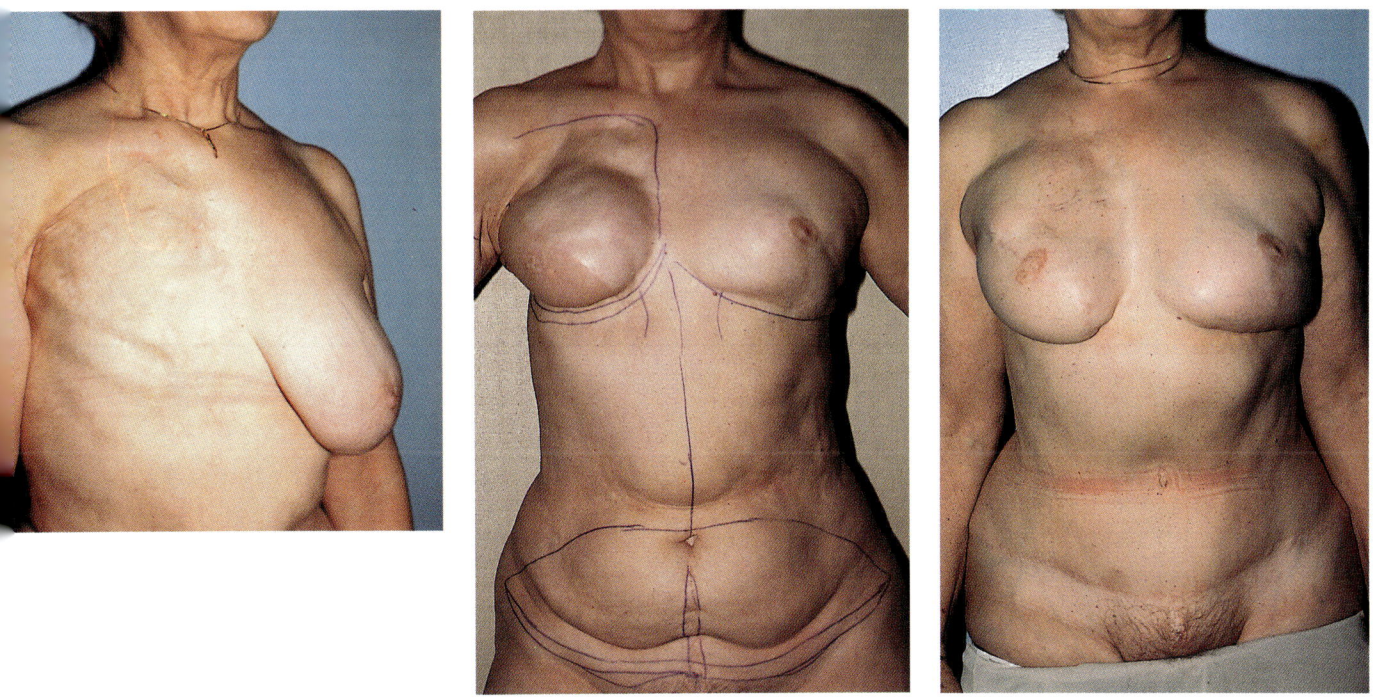

This woman had breast reconstruction with a latissimus dorsi flap and a breast implant. Capsular contracture developed along with unsatisfactory symmetry. She had a staged reoperative breast reconstruction to correct this problem: the implant was removed, the latissimus dorsi flap was deepithelialized and used for upper breast reconstruction, and the TRAM flap was transferred to reconstruct the lower breast region.

Tightness or Contracture of Donor Site

When there is tightness or contracture of the donor site of the latissimus dorsi flap, at the time of the finishing touches the thoracodorsal pedicle is dissected and a segment of the thoracodorsal nerve is removed. When the tightness extends laterally and the patient complains of difficulty when she brings the arm around to the opposite side, then the insertion and the proximal portion of the latissimus dorsi muscle are dissected and the latissimus dorsi muscle is separated from the teres major muscle.

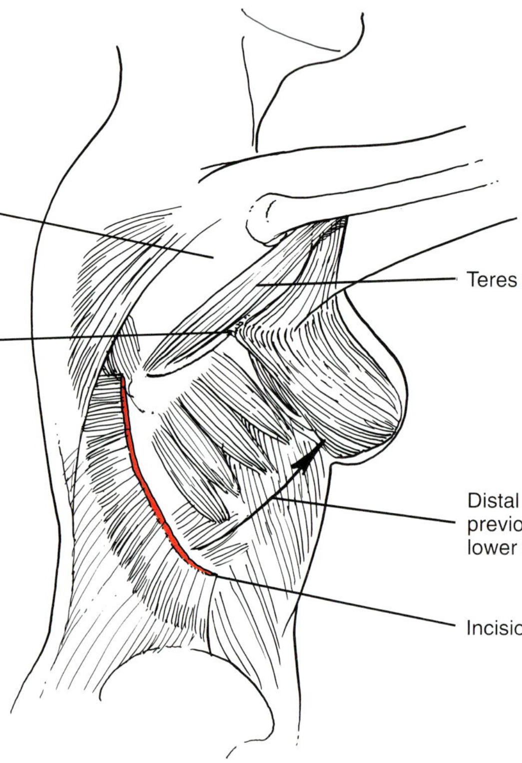

Other donor site revisions may be needed after a latissimus dorsi flap transfer. When the latissimus dorsi flap has been elevated incompletely at the time of the breast reconstruction and is still attached laterally to the teres major muscle and other lateral structures, the patient often complains of tightness of the chest wall. This tightness can be alleviated during a secondary procedure by releasing the latissimus dorsi flap from the teres major muscle and dividing the latissimus dorsi tendon from the insertion. The patient may also have symptoms related to muscle pull and silicone breast implant distortion after latissimus dorsi flap reconstruction because the latissimus dorsi muscle is contracting too much and thereby distorting the breast reconstruction. In this situation the latissimus dorsi muscle can be denervated by dividing the thoracodorsal nerve at the time of the secondary procedure.

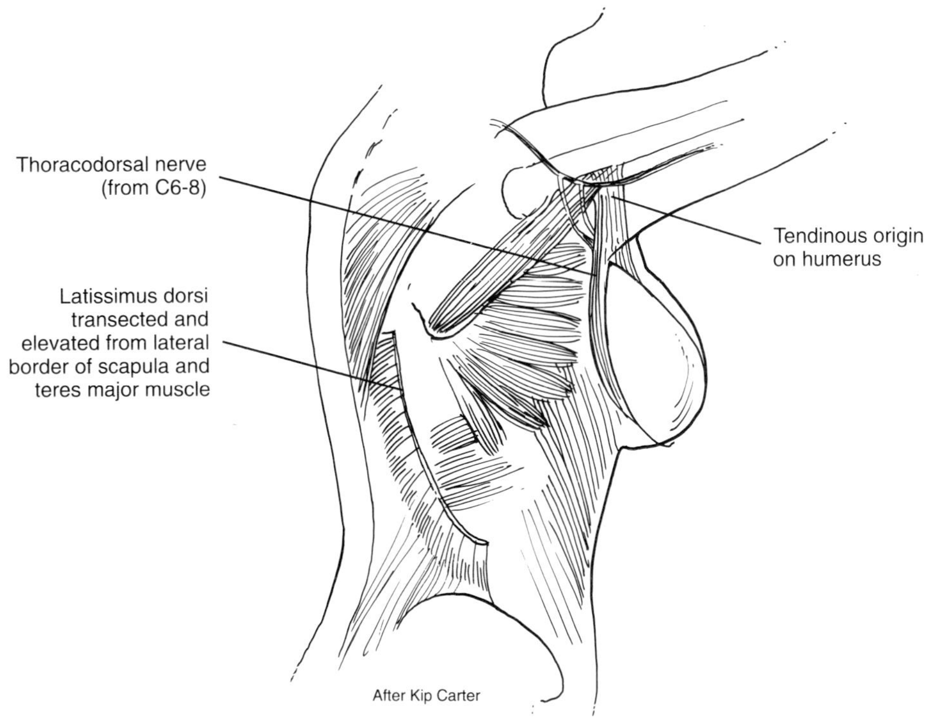
Thoracodorsal nerve
(from C6-8)
Tendinous origin
on humerus
Latissimus dorsi
transected and
elevated from lateral
border of scapula and
teres major muscle
After Kip Carter

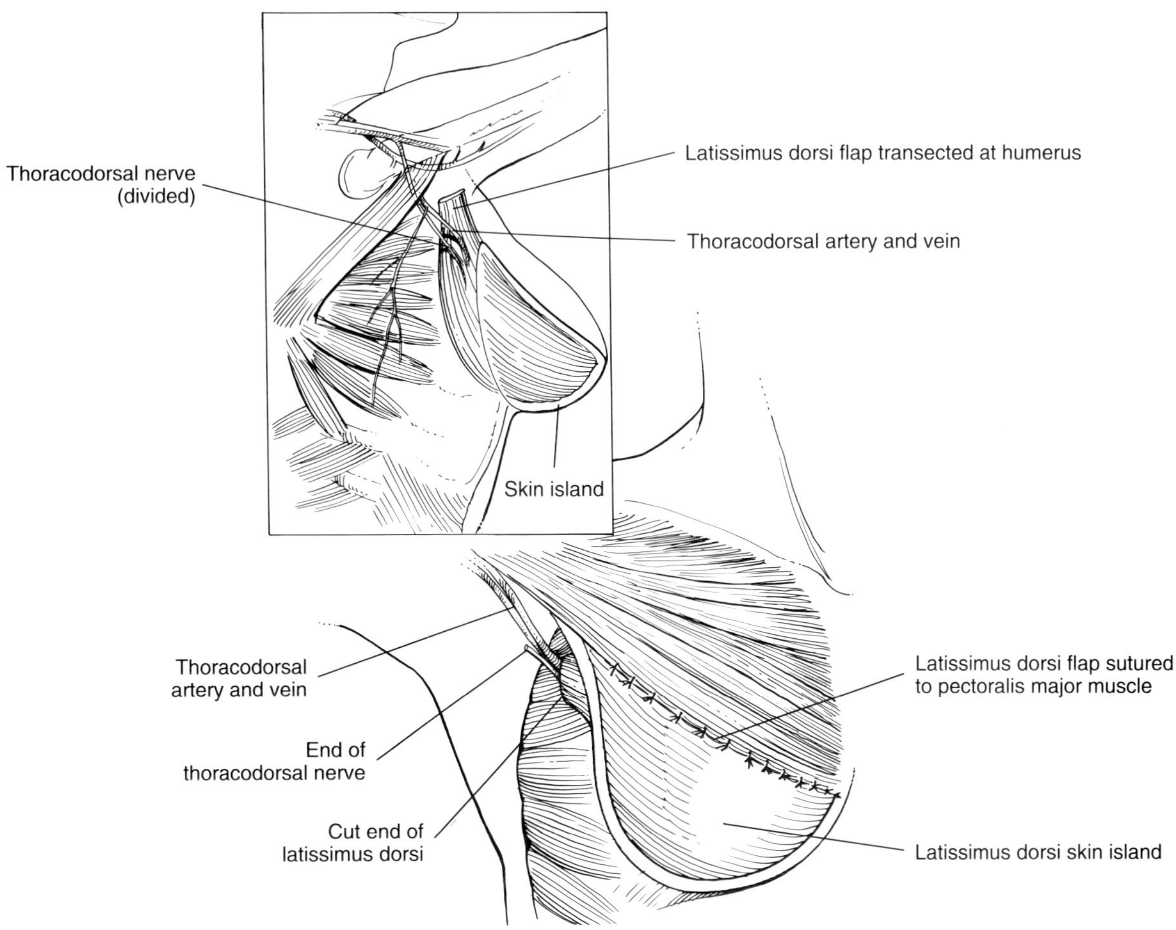
Thoracodorsal nerve
(divided)
Latissimus dorsi flap transected at humerus
Thoracodorsal artery and vein
Skin island
Thoracodorsal
artery and vein
End of
thoracodorsal nerve
Cut end of
latissimus dorsi
Latissimus dorsi flap sutured
to pectoralis major muscle
Latissimus dorsi skin island

Missing Anterior Axillary Fold

When the anterior axillary fold is missing as the result of radical mastectomy or Poland's syndrome, the best correction is the transfer of the latissimus dorsi tendon anteriorly to the insertion of the pectoralis major muscle on the humerus. If this transfer is not performed at breast reconstruction, it may be needed at the time of the finishing touches.

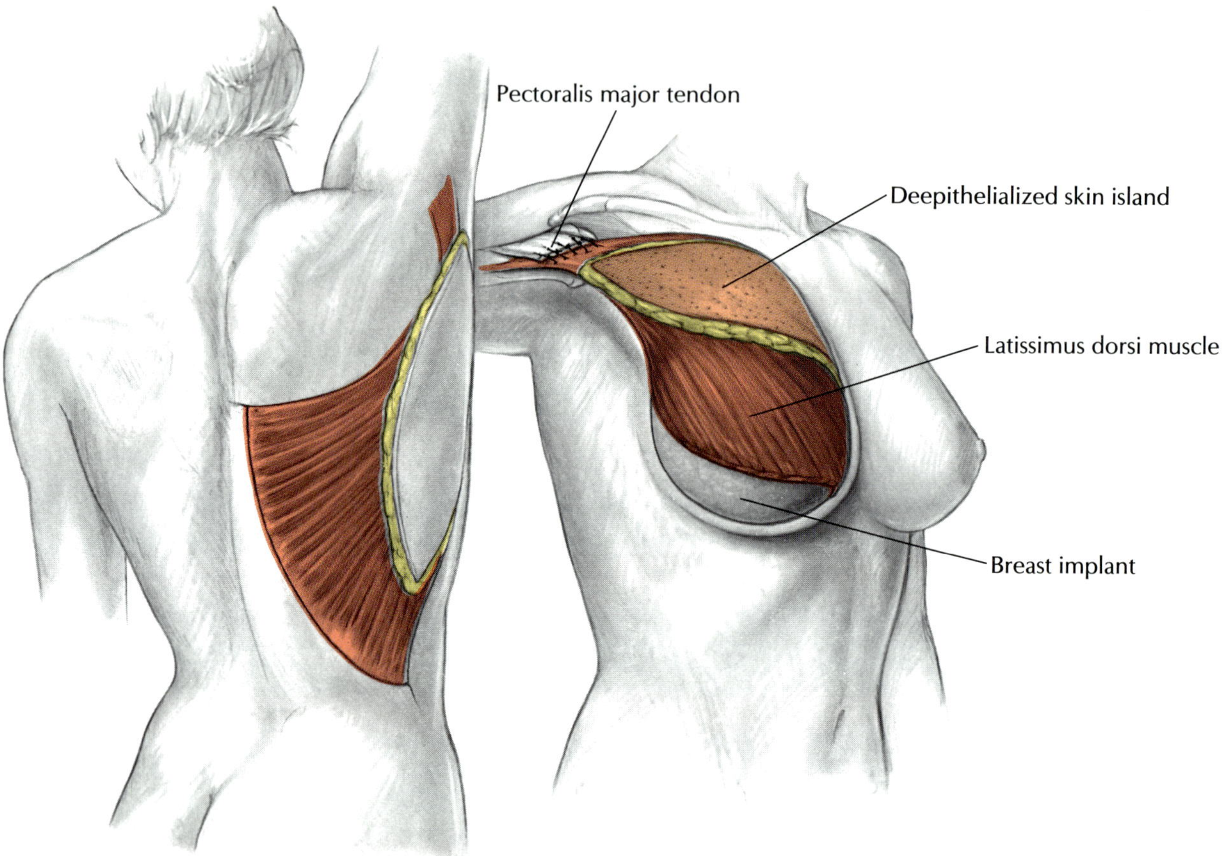

The deepithelialized skin island provides the best fill; however, the transposed muscle can also give effective improvement.

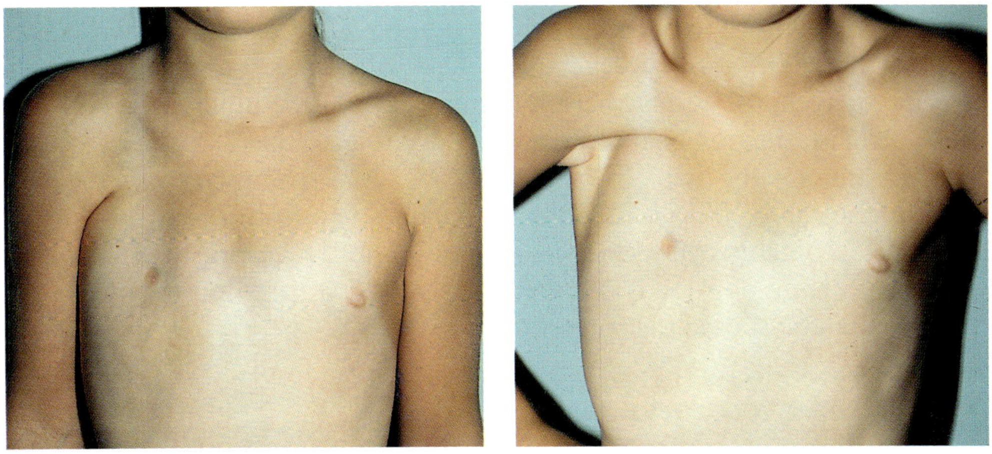

Reconstruction in young patients with Poland's syndrome is usually a staged procedure, with necessary changes made over the years to accommodate growth and development. This was the case for this 9-year-old girl with Poland's syndrome: she exhibited absence of the pectoralis major muscle, anterior axillary fold, and breast.

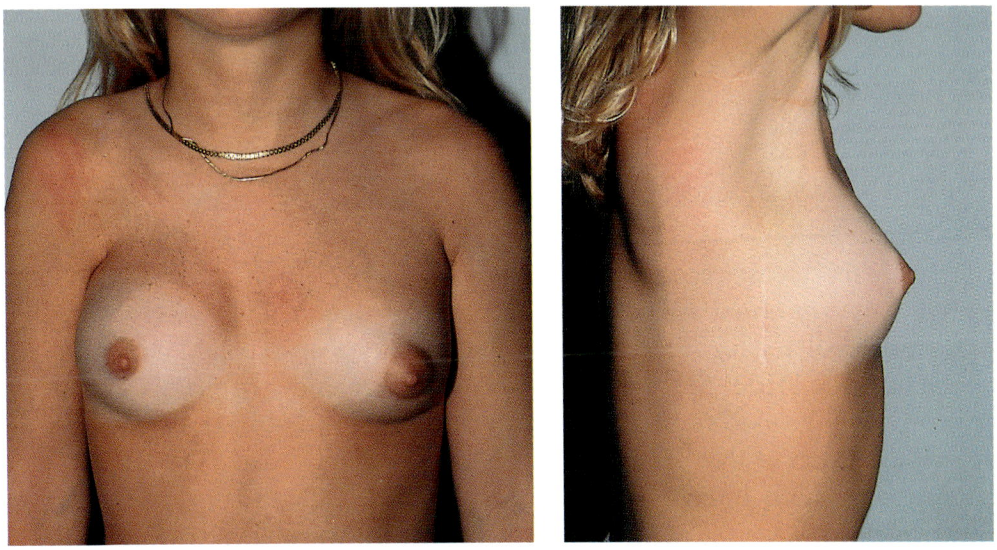

The pectoralis major muscle was reconstructed with the transfer of the latissimus dorsi muscle. As she grew and developed, the breast was reconstructed with a breast implant. For symmetry, a breast implant was also placed in the opposite breast via an axillary incision. Today, rather than fixed-volume breast implants, a permanent expander-implant with a valve for adjustment with saline solution is the preferred device for reconstruction in young women.

Axillary Hollowness

Some patients who have had an axillary lymph node dissection complain of axillary hollowness; correction of this defect poses an aesthetic and functional problem for patients. When there is significant axillary hollowness, the latissimus dorsi insertion can be divided and rotated to give the fill, or in a secondary procedure autogenous tissue from the TRAM flap can be used to fill the axilla. This area also can be filled with a fasciocutaneous flap from the area of subaxillary fullness, which usually exists along the lateral border of the mastectomy site. When a large dog ear is present laterally, a flap based on a subcutaneous pedicle can be transposed for correction.

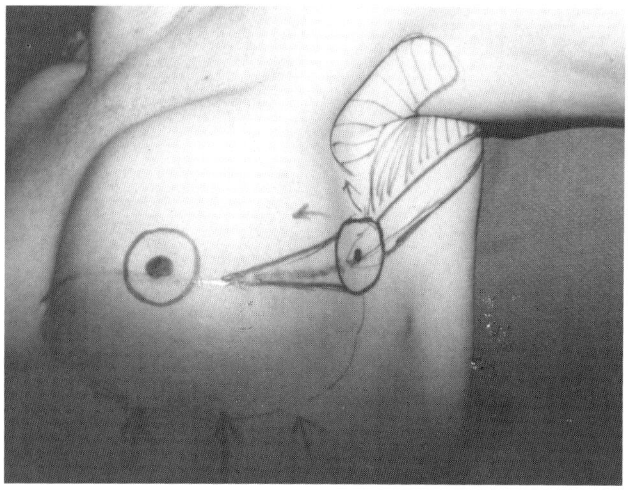

After primary breast reconstruction this patient had good volume symmetry, but she was concerned about the hollowness of the left axilla and the fullness beneath the axillary region. To correct this problem, an areola donor skin graft will be harvested from this axillary region. The remainder of the excess subaxillary tissue will be used to fill the axilla. In addition to the full-thickness graft, an internal elevation of the inframammary crease is also needed. This correction is accomplished with internal capsulorrhaphy of the inframammary crease (arrows).

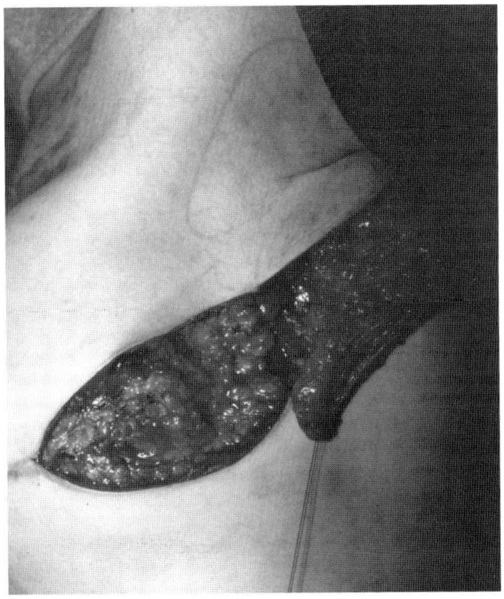

The full-thickness graft is harvested and will be used to reconstruct the areola. The skin lateral to the areola donor site is deepithelialized. A fasciocutaneous flap based on the subcutaneous tissue and fascia from the axilla is mobilized toward the axilla.

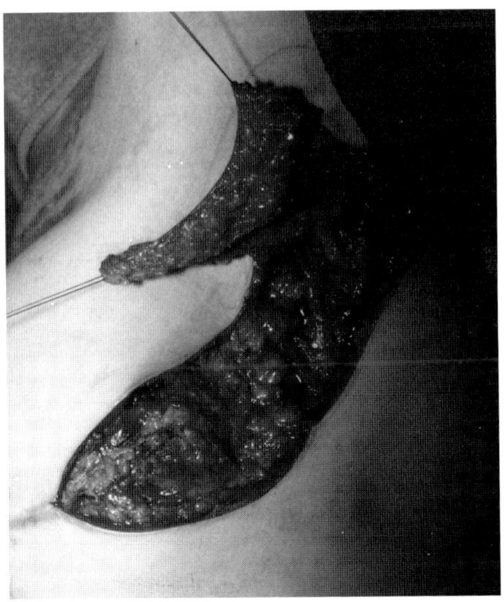

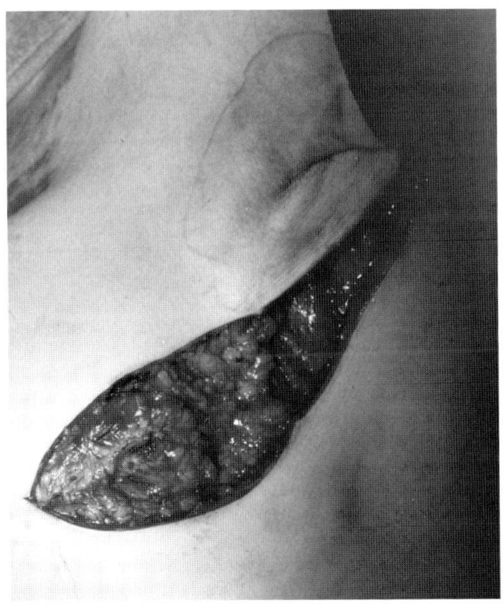

This subcutaneous tissue is then mobilized and the axillary skin is undermined. The flap is turned on itself (like a page in a book), placed into the axillary defect, and sutured. The remainder of the incision is closed directly. This technique fills the axillary concavity and provides donor skin for the areola. An open capsulotomy is performed through this incision. The implant is removed, a lower capsulectomy is performed, and the lower incision is resutured using a lighted retractor and long instruments.

FINISHING TOUCHES AND SECONDARY NIPPLE-AREOLA RECONSTRUCTION

After the initial breast reconstruction, nipple-areola reconstruction is usually performed once the breasts are symmetric. In the past, when nipple-areola reconstruction was performed at the time of the breast reconstruction or before symmetry of the breasts was obtained, the nipple-areolae often were not symmetric and their positions were not ideal. It is better to wait than to have the areolae placed and reconstructed in the improper positions or to have the tissues stretch beneath them and cause asymmetry of the diameter of the nipple-areolae.

The nipple-areola position is determined initially. Nipple-areola reconstruction is usually now performed with available local tissues and without the need for specialized tissues from the opposite nipple or the upper inner thigh crease.

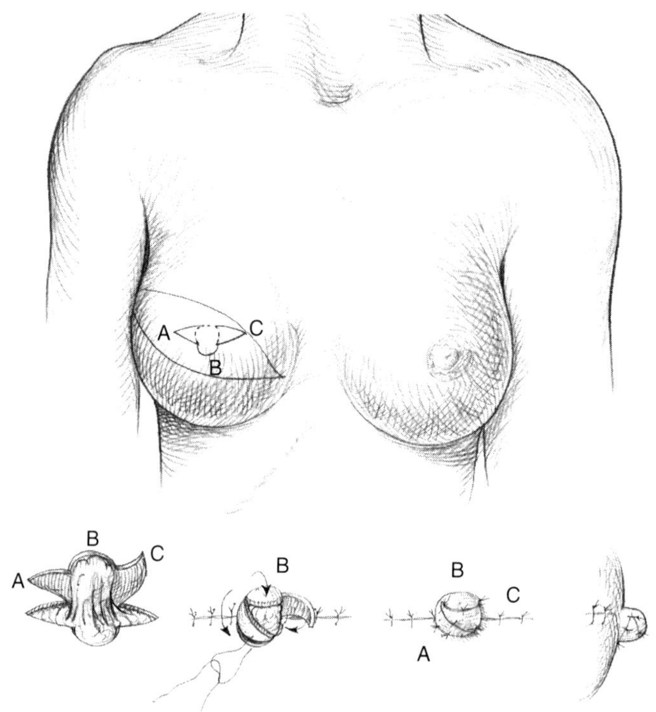

The C-V flap

I prefer the modified star flap (C-V flap) with the areola tattooed.[2] With this technique a layer of skin and fat on the reconstructed breast is shifted to the center of what will be the future nipple-areola area and formed into a nipple. The skin is used to create the nipple and the underlying fat is used to add bulk, fullness, and permanent shape. This technique permits closure of the donor sites for the nipple reconstruction.

When there is tissue available for a full-thickness skin graft, then the skate flap or the modified star flap can be used.[1,3,4] The areola diameter and shape are determined and drawn on the site to be reconstructed.

When the nipple-areola reconstruction is malpositioned or unattractive, the best strategy is usually to remove the reconstructed nipple-areola with direct excision, reconstruct a new one as a primary reconstruction with the C-V or skate flap, and either use a tattoo to provide a semblance of an areola or reconstruct the areola with a full-thickness graft. When the areola diameter is so large that the areola cannot be excised without distorting the breast, then I remove it with a tangential excision and allow the site to reepithelialize.

In some situations following nipple-areola reconstruction when there is not enough nipple projection and the opposite nipple is large, a composite graft can be considered.

Postoperative Care

Postoperative care after reoperation focuses on general as well as local considerations. When there has been a major flap reconstruction, the ideal combination of blood flow and oxygen delivery is obtained with a hematocrit level of about 30% to 32%. When the hematocrit level is higher, there can be sludging of the erythrocytes; when it is lower, poor oxygen delivery results. This titration of the blood count is facilitated by having autologous blood available for these procedures.

After TRAM flap reconstruction, it is important to consider the possibility of deep vein thrombosis and pulmonary embolism. These complications are related to the patient's history of pulmonary embolism as well as to the length of the procedure (the risk of deep vein thrombosis is increased when the procedure lasts more than 4 hours). For these patients, intermittent lower extremity compression devices are used and the patient is instructed to get out of bed and begin walking the day after the operation.

Following a primary TRAM flap procedure or correction of an abdominal wall hernia, the patient should not lift over 5 kg for 2 to 3 months. I also suggest that she avoid other strenuous activities for 3 months.

AESTHETIC POSSIBILITIES AND LIMITATIONS OF REOPERATIVE SURGERY

Reoperation and secondary surgery in the breast region offer the potential for significant improvement in most instances. Usually the surgeon has several options to choose from when planning corrections or improvements. Modification of the opposite breast can also be considered to improve breast symmetry. Breast implants offer the possibility of obtaining additional breast volume beyond what is ordinarily possible with pedicled flaps alone. The patient needs to make a decision, however, as to whether she wants a breast implant or prefers only autogenous tissue. When autogenous tissue is insufficient and a breast implant is not used, the limitations are obvious.

The use of a second pedicled flap should be considered when the first procedure falls short of the expected result and a volume deficit remains. In this situation the latissimus dorsi flap can often enhance the upper breast reconstruction once a TRAM flap restores the lower breast contour. A free flap is also a consideration but involves another major surgical intervention, which a patient may not be willing to undergo unless the defect is extensive and only an autogenous tissue reconstruction is desired.

The expected result following reoperation after pedicled flap reconstruction is often related to the condition of the reconstruction before this correction. The reconstructive surgeon must know the realistic possibilities for these corrections and should be sure that the patient understands and accepts them.

When a textured-surface implant or expander is used, the capsular contracture rate for these devices, which have been available for only a few years, is reported to be low. Realistically, however, I believe that the capsular contracture rate for reoperation in the situations described in this chapter could be higher.

The anticipated outcome after reduction of an autogenous breast reconstruction with either direct excision or suction-assisted lipectomy is more predictable. The patient should know, however, that the final result can take months or even up to 1 year to evolve because of the hematoma, bruising, and swelling that follow every instance of suction-assisted lipectomy.

The key to producing a satisfactory result is scrupulous technical execution and realistic expectations. The best approach to the anticipated outcome after reoperation is to promise less than the ideal result because this is most often the true outcome.

References

1. Bostwick J III. Plastic and Reconstructive Breast Surgery. St. Louis: Quality Medical Publishing, 1990.
2. Berger K, Bostwick J III. A Woman's Decision, 2nd ed. St. Louis: Quality Medical Publishing, 1994.
3. Little JW III. The nipple-areolar reconstruction—Skate technique [abstract]. Plast Reconstr Surg 76:806, 1985.
4. Little JW III, Spear SL. The finishing touches in nipple-areolar reconstruction. Perspect Plast Surg 2(1):1, 1988.

31

Reoperation Following Free Flap Breast Reconstruction

James C. Grotting, M.D.

Reoperative Problems

Failing free flap
Donor site contour irregularities
Hernia
Breast contour deficiencies or excesses
Scars
Peripheral nerve injuries
Inframammary fold irregularities
Missing axillary fold
Inadequate central breast projection
Breast mound asymmetry
Nipple-areola deformities
Partial or total flap failure

Breast reconstruction is like a love affair:
any fool can start it, but it takes a genius to end it.
Robert Goldwyn, M.D.

Despite the advantages offered by free flap breast reconstruction, it remains a staged procedure in most surgeons' hands. Therefore reoperations and revisions play an important role in the planning and execution of microsurgical breast reconstruction. There is considerable wisdom in Dr. Goldwyn's quotation. Many surgeons find it easier to successfully accomplish the free tissue transfer to the chest wall than to secondarily mold the tissue into an aesthetically pleasing breast shape.

Microsurgical breast reconstruction encompasses not only microsurgical skills but also principles of aesthetic surgery, oncologic surgery, and general reconstructive surgery. As such, it is one of the most challenging yet satisfying areas of our specialty. It demands great attention to aesthetic details, yet the surgeon must not lose sight of the fact that the patient has or has had breast cancer and is at risk for recurrence and death. The surgeon must keep the "big picture" in mind because some patients may escape from the concern about the cancer by becoming deluded by false expectations or by inappropriately worrying about minute details of the reconstruction. One must resist the urge to perform any procedure that is oncologically ill-advised only to achieve a small improvement in aesthetics of the reconstructed breast.

During the initial consultation, each patient should be counseled regarding the staged nature of microsurgical breast reconstruction. Patients presenting for delayed breast reconstruction are psychologically prepared for a second procedure, having recovered from the initial mastectomy. However, patients who undergo immediate breast reconstruction may have never had any previous surgery and, unless well counseled beforehand, may be reluctant to proceed with revisions and secondary surgery. Many times the extent of secondary surgery following microsurgical breast reconstruction can be accurately estimated by careful examination of the flap donor site before breast mound construction. Although we strive to achieve as accurate symmetry as possible in the primary operation, sometimes a flap cannot be safely trimmed to match the opposite breast without risking compromise of the circulation to portions of the flap. For example, a thick free TRAM flap, in which overcorrection of the upper pole is necessary because the flap is simply too thick in this area, must be trimmed secondarily. In order to preserve the venous drainage of random portions of the flap, thinning should be confined to the region beneath Scarpa's fascia. However, occasionally the amount of tissue beneath Scarpa's fascia is limited, thereby necessitating second-stage thinning rather than primary contouring. With careful preoperative examination of the thickness of the various zones of the flap compared to the contour of the opposite breast, this problem can be minimized by carefully planning which portion of the flap will be used to reconstruct each segment of the breast.

The causes for reoperation in microsurgical breast reconstruction generally fall into the following categories: (1) acute complications usually involving flap viability or bleeding, (2) donor site problems, (3) revisions for improving the breast mound shape or contour, (4) nipple-areola complex reconstruction, (5) malpositioned or hypertrophied scars, and (6) miscellaneous problems including peripheral neuropathy and masses caused by fat necrosis.

Each flap has an intrinsic set of potential problems and complications related to harvesting and insetting of the flap based on donor site, recipient site, and flap characteristics. For example, revisional breast mound surgery following a free TRAM flap might include attempts to increase projection. Conversely, the gluteal flap, because of its inherent thickness, may actually overproject but fail to fill the infraclavicular hollow as well as the free TRAM flap might. These compromises are taken into consideration when the choice of the initial flap is made and will impact the type and extent of secondary surgery required.

Most microsurgeons would now agree that the free TRAM flap is the flap of choice for the majority of patients undergoing microsurgical breast reconstruction. Although many other flaps have been used (see box), the free TRAM flap remains the most suitable and readily available. For this reason most of the comments regarding revisional surgery in this chapter relate to the free TRAM flap. Specific problems related to the other more common flaps are discussed under separate subheadings.

Free Flap Options for Breast Reconstruction

Transverse rectus abdominis musculocutaneous (TRAM) flap[1-6]
Tensor fascia lata flap[7]
Lateral transverse thigh flap[8]
Lateral vertical thigh flap[7]
Superior gluteus flap[9-12]
Inferior gluteus flap[13,14]
Extended inferior gluteus (trefoil) flap[15]
Superficial inferior epigastric artery (SIEA) flap[16,17]
Deep inferior epigastric perforator flap[18,19]
Groin flap[20,21]
Rubens' flap[22,23]
Transverse gracilis flap[24]
Contralateral latissimus dorsi flap[21,25]
Lateral thoracic opposite breast flap[26,27]
Omental flap[5]

TIMING

Timing of revisional surgery in microsurgical breast reconstruction is dictated by several factors. If the original operation was performed as an immediate breast reconstruction, then factors such as the adjunctive treatment of the breast cancer must be considered. Our oncologists prefer to begin chemotherapy approximately 4 weeks following the mastectomy/reconstruction. It is unnecessary for all wounds to be totally healed for chemotherapy to be initiated. Proceeding with adjunctive treatment is more important than waiting for healing of all areas. As long as an open wound is kept well debrided and clean with dressing changes, the wound will continue to heal even in the patient immunosuppressed by chemotherapy.

If a patient is a candidate for postoperative chemotherapy, we prefer to delay all revisional surgery until at least 1 month following completion of the treatment. This allows time for the blood cell counts to return to normal levels before elective revisional surgery is performed.

Postoperative radiotherapy to the chest wall is much less common in the immediate reconstruction group. In fact, it is my preference to not perform immediate reconstruction in any patient who might be a candidate for radiation to the chest wall following mastectomy. However, if a flap reconstruction has been performed and postoperative radiotherapy is required, revisional surgery should be delayed until all visible evidence of the acute effects of radiation have disappeared. As a general rule, when the tissues are soft with no visible swelling and all erythema has disappeared, it is safe to proceed with secondary surgery on the breast mound.

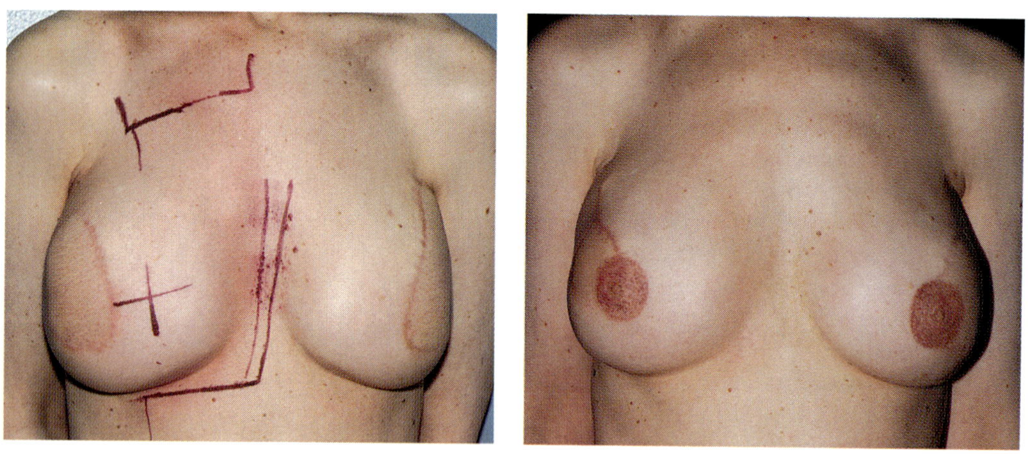

This 40-year-old patient is an example of how radiation influences the timing of secondary surgery. She required postoperative radiotherapy following mastectomy and immediate bilateral reconstruction using lateral vertical thigh flaps.

Once the radiotherapy had been completed and the erythema and edema had subsided, mound revision and nipple-areola reconstruction were performed during secondary surgery.

In immediate reconstruction patients who do not receive postoperative chemotherapy or radiation, secondary revisions are timed much like those for patients undergoing delayed reconstruction. When the tissues have reached "equilibrium"—are soft, pliable, and maximally elastic—they are maximally responsive to reoperative maneuvers. ***In microsurgical breast reconstruction, I find that about 3 months after the first operation the patient is psychologically ready and the tissues have settled enough to allow for accurate planning and execution of secondary procedures on the breast mound.***

I prefer to plan to complete a microsurgical breast reconstruction in two operations. In the first procedure the flap is transferred and shaped to obtain symmetry as close as possible to the opposite side. I prefer to perform opposite breast revisions at the time of the initial reconstruction because it is easier to match a corrected opposite breast than it is to later modify it to match a reconstructed breast mound. One of the advantages of microsurgical breast reconstruction is that flaps can be liberally shaped, sutured, and folded to gain symmetry in the first operation. However, it is a rare event in my practice to have a reconstructed breast mound that is so perfect that it would not benefit by any secondary revision no matter how minor. The planned second-stage revision plays a key role in achieving excellent results in microsurgical breast reconstruction. Small alterations in shape and contour of the breast mound, nipple-areola reconstruction, and opposite breast revisions in a second operation often can elevate a good reconstruction to a superior one.

PLANNING

The principles of planning any reoperation are problem specific: the goal of the procedure dictates the approach. For example, if faced with a failing free flap, the surgeon must anticipate the possible need for vein grafts and discuss this option with the patient as well as prepare a donor site in the operative field.

Also, the surgeon must anticipate how one maneuver might affect another. For example, if the revision of a widened superior mastectomy scar and a nipple-areola reconstruction are planned, the latter procedure must be done second. If the nipple-areola reconstruction were performed first followed by the excision of a widened scar in the superior pole, the final position of the nipple-areola would necessarily be raised by the amount that the scar is narrowed and unacceptable symmetry may result. Whereas if the scar is revised first followed by siting of the nipple-areola complex, then the nipple will almost always be in the correct location. As a rule, all breast mound revisions must be completed before the nipple-areola complex is sited.

One additional judgment that must be taken into consideration is whether nipple-areola reconstruction can be accomplished at the same time as a major revision of the breast mound. ***If mound revision requires major alterations such as the placement of an implant beneath the free flap or a considerable reduction in size, it is often better to delay nipple-areola reconstruction until final settling of the mound has occurred.*** However, with proper attention to the details of shaping in the first operation, the need for major revisions and third-stage procedures can be minimized.

GOALS OF TREATMENT

When acute complications occur, the patient is usually faced with an emergent return to the operating room to salvage a deteriorating situation. She must yield to the judgment of her surgeon entirely. Conversely, when it comes to refinements and revisions, the patient plays a much greater role in determining the reoperative plan. Usually, after the patient has lived with the newly reconstructed breast for several months, she can very specifically point out areas that continue to trouble her. The surgeon must listen carefully to these concerns as they should be the primary influence on the approach that is ultimately taken. Imperfections that the surgeon notices may cause the patient little concern. She may have no interest in undergoing additional procedures simply to enhance the surgeon's postoperative photographs! However, after the patient explains what she would like reoperative surgery to achieve and the surgeon has evaluated his goals and capabilities, a shared understanding of the expected result can be agreed upon.

SPECIFIC PROBLEMS

The Failing Free Flap

Unfortunately, microsurgery and occasional microvascular thrombosis go hand in hand. A failing free flap breast reconstruction represents a plastic surgical emergency. A return to the operating room is virtually always indicated. Understandably, this event is unnerving for both surgeon and patient. Yet, at the present time, there is no other way to salvage a flap that is failing due to either microarterial or venous thrombosis.

However, the situation can be viewed optimistically: with timely return of the patient to the operating room, failing free flaps can virtually always be salvaged. In our series of over 220 free flap breast reconstructions, nine patients required reexploration because of evidence of arterial or venous thrombosis. The flaps were salvaged in every case. We attribute this success in part to vigilant postoperative monitoring; however, other important factors played a role. Because flaps used for breast reconstruction are largely fat and skin, the flaps can tolerate a long ischemic period without irreversible tissue death. The muscle contained within these flaps generally serves as a conduit for the major vascular pedicle.

Portions of the muscle carrier can experience ischemic necrosis without the vascular pedicle that traverses it being compromised. For this reason, a microsurgeon reexploring a failing free flap breast reconstruction can be optimistic that he will be able to correct the problem in the majority of cases.

Flap Monitoring:
- Color
- Turgor
- Temperature
- Capillary refill
- Doppler ultrasonography (artery and vein)

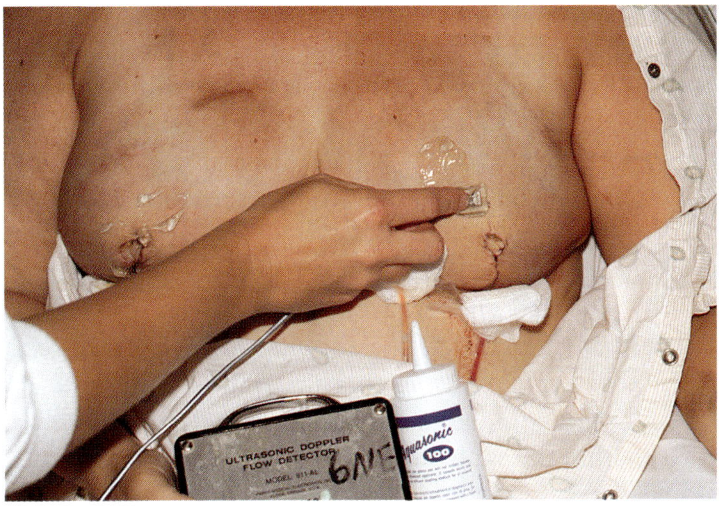

Our most reliable monitoring system continues to be a combination of visual and tactile inspection coupled with monitoring with a handheld conventional Doppler device. Flaps are inspected visually and with Doppler ultrasonography at hourly intervals for the first 24 hours postoperatively, at 2-hour intervals for the next 24 hours, and then every 4 hours for the next 2 days. The examiner inspects the color, temperature, capillary refill, and turgor of any exposed skin island. The Doppler device is then used to detect the typical sound of arterial flow, but more important, that of venous outflow. If the typical undulating continuous flow sound of the venous outflow of the flap is heard, one can be assured that both the artery and vein are open. If only the arterial signal is detected, the vein may have failed. Fortunately, when a skin island is left exposed, flap circulation can be easily assessed visually and tactilely. For this reason we always leave at least a small skin island or area of the flap exposed so that if the circulation is in doubt, active bleeding can be verified with a needle prick or No. 11 blade stab wound.

In our experience, flaps that are most likely to thrombose postoperatively are those that for one reason or another developed intraoperative technical problems. For instance, the arterial or venous anastomosis may have had to be revised intraoperatively to establish initial flow. Sometimes mechanical factors play a role, such as a small branch off the pedicle that was divided and is producing localized vasospasm. An anastomosis under tension will have a high rate of failure. Sometimes kinking of the vessels will occur following flow restoration, causing turbulence and platelet aggregation. Also, pressure from a tight dressing or patient positioning could potentially cause compression of the pedicle and lead to thrombosis. I am aware of two cases of axillary pedicle avulsion in the early postoperative period apparently caused by patients reaching with the ipsilateral arm. None of our patients has experienced this complication; however, as a precaution we instruct our patients to maintain the shoulder between 20 and 90 degrees of abduction for the first 10 days postoperatively.

Our approach to treating a failing free flap breast reconstruction is to immediately return the patient to the operating room. We usually heparinize the patient systemically with a bolus of 3000 to 5000 U of intravenous heparin. If the flap is pale and cool, an arterial thrombosis is suspected. If the flap is edematous and cyanotic, a venous thrombosis is usually the cause. Dark venous blood exiting from the suction drains is also suggestive of a venous outflow problem.

The patient is positioned much like she was for the initial free flap transfer, with the ipsilateral arm prepared and draped free on an arm board. It is helpful to place an additional pad posterior to the shoulder to elevate the axillary contents slightly. Since microvascular revisions might require a vein graft for replacement of the thrombosed segment, we usually prepare a donor site for vein grafts as well. In most cases I use the saphenous vein at the ankle or one of the tributaries to the saphenous system in the upper medial thigh. The ipsilateral cephalic vein might also be considered as either a graft or as an alternate recipient vein.

The vascular pedicle can usually be accessed by simply opening the lateral portion of the wound. Oftentimes, it is necessary to open the entire incision in order to adequately place retractors to reach the segment of the pedicle that requires repair. If the problem is a venous thrombosis, occasionally the second deep inferior epigastric vein can be used (if it exists) to immediately vent the built-up venous pressure; the end of the clip is simply cut off while the pedicle is examined under the microscope. If the flap pedicle has been thrombosed for many hours, a longer segment of thrombosis may be encountered in either the artery or the vein. Under these circumstances it is better to resect the segment and replace it with a vein graft than risk placing any tension on the repair. The microvascular repairs are completed, the incision is reclosed, and the patient is kept heparinized for 2 to 4 days postoperatively, depending on the level of the surgeon's concern about the patient's coagulation status.

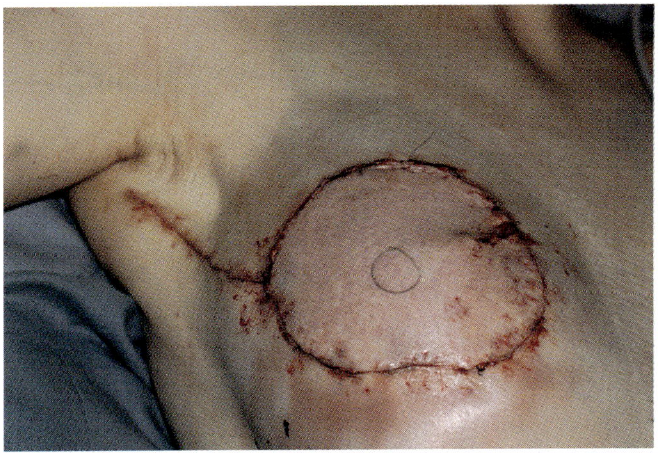

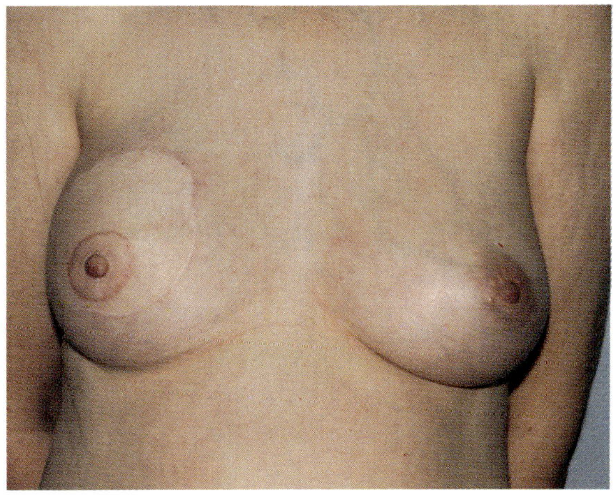

Twenty-four hours after undergoing immediate reconstruction of the right breast using a free TRAM flap, this patient presented with the cyanotic discoloration of the flap. She was returned to the operating room to correct venous outflow obstruction. Interestingly, the patient had had a venous thrombosis intraoperatively during the primary procedure that required a revision of the anastomosis. On reexploration, the vein was found to again be thrombosed; it was replaced with a segment of reversed saphenous vein graft from the ankle. Postoperatively, she had an uneventful course and healing ultimately occurred.

If the ischemic interval has been long, some degree of fat necrosis or fat atrophy can be anticipated over the next 3 to 6 months. Secondary revision in these patients is best postponed until the flap has maximally settled and softened.

Hematoma

Hematomas can occur following free flap breast reconstruction just as they can following virtually any surgical procedure. Although most hematomas are considered minor complications, one of the consequences of a hematoma in a free flap breast reconstruction might be critical compromise of the vascular pedicle. In addition, the cause of the hematoma could be leakage from the microvascular arterial or venous anastomosis or small branches therefrom. Therefore it is usually best to return these patients to the operating room for operative exploration. The hematoma may be heralded by increased output from either the donor site or recipient site drains. If a drain under or near the flap is collecting dark venous blood, a venous outflow obstruction may be present. For this reason the microvascular anastomosis must be examined carefully at reexploration.

Not uncommonly, the source of the hematoma cannot be found when the area is reexplored. It is best to take down all of the incisions and to carefully mobilize the undersurface of the flap to make certain that a "pumper" is not found. There is nothing more frustrating than to drain a hematoma, reclose the wound, and return the patient to the ward only to find that the bleeding recurs.

Deep Vein Thrombosis and Pulmonary Embolus

Deep vein thrombosis and pulmonary embolus are only very rarely reoperative conditions, but their recognition and treatment could be lifesaving. The spectrum of presentation can be unnerving. The condition can be totally asymptomatic, progressing in a very short period of time to cardiovascular collapse and respiratory arrest. The most common presentation of deep vein thrombosis is a gradual unilateral swelling of the leg, which may become tender to deep palpation. Proximal thigh deep vein thrombosis is serious because of its propensity for producing emboli. Doppler ultrasonography is the best diagnostic test to use initially because it is noninvasive and reliable. If Doppler studies are equivocal, phlebography should be considered.

Pulmonary embolus classically presents with a pleuritic-type chest pain, hyperpnea or dyspnea, and left-axis shift on ECG. Pulmonary angiography is definitive for diagnosing pulmonary embolus and may also be used for infusion of clot-lysing substances. A ventilation perfusion scan is indicated as a first-line diagnostic procedure.

Prevention is the key to avoiding these two life-threatening complications. A surgical team must be ever mindful to the recognition of these problems as well as to maneuvers that can reduce their incidence. ***The patient is most vulnerable to the development of a nidus of thrombus in the venous sinuses of the lower extremity while anesthesia is being induced.*** For this reason prophylaxis is begun preoperatively with the administration of 5000 U of heparin subcutaneously 30 minutes before induction of anesthesia. The patient is fitted with long leg-support stockings and a sequential pneumatic compression pump device that must be activated during induction. Pneumatic compression is continued until the third postoperative day when the patient is spending long periods of time up and around at the bedside. She is encouraged to be up at the bedside during the first 24 hours; while in bed, she is told to flex and extend the feet to maintain the normal pumping action of the calf muscles. Subcutaneous heparin administration is not continued postoperatively because of concern about bleeding complications. Aspirin (325 mg) is given once daily and continued as antiplatelet therapy for 2 months.

Seroma

Persistent seromas rarely occur with free flap breast reconstruction as long as adequate drains are inserted initially and left in place until output is minimal. Two drains are positioned beneath the flap with at least one in the axilla. We usually insert at least two drains in the donor site as well. When a recurrent seroma does develop, repeated aspiration is not as effective as simply placing another drain. Persistent seromas are much more common with the latissimus dorsi or lateral thigh donor sites.

We encountered one extremely unusual complication from the simple drainage of an axillary seroma. A 38-year-old patient underwent bilateral simple mastectomy with immediate reconstruction using bilateral microvascular free TRAM flaps. She recovered exceedingly well and was discharged on the fifth postoperative day. Drainage from the axillary area and all of the other drains diminished to less than 30 cc per day and so the drains were removed by the tenth postoperative day. She returned for follow-up 1 week later at which time it was noticed that an obvious seroma in the right axilla had developed. A Penrose drain was placed under sterile conditions in the office, with drainage of approximately 60 cc of straw-colored fluid. Six days following placement of the drain, the patient presented with a short history of fever to 104° F and shaking chills. On examination in the office, the patient was lethargic, mildly hypotensive, and tachycardic. She had no other symptoms of pain or tenderness in any location. She was admitted to the hospital, a full range of culture studies was performed, and administration of broad-spectrum antibiotics was instituted. *Staphylococcus aureus* was eventually recovered from both the blood and drainage from the right axillary seroma; a diagnosis of staphylococcal toxic shock syndrome was made. The patient ultimately recovered without sequelae.

Infection

Infection following free flap breast reconstruction is unusual. Nevertheless, infection will present from time to time as cellulitis involving either the breast or the abdomen. Interestingly, most cases of cellulitis occur late (>30 days) after flap transfer.

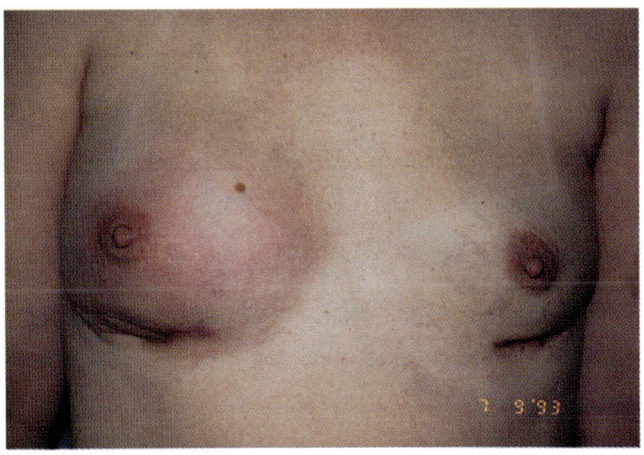

This 32-year-old patient had previously undergone subcutaneous mastectomies and implant reconstruction but suffered from recurrent deformity and implant rupture. She underwent bilateral implant removal and reconstruction using bilateral buried free TRAM flaps. Two months postoperatively she presented with swelling and erythema of the right reconstructed breast. Most likely this situation represented infection from either retained foreign material from the previous implant or possibly inadequate deepithelialization of the buried flap. The patient responded quickly to systemic antibiotic administration.

Patients who are undergoing chemotherapy following immediate free flap breast reconstruction seem to be slightly more susceptible to infection. Fortunately, such patients generally respond rapidly to the administration of intravenous antibiotics and local care if an open wound is present. In rare instances a collection may need to be drained.

Alloplastic mesh used to reinforce the abdominal wall closure following the free TRAM flap transfer may also serve as a nidus of infection. Infection usually results when exposure of the mesh occurs following partial loss of the random abdominal skin flap. In this situation, it is not always essential that the Marlex mesh be removed. In fact, most of the mesh may already be well incorporated; simply treating the wound open with dressing changes and antibiotics will allow it to granulate. Any excess edges or loose pieces of mesh should be debrided like any other foreign body.

On rare occasions, the Marlex mesh may be completely involved with the infection. Loosening of the sheet or purulence involving the entire surface of the mesh is an indication for its removal. It is usually best to remove the mesh and leave a temporary hernia until the infection is under control and the tissues are again healed and soft. At that point, elective repair with autogenous tissue is preferred. If inadequate local tissue is available, a fresh sheet of clean mesh can be inserted.

Fat Necrosis

Fat necrosis following free flap reconstruction has not been observed to the same extent as that following pedicle flaps. The incidence of fat necrosis among free TRAM flap breast reconstruction patients is less than 2%.[23,28] However, when fat necrosis does occur, it usually results from one of the following reasons: (1) inadequate trimming of the flap at the time of initial transfer (occurs in the most distal random portions of the flap), (2) attempts to preserve flap tissue on the opposite side of a previous scar that divides the flap, (3) postoperative thrombosis that requires a flap salvage procedure.

Some degree of firmness may be observed in free flap breast reconstruction patients in the first 2 months. However, with time, these firm areas virtually always soften and nothing surgical needs to be done. A few patients, however, will be left with varying degrees of "stoney-like" firm areas that may benefit from excision. The main problem with not excising these areas is that the patient continues to be concerned and fears the return of breast cancer. Similarly, oncologists and other examining physicians may be confused by the presence of these areas and not understand the rationale in leaving them alone. Therefore excision is usually the best option and can be accomplished at the time of nipple-areola reconstruction or mound revision.

Baseline mammography of the reconstructed breast may reveal other areas of microscopic fat necrosis as indicated by typical calcifications. However, these calcifications are not clinically significant and need not be further treated.

Partial or Complete Flap Loss

Although partial flap loss is much more common with pedicle flaps, it may occur with free flaps as well. The incidence of both fat necrosis and partial flap loss has been considerably reduced in our experience using the microvascular free flap procedure vs. the pedicle flap procedure. Depending on the degree of flap loss, various treatments might be required. If the tissue loss is minor, it can usually be treated conservatively and allowed to heal secondarily. For minor deficiencies, it is often possible to shift excess flap tissue from another quadrant into the area of deficiency to gain symmetry.

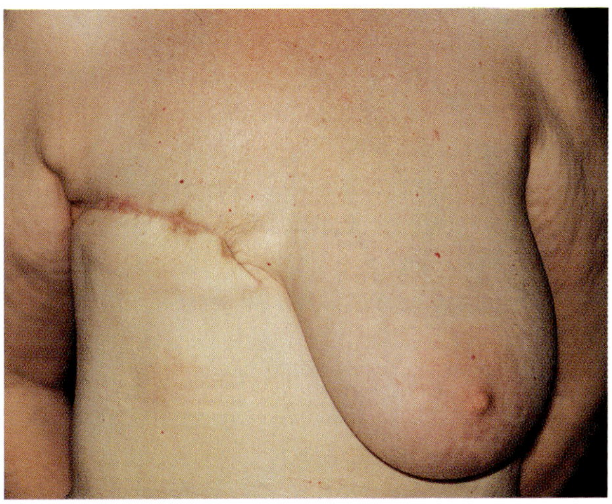

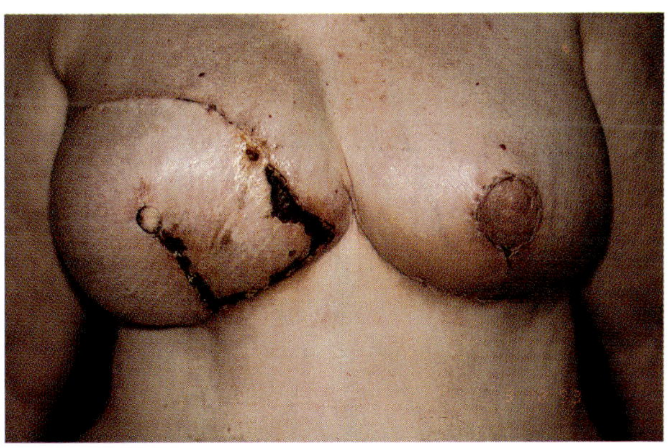

This patient underwent delayed breast reconstruction using the microvascular free TRAM flap. No previous abdominal surgery had been performed. Nevertheless, circulation was marginal to the distalmost aspect of the flap, resulting in marginal necrosis of the TRAM skin island with an area of fat necrosis beneath it as shown 2 weeks postoperatively.

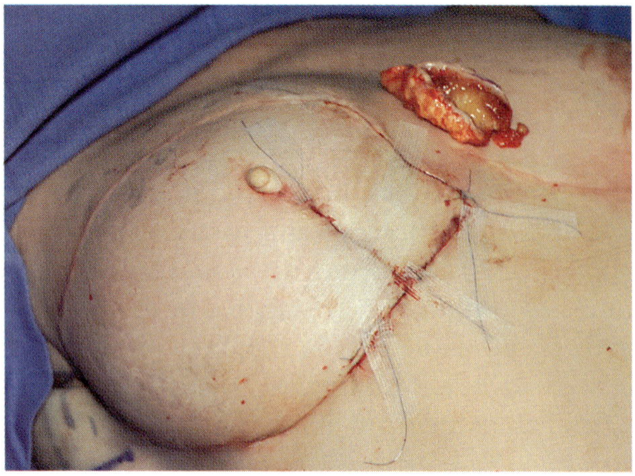

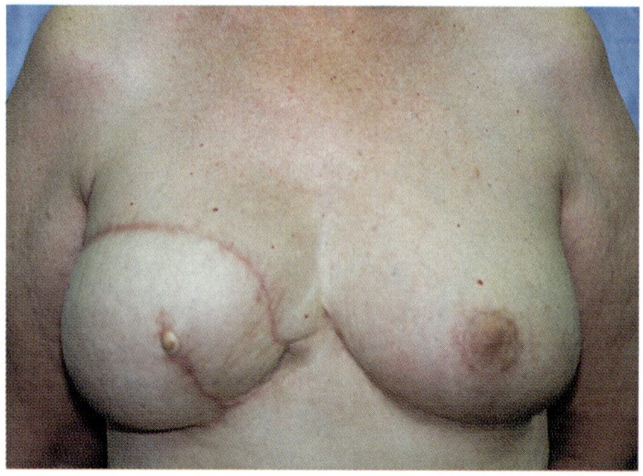

Eight weeks postoperatively the firm area of fat necrosis was excised and the flap was advanced, creating a satisfactory result.

If flap loss is major, either an implant or a second flap may be required to round out the breast mound. These techniques are discussed in Chapter 30 in detail; the techniques for pedicle flaps and free flaps are similar. However, consideration must be given with regard to the use of the ipsilateral latissimus dorsi flap based on which recipient vessels have been used for the free flap transfer. My preference has been to use the thoracodorsal vessels end to end for the free flap transfer. This vessel configuration preserves the serratus collateral branch, which is known to be able to provide axial flow to the latissimus dorsi muscle following division of the thoracodorsal pedicle. Therefore, if I am certain that this collateral artery is intact, I do not hesitate to use the ipsilateral latissimus dorsi flap to fill out a deficient mound when required. Either color-laser Doppler examination or arteriography might be considered for clarifying the vascular anatomy.

Total flap failure is and should be an exceedingly rare event. Nevertheless, the possibility must be carefully discussed preoperatively with each patient. In the event that this were to occur, there is little choice but to debride the flap and attempt secondary wound closure. I prefer to delay a secondary attempt of breast reconstruction until the chest wall tissues have been allowed to completely heal and soften. The secondary alternatives for flap reconstruction discussed in Chapter 30 also apply here. However, the factors that led to the choice of the free tissue transfer for the primary operation might influence the choice of a secondary procedure. A second microvascular transfer may need to be considered if the medical and psychological condition of the patient would allow it.

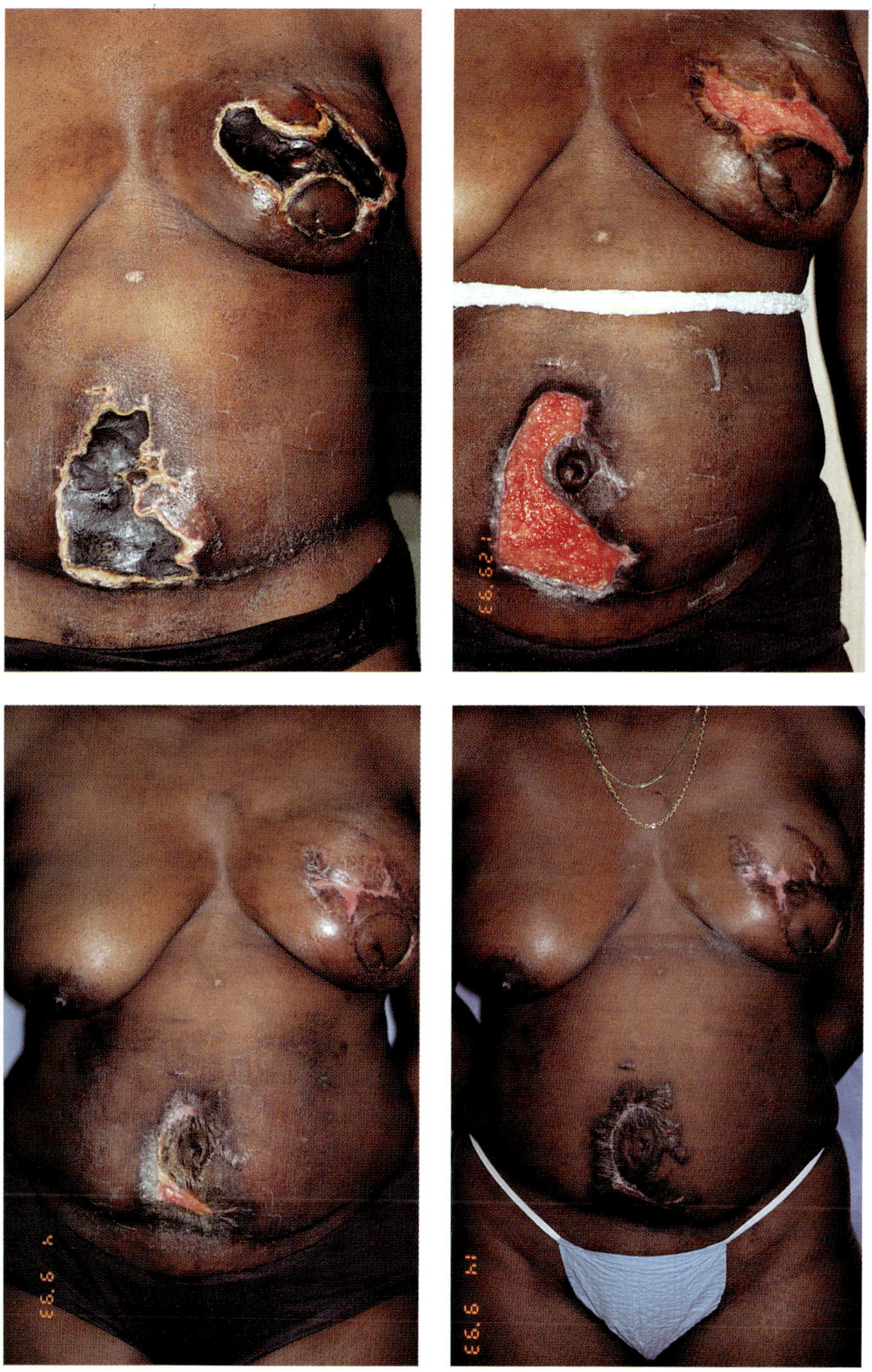

This patient represents the worst case of random flap necrosis that I have encountered. Because of her history of steroid-dependent mixed connective tissue disease, we elected immediate reconstruction using autogenous tissue. A microvascular free TRAM flap was performed with complete flap survival. However, the random flaps including both the superior mastectomy flap and the abdominal flap underwent full-thickness ischemic necrosis. This wound gradually healed over the next 6 months.

Mastectomy Flap Necrosis

This is an untoward event almost entirely limited to immediate reconstruction. In some patients the plane between the breast tissue and subcutaneous fat is so superficial that following mastectomy long skin flaps simply will not survive as random flaps. General surgeons who are unaccustomed to skin-sparing techniques may leave skin flaps that are nonviable. It can be a difficult judgment to decide how much of this skin to debride at the time of the inset of the free flap. In the reconstructive surgeon's zeal to preserve natural breast skin, which is a perfect color and texture match with the opposite breast, it may be easy to misjudge the perfusion of the mastectomy flaps, and nonviable portions may be left behind. The price for this judgment error is partial-thickness or full-thickness loss in these portions of the mastectomy flaps. Usually, the underlying free flap is healthy and viable.

Treatment should be conservative. The extent of the loss can never be accurately predicted, and sometimes only a minimal or partial-thickness slough rather than an entire discolored area will occur. As long as infection does not intervene and the underlying free flap is healthy, I treat these mastectomy flap sloughs with topical Betadine once the eschar has stabilized. When the skin has clearly demarcated and the eschar begins to spontaneously separate, a judicious trim of the nonviable area followed by dressing changes will enhance wound contraction, granulation, and healing. Unfortunately, this process may take several months. I still believe that allowing these areas to heal spontaneously is the better choice than placing a skin graft. Healing by secondary intention allows greater forces of wound contracture, facilitating secondary revision.

On occasion some patients will simply not accept an open wound for this period of time. In this case skin grafting or debridement and closure with local tissues may be the best decision. Some oncologists may insist on this treatment option before initiating chemotherapy. However, open wounds will continue to contract and heal despite the initiation of chemotherapy.

Abdominal Flap Necrosis

Following the harvest of the TRAM flap, necrosis of the random abdominal skin flap can occasionally occur. This problem is most common in patients who have had previous Kocher-type incisions in the right subcostal area. However, necrosis can develop in the absence of this previous scar in smokers, chronically obese patients, or patients in whom the amount of tension on wound closure has been misjudged. In addition, wide undermining above the costal margins and beyond the anterior axillary line will divide the collateral circulation to the superior abdominal flap and precipitate necrosis.

Management is similar to that described for mastectomy flap necrosis. Early suture removal does not result in the release of enough tension to prevent partial-thickness or full-thickness loss of the central part of the abdominal flap. Again, the best course of action is conservative treatment until the eschar is clearly demarcated and beginning to spontaneously separate. Usually, the underlying fascial repair will not be affected and will simply granulate over. Ultimately the wound will heal.

Clearly the key to avoidance of this complication is prevention. A previous right subcostal incision is a "red flag" and demands extreme care in determining the correct amount of abdominal skin undermining. ***If the flap design can be shifted superiorly to include at least the lateral portion of the subcostal incision in the flap outline, the area at risk can be diminished.*** Very limited undermining, if any, should be performed. Release of only the left side of the abdominal wall and enough release centrally to allow closure is the preferred method, even if the result is at first somewhat unaesthetic.

If the umbilicus has necrosed, little can be done early on except to perform conservative debridement as necessary to allow healing by secondary intention. A delayed umbilicoplasty can be performed at the time of nipple-areola reconstruction (see pp. 1150 and 1151).

Breast Mound: Problems and Solutions

Lack of Projection

Of the various free flaps available for breast reconstruction, the TRAM flap is the most often used, yet it does not offer the natural projection of flaps from either the thigh or the buttock region. The thickness of the subcutaneous fat of the abdomen is often inadequate to project the reconstructed breast to match the opposite breast. However, the free TRAM flap is robust and it permits placement of plication sutures or flap molding at the initial operation to achieve reasonably good projection. If, however, projection is inadequate, several maneuvers can be performed secondarily. I usually perform these procedures at the time of nipple-areola reconstruction: 3 months following initial flap transfer or 1 month following the completion of chemotherapy.

Most patients at the present time want to avoid the use of a breast implant to improve projection. Therefore, if the revision can be done with local tissues alone, this approach is preferred.

Decreased lateral fullness and increased projection can be achieved by V-Y advancement of the lateral portion of the reconstructed breast. With this technique, precise skin excision and plication of lateral fat improve both contour and projection.

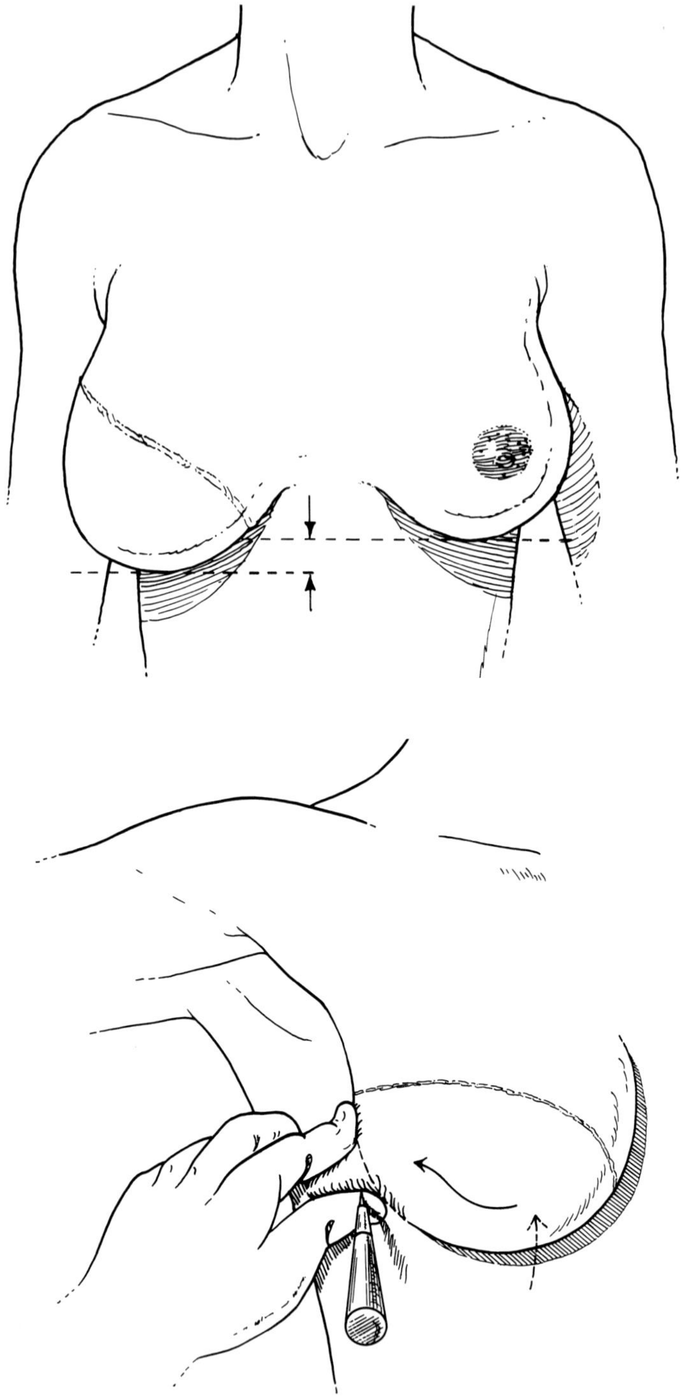

I mark the patient while she stands in front of me. Often the breast is too full laterally, appears slightly ptotic, and lacks projection. By digitally pinching the skin laterally, one can examine the contour of the inferior lateral portion of the breast on both sides. In this way the amount of skin that needs to be resected to elevate the breast and to reduce the lateral fullness can be estimated.

A triangle of TRAM skin flap or mastectomy skin flap is marked for excision. If nipple-areola reconstruction is to be performed concomitantly, it is helpful to mark the estimated position of the nipple-areola reconstruction on the corrected breast mound while this correction is simulated manually. The midline should also be marked for placement of pendulum sutures to help to verify the nipple position intraoperatively.

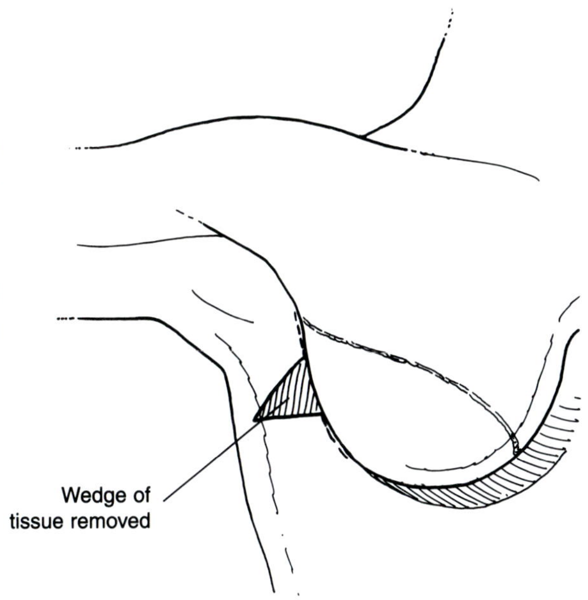

I usually perform these corrections with the patient under general anesthesia on an outpatient basis, although local anesthesia is also an option. The patient is positioned with her arms abducted on arm boards at approximately 90 degrees. Careful padding and positioning of the forearms are essential to prevent nerve injury (see p. 1155). Plans are made to sit the patient up intraoperatively to confirm the accuracy of the revision; it is helpful to rehearse this maneuver with the anesthesiologist before preparing and draping the patient for surgery.

With the V-Y advancement technique, the incisions are reopened and the mastectomy skin flaps are undermined to the predetermined level. If the reconstructed breast is too full laterally, the surface of the TRAM flap fat can be shaved down to the right size. However, to use this additional tissue to increase projection, plication sutures are placed to imbricate the lateral portion of the fat, forcing it to shift centrally and thus further project the reconstructed breast mound.

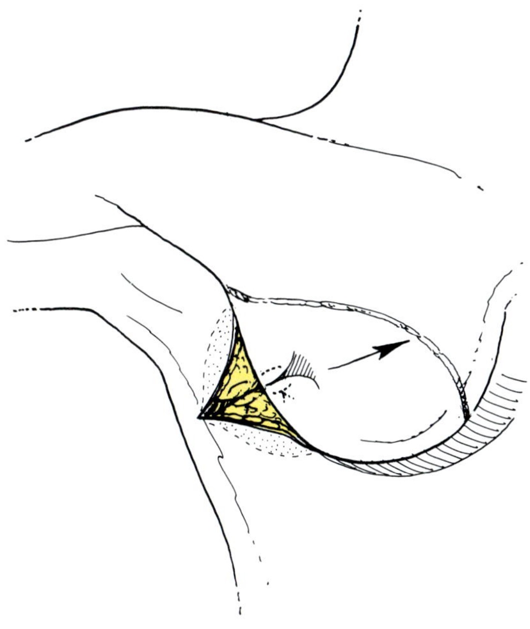

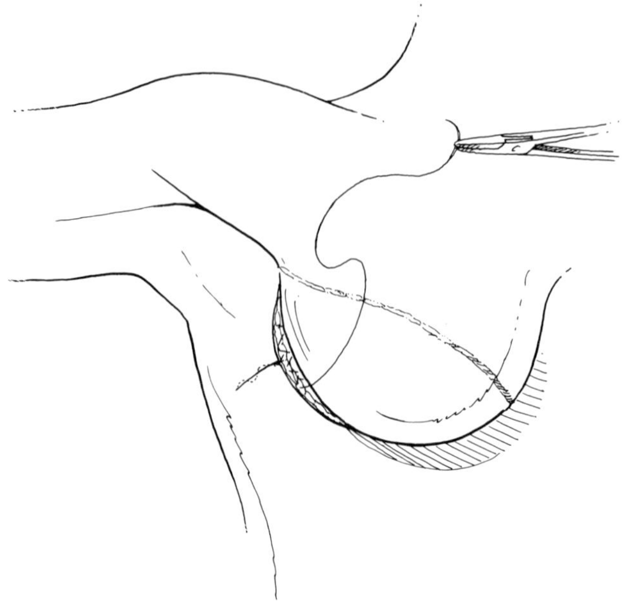

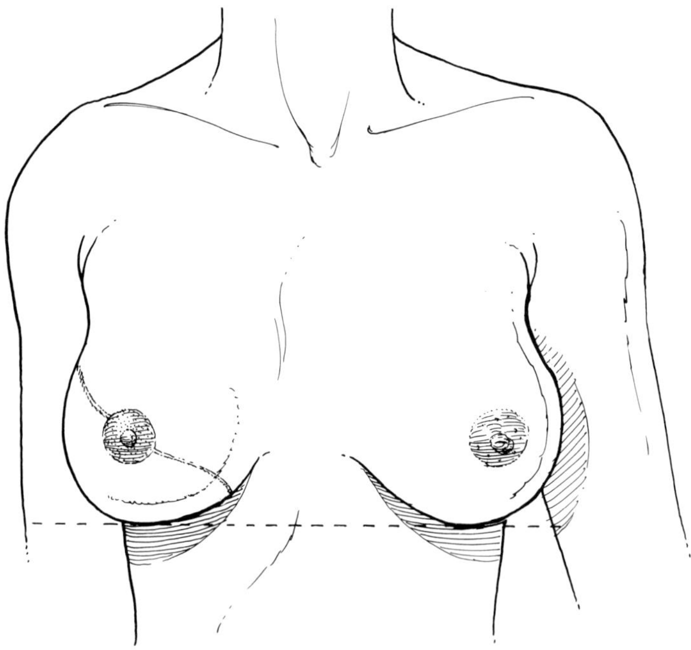

The mastectomy skin flaps can then be reapproximated over the TRAM skin island temporarily as the amount of skin island to be trimmed is marked. The TRAM skin island is then trimmed and final closure is carried out.

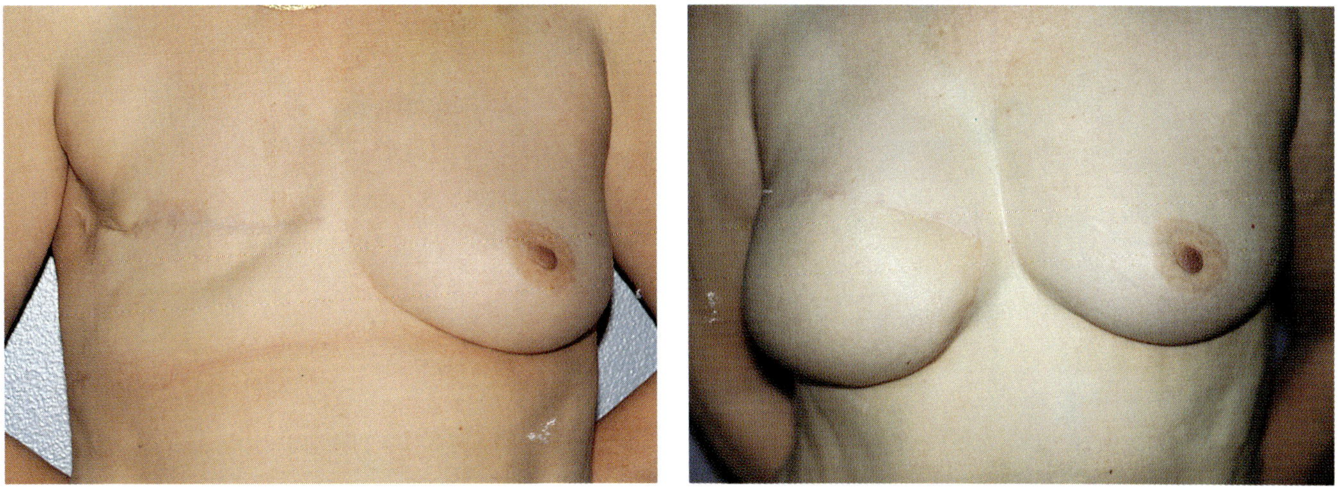

In this patient a delayed microvascular free TRAM flap reconstruction was performed. Three months postoperatively, the breast mound appeared too low and large and lacked projection.

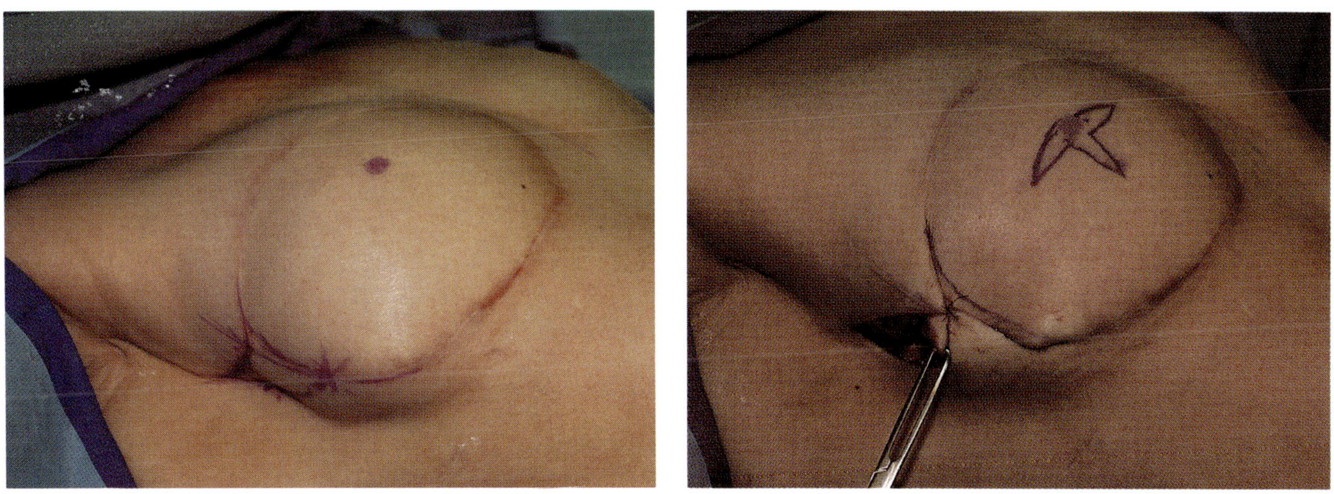

The correction was marked for a V-Y advancement of the lateral breast with plication sutures in the breast mound. The excess TRAM skin island was drawn beneath the lateral mastectomy flaps, marked, and excised.

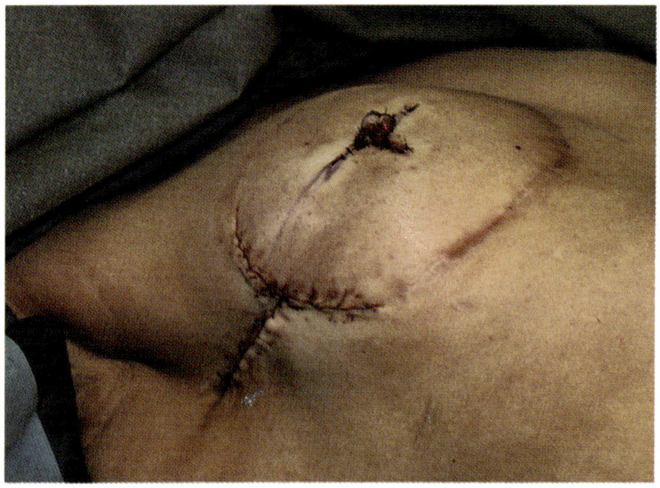

Nipple-areola reconstruction was performed using the star flap technique. Tattooing of the areola was completed 6 weeks later.

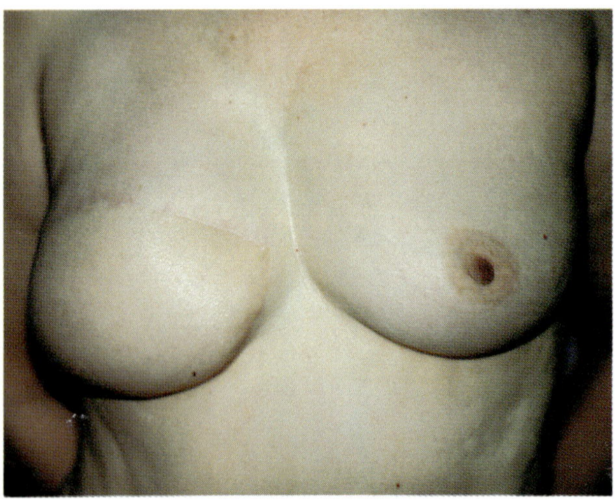

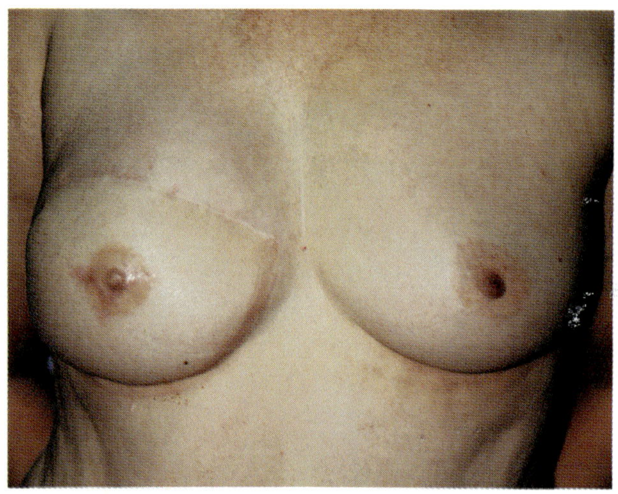

Comparison of the postoperative views following primary reconstruction and postrevision demonstrates a noticeable improvement in symmetry.

For larger discrepancies in volume as well as projection, an implant is the simplest option if the patient will accept it. I prefer to use a small saline implant placed in the subpectoral position. An excellent increase in projection can usually be achieved with the insertion of only a small 100 to 150 cc implant. Small implants can also be used to fill areas of deficiency (e.g., medial or lower lateral pole) or to provide additional bulk in the inferolateral portion of the reconstructed breast.

Large discrepancies in breast size in the presence of complete flap survival usually are indicative of a planning error (i.e., insufficient donor tissue was available to match the opposite side). However, if the patient concurrently underwent reduction mammaplasty on the opposite breast, occasionally size discrepancy can result from inadequate breast reduction. If this is the case, a revision of the reduced breast to decrease projection or bulk is the best way to gain symmetry (see Chapter 27).

Upper Pole Fullness

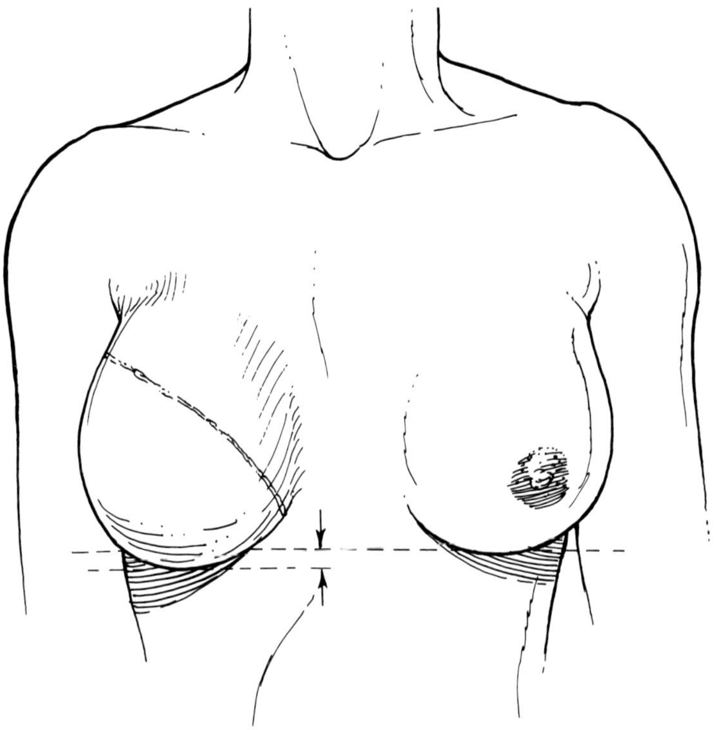

Failure to adequately trim the TRAM flap at the initial operation will result in a breast that is simply too large. This is the most common mistake that surgeons make in their earliest experience with autogenous breast reconstruction. Occasionally, however, the TRAM flap is deliberately left bulky. In these cases the flap cannot be safely trimmed to match the opposite side at the initial operation because of the risk of damaging the blood supply to the random portions of the flap. This situation commonly occurs in patients with an opposite breast that has a flat upper pole and only minimal ptosis. In addition, if the abdominal subcutaneous tissues are thick, then it may not be possible to safely thin the upper portion of the TRAM flap to match the opposite side. However, after 3 months, the flap can be safely suctioned or trimmed in any fashion desired as long as the blood supply is preserved.

I attempt to preserve the main vascular pedicle to the free flap during revisional surgery. I have had one case in which although I was quite confident that the flap was receiving adequate collateral circulation from the surrounding wound bed, the flap became pale after secondary division of the pedicle. Although the entire flap survived, I observed some slight atrophy in the flap that I do not believe would have occurred otherwise (see pp. 1142 and 1143).

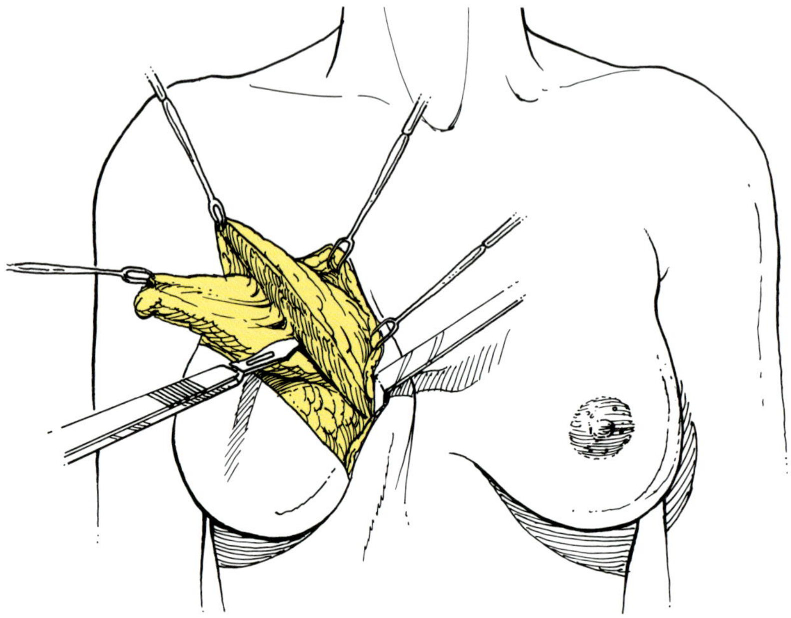

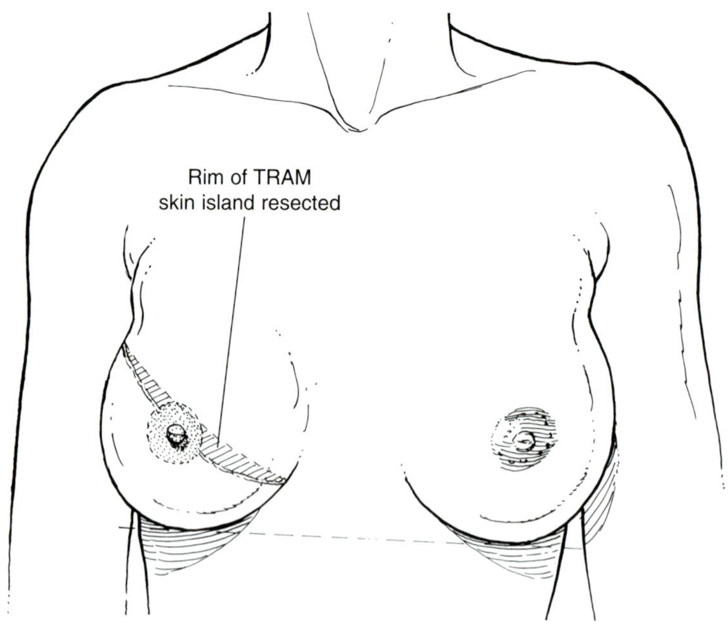

A bulky flap can be trimmed by simply cleaving the excess surface bulk from the flap. This excision is most commonly done in the superior portion of the reconstructed breast, particularly if the breast mound is also somewhat ptotic. The flap is reentered at the superior mastectomy scar incision and the mastectomy flap is undermined to the subclavicular area. The surface of this flap is trimmed to match the opposite side.

If necessary, the TRAM skin island can then be elevated beneath the superior mastectomy flap, temporarily stapled, marked, trimmed, and resutured so that both the fullness and the ptosis are corrected simultaneously. If the breast is nonptotic but simply too full superiorly or laterally, suction-assisted lipectomy is both a simple and safe method of secondary correction. In the absence of fat necrosis, the vascularized fat can be easily suctioned. In fact, care must be taken not to overreduce the breasts in this technique.

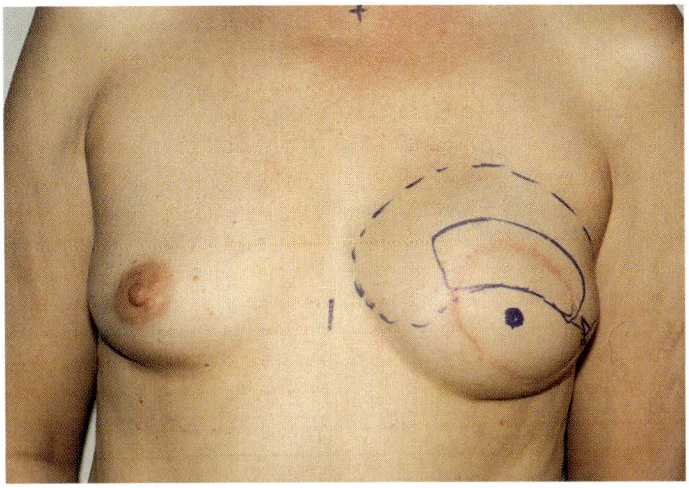

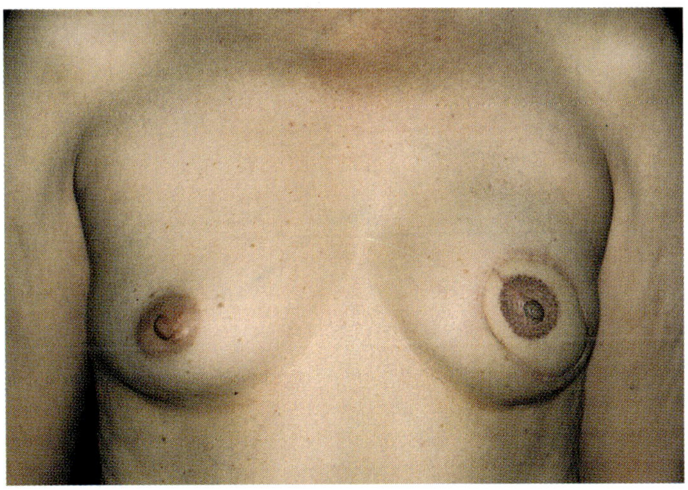

This 46-year-old patient underwent modified radical mastectomy and immediate reconstruction of the left breast using a microvascular free TRAM flap. The flap was too thick to be safely trimmed in the primary operation. She was thus left with a reconstruction that was too large and full superiorly. Liposuction of the left breast was performed to make it symmetric with the right breast. Nipple-areola reconstruction was performed concomitantly. Although augmentation of the right breast might have been an option in this patient, most patients prefer that the unoperated breast not be altered. Therefore we are now attempting to reconstruct smaller breasts with autogenous tissue.

Excessive Ptosis

If the breast is the proper size but is simply too low, the easiest way to correct this problem without lengthening the scars is to imbricate the lateral portion of the mastectomy flaps. This correction is best judged preoperatively while the patient stands. Very slight overcorrection is recommended as recurrent settling may cause the ptosis deformity to recur after 1 year.

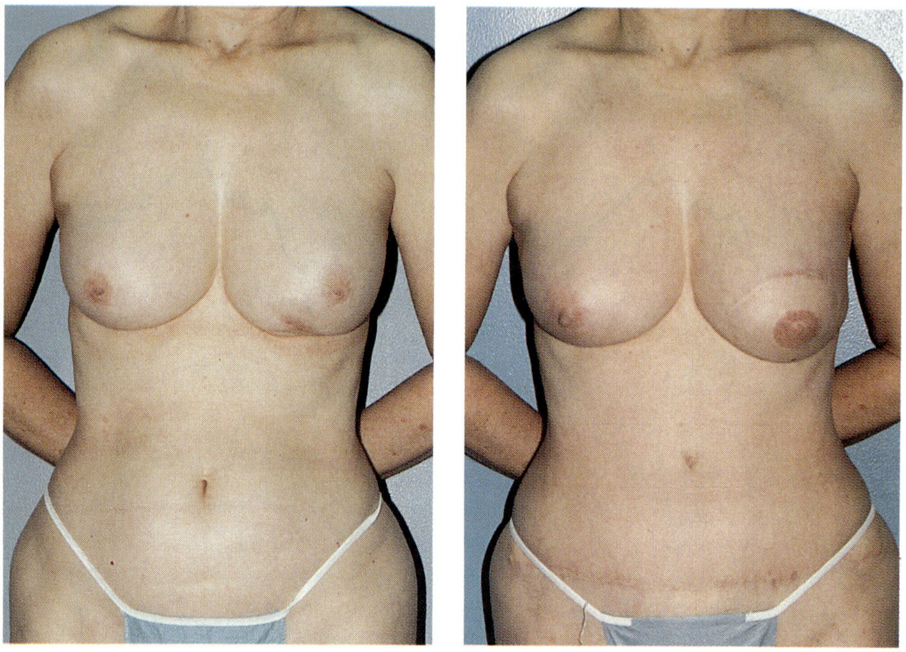

This patient underwent immediate free TRAM reconstruction of the left breast. Although the reconstruction was symmetric at the time of the secondary revision, by 1 year postoperatively gradual continued settling led to recurrent ptosis.

The other method of dealing with ptosis is to simply excise excess TRAM skin island either at the superior mastectomy incision or in the inframammary fold if the TRAM skin island was inset at that level. If the umbilicus was previously inset at the 6-o'clock position, resulting in a vertical scar in the median of the reconstructed breast, both a horizontal and a vertical excision can sometimes be advantageous to increase projection and decrease ptosis much like would be done in a conventional mastopexy.

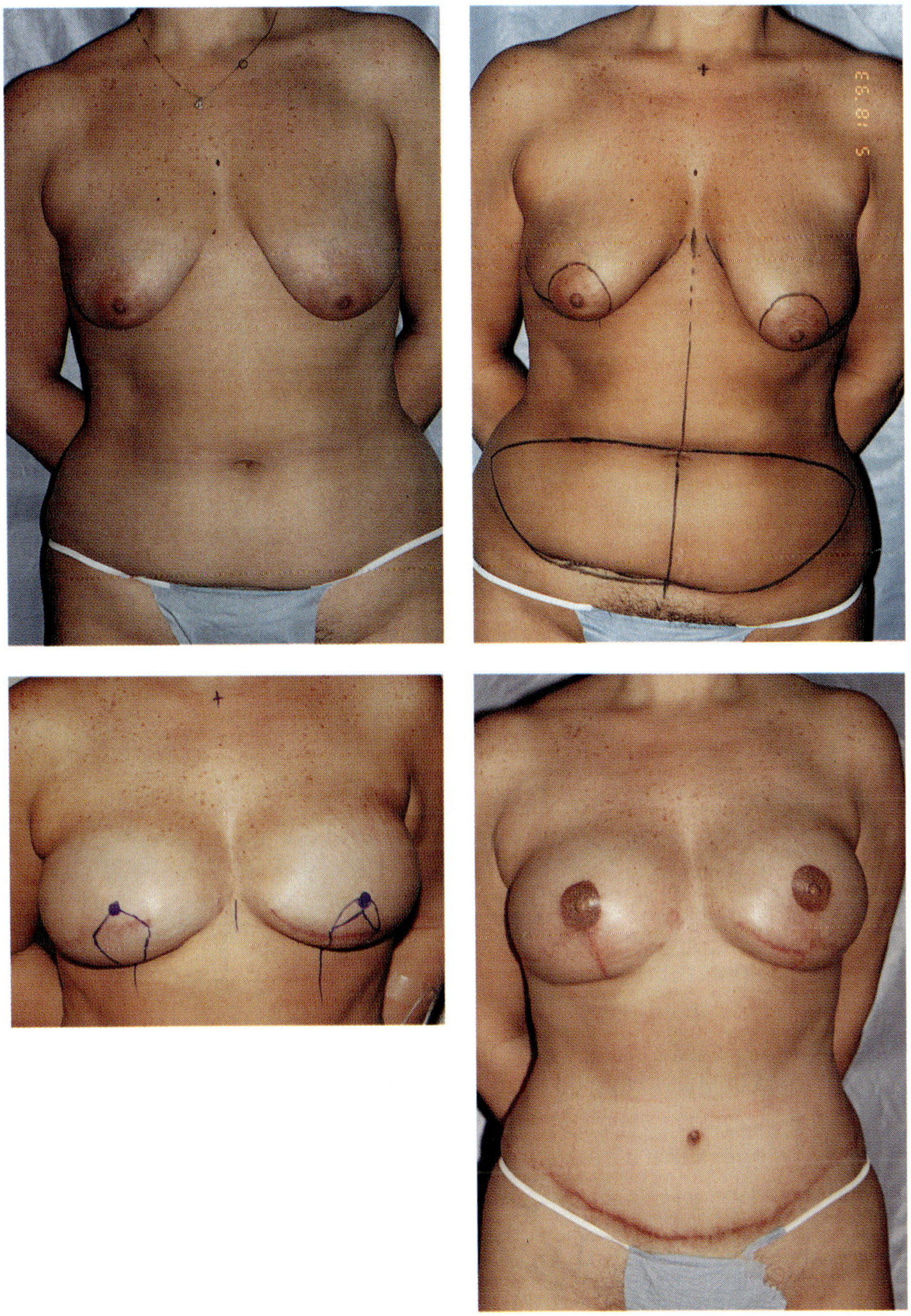

This patient underwent bilateral simple mastectomy and immediate reconstruction for premalignant mastopathy. Because of a previous appendectomy incision, which had divided the deep inferior epigastric artery on the right, a pedicled TRAM flap was rotated on the right and a microvascular free TRAM flap was transferred on the left. Postoperatively, the patient requested correction of the flat appearance and wide base of the breasts. In order to correct the broad base, a V-shaped excision of skin was designed in the midline of the inferior pole of each breast as in a conventional mastopexy. Nipple reconstruction was carried out simultaneously followed by nipple-areola tattoo.

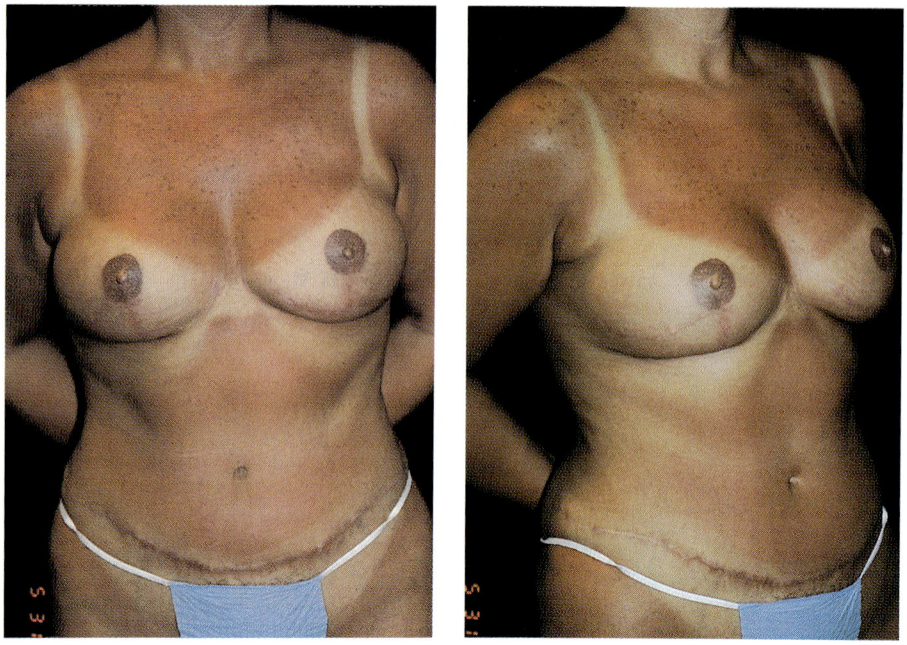

The final result is shown at 1½ years postoperatively.

Inframammary Fold Irregularities

These problems were more common before general surgeons began preserving the inframammary fold at the time of the initial mastectomy. With the natural fold preserved, one can be assured that the lower pole will project symmetrically from the proper position on the chest wall. However, when the fold has been obliterated or needs to be reset as with delayed reconstruction, irregularities can occur. A common example is when one attempts to fill the reelevated inferior mastectomy flap in delayed reconstruction rather than remove it. Shrinkage of the lower mastectomy flap after mastectomy alone will cause there to be not enough fill to project the reconstructed breast or to allow ptosis. Similarly, the fold will not form at the proper level. To prevent this problem in delayed reconstruction, we usually debride the inferior mastectomy flap to within approximately 1 cm of the projected inframammary fold so that the free flap can be inset in the fold and project naturally from this point.

If the inframammary fold ends up being too low because of too extensive undermining or excessive debriding of the inferior mastectomy flap, the fold must be secondarily elevated. This can be done by reentering the inferior mastectomy incision and plicating the remnant of the inferior mastectomy flap at a higher level. A rim excision of the inferior curve of the reconstructed breast must accompany this maneuver in order to convert breast skin to abdominal wall skin and thereby raise the fold level.

If the fold is simply indistinct, fold definition can be improved by the percutaneous suture technique coupled with suction-assisted lipectomy. In this technique percutaneous sutures secure the skin of the inferior mastectomy flap to the chest wall fascia, creating a discrete inframammary fold.

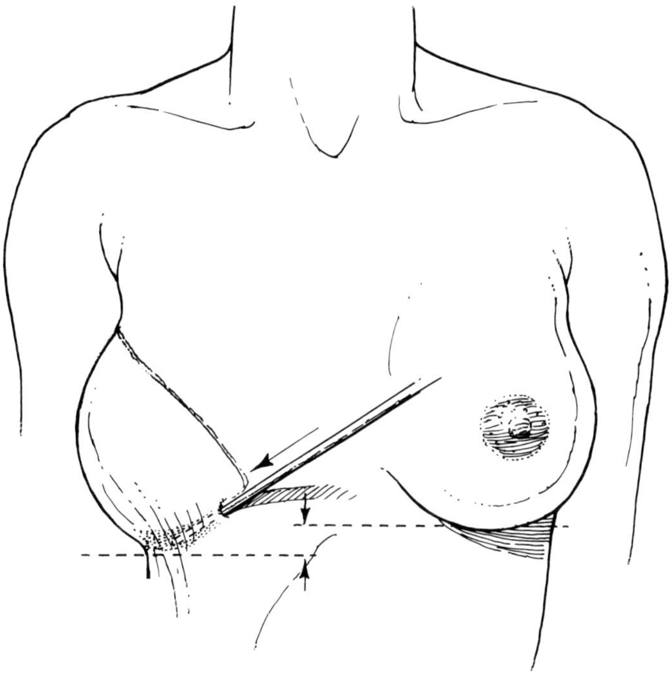

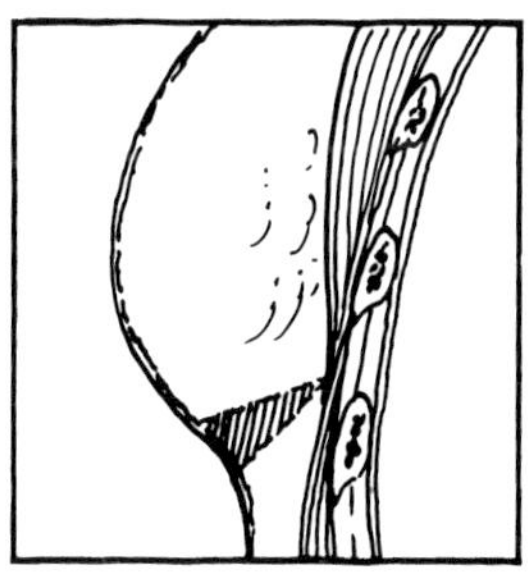

With the patient in the standing position, the inframammary fold is marked at the proper level. The area to be suctioned is also marked. At operation, several small stab wounds are made with a No. 15 blade in the marking for the new inframammary fold. Liposuction via a small cannula can be performed at this point to remove fat and thus help to further define the fold.

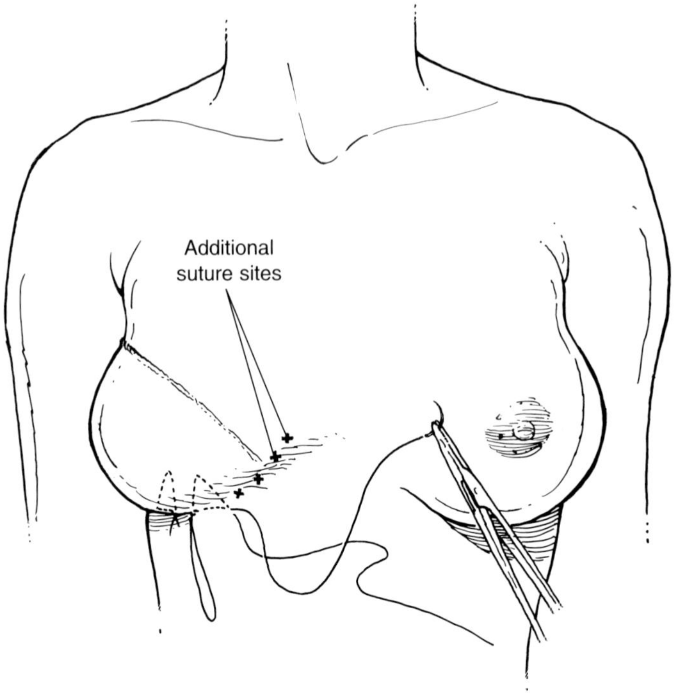

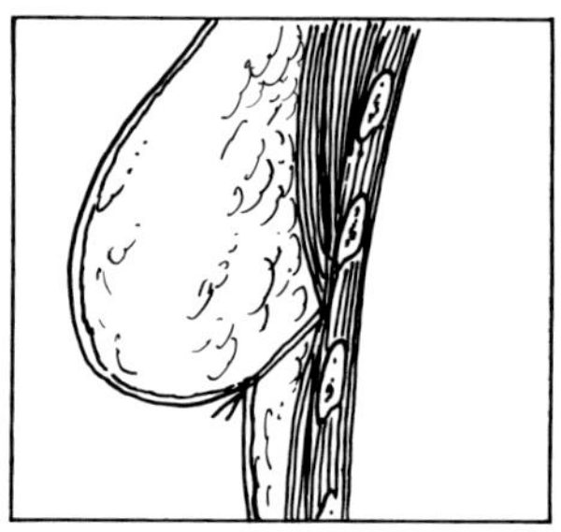

A 2-0 Prolene suture on a large needle is passed through a stab wound and then through the chest wall fascia; the needle is brought out through the adjacent stab wound. The needle is then passed back through the stab wound it just exited, catching the dermis of the mastectomy flap. The needle is then brought out through the original stab wound and the suture is tied down. The knot is dropped through the percutaneous stab wound, and a small suture is placed in the skin. A series of these sutures can be placed adjacent to one another to give much improved definition of the inframammary fold without reopening the entire fold.

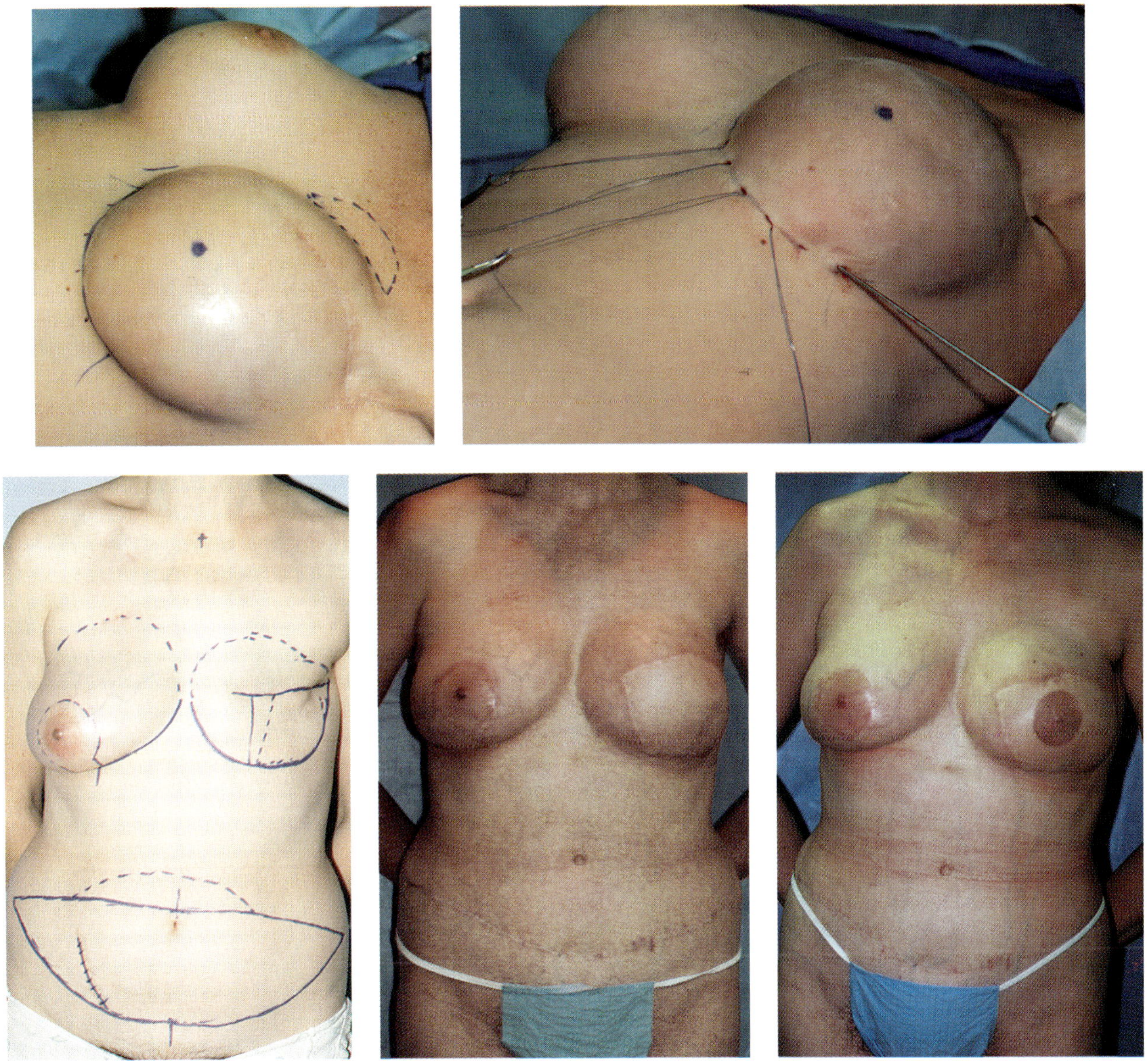

In this patient, the inframammary fold was slightly low. Improved definition of the fold was obtained via liposuction followed by the placement of percutaneous sutures. The corrugations apparent postoperatively disappear with time, but the fold improvement persists. The area marked in the upper pole was filled out with fat injection.

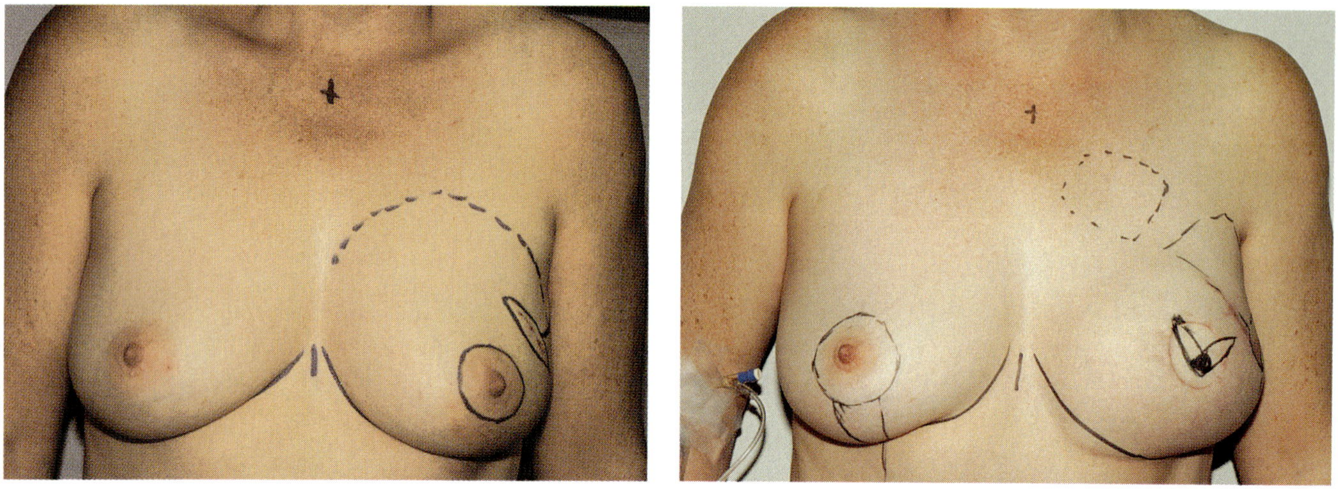

The postoperative result following immediate free TRAM flap reconstruction demonstrates asymmetry of the medial part of the inframammary fold and slight ptosis of the opposite breast. The patient desired a modest mastopexy in conjunction with the correction of the inframammary fold irregularity, nipple-areola reconstruction, and fat injections into a subtle hollow in the infraclavicular region.

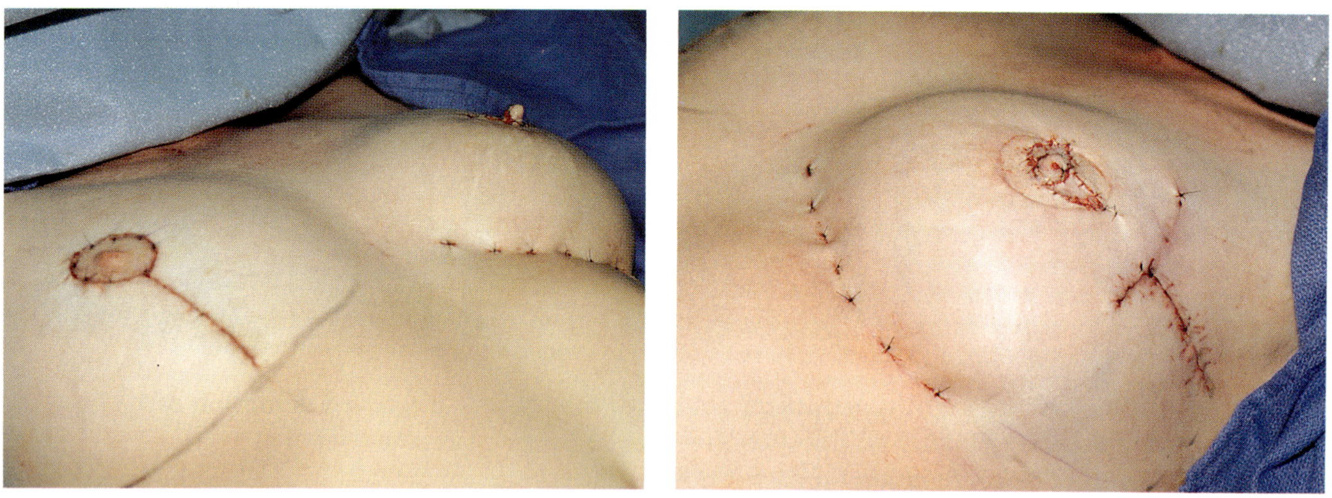

During the procedure, the inframammary fold was corrected by liposuction and the percutaneous suture technique. A correction of the lateral contour of the breast was accomplished by V-Y advancement and nipple reconstruction using the modified fish tail flap.

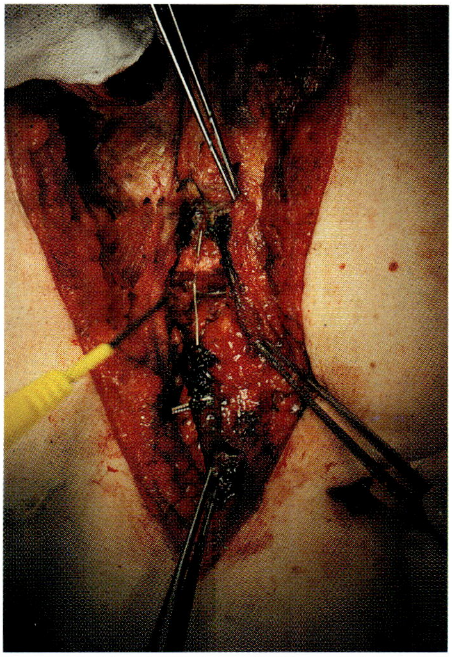
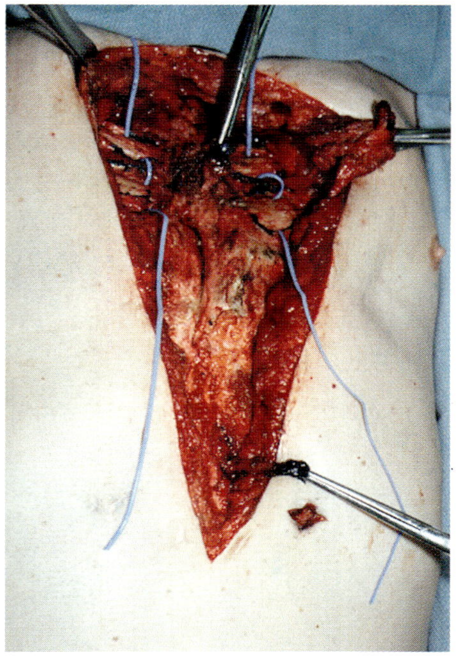

A close-up view of this inferior portion of the wound demonstrates the unroofed sinus tract and reveals a long pacing wire that had been the focus of the multiply recurrent inferior component of the infections. After this wire was fully excised, the surrounding diaphragmatic and inferior cardiac surfaces were curetted, with the contiguous xiphoid being resected as well.

Attention was then turned to the superior of the two tracts, the orifice of which had already been excised with reincision of the sternotomy scar and kept in continuity with its deeper origins. Once it became obvious that the midsternal tract extended through the old manubrial portion of the sternal split, it became necessary to remove a block of bone. If the sinus were arising from this segment of bone itself, segmental ostectomy of the manubrium would be curative. If this segment of bone were not the origin of the infection, its removal would be required for adequate exposure of any underlying extension of the tract.

To facilitate safe resection of the manubrium in the setting of multiple prior surgical debridements and dense retrosternal adhesions while still preserving the encased sinus tract, the previously unviolated adjacent second and third costal cartilages were subperichondrially resected bilaterally. Thus the manubrium could be progressively elevated in a centripetal fashion from a more peripheral, safer, and better defined area. The vessel loops are seen passing beneath the subperichondrially dissected cartilages just before segmental resection. The Kocher clamp is holding the manubrial segment to be lifted subperiosteally from the underlying heart.

Once the manubrium was resected, the body of the sternum was split cautiously with the oscillating saw. It became apparent that the tract continued relatively far posteriorly alongside the heart through unusually dense fibrous tissue. Continued attempts at following the blue-stained tract toward its origins were frustrated by an inability to define a safe plane. It could be determined, however, that the tract likely extended to the area in which troublesome bleeding had been encountered at the atrial cannulation site during the original coronary artery bypass surgery. This area had been controlled, according to the original operative note, with Teflon-pledgeted sutures. It seemed highly likely that these pledgets were the origin of the continued recurrent contamination.

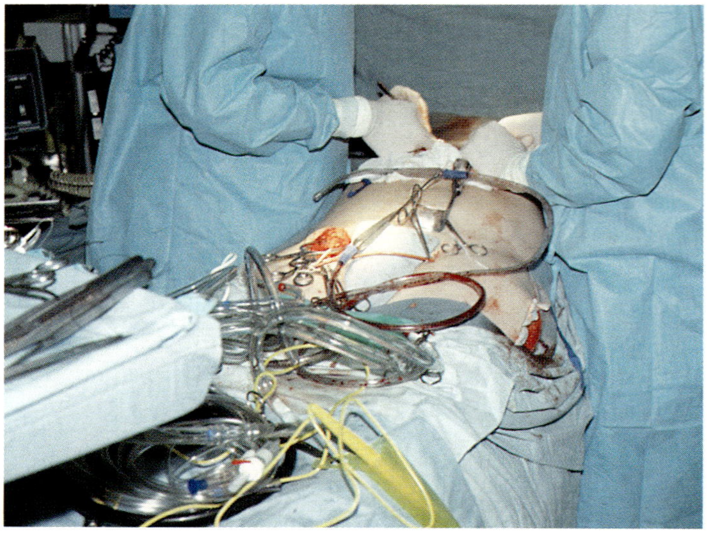

To achieve safe access to this area, it was decided that an internal counterincision would be helpful in establishing safe anatomic landmarks. Accordingly, the second right intercostal space was opened into the previously unviolated right pleural space (traditional right thoracotomy is an accepted approach for cannulating the atria and cavae) via the existing wound. This was an internal thoracotomy of sorts, which did indeed greatly improve and make safer the exposure of the area of concern in the posterior pericardial sac, although it divided the right internal mammary artery. It was also believed that, even with improved exposure, there was a significant risk of hemorrhage or possibly of the need to resect a segment of the atrium containing the offending foreign bodies. For this reason the right femoral artery (the aorta was not readily accessible due to fibrosis) and the inferior right atrium were cannulated for the contingency that rapid institution of cardiopulmonary bypass and reinfusion of shed blood would be necessary. Furthermore, a patch of left fascia lata was harvested should expeditious atrial resection and autologous patch repair be necessary.

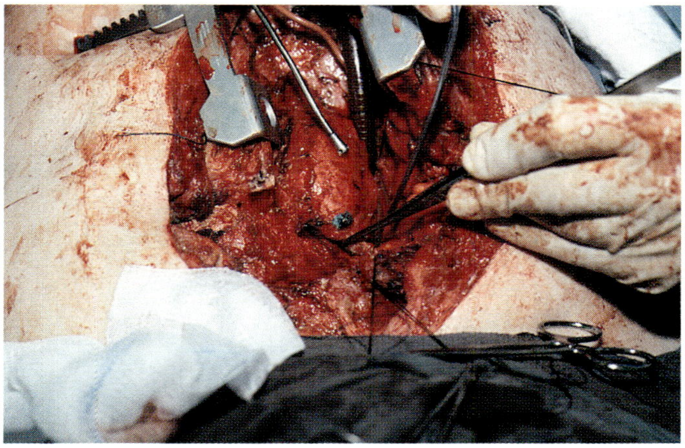

Once the cannulas were in place and the internal thoracotomy provided improved access, the blue-stained tract was followed tediously down to the area indicated by the forceps near the former atrial cannulation site. At this site numerous blue-stained Teflon pledgets with associated debris and purulent drainage were located and removed.

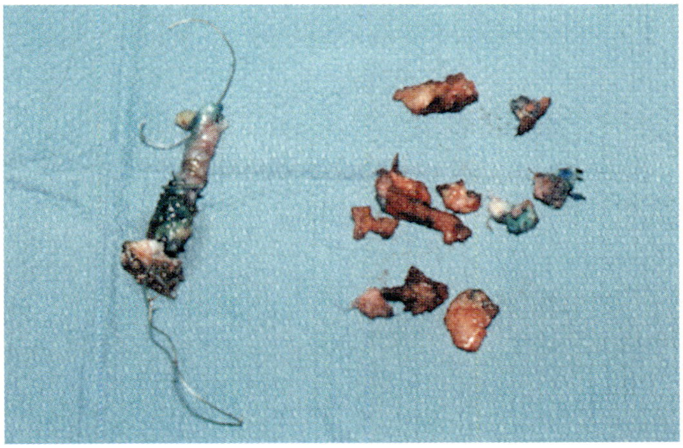

Any portion of the tract that could not be excised (i.e., that part abutting the heart) was curetted. The removed infected pledget material is demonstrated on the right, and the excised sinus tract and accompanying lengthy segment of pacing wire are on the left. The margins of the residual body of the sternum that was split were pristine and clearly uninvolved with infection. The wound was jet lavaged with dilute hypochlorite solution in preparation for closure.

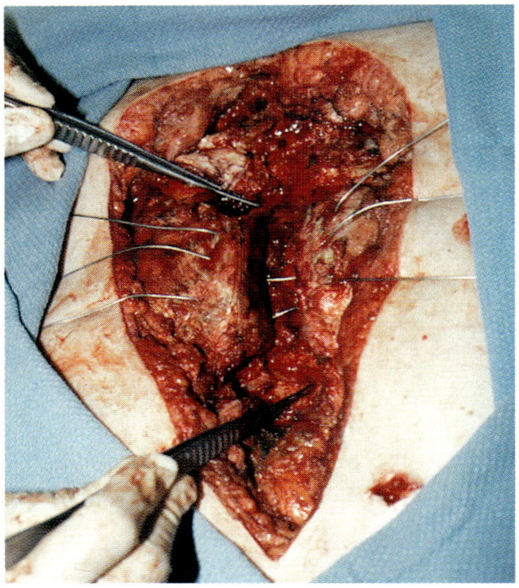

The residual sternum was reapproximated with sternal wires. Wound cavities persisted superiorly and inferiorly at the sites of the manubrial and xiphoid resections, respectively. The superior cavity was obturated by segmental elevation and readvancement of the previously advanced upper left pectoralis major muscle (upper forceps). The lower space was filled with an inferiorly based right rectus abdominis muscle transposition flap (lower forceps). The remainder of the pectoralis major flap was reapproximated in the midline as before, and advancement of the pectoral cutaneous advancement flaps completed the closure. In light of the multiply recurrent 7-year history of infection, the patient was treated with a 6-week course of parenteral, culture-specific antibiotics.

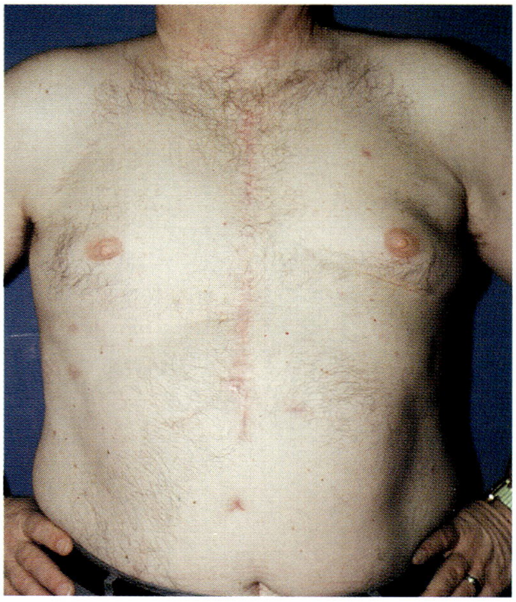

The patient is shown 6 months postoperatively. There were no short- or long-term complications.

Thus counterincisions are especially useful when foreign bodies extend deep to the bone or cartilage and give rise to a recurrent pathologic condition that must be eradicated. An example would include an internal intercostal extension or counterincision beneath an already elevated cutaneous and/or muscle flap at the site of a prior sternotomy. This allows the surgeon to alternately approach an area that must be resected at the level of the atria, ventricles, great vessels, or pulmonary hila at the site of prior procedures and resultant fibrosis. The margin of resection is extended beyond what is grossly involved to ensure cure of the persistent or recurrent problems that tend to present in this area. This resection would include all cartilage of any rib involved or that becomes exposed adjacent to the involved area or during the surgical resection. Such exposed cartilages are very susceptible to recurrent desiccation, contamination, and/or drainage. In this way the patient is more likely to be cured of the problem that led to reoperation. This philosophy of debridement also prevents exposure of cartilage or bone in the event of subsequent dehiscence or if drainage and packing of a new fluid collection become necessary.

After resectional debridement of involved and adjacent tissues, any vital organs bordering the area of resection are lightly curetted if resection is not possible. If the sinus tract or recurrent infection appears to arise from infected synthetic patches, vascular conduits, or other synthetic material, it is extremely difficult to eradicate such an infection solely with debridement and coverage unless the infected material itself is removed and replaced with the patient on cardiopulmonary bypass if necessary. As previously stated, biologic prostheses such as pericardial autografts, homografts, or heterografts tolerate such contamination or infection better than synthetic materials and usually do not need to be replaced. If the indication for the reoperation is dehiscence, inability to close the chest, or tumor as opposed to recurrent infection, such synthetic materials need not be removed.

If synthetic materials must be removed, replacement with autogenous materials is desirable. Depending on the tissues needed, small fascial or muscular fragments can be used for pledgets, whereas fascia lata or epithelialized dermal grafts can be used as a synthetic patch. Pericardium may not be available in the reoperative situation due to fibrosis. Vascular conduits are ideally replaced with homografts. If a synthetic replacement is absolutely necessary, the less porous synthetic graft materials are less likely to harbor or retain bacteria than the more porous materials.

After debridement is completed, jet lavage of the wound is performed using the water pik or a large syringe and plastic catheter with dilute hypochlorite irrigant to further reduce the wound bacterial count. At that point previously used muscle flaps can be carefully elevated, readvanced, and effectively used to augment or complete the soft tissue reconstruction.

As with primary chest wall reconstruction, pectoralis major muscles and/or rectus abdominis muscles are prime donor tissues for reconstruction of soft tissue deficits resulting from debridement. As previously mentioned, the greater omentum can be used as a new flap or a readvancement flap to help to fill a defect with vascularized tissue. The greater omentum is usually easily elevated from the mediastinal contents with fewer adhesions than would otherwise have been expected.

Another source of pedicled tissue for this site includes the latissimus dorsi muscle, as mentioned previously. Transposition of the latissimus dorsi muscle to the anterior midline usually requires division of the tendinous insertion of the latissimus dorsi muscle if not skeletonization of the pedicle to deliver adequate bulk to the arc lengths desired. It should be noted, however, that the attachment of the serratus collateral vessel to the thoracodorsal pedicle is best preserved in the case of prior axillary radiation or if there is any concern about preservation of the thoracodorsal pedicle when axillary dissection has been previously performed.

Once adequate vascularized tissue bulk has been delivered to the wound, all possible geometric combinations of flap inset are evaluated. When possible, the most hearty, dependable, and robust portion of the flap should be placed in the area that most critically needs coverage. The bony margins of resection are ideally covered by well-perfused portions of the flap by interposing these portions between the bony margins and cutaneous margins. This method of flap inset also prevents exposure of bone or cartilage if fluid collections must be drained or if small dehiscences occur.

Once the flaps are positioned as desired, sutures of absorbable material are placed in such a way to secure the flaps to stout adjacent tissue, such as periosteum, nearby muscle fascia, or occasionally fellow flaps. This inset should maintain adequate tissue bulk in the cavities created by the debridement or resection and prevent undue tension on the flaps. Before closure each tissue plane should be generously and aggressively evacuated and drained with large suction catheters exiting through distant separate stab wounds. Closed systems with controlled suction are used for connection to drains placed directly on the heart or great vessels. Otherwise drains in the submuscular or subcutaneous planes are placed directly to wall suction.

When possible, it is desirable to use cutaneous advancement flaps to complete skin closure. Possible contraindications to extensive cutaneous advancement flaps include the presence of pendulous breasts (which place undue tension on the suture line), obesity and diabetes (which can contribute to ischemia of overlying breasts), and prior surgical incisions (which must be released [e.g., with Z-plasty] or at least considered in the placement of any new incisions and evaluated in terms of possibilities for safe cutaneous flap elevation).

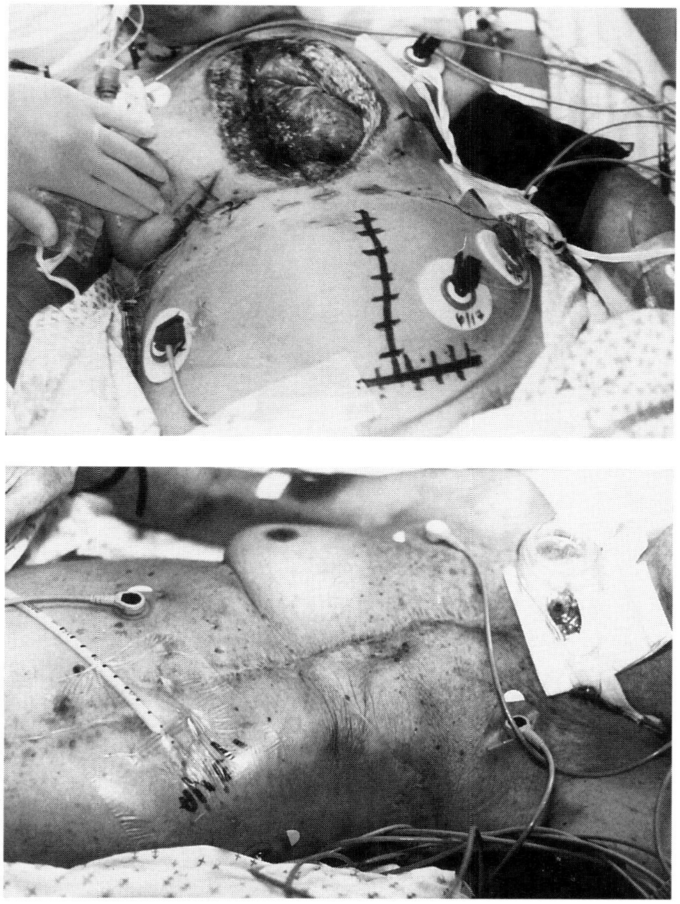

This 80-year-old woman had undergone urgent mitral valve replacement and had been reexplored for bleeding. Postoperatively mediastinitis developed, resulting in a sternal wound. She had multiple thoracic and abdominal incisions including a left mastectomy scar and a right thoracotomy scar. She underwent sternal wound reconstruction with a left rectus abdominis flap and a right pectoralis major muscle advancement flap after extensive debridement. Closure was completed with bilateral cutaneous advancement flaps. Both cutaneous advancement flaps required Z-plasty releases of the prior thoracic incisions. Four weeks postoperatively the wound was well healed; the healed wound is shown 3 months postoperatively.

Care must be taken to ensure that the wound edges do not invert and that all cutaneous surfaces are well apposed, making the closure airtight and watertight. Even a 1 or 2 mm loss of incisional integrity early in the postoperative course can lead to open communication with large subcutaneous or submuscular planes created in the dissection. Such a small breach of the closure can be a cause of persistent contamination or preclude adherence of the undersurface of flaps to the tissues beneath. Occasionally even this small technical indiscretion can result in the need to pack the entire wound open or in a significant complication or reconstructive failure. If the skin cannot be closed, alternatives include closure with musculocutaneous flaps or skin grafts.

PLEURAL SPACE PROBLEMS

The factors that predispose to recurrent fistula or empyema—inadequate debridement of the wound margins, inadequate closure of fistula, residual inflammation, malignancy, and prior radiation therapy—make reoperative reconstruction of the pleural space more challenging. In the reoperative setting flap donor units often have already been violated by the reconstructive needs in the primary reconstruction or by a prior thoracotomy, injury, illness, or radiation therapy.

Other indications for reoperation in chest wall reconstructive surgery involving the pleural space include infection or dislodgment of previously placed Prolene mesh, Prolene-methacrylate "sandwich," and rib grafts. Reoperation can also be necessitated by flap failure due to ischemia, undue tension, or poor flap design.

Empyema

Empyema is defined as a purulent collection within the pleural space. In the preantibiotic era it was a common sequela of pneumonia. The development of antibiotics, however, has rendered this disease a much less common entity. Empyema now more commonly presents as a thoracic surgical complication. Typical symptoms of pleural empyema include pleuritic chest pain, fever, tachypnea, tachycardia, decreased respiratory excursions, cough, and friction rub. These symptoms might occur, as previously mentioned, in the setting of recent surgical or percutaneous violation of the pleural space; bacterial, fungal, or tuberculous pneumonic process; or endobronchial tumor or aspirated foreign body. Radiographs of the chest usually demonstrate a pleural effusion or opacification, sometimes superimposed on a pulmonic infiltrate.

Early intervention consisting of evacuation of the offending fluid and antibiotic treatment achieves lung expansion before fibrosis fixes and permanently restricts lung expansion. The morbidity of empyema is greatly increased when such a fixed cavity is established. These cavities sometimes may "point," eroding the subcutaneous tissues and draining spontaneously (empyema necessitatis). An erosive process may extend centrally into the bronchial tree, giving rise to a bronchopleural fistula with increased production of foul sputum and possibly an air fluid level visible on x-ray film.

It is critical not to mistake a pulmonary abscess for empyema since the former is an intrapulmonary lesion and its treatment differs from that of empyema or bronchopleural fistula. Chronic empyema typically occurs approximately 6 weeks after the offending process begins and results in a fibrinous exudate or peel that restricts simple reinflation or expansion of the lung that could otherwise be achieved with thoracentesis or dependent tube thoracostomy. In the chronic phase the fixed lung and the abscess cavity require open drainage, often with rib resection, chronic drain placement, and irrigation.

At times, well-drained empyema may gradually and spontaneously diminish in size and proceed to ultimate healing. Large empyema cavity size, residual malignancy, large persistent air leak (bronchial fistula), prior radiation therapy, inadequate dependent drainage, ongoing contamination, and persistent malignancy hinder successful spontaneous healing of such cavities. In these situations the cavity margins become increasingly fibrotic and unyielding with a poor blood supply, which results in prolonged unsuccessful courses of tube drainage or dressing changes.

Fistula

Fistulous tracts between the tracheobronchial tree and the pleural space (bronchopleural fistula), skin (bronchocutaneous or pleurocutaneous fistula), or other adjacent structures (e.g., bronchobiliary) may develop as a result of not only aspiration pneumonia or surgical or nonsurgical empyema but also bacterial infection of a pulmonary infarct or traumatic or iatrogenic invasions of the pleural space. These entities include transbronchial lung biopsy or pleural biopsy, errant thoracentesis or thoracostomy tube insertion, and inadequate bronchial closure or healing following pulmonary resection. The risk factors for poor bronchial stump healing include preoperative radiation therapy, residual bronchitis or carcinoma at the site of the bronchial stump closure, or inadequate tissue for bronchial stump closure.

Surgical closure of the fistulae is important for repair unless the air leak merely results from multiple small peripheral air leaks in a poorly drained cavity, which often will respond to improved pleural drainage. Otherwise the fistulae must be closed with thorough debridement or resection of abnormal tissue, meticulous dissection of the fistula tract, and elimination of the related cavity.

When the surgeon prepares to perform a thoracic reoperation for treatment of empyema or bronchopleural fistula, the treatment options include a combination of resection and collapse of the chest wall with closure of any bronchial leak (by alternate exposure if necessary) and obturation of the wound with as much vascularized tissue as possible. Thus the size, geometric shape, and location of the cavity as well as the reconstructive units still available help to determine which combination of options is chosen for such treatment.

Thoracoplasty obliterates empyema cavities by collapsing the chest wall into the cavity. Decortication or empyemectomy allows expansion of the restricted lung. The cavity can also be obturated with well-vascularized tissue or flaps. Thoracoplasty, although effective in some cases, has the disadvantage of producing a severe deformity and fails to recruit as well-vascularized tissues to the cavity walls, particularly when they have been previously damaged by radiation therapy. Thoracoplasty, however, is quite useful as an adjunct to muscle flap reconstruction in that it helps to achieve adequate exposure for reexploration, resectional debridement, fistula repair, flap tunneling, flap access and inset, and modest cavity size reduction.

Empyemectomy or decortication is tedious to perform and can result in significant blood loss and multiple iatrogenic peripheral pulmonary air leaks. It does, however, reduce contamination and allow lung expansion. In this way it is a valuable adjunct to the obliteration of empyema cavities. Instillation of broad-spectrum antibiotic solutions into such cavities (e.g., Clagett procedure) has shortcomings in that it cannot neutralize unreasonable levels of bacterial contamination or achieve what aggressive resectional debridement and vascularized tissue reconstruction can provide. It can be an adjunctive maneuver, however, in the staged closure of large bronchopleural fistulae or empyema cavities. In cases in which there is a profound mismatch between cavity size and tissue available for reconstruction, a second-stage closure of the large cavity can be achieved once fistula closure is accomplished.

The preoperative analysis of the particular problem or problems culpable for the recurrent or persistent disease process will also determine the extent to which each of these issues must be addressed. In cases of reoperation for chest wall malignancy, an assessment of the extent of disease and the palliative vs. curative nature of the operation will determine the degree of aggressiveness that will characterize the proposed operation.

In addition to surgical options reviewed before the planned procedure, thought must be given to options for adjuvant treatments that are available such as external beam or interstitial seed radiation therapy. Another consideration that may need to be addressed, especially in instances of multiple reoperation and/or radiation therapy for recurrent or persistent malignancy, is whether to replace or bypass involved or threatened vascular structures.

Flaps available for reconstruction of defects in this region typically include the pectoralis major, latissimus dorsi, serratus anterior, trapezius, rectus abdominis, external oblique, greater omentum, and free flaps. In reoperative cases, of course, one or more of these units, in whole or in part, typically will have been rendered unusable.

In cases in which the extent of the defect resulting from the resection exceeds the ability of available tissues to readily fill it, reconstruction with microvascular free flaps or a combination of newer flap techniques and older techniques such as thoracoplasty or staged closure over instilled antibiotic solution can be helpful.

Preoperative Preparation

The anesthesiologist must have a working knowledge of a number of relevant techniques in addition to the usual general anesthetic and perioperative critical care. A familiarity with the use of differential lung ventilation, double-lumen endotracheal tubes, and high-frequency ventilation is necessary.

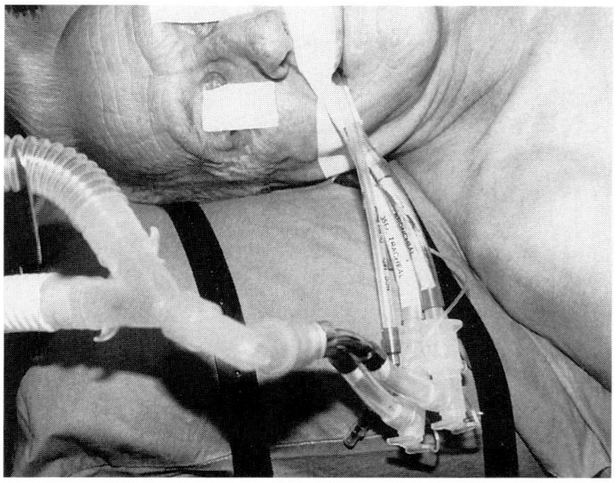

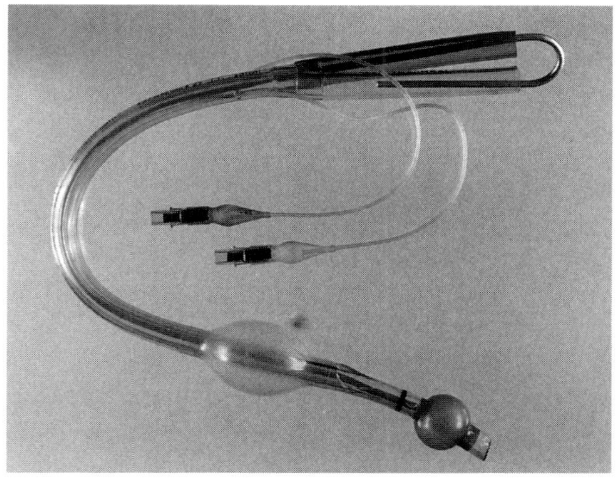

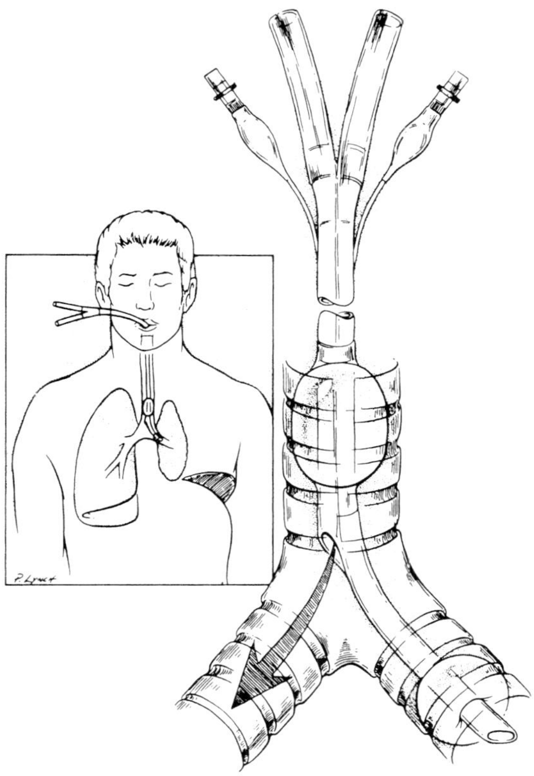

The double-lumen endotracheal tube is invaluable for differential lung ventilation. With this device exposure can be maximized by single-lung ventilation while an operative intervention is proceeding within the contralateral pleural space. Furthermore, intraoperative air leaks and cross tracheal bacterial contamination of the lungs can be minimized in this manner. Postoperatively, differential lung ventilation may be maintained with this tube as well.

Photographs and illustration from Stahl RS, Sando WC. Reconstruction of defects of thorax and spine. In Jurkiewicz MJ, Krizek TJ, Mathes ST, Ariyan S, eds. Plastic Surgery: Principles and Practice. St. Louis: Mosby, 1990.

This modality is employed when it is desired to prevent contamination by the spillage of secretions from the abnormal to the normal lung or to differentially deflate the involved lung to achieve improved exposure. Furthermore, the high-frequency ventilation can help to maintain adequate ventilation and at the same time minimize the escape of air through the problematic bronchial fistula or bronchial closure.

Epidural catheter placement for postoperative analgesic administration helps to minimize postoperative pain and splinting, thus preventing postoperative pulmonary complications. At times the assistance of the perfusion team may be needed to make partial or total cardiopulmonary bypass available or to reinfuse shed blood in select difficult cases. Reinfusion of shed blood is to be avoided in a contaminated wound. Thus this technique is problematic in cases of empyema and bronchopleural reconstruction.

Patient positioning is critical to trouble-free reconstructive sequence. Access to all necessary reaches of the thorax must be ensured for resection, debridement, flap elevation, and inset. Use of the beanbag is invaluable to satisfactory positioning when lateral decubitus positions are required intraoperatively. In some operations it may be necessary to prepare for the possibility that multiple positions may be required at the same operative setting. In these cases appropriate cleansing of the patient, draping, and positioning must be performed to allow for intraoperative changes in position with a minimum of encumbrances or disruptions to the procedure.

Achieving this end requires that the anesthesiologist avoid placing intravenous or arterial lines or other monitoring devices at sites that may need to be used during the procedure. It is preferred to prepare and expose entire extremities, which thus allows for monitoring of hand perfusion when the subclavian-axillary axis is involved, availability of vein graft donor sites if vascular reconstruction is a possibility, and harvesting of skin grafts when necessary. In addition, the groin is left exposed and femoral pulses are verified to prepare for the contingency that partial femoral bypass may need to be implemented.

When combinations of anterior, lateral, and/or posterior trunk exposure are necessary, it is most helpful to prepare the areas that may be required during the secondary portions of the procedure, secure the drapes with staples or skin sutures, and then turn the patient to the position that will be needed for the initiation of the procedure. This preparation can be performed completely with the patient on the beanbag so that turning of the patient can be accomplished intraoperatively with a minimum of disruption or redraping. Care should be taken, of course, to secure the endotracheal tube—if necessary, to a tooth—and suture sterile cardiogram leads into place as well as the other lines so that they will be maintained during the position change.

In certain reoperative or complex operative procedures it may be necessary to have virtually the *entire* thorax exposed at one time or another during the procedure. In these cases it is feasible to prepare the patient circumferentially while awake and standing before the administration of the anesthetic. The patient then reclines on a sterile sheet, beneath which a second impervious sheet has been placed. Next another sterile sheet is placed over the patient, and towel clips are used to secure the cuffs of the two sheets to each other at the neck for the induction of anesthesia. The patient is then uncovered, with the superficial sheet being folded up to the anesthesiologist.

Transvenous (i.e., jugular) catheters can be placed above the cuffed drapes at this time. Sterile arterial lines can be inserted aseptically after preparation and draping. Also, a groin cloth is secured with sutures or clips. Any extremities that may not require exposure during the operation and whose draping will not encumber the turning of the patient or intraoperative exposure can then be draped out of the field with appropriate cuffed sheets or stockinettes.

Technique

At this point, with provisions for comprehensive exposure and monitoring executed, the necessary antibiotics are administered and the operation is commenced. In tumor cases the desired margin of resection is outlined and circumscribed with a margin of 4 to 6 cm in the soft tissue and one to two ribs and interspaces beneath.

It is particularly useful to enter the underlying pleural space—if it is not obliterated by adhesions in the setting of prior operations—early in the resection to assess the underlying anatomy, pulmonary adhesions, or intrapleural or parenchymal spread of tumor. The surgeon's bidigital or bimanual examination can thus also facilitate an expeditious, effective, and safe extirpation by "cutting down" toward the underlying hand at each margin. At this point any central resectional adhesions or tumor involvement can be evaluated, and if necessary, pulmonary resection can be performed with improved exposure in an en bloc fashion.

Often in reoperations in this setting, adhesions to underlying lung or neurovascular structures necessitate careful dissection to and exposure of those structures at the peripheral margin of resection, with the subsequent painstaking separation of the underlying vital structures from the overlying tumor. When it seems evident that the tumor invades the underlying structures, vascular resection with bypass or placement of interstitial radioactive seeds may be indicated. It is next advisable to examine the specimen personally with the pathologist so that the complex three-dimensional anatomy and orientation can be maintained and appropriate frozen section studies can be obtained to further assess the diagnosis and adequacy of resection.

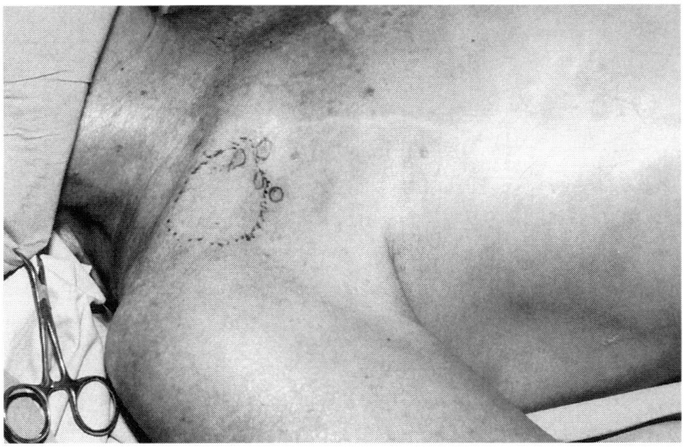

Twenty-five years earlier this 71-year-old woman underwent radical mastectomy for carcinoma of the breast. She was without evidence of disease until an infraclavicular local recurrence was excised locally 2 years before referral. External beam radiation therapy to the entire mastectomy site including the clavicular region was administered.

For 2 months she had noticed a new 2.5 cm area of dense nodularity adherent to the clavicle. There were also found to be multiple 2 to 3 mm superficial nodules overlying this area. There was no evidence of other local, regional, or systemic disease. Vascular examination of both upper extremities was normal. The ipsilateral latissimus dorsi muscle was innervated. Other than the clavicular mass, a CT scan of the chest and arteriogram were unremarkable; the thoracodorsal artery was patent.

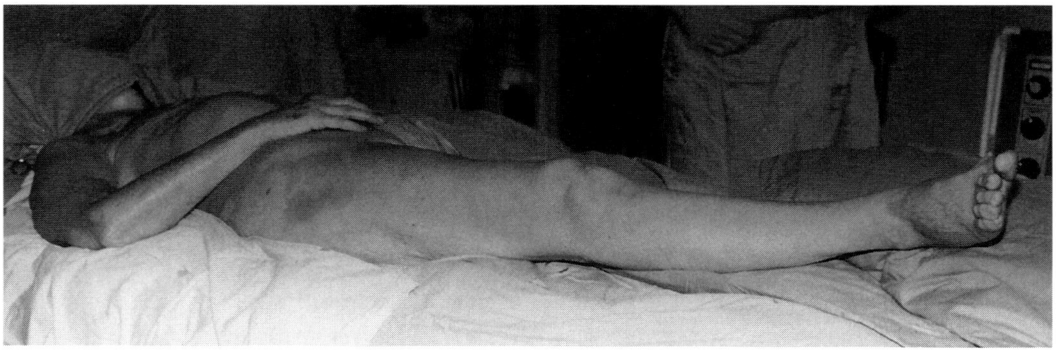

At operation the patient was placed on the beanbag and the chest, abdomen, back, and the upper and lower extremities were prepared. The drapes were stapled to the posterior midline of the trunk. In this manner the area of resection; latissimus dorsi, rectus abdominis, and omental flap donor sites; and skin and vein graft donor sites were all readily available without redraping. Furthermore, the right arm and axilla availability allowed for ongoing intraoperative vascular examination or upper extremity bypass contingencies.

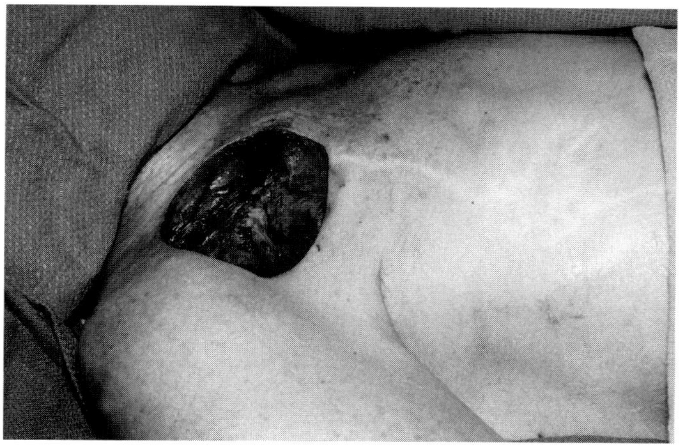

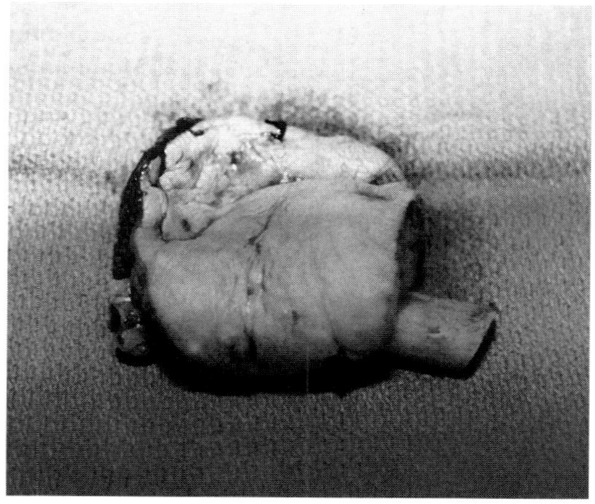

She was treated with wide resection of the recurrent breast carcinoma with claviculectomy and a difficult dissection of the subclavian vessels. The frozen section margins at the subclavian vessels were positive for tumor. Because of the dense radiation fibrosis, the vessels were not excised. Instead, iodine 125–radioactive seeds were implanted on the areas of positive margins.

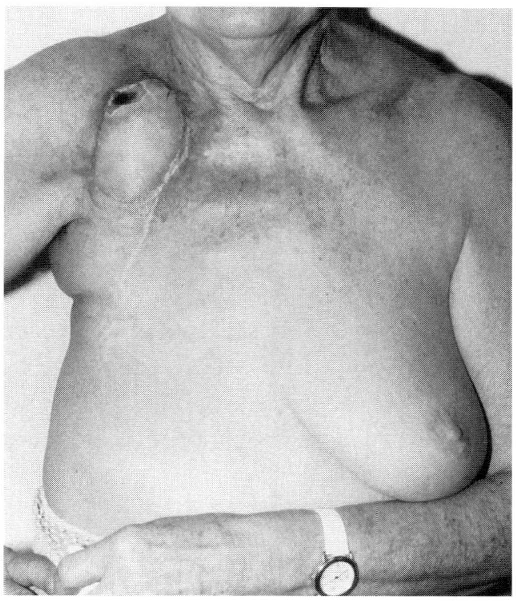

The wound was then reconstructed with a right latissimus dorsi musculocutaneous flap, preserving the serratus collateral vessels. Despite interval escharification of the distal tip of the skin island in the setting of prior and ongoing radiation, the wound healed well. The patient is doing well without clinical evidence of disease 3 years later.

When possible, prior incisions should be used, specifically thoracotomy incisions, to unroof the musculoskeletal structures overlying the empyema cavity. A central bony-cartilaginous window is made into the underlying defect, and an assessment is made of the extent of the cavity and the number and extent of rib resections that must be performed.

It is crucial to adequately expose the cavity just to and slightly beyond its margins by adequately removing the overlying ribs. This maneuver allows adequate exposure of the cavity for debridement and repair of any contamination, debris, or fistulae that may be present. Furthermore it exposes the cavity adequately enough to facilitate comfortable flap inset and to completely obturate the defect with vascularized tissue and prevent the persistence of potential spaces beneath the bony margins of the wound.

This resection of bone and cartilage and unroofing of the defect is performed in a rib-by-rib piecemeal fashion with subperiosteal and subperichondrial dissections, preserving the periosteal and intercostal flaps above and below the old thoracotomy site. Likewise, the sites of prior division of the latissimus dorsi, serratus anterior, and the pectoralis major muscles from prior thoracotomies are preferentially reincised to preserve any remaining bulk of these muscles' remnants for possible reconstructive use as they are elevated for the debridement or resection.

Any exposed rib or clavicular margins, especially when they are cartilaginous, are debrided beyond the wound margin so that they are adequately covered by surrounding soft tissue because they are particularly prone to desiccation, smoldering contamination, or radionecrosis. Any underlying granulations are curetted when they lie on vital organs, but the more peripheral wound surfaces are definitively resected back to normal tissue to reduce contamination and to achieve better potential for healing.

To successfully close any thoracic wound, the issue of bronchial fistula or peripheral air leaks must be definitively addressed. Otherwise, fistula, infection, subcutaneous emphysema, and/or recurrent wound will usually occur. Severe obstructive pulmonary disease will also predispose to recurrence of peripheral air leaks.

Fistulae of the large airways will seldom heal without definitive dissection and repair. Aside from inadequate primary technical closure of the airway, common causes include persistent inflammation or infection at the bronchial margin, residual tumor, and residual foreign body, especially in the presence of contamination. These problems must be ruled out at the time of closure.

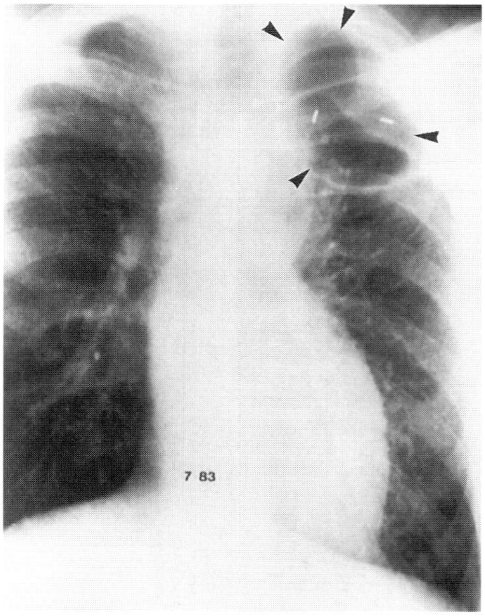

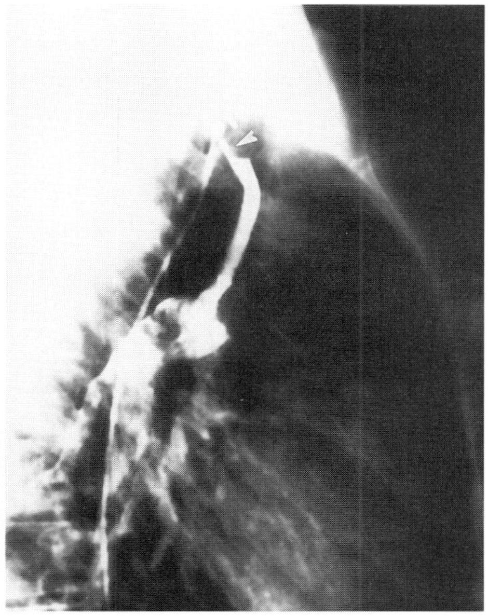

The 20-year-old man whose x-ray film is shown above had undergone multiple procedures since birth for tricuspid atresia. The most recent operation had been a Blalock-Taussig (left subclavian to pulmonary artery) shunt with Gore-Tex at the age of 15 years. He was left with an initially asymptomatic left apical pleural cavity measuring approximately 10 × 8 cm on chest x-ray film since the time of this procedure, which had been performed by another cardiac surgeon. The operative note of the last procedure reported that there had been numerous bloody adhesions and multiple air leaks encountered in the then difficult reoperative thoracotomy.

Although asymptomatic for a number of years, he had been more recently experiencing an increasingly severe chronic cough with occasional episodes of hemoptysis and coughing up of surgical hemoclips. Radiographically the cavity had diminished in size slightly during the past 1 to 2 years. Based on these clinical and more recent radiographic findings (an associated air bronchogram), the diagnosis was considered to be a chronic bronchopleural fistula.

The prior operations had been performed through a right anterior thoracotomy extending to the midsternum. This approach violated the right pectoralis major muscle and the right internal mammary artery. He also had previously undergone two procedures via a posterolateral thoracotomy on the left that violated the latissimus dorsi and serratus anterior muscles. A preoperative angiogram (right) revealed partial proximal occlusion of the Gore-Tex subclavian–pulmonary artery bypass graft.

It was decided to explore the left apical pleural cavity and attempt to debride and reconstruct it with vascularized tissue. At operation the left apical pleural cavity was exposed through the previous posterolateral thoracotomy. There was dense adhesion formation, and the dissection required to expose the cavity was quite difficult, with continuous bleeding from multiple chest wall collateral vessels and multiple small peripheral air leaks from the pulmonary dissection.

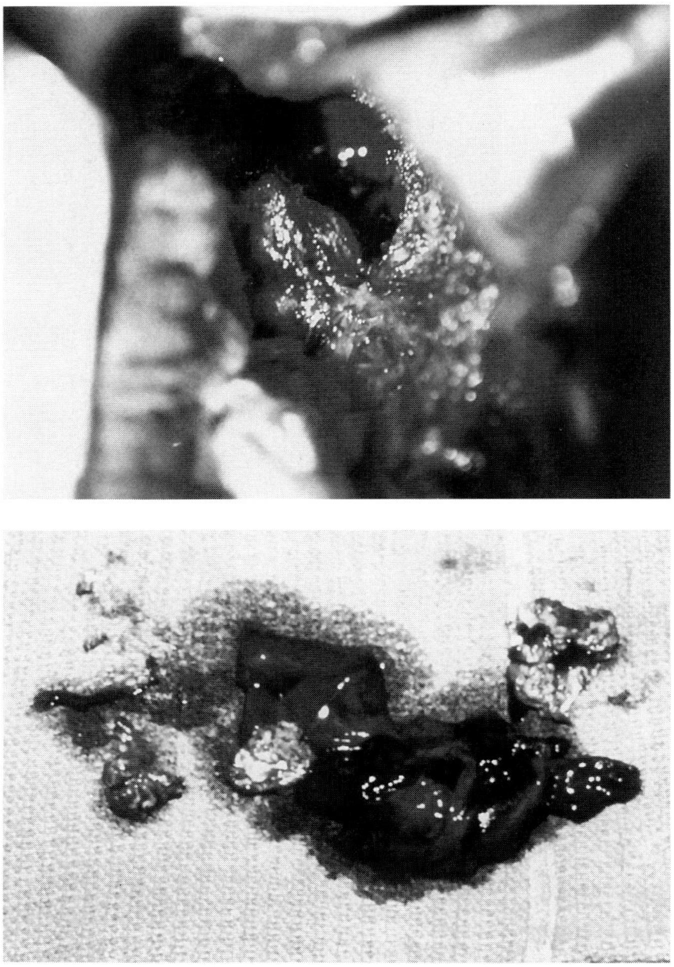

Once the distant apical cavity was exposed, a fungus ball (bottom) was encountered that ultimately cultured *Aspergillus.* A small segment of the Gore-Tex Blalock-Taussig shunt was visualized at the medial margin of the cavity; however, it was feared that the patient's marginal pulmonary function would not tolerate the removal of the graft. Furthermore, it was also thought that gaining access to the entire length of the graft as well as the proximal and distal anastomoses would have a high likelihood of resulting in exsanguinating hemorrhage or at least result in a pneumonectomy.

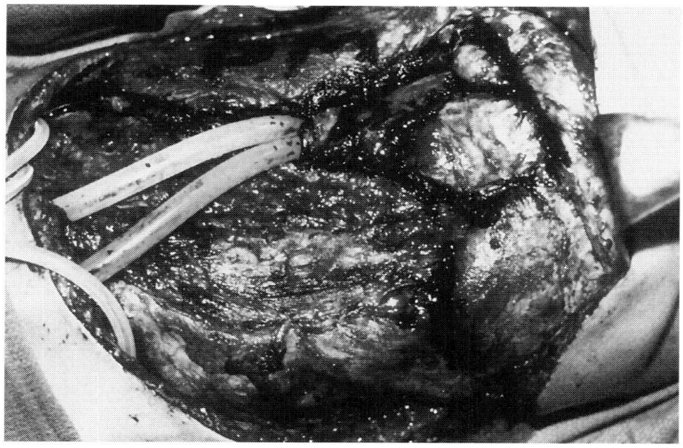

This cavity was debrided extensively and jet lavaged. Many small broncho-pleural fistulae within the cavity and in the area of dissection of the lung were closed with small absorbable sutures and in some cases with small pledgets of autogenous tissue. The cavity was well obturated with the serratus anterior and the latissimus dorsi remnants. These tissues were secured around large chest tubes, which were placed on the areas of air leak that could not be effectively sutured.

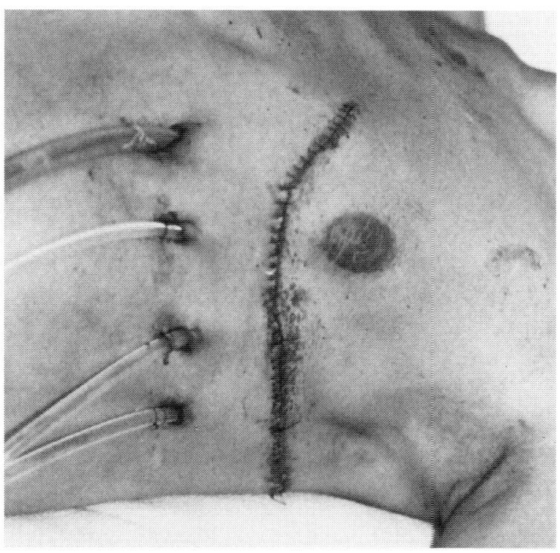

The cutaneous flap that had been elevated for access was closed over the inset muscles with subcutaneous suction catheters in place to complete the closure. The wound went on to heal externally with obliteration of the cavity. Not surprisingly, the air leak did persist, requiring maintenance of one of the chest tubes in place within the subtotally obliterated cavity. Approximately 7 weeks postoperatively the patient suffered a fatal episode of hemoptysis.

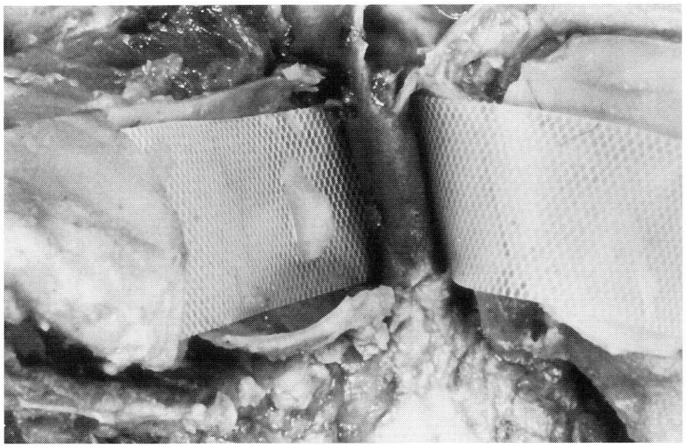

At postmortem examination the cavity itself was well obliterated. It was found that the hemoptysis resulted from a ruptured, previously unappreciated false aneurysm at the subclavian–Gore-Tex anastomosis. This anastomosis had been wrapped with a Silastic sheet at the time of the previous operation, resulting in even more foreign body material present than appreciated and further isolating the vascular prosthesis from inspection, debridement or removal, and from the muscle flaps used to fill the cavity. Successful healing of this contaminated wound and vascular prosthesis was unlikely without the removal of all foreign material and probably would have resulted in a pneumonectomy.

▪ ▪ ▪

Dissection of the airway through the wound in the pleural space should proceed until enough of a bronchial stump margin is available for repair. In reoperative and/or irradiated cases the safe but definitive dissection of stump margins adequate for repair can be challenging given the close proximity of vital organs usually encased in a block of fibrotic scar. One alternative to dissecting the mainstream bronchus in such cases is the transpericardial ligation of the bronchus through a midline sternotomy counterincision.

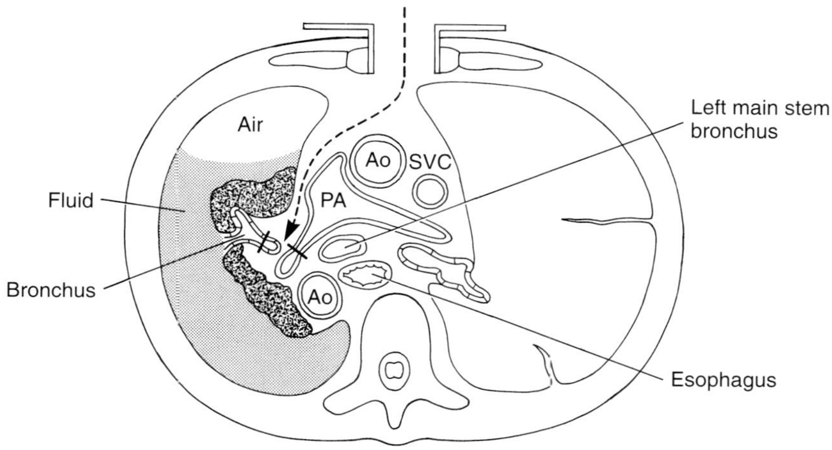

Adequate closure of a bronchopleural fistula can be difficult and dangerous in reoperative cases given the intense fibrosis that surrounds the air leak at the pulmonary hilum. Ideally the airway can be adequately dissected to allow a sufficient margin for delayed primary repair, flap repair, or a combination thereof. In select cases, especially chronic ones or those in which reoperation is indicated, control of the bronchial leak can be more safely achieved via median sternotomy and a transpericardial approach. The dissection proceeds lateral to the aorta and pulmonary artery in the pericardial space without the hindrance of the hilar and perihilar fibrotic tissue, which would impede visualization.

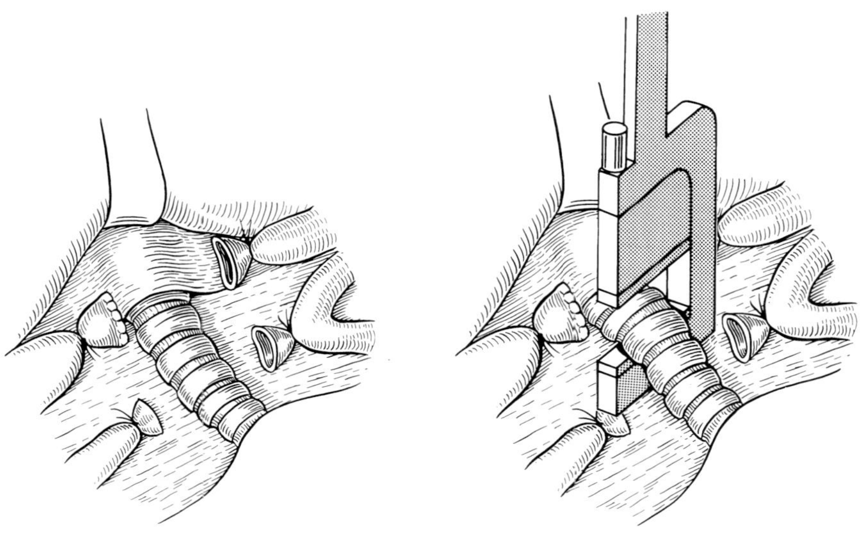

The pulmonary vessels are first ligated, and the bronchial stump is isolated for stapling central to the original bronchial suture line. Ideally the distal stump is resected to eliminate this site as a possible source of future collections or infection. Furthermore, the stump can be sent for histopathologic examination since one cause of persistent or recurrent bronchial fistula is residual tumor at the suture line.

Peripheral air leaks occurring in the reoperative setting, with the implied increased degrees of contamination, prior radiation therapy, and obstructive disease, have a high risk of not sealing or healing. If the tissues are in reasonable condition, primary suture with fine, absorbable material on a tapered, noncutting needle, with the suture carefully tied, can secure most minor leaks. When this method is impractical, pledgeted absorbable sutures with bits of autogenous pledget material such as muscle or fascia can be used to help to secure these small areas of air leak.

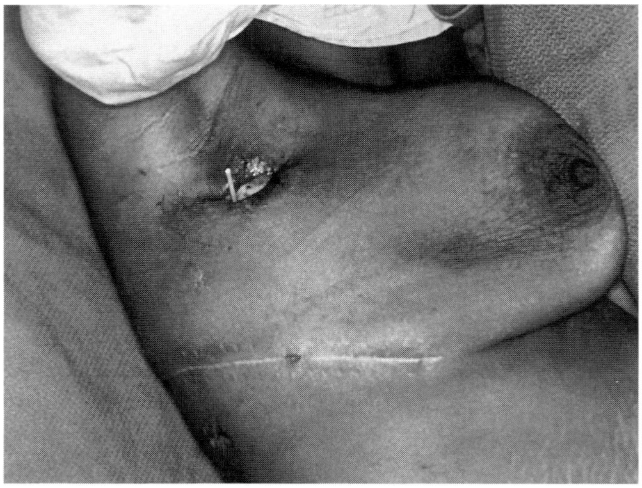

This alternative approach was taken with this patient who had a postlobectomy bronchopleural fistula refractory to local care. A cotton-tipped applicator had been placed in the wound.

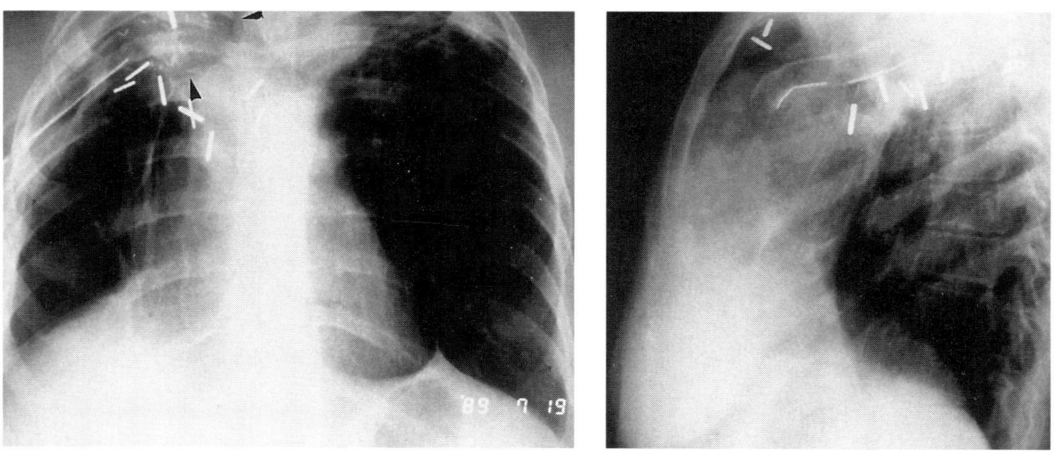

Posteroanterior and lateral chest x-ray films show the superior location of the associated cavity with the indwelling tube and surrounding hemoclips.

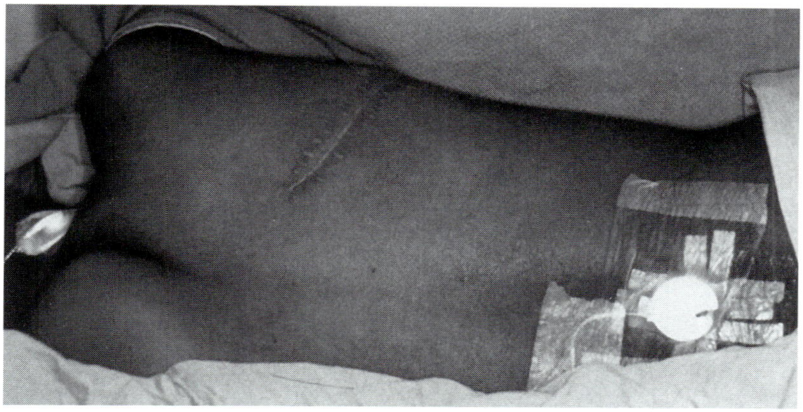

The patient was positioned in the lateral decubitus position on a beanbag device with the right arm prepared in the operative field. Before initiation of the operative procedure, an indwelling epidural catheter was placed for perioperative-intraoperative administration of narcotics. Narcotic administration minimizes the depth of anesthesia required for the operation, and the catheter may be left in place for postoperative delivery of narcotics to minimize splinting and associated pulmonary complications.

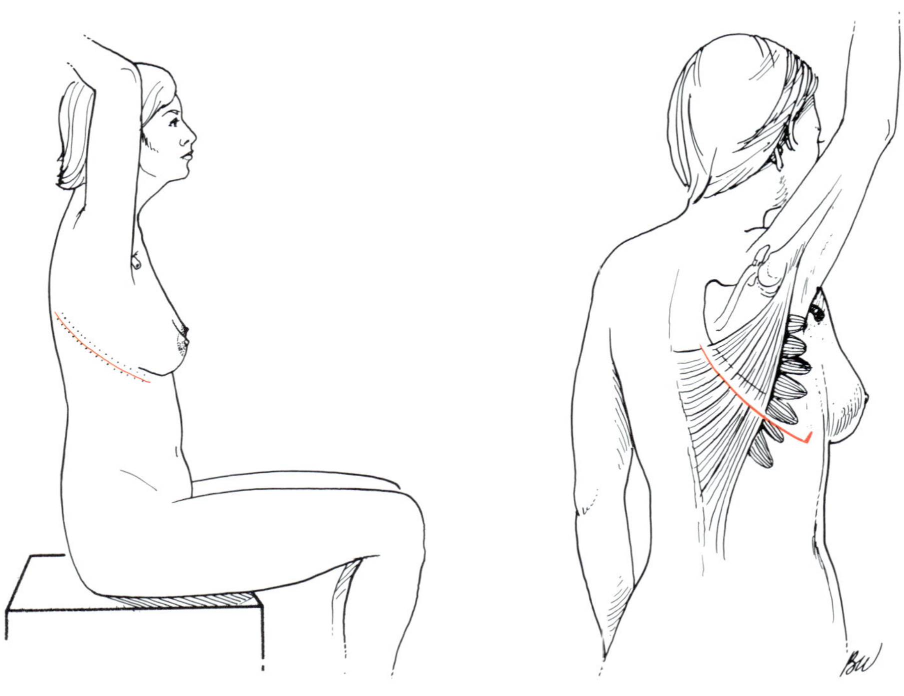

The locations of the posterolateral thoracotomy incision and empyema-fistula tube are illustrated. The former incision was used with a superoanterior extension, and a counterincision was used around the fistula site. The cutaneous flap was fully elevated to the axilla.

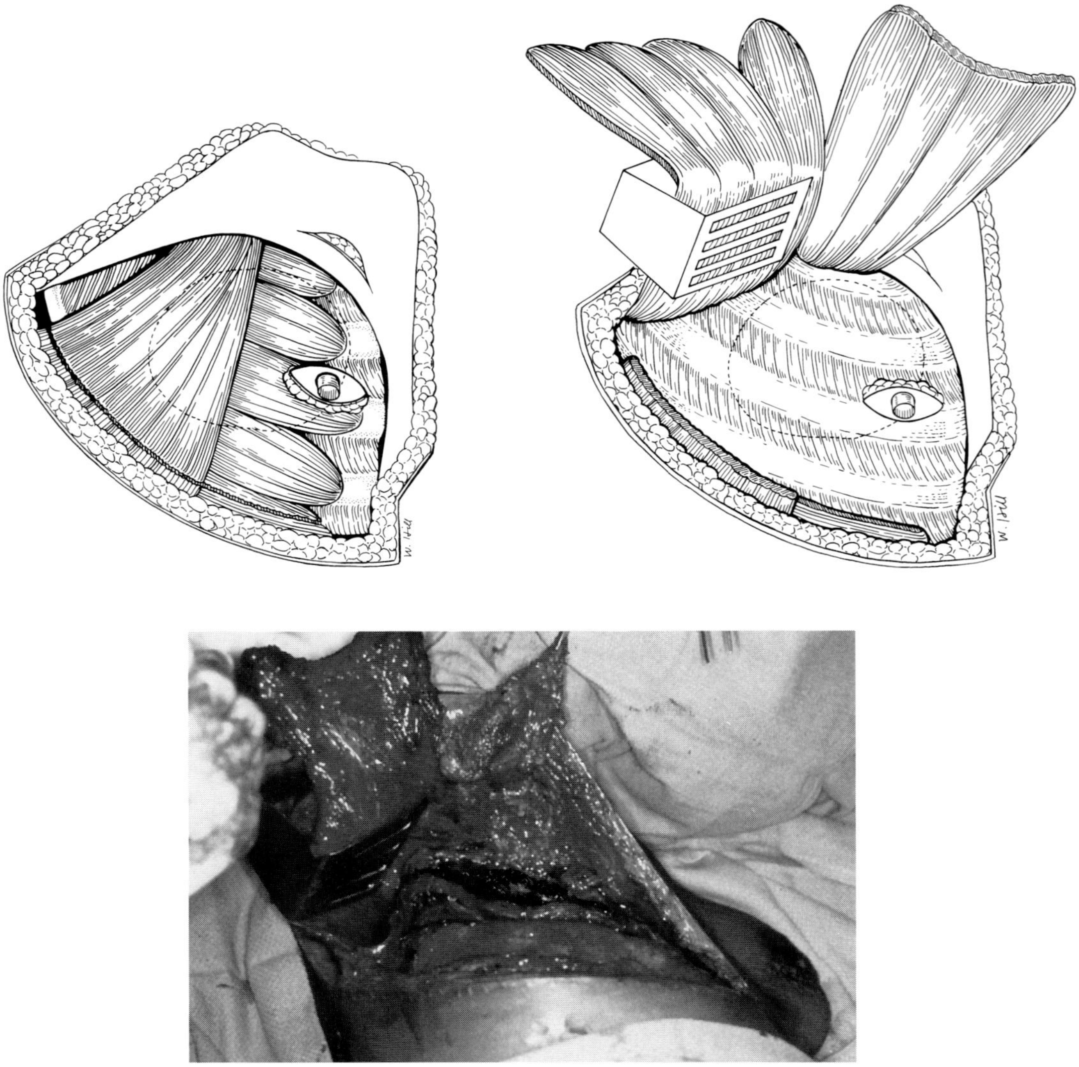

On the top left, the underlying, previously divided latissimus dorsi and serratus anterior muscles are visualized. The cutaneous flap has been elevated. Note the fistula counterincision and excision site. The previously divided and repaired latissimus dorsi and serratus anterior muscles are seen with the extent of the underlying cavity indicated by the dotted line. As a prelude to exposure of the underlying cavity, the latissimus dorsi and serratus anterior remnants are elevated and preserved for later use (top right). Again, the underlying cavity is demarcated with the dotted line. The latissimus dorsi and serratus anterior flaps have been elevated. The scapula is held with the scapular retractor. The site of the fistula is outlined in methylene blue (bottom).

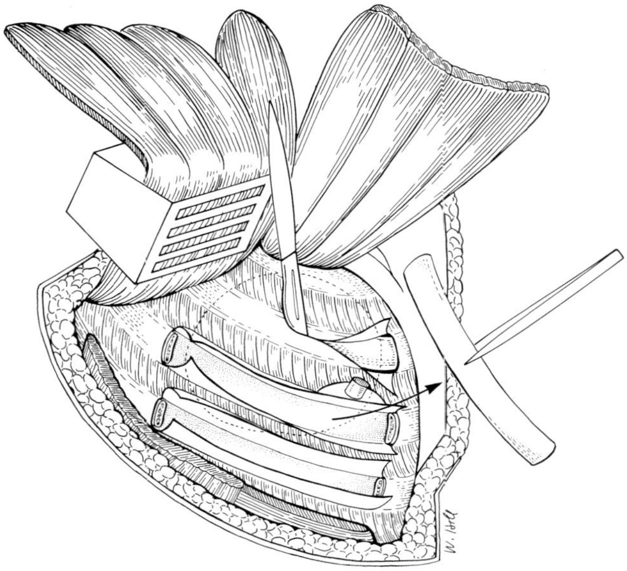

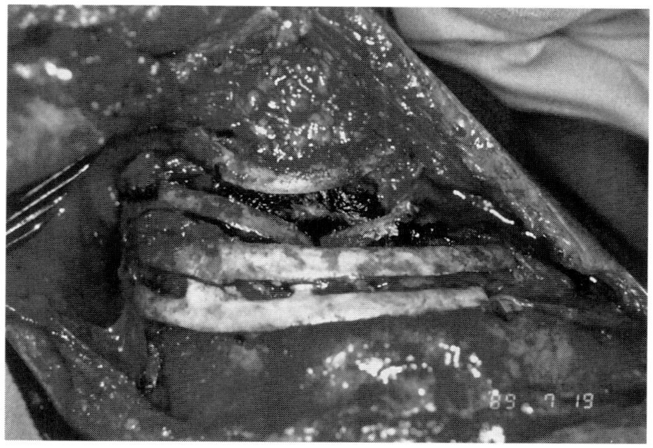

The overlying rib segments were subperiosteally resected, preserving both the superior and inferior intercostal flaps that may be used to buttress the repair. The subperiosteally resected rib segments are visualized in situ. The second visualized rib fractured at the fistula site and resultant segments are seen protruding into the fistula cavity.

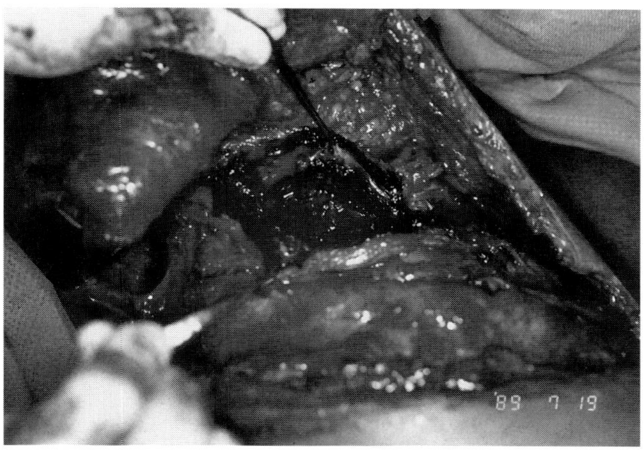

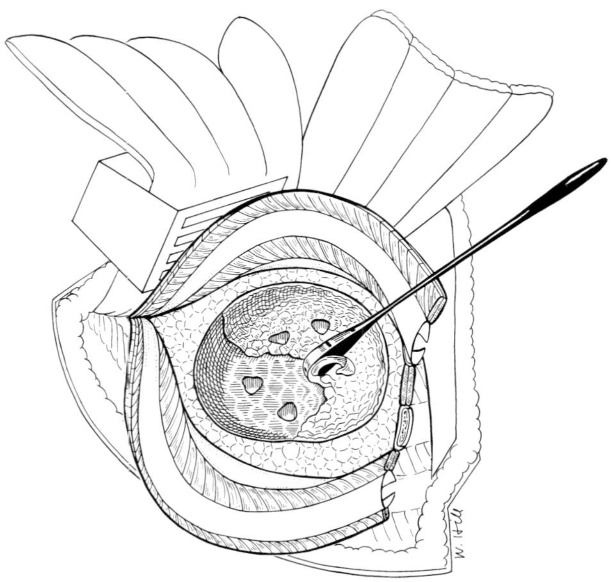

The ribs were removed to fully expose the underlying cavity. Intercostal flaps were held away from the wound with the forceps, both superiorly and inferiorly. The cavity was marked with methylene blue. Several small fistulae were discovered within the wound. Any areas that could not be safely debrided sharply were curetted to remove the exudative peel and debris so that fresh tissue margins could be attained for repair without further injury to the lung.

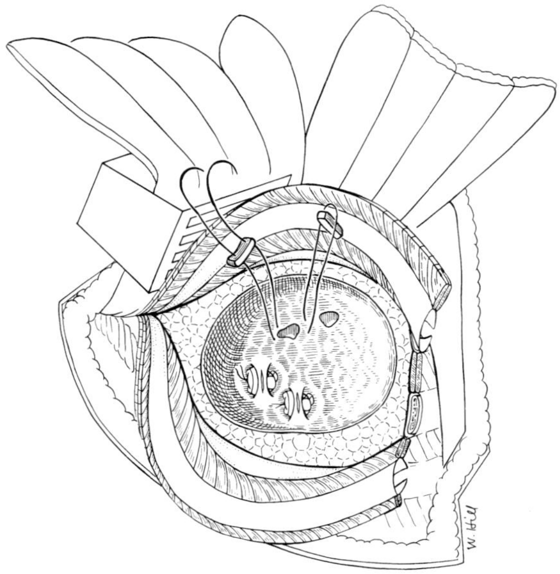

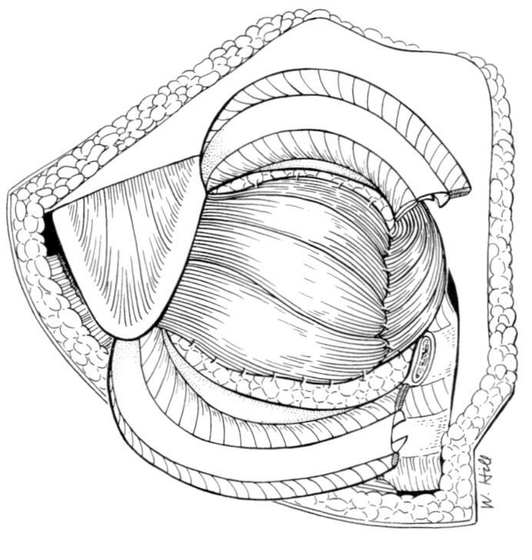

Each fistula was repaired with a pledgeted suture using small pieces of adjacent muscle as autogenous pledget material. An airtight repair was formed and verified before wound closure. The resultant cavity was filled with latissimus dorsi and serratus anterior remnants. The flaps were inset and secured with absorbable sutures.

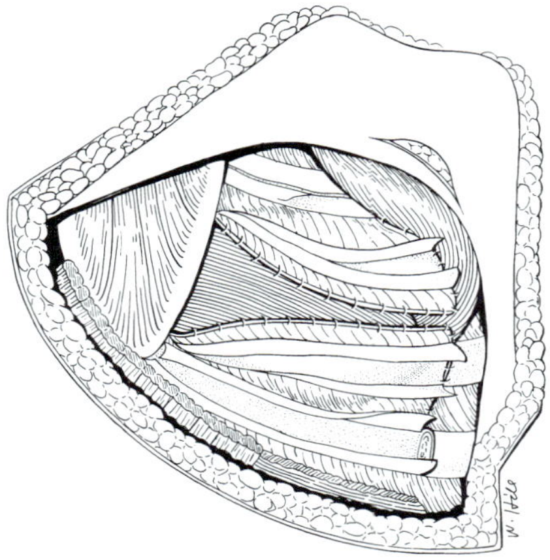

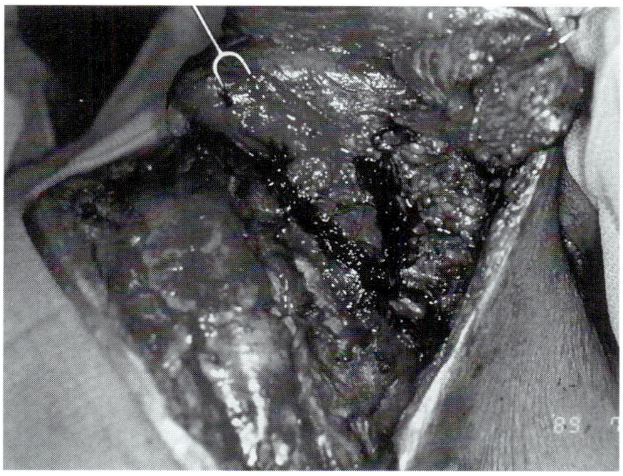

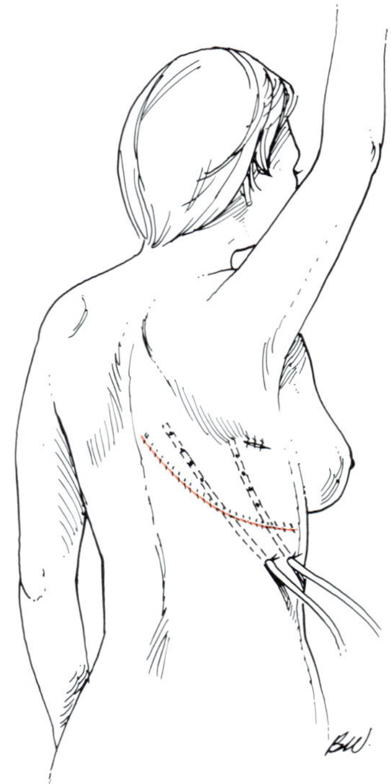

The intercostal flaps were then sutured to firmly secure and buttress the underlying latissimus dorsi and serratus anterior muscles. The inset muscle flaps can be seen with methylene blue outlining the muscle repair margins. The cutaneous wound was closed in a meticulous fashion over suction catheters placed in the subcutaneous plane. Since the lung was adherent to the pleura in the area surrounding the cavity, there was no risk of lung collapse. The use of a pleural catheter or thoracostomy tube was avoided to prevent predisposing to a recurrent air leak by the suction. The patient was placed on high-frequency ventilation postoperatively to minimize recurrent air leak until extubation.

If the air leaks are refractory and the prognosis for healing is considered small, they should be treated more centrally with a preemptive wedge, segmental, or lobar resection to achieve adequate tissue for a more secure bronchial repair.

Regardless of the technique of closure, the risk of breakdown is minimized by buttressing and protecting the repair with vascularized tissue.

Photograph and illustrations from Stahl RS, Seyfer AE. Chest wall reconstruction. In Russell RC, ed. Plastic Surgery Educational Foundation Instructional Courses, vol 3. St. Louis: Mosby, 1990.

In total pneumonectomy defects or in situations in which a secure bronchial closure is not ensured, especially when prior radiation has not been delivered to the site, it may be desirable to stage the wound closure. Open packing of the residual pleural space can be used to maintain wound hygiene as the airway repair suture line heals. If necessary, the patient can subsequently be returned to the operating room for definitive staged closure of the persistent or remaining cavity. The reconstructive problem is thus less complicated, with secure closure of the airway having been achieved.

In the case of a large thoracic defect, such as a pneumonectomy wound in which it is occasionally impractical or impossible to adequately obturate or fill the wound with vascularized tissue, a second-stage Clagett procedure can complement the achievement of the limited but critical goal of airway closure by completing the closure, as demonstrated by Arnold and Pairolero.

The Clagett procedure eliminates the need to eradicate the empyema space if wound contamination can be reduced adequately and there is no underlying bronchopleural fistula. It is performed by the sequential debridement, interval open drainage and wound care, and instillation of antibiotic solutions, with the open wound surface being sutured and closed over the pneumonectomy defect surgically.

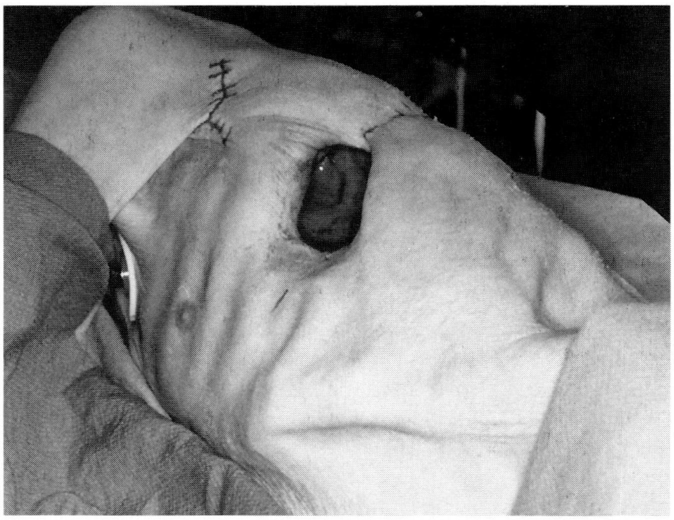

This cachectic 72-year-old man presented 1 year following pneumonectomy for carcinoma of the lung. His recovery was complicated by bronchopleural fistula formation refractory to attempted repair by the original thoracic surgeon. After evaluation, two-stage reconstruction was planned: (1) suture repair of the bronchial stump by the transpericardial approach (see p. 1261) and (2) closure of the remaining total unilateral/hemithoracic empyema cavity after an interval of local wound care and nutritional support.

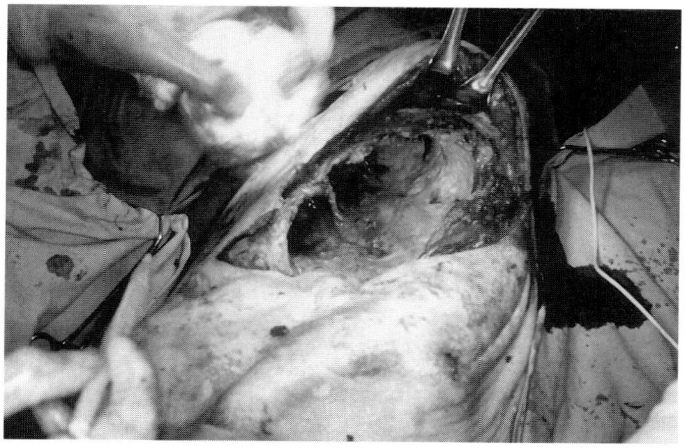

At the final stage further collapse of the cavity was achieved by multiple rib resection and debridement of the cavity. Given the lack of flap donor sites with suitable bulk, the cavity was filled with antibiotic solution and the orifice was closed with local muscle and skin flaps (modified Clagett procedure).

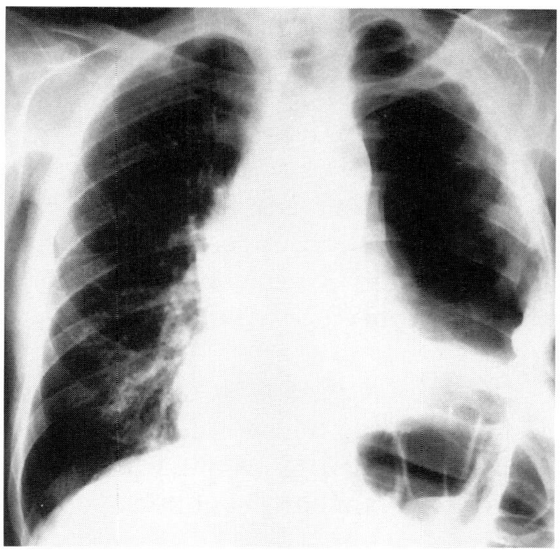

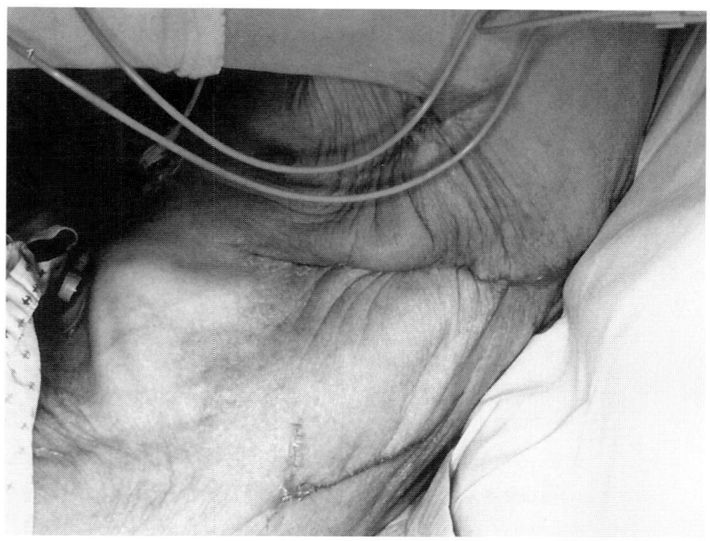

The postoperative chest x-ray film and the healed wound are shown 2 months postoperatively. The patient later required open packing after recurrent drainage from a much smaller cavity following hip fracture and bacteremia from contralateral pneumonia.

Bony Reconstruction

When more than two or three rib segments are to be resected, consideration should be given to reconstructing the bony skeleton. This is especially true if the segments are lengthy, if they do not lie beneath the support of the scapula (obviating the need for bony reconstruction), or if there is limited pulmonary reserve.

Significant pulmonary air leak also has the potential for contaminating any bone grafts or prosthetic mesh. It is usually true that bony resection is better tolerated than anticipated. The exception is young children in whom the thoracic skeletons are cartilaginous and prone to baseline paradoxical motion.

In patients who have had radiation or in whom future radiation therapy is indicated and in those in whom there has been significant contamination or intraoperative air leak, it is preferred that skeletal reconstruction be deferred or omitted. These patients have a high incidence of infection or nonunion of the skeletal reconstruction. However, when resection is performed in the absence of contamination or when the bony defect is quite large, resulting in a problematic respiratory paradox, skeletal reconstitution must be undertaken.

Options for skeletal reconstruction include free rib grafts or split rib grafts in which the residual split ribs are returned to their donor sites to minimize resultant or secondary donor site paradox. Another option is prosthetic mesh secured in a very taut manner to the margins of the wound via sutures to the periosteum or to holes punched in the marginal rib or sternum. The mesh must be secured tautly or respiratory paradox will certainly persist.

Prosthetic mesh incorporated into a "sandwich" with methacrylate, custom-made at the time of the operation, is another option for the reconstruction of skeletal defects. Some have reported difficulty with migration or loosening of this material postoperatively, and there is the additional problem of the presence of a significant foreign body in contaminated cases.

One final option for bony reconstitution in select cases is the transposition of marginal pedicled ribs. This reconstruction can be performed by transecting ribs adjacent to the defect, maintaining the opposite end of the rib in bony continuity with its intercostal bundle, and securing it to a transected margin of the adjacent rib that has been resected. Thus the rib is maintained as a vascularized rib flap and more evenly distributes the respiratory paradoxical tendencies over a larger area. This reconstruction can be performed both inferior and superior to the resection.

Any bony reconstitution must be accomplished in a way that is mindful of the need to drape muscle flaps over or tunnel muscle flaps beneath these firm grafts. Thus circulatory embarrassment of the grafts can be avoided and enough three-dimensional space can be allowed for all necessary bony and soft tissue reconstruction to coexist without one jeopardizing the other.

Soft Tissue Reconstruction

At this point the soft tissue deficit must be addressed. After soft tissue flaps are elevated and placed into these typically concave defects, they must be secured in the wound to prevent the recurrence or persistence of a significant potential space. Usually one is confronted with a paucity of structures at the depths of the wound that can tolerate anchoring sutures.

Techniques that can compensate for this problem include suturing superiorly and inferiorly based intercostal flaps to the tissues and obturating the defect under slight tension so that their elasticity and tension secure the soft tissues in the depths of the wound. Similarly the fascia overlying any muscles whose bases geometrically oppose each other can be sutured together, thus indirectly securing the infolding of these muscles in their new location in the wound. Peripheral suturing of inset flaps to the margins of the reconstructed wound also helps to achieve this goal.

It must be remembered that large potential spaces that result from the extensive dissection of cutaneous and other flaps must be adequately drained since they tend to form significant fluid collections. The aggressive use of suction drains is favored, although care must be taken to avoid the placement of drains near areas of repaired air leaks since this proximity will encourage a recurrence of the air leak. These drains are brought out through separate stab wounds and firmly secured with sutures.

Meticulous cutaneous closure must be ensured to complete a successful thoracic reconstruction. At times, additional cutaneous flap dissection may be necessary to accomplish tension-free closure, and local flaps must be designed as needed for this purpose. A thorough knowledge of prior incisions helps to ascertain that cutaneous flap circulation will be adequate. Once appropriate cutaneous flaps have been identified or selected, meticulous attention is paid to achieving layered, watertight, and airtight wound closure. Even a small technical indiscretion, causing what would otherwise be an insignificant breach in the incision, can lead to contamination of a massive subcutaneous space due to an air leak or can extend leakage of a fluid collection with resultant contamination, prolonged morbidity, and possibly indication for further reoperation.

DEPRESSION AND PROTRUSION DEFORMITIES: PECTUS CARINATUM AND PECTUS EXCAVATUM

The primary correction of protrusion and depression deformities usually requires dramatic resection of costal cartilages with sternal osteotomy and repositioning. These extensive maneuvers must then be followed by adequate stabilization of the repositioned osseous structures. Many methods have been described for this bony stabilization including suture fixation and a variety of hardware devices, metal bars, and pins.

Reoperation in these patients is usually indicated for recurrence or nonunion. An analysis of each case must be performed to formulate a surgical plan based on the etiology of the patient's problem and the surgical anatomy.

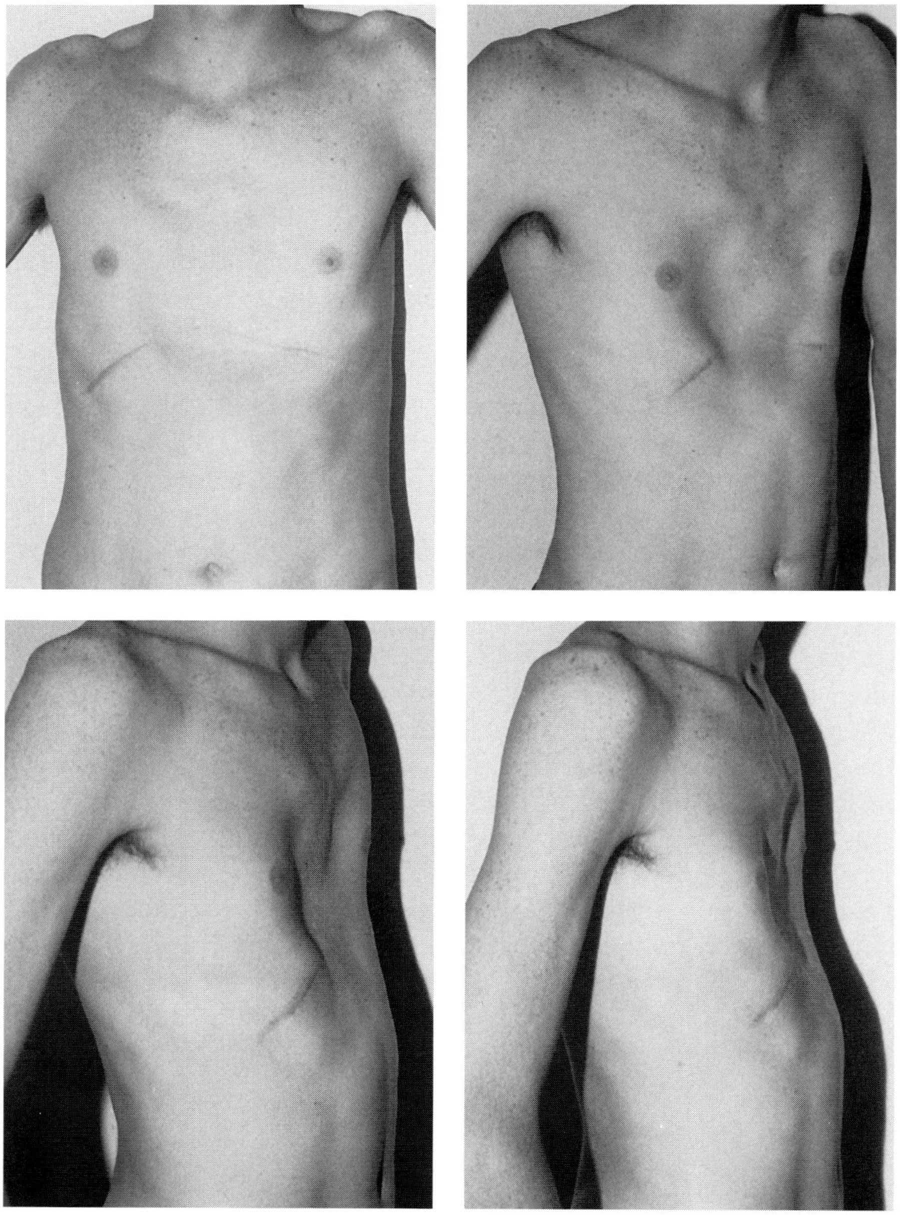

A three-dimensional CT scan or MRI can be helpful in the preoperative evaluation of these complex problems and in planning surgical intervention. Several years after having undergone correction, this teenager presented with recurrent pectus excavatum. Examination revealed a marked depression in the epigastric–lower sternal region. The presence of bone between the respective costal margins and in the entire area of concavity could not be confirmed on palpation.

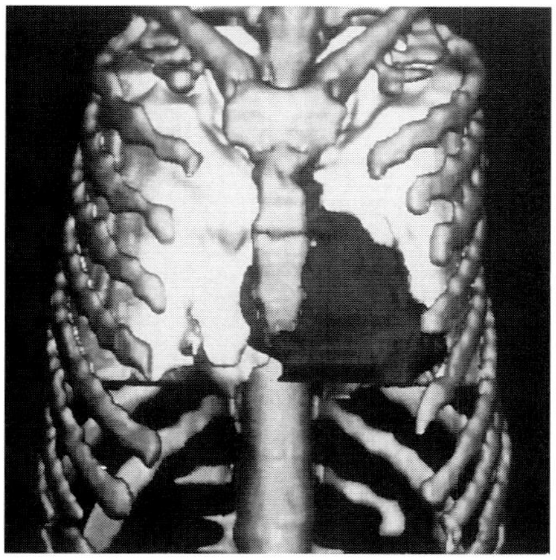

A three-dimensional CT scan reveals the presence of all sternal fragments. They were freely mobile such that it was not possible to definitively palpate them. This finding highlights the importance of adequate bony stabilization and the degree to which inadequate fixation leads to recurrence.

Technique

Although midline incisions can be employed for such procedures, the primary procedure usually requires a long transverse incision in the infrasternal or midsternal region. This incision is usually used again for reoperation, but it may need to be extended to allow for adequate cutaneous and muscular flap elevation since total exposure of the defect is essential.

Adequate bony margins are identified and prepared for stabilization. Subperichondrial dissection of these cartilages is performed to remove the cartilages during the repositioning. The perichondrium is left in place to allow for regeneration of cartilage as a means of achieving a new cartilaginous contour. Internal fixation plates with or without split rib grafts can offer an effective means of stabilizing the reoperative correction of the depression or protrusion deformity if adequate ossification has occurred. To avoid fragmenting the rib grafts or sternum, drill holes must be created and plates secured in a cautious manner, with plates and screws of the appropriate size. Circumcostal wires can also help to augment fixation of rib grafts.

The patient and his family must be alerted to the difficulties of achieving a perfect thoracic contour in reoperations of this area since some rib or cartilage margins may not perfectly regenerate or have the exact or curvilinear contour when the ultimate result is achieved. In many cases subsequent revisions can help to refine this contouring.

As with other thoracic reoperations, adequate, vascularized, musculocutaneous coverage and suction drainage minimize postoperative complications and must be tended to meticulously.

LATERAL CHEST WALL DEFORMITIES: POLAND'S SYNDROME

Reoperation for lateral congenital chest wall deformities is most commonly required for inadequate soft tissue and/or bony reconstruction. In severe thoracic defects, adequate bulk must be transferred to the recipient site in the most anatomic manner possible, with the transfer of both the origin and insertion of any muscle units used. For example, in the case of Poland's syndrome, the latissimus dorsi muscle is transferred to mimic the absent or hypoplastic pectoralis major muscle. When the entire muscle is not transferred as a neuromuscular unit with preservation of motor activity and when both the origins and insertion of the muscle are not transferred, an inadequate correction is achieved. Even when the muscle is transferred in toto in this manner, additional soft tissue bulk may be necessary in severe cases, especially in the infraclavicular region. To augment persistent deficits, free flap transfer of donor units such as the omentum, opposite latissimus dorsi or rectus abdominis is helpful.

This 16-year-old teenager requested evaluation for a persistent Poland's syndrome–variant chest wall deformity. Nine years earlier he had undergone multiple rib grafts and segmental latissimus dorsi transfer. Examination revealed a complex sternocostal and soft tissue deformity. The sternal portion of the deformity had both asymmetric protrusion and depression components. There were multiple segmental rib deficiencies at and lateral to the left midsternal border. Although an anterior axillary fold was established by the margin of the transferred latissimus dorsi muscle, it was suboptimal because the insertion was not transferred anteriorly and the amount of bulk delivered was deficient to mimic the aplastic pectoralis major muscle. For similar reasons a marked infraclavicular hollow was evident as well. The patient's ipsilateral nipple was hypoplastic, and there was an abnormal superior extension of the rectus abdominis muscle into the chest—a persistent rectus thoracis.

"Corrected" patients may also complain of residual bony deficits that may be difficult to remedy. The thoracic skeleton serves as a platform for overlying soft tissues, and unless this platform is elevated or corrected to adequately support and project the overlying musculocutaneous cover, it can further accentuate soft tissue deficits.

Segmental rib absence can be corrected by placement of bone grafts to bridge the resultant gaps. At times, however, adequate correction of the thoracic skeleton can require very significant takedown and dissection of many levels of the sternocostal region. A very stable repositioning akin to that for sternal depression and protrusion deformities must be performed. It is equally critical to the success of the result to adequately stabilize these structures as well.

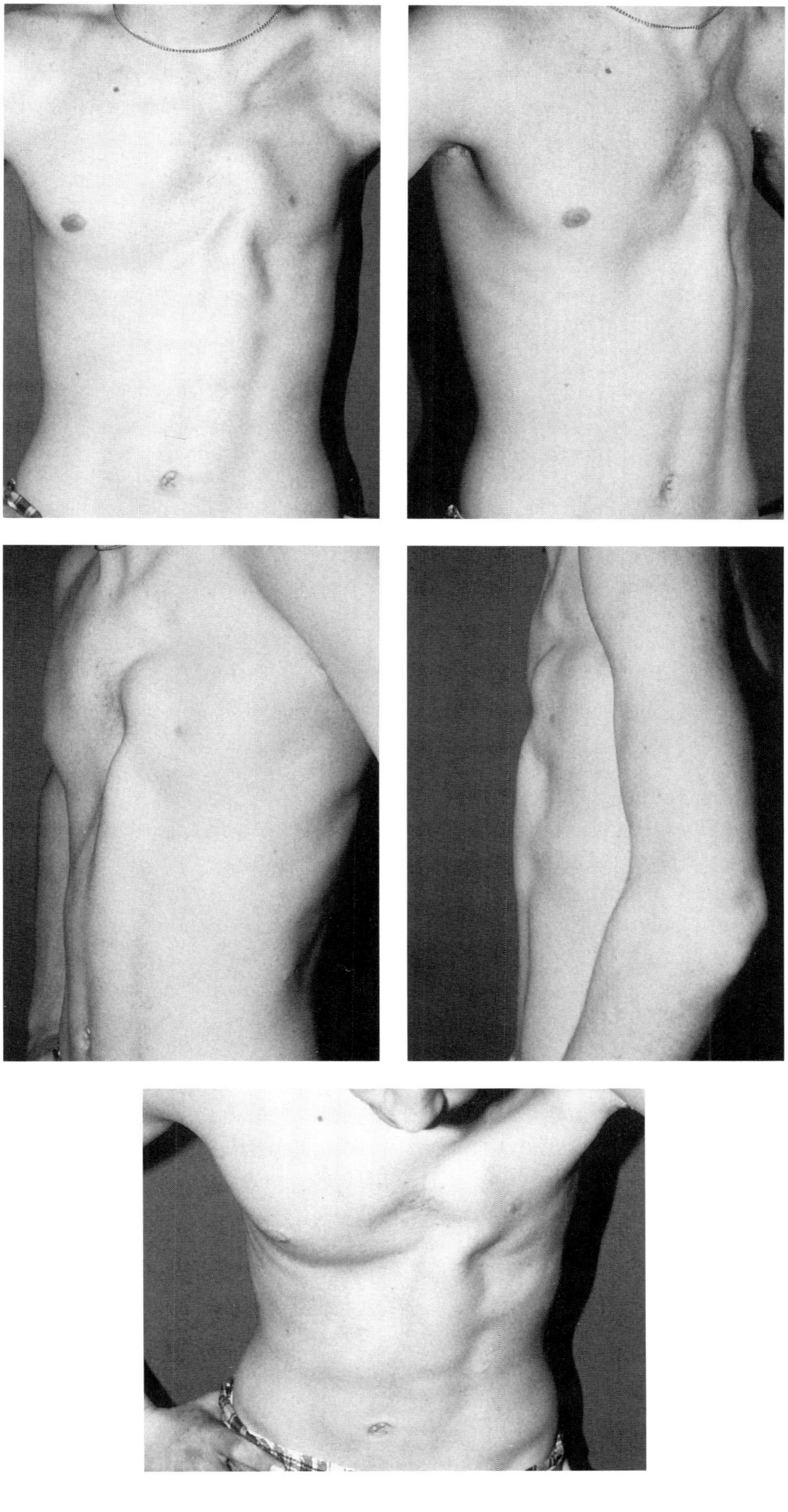

It is difficult, however, to anticipate every operative maneuver that will be necessary until the actual anatomic structures are exposed. Accordingly, it should be remembered that individualized surgical plans cannot be completed or executed until the procedure is under way. Both surgeon and patient must be comfortable with this aspect of the correction to allow for selection from a wide range of reconstructive techniques to achieve the best possible result.

In every case, to avoid unrealistic expectations, the patient must understand that perfect correction of these deformities is impossible. However, the patient should be encouraged to understand that significant or great improvement can be achieved in most instances.

POSTOPERATIVE CARE

In the postoperative period careful attention must be paid to not only general critical care issues but also those matters relating directly to the care of the reconstructed wound. Extubation should be achieved as early as the patient's condition will permit since positive pressure ventilation places stress on airway suture line closure and also increases the degree of air leak that may be present. These spaces are thus more likely to collect air or become contaminated. Pulmonary toilet, especially with vigorous voluntary forced inspirations, is the safest way to combat tendencies toward atelectasis or pneumonia and yet maintain the lowest possible airway pressures and minimize stress on bronchopulmonary wound margins.

Patients must be adequately monitored for maintenance of fluid balance and circulation. These patients are at risk for pulmonary embolism, and a combination of intermittent antiembolic compression devices and minidose heparin administration can minimize this risk. As early as possible, the patient should be mobilized and adequate nutrition should be initiated. When necessary, aggressive nutritional support with central hyperalimentation or nasogastric feedings are instituted early in the postoperative period without waiting to see "if the patient takes enough food orally."

Certain issues of postoperative care also depend on the particular flaps selected for soft tissue reconstruction. For example, it may be desirable to minimize shoulder motion in the first few days after reconstruction if pectoralis major flaps have been inset in a relatively taut manner, especially if the muscular insertions have been preserved. The most important issue of postoperative management relative to specific flap selection involves the greater omentum. Patients are particularly prone to prolonged gastric ileus after the greater curvature gastric dissection required for omental harvest. Accordingly, it is crucial to maintain nasogastric suction long enough for definitive gastrointestinal function to resume.

Specific antibiotic coverage is maintained for 24 hours postoperatively in clean cases such as when bone grafts or prosthetic material is used. In contaminated cases culture-specific antibiotic coverage is continued for 1 to 2 weeks depending on the extent of resection debridement possible during the procedure and the resultant confidence of the surgeon in the clearance of contamination from the wound and its margins. In some cases the location of vital organs can preclude aggressive debridement or resection of some portions of the wound. In these cases and in patients who are immunocompromised or who have had protracted, multiply recurrent courses of infection, antibiotic coverage will occasionally need to be continued for 4 to 6 weeks.

Observation and maintenance of the suction catheters is crucial, especially in the first few days postoperatively. Failure to establish or maintain adequate suction drainage is a significant cause of recurrent wound complications.

It is helpful to mobilize the patient even if it involves merely a move to a cardiac chair or a few steps at the bedside for an intubated patient. Intermittent antiembolic pneumatic compression stockings are kept in place until the patient is reasonably mobilized.

Depending on the circumstances and technique of incisional closure, sutures are removed at approximately 2 weeks postoperatively, but only if it appears that wound edges have adequately healed. Otherwise the surgeon should be prepared to leave sutures in place for longer periods of time in patients with risk factors for poor wound healing.

Reconstructed thoracic wounds must be watched carefully for the first 3 to 4 weeks postoperatively since it is not uncommon for wound complications to arise as late as 1 month postoperatively after such complex procedures. In the setting of prior radiation therapy, obesity, diabetes mellitus, or immunocompromised states the critical period of complication-free wound healing should be considered to extend this surveillance period to 6 to 8 weeks postoperatively.

FUTURE CHALLENGES

Major advances have been achieved in the surgical treatment of diseases and deformities of the thorax. Yet with each new development, new demands and challenges arise in primary and secondary reconstructive thoracic surgery. Although improved plastic surgical techniques have increasingly met these demands, many problems could be solved more elegantly and practically. Further improvement is needed in restoring an adequately rigid yet physiologically pliable and dynamic thoracic skeleton in cases of resection or anomaly. Improvements are needed in methods of debridement of wounds involving vital organs. Dynamic imaging or other monitoring during the debridement—or perhaps a topical, enzymatic, or more selective technique—would help to expedite what can be a tedious and treacherous wound resection.

Reconstructive efforts can achieve the restoration of thoracic form, a protective cover, and some physiologic functions. Early efforts are under way to perform functional although primitive cardiac reconstruction, for example, with neuromuscular transfers and cardiac muscle augmentations. Not only should these efforts be redoubled, but further efforts should be made to dramatically improve respiratory function with reconstructive methods. Similarly, tracheobronchial reconstruction with autogenous tissue is by no means perfected.

Finally, closer monitoring of all children with cardiothoracic interventions will allow us to understand and classify better the growth disturbances that follow such surgery. Only then can analysis and appropriate intervention—or even prevention—be possible.

Bibliography

Alday ES, Goldsmith HS. Surgical technique for omental lengthening based on arterial anatomy. Surg Gynecol Obstet 135:103, 1972.

Arnold PG. Abdominal and Chest Wall Reconstruction. Atlanta: Medical Association of Georgia, 1982.

Arnold PG, Witzke BJ, Ironis GB, et al. Use of omental transposition flaps for soft-tissue reconstruction. Ann Plast Surg 11:508, 1983.

Arnold PG, Irons GB. The greater omentum: Extension in transposition and free transfer. Plast Reconstr Surg 67:169, 1981.

Arnold PG, Pairolero PC. Intrathoracic muscle flaps: An account of their use in the management of 100 consecutive patients. Ann Surg 211:656, 1990.

Arnold PG, Pairolero PC. Surgical management of the radiated chest wall. Plast Reconstr Surg 77:605, 1986.

Arnold PG, Pairolero PC. Use of pectoralis major muscle flaps to repair defects of anterior chest wall. Plast Reconstr Surg 63:205, 1979.

Arnold PG, Pairolero PC, Waldorf JC. The serratus anterior muscle: Intrathoracic and extrathoracic utilization. Plast Reconstr Surg 73:240, 1983.

Bryant LB, Spencer FC, Trinkle JK. Treatment of median sternotomy infection by mediastinal irrigation with an antibiotic solution. Ann Surg 169:914, 1969.

Chicarilli ZN, Ariyan S, Stahl RS. Costochondritis: Pathogenesis, diagnosis, and management considerations. Plast Reconstr Surg 77:50, 1986.

Chicarilli ZN, Ariyan S, Glen WWL, et al. Management of recalcitrant bronchopleural fistulas by muscle flap obliteration. Plast Reconstr Surg 75:882, 1985.

Clagett OT, Geraci JE. A procedure for the management of postpneumonectomy empyema. J Thorac Cardiovasc Surg 45:141, 1963.

DeMeester TR, Lafontaine E. The pleura. In Sabiston DC, Spencer FC, eds. Gibbon's Surgery of the Chest, 4th ed, vol 1. Philadelphia: WB Saunders, 1983.

Dotty DB, Hawkins JA. A turnover operation for pectus excavatum at the time of correction of intracardiac defects. J Thorac Cardiovasc Surg 86:787, 1983.

Eloesser L. An operation for tuberculous empyema. Surg Gynecol Obstet 60:1096, 1935.

Gray SW, Skandalakis JE, eds. Embryology for Surgeons. Philadelphia: WB Saunders, 1972.

Haller JA. Pectus excavatum: A 20-year surgical experience. J Thorac Cardiovasc Surg 60:375, 1970.

Haller JA, Turner CS. Diagnosis and operative management of chest wall deformities in children. Surg Clin North Am 61:216, 1982.

Haller JA Jr, Shermeta EW, Tepas JJ, et al. Correction of pectus excavatum without prosthesis or splints, objective measurement of severity and management of asymmetrical deformities. Ann Thorac Surg 26:73, 1978.

Hartrampf CR, Scheflan M, Black PW. Breast reconstruction with a transverse abdominal island flap. Plast Reconstr Surg 69:216, 1982.

Hawkins JA, Ehrenhaft JL, Doty DB. Repair of pectus excavatum bisternal eversion. Ann Thorac Surg 38:368, 1984.

Herrera HR, Mijangos J, Weiner RS, et al. Mediastinal cutaneous fistulae arising as a complication of major cardiac surgery: The value of sinography and injection of methylene blue in their radical excision and immediate repair. Br J Plast Surg 36:421, 1983.

Higgins R, Stahl R, Baldwin JC. Skin grafting for repair of a cardiac laceration. Ann Thorac Surg 52:1161, 1991.

Hodgkinson DJ, Arnold PG. Chest-wall reconstruction using the external oblique muscle. Br J Plast Surg 33:216, 1980.

Jurkiewicz MJ, Arnold PG. The omentum: An account of its use in the reconstruction of the chest wall. Ann Surg 185:548, 1977.

Jurkiewicz MJ, Bostwick J, Hester TR, et al. Infected median sternotomy wound: Successful treatment by muscle flaps. Ann Surg 191:738, 1980.

Kiricuta I. L'emploi du grand epiplois dans la chirurgie du sein cancéreux. Presse Med 71:15, 1963.

Lemmer JH, Gomez MN, Symreng T, et al. Limited lateral thoracotomy. Arch Surg 125:873, 1990.

Nahai F. Personal communication, 1983.

Nahai F, Rand RP, Hester TR, et al. Primary treatment of the infected sternotomy wound with muscle flaps: A review of 211 consecutive cases. Plast Reconstr Surg 84:434, 1989.

Ochsner A, DeBakey M. Chone-chondrosternon: Report of a case and review of the literature. J Thorac Surg 8:469, 1939.

Pairolero PC, Arnold PG. Management of infected median sternotomy wounds [editorial]. Ann Thorac Surg 42:1, 1986.

Pairolero PC, Arnold PG. Bronchopleural fistula treatment by transposition of pectoralis major muscle. J Thorac Cardiovasc Surg 79:142, 1980.

Price G, Stahl RS. Reconstruction of penetrating cardiac injuries in infected sternal wounds. International Forum on Plastic Surgery, Florence, Italy, 1994.

Ravitch MM. Asymmetric congenital deformity of the ribs: Collapse of the right side of the chest. Ann Surg 191:534, 1980.

Ravitch MM. Repair of pectus excavatum in children under 3 years of age: A 12-year experience. Ann Thorac Surg 23:4, 1977.

Ravitch MM. Congenital Deformities of the Chest Wall and Their Operative Correction. Philadelphia: WB Saunders, 1977.

Ravitch MM. The operative corrective of pectus carinatum (pigeon breast). Ann Surg 162:29, 1965.

Ravitch MM. Unusual sternal deformity with cardiac symptoms operative correction. J Thorac Surg 23:138, 1952.

Ravitch MM. Pectus excavatum and heart failure. Surgery 30:178, 1951.

Ravitch MM. The operative treatment of pectus excavatum. Ann Surg 129:429, 1948.

Shumacker HB Jr, Mandelbaum I. Continuous antibiotic irrigation in the treatment of infection. Arch Surg 86:384, 1963.

Smith DE, Karish AF, Chapman JP, et al. Healing of the bronchial stump after pulmonary resection. J Thorac Cardiovasc Surg 46:548, 1963.

Stahl RS, Kopf GS. Reconstruction of infant thoracic wounds. Plast Reconstr Surg 82:1000, 1988.

Stahl RS, Sando WC. Reconstruction of defects of thorax and spine. In Jurkiewicz MJ, Krizek TJ, Mathes SJ, Ariyan T, eds. Plastic Surgery: Principles and Practice. St. Louis: Mosby, 1990, p 1169.

Stahl RS, Seyfer AE. Chest wall reconstruction. In Russell RC, ed. Plastic Surgery Educational Foundation Instructional Courses, vol 3. St. Louis: Mosby, 1990, p 258.

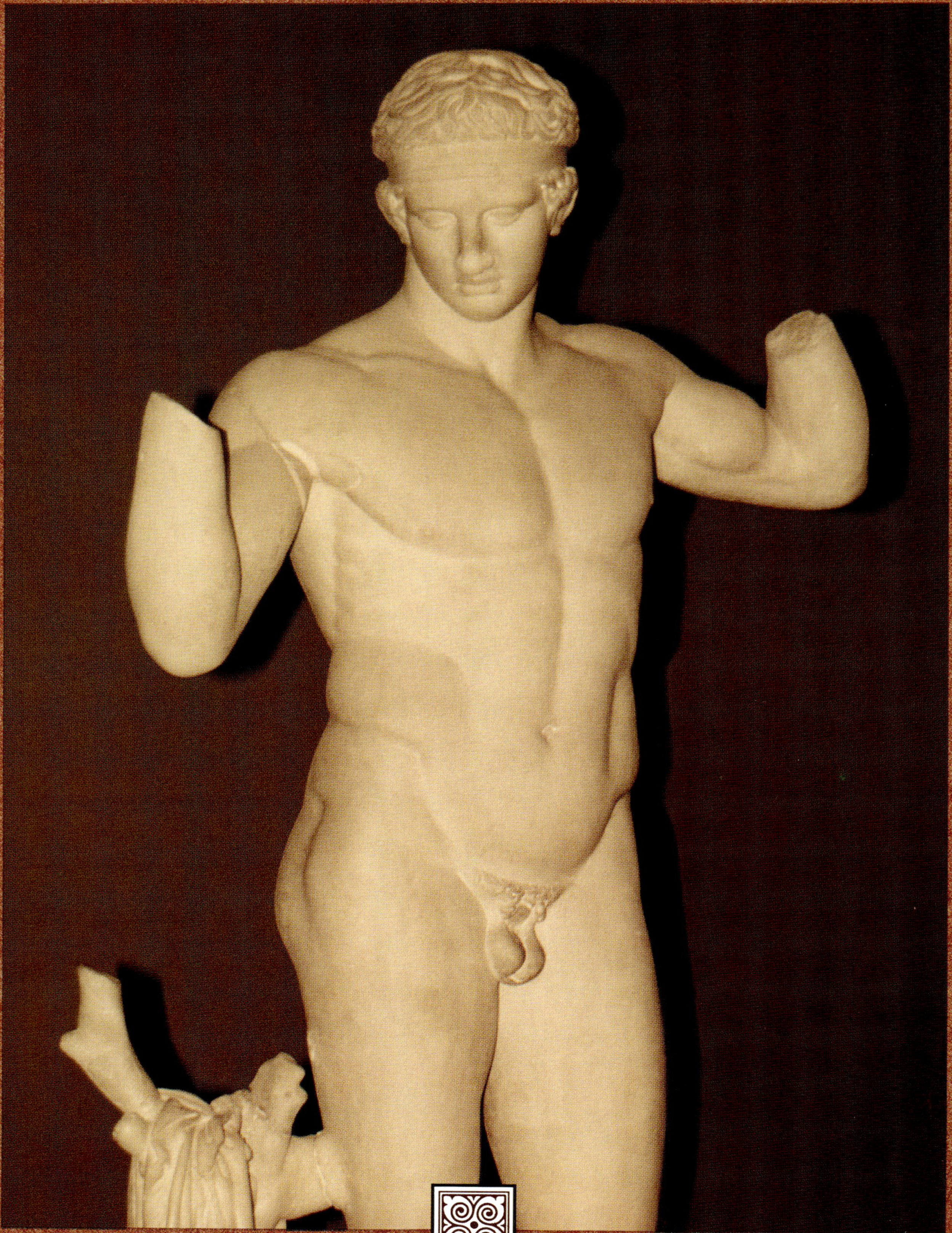

V

Reoperative Surgery of the Trunk

35

Reoperation After Liposuction and Body Contour Surgery

Ricardo Baroudi, M.D.

Reoperative Problems

Insufficient or excessive fat removal	Bulging
Skin irregularities	Incorrect placement of umbilicus
Skin laxity	Scar malposition

Body contour surgery most frequently involves the breasts, abdomen, flanks, buttocks, thighs, and arms. Although this surgery produces the necessary body contouring, the associated sequelae, particularly the long, unpredictable scars, are often objectionable and a lingering problem for patient and surgeon. The results of body contour surgery have improved significantly with the introduction of liposuction for fat removal. This technique leaves inconspicuous scars and offers patients an excellent option for body sculpturing. Liposuction and traditional aesthetic surgery operations can be staged or performed in combined procedures to improve postoperative results and to accommodate anatomic and histologic characteristics and aging changes encountered in each body region.

In body surgery the possible need for a minor or a major reoperative procedure always exists. The effect of aging on the human body is unpredictable. One might ask why healthy people in the same decade of life, even at the same age, look so different and have such diverse body configurations. We know that genetics, life-style, disease, and diet can influence body appearance. We also know that body shape and skin quality, musculoaponeurotic texture, and fat deposits can also affect the appearance of the body. When surgery is performed, these same factors will influence the success of the final result. Even without the occurrence of complications (e.g., necrosis, hematoma, infection) natural factors beyond the surgeon's control may compromise the final surgical result and bring about the need for reoperation. The need for reoperation can be attributed to improper surgical planning, anatomic and tissue failure, poor patient selection, incorrect choice of procedure, poor technique, and complications beyond the surgeon's control. In some cases the patient's unique body structure can be responsible for poor results even when a well-qualified expert has performed the operation. No surgeon achieves 100% success; reoperation is always a possibility.

PATIENT-PHYSICIAN RELATIONSHIP IN THE REOPERATIVE ENVIRONMENT

There are no specific rules for treating an unsatisfactory result or for anticipating the response of an unsatisfied patient. Each patient's expectations and emotional behavior will vary according to personality, education, or family involvements.

The surgeon should be careful to offer the patient the feeling of absolute understanding during the healing period. If the surgeon fails by overlooking a significant detail or by tactless, negligent, or imprudent behavior, this patient-physician equilibrium can be easily disrupted. Reoperative candidates are highly insecure. Most likely their first surgical experience was disappointing and has made them unhappy and anxious. Setting a deadline for the completion of projected corrections is recommended to encourage the patient to persevere with the surgery in order to achieve a definitive solution to the problem.

Patients who present with a still unresolved complication from a previous surgical procedure are anxious to have the problem corrected as quickly as possible. Very often they do not understand the extent of the complication and its possible consequences. Whatever the situation, the surgeon should display an optimistic outlook. In dangerous situations or in those in which the surgeon recognizes that there are limitations to solving the problem, providing accurate information and documentation to the patient is important for ethical and legal reasons. The patient should be informed of the expected result, number of surgical stages required, length of postoperative recovery, and cost.

Patients without complications but with suboptimal results can also become frustrated with their surgeon. Refusing to tolerate another disappointment, they frequently search for another surgeon who can improve the result. With these patients it is imperative to establish what improvements can be realistically achieved. It is better to offer less than more. If the results exceed the patient's expectations, the patient will be happier.

In complex primary operative situations in which suboptimal or poor results could occur, the patient should be informed of this possibility. Difficult cases often require second procedures at a later date. This concept—that any secondary procedure is part of a surgical plan—should be clearly indicated on the surgery consent form, and the patient should understand that to attain the desired effect, a second or even a third stage may be necessary. The patient also is informed that no fee will be charged for additional procedures; he will be responsible for only hospital charges and in certain situations for the anesthetist's fee. The secondary procedure is usually performed 6 months to 1 year later.

Even with the best communication there is a small group of patients who demand results beyond those which can be attained surgically. Given the negligible improvement that can be achieved and the unreasonably high patient expectations, for these difficult patients reoperation should not be recommended. The surgeon must be able to distinguish which patients will benefit from revisional surgery and which chronically dissatisfied patients will never be pleased. For this latter group it is better to refuse reoperation.

LIPOSUCTION

With liposuction the final result is a combination of fat removal and skin retraction. Determining the correct amount of fat removal to obtain a perfect result is difficult because liposuction is a blunt and inexact procedure that always results in some injury to the subcutaneous fat. Furthermore, skin elasticity, scarring, and the extent of injury to the subcutaneous fat are unpredictable at best. The patient's age, skin turgor, body shape, and the surgeon's experience also influence the final result.

The following basic questions need to be addressed: How much fat should be removed? Are one or two stages needed? When is liposuction not needed and skin excision preferable? When should liposuction be used alone? When should liposuction be used in combination with traditional aesthetic surgery procedures?

In an attempt to clarify the indications for specific procedures, I have developed a classification of liposuction candidates (Table 35-1). Regardless of the classification, it is essential for the surgeon to determine the type of procedure indicated and how it should be performed.

Table 35-1 Patient Classification for Liposuction

	Characteristics	*Type*	*Treatment*
Group 1	Good skin turgor, no flaccidity, moderate fat deposit	Young patients	Liposuction in one stage
Group 2	Moderate or voluminous fat deposit, no flaccidity, mild skin turgor	Patients over 35 years of age; young patients with weight fluctuation problems; patients with excessive skin laxity	Liposuction in one or two stages (depends on degree of flaccidity after first procedure)
Group 3	Skin flaccidity, fat deposits	Patients in their forties or older; young patients with structural or metabolic problems	Liposuction and surgery in one operation or staged
Group 4	Skin flaccidity		Traditional surgery alone (no liposuction)

Problems Following Liposuction

Patient complaints after liposuction most commonly are related to insufficient or excessive fat removal, skin irregularities, and skin laxity due to poor skin retraction. Following liposuction of the abdominal wall, even when indicated, these problems can be compounded by body weight variations after the surgery. The unpredictable capacity of the skin to shrink with more than 6 kg of weight loss may affect skin turgor. It is unclear why, in patients of similar age, the skin reacts differently when suctioned.

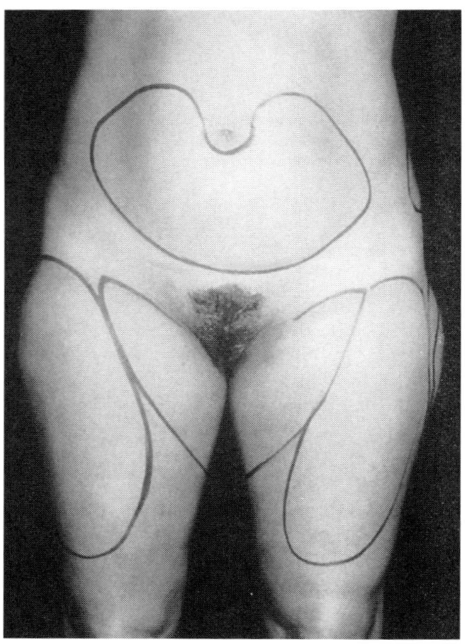

The effect of weight fluctuations after liposuction is illustrated by this 37-year-old patient who had prior liposuction in the hypogastrium and the thighs. Four years later she returned with abdominal skin flaccidity subsequent to several episodes of weight loss and gain.

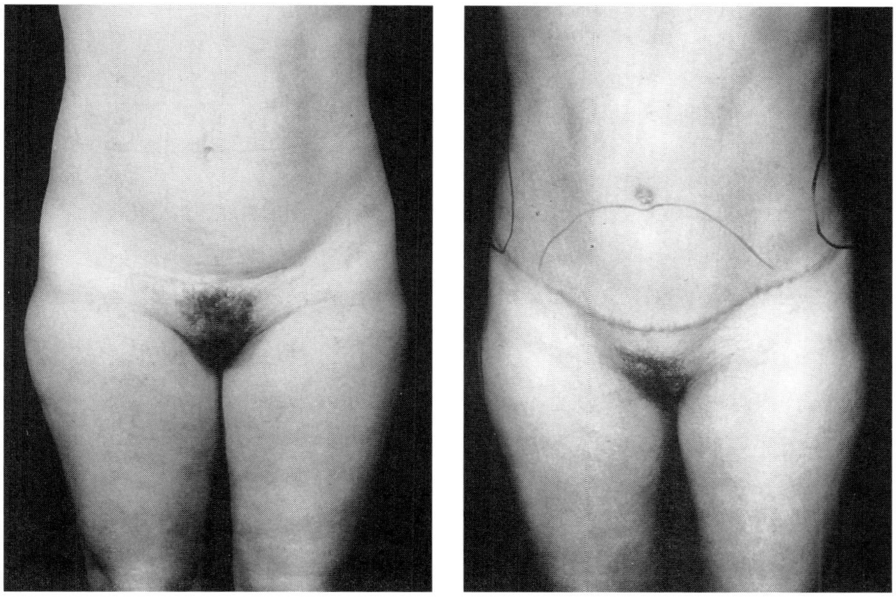

She is shown preoperatively and 8 months postoperatively after routine abdominoplasty. Because she was unhappy with scar quality and the residual flank and hypogastrium fat deposits, scar revision and secondary liposuction were performed.

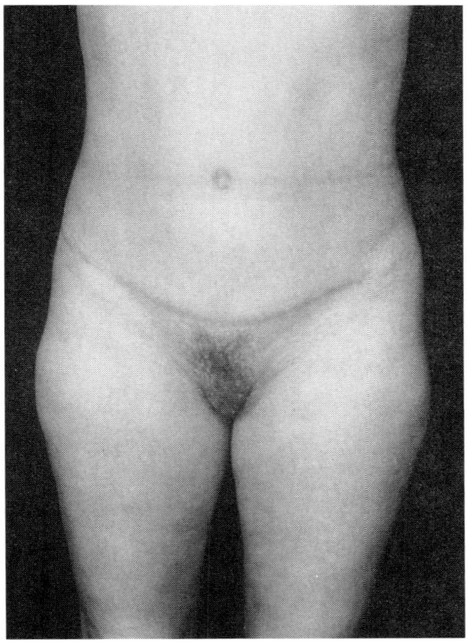

Four months after these reoperative procedures, a handlebar-shaped scar remains. The scar is sufficiently high at the inguinal regions and low at the pubis to remain hidden under a bikini.

Insufficient fat removal occurs when the surgeon does not accurately estimate preoperatively the volume to be suctioned, when the patient has excessive fat volume, or when liposuction has to be terminated before the desired amount of fat is removed because of possible secondary laxity due to limited skin retraction.

In the case of insufficient liposuction, a minimum of 6 months should elapse before additional fat removal is attempted. When skin retraction is poor, as in patients in group 2, secondary liposuction should not be attempted. Patients in group 1 have excellent skin for suctioning. This is also true of patients in group 3 whose skin turgor tends to improve after the surgery and becomes similar to that of patients in group 1.

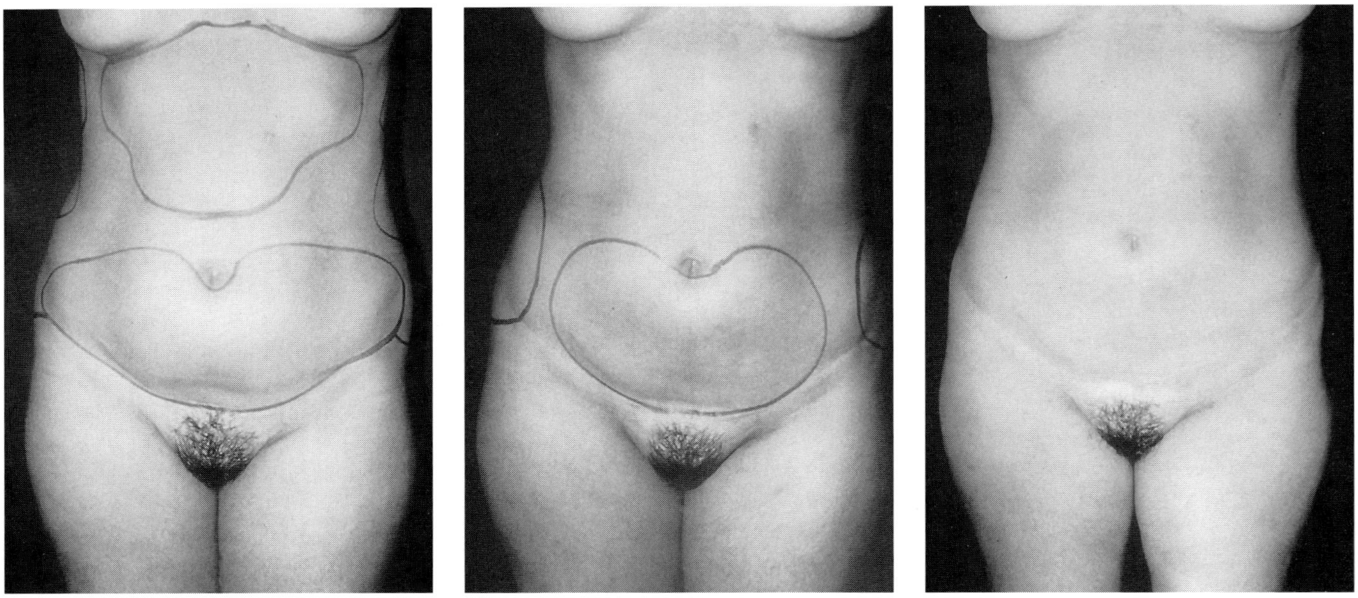

This 34-year-old woman had moderate fat deposit and skin flaccidity in the supraumbilical regions, flanks, and lateral trunk areas. Liposuction was performed. Eight months postoperatively the patient still complained of residual bulges in the hypogastrium and flanks. Reoperative liposuction was performed to complete the treatment.

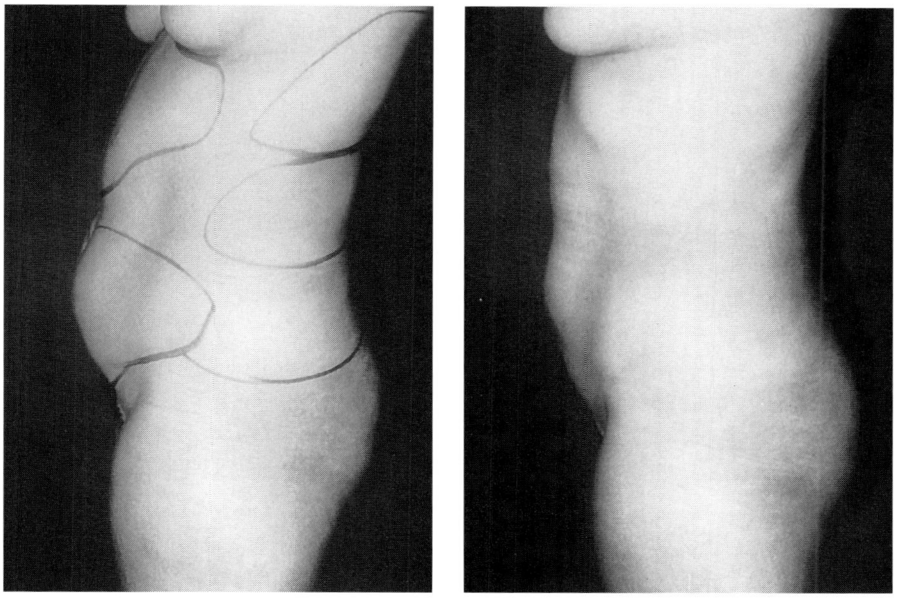

No flaccidity or indentations were evident after the second liposuction. Natural skin retraction occurred. The improvement in contour can be observed on comparison of the preoperative and postoperative lateral views.

Excess fat removal causes localized skin irregularities, indentations, and skin flaccidity, which are difficult to correct. Treatment for excessive fat removal is based on a logical approach: the indentations are refilled by fat injection,* the undulations are removed with secondary localized liposuction, and/or surgical skin resection is performed to stretch the skin to restore turgor. A single region may receive any combination of treatments.

*Despite the use of fat injection by many specialists to correct indentations, treat cellulite, and restore body contour, this practice is still controversial. Extensive research is still needed to ensure predictable results.

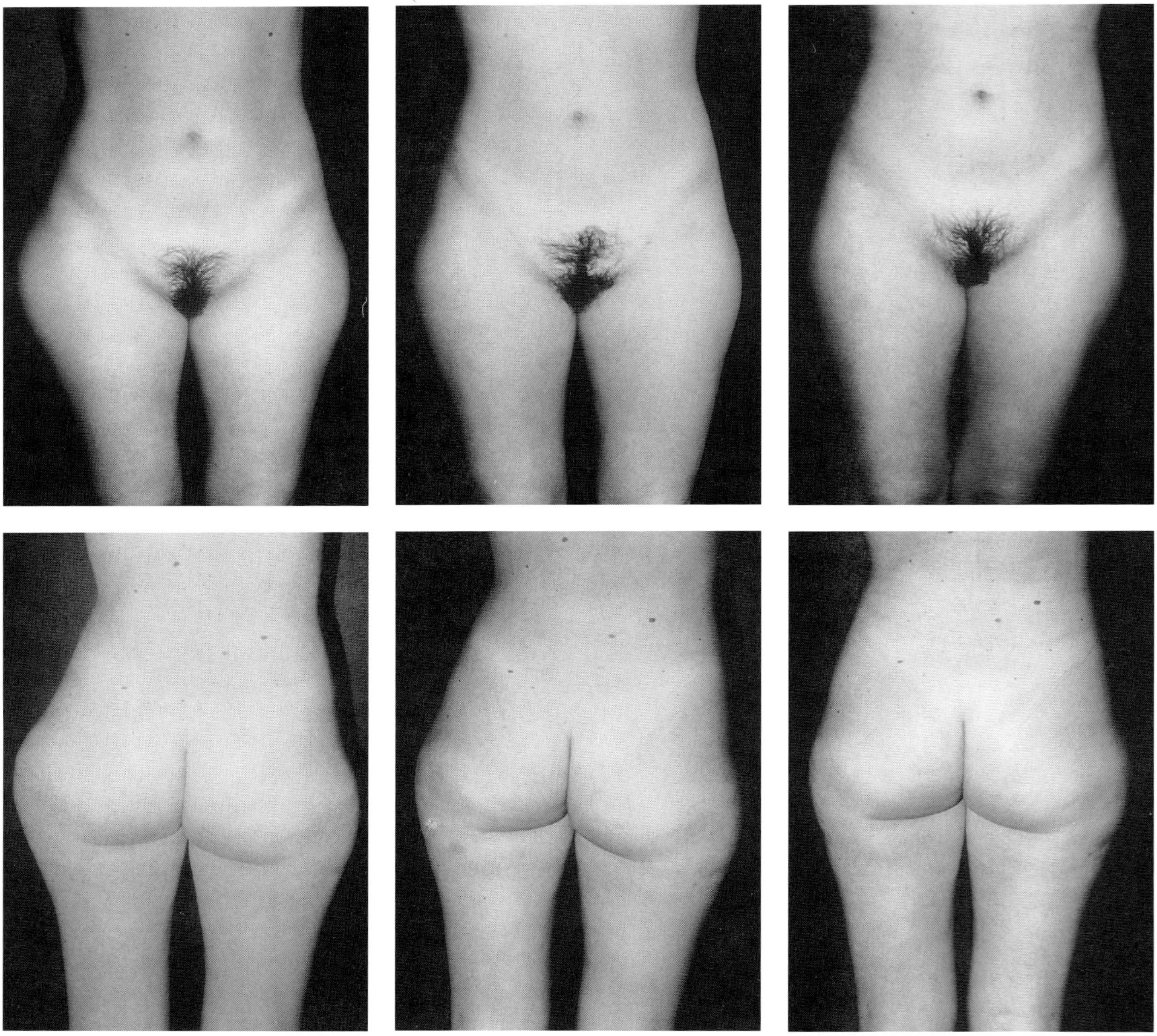

This 23-year-old woman had extensive bilateral femoral fat deposits with evident asymmetric volume. Despite good skin turgor, liposuction was performed in two stages because of the difficulty in predicting the amount of skin retraction that would occur postoperatively and in order to avoid causing skin laxity and/or undulations. This conservative approach obviated secondary problems. The volume reduction is evident, and body contour now appears normal. The patient is shown after the first liposuction and 8 months later after the second liposuction.

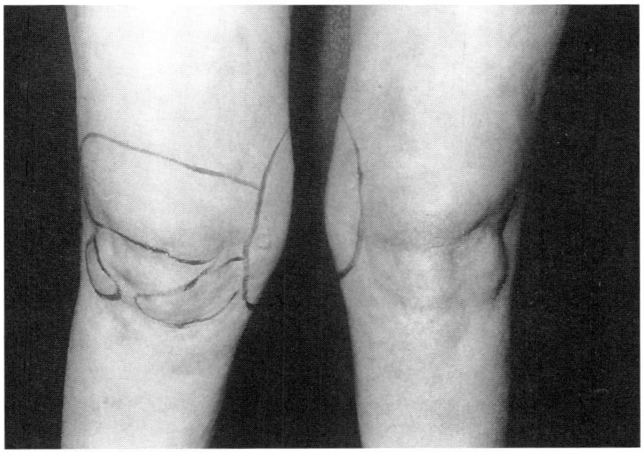

This 57-year-old patient represents a case of insufficient liposuction with a suboptimal final result despite liposuction being performed in two successive stages. She had bulging inner knee fat deposits combined with multiple small fat deposits around the knee.

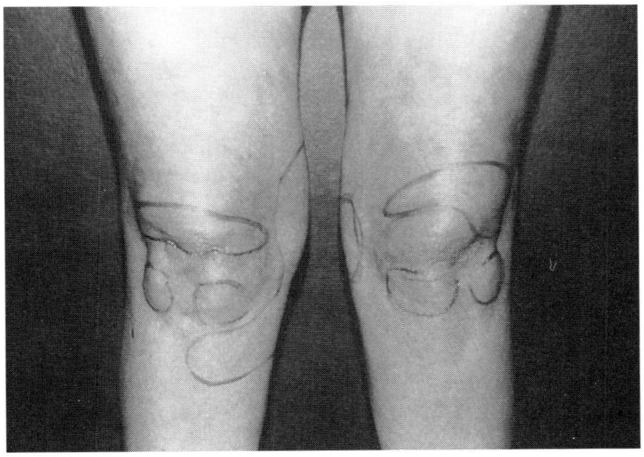

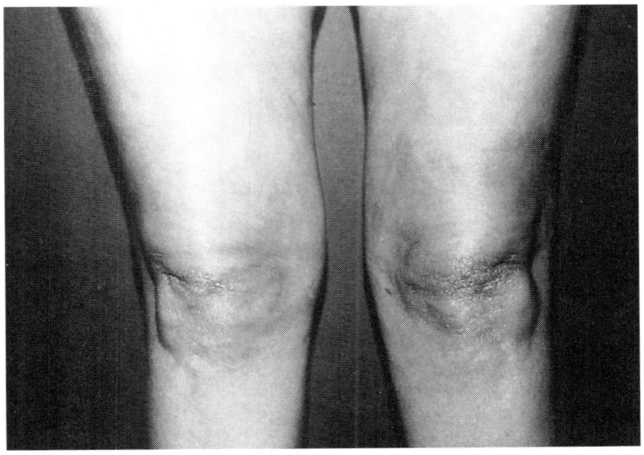

Postoperatively the patient still has residual fat collections. A second liposuction procedure was performed. Six months following the second conservative liposuction procedure the patient still demonstrates residual fat deposits.

Insufficient liposuction is a difficult problem to solve completely. Patients should be advised about these possible limitations. A third localized liposuction may still be indicated for one or two specific small bulges if the patient demands further treatment.

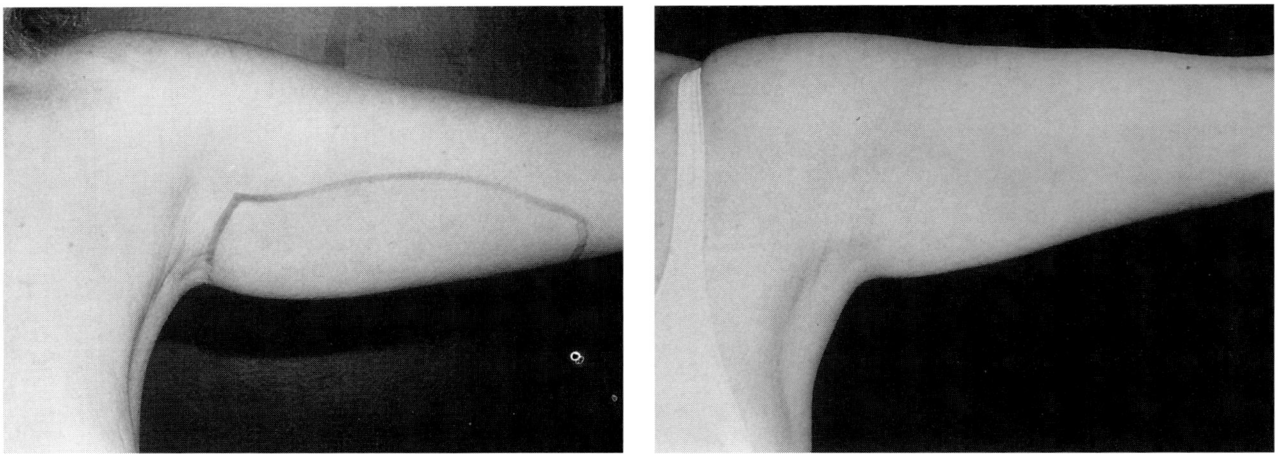

This 45-year-old patient had moderate fat deposits in the lower segment of the upper arm and mild skin laxity. Routine liposuction was performed. Although there was volume reduction, the patient complained of skin laxity.

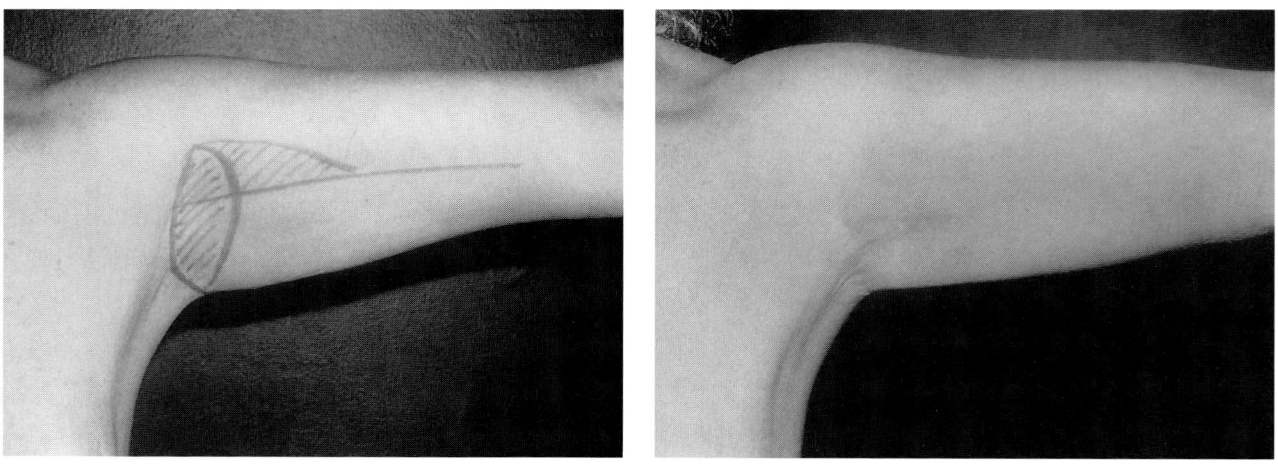

A reduction brachioplasty near the axilla was performed. A fusiform skin resection combined with a half triangle resection (with the base of the triangle at the axillary line) removed the skin excess, leaving an L-shaped scar.

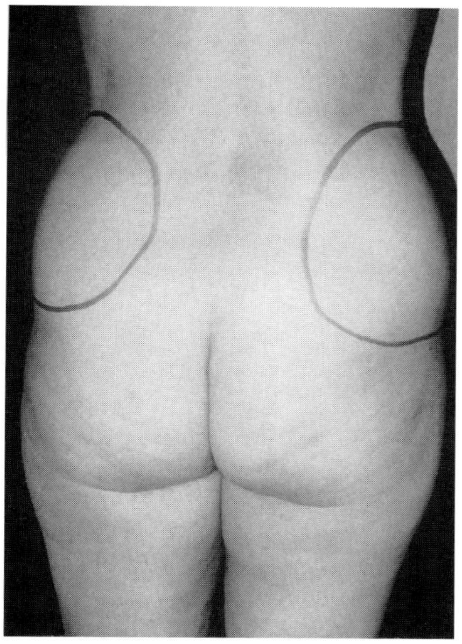

This 45-year-old patient had fat bulges in the flanks with good skin turgor. The patient's main complaint related to the need for flank reduction. Liposuction was performed specifically in these areas.

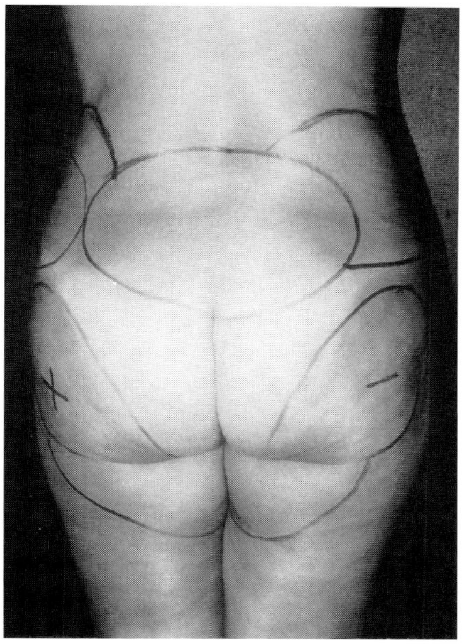

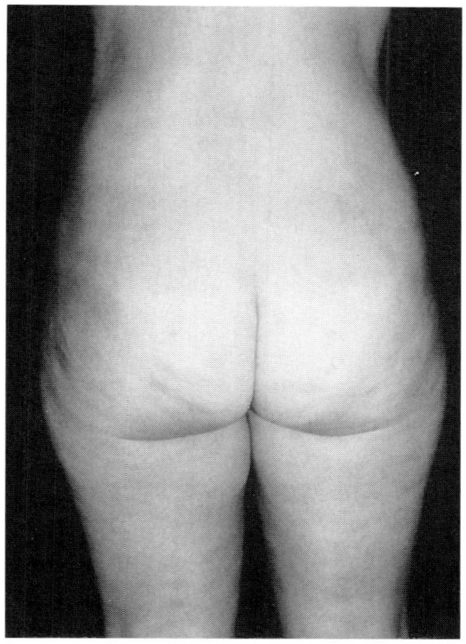

Two years later the patient returned 6 kg overweight, indicating that she was trying to return to her normal weight. The flanks did not show fat recurrence, whereas the hip regions and the posterior upper thighs were voluminous. All of the demarcated regions were suctioned again, including the flanks. The final result is shown 4 months postoperatively. Since the second liposuction the patient has lost 4 kg. It is interesting to note the nonrecurrence of the previously suctioned fat deposit after limited weight gain.

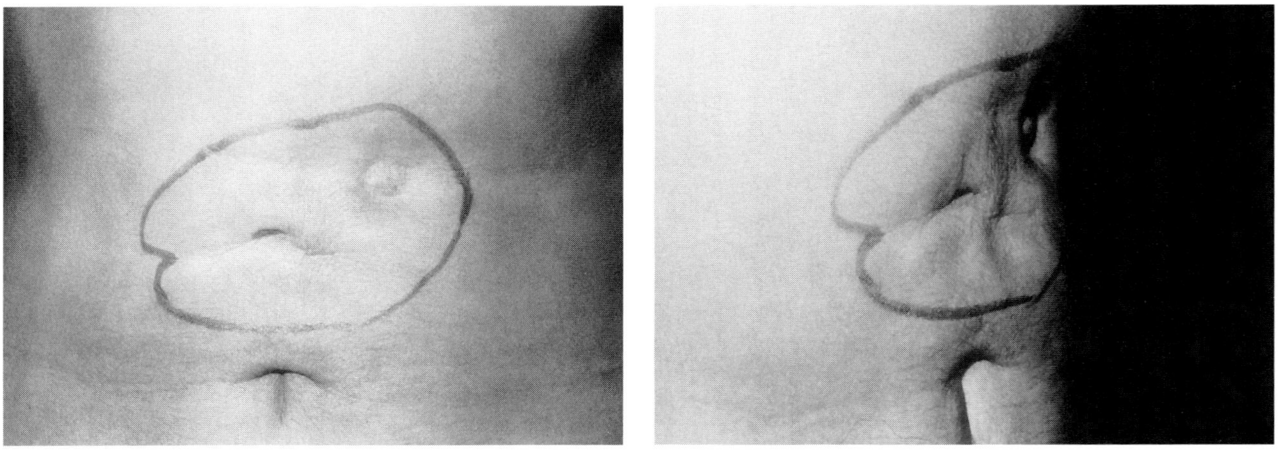

This 37-year-old patient presented for consultation after liposuction of the abdominal wall (epigastrium) with resilient depressions and two small necrotic skin spots after triamcinolone injections for local indications.

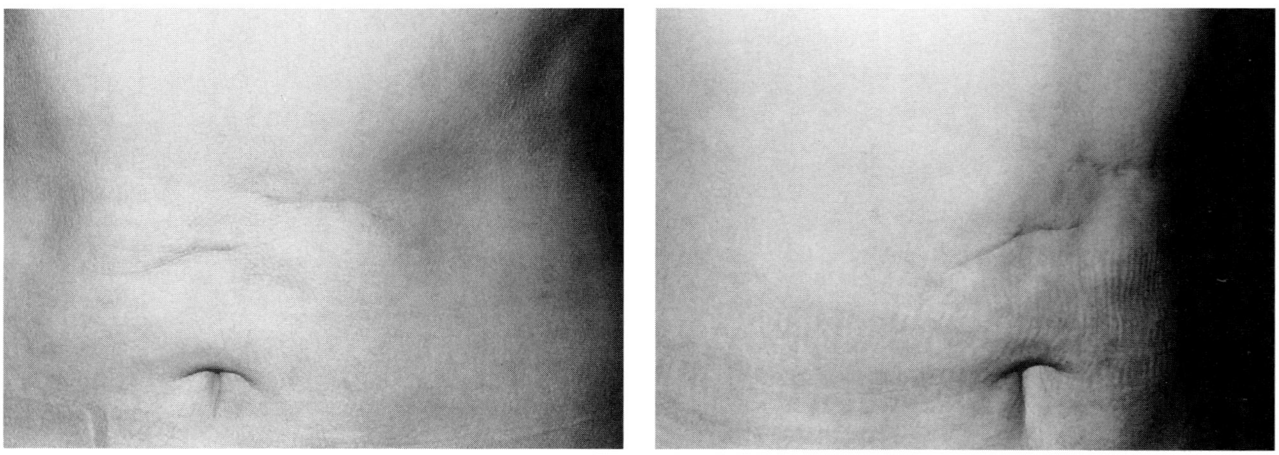

The results are shown 6 months after two consecutive fat injections were performed (with a 4-month interval between) and skin resection for the removal of the necrotic sites. Limited but more acceptable results were obtained.

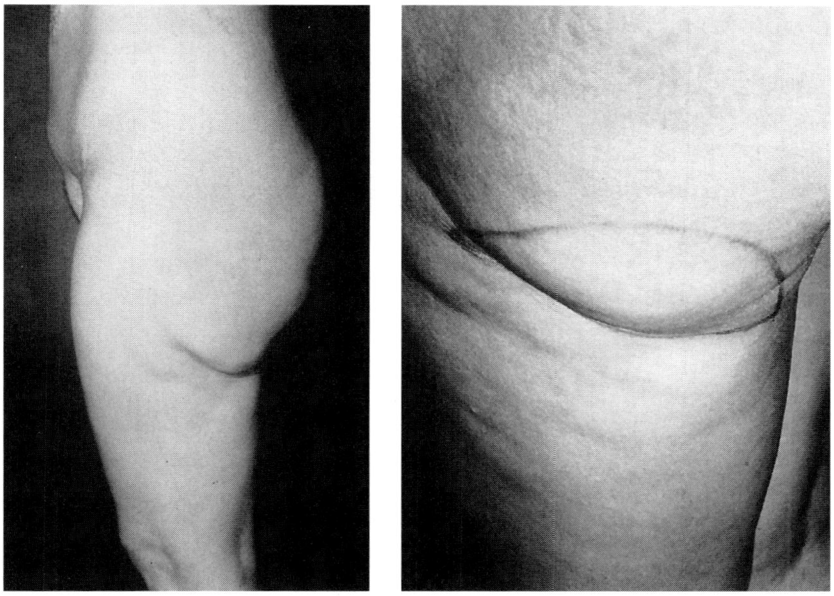

This 39-year-old patient operated on elsewhere presented with lipodystrophy combined with a specific deformity in the femoral lateral region near the lateral gluteal aspect after excessive liposuction. The preoperative profile view shows the skin apron with skin flabbiness evident.

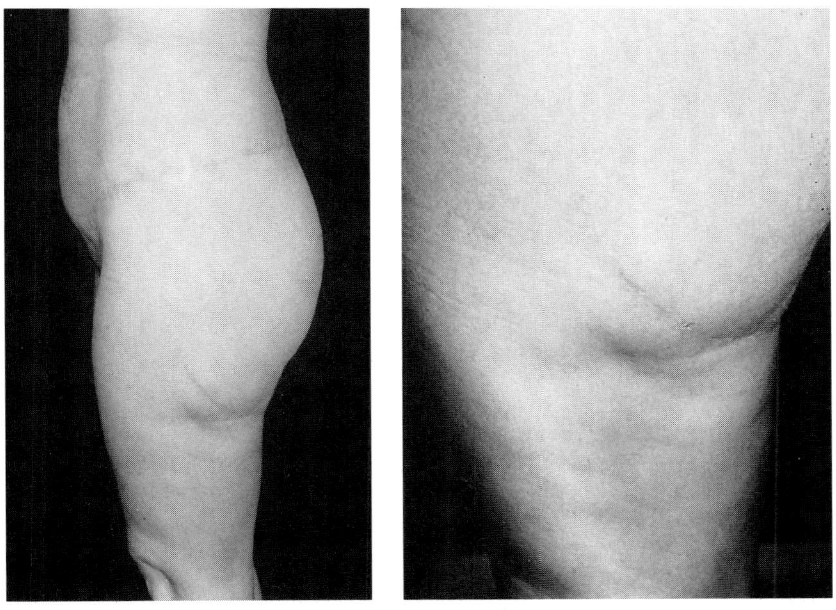

The patient underwent an upper inner thighplasty combined with flankplasty and elliptic skin resection around the deformity. Despite the local skin resection, a residual dimple remains below the suture line. Secondary resection or fat injection could possibly fill the deformity.

PRIMARY OPERATIVE APPROACHES TO ABDOMINAL CONTOURING

Candidates for primary abdominoplasty exhibit fat deposits localized in one or more regions of the anterior abdominal wall, abdominal skin flaccidity, or both. Liposuction, conventional abdominoplasty, or a combined procedure, performed in stages or concurrently, is indicated.

Patients with abdominal fat deposits who have good skin turgor are good candidates for liposuction performed in one stage. The good results are obtained without scars or residual flabby skin. When the fat volume is more significant and there is a moderate degree of skin turgor, the capacity of the skin to retract is reduced. Although volume reduction will be achieved, flabby abdominal skin will result. The extent of liposuction performed should be based on the amount of fat removal possible, not on the surgeon's desire. The skin should retract over the new fat frame within the natural limits. A second liposuction procedure will be indicated if the skin retracts properly; otherwise a miniabdominoplasty or traditional abdominoplasty, perhaps combined with liposuction, is recommended. This determination of future treatment is based on the final result after the first liposuction.

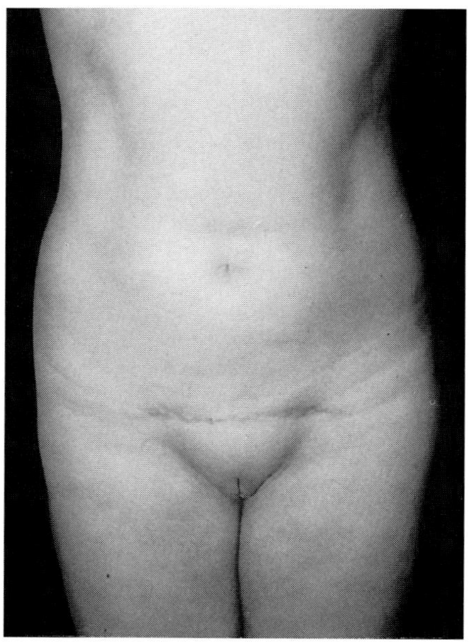

This 33-year-old woman had moderate fat deposits in the anterior abdominal wall combined with mild skin flaccidity at the hypogastric regions and a previous cesarean scar. Liposuction of the entire abdomen and a miniabdominoplasty without umbilical mobilization and an infraumbilical recti plication of the rectus abdominis were performed.

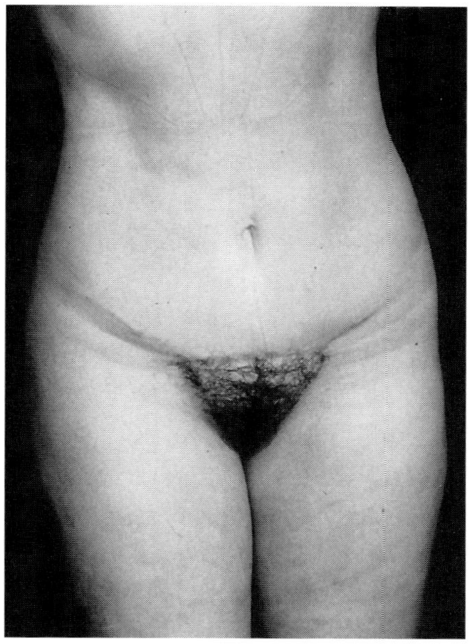

Postoperatively the patient still complained of residual fat left in the hypogastrium and some dog ears at the end of the scar. The dog ears had resulted because we were trying not to extend the incision.

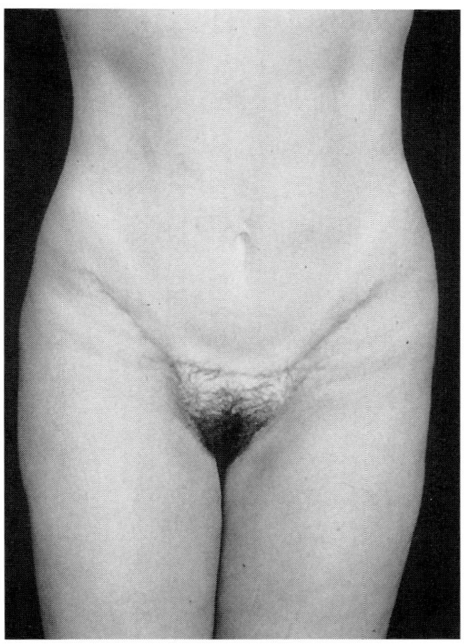

Patient satisfaction was achieved after reoperation with secondary liposuction and resection of the skin excess, leaving a handlebar scar that is hidden under a bikini.

When the abdomen has fat deposits and flabby skin, miniabdominoplasty or traditional abdominoplasty is required. The extent of the problem determines which technique is selected. The miniabdominoplasty, with or without liposuction, offers a moderate resection of excess skin; liposuction can be performed in the same stage. The extended miniabdominoplasty allows plication of the rectus abdominis muscles, which requires umbilicus mobilization.

The umbilicus may be placed in the same position, moved 1 to 2 cm below its original position, or even be amputated. In this last situation, when downward migration of the umbilicus would result in an unaesthetic appearance, neo-umbilicoplasty is performed in the ideal position.

Traditional abdominoplasty is indicated when an excessive amount of skin needs to be resected to obtain good skin turgor. This surgery may be combined with liposuction of the epigastrium and hypochondrium in the same surgical stage. Liposuction should be moderate to preserve the good condition of the skin flap's blood supply. Scar lengthening and the quality of the result should compensate for the previous aesthetic appearance of the abdomen.

Problems Following Abdominal Contouring

Despite the continuous refinements in the surgical treatment of the abdominal wall, several secondary problems can occur that require reoperation. These problems include scarring, residual fat deposits, umbilical distortions, and residual bulges. Very often, liposuction, scar repositioning, and umbilicoplasty are required to remedy these deformities.

Bulging Epigastrium, Hypogastrium, Periumbilicus, and Flanks

All of these regions alone or combined may exhibit residual bulges after miniabdominoplasty or traditional abdominoplasty with or without liposuction performed in the same surgical setting. Although patients often report that no protrusion existed preoperatively, in fact the bulging epigastrium, hypogastrium, and flanks were always present. The abdominoplasty removes only the skin and fat from the umbilicus downward to the pubis in an elliptic-shaped resection. After rectus abdominis muscle plication and the caudal slide of the skin flap, the upper abdominal region (epigastrium) retracts backward mildly compared to the position of the infraumbilicus segment. As a result the epigastrium and the flanks become more protruded and their contour becomes more obvious to the patient. In this situation flankplasty and abdominoplasty are performed in the same stage, which offers the patient an improved contour.

The epigastrium, even after moderate liposuction and before skin undermining during abdominoplasty or after resection of fat excesses below Scarpa's fascia, is still thicker than the area below the incision at the pubis and the inguinal segments. Residual moderate lymphedema of the skin flap can occur, causing the flap to remain swollen for several months postoperatively. This state manifests as an unaesthetic step over the scar line.

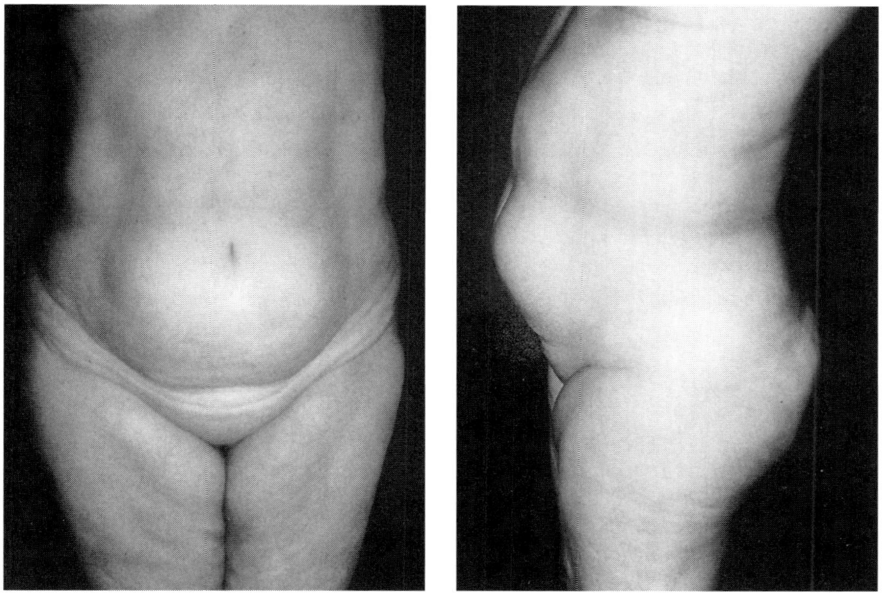

This 61-year-old patient with a thick, adipose panniculus and a protruding abdomen underwent routine abdominoplasty having been informed about the necessity of a complementary liposuction procedure at a minimum of 6 months postoperatively.

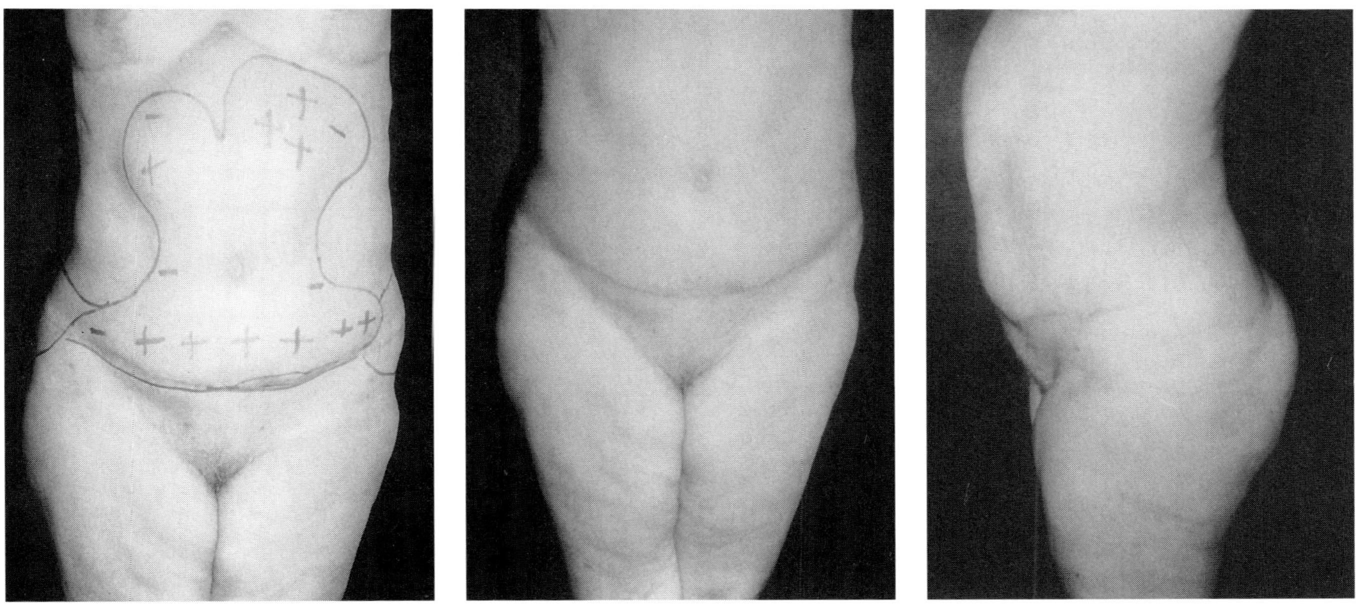

Eight months later the patient underwent liposuction as marked and scar revision. The final result is shown 6 months following the second surgery.

Skin Laxity, Fat Deposits, Scars, and Umbilical Malposition

Secondary skin laxity in the anterior abdominal wall usually occurs after excessive liposuction. Residual and localized fat deposits, as well as unacceptable scars and unaesthetic umbilical position or shape, also may be present after primary abdominoplasty.

Miniabdominoplasty or traditional abdominoplasty, alone or in combination with other procedures, is indicated to solve these problems. The nonextended miniabdominoplasty is performed without umbilicus mobilization. It affects only the hypogastrium where rectus abdominis muscle plication may or may not be performed. With miniabdominoplasty the entire region is undermined to the umbilical level for fascia plication. With traditional abdominoplasty undermining is performed up to the xiphoid. In both procedures a transverse elliptic skin resection is performed at the suprapubic level. Suturing is performed in a straight or arcuate line 13 to 18 cm in length, depending on the amount of skin resection.

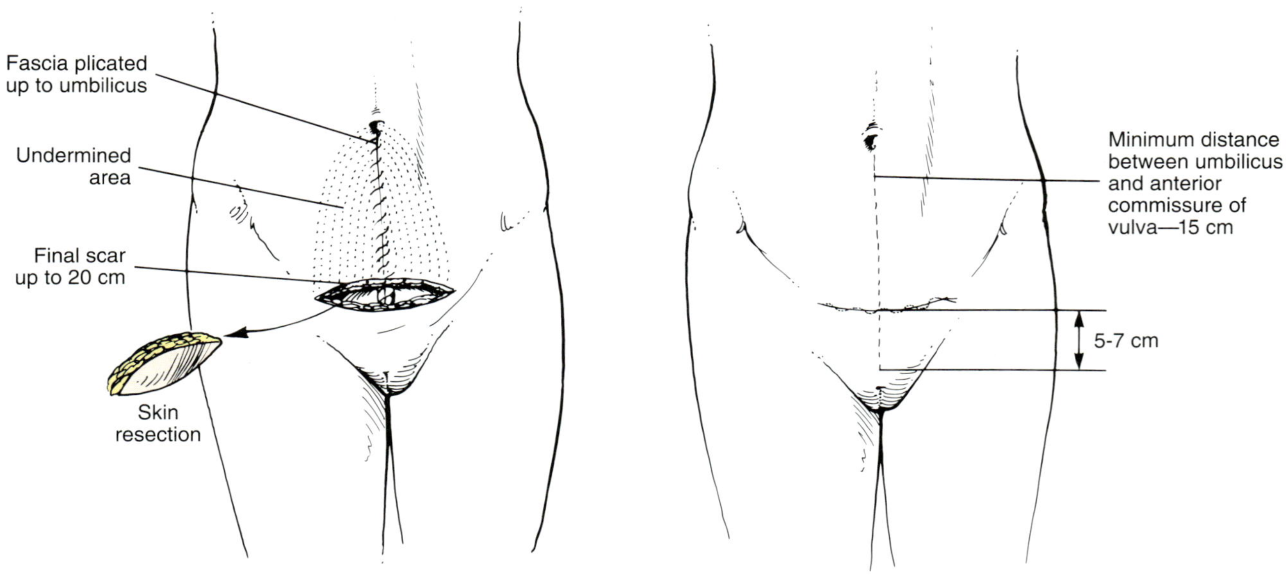

Nonextended miniabdominoplasty

The nonextended miniabdominoplasty is performed in patients undergoing primary and secondary abdominoplasty in whom liposuction in one or more abdominal wall regions is indicated. A small skin ellipse is resected transversely at the pubis level. In some situations undermining up to the umbilicus with or without rectus abdominis muscle plication can be combined. The final scar (up to 20 cm in length) is placed transversely in the pubis no more than 7 cm above the anterior vulvar commissure.

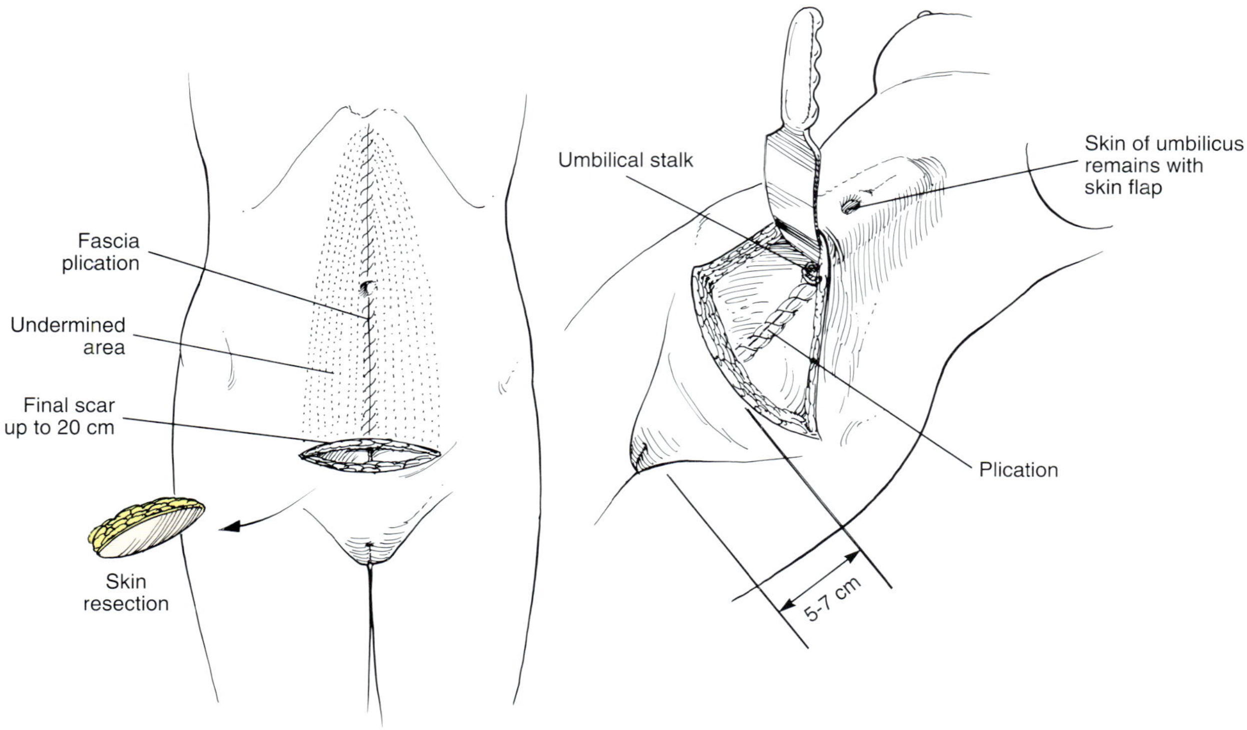

Extended miniabdominoplasty

The extended miniabdominoplasty is performed in patients undergoing primary and secondary abdominoplasty. The skin incision is similar to that used in the nonextended miniabdominoplasty. Indications for liposuction in the abdominal wall regions are also similar to those that apply to the nonextended miniabdominoplasty. Undermining is performed in a triangular area and extends to the xiphoid level. The umbilicus is sectioned from its pedicle to facilitate plication. A special retractor with a long sheet is placed to expose the extended tunnel. With the tunnel open, plication is performed in two planes. Isolated 2-0 nylon stitches are placed from the xiphoid to the pubis. A second continuous suture line, also with 2-0 nylon, is placed over the first. The skin is stretched caudally, the excess skin is resected, and two suction drains are placed in the dissected area and through the pubis. The umbilicus may be replaced in its original position or 1 to 2 cm below it. Two transfixion stitches are made to bite the umbilical skin and the fascia below and to emerge again through the umbilical skin. When the stitches are tightened, the umbilical depth is obtained again. A gauze pad is placed over the stitches to aid in cicatrization during the first 5 postoperative days.

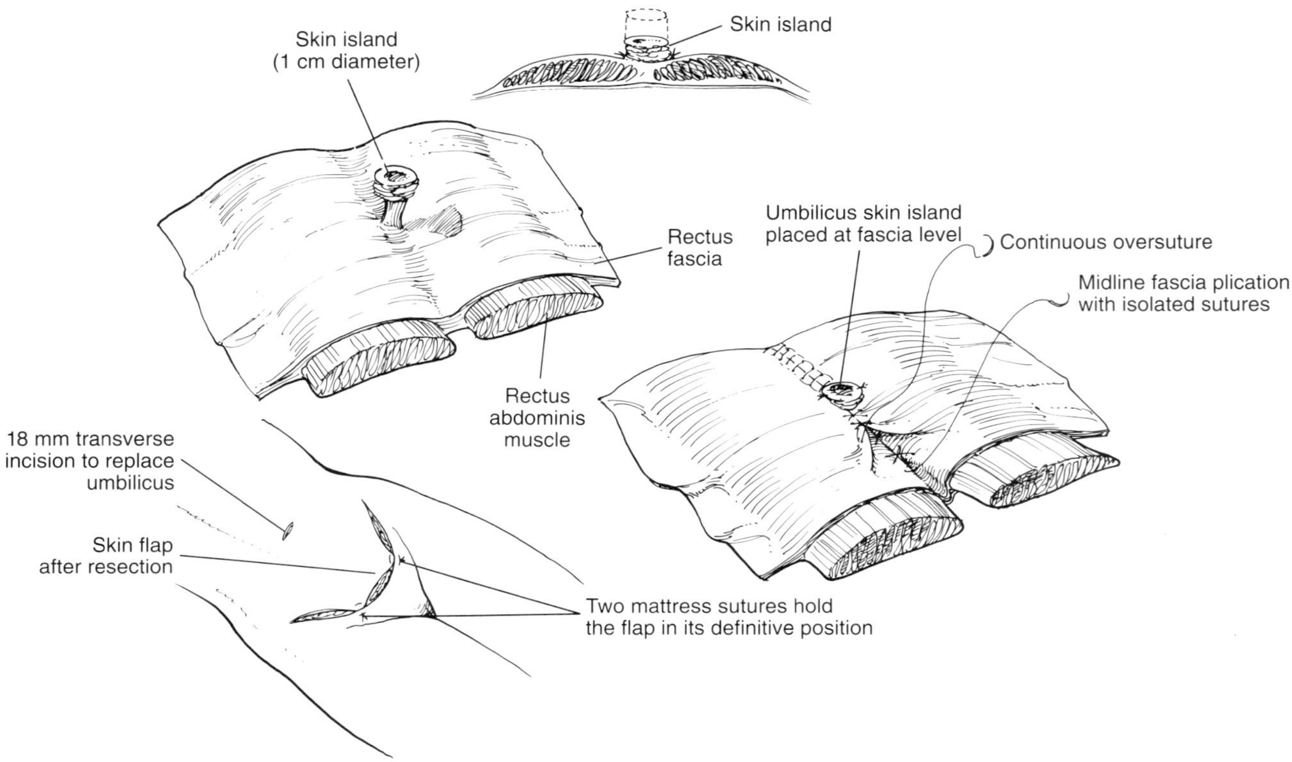

Umbilicoplasty

In patients in whom the umbilicus remains below the aesthetic level (less than 15 cm from the anterior vulvar commissure), reoperative umbilicoplasty is indicated. The umbilicus is resected from the abdominal skin flap through an elliptic vertical incision. The umbilical stalk is dissected, and a skin island 1 cm in diameter is left in its free extremity. Fascia plication shortens the stalk and places the skin island at the level of the umbilicus. The umbilical hole at the skin flap is sutured in three planes, leaving a vertical suture 3 to 5 cm in length. The skin flap is stretched caudally and the excesses are resected. Between 15 to 18 cm from the anterior vulvar commissure an 18 mm transverse skin incision is made at the xiphoid-pubic line to place the umbilicus in its final position. Below this incision, fat is resected in a circular fashion. Four stitches are placed in the cardinal positions around the skin incision. These sutures are isolated 2-0 nylon stitches that bite the skin edge, go deep and bite the fascia and umbilicus skin island, and then emerge through the skin incision. When the stitches are tightened, the wound closure becomes circular. Another eight isolated 4-0 nylon stitches are placed around the umbilicus to complete the closure. A natural invagination is obtained with the skin island placed below. A gauze bolster covered with ointment is placed on the umbilicus in a Brown-type pad and remains in place for the first 5 postoperative days.

The pubic incision is closed in three suture planes: subcutaneous plane with isolated 2-0 Vicryl sutures, dermal plane with isolated 3-0 Vicryl sutures, and intracuticular plane with running 4-0 Vicryl sutures. Vacuum drains that emerge through the pubis are placed in the undermined area. Micropore material is placed over the suture and ABD pads are placed on the abdominal wall. The patient leaves the surgical room wearing an elastic girdle.

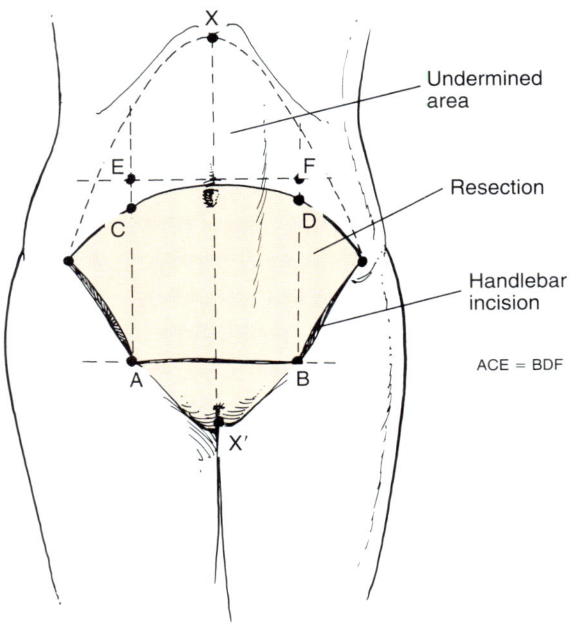

Traditional abdominoplasty

Traditional abdominoplasty is indicated when skin flaccidity of the entire anterior abdominal wall is evident and when skin resection involves the entire hypogastrium. For this procedure I have been using a new type of low transverse pubic-inguinal incision rather than the handlebar incision used previously. The skin is marked in the following manner: A vertical line from the xiphoid to the vertex of the anterior vulvar commissure (X-X^1) determines the abdominal midline for the future position of the umbilicus. Two transverse and parallel lines are placed perpendicular to this line, one at the upper level of the umbilicus (E-F) and the other 5 to 7 cm above the anterior vulvar commissure (A-B). According to the pubis volume and limits, two reference points (A and B) are marked at the transverse pubic line and are placed 5 to 7 cm from the central vertical line bilaterally. Similar reference points (E and F) are bilaterally placed at the transverse line at the umbilical level. The distance of A-E should equal that of B-F. The length of these lines is usually 10 to 14 cm and varies according to the shape of the pubis and the volume of the patient's hips. At this point the assistant stretches the lower abdominal skin upward with both hands and with equal tension. This maneuver eliminates all skin flabbiness in the hypogastrium and inguinal regions. From points A and B a line is drawn toward the anterior superior iliac spine on each side. These lines have a concave, curved configuration. Small variations in this marking may exist and are acceptable if this curved line extends only a few centimeters inside or outside the iliac spine. A concave, curved line is drawn from the extremities of the iliac spine on each side and up to above the umbilicus. These lines intersect the lines A-E and B-F at points C and D bilaterally. The distance A-C-E and D-B-F should be equal for symmetric resections and for aesthetic scar positioning. Temporary key stitches during the surgery are placed at points A, B, C, and D to serve as reference points in case the ink markings become smeared. These stitches are removed at the end of the operation.

The demarcated ellipse represents the skin segment to be resected. The triangular shadowed area from the xiphoid to the iliac spines represents the region to be undermined. The iliac spines, A-B and C-D, represent the area to be resected.

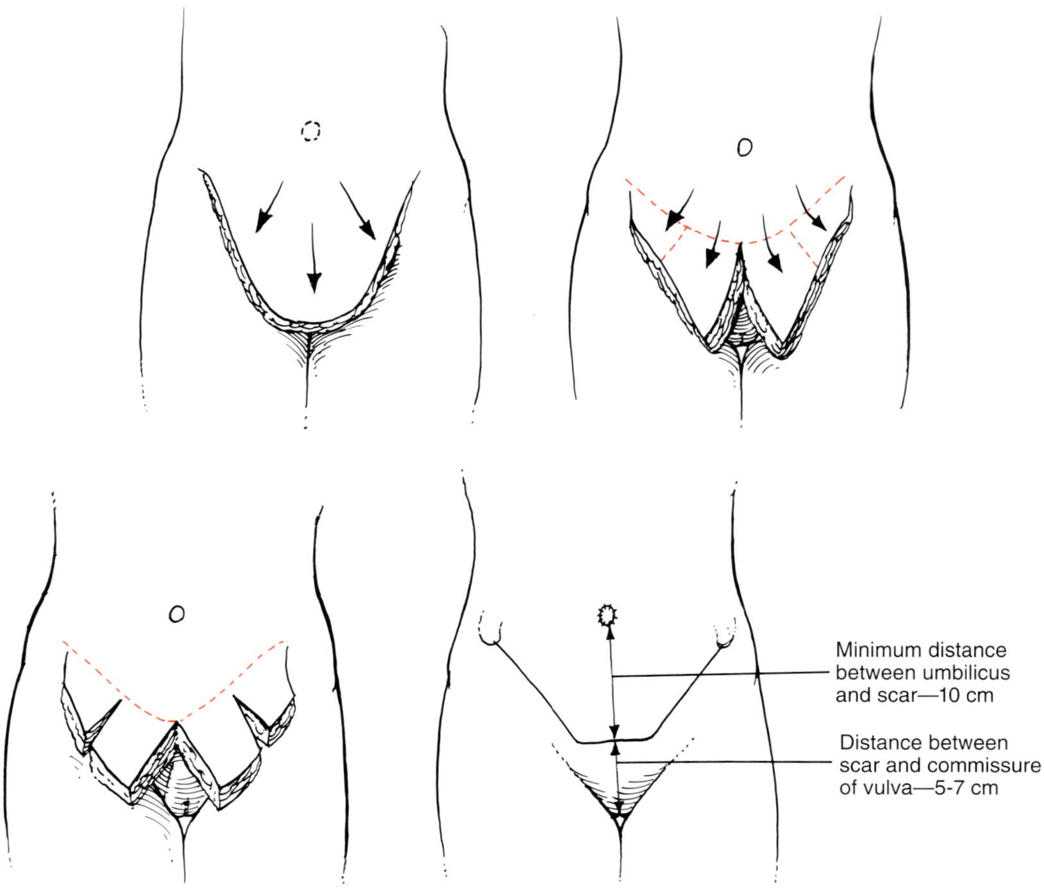

After rectus abdominis muscle plication, the abdominal skin flap is stretched caudally. The flap is divided in two parts along the central vertical line (X-X[1]), and a mattress stitch is placed to fixate the pubis to the upper umbilical hole after its dissection from the abdominal skin flap. Each half of the skin flap is incised along the lines A-C-E and B-D-F equally. Two mattress stitches are placed, one at point A and one at point B. The four flaps are resected. Finally the wound is closed in three planes as has been described earlier. Umbilicoplasty is performed according to the previously described technique before the final closure.

Reoperative abdominoplasty follows the routine procedure: skin undermining, rectus abdominis muscle plication, excess skin resection, umbilicoplasty, and placement of the final sutures. ***Based on personal experience, an important point to remember is that skin flap undermining should be as conservative as possible to reduce the extent of the resulting dead space.*** The area of the flap that is undermined has a triangular configuration: the base is positioned along the lower transverse incision and the vertex is at the xiphoid appendix. With this pattern of undermining the skin flap blood supply remains better preserved and the risk of postoperative hematoma or seroma is reduced. Umbilicoplasty is performed as described for extended miniabdominoplasty and traditional abdominoplasty.

The excess skin flap resection and suturing are also performed routinely. The final closure resembles a handlebar. The pubic low transverse suture segment is 10 to 14 cm in length (or longer depending on its volume), placed 5 to 7 cm above the anterior vulvar commissure. The two lateral segments that run above the inguinal crest toward the iliac crest bilaterally can be of variable length depending on the volume of the hips.

Scar Malposition

Abdominoplasty through a traditional low transverse pubic-inguinal incision as was performed before liposuction was introduced is now the third most popular option for aesthetic abdominal treatment, with liposuction being the first choice and miniabdominoplasty the second. The presence of vertical scars in the abdominal wall or transverse scars in the epigastrium or hypogastrium from previous surgical procedures will influence the type of procedure chosen: liposuction, surgery, or both.

The most common secondary problems observed after routine abdominoplasty are scar malposition and unacceptable scar quality (e.g., broad, hypertrophic, keloid). Often the scar is too high in the hypogastrium, placed 10 to 14 cm above the anterior vulvar commissure, and runs transversely to the root of the thighs instead of toward the anterior superior iliac spine bilaterally. Very often the scar appears as an open W and is exposed when the patient wears a bathing suit. The pubic scar becomes exposed because it is too high, and the lateral scar segments are also exposed because they are too low at the thigh root. It is the exact reverse of the ideal scar, which is high laterally and low in the pubis so that it remains hidden by the V shape of a bikini.

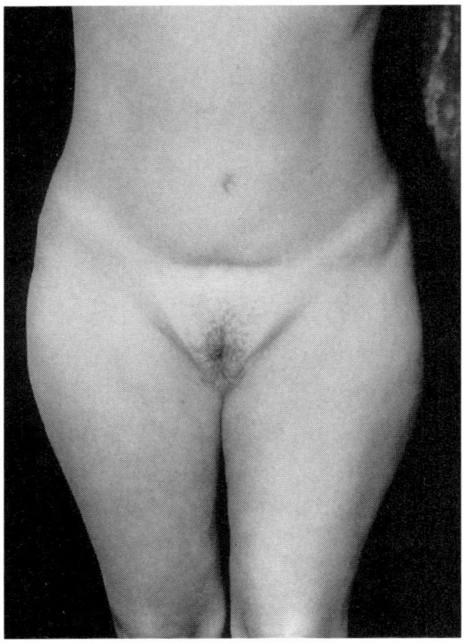

Following abdominoplasty this 45-year-old patient was left with a scar that extended as a straight transverse line, very high at the pubis and running to the root of the thighs. The tan lines reveal that the scar remains exposed. The umbilicus is also dislocated laterally.

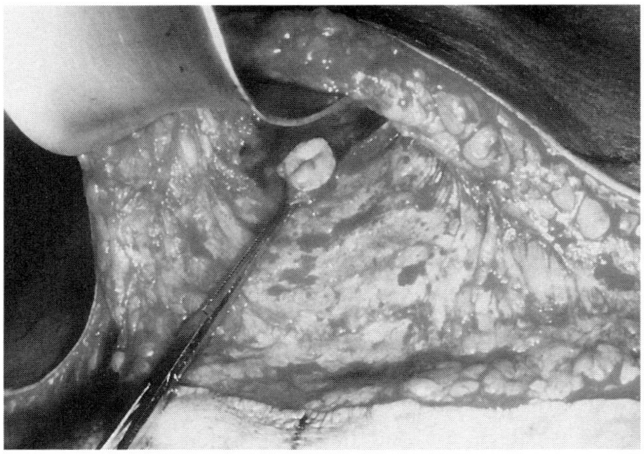

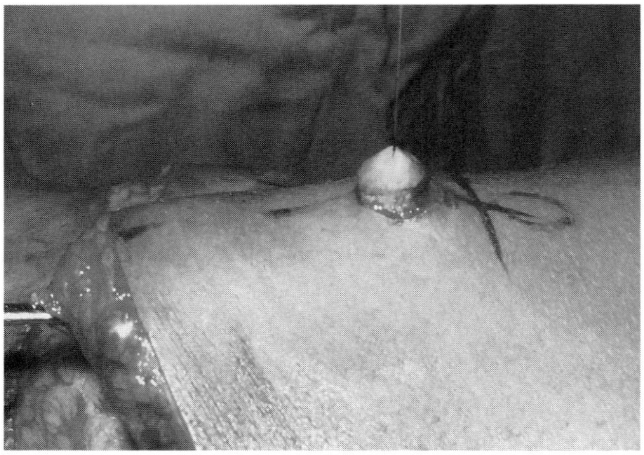

The scar was revised by a handlebar incision so that the scar is now completely hidden by the bathing suit. The incision was extended toward the iliac spine to allow resection of skin flabbiness near the flanks. The umbilical pedicle was dissected from the skin flap and a small skin island was left in its free extremity.

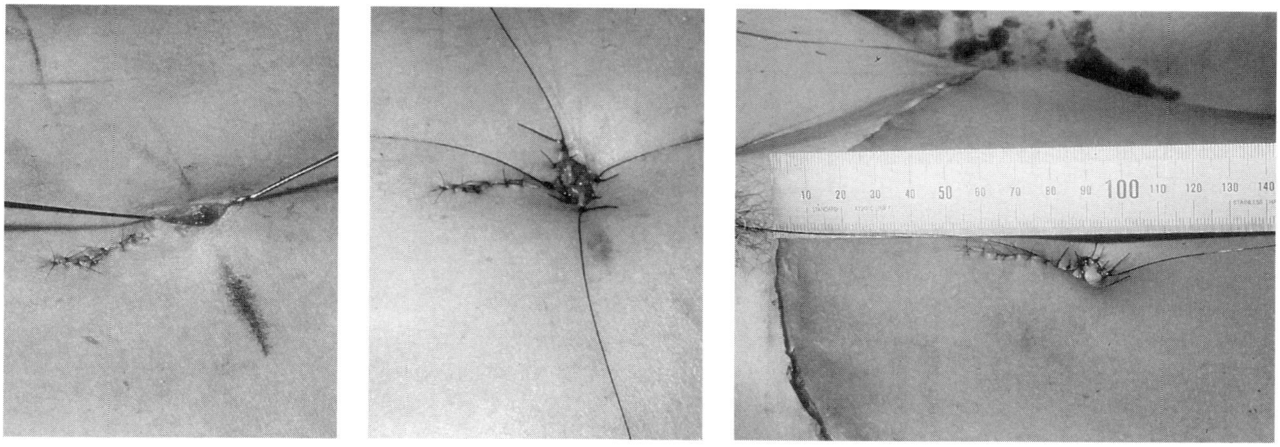

To correct the excessively low umbilical pedicle position (less than 10 cm from the vulvar anterior commissure), the primitive umbilical skin hole was sutured and a new opening a few centimeters above was made. Routine umbilicoplasty was performed. The distance of the new position of the umbilicus remains 9 cm from the pubic incision. Transversely it is not the ideal distance, but the position is acceptable in this case.

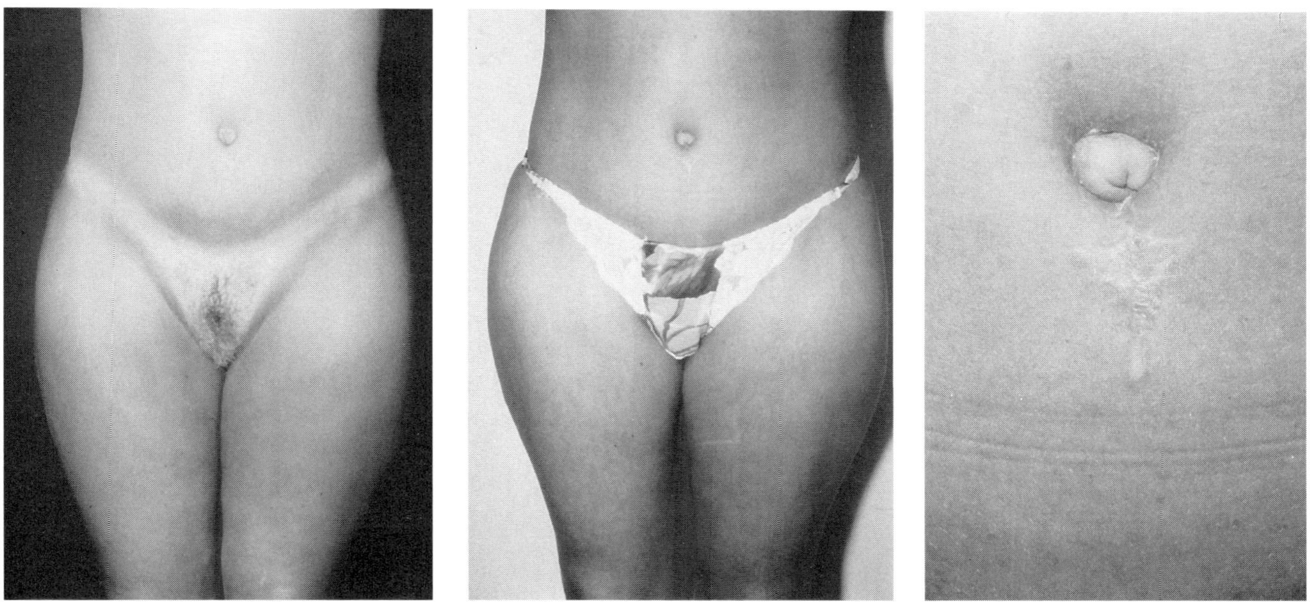

Eight months after reoperative surgery the scar and overall abdominal appearance are much improved. The scar is now hidden by the bikini. There is an inconspicuous scar below the final umbilicus. The disadvantage of this small scar is more than offset by the advantage of a well-placed umbilicus.

Incorrect Placement of Umbilicus

The umbilicus is the only natural scar in the body that is acceptable aesthetically. Distortions in its shape and position can draw negative attention. Several types of surgical umbilicoplasty attempt to reproduce the natural aspect of the umbilicus. The surgeon should select the technique that can offer the best result. Unfortunately, aesthetic problems secondary to umbilical surgery are common. Stenosis, resulting in a big umbilical hole, and malposition are the most common complaints associated with the umbilicus and are usually due to keloid reaction, necrosis, infection, or dehiscence.

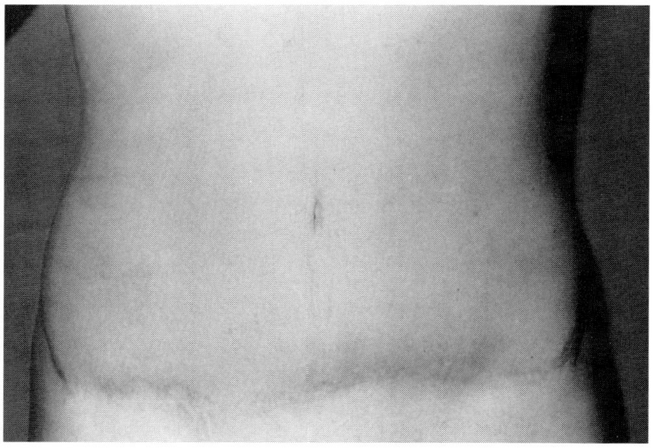

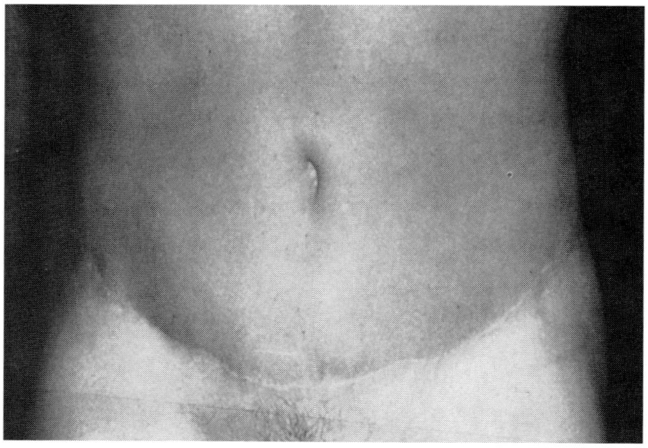

This 47-year-old patient exhibited a combined problem of unacceptable scar position and a stenotic umbilicus following a previous surgery. During reoperative surgery the scar was revised to resemble a handlebar shape and umbilicoplasty was performed in the same stage. The result is shown 1 year postoperatively.

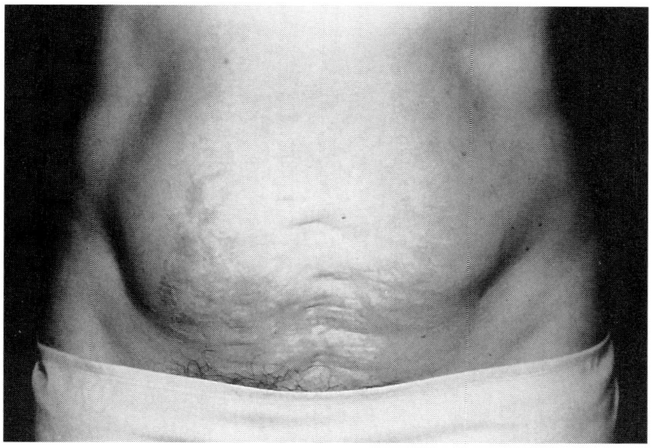

Following an abdominal procedure this patient was left with several scars located in the hypogastrium after secondary healing of an infection in the abdominal wall. The umbilicus had been completely lost.

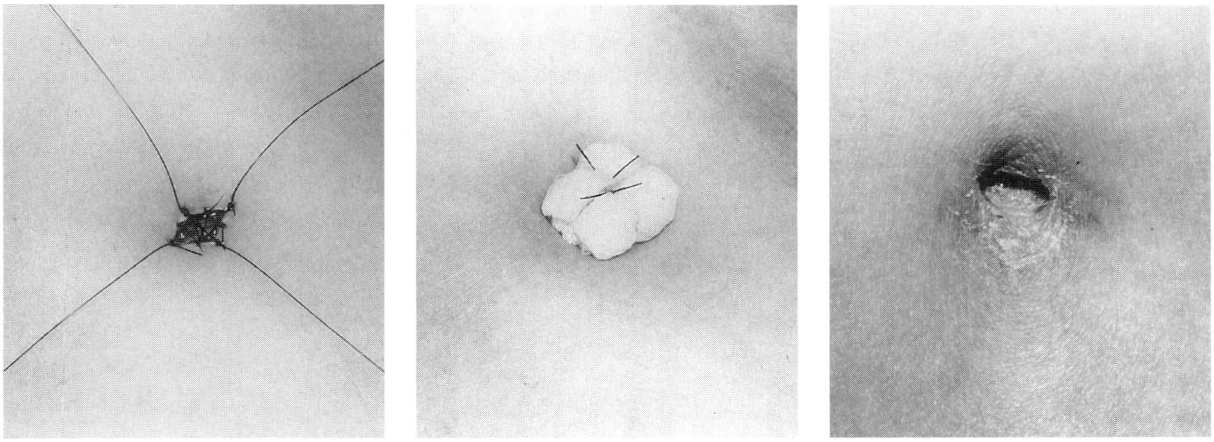

To correct this problem, routine abdominoplasty was performed with complete skin resection of the hypogastrium. Neoumbilicoplasty was performed in the same surgical stage. A transverse skin incision was made and a defatting maneuver was performed. Several stitches fixed the skin incision edges to the deep fascia. A Brown-type bandage was placed over the neoumbilicus and removed 5 days postoperatively. The wound was allowed to heal by secondary intention.

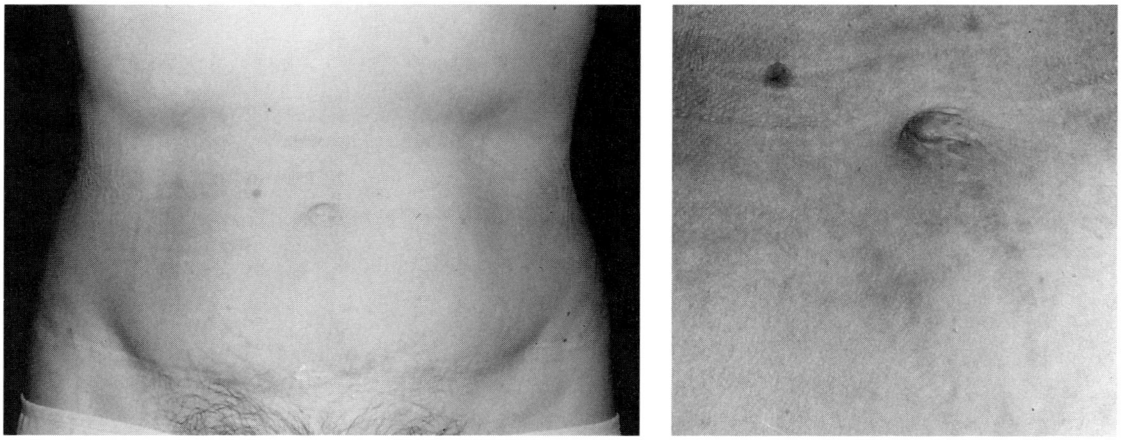

The final postoperative result is shown.

FLANK PROCEDURES

Well-proportioned flanks contribute to an aesthetic body contour. Often these regions have large fat deposits and skin flaccidity, causing unattractive bilateral bulges. When too voluminous, these bulges disrupt the harmony of the female curves and buttocks, creating square-appearing hips. Liposuction has become the elective treatment of choice for large flanks without skin flaccidity. In patients with large fat deposits and flaccid skin in this area, flankplasty based on an extended fusiform skin resection is still the only operative solution. This surgery leaves long bilateral scars that run from the anterior superior to the posterior superior iliac spine. When fat deposits and flaccid skin are present, lipoplasty is combined with flankplasty in the same surgical stage.

After traditional abdominoplasty, bulging flanks may appear more prominent. Removal of the hypogastrium skin makes the abdomen flat, exposing the flank excesses. These fat deposits always existed but were less evident preoperatively. In this situation flankplasty and abdominoplasty should be performed in the same stage, which offers the patient a better contour.

Flankplasty is a fusiform skin and fat resection from the anterior superior to the posterior superior iliac spine. The amount of resection necessary is estimated by the pinch test. The surgery starts with the patient in a prone position. The skin ellipse is resected in its posterior and lateral segments. Closure is performed in three planes: deep sutures with isolated 2-0 Vicryl stitches to eliminate the dead space, dermal sutures with isolated 3-0 Vicryl stitches, and running intracuticular sutures with 4-0 Vicryl. The residual skin redundancy above the sacral region requires that the excess be resected and the suture lines be joined, leaving a V-shaped closure. The skin excesses at the lateral aspect of the flanks are protected by ABD pads while the patient is turned to the supine position. The excesses are then resected. The final closure is performed in three planes as described earlier. The final suture is placed along or a few centimeters below the iliac posterior crest up to the anterior superior iliac spine. No drains are required.

Problems Following Flank Procedures

The most common secondary aesthetic problems after flankplasty are related to insufficient fat removal and skin flaccidity. Insufficient fat removal requires secondary liposuction, whereas skin resection alone is indicated to treat flaccid skin.

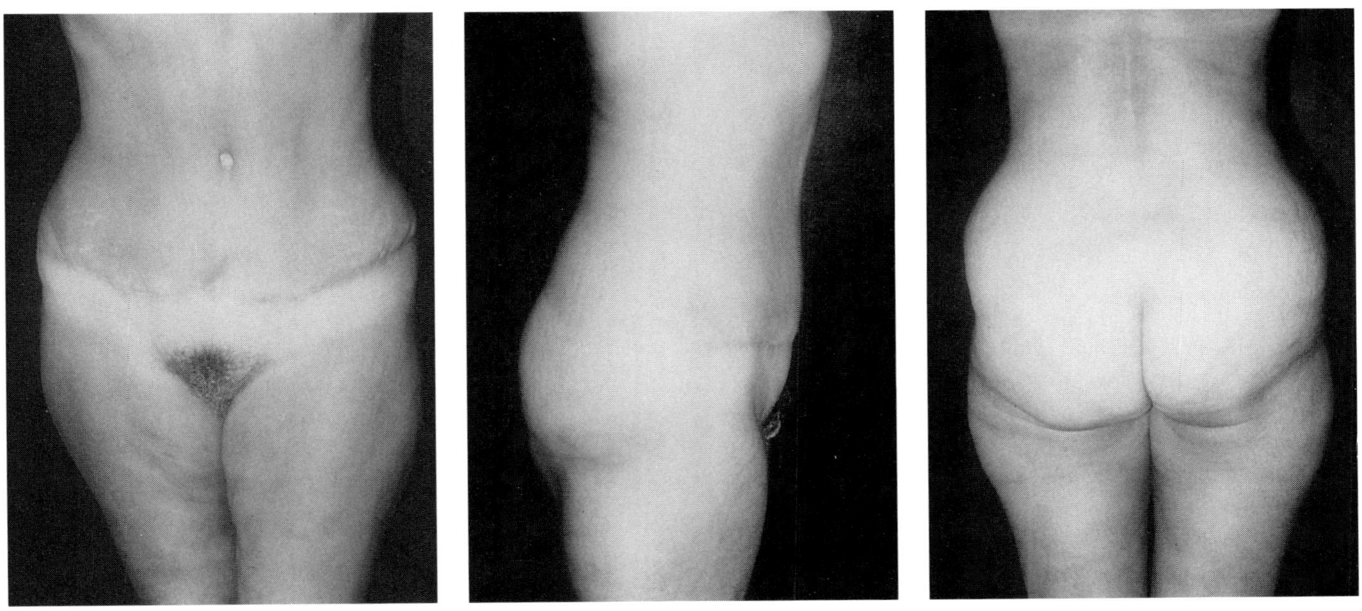

A 55-year-old patient on whom we performed a routine abdominoplasty returned 1 year later complaining of bulges and irregularities in the anterior abdominal wall and in the flanks.

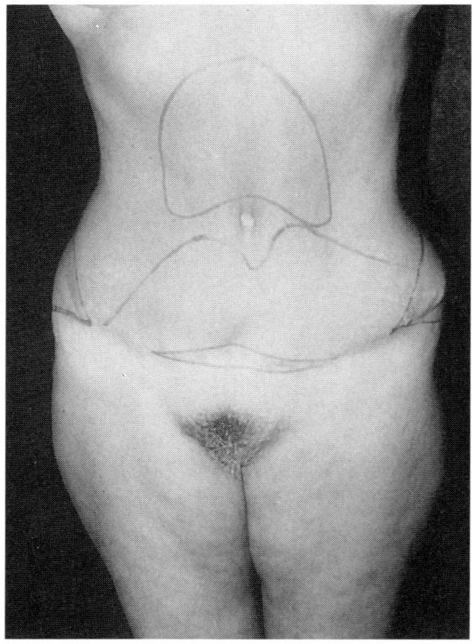

Scar revision combined with flankplasty and liposuction of the epigastrium and hypogastrium were proposed. No undermining or umbilical mobilization was necessary.

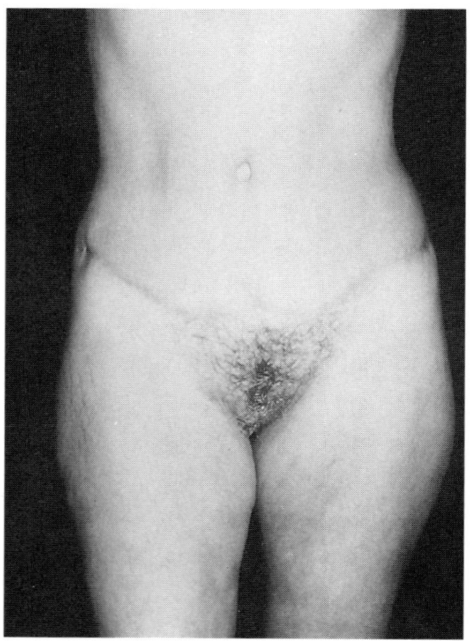

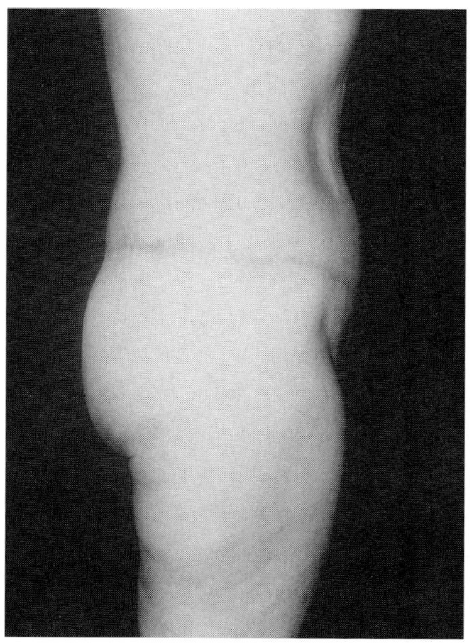

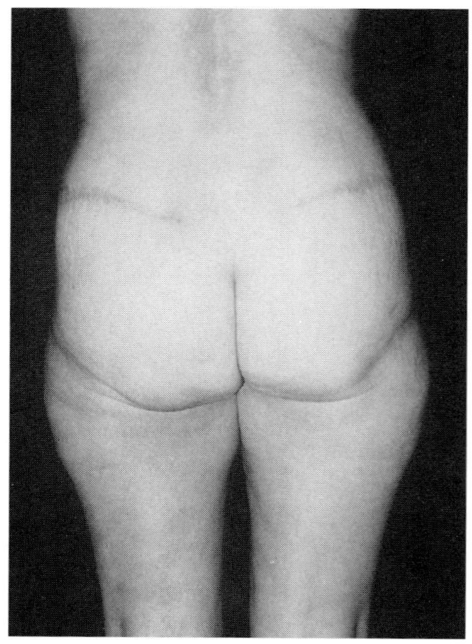

The result 6 months postoperatively shows the improved body contour. The new scar, along the flanks and the pubic-inguinal lines, can now be hidden by a bathing suit. The flank bulge excesses have been eliminated.

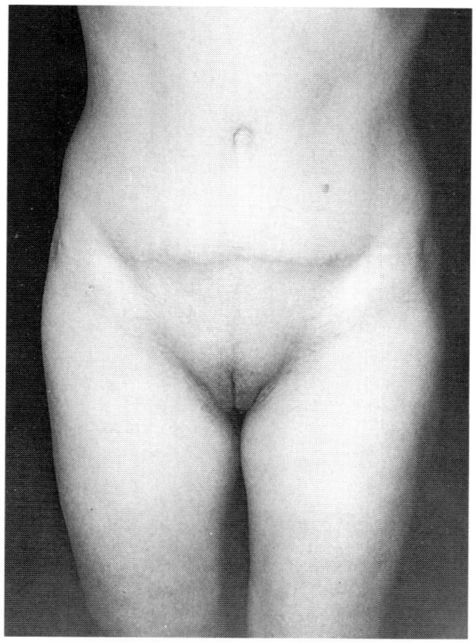

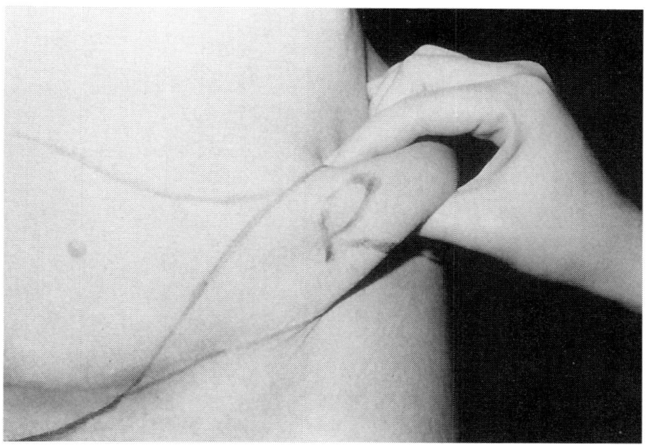

We performed abdominoplasty on this 50-year-old patient 8 years earlier. The final scar remained too high and was placed transversely up to the root of the thighs. The patient wanted the scar to be hidden by her bathing suit and she requested the removal of the skin excesses at the iliac crest roll.

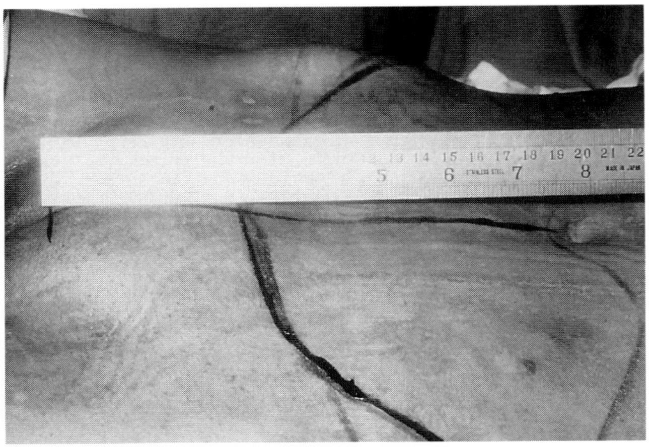

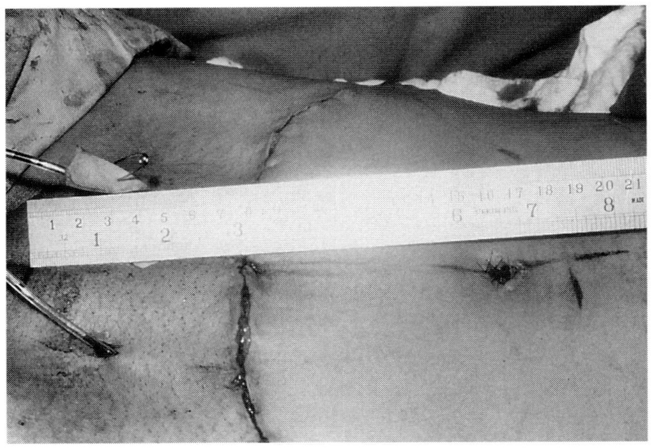

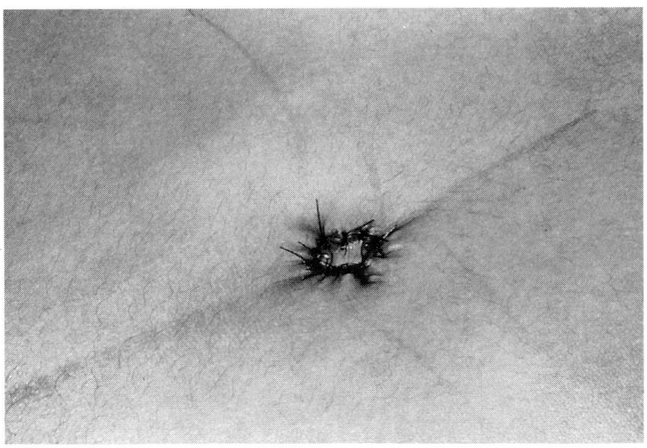

The distance from the pubic scar to the anterior vulvar commissure was 11 cm. To correct this problem, the abdominal wall skin was dissected up to the xiphoid; the umbilicus was also dissected from its position. The skin flap was slid caudally and the original scar was resected. The final suture line was 8 cm from the anterior vulvar commissure and 16.5 cm from the umbilicus, placing the umbilicus in a normal aesthetic position. The umbilicus was sutured in place to the abdominal skin flap.

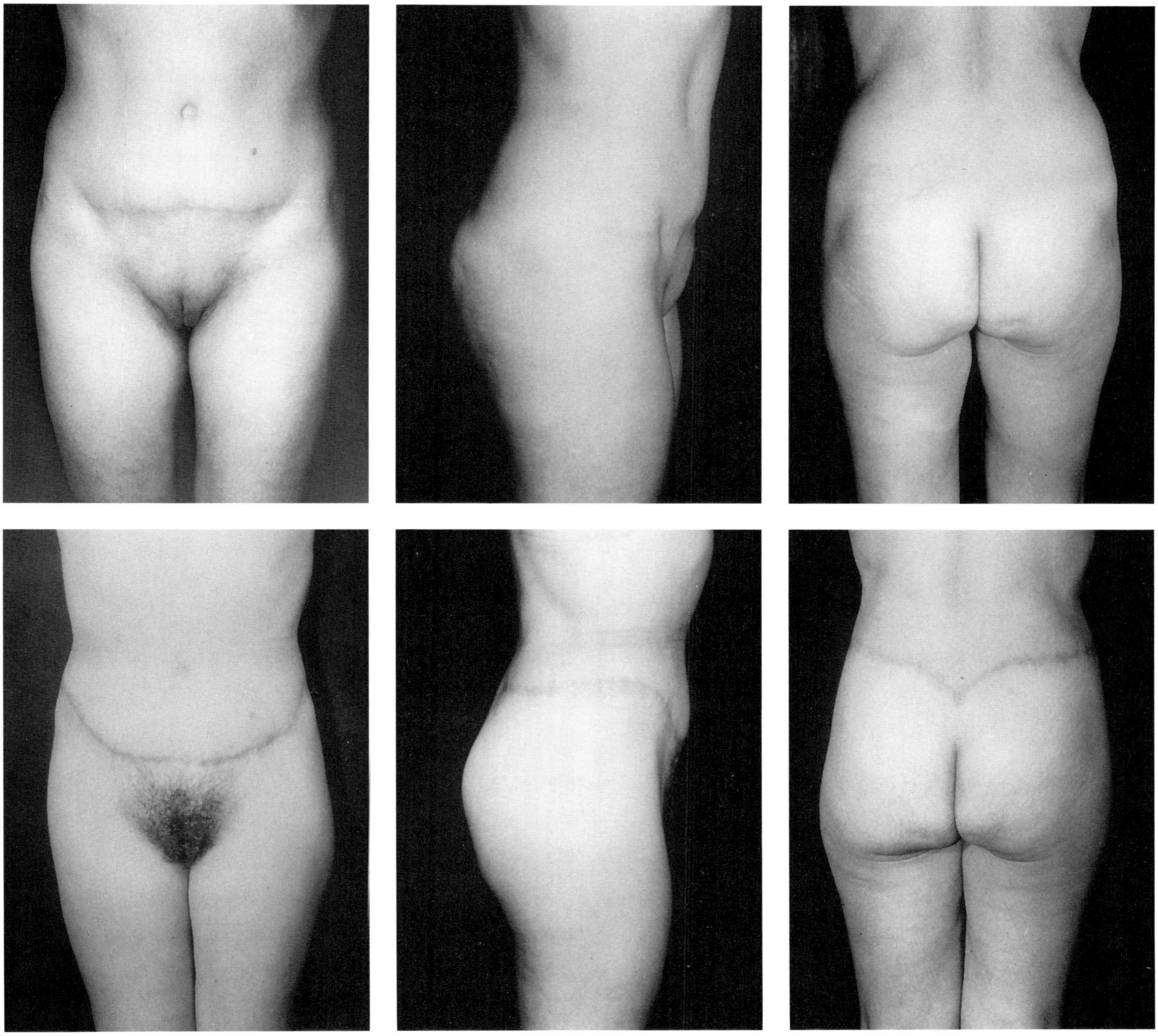

Three months postoperatively the patient now has a handlebar-shaped scar that extends around the flanks. The scar lines run along the flank regions and extend to the anterior superior iliac spine and posterior iliac crest projection. The body contour reveals a new shape; the flank bulges, skin flaccidity, excessive skin laxity over the sacral region, and the buttocks ptosis have been eliminated. Although the resection was performed in a belt shape, the final scar is shaped like a V.

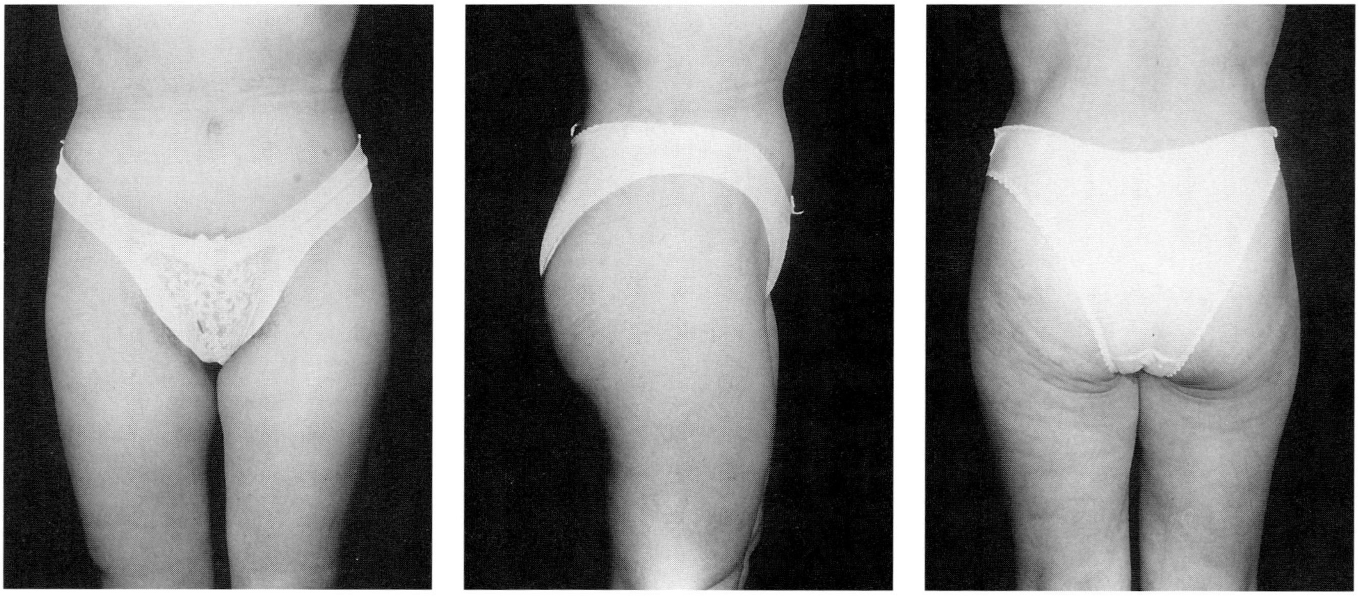

The patient's underwear now completely hides the scar that encircles her body.

COMBINED FLANKPLASTY AND ABDOMINOPLASTY

A number of different types of surgical procedures can be performed on the flanks and abdomen depending on the specific secondary problems. Liposuction and surgery, alone or in combination, are routinely performed on these regions.

When flankplasty and abdominoplasty are performed in the same stage, flankplasty is performed first with the patient in a prone position. An extensive fusiform skin resection is undertaken as was described earlier. The patient is then placed in a supine position and abdominoplasty is performed.

With these combined procedures some precautions are necessary. Skin undermining of the epigastrium and hypogastrium should be conservative to avoid severing the skin flap blood supply. In addition, at the point at which the flanks meet the abdomen, excess skin should be dissected as little as possible; any dissection that is performed should be as symmetric as possible.

The final suture line follows the transverse pubic and inguinal lines to a few centimeters above the anterior superior iliac spine, runs parallel to the posterior iliac line, and ends before reaching the intergluteal sulcus. When the incision extends to the other side, the closure is V shaped. Steri-Strips are placed over the entire suture line, and suction drains are inserted in the abdominal area and are left in place up to 3 days. ABD pads are used to cover the suture line, and an elastic girdle is worn by the patient for 1 month postoperatively.

BUTTOCKS PROCEDURES

The buttocks is one of the body regions that exhibits significant shape and volume variations among individuals. Genetics, aging, body weight changes, and life-style contribute to these variations. Skin retraction of the buttocks is more limited when compared to other regions of the body; this limited retraction capacity becomes progressively evident with the aging process. The buttocks may be flat, protruded, voluminous, drooped, or small. Liposuction, volume reduction, and volume augmentation with silicone implants can be used to improve the appearance of the buttocks. Regardless of the procedure used, secondary problems requiring reoperative solutions can occur.

Problems Following Buttocks Procedures

The most common problems in the buttocks that call for reoperation are flabbiness and drooping subsequent to excessive fat removal via liposuction with poor skin retraction. In this situation the buttocks may become flaccid and drooped with a deep gluteal fold. Liposuction is indicated only when good skin turgor is present and there is only moderate fat volume. Flabbiness can be corrected by two methods: skin resection at the gluteal fold and/or flankplasty in which a more extended incision is made up to the lateral portion of the gluteal fold. Flankplasty in which the incisions on the sacral projection are not joined may be indicated to improve buttocks shape, volume, and skin turgor.

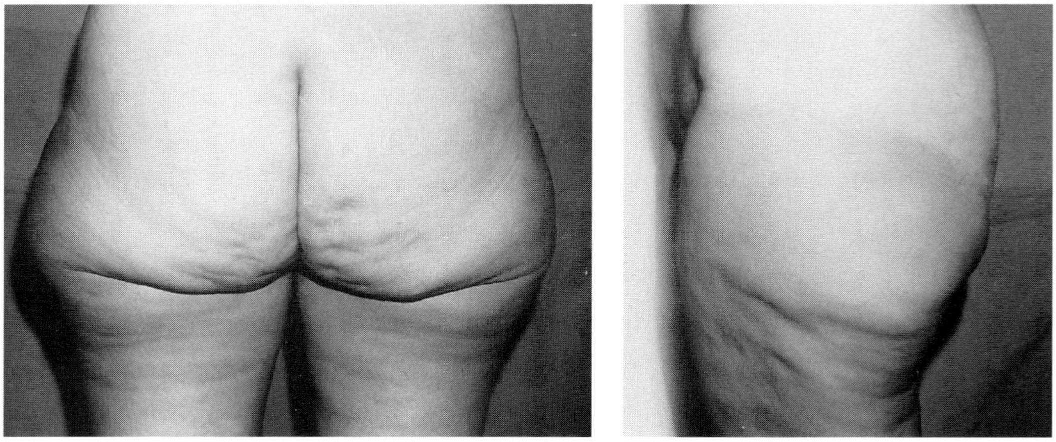

This 54-year-old patient had sagging buttocks after excessive liposuction. A deep gluteal fold combined with skin flaccidity and lateral femoral fat deposits also contributed to the body contour distortions. A semicircular Pitanguy technique was performed.

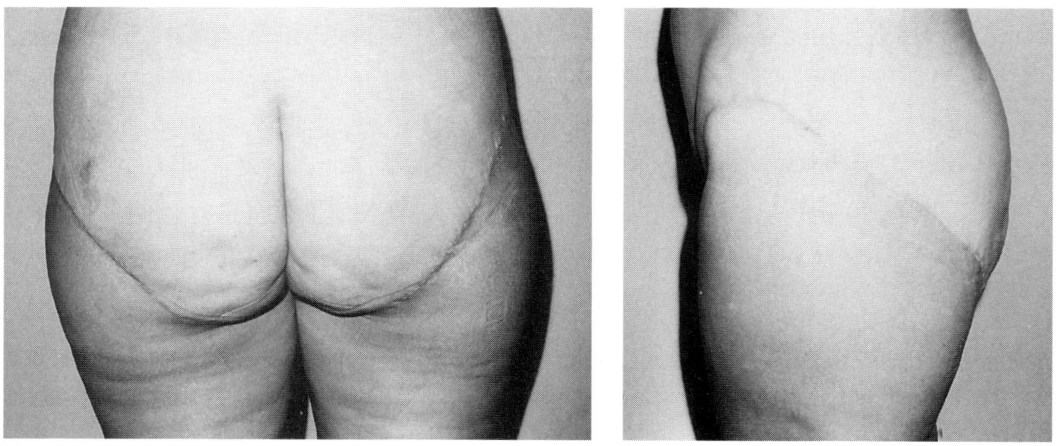

Despite the improvement in contour, the scar is quite evident. The skin does acquire improved turgor with this procedure, making this surgery acceptable for certain cases.

Surgical augmentation of the buttocks became an acceptable procedure after the introduction of the Roble technique in 1984 in which a silicone implant is placed into a pocket between the muscular plane of the hip and the gluteus maximus muscle.

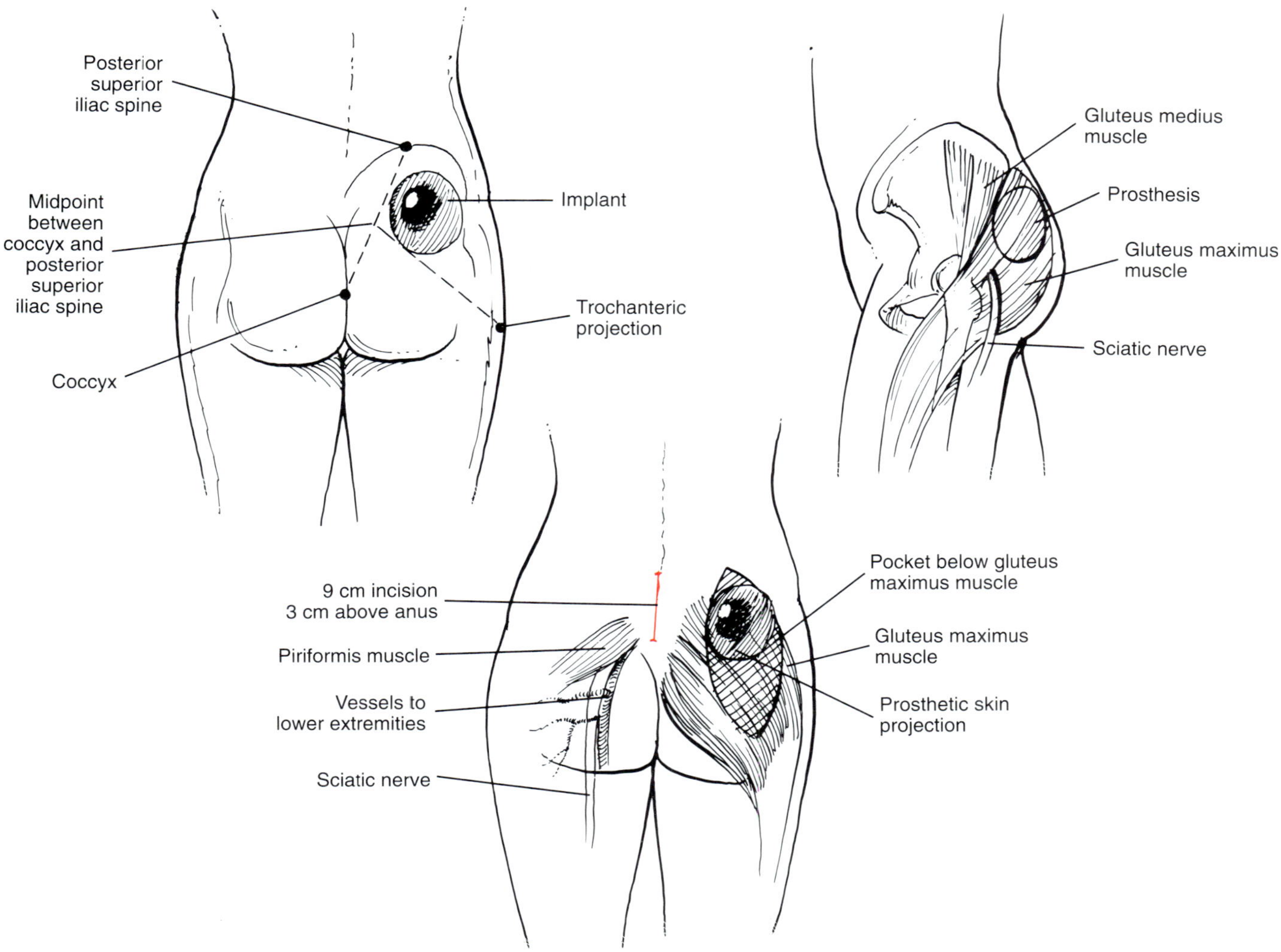

With this procedure access is gained through a 9 cm incision placed vertically along the intergluteal sulcus 3 cm above the anus. The dissection goes deep to the aponeurotic plane and then bilaterally above the gluteus maximus fascia. The gluteus maximus muscle is opened along its fibers, and the dissection transects the muscle to the subgluteal space where the pocket for the implant is prepared. No dissection should be performed below the cutaneous projection of the piriformis muscle where the sciatic nerve and the vessels for the lower limbs merge. No muscular opening at the lateral portion of the gluteus maximus muscle should exist. The prosthesis must be placed completely beneath the gluteus maximus muscle and above the gluteus medius muscle and all of the other deep muscles. The musculocutaneous tissue above the implant maintains the prosthesis in position with a low incidence of capsular contracture.

Despite the superior results that can be achieved, occasional problems may occur if the prosthesis is not inserted exactly into the submuscular pocket. In addition, if a muscular opening exists in the dissected limits, malpositioning can occur and distortions and asymmetries can become evident.

Distortion of the buttocks shape is the most common problem observed when the implant is placed in an abnormally high position. An unnatural curved appearance becomes evident. The lower portion of the buttocks remains drooped or flat with some skin excess visible at the gluteal fold. Sagging at the gluteal fold also may occur. On posterior view an artificial bulging projection in the upper middle buttock segment created by the prosthesis is apparent. And if hard spherical contracture of this implant occurs, an unaesthetic localized bulging results.

Buttocks distortion secondary to implant placement can occur unilaterally or bilaterally. The possible reoperative options are (1) skin resection at the gluteal fold and/or (2) repositioning the implant in a lower position. In the latter situation the same sacral access approach is used and the implant is removed. The pocket is reconstructed as is appropriate to correct the problem. Localized sutures in the upper and lateral aspects to obtain an improved shape or a new dissection in the lower edge of the pocket to correctly position the implant may be necessary. Special care must be taken with the vessels and the sciatic nerve.

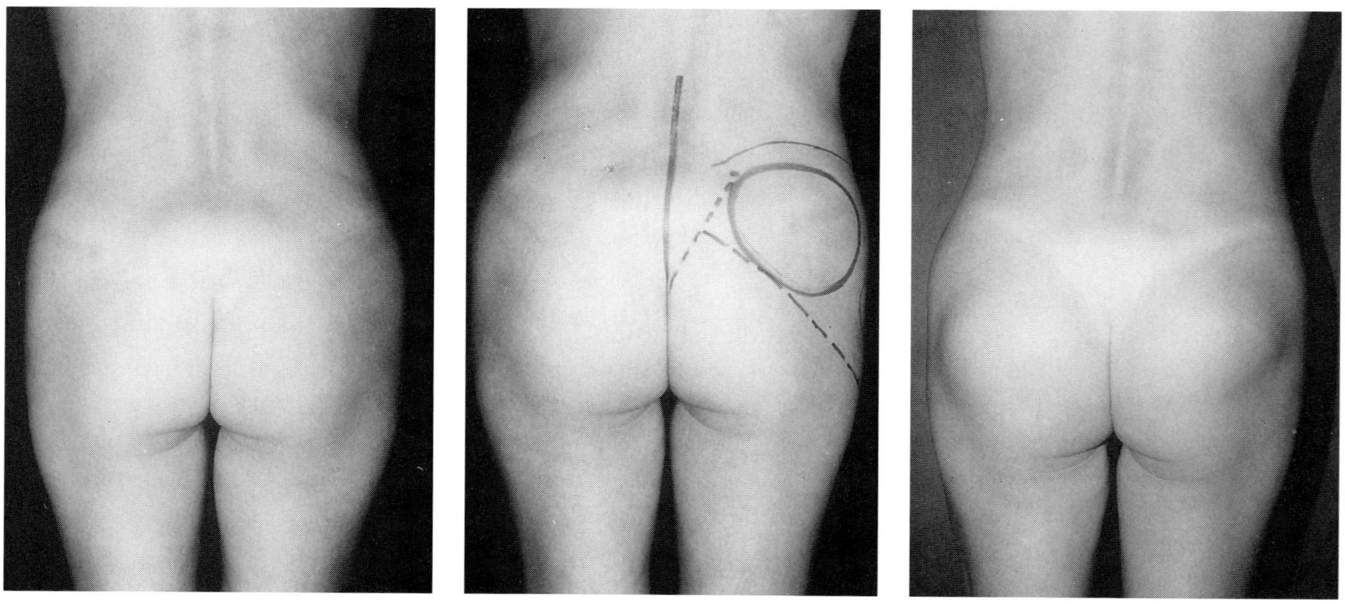

This 42-year-old patient had flat buttocks. Silicone implant placement with the Roble technique was planned. The prostheses were inserted in submuscular pockets under the gluteus maximus muscle. The circular skin demarcation shows how the implant bulges bilaterally. This bulge was more evident on the right side. Postoperatively the prostheses were too high. During reoperation the pockets on both sides were rebuilt.

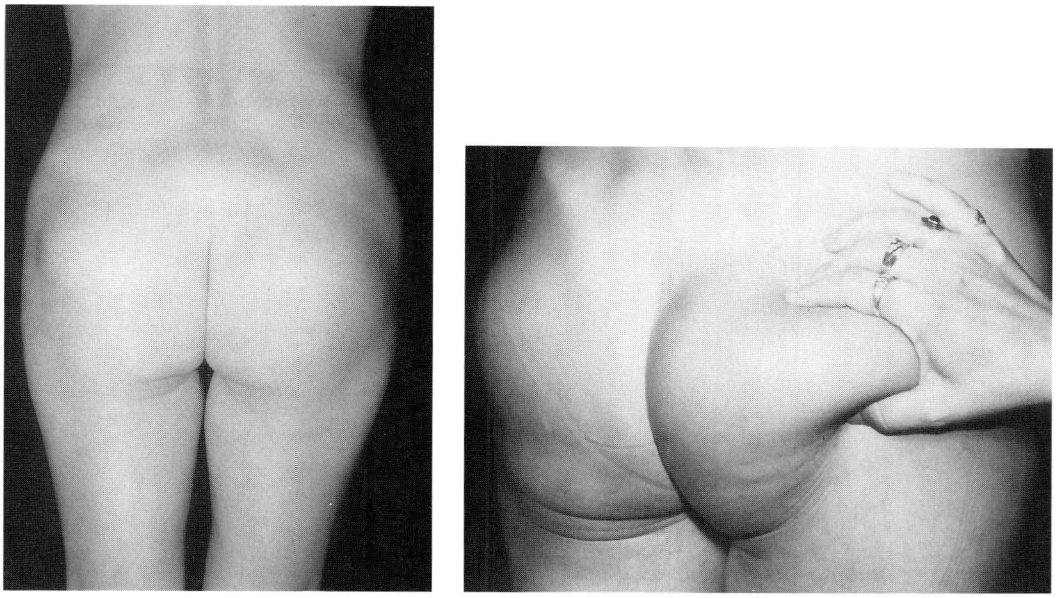

Despite the new pocket shape created by undermining the lower aspect of the pocket and closing the capsule in the upper lateral segment, the implant position was still not completely correct and a bulge projected in the left buttock. The patient chose not to undergo further revision. No capsular contracture was palpable.

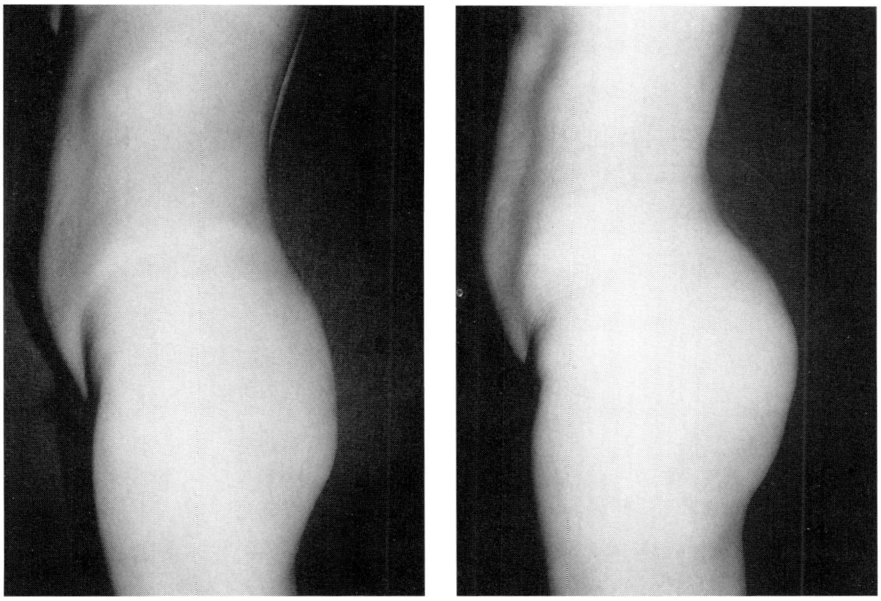

Comparison of preoperative and postoperative lateral views shows the improvement of the buttock's contour. No implant bulge can be detected.

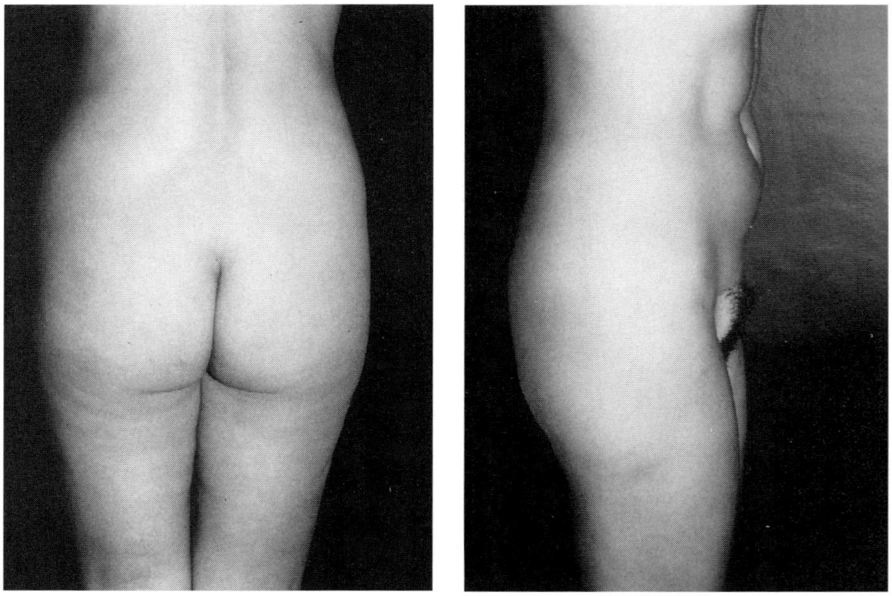

This 35-year-old patient complained of flat buttocks and was a candidate for a silicone implant inserted with the Roble technique.

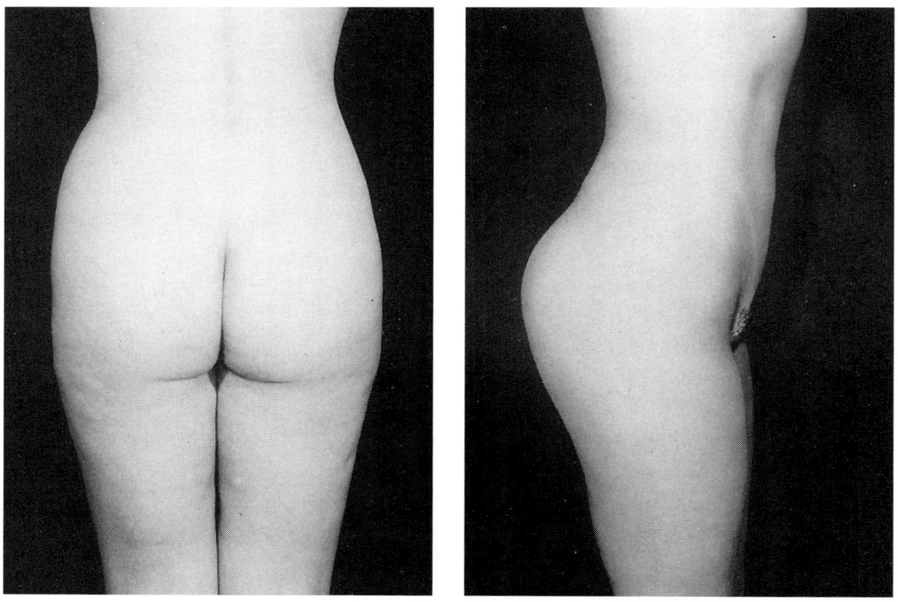

Nine months postoperatively improvement in the buttocks volume can be seen, but the patient still complained about the small size of the prosthesis and its high position, which created a flattened appearance in the lower middle portion of the buttocks.

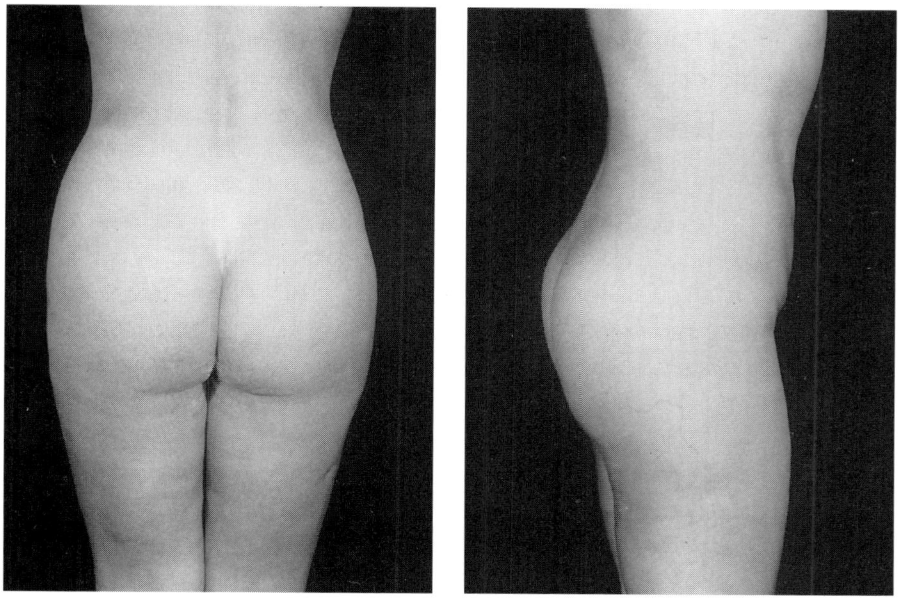

In a second procedure the prosthesis was replaced with a larger one and the implant pocket was rebuilt in order to place the implant in a lower position. Following this secondary procedure the contour was improved and the patient was satisfied with the volume augmentation.

Combined Procedures

The most common combined reoperative procedures in body contouring are flankplasty and abdominoplasty; flankplasty and upper inner thighplasty; and flankplasty, thighplasty, and abdominoplasty performed in the same surgical stage. These combined procedures may be indicated for primary cases and for secondary situations in which there are localized problems. Patients who have undergone abdominoplasty may also undergo a secondary abdominoplasty combined with primary flankplasty and/or upper inner thighplasty. Whatever combination of procedures is performed, the final objective is improvement of body contour and skin turgor. Liposuction may also be integrated into the surgical program in these areas or in neighboring regions.

Intraoperative and Postoperative Care

Surgery is performed with the patient under epidural or general anesthesia and with endotracheal intubation. Intravenous antibiotics (cephalosporin, 2 gm) are administered intraoperatively. The bladder is catheterized at the end of the surgery. No permanent catheter is used. In patients for whom epidural anesthesia is planned, enteroclysis is performed the night before. Routine monitoring is performed.

No significant dead space should exist after the tissue resection except following extended miniabdominoplasty and traditional abdominoplasty. In almost all cases a running intracuticular suture is placed. The confluent incisions are closed with isolated stitches in the skin. Two vacuum drains that merge through the pubis are placed in the undermined area of the abdomen. Drainage is checked each 24 hours. In general, the average volume the first day is around 180 to 240 cc. After 48 hours drainage is reduced to 110 cc, and by the third day it falls to 40 cc. In almost all cases the drains are removed when drainage falls to this volume. Patients leave the hospital with the drains in place. They are removed several days later depending on the drainage level. Micropore and ABD pads are used to cover the surgical area. Postoperatively the patient is placed in an elastic girdle.

Depending on the procedure performed patients are hospitalized for a minimum of 24 hours and a maximum of 3 days. Drains are removed before the patient leaves the hospital.

Ambulation is encouraged 12 to 24 hours after the surgery. To avoid thrombosis, early ambulation, massage, and leg movements are encouraged. Bandages on the legs are indicated during the intraoperative period only in patients with known circulatory problems. The administration of symptomatic medications and antibiotic therapy are continued for 3 to 7 days postoperatively.

Stitches are removed between the sixth and tenth postoperative days. Stitches are removed from the umbilicus on the fourteenth postoperative day. Patients who were operated on in the upper thigh region are told to wash the pudendal area two times a day and after physical activities. No bandages are used in these regions. Postoperatively the patient may rest in the supine position or even in the free decubitus position depending on the type of surgery; the patient will find the ideal position. The prone position is not recommended after abdominoplasty. Anti-inflammatory, hypnotic, and ansyolitic medications are prescribed routinely for the 2-week postoperative period according to patient requirements. An elastic girdle is worn continuously during the first 10 to 30 postoperative days depending on the surgical program: simple reoperative liposuction requires the use of a girdle for no more than 1 week, whereas complete body contouring or abdominoplasty necessitates girdle use for 1 month.

Based on the extent of the surgery, patient age, and physical condition, the patient is permitted only a moderate degree of activity at home during the first postoperative week. Ambulation beyond the home and visits to the surgeon's office may be restricted during this first week. During the second postoperative week, based on the extent of the surgery, the patient is freer to participate in activities.

Extensive combined surgeries require a minimum of 2 to 3 weeks before driving and return to work are permitted. Limited domestic activities are allowed. Sunbathing is allowed only after the bruises have disappeared (usually after 2 to 3 weeks). Patients should wear bathing suits that cover the operated areas. Participation in sports activities is permitted after 6 weeks. Pain, swelling, and fatigue are the main signs that the patient is engaging in overly strenuous activities too early. The surgeon should evaluate and monitor the patient in this regard.

Bibliography

Baroudi R. Umbilicoplasty. Clin Plast Surg 2:431, 1975.

Baroudi R. Body sculpturing. Clin Plast Surg 11:419, 1984.

Baroudi R, Carvalho C. Neoumbilicoplastias: Un procedimiento eléctico en el transcurso de las abdominoplastias. Cir Plast Iberolat 7:391, 1981.

Baroudi R, Moraes M. Philosophy, technical principles, selection and indication in body contouring surgery. Aesthetic Plast Surg 15:1, 1991.

Baroudi R, Keppke EM, Tozzi Neto F. Abdominoplasty. Plast Reconstr Surg 54:161, 1974.

Gonzalez-Ulloa M. Circular lipectomy with transposition of the umbilicus and aponeurotic technique. Cirurgia 27:394, 1959.

Gonzalez-Ulloa M. Torsoplasty. In Gonzalez-Ulloa M, Meyer S, Smith J, Zaoli G, eds. Aesthetic Plastic Surgery, vol 5. Padova: Piccin Nuova, 1988, p 87.

Grazer FM, Klingbeil J. Body Image: A Surgical Perspective. St. Louis: Mosby, 1980.

Guerrerosantos J. Hip-buttock-thighplasty. In Goldwyn R, ed. The Unfavorable Result in Plastic Surgery, 2nd ed. Boston: Little, Brown, 1984, p 865.

Hetter GP. Lipoplasty. The Theory and Practice of the Blunt Suction Lipectomy, 2nd ed. Boston: Little, Brown, 1990.

Illouz Y-G. Surgical remodeling of the silhouette by aspiration lipolysis or selective lipectomy. Aesthetic Plast Surg 9:7, 1985.

Lewis CM. Early experience of aspirative lipoplasty of the abdomen. Aesthetic Plast Surg 11:33, 1987.

Lockwood TE. Superficial fascial system (SFS) of the trunk and extremities: A new concept. Plast Reconstr Surg 87:1009, 1991.

Lockwood TE. Transverse flank-thigh-buttock lift with superficial fascial suspension. Plast Reconstr Surg 87:1019, 1991.

Pitanguy I. Thigh lift and abdominal lipectomy. In Goldwyn RM, ed. The Unfavorable Result in Plastic Surgery: Avoidance and Treatment. Boston: Little, Brown, 1972, p 387.

Regnault P, Baroudi R, Carvalho CGS. Correction of the lower limbs lipodystrophy. Aesthetic Plast Surg 4:215, 1980.

Robles JM, Tagliapietra JC, Grandi MA. Gluteoplastia de aumento: Implante submuscular. Cir Plast Iberolat 4:365, 1984.

36

Reoperative Surgery of the Abdominal Wall

Grady B. Core, M.D., and James C. Grotting, M.D.

Reoperative Problems

Seroma	Radiation injury
Hematoma	Impaired vascularity and/or innervation
Acute abdominal wound dehiscence	Recurrent neoplasm
Infection	Improper placement of stoma site
Hernia	Contour deformities
Fistula	Hypertrophic scarring
	Improper position of umbilicus

It is fortunate that in most plastic and reconstructive procedures the development of complications rarely results in a serious threat to the patient's life. However, the abdominal wall is one area where a major complication can pose such a threat. For this reason, among others, the reoperative surgeon must have a sound knowledge of the full spectrum of diagnostic and surgical approaches to the abdomen. Optimally he should be well versed in general surgical principles and be thoroughly confident of his ability to properly assess, approach, and repair any intra-abdominal injury that may occur. The plastic surgeon, fully trained in general surgery, obviously has an advantage in this area. Within the context of the following chapter, however, we review a body of information that allows any plastic surgeon contemplating reoperative abdominal surgery to proceed safely through this potentially disastrous and unforgiving area.

ANATOMY

Knowledge of anatomy is the key to success in reoperative surgery of the abdomen. Although the topic of this chapter is reoperative abdominal wall surgery, the intimate relationship of the abdominal wall with the intra-abdominal cavity mandates a thorough review of the anatomy of both regions.

Reoperative surgery of the abdominal wall implies that the anatomy is already distorted. This distortion may be in the form of derangements of the aesthetic appearance of the skin and subcutaneous tissue, integrity or location of the musculofascial structures, impaired vascularity or innervation, or abnormal location of intra-abdominal contents outside the abdominal cavity.

Skin and Subcutaneous Tissue

The anatomy of the skin envelope is directly related to body habitus. For example, obese patients have an excess of abdominal skin due to a thick underlying subcutaneous layer. Patients undergoing tissue expansion will also have changes in skin anatomy not only with regard to shape but also with increased vascularity to the overlying skin, which may even aid in flap planning.[1] Obviously, previous abdominal incisions will also change the anatomy of the skin with regard to orientation of blood supply.

The underlying subcutaneous tissue has been studied extensively and is noted to consist of two layers: superficial and deep. The two layers are separated by Scarpa's fascia.[2] The deep layer is located in the lower abdomen below an imaginary line extending from one iliac crest to the other and passing through the umbilicus. Between the skin and the anterior fascia of the abdominal wall is a subcutaneous fascial system that has been shown to contribute to the aesthetic appearance. Attention to detail and proper management of this fascial system can prevent later aesthetic complications.[3]

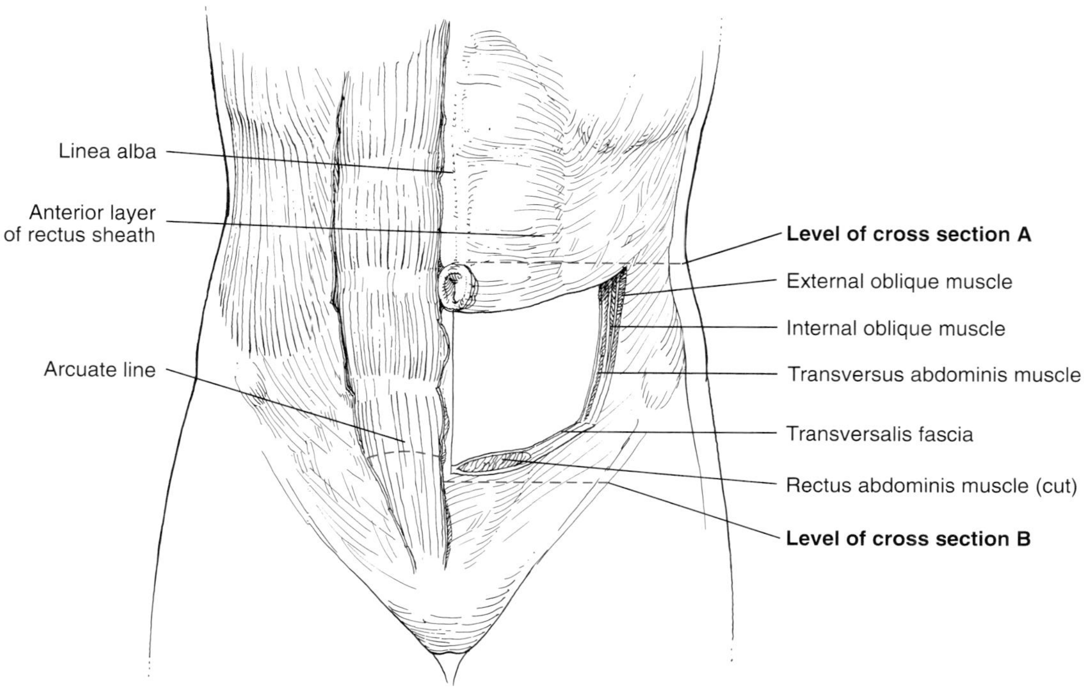
Linea alba
Anterior layer
of rectus sheath
Arcuate line
Level of cross section A
External oblique muscle
Internal oblique muscle
Transversus abdominis muscle
Transversalis fascia
Rectus abdominis muscle (cut)
Level of cross section B

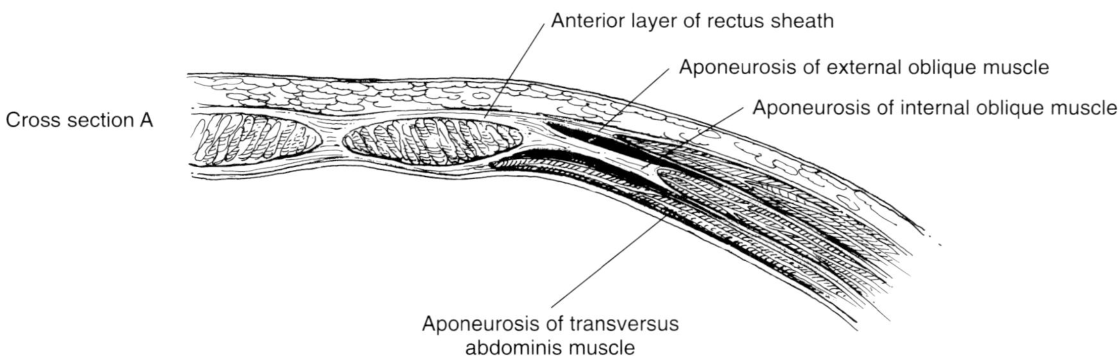
Cross section A
Anterior layer of rectus sheath
Aponeurosis of external oblique muscle
Aponeurosis of internal oblique muscle
Aponeurosis of transversus
abdominis muscle

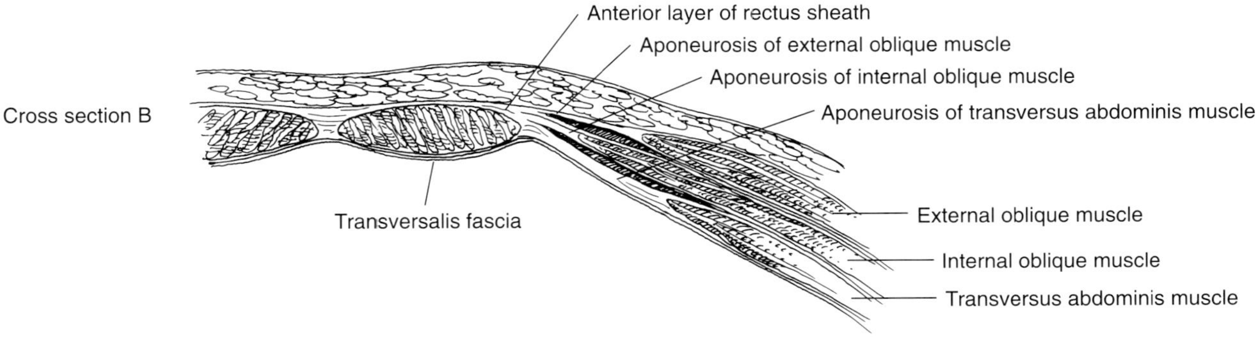
Cross section B
Anterior layer of rectus sheath
Aponeurosis of external oblique muscle
Aponeurosis of internal oblique muscle
Aponeurosis of transversus abdominis muscle
Transversalis fascia
External oblique muscle
Internal oblique muscle
Transversus abdominis muscle

Musculofascial Layers

The musculofascial layers of the abdominal wall and their respective transition zones differ in composition based on the level. These differences in composition are clinically important in terms of the structural integrity of the layers available for closure. Fusion of the fascial layers forms three important vertical lines on the anterior abdominal wall: midline linea alba and bilateral semilunar lines. The muscles of the abdominal wall are divided into three regions: anterior, anterolateral, and posterior. Posteriorly is the quadratus lumborum muscle, anteriorly are the rectus abdominis and pyramidalis muscles, and anterolaterally are the external oblique, internal oblique, and transversus abdominis muscles. The anterolateral muscles have extensive fascial aponeuroses, which contribute to the anterior and posterior rectus sheaths. Below the arcuate line, the transversus abdominis aponeurosis and the internal oblique aponeurosis pass anteriorly to the rectus abdominis muscle such that the transversalis fascia is the only layer of structural integrity posterior to the rectus abdominis muscle.[4] The transversalis fascia is continuous with the endoabdominal fascia (which lines the entire abdominopelvic cavity) and is particularly important in anatomic repair of the lower abdomen. Laterally and superiorly it covers the internal surface of the transversus abdominis muscle and aponeurosis, separating them from the underlying fat and peritoneum.[5]

No area of the abdominal wall has undergone as many variations in surgical techniques as the inguinal region; therefore this area offers the widest variety of anatomic distortions from prior surgery. The area of transversalis fascia below the discontinuation of the transversus abdominis muscle and yet above the iliopubic tract and Cooper's ligament is known as the "weak area."[5] Direct hernias occur medially through the posterior floor of the inguinal canal, and indirect hernias occur laterally through the internal inguinal ring. Femoral hernias, of course, occur through the femoral canal.

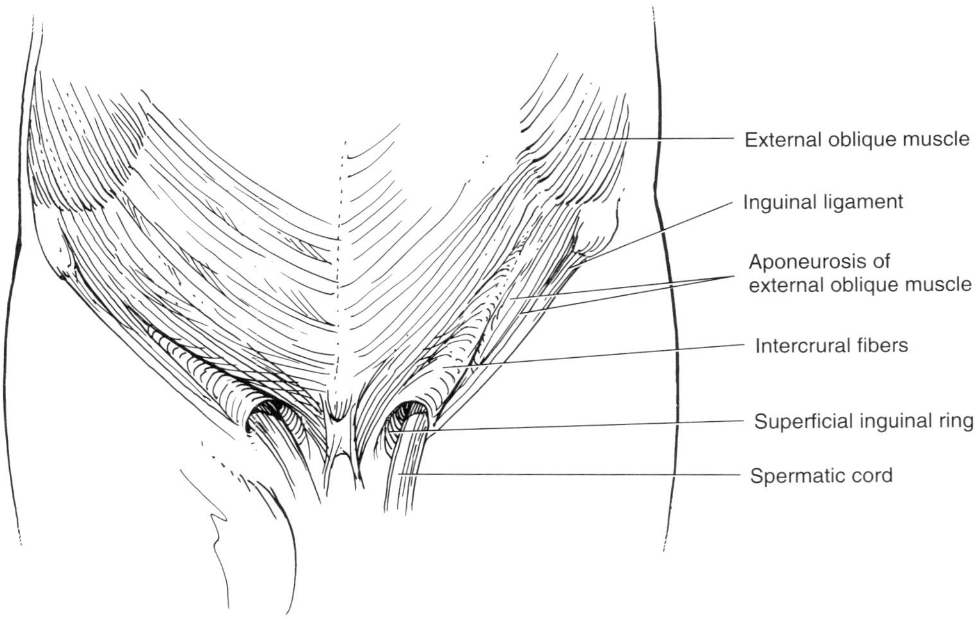
External oblique muscle
Inguinal ligament
Aponeurosis of
external oblique muscle
Intercrural fibers
Superficial inguinal ring
Spermatic cord

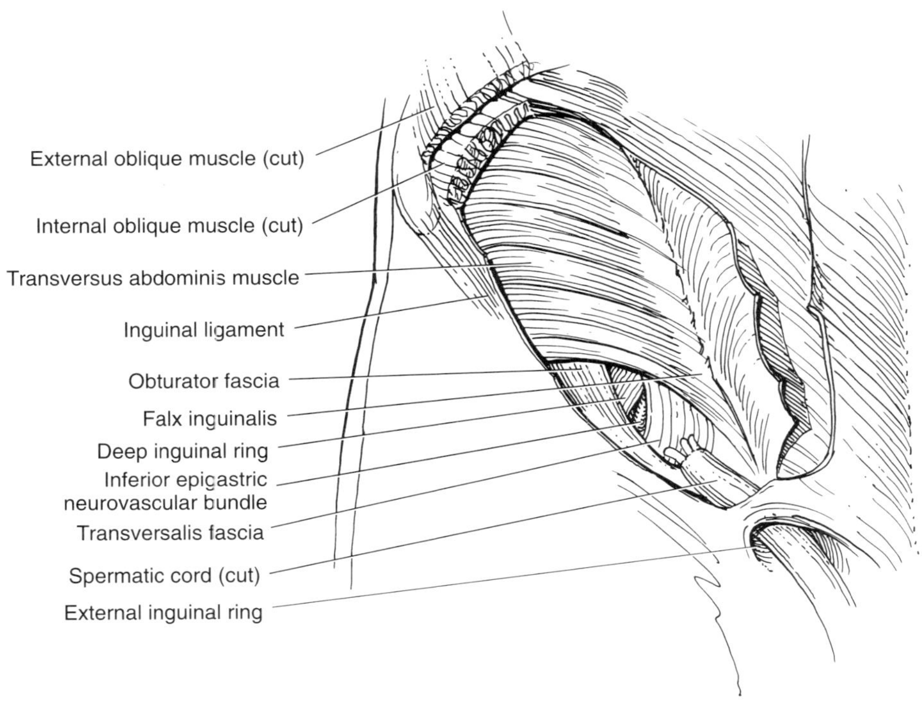
External oblique muscle (cut)
Internal oblique muscle (cut)
Transversus abdominis muscle
Inguinal ligament
Obturator fascia
Falx inguinalis
Deep inguinal ring
Inferior epigastric
neurovascular bundle
Transversalis fascia
Spermatic cord (cut)
External inguinal ring

Vascular Supply

The vascular supply of the abdominal wall consists of a rich network of vessels that approach from all directions. This network allows the abdominal wall to be resilient to repeated insults but at the same time dictates a set of surgical parameters that cannot be violated lest ischemia and necrosis result. The vertical axis of blood supply to the abdomen is represented by the superior epigastric arteries in the cephalad region and caudally by a deep and superficial system formed by five major branches of the iliac system: deep inferior epigastric, deep circumflex iliac, superficial inferior epigastric, superficial circumflex iliac, and superficial external pudendal branches. The horizontal axis is represented by the intercostal arteries (10th and 11th), subcostal arteries, and four paired lumbar arteries.[4]

Because of this multiaxial inflow, it is difficult to design an abdominal flap not based on a significant artery. Injection studies have demonstrated that the deep inferior epigastric artery is more significant than the superior epigastric arteries in supplying the skin of the anterior abdominal wall.[6] Perforating arteries that emerge through the anterior rectus sheath feed into a subcutaneous vascular network that has its highest concentration of perforators in the periumbilical region. Within this subcutaneous space there are connections (choke vessels) with adjacent vascular territories: inferiorly with the superficial inferior epigastric artery, inferolaterally with the superficial circumflex iliac artery, superiorly with the superficial superior epigastric artery, and superolaterally (and most dominant) with the lateral cutaneous branches of the intercostal arteries. It should be kept in mind therefore that there are two levels of an interconnecting vascular supply, one being in the deep muscular plane (where all inflow vessels also have an anastomotic network through "choke connections") and the other in the more anterior subcutaneous plane.

The course of venous drainage essentially parallels that of the arterial inflow. However, venous drainage is controlled by the presence of valves that direct the flow from the superficial to the deep system. In certain flaps it has been shown that retrograde flow can occur despite the presence of valves, although it may require greater pressure to overcome valvular resistance.[7] In addition to understanding the importance of collateral blood flow to the abdomen as it pertains to reoperative surgery of the abdominal wall, one should especially respect this collateral system in patients who have atherosclerotic stenosis of the abdominal aorta and thus rely on this anastomotic network for bypass to the lower extremities since the epigastric artery arcade can supply an important communication between the left subclavian and internal iliac arteries.[8]

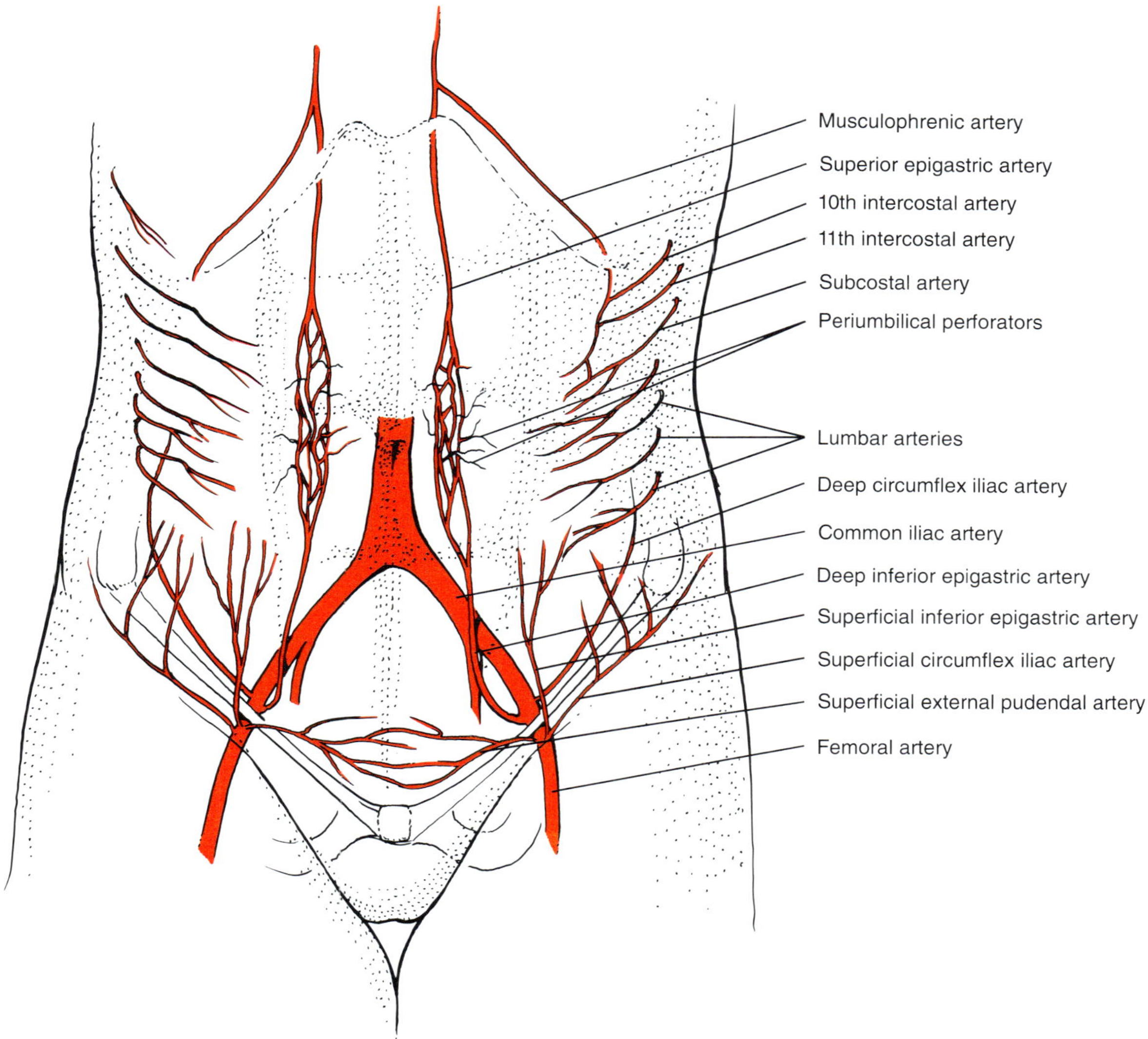
Musculophrenic artery
Superior epigastric artery
10th intercostal artery
11th intercostal artery
Subcostal artery
Periumbilical perforators
Lumbar arteries
Deep circumflex iliac artery
Common iliac artery
Deep inferior epigastric artery
Superficial inferior epigastric artery
Superficial circumflex iliac artery
Superficial external pudendal artery
Femoral artery

Nerve Supply

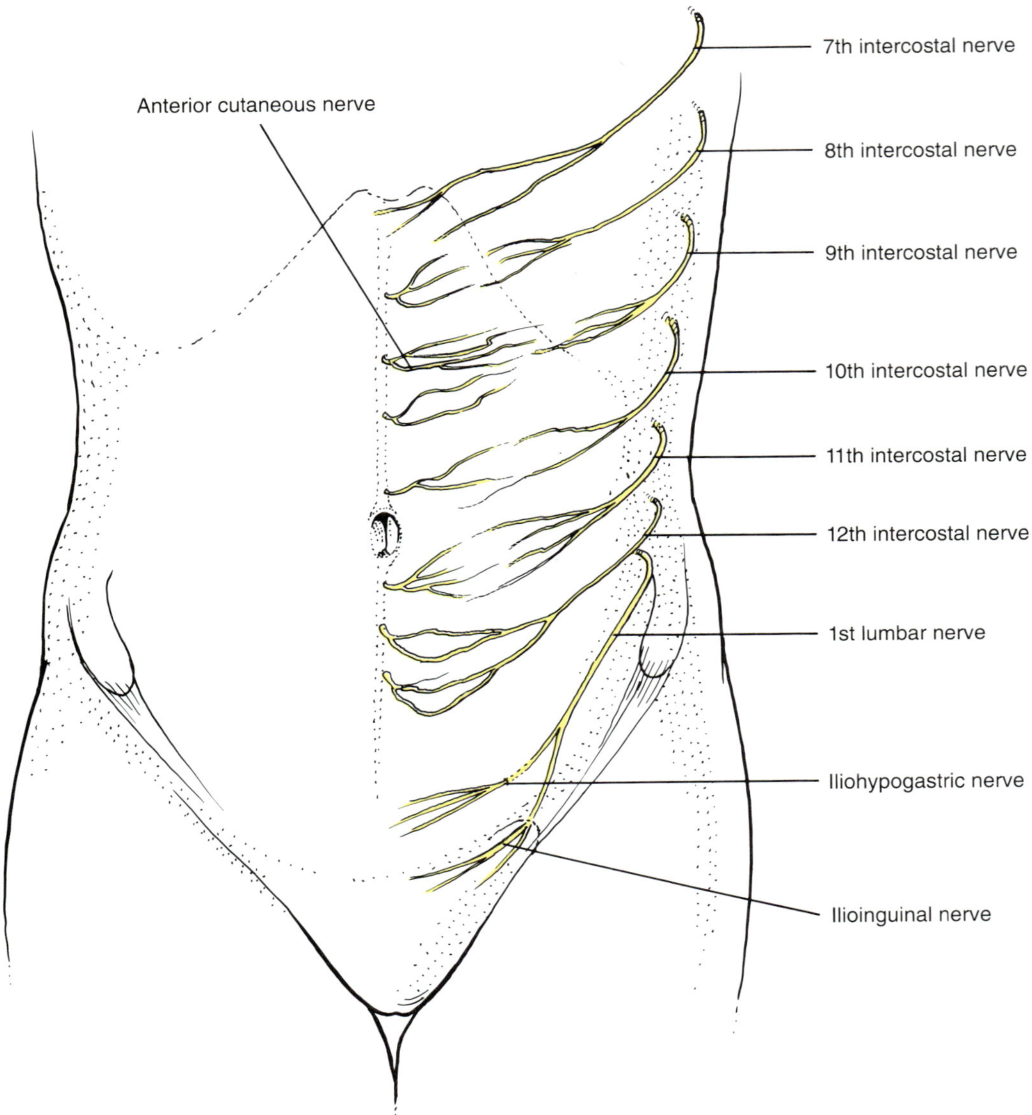

The nerve supply to the abdominal wall is derived from the roots of spinal nerves T-7 through L-4, which give rise to the intercostal (7-11), subcostal, iliohypogastric, and ilioinguinal nerves. When possible, it is important to preserve these nerves not only for sensation but also for motor preservation to the abdominal musculature. The rectus abdominis muscle is innervated by the lower five intercostal nerves and the subcostal nerve. The external oblique muscle is innervated by intercostal nerves (7-11), subcostal, and iliohypogastric nerves. The internal oblique and transversus abdominis muscles are supplied by intercostal nerves (8-11) and the subcostal, iliohypogastric, and ilioinguinal nerves. Interruption of motor nerves results in defunctionalized muscle units, which causes atrophy and areas of weakness in the abdominal wall.

Lymphatics

The lymphatic drainage of the abdominal wall flows cephalad and caudad in a vertical axis as well as from anterior to posterior, with the horizontal axis thus following a similar pattern of the venous drainage. If the vascular architecture in the reoperative field is not compromised, lymphatic drainage is rarely a problem.

SPECIFIC PROBLEMS

In this section we review the wide variety of secondary problems that may be encountered by the reoperative surgeon. Although these problems may have infinite variations, it is important to be familiar with the more common presentations in order to proceed with proper planning for management.

Acute Wound Dehiscence

The incidence of acute abdominal wound dehiscence is approximately 1.8%[9,10] and is similar regardless of the technique of abdominal wall closure (whether running or interrupted). Risk factors include age over 50 years, poor nutrition, pulmonary disease, ischemia, male sex, emergency surgery, and bacterial contamination with wound infection.[11]

The very nature of dehiscence implies that the abdominal wall has lost its integrity completely by rupture of the musculofascial layers. At initial presentation the wound may appear normal if the skin is still intact. The patient may complain of a sudden sensation of "tearing" or "popping," usually precipitated by vomiting, coughing, or sneezing. A high level of suspicion needs to be maintained. Serosanguineous drainage may be the only hailing sign, although the initial presentation may also be complete evisceration. Dehiscence most commonly occurs approximately 1 week after the initial surgery.[11,12] The plastic surgeon is rarely called upon to treat abdominal wounds in the acute phase but is usually summoned after many days or weeks of failure of wound healing to progress. By this time the layers of the abdominal wall may be widely separated and the viscera exposed. Frequently debridement has already been carried out. These patients often have associated intra-abdominal infectious complications. There is also a high incidence of associated disease states such as diabetes mellitus, renal disease, and poor nutritional states, which reflects impairment in host defense function. Recurrent dehiscence in such patients is high.[11]

Other common causes of large, acute, open defects are radical debridement secondary to necrotizing soft tissue infection, abdominal wall trauma, and en bloc tumor resection.[13] On occasion, prolonged abdominal surgery will result in an open defect due to bowel distention and inability to close the wound primarily.

Abdominal Wall Hernia

For most surgeons who reoperate frequently on the abdominal wall, herniation is one of the most common presentations, especially incisional hernias and groin hernias. The incidence of incisional herniation is approximately 1% to 11%, with most studies showing a range of 2% to 4%.[14]

Incisional herniation has a multifactorial etiology. Contributing factors can be divided into those that are mechanical (local wound factors or technical factors) and constitutional problems with the patient. Among the latter, the most commonly noted are obesity, advancing age, malnutrition, male sex, pulmonary disease, and sepsis.[14] Mechanical factors include local wound problems (e.g., decreased blood supply from prior surgery or radiation), abdominal distention (e.g., from ascites or paralytic ileus), wound infection, hematoma, or local tissue deficiency resulting in increased tension. Technical factors consist of inadequate suture technique, improper placement of the incision, use of absorbable sutures, use of drains, enterotomies, long duration of operation, and excessive tension during closure.

Of these contributing factors, the most important is proper technique. Since the adoption of the mass closure technique by Jones, Newell, and Brubaker,[15] which supplanted the layered closure of Halsted, a significant reduction in the incidence of wound dehiscence and incisional hernia has occurred. However, still today many surgeons insist on closing the abdomen in layers. Whether or not to close the peritoneum as a separate layer remains controversial. The peritoneum has been shown by one group to be particularly prone to adhesions if closed as a separate layer or included in the mass closure method.[16] In addition, overzealous suturing techniques can result in ischemia and tissue necrosis. Sutures that are too tight may cut through tissues, resulting in localized areas of weakness. Placement of sutures in infected or necrotic wound margins also constitutes a technical error.

The most common presentation of incisional hernia is caused by a secondary subclinical fascial dehiscence occurring late (usually within 6 months) after a previous operation[17] and may be asymptomatic in some patients. The natural history of this type of hernia is one of continued enlargement. As the hernia ring enlarges, the threat to the patient's life becomes less since the risk of incarceration or strangulation decreases. It is recommended that these hernias be repaired unless the patient's medical condition prevents it. In obese individuals small incisional hernias may be camouflaged, presenting as only a localized area of abdominal wall tenderness. If incarceration or strangulation occurs, frank bowel obstruction may result, with vomiting, intermittent cramping, abdominal pain, distention, and obstipation.

Large ventral hernias cause the intestinal viscera to become displaced to some degree outside the abdominal cavity. This in turn causes secondary sequelae such as paradoxical respiration, problems with micturition, back pain, splanchnic venous stasis, and distention and atony of the hollow viscera. In addition, the skin may become atrophic, hypoxic, and devoid of subcutaneous fat. Spontaneous ulcerations may occur in the thin overlying skin.[18]

The most formidable challenge in treating ventral hernias is the patient who presents with inadequate tissue peripherally for primary closure. Many times previously these patients have had open wounds that began initially as acute wound dehiscences or infections. These wounds usually were treated open and by the time the plastic surgeon is consulted, the abdominal wall components are widely separated, with thin skin grafts over the abdominal viscera. The skin grafts may even have prosthetic mesh underneath. Associated problems may include bowel fistula, mesh extrusion, and reherniation around the edge of the mesh from improper closure. These complications are more common in patients repaired with Marlex mesh; these patients may present to the reconstructive surgeon with such problems years after placement of the mesh.[19] Options for reclosure in patients who have tissue deficiency are discussed later.

Recurrent Groin Hernia

The most common complication of inguinal hernioplasty is recurrent herniation,[20] with a rate from 1% to 10% depending on technique and length of follow-up. Patients with bilateral hernias and/or direct hernias have a higher chance of recurrence than patients with unilateral or indirect hernias. A patient with a recurrent groin hernia often will present with pain or with an obviously visible recurrence in the previous repair site. Recurrences tend to be the same type of hernia as the previous one. Most recurrences also tend to occur after the first postoperative year, although there is a wide variability in terms of time to recurrence.[21,22] Recurrence after groin hernia repair is often attributed to technical error, and in the cases of early recurrence, this may be particularly true. However, in the late recurrence the same dynamic forces that led to the original herniation often are still at work and thus again incriminated.[23] Whatever the cause for recurrence—technical error, nonanatomic repair, inherent tissue weakness, wound infection—it is apparent that the etiology of recurrences is multifactorial.[24] Numerous other risk factors for recurrence of inguinal hernia have been proposed and range from obesity, pulmonary disease, ascites, other causes of increased intra-abdominal pressure, and even smoking.[25] Inguinal hernia procedures performed in the United States account for approximately 15% of all general surgery operations; therefore in light of the recurrence rates mentioned earlier, this procedure is a common operation for the reoperative abdominal surgeon. Familiarity with not only the anatomy of this area but also the various techniques of primary repair is essential in order to plan a reasonable secondary reconstructive approach. McVay and Chapp,[26] Bassinni,[27] Iles[28] (Shouldice technique), and others[23] describe the most common types of autogenous primary repair used in the United States. With the recent advent of endoscopic abdominal surgery, recurrences around prosthetic mesh plugs or patches placed from an intra-abdominal approach in addition to other problems such as infected prosthetic mesh will now be encountered.[29]

Parastomal Hernia

Stoma formation is complicated by parastomal herniation, with an incidence of approximately 10%.[30] Most parastomal hernias at presentation are not symptomatic and usually consist of an unsightly bulge adjacent to the stoma. However, in 10% to 20% of patients, the symptoms become severe enough to warrant operative correction. These hernias can be annoying since the hernia will reduce itself when the patient reclines but then recur when the patient stands and may dislodge the stoma appliance, resulting in soilage. Eventual interference with the function of the ostomy as well as pain referable to the hernia site can also occur. Ultimately one must also consider the possibility of incarceration or strangulation as is a problem with any other abdominal wall hernia.

The etiology of these hernias is likely secondary to technical errors as well as obesity, malnutrition, postoperative sepsis, abdominal distention, ascites, ambulatory dialysis, chronic cough, or obstructive uropathy.[30] The most common technical error is placement of the ostomy lateral to the rectus abdominis muscle or through an operative incision. Indications for repair include cosmesis, persistent pain, stoma dysfunction, enlargement, and intestinal complications.

Prosthetic Material

For patients presenting with complications secondary to previously placed prosthetic material, the most common problems include infection, extrusion, fistula formation, and hernia recurrence.[19] Periprosthetic seroma or hematoma may also occur. Infected patients may present with pain and erythema over and around the implanted material. When the process is of a chronic nature, they may present with draining sinus tracts to the skin. Recurrent herniation around prosthetic mesh is usually caused by excessive tension at the original surgery site or by the use of an insufficient suture technique around the perimeter of the mesh.[31]

There have been a wide variety of prosthetic materials utilized in abdominal wall repair. These materials can be classified as either meshed or nonmeshed materials or as absorbable or nonabsorbable. Most problems experienced with these materials in the United States were associated with the use of tantalum mesh in the

Prosthetic Materials Commonly Used in Abdominal Wall Repair

Type	Material	Absorbability
Meshed	Vicryl (polyglactin-910)	Absorbable
Meshed	Dexon (polyglactic acid)	Absorbable
Meshed	Marlex (monofilament polypropylene)	Nonabsorbable
Meshed	Prolene (monofilament polypropylene)	Nonabsorbable
Meshed	Surgipro (monofilament polypropylene)	Nonabsorbable
Meshed	Mersilene (polyester Dacron)	Nonabsorbable
Nonmeshed	Gore-Tex (PTFE)	Nonabsorbable
Nonmeshed	Dura mater	Nonabsorbable
Nonmeshed	Silastic (silicone sheeting)	Nonabsorbable

early years and by Marlex—to a lesser degree—in more recent years. Marlex is a polypropylene mesh that has been for the most part replaced by Prolene, which, although made of the same material, is not as stiff and has been found to have a lower complication rate.[31] Absorbable mesh, such as Vicryl or Dexon, is made of polyglycolic acid, which absorbs in 4 to 6 weeks. Indications for this material in hernia repair are limited since after absorption, the ventral hernia still remains. Of the nonmeshed materials, expanded polytetrafluoroethylene (PTFE) has come to be the most popular. PTFE has been extensively used in vascular surgery, but its use in abdominal wall repair is fairly recent.

Fistula

The treatment of patients presenting for abdominal reconstruction who have an active fistula require the cooperative involvement of both the general and reconstructive surgeons. These patients may also have an absolute deficiency of tissue of the abdominal wall with very superficial bowel, which has subsequently opened to the surface. Of course, other causes of fistulization may come from deep in the abdomen such as radiation injury, malignant tumors with extension to the abdominal wall, traumatic injuries, infectious wound complications, inflammatory bowel disease, and iatrogenic injury. Many fistulae close spontaneously with appropriate dietary restrictions and if necessary with complete bowel rest and parenteral nutrition. However, if the fistula persists, the cause should be reevaluated and the contribution of such problems as distal bowel obstruction, bowel discontinuity, malignancy, foreign body, radiation injury, epithelialized tract, or inflammatory bowel disease should be considered.[32] Optimally a fistula should be closed before any reconstructive surgery is attempted; cooperation with the general surgeon is imperative. Such patients will also frequently have associated nutritional deficiencies or electrolyte imbalances that should be thoroughly evaluated before reconstructive surgery is undertaken.

Traumatic Injury

Trauma patients have a wide spectrum of presentations. For our purposes the etiology is categorized as blunt or penetrating trauma.

Traumatic rupture of the abdominal wall usually results in an abdominal hernia.[33,34] Traumatic abdominal hernias are most commonly secondary to blunt trauma with small objects such as bicycle handlebars. These hernias will usually present as small abdominal wall defects. Large traumatic abdominal wall defects are usually secondary to motor vehicle accidents.

On physical examination, a reducible mass, which on palpation feels like bowel, may be the initial finding. In large hernias with subcutaneous bowel, the skin will assume a nodular appearance, conforming to the underlying bowel. On the initial examination the patient may appear entirely normal. Therefore a high index of suspicion should be maintained in the patient who has suffered blunt abdominal trauma. Lateral or oblique plane x-ray films of the abdomen may help reveal gas-filled loops outside the abdominal cavity. CT scans have also been shown to accurately depict internal injury resulting from blunt abdominal trauma and should be employed if the diagnosis is questionable.[34] Other findings that may mimic abdominal wall hernias are rectus sheath hematomas or preexisting abdominal wall hernias or tumors.

The overall incidence of associated intra-abdominal injury has been estimated at approximately 30%, and the incidence of such injury appears much higher when the hernia is superior to the umbilicus.[33,34] Again this is a situation in which cooperation with the general surgeon is necessary. Although early repair is recommended, in some instances the patient's overall condition may mandate delay.

Penetrating abdominal injuries are generally not managed by plastic surgeons since the need for abdominal wall reconstruction is rare. However, in some cases of prolonged surgery for intra-abdominal trauma, problems with primary closure can be encountered and the reconstructive surgeon may be called upon to aid in the closure.

Fasciitis

The abdominal wall may be the site of necrotizing fasciitis, which is usually caused by clostridial organisms and can result in extensive myonecrosis. These patients usually present after undergoing a recent abdominal procedure with wound swelling, erythema, and tenderness in association with serosanguineous drainage from the wound. These infections may commence within hours of an operation and progress very rapidly.[35] The patients are frequently elderly, although patients of all ages are susceptible. The infections are often associated with open bowel procedures, perirectal abscesses, or procedures involving urinary extravasation. The appearance of the patient may initially be unalarming, although the temperature elevation can be marked. However, rapid deterioration in the patient's condition is likely unless diagnosis and treatment are prompt. Surgeons performing reoperative abdominal surgery should be aware of the possibility of this complication in their own reoperated patients, although they most likely will be consulted to treat such patients for debridement and eventual wound closure.[35,36] Mortality rates for necrotizing fasciitis are reported to range from 9% to 70%.[36]

Prior Incision

It is well known that an incision creates a wall of scar tissue that interrupts the normal neurovascular pathways. However, there is regeneration of vascular supply across a previous incision as proved by the ability of transferred tissue to remain vascularized after transection from a primary vascular pedicle.[37] At the same time it is wise not to create areas of relative ischemia by acutely intersecting previous incision lines. Therefore the orientation of previous incisions should be noted and well documented by any surgeon reoperating on the abdominal wall. Consideration of the effects of all previous incisions regarding vascularity and nerve supply, as well as examination of the patient for defunctionalized muscle segments, should be performed. Incisions particularly prone to such problems are the paramedian and chevron (or "bucket-handle") incisions.

Neoplasia

Neoplastic problems of the abdominal wall are of both a primary and secondary nature. Primary tumors of the musculofascial abdominal wall consist of desmoid tumors and sarcomas. The desmoid tumor is considered to be a low-grade malignant neoplasm, which, according to the American Joint Committee for Cancer Staging and Results Reporting, is a nonmetastasizing, low-grade fibrosarcoma.[38] The most common presentation of a primary tumor of the abdominal wall is a painless mass. This is especially true of desmoid tumors; however, with a nondesmoid sarcoma, associated pain is described by approximately one half of these patients. The location of the tumors on the abdominal wall may be variable, and the size may range from 1.5 cm to an excess of 30 cm in diameter. On physical examination these masses are characteristically very hard and nontender. They will appear to be contained within the musculoaponeurotic portion of the abdominal wall itself. Desmoid tumors most often occur in women of childbearing age, but men can become affected, as can older female patients.

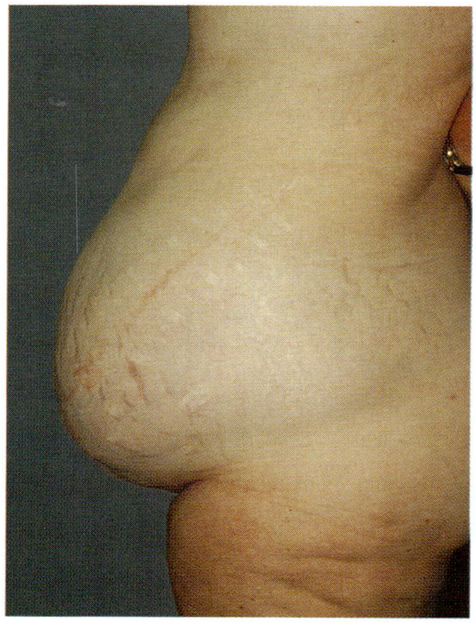

This 56-year-old woman was referred for abdominal wall reconstruction 9 years after the resection of a huge desmoid tumor of the abdominal wall. She was free of recurrence but had a hernia that involved approximately 60% of the anterior abdominal wall.

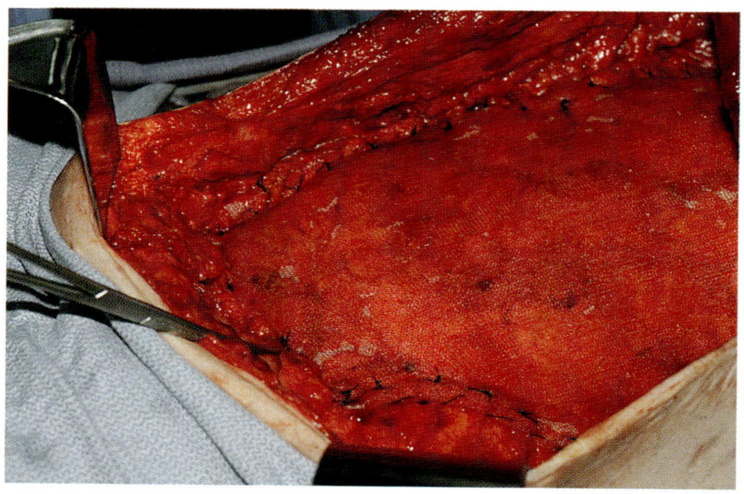

Intraoperatively the abdominal viscera and hernia sac were dissected from the subcutaneous fat, leaving an enormous musculofascial defect. The inguinal ligament had been previously resected. A sheet of Prolene mesh was sutured to the undersurface of the surrounding fascial rim medially and laterally, the costal margin superiorly, and the iliac periosteum inferiorly. The repair was pulled taut to reduce the circumference of the residual defect.

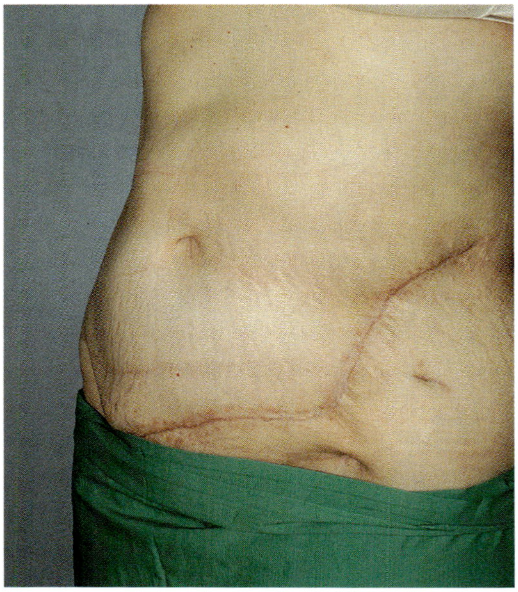

Three months postoperatively the patient was well healed and considerably more comfortable.

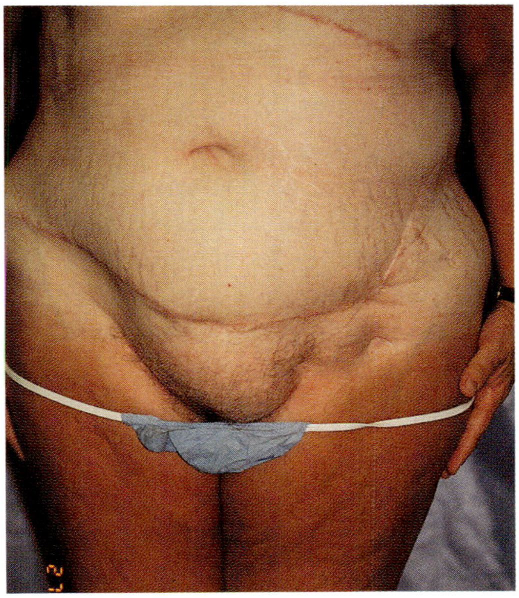

However, 3 years postoperatively after considerable weight gain she presented with a small hernia in the left groin, which was intermittently tender. This defect was repaired by resuturing the mesh to periosteum of the ilium. Correction has been maintained.

Desmoid tumors have been reported to present in preexisting surgical incisions and can be associated with Gardner's syndrome.[39] Nondesmoid sarcomas, however, seem to have little association with sex or age but can be associated with sites of previous radiation.[40] In addition to cases of primary lesions in which reconstruction is being considered, the reoperative surgeon may also be called to examine patients with local recurrences of these tumors. A high index of suspicion should be maintained when examining patients with an abdominal wall mass that may appear small and innocuous.

Another primary neoplastic lesion that should be considered is trunk melanoma, which may or may not appear typical. Again in this setting a high index of suspicion must be maintained.

Large, open chronic wounds, especially secondary to radiation, may give rise to primary malignant tumors of the abdominal wall such as squamous cell carcinoma. Chronic burn scars on the abdomen can also develop scar carcinoma.

Secondary neoplasia usually implies direct extension from an intra-abdominal tumor; however, foci of malignant cells can also reach the abdominal wall by the blood-borne or lymphatic route. In addition, peritoneal seeding of intra-abdominal tumors can result in a diffuse involvement of the abdominal wall.

Radiation

Radiation injury of the abdominal wall is less common than radiation injury in other regions where radiation therapy is more often employed as primary therapy such as the head and neck, chest wall, and extremities. In addition, when radiation is applied to the abdomen, the abdominal viscera are more susceptible to acute and chronic injury than the abdominal wall itself. The problem of radiation enteritis is beyond the scope of this chapter; however, in patients presenting with acute onset of abdominal pain, bleeding, or nausea and vomiting, the diagnosis of radiation enteritis should be kept in mind.[40]

In regard to the overlying abdominal wall, chronic radiation injury may present many years after treatment and may consist of only skin changes with telangiectasis and induration from fibrosis or there may be an open, nonhealing ulcer due to local tissue hypoxemia.[41] Many times these patients are very frustrated, can have significant social problems secondary to foul odors and soilage of their clothes, and often present with chronic pain as well. It should be remembered that the end result of radiation injury and the cause of the patient's wound is essentially a vascular injury at the microscopic level; therefore overall blood flow and oxygen delivery into such a region is significantly reduced. Even in patients who present for reoperative surgery whose indication is not the previous radiation, one must consider the compromised nature of this tissue and how it will affect the planning of the reoperative procedure.

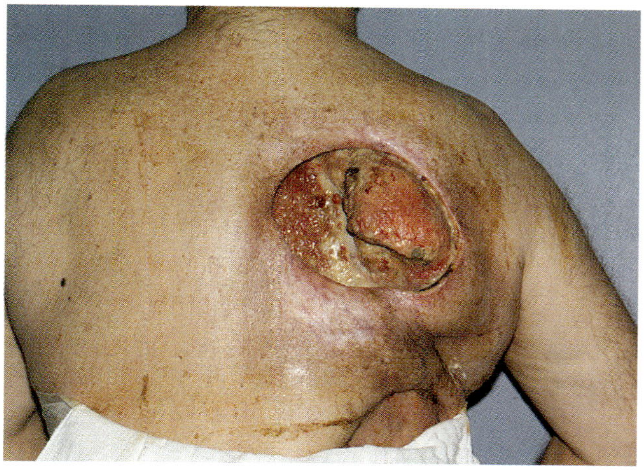

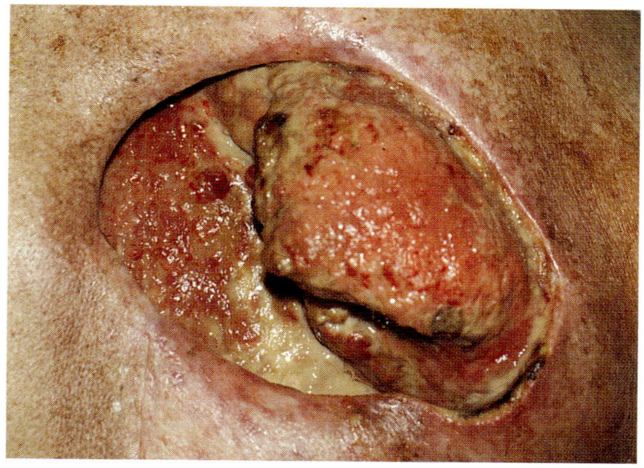

This 67-year-old patient is a good example of the problems associated with neoplasia, heavy radiation, and failed previous reconstructive surgery. A mass developed on his back and was originally thought to be a lipoma. However, following excision this lesion was noted to be a malignant fibrous histiocytoma. A secondary wide local excision was performed and was followed by the delivery of 6600 rads of radiotherapy over 50 days. A large radionecrotic wound in the area of the right trapezius with an exposed scapula resulted. At the time of referral he had undergone an attempt to transpose the ipsilateral latissimus dorsi muscle to cover the defect, but the flap had failed and required debridement.

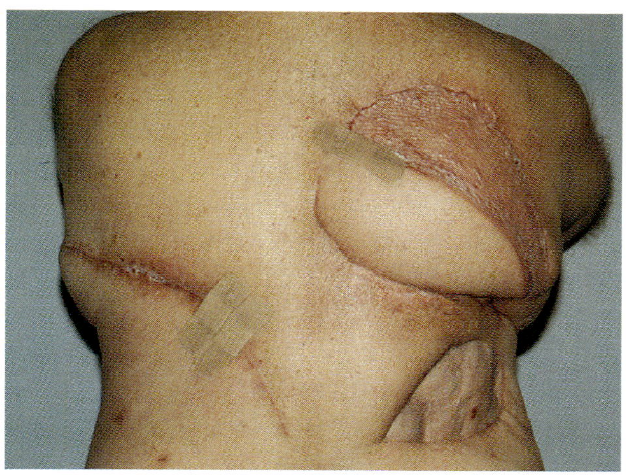

Without any good local options for coverage, a free tissue transfer was selected. The opposite latissimus dorsi muscle was considered to be the most reliable option; however, we did not believe that it would completely cover the defect if used as a turnover flap. We therefore elected to perform a free tissue transfer anastomosing the contralateral latissimus dorsi muscle to the thoracodorsal pedicle from the previous failed ipsilateral latissimus dorsi muscle.

Photographs from Grotting JC. Latissimus dorsi musculocutaneous flap for repair of radionecrotic scapular wound. Perspect Plast Surg 6(1):146, 1992.

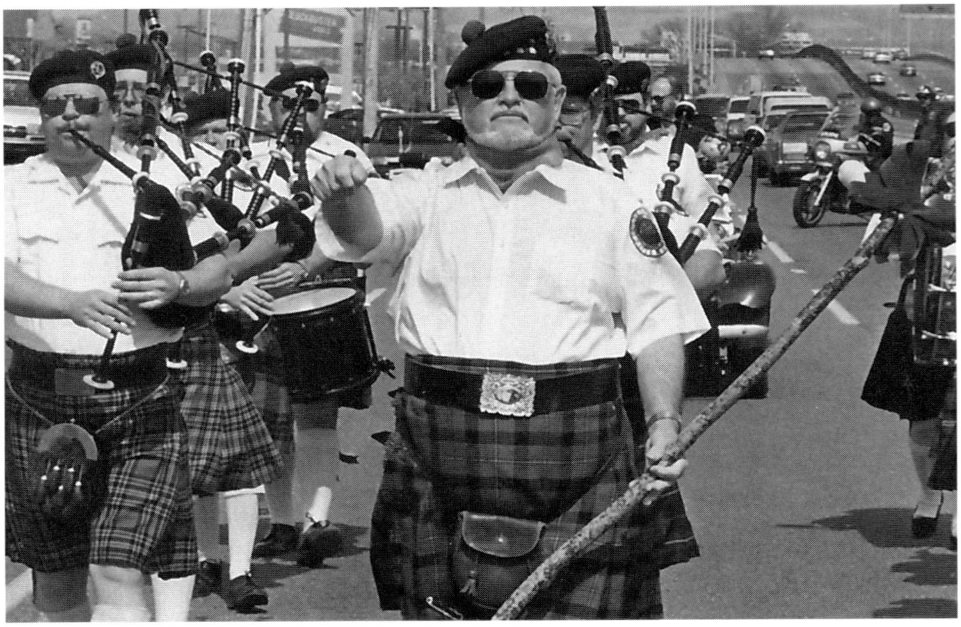

Photo by Dave Dieter, *The Huntsville Times*

The wound healed uneventfully, and the patient has returned to his vital, active lifestyle.

Failed Aesthetic Surgery

Patients who have undergone previous abdominoplasty and/or suction-assisted lipectomy can frequently be the most frustrating patients because their expectations are the highest of all who present for reoperative abdominal wall surgery. The most common problems in these patients presenting for reoperation are seromas,[42,43] which are not normally serious problems. However, other complications of previous abdominal aesthetic surgery can be more difficult: skin loss, irregular or hypertrophic scarring, improper position of the umbilicus or mons pubis, significant contour deformities, and sclerolipomatosis resulting from panniculitis. Illouz[44] defines sclerolipomatosis as fatty infiltrates permeating scarred tissue from prior surgery or liposuction. The fat is likely produced from multipotential cells present in the sclerotic tissue and can give rise to irregularities. The most serious complication in the acute setting is bowel perforation from a liposuction cannula, although fortunately this is quite rare. Another serious complication is enlarging hematoma with secondary volume depletion.[43]

PLANNING

Goals

A clear understanding of the obtainable goals is essential and at the minimum, these should include (1) coverage of the intra-abdominal contents, (2) restoration of the function and integrity of the musculofascial abdominal wall, (3) eradication of preexisting factors that contributed to the patient requiring the reoperation (e.g., poor technique, inadequate debridement, inadequate tumor resection, infection), (4) reconstruction with like tissue, and (5) attention to aesthetic detail.

Assessment

In the preoperative setting there are many factors to be considered before selecting the type of reconstructive procedure. First and foremost is the overall condition of the patient. The extent of reconstructive effort will obviously depend on what the patient can tolerate medically. Patients who are too ill to undergo immediate reoperation for a serious problem such as an acute wound dehiscence should be managed nonoperatively.[44]

For those patients able to tolerate reoperation, an acute assessment of the problem at the local wound level is essential. One must understand the factors that created the initial failure and take steps to avoid them. In addition, one must consider the quality and amount of available tissue for reconstruction, location of the defect, and type and amount of tissue (or prosthetic material) needed to correct the problem. One must then match the technique to the above considerations.

Preoperative Care

In the preoperative period there are several adjuvant therapies that can be beneficial such as placement of a nasogastric tube for preoperative bowel decompression. Appropriate skin preparation and preoperative antibiotic therapy are essential. A broad-spectrum antibiotic regimen is desirable; usually one agent is adequate.[31] However, certain special circumstances, such as intraluminal stasis of bowel contents, or perhaps an emergent infectious problem, such as fasciitis or gangrenous bowel, may require expanded coverage. In such cases broad-spectrum Gram-negative and Gram-positive coverage is indicated as well as strong anaerobic coverage.

In elective cases bowel preparation should be performed if any encroachment on adjacent bowel is a possibility. In addition, one should always remember that in the obese ventral hernia patient, weight reduction will vastly lower the chances of recurrence. Appropriate antiembolic therapy such as intermittent pneumatic compression stockings should also be considered. Attention to the preoperative correction of other underlying problems such as nutritional deficits, pulmonary disorders, and fluid and electrolyte disorders is important. Acute dehiscence will require appropriate overall resuscitation methods and protection of exposed bowel until closure can be obtained.

Incisions

It is important to begin the reoperative procedure with incisions that are designed with regard to relaxed skin tension lines as well as underlying neurovascular and muscular structures. A midline incision is the least damaging from a functional standpoint, although it does place the wound under tension because the lines of tension extend horizontally. No significant difference in dehiscence rates has been found between vertical, horizontal, or oblique incisions.[17] However, the dehiscence rate is not the only factor that should be considered in selecting an incision.

Paramedian incisions are to be avoided if possible since they interrupt neurovascular structures entering from the lateral abdomen and create a defunctionalized segment of abdominal wall between the incision and the midline. Consideration should be given also to vascular inflow, and, to prevent ischemia, acute angles of incision should be avoided. Extreme care should be taken to avoid causing bowel injury when making the incision. However, if bowel perforation occurs, it can usually be managed with simple oversewing of the enterotomy in the case of a patient who has had an adequate bowel preparation. In the unprepared bowel, enterotomies in the small bowel and colon enterotomies with minimal contamination can still be oversewn. However, with more extensive contamination from a colon enterotomy, the creation of a colostomy or an exteriorization of the injured bowel may be indicated.[45] Copious localized irrigation of the areas involved with spillage of enteric contents should be performed.

MANAGEMENT

Acute Wound Dehiscence

Decisions for operative management in stable patients are based primarily on the adequacy of the available tissue as well as on basic surgical principles that relate to infected, contaminated, or clean tissue (Table 36-1). Other issues such as constitutional factors and local wound factors obviously also play a role in the operative plan.

A close inspection of the opened wound in the operating room may reveal factors that directly contributed to the dehiscence. In addition to inspection of the wound itself, if there is a suspicion of associated intra-abdominal problems, then exploratory laparotomy should be performed in conjunction with the general surgeon. The optimal situation is when *adequate tissue* is present and primary fascial closure can be obtained without undue tension. The proper technique of fascial closure is the placement of nonabsorbable sutures at intervals at least 1 cm

Table 36-1 Operative Planning for Abdominal Wall Closure After Wound Failure in Stable Patient

Reconstructive Limitations	*State of Wound*	*Plan in Acute Setting*	*Plan in Nonacute Setting*
Adequate available tissue	Clean	Primary fascial closure including skin and subcutaneous tissue.	Obtain primary fascial closure in small defects. Consider prosthetic material in large defects, especially if recurrent.
	Contaminated	Primary fascial closure. Delayed primary closure of skin.	Primary fascial repair after wound converted to clean wound as possible (stoma closure, debridement, etc.). Avoid prosthetic materials, if possible.
	Dirty	Primary fascial closure. Allow wound to heal by secondary intention.	
Relative tissue deficiency	Clean	Relaxing incisions. If excess tension, use prosthetic material, which is removed when distention resolves.	Release scarring. Remove prosthetic material or skin grafts as necessary. Relaxing incisions. Should not need flaps. May consider prosthetic material if closure under tension.
	Contaminated	As above. Leave skin open if contamination is heavy.	Convert to clean wound as much as possible prior to closure.
	Dirty	As above. Leave skin open.	
Absolute tissue deficiency	Clean	Relaxing incisions. Consider local flaps, then regional flaps, then free flaps. Prosthetic material with simultaneous coverage with vascularized tissue.	Release scarring. Remove prosthetic material and/or skin grafts as necessary. Early consideration for use of prosthetic material. Autogenous methods in selected cases (e.g., radiation).
	Contaminated	As above. Avoid placing foreign material in contaminated wound if possible to avoid the need for secondary surgery for removal. If unavoidable, cover Prolene mesh material with well-vascularized tissue.	Convert to clean wound as much as possible prior to closure.
	Dirty	Complete debridement. Prosthetic material for fascial integrity. *Absorbable:* STSG to granulation tissue. Late repair of ventral hernia. *Nonabsorbable:* (1) STSG to granulation tissue with later removal of material and replacement with coverage using well-vascularized tissue, *or* (2) may be able to cover indwelling mesh with flaps if wound clean. Some risk for late infection.	

STSG, split-thickness skin graft.

apart and 1.5 cm away from the fascial edge.[17,46] No clear advantage to running vs. interrupted suturing techniques has been identified, although running suturing techniques have shown a slightly lower dehiscence rate in recent studies.[17] The use of absorbable sutures has been shown to increase the rate of late incisional hernia formation.[47] In addition, the closure technique should not include the peritoneum since involvement of this structure in the closure increases the risk of intra-abdominal adhesions.[15] In clean wounds the skin and fascia can be approximated primarily. However, in contaminated wounds either the skin should be left open or a subcutaneous irrigating catheter should be used.[48] If the contamination is heavy, the skin and subcutaneous tissue should be left open. In heavily contaminated or infected wounds, delayed primary skin closure can be performed once the wound is clean (bacteria $<10^5$/gm of tissue) or the wound can simply be allowed to heal secondarily.[49]

In wounds that have a tissue deficiency, it should be determined whether this deficiency is relative or absolute. An example of relative tissue deficiency is excessive bowel distention with inability to close the abdomen. Absolute tissue deficiency would be the case when tissue has been resected and even in the presence of decompressed bowel primary closure cannot be obtained because of excessive tension. Relative tissue deficiency can sometimes be managed with the use of relaxing incisions designed strategically to avoid eventration[50,51]; however, if excessive tension still exists, prosthetic material should be placed for temporary fascial support until the distention improves. When the relative tissue deficiency has resolved by decompression of the bowel, the wound can be closed primarily and the heavily contaminated or infected wound can undergo fascial closure via either secondary healing of the skin or delayed primary skin closure.

In the case of absolute tissue deficiency in a clean wound, local autogenous tissue should be employed to obtain closure if the defect is not large. For a vertical midline incision, one can again try a relaxation technique such as the components separation method or fascial/partition release.[50,51] These techniques are similar in that they use parasagittal relaxing incisions through the external oblique muscle and create a dynamic, vascularized, and innervated bipedicled rectus abdominis (RA) flap that can be advanced medially. They differ in the location of the posterior fascial release. Care must be taken not to extend the relaxing incision in the external oblique muscle into Hesselbach's triangle; otherwise groin herniation may occur. Long-term follow-up of patients who have undergone these techniques is not available, but the early experience is encouraging. Turnover flaps of rectus fascia can also be used above the arcuate line for the repair of small defects; however, it should be remembered that the lower abdomen has no posterior rectus sheath, and the anterior sheath should not be used for a local fascial flap because abdominal wall eventration can result.

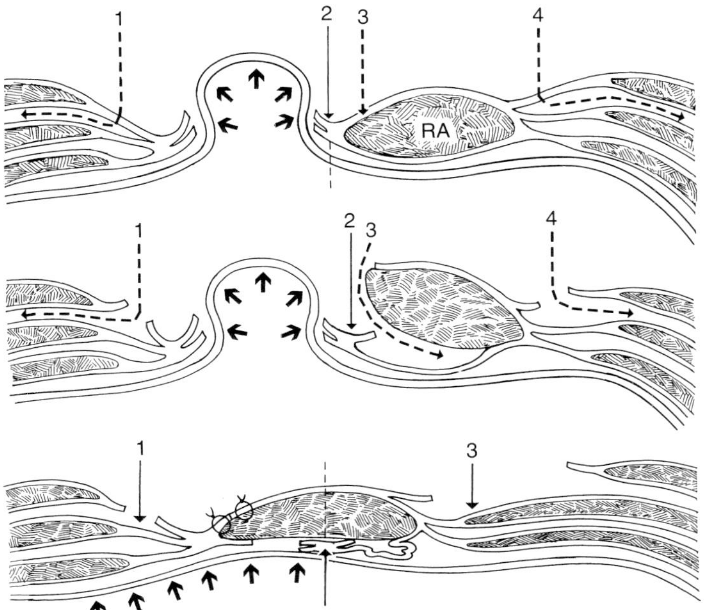

Components separation method

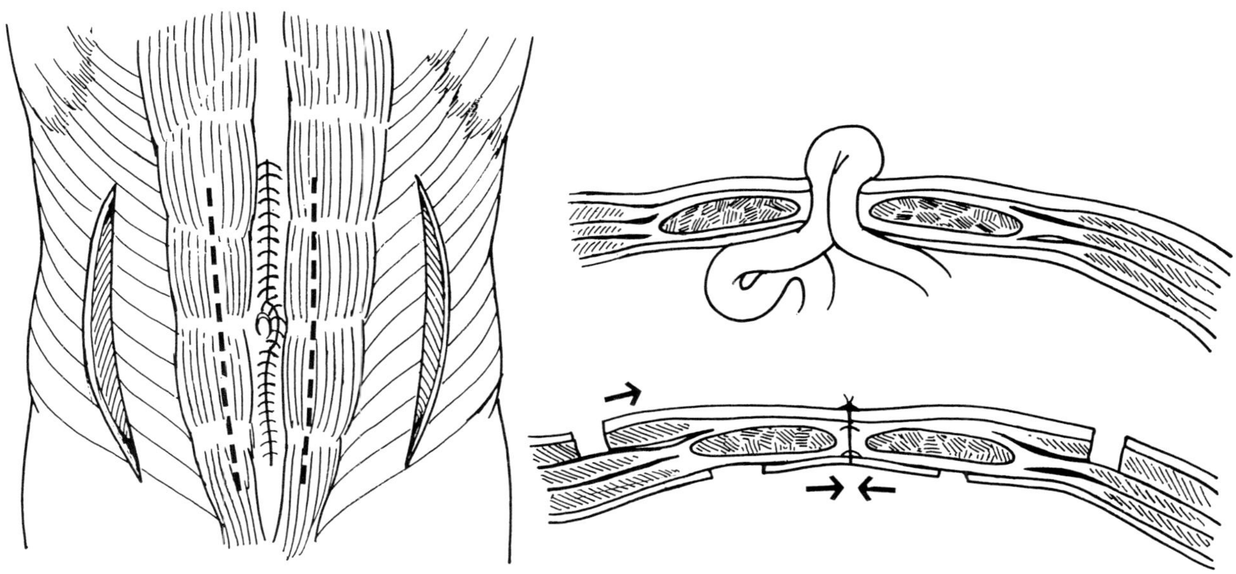

Fascial partition release method

If local autogenous tissue is not available for achieving a low-tension closure, then prosthetic material for fascial repair should be used, with simultaneous coverage with vascularized tissue of adjacent skin and subcutaneous tissue or local or regional flaps.[52,53] If prosthetic material is selected, it is best to use permanent material since the use of absorbable material tends to result in late incisional hernia.[54] Prosthetic material should be placed using an inlay, not onlay, method, with secure, permanent fascial sutures.[31,52] Regional flaps may be used in this setting as well, although often the patient with acute wound dehiscence is in need of rapid reclosure with minimal associated donor site morbidity, thus making regional flaps less desirable in most cases.

In heavily contaminated or infected wounds with absolute tissue deficiencies, one should avoid the use of local or regional flaps since opening tissue planes elsewhere in the body can predispose to the spread of infection. Early consideration should be given to the use of prosthetic material. Controversy exists regarding the use of absorbable vs. nonabsorbable material in this setting. In the infectious setting, prosthetic material may be absorbable or nonabsorbable and meshed or unmeshed. Prolene mesh has been associated with the best results in this group.[13,31,52,53] Mesh material is also advised by some surgeons who claim that the interstices allow drainage from a septic abdominal cavity, and a zipper can be placed for repeated access when serial debridements are anticipated.[55] However, others argue that the abdominal cavity seals within 12 hours and becomes impermeable to drainage even when mesh is used.[56] What really is most important is to provide a fascial substitute for coverage and support of the intestinal viscera. Unmeshed prosthetic material such as human dura mater or polytetrafluoroethylene (Gore-Tex)[57,58] also has its proponents. Gore-Tex, which is a solid sheet of microporous PTFE, has been shown to produce fewer adhesions than any other prosthetic material and also has been demonstrated to provide a less adherent surface for bacteria.[59] However, because it also does not allow bacterial egress through the small pores,[60] its use should be restricted to clean wounds or cases in which it is intended only as a temporary prosthesis. Other surgeons have recommended using absorbable mesh in the infected setting because nonabsorbable materials, particularly polypropylene (Marlex), have been associated with a high complication rate in some series.[54] The absorbable mesh can provide good fascial support as long as it is not necessary for the long term; otherwise, the absorbable mesh will eventually disappear and the patient will be left with a ventral hernia. A rationale for using absorbable mesh is that the eventual hernia is the price one has to pay to avoid the complications associated with permanent mesh such as extrusion and possible erosion into bowel.[54] The etiology of these problems with permanent mesh is presumed to be that the application of skin grafts to the granulation bed growing through the mesh results in relatively ischemic coverage. As the wound then heals and contracts, wrinkling occurs, contributing to loss of coverage, extrusion, or erosion into bowel. Although absorbable mesh thus avoids these problems, the loss of the fascial support is imminent. It should be mentioned that Prolene mesh has not had the problems attributed to Marlex and has performed well in the infectious setting. Whichever material is used, a second procedure will likely be required, either to replace or cover the nonabsorbable material or to reconstruct the ventral hernia that will result from the use of absorbable mesh.

Patients who are medically unstable require an entirely different approach since early closure of the wound is of lesser priority. The use of a wound pack with an abdominal binder can be used in cases when necessary to prevent acute evisceration.[53] Wounds with granulation tissue in the base where the viscera have already become "fixed" may be covered with a split-thickness skin graft even in the intensive care unit. These methods will help to reduce fluid and protein loss through the wound as well as give some degree of protection to the underlying viscera.

Ventral Hernia

Since ventral hernias occur late in the postoperative course, they can be repaired in an elective fashion. If a temporary colostomy or draining fistula site is present in association with a stable ventral hernia, then this problem should be addressed first if possible to eliminate the risk of contamination.

The determination of relative vs. absolute tissue deficiencies in stable ventral hernias is more difficult, and many times what appears to be a deficiency of tissue peripherally is nothing more than widely separated fascial layers with contraction and scarring.[50] Consequently attempts to release scarred tissues and advance fascial edges for a low-tension, primary closure should be made. Many times the determination of absolute tissue deficiency cannot be made until the actual surgery. If necessary, tissue expansion preoperatively can be used to increase tissue availability peripherally. Tissue expansion is not recommended in the presence of open wounds, enterocutaneous fistulas, or enterostomies. Also, the time and expense of staged reconstruction with tissue expanders must be weighed against the one-stage application of a mesh inlay repair.

If possible, a low-tension closure with autogenous tissue is preferred; therefore local fascial flaps or a relaxation method is optimal. However, if necessary to obtain a low-tension closure, one should not hesitate to use prosthetic material that is covered with well-vascularized tissue.[53] Local, regional, or distant flaps may be necessary to cover the inlaid material. The use of drains in association with prosthetic material should be minimized and removed early to avoid possible contamination through the drain tract.

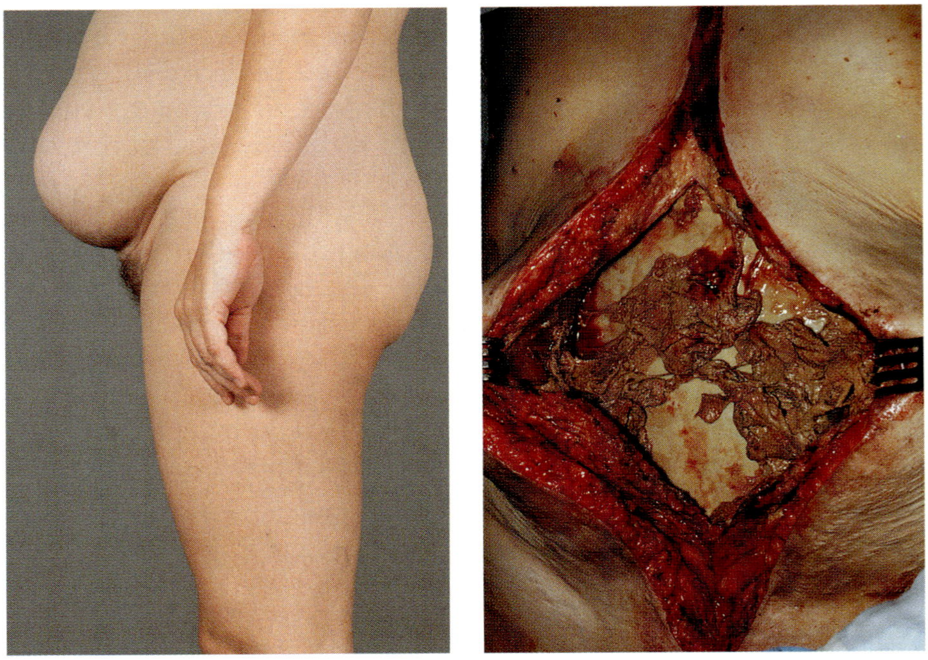

Following aortofemoral graft placement and closure with a Gore-Tex patch, this patient presented with a ventral hernia. Intraoperatively a periprosthetic collection of old blood was found.

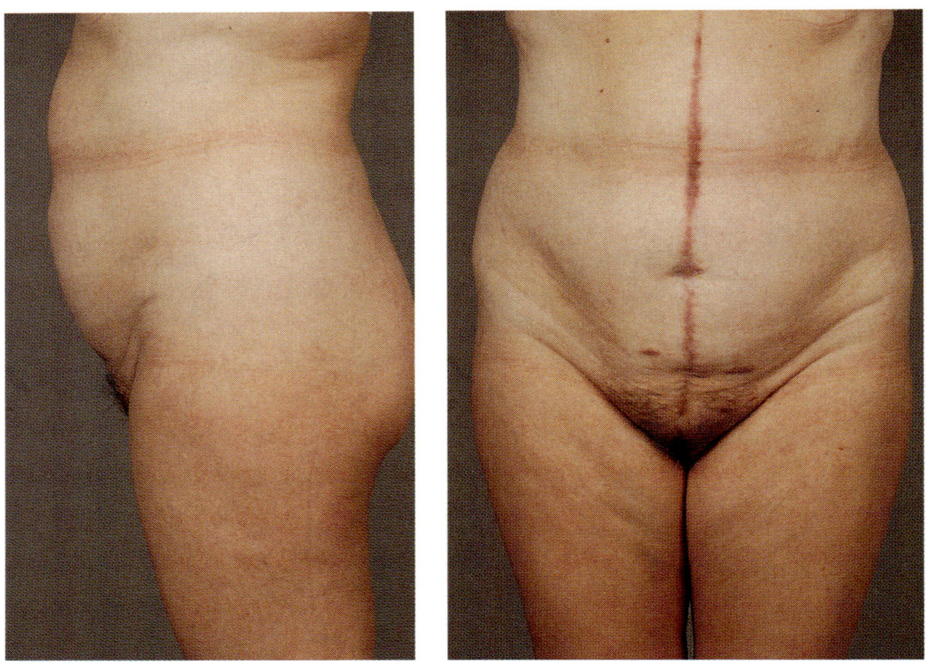

After removal of the Gore-Tex patch, correction of a diastasis recti was achieved with fascial plication, resection of redundant underlying tissue, and closure.

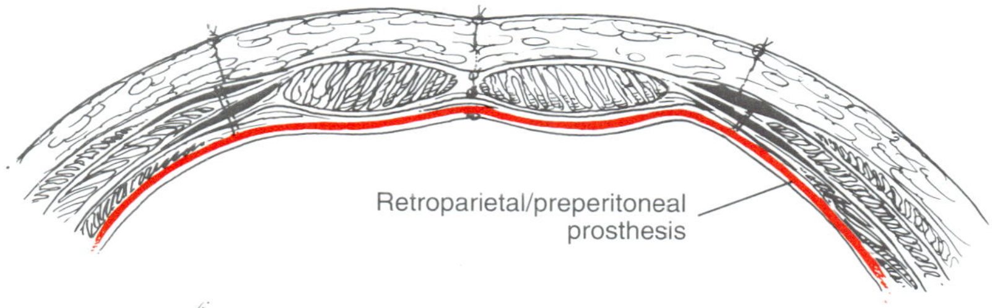

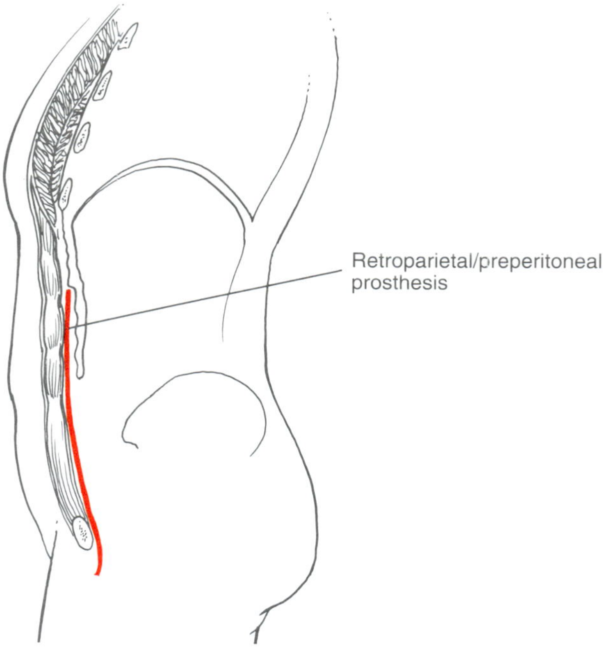

An alternative method of prosthetic material reconstruction for ventral hernias and groin hernias has been described by Stoppa[61,62] and reportedly has a much lower recurrence rate than autogenous repair. This method is termed "giant prosthetic reinforcement of the visceral sac" (GPRVS) and consists of the placement of a large sheet of Mersilene mesh within the abdominal wall such that the mesh lines the abdominal cavity for an extensive distance around the defect. The intra-abdominal pressure holds the mesh against the inside of the abdominal wall anterior to the peritoneum or posterior rectus sheath. The need for extensive peripheral sutures is therefore unnecessary; the only ones used are in areas in which a strategic anchor for an edge is needed. The portion of the material extending across the defect provides a secure barrier against herniation of intra-abdominal contents. Excellent results have been reported with this technique with recurrence rates much lower than with standard mesh inlay techniques or autogenous methods.[61,62] Although described initially for recurrent groin hernias, it is applicable to isolated areas of abdominal wall herniation where the visceral sac may need reinforcing. It addition, by placing the mesh below a complete repair of a hernia, one may still gain the mechanical advantage of GPRVS in relation to decreasing tension on the repair postoperatively.

Illustration from Stoppa R. Advances in the care of large incisional hernias. Hospimedica 10:43, 1992.

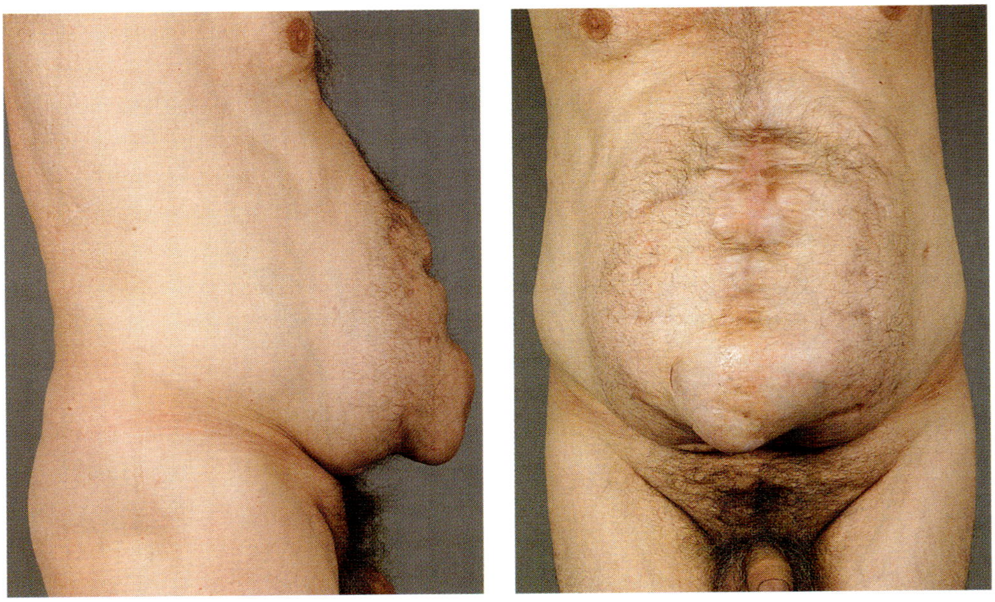

In our limited experience with this technique for ventral herniation we have observed no complications and no recurrences. This patient presented with an extensive ventral hernia from a previous laparotomy that was performed for abdominal trauma and splenectomy.

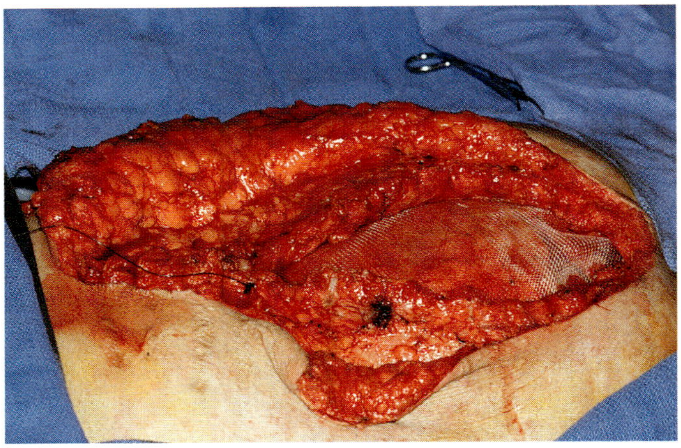

At surgery giant prosthetic reinforcement of the defect was obtained with the placement of Prolene mesh.

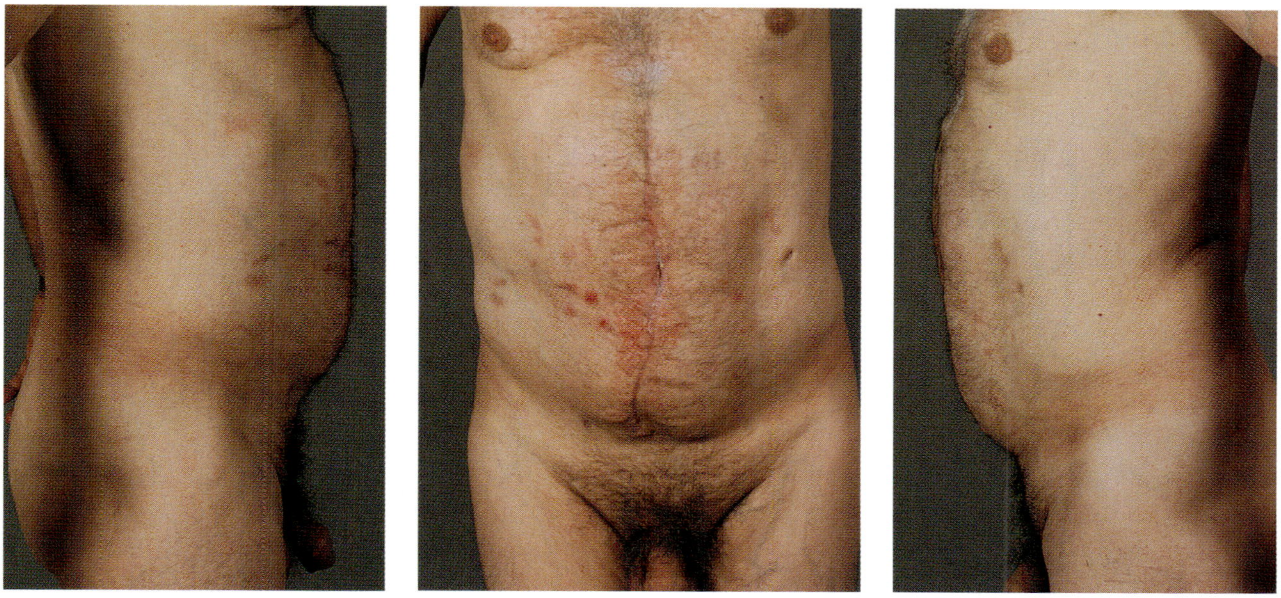

Eight months after the repair there is no evidence of recurrence.

Although the mesh should be placed preperitoneally or in front of the posterior rectus sheath if possible, Larson and Vandertoll[52] have reported intraperitoneal Marlex closure of the abdominal wall without any problems. Our experience has been with Prolene mesh, and we also have not encountered any problems if intraperitoneal placement is required. Others have noted occasional recurrence with Prolene mesh and believe that, unlike Mersilene mesh, it is not adherent enough for GPRVS.[63]

Inlay methods of mesh repair when the abdominal wall is not reapproximated and the mesh is used to fill the defect also appear to be effective compared with autogenous repair in larger defects.[53] No direct comparative studies of GPRVS vs. inlay mesh repair have been reported.

If the use of mesh is undesirable and local methods are not sufficient to close the ventral hernia, the use of regional or distant flaps of autogenous tissue is required (see p. 1364).

Recurrent Groin Hernia

The recurrent groin hernia has been a source of controversy concerning its proper management. Classic hernioplasty, which consists of an anterior approach using autogenous tissue for repair, has had recurrence rates that range from 4% to 21%.[64] Lower recurrence rates have been reported following the use of prosthetic mesh and the Shouldice technique.[63] Many surgeons now believe that repairing a recurrent hernia using endogenous tissue alone results in a higher recurrence rate than prosthetic mesh repair since underlying factors that possibly contributed to the recurrence may still be in play such as deficiency in collagen synthesis due to an underlying metabolic, biochemical, or toxic process.[14] With the use of prosthetic mesh for the repair for a recurrent inguinal hernia, the reasons for failure are reduced to exclusively that of technical error.[61]

Several techniques have been described for the prosthetic mesh repair of a recurrent inguinal hernia,[29,61,65,66] including standard inlay techniques, GPRVS, preperitoneal approach, and laparoscopic approach. Nyhus et al.[65] choose the preperitoneal approach and anchor the mesh in place with sutures. Laparoscopically, rolled strips of polypropylene mesh have been used to plug the recurrent hernia defect.[66] Prosthetic material has also been placed laparoscopically as a sheet across the inguinal floor and stapled at its edges in order to prevent movement of the material. Many of these techniques are at present experimental; however, it is becoming quite clear that recurrence rates for techniques using prosthetic material are lower than those for techniques involving autogenous tissue.[63] Only the Shouldice repair has matched the low recurrence rates of prosthetic material in the treatment of recurrent groin hernia. However, it should be remembered that these results were obtained by the originators of that technique and therefore reflect their vast experience and careful patient selection.[67] These results cannot necessarily be translated to any surgeon who employs the Shouldice technique. This technique may be the method of choice in situations in which prosthetic material repair is undesirable due to infectious risk factors already in place.[63] Muscle transposition in patients with infectious risk factors should also be considered an option, especially if there is an absolute tissue deficiency[68] (see p. 1364).

Parastomal Hernia

Recurrent parastomal hernias should not be managed by attempts at local fascial reconstruction without moving the stoma to a new location, preferably within the rectus abdominis muscle.[30] Once the stoma is relocated, local autogenous repair can be employed. Attempts to use prosthetic mesh for parastomal hernias without moving the stoma should also be avoided since there is potential for bowel erosion and infection. However, with movement of the stoma and absence of contamination, prosthetic material can be a useful adjunct when the defect is large and can be employed as described for ventral hernia repair.

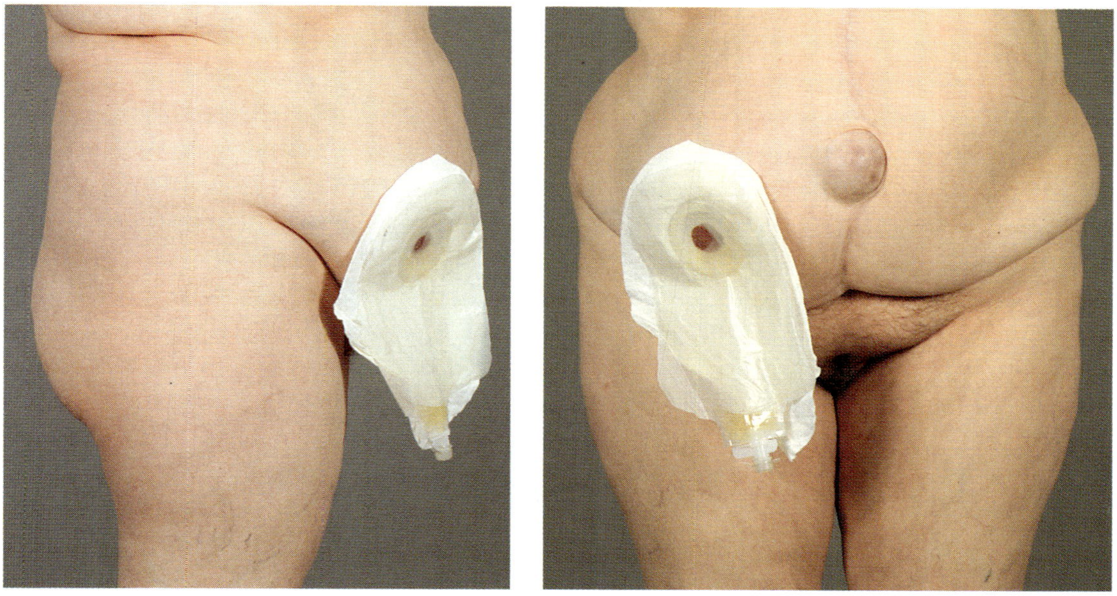

A massive parastomal recurrent ventral hernia developed in this patient due to the improper placement of the stoma site lateral to the rectus abdominis muscle.

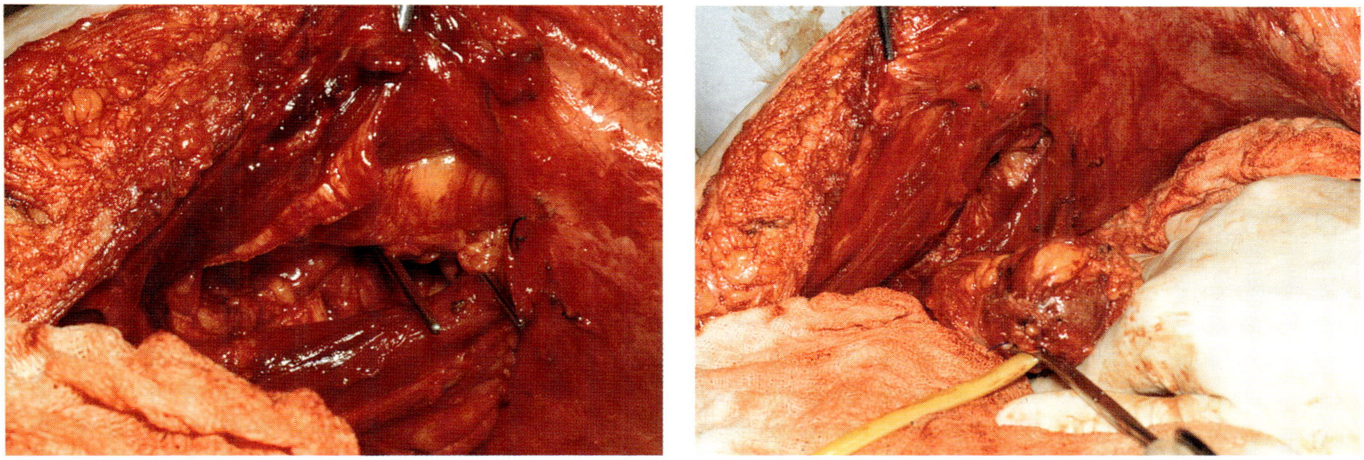

After takedown of the ureterostomy, the extent of the parastomal hernia was apparent.

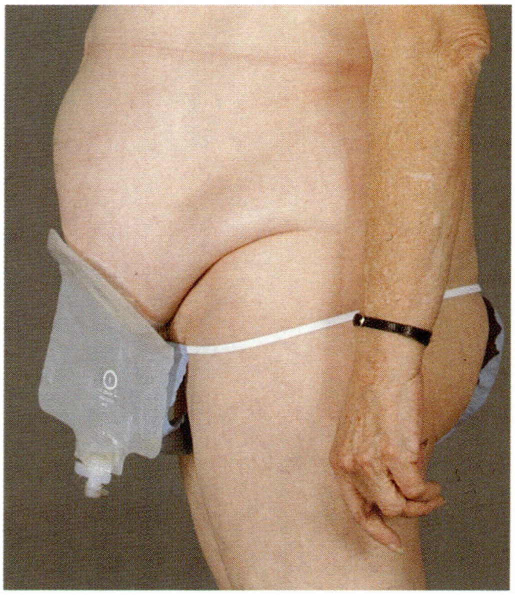

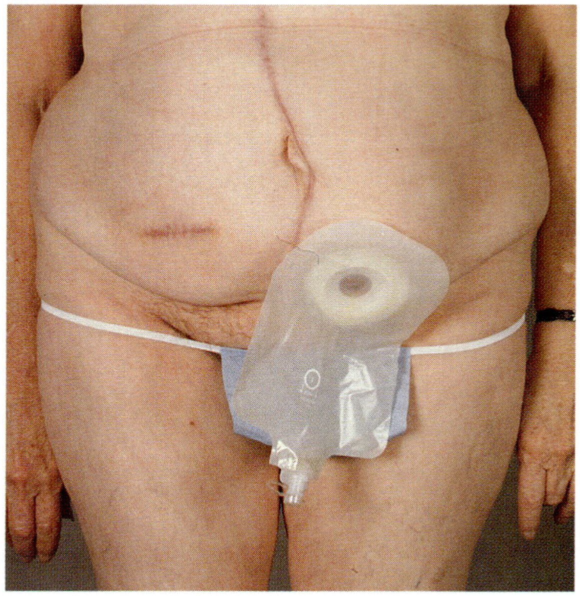

The patient is shown 1 year postoperatively. The parastomal hernia was repaired using right unilateral giant prosthetic reinforcement with Prolene mesh. The stoma was moved to the opposite side of the abdomen and placed through the rectus abdominis muscle. There is no evidence of recurrence.

Lumbar Hernias

Recurrent lumbar hernias are uncommon and require reconstruction based on the etiology of the recurrence. Most recurrences involve previously placed prosthetic mesh, which is indicated for the initial repair of lumbar hernia.[69] However, again, in patients with infectious risks in whom prosthetic material should be avoided, an autogenous fascial substitute is preferable and can be obtained from local, regional, or distant flaps.

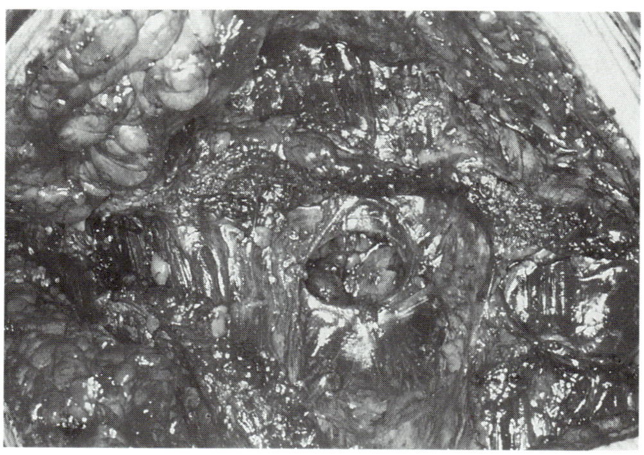

Courtesy R. Read, M.D.

In this patient a Grynfelt-type lumbar hernia was present.

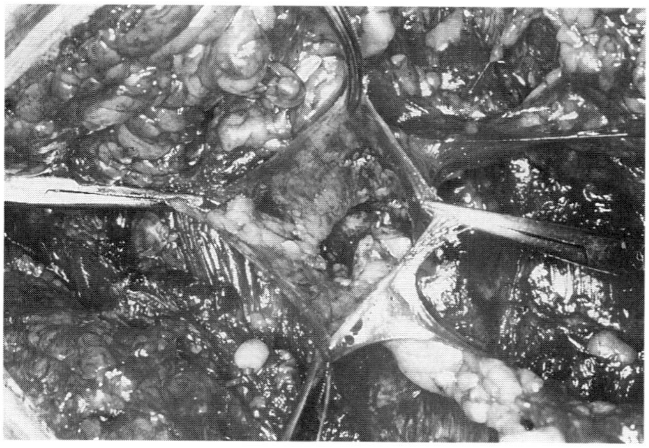

Delineation of the peritoneal sac is shown. It was ligated and reduced.

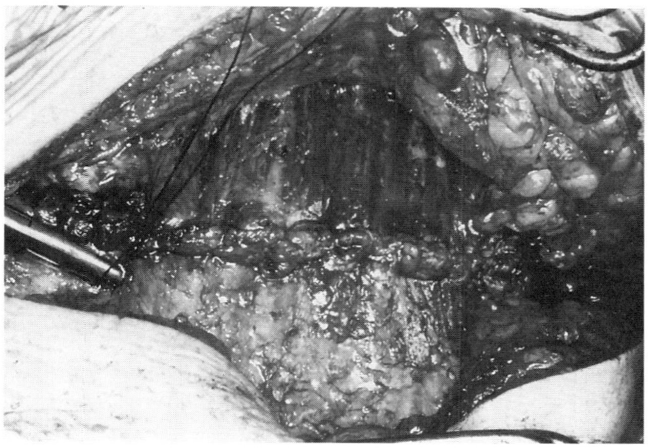

A Marlex mesh inlay patch was used to repair the fascial defect. The latissimus dorsi muscle flap was reapproximated over the patch to complete the reconstruction.

Neoplasia and Radiation

The reconstruction of abdominal wall defects secondary to the ablation of neoplastic lesions may occur in association with a primary tumor or in the case of a recurrence. In either situation reconstruction is aimed at replacing the loss of large blocks of tissue in order to obtain coverage and integrity of the abdominal wall. In the setting of a primary tumor, the reconstructive nomogram follows the order of preferential options as applies to the treatment of any clean abdominal wound (see Table 36-1). This implies one should first consider primary closure if possible, followed by local flaps or a component separation method, followed by regional or distant flaps. The use of prosthetic material may be indicated in order to obtain abdominal wall integrity in large resections. The use of prosthetic material in this setting is favored by most oncologic surgeons since it avoids the possibility of donor site morbidity.[38] However, each case should be individualized, and one should always keep in mind the options for reconstruction with dynamic innervated muscle flaps.

In the case of recurrent tumor, one may be faced with scarring, fibrosis, impaired blood supply, and possible radiation injury. In this setting, especially one involving radiation injury, the use of primary closure and/or local tissue may not be the best option because of the compromised blood supply. Consideration should be given to bringing in new, well-vascularized tissue from outside the region. Fascial integrity may be obtained in these cases with either the transfer of an appropriate flap or prosthetic material covered with flap tissue. Areas of chronic radiation injury should be completely excised before reconstruction.[70] Irradiated tissue that does not demonstrate the sequelae of radiation injury, however, may tolerate limited local procedures with careful handling of tissue.[71]

Fasciitis

The appropriate treatment of fasciitis is based on early recognition and resuscitation of the patient followed by early, thorough debridement. The most common cause of mortality from necrotizing fasciitis is delay in diagnosis and inadequate debridement.[35] Planning the reconstruction of the abdominal wall after necrotizing fasciitis follows protocol involving dirty wounds with an absolute deficiency of tissue (see Table 36-1). In some situations there may be some available tissue locally; however, in most cases any residual tissue is too inflamed to tolerate primary repair and thus prosthetic material is commonly employed.

Prosthetic Material

The reoperative management of infected, foreign material commonly involves its removal either completely or partially. In the case of meshed material, removal can be a painstaking procedure, especially when it is in contact with underlying viscera. PTFE, however, is usually easily removed due to its low degree of tissue ingrowth.

Some surgeons have reported being able to resurface meshed material after granulation tissue has grown through it and the wound is exceptionally clean. However, salvage of the original mesh in such a setting requires coverage with well-vascularized tissue. Skin grafts alone have not been highly successful. Although some have reported PTFE to perform well in a contaminated or infected setting,[58] others have reported poor clinical outcomes.[60] Experimental evidence in support of the use of PTFE in the contaminated wound has also been conflicting.[57,60] The most recent reports have hypothesized that the small pore size of the PTFE soft tissue patch inhibits early ingrowth of fibrous tissue and, although this permits ease of removal, it also allows for the existence of potential space between the implant and the surrounding tissue, which can continue to be colonized by bacteria. This patch also creates a physical barrier to underlying bacteria and prevents their egress from the wound. In addition, it acts as a barrier to granulation tissue, which is unable to grow through the material and instead forms beneath the PTFE patch. These recent reports suggest that PTFE is not suitable for use in the contaminated or infected wound. In fact, when used in an uncontaminated wound that later becomes infected, PTFE should be removed. After removal, the wound should be thoroughly irrigated and, depending on the degree of contamination and whether or not the wound has become "fixed" due to fibrosis and granulation tissue, one may choose several reconstructive options. If fascial integrity is absolutely necessary, one may replace the PTFE with Prolene or absorbable mesh; if contamination is heavy, it may be necessary to leave the wound open. If the wound does not need immediate fascial integrity, then the wound may be skin grafted directly onto the underlying granulation bed, the wound may be left open, or if relatively clean, local tissue may simply be advanced for closure over drainage catheters. Ventral herniation may result, which will require later repair in a clean setting.

In contrast to PTFE, meshed material, especially Prolene, seems to have a higher salvage rate in the contaminated setting.[19,53,60] Exact statistics on the percentage of success in the salvage of mesh in a previously contaminated wound are not available. If the infection is detected early postoperatively and the mesh is vital for abdominal wall integrity, then the mesh should be exposed by opening the wound. Dressing changes should then be instituted to help to rid the wound of infection. Later coverage with well-vascularized tissue can then be achieved in most cases. However, it should be remembered that there may be a delayed occurrence of infection or sinus tracts in association with a previously contaminated foreign body that may not present until years later. For this reason some surgeons recommend either (1) complete removal of the contaminated mesh whenever possible with reconstruction performed at a later date or (2) staged removal.[36]

Others believe that complete removal of mesh should be performed only when infection is detected early postoperatively. When infection is encountered late in the postoperative course, only the isolated part contributing to a sinus tract needs to be removed and the integrated uninvolved part may be left in place.[18] For the purpose of late reconstruction, it is recommended that prosthetic material not be replaced into a wound associated with contamination unless absolutely necessary.

Failed Aesthetic Surgery

Reoperative techniques for failed aesthetic surgery usually involve corrections of asymmetry, scar revisions, liposuction of residual fat deposits or dog ears, and drainage of seromas or hematomas. In addition, skin necrosis at the apex of the abdominal flap due to ischemia may require significant debridement and conversion of the area to an open wound. Although this wound may be skin grafted, it is best to manage this defect as an open wound since it will contract over a period of time, reducing the size of the wound and thus the secondary scar. After the wound softens months later, secondary revision is much easier than if the entire area had been initially skin grafted. Other common problems of abdominoplasty, such as the superior displacement of the pubic mound and suprapubic scar depression (due to contraction of the unrepaired superficial fascial system), can be repaired by excision of the lower abdominal scar and proper attention to the repair of the superficial fascial system followed by skin repair.[3] Sclerolipomatosis, according to Illouz,[44] must be treated by liposuction to smooth out irregularities. Drastic complications of abdominoplasty such as bowel perforation, necrotizing fasciitis, or massive hernia are fortunately uncommon.

FLAPS

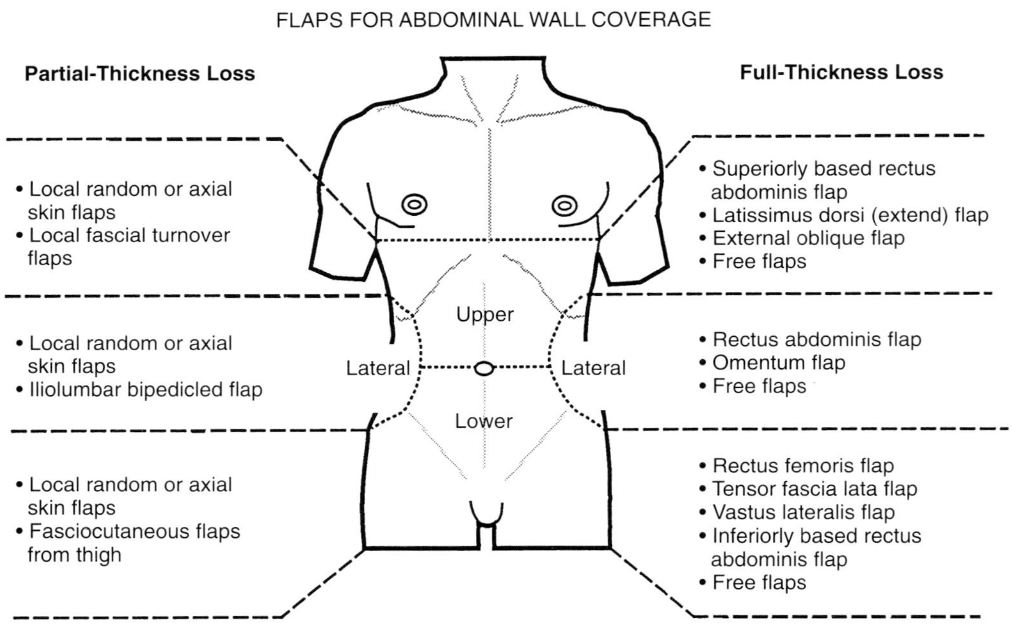

For repair in the mid to upper abdomen, the extended latissimus dorsi flap has been shown to be effective.[72] This reconstructive technique involves an incision that extends along the lateral border of the latissimus dorsi muscle and then over the gluteal region. The pregluteal fascia and the lumbodorsal fascia are exposed, and a section of this fascia is raised in continuity with the muscle flap. This enlarges the arc of rotation of the muscle, enabling it to contribute to the fascial closure of the abdomen. The flap is usually passed through subcutaneous tunnels to the anterior abdominal wall. A skin island can be transferred with the flap if necessary, or the muscle or pregluteal fascia can be skin grafted, which allows the defect to contract. Experience with this flap is limited but the results are encouraging. It should be kept in mind that the pregluteal fascia is very thin, and the dissection over the gluteus maximus can be very tedious; however, this fascia has been found to be fairly resilient and capable of adding strength to the abdominal repair. In addition, it can also be folded if necessary.[73]

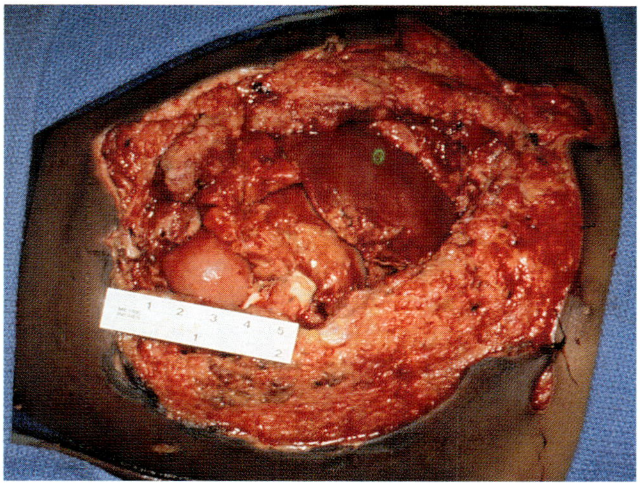

This patient suffered a gunshot wound, which resulted in an extensive left upper quadrant defect with exposed viscera.

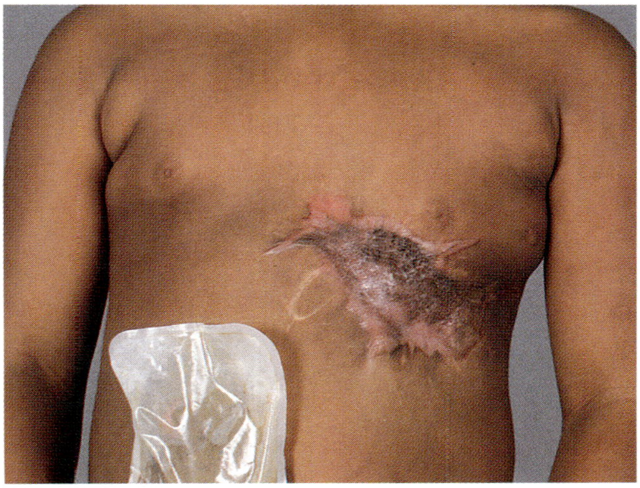

Wound closure was achieved with an extended latissimus dorsi flap covered with a skin graft. The result is shown 3 months postoperatively. Excellent abdominal wall competence has been obtained. Future tissue expansion for aesthetic refinement is planned.

For defects of the upper and lateral abdominal wall, an iliolumbar bipedicle flap has been described.[74] This flap involves a large segment of lower, lateral abdominal wall and is vascularized by the superficial circumflex iliac vessels anteriorly and perforating cutaneous branches of the lumbar vessels posteriorly. This area is incised down through skin and subcutaneous tissue to the musculofascial layer. This tissue can then be transposed cephalad over a fascial graft or prosthetic material and the donor site skin grafted. This flap does not aid in the transposition of fascial tissues, only in coverage.

Another source of tissue useful for reconstruction in the upper abdominal wall (as well as anywhere else in the abdomen) is the omentum.[75] The advantage of this tissue is that it can reach almost anywhere and conform to almost any defect. In addition, because it is exceptionally well vascularized, it covers prosthetic mesh well and supports skin grafts easily. The disadvantage, of course, is that it has no intrinsic support and because support is necessary, the use of prosthetic material is inevitable. Also, omentum tends to weep significantly after transposition, which can be a nuisance postoperatively.

The superiorly based rectus abdominis flap with transfer of anterior rectus sheath from above the arcuate line can be used for the closure of upper abdominal wall defects.[75] This technique provides good fascial support with well-vascularized tissue. Care should be taken not to extend the fascial donor site below the arcuate line or else lower abdominal wall weakness will result.

The external oblique musculocutaneous flap has also been used for transposition to upper abdominal wall defects.[76] This muscle flap can provide good support and coverage; however, the degree of rotation obviously is quite limited and is indicated only in selected cases.

In the mid to lower abdomen the flaps of choice are usually taken from the thigh.[75] In recent years the flap of choice has become the rectus femoris muscle due to its reliability, arc of rotation, innervation, and minor donor site morbidity.[76] This flap can be raised as a muscle flap alone or as a musculocutaneous flap. There is a posterior fascial element on the muscle that aids in reconstructing the fascial defect of the lower abdomen. The fasciocutaneous territory overlying the muscle can be used alone for coverage of partial-thickness defects.

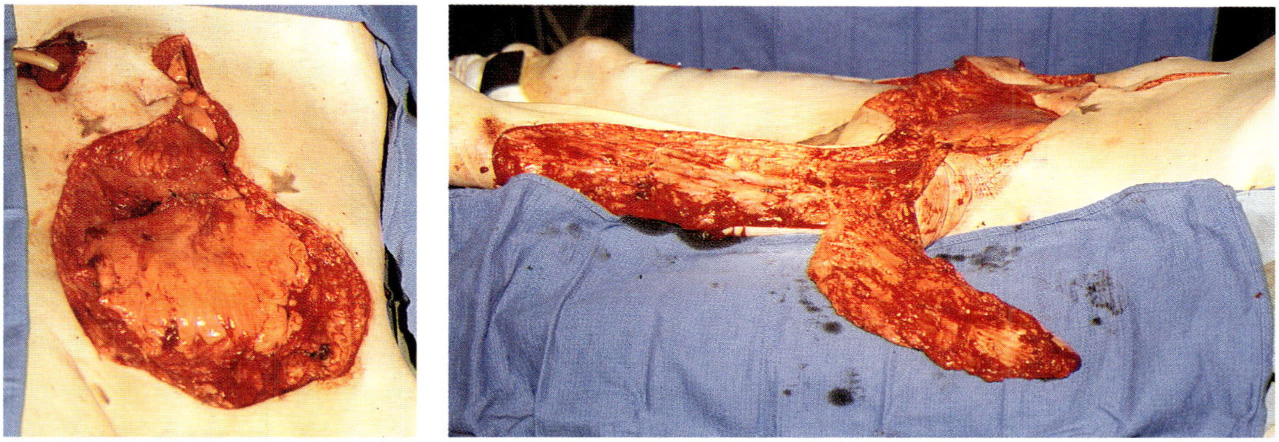

This patient was left with a massive lower abdominal wall defect after the resection of bladder carcinoma that involved the abdominal wall. Rectus femoris musculocutaneous flaps were elevated for transfer into the abdominal defect.

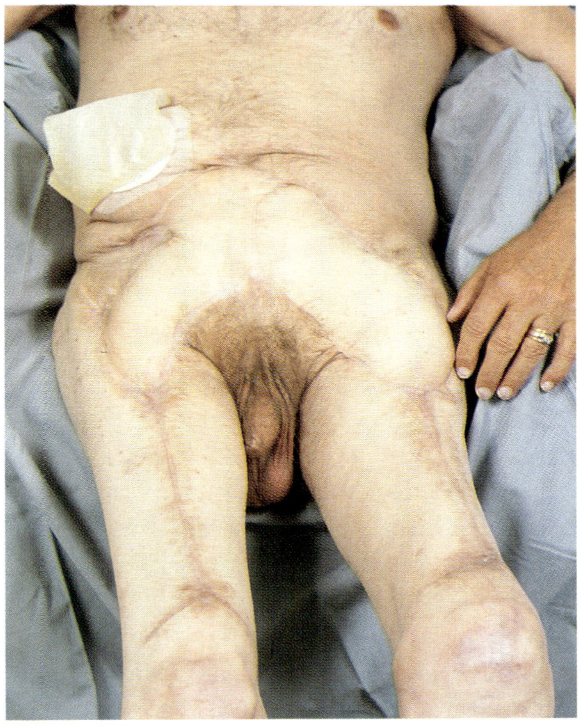

Complete abdominal wall competence was obtained as shown 9 months postoperatively.

The tensor fascia lata has also been used successfully in the closure of defects of the lower abdomen and midline.[75] The arc of rotation is similar to that of the rectus femoris muscle except that defects in the lower lateral abdomen are more difficult to cover with this flap. There is an extensive fascial component associated with this flap, which can aid in fascial repair of the abdomen. Although the muscle can be transposed as a musculocutaneous flap, care should be taken not to extend the skin island distally into the lower one third of the upper thigh since this will result in necrosis of the distal skin island in many cases.

Inferiorly based rectus abdominis flaps can also be a good choice for closure of lower abdominal wall defects in selected cases. However, bringing in tissue from outside the abdomen is usually the optimal choice since making a donor site from the remaining functional abdominal wall may create more extensive problems if complications occur.[77]

The sartorius flap has also been described for closure of lower abdominal wall defects.[78] However, since the blood supply is segmental (type IV), the distal portion of this flap is not as reliable and is not recommended as a first-line choice.

The gracilis musculocutaneous flap has fallen into disfavor due to the unreliability of the distal skin island. It is primarily of use for reconstruction in the perineal region as opposed to the lower abdomen. However, this situation may change due to recent descriptions demonstrating the ability to extend the distal skin island by turbocharging.[79]

The vastus lateralis flap could be used to repair the lower abdomen; however, there is no significant fascial component with this flap, and due to the success of other muscle flaps, experience with this particular flap for abdominal wall closure is uncommon.[76]

At times, free tissue transfer to the abdomen may be the only remaining method available. Although there is now a variety of free flaps available that could be used for free tissue reconstruction successfully, experience with the tensor fascia lata has been reported most commonly.[80,81] When recipient vessels are unavailable, the omentum has been described as a vascular supply for a free flap transfer.[82] Another alternative is the use of a long saphenous vein graft loop, which can supply inflow as well as outflow for free flaps to the abdominal wall.[83] In this technique the long saphenous vein is freed up along its entire course and transected distally at the ankle. Its attachment to the common femoral vein is left in place, and it is then sewn to the femoral artery below the deep femoral artery. In this manner, an arteriovenous loop is created, which can be tunneled up into the abdominal area adjacent to the defect. The free flap can then be sewn into position over the defect and the loop divided, providing arterial inflow and venous outflow. It should be remembered that when free tissue transfers to the abdomen are performed, muscles associated with strong fascial elements are preferable. However, a reasonable second choice would be to place the muscle flap over prosthetic material.

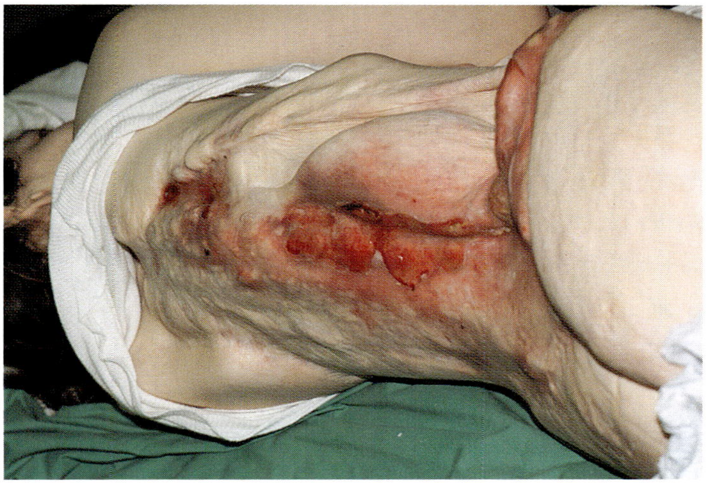

Although this case represents an enormous wound of the back rather than the abdomen, it illustrates several of the important principles regarding free tissue transfer in the trunk. This unfortunate, previously healthy 15-year-old girl developed necrotizing fasciitis involving the back. Extensive debridement of back and paraspinous muscle all the way to peritoneum was required. The patient survived this episode but was left with an unstable skin graft overlying the kidney and colon. An attempt was then made to place Harrington rods because of spinal collapse. The procedure was complicated by the development of permanent paraplegia. When referred to us, the patient was bedridden with a huge lumbar hernia and chronic superficial infection.

Photograph from Stephens DR, Grotting JC. Coverage of the chest wall and spine. Orthop Clin North Am 24:449, 1993.

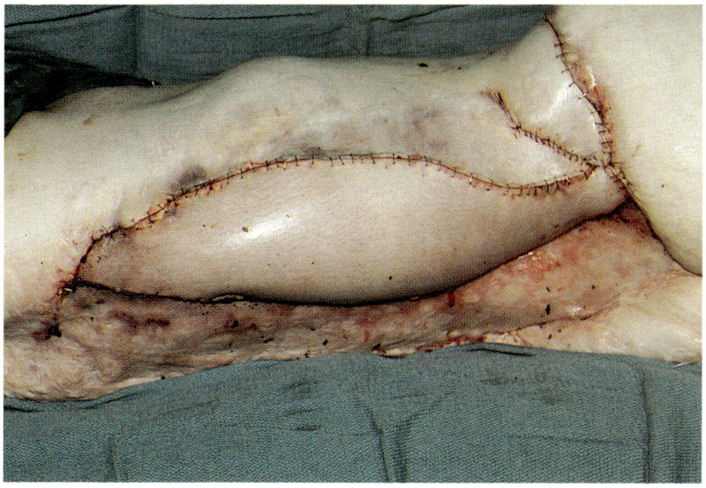

The only segment of tissue available for coverage of this area was the TRAM flap. We elected to transfer this flap using an arterial venous loop from the right groin. The saphenous vein was dissected nearly to the ankle, used as a reverse loop, and anastomosed to the superficial femoral artery. The flap survived in its entirety.

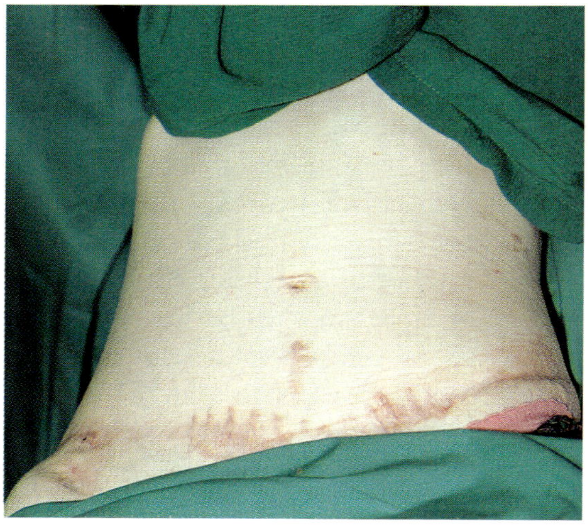

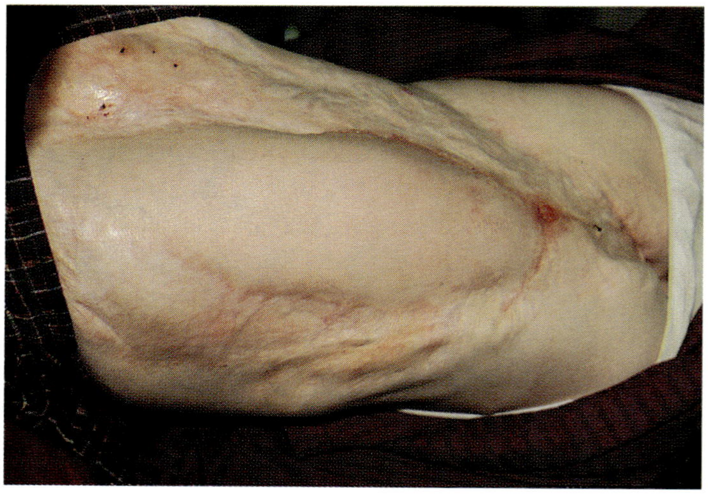

Ultimately this patient was found to have a white cell maturation defect which responded to neutrophil colony–stimulating factor. Three years postoperatively the wound remains stably healed.

Photographs from Stephens DR, Grotting JC. Coverage of the chest wall and spine. Orthop Clin North Am 24:449, 1993.

TISSUE EXPANSION

Tissue expansion should be kept in mind as a primary or adjuvant procedure. Although experience with tissue expansion in the abdominal wall is limited, it has been shown to have promise provided the defect is not grossly contaminated or infected and closure can be delayed until expansion is complete.[84] Advantages are that reconstruction can be performed with well-vascularized, innervated autogenous tissue that is a good color match and "like" tissue.[1] If tissue expansion is chosen as the reconstructive option, it is preferable to place the expanders into planes where they will not interfere with the neurovascular supply of the abdominal wall. One option is anterior to the musculofascial wall so that only skin and subcutaneous tissue is expanded. Alternatively, a safe place within the abdominal wall is in the plane between the internal oblique and the transversus abdominis muscles.[85] It should be noted that during expansion the internal organs provide such a soft cushion to the expander that although most of the expansion is anterior, there is also some expansion of the posterior layers of the abdominal wall and peritoneum. In congenital defects, defects in excess of 50% of the abdominal surface can be repaired.[85]

UNSOLVED PROBLEMS

The ultimate goal of surgical research is to find ways in which surgery is not only more successful but also less harmful to the patient. With the exploration of less invasive methods of surgical repair, hopefully the application of some of these methods can be focused to the abdominal wall. The use of the endoscope is being aggressively studied as a method of hernia repair in many centers, although its application has been reported only for primary hernioplasty at the present time.[66] It remains to be seen if this technique will have applications in recurrent hernia repair.

For reconstruction of abdominal wall defects, although tissue expansion offers some promise of reconstruction with like tissue, its technical limitations restrict its use. Optimally reconstruction with like tissue would be best if new tissue could actually be generated without use of the body as a donor site. Although primitive at this time, experimental research involving attempts to grow specific tissue types is being carried out.[86]

Further investigation is necessary into the actual importance of the abdominal wall in abdominal physiology.[87] Certainly replacement of defunctionalized segments with functioning muscle with a microneurovascular technique needs to be explored further.

Also further attention to the aesthetic refinement of abdominal wall reconstruction is important since the optimal goal of all reconstructions is to re-create the normal, both in function and in appearance. Certainly all the techniques described in this chapter will continue to be refined and improved for the benefit of our patients.

References

1. Bengtson BP, Ringler SL, George PR, et al. Capsular tissue: A new local flap. Plast Reconstr Surg 91:1073-1079, 1993.
2. Scarpa A. Sull'ernie Memorie anatomico-chirurgiche mellon: della Reale, 1809.
3. Lockwood TE. Superficial fascial system (SFS) of the trunk and extremities: A new concept. Plast Reconstr Surg 87:1009-1018, 1991.
4. Woodburne RT. Essentials of Human Anatomy, 5th ed. Oxford, England: Oxford University Press, 1973.
5. Condon RE. Surgical anatomy of the transversus abdominis and transversalis fascia. Ann Surg 173:1-5, 1971.
6. Boyd JB, Taylor GI, Corlett R. The vascular territories of the superior epigastric and the deep epigastric systems. Plast Reconstr Surg 73:1-16, 1984.
7. Carramenha e Costa MA, Carrequiry C, Vasconez LO, et al. An anatomical study of the venous drainage of the transverse rectus abdominis musculocutaneous flap. Plast Reconstr Surg 79:208-217, 1987.
8. Krupski WC, Sumchai A, Effeney DJ, et al. The importance of abdominal wall collateral blood vessels. Arch Surg 119:854-857, 1984.
9. Fagnieze PL, Hay JM, Lacaine F, et al. Abdominal midline incision closure. Arch Surg 120:1351-1353, 1985.
10. Wissing J, VanVroonhoven ThJMV, Schattenkerk ME, et al. Fascia closure after midline laparotomy: Results of a randomized trial. Br J Surg 74:738-741, 1987.
11. Greenberg C, Saik P, Peskin GW. Wound dehiscence—Pathophysiology and prevention. Arch Surg 189:345-352, 1979.
12. Guiney EJ, Morris PJ, Donaldson A. Wound dehiscence: A continuing problem in abdominal surgery. Arch Surg 92:47-51, 1966.
13. Stone HH, Fabian TC, Turkelson ML, et al. Management of acute full-thickness losses of the abdominal wall. Ann Surg 193:612-618, 1981.
14. Mudge M, Hughes LE. Incisional hernia: A 10-year prospective study of incidence and attitudes. Br J Surg 72:70-71, 1985.
15. Jones TE, Newell ET, Brubaker RE. The use of alloy steel wire in closure of abdominal wounds. Surg Gynecol Obstet 72:1056-1059, 1941.
16. Ellis H. The causes and preventions of intestinal adhesions. Br J Surg 69:241-243, 1982.
17. Richards PC, Balch CM, Aldrete JS. Abdominal wound closure. Ann Surg 197:238-243, 1983.
18. Wantz GE. Abdominal wall hernias. In Schwartz SI, Shires GT, Spencer FC, eds. Principles of Surgery, 6th ed. New York: McGraw-Hill, 1994, pp 1538-1539.
19. Voyles CR, Richardson JD, Bland KI, et al. Emergency abdominal wall reconstruction with polypropylene mesh. Ann Surg 194:219-223, 1981.
20. Goris RJA. Oglivie's method applied to infected wound disruption. Arch Surg 115:1103-1107, 1980.
21. Quillinan RH. Repair of recurrent inguinal hernia. Am J Surg 118:593, 1969.

22. Thieme ET. Recurrent inguinal hernia. Arch Surg 103:238, 1971.
23. Lichtenstein IL, Shore JM. Exploding the myth of hernia repair. Am J Surg 132:307-315, 1976.
24. Greenburg AG. Revisiting the recurrent groin hernia. Am J Surg 154:35-40, 1987.
25. Read RC, White HJ. Inguinal herniation 1777-1977. Am J Surg 136:651-654, 1978.
26. McVay CV, Chapp JD. Inguinal and femoral hernioplasty. Ann Surg 148:499, 1958.
27. Bassinni E. Nuova tecnica per la cura delle ernie inguinal. Soc Ital Chir 40:380, 1887.
28. Iles JDH. Specialization in elective herniorrhaphy. Lancet 1:751, 1965.
29. Shulman AG, Amid PK, Lichtenstein IL. The "plug" repair of 1,402 recurrent inguinal hernias: A 20-year experience. Arch Surg 125:265-267, 1990.
30. Pearl RK. Parastomal hernias. World J Surg 13:569-572, 1989.
31. Fry DE, Osler T. Abdominal wall considerations and complications in reoperative surgery. Surg Clin North Am 71:1-11, 1991.
32. Metcalf A, Maher JW. Small bowel trauma, fistula, and radiation injury. In Hardy JW, ed. Hardy Textbook of Surgery, 2nd ed. Philadelphia: JB Lippincott, 1988, p 553.
33. Wood RJ, Ney AL, Bubrick MP. Traumatic abdominal hernia: A case report and review of the literature. Am Surg 54:648-651, 1988.
34. Metztorff MT, Miller SH, Smiley P, et al. Blunt traumatic rupture of the abdominal wall musculature. Ann Plast Surg 13:63-66, 1984.
35. Howard CA, Turner MW. Successful treatment of early postoperative necrotizing fasciitis of the abdominal wall. Crit Care Med 17:586-587, 1989.
36. Casali RE, Tucker WE, Petrino RA, et al. Postoperative necrotizing fasciitis of the abdominal wall. Am J Surg 140:787-790, 1980.
37. Hallock GG. Skin recycling following neovascularization using the rat musculocutaneous flap model. Plast Reconstr Surg 88:673-680, 1991.
38. Shiu MH, Winestein L, Haju SI, et al. Malignant soft tissue tumors of the anterior abdominal wall. Am J Surg 158:446-451, 1989.
39. Gardner EJ, Richards RC. Multiple cutaneous and subcutaneous lesions occurring simultaneously with hereditary polyposis and osteomatosis. Am J Human Genet 5:139, 1953.
40. Nussbaum ML, Campana TJ, Weese JL. Radiation-induced intestinal injury. Clin Plast Surg 20:573-580, 1993.
41. Kuske RR. Personal communication. New Orleans, La.: August 1993.
42. Matarasso A. Abdominolipoplasty. Clin Plast Surg 16:289-303, 1989.
43. Bazola R, Psallikas JM. Abdominoplasty: A new concept in classification for treatment. Plast Reconstr Surg 82:983-993, 1988.
44. Illouz G. Personal communication. New Orleans, La.: September 1993.
45. Flint LM, Vitale GC, Richardson JD, et al. The injured colon. Relationships of management to complications. Ann Surg 193:619, 1981.
46. Jenkins TPN. The burst abdominal wound: A mechanical approach. Br J Surg 63:873-876, 1976.
47. Bucknell TE, Cox PJ, Ellis H. Burst abdomen and incisional hernia: Prospective study of 1129 major laparotomies. Br Med J 184:931-933, 1982.
48. Farnell MB, Worthington-Self S, Mucha P Jr, et al. Closure of abdominal incisions with subcutaneous catheters. Arch Surg 121:641-648, 1986.
49. Robson MC, Shaw RC, Heggers JP. The reclosure of postoperative incisional abscesses based on bacterial quantification in the wound. Ann Surg 171:279-282, 1970.
50. Thomas WO, Parry SW, Rodning CB. Ventral/incisional abdominal herniorrhaphy by fascial partition/release. Plast Reconstr Surg 91:1080-1086, 1993.
51. Ramirez OM, Ruas E, Dellon AL. "Components separation" method for closure of abdominal wall defects: An anatomic and clinical study. Plast Reconstr Surg 86:519-526, 1990.
52. Larson GM, Vandertoll DJ. Approaches to repair ventral hernia and full thickness losses of the abdominal wall. Surg Clin North Am 64:335-349, 1984.
53. Read RC. Recurrent and incisional hernias. In McQuarrie DG, Humphrey EW, eds. Reoperative General Surgery. St. Louis: Mosby, 1992, pp 485-494.

54. Tyrell J, Silberman H, Chandrasoma P, et al. Absorbable versus permanent mesh in abdominal operations. Surg Gynecol Obstet 168:227-232, 1989.
55. Hedderich GS, Wexler MJ, McClean APH, et al. The septic abdomen—Open management with Marlex mesh with a zipper. Surgery 99:399-408, 1986.
56. Boyd WC. Use of Marlex mesh in acute loss of the abdominal wall due to infection. Surg Gynecol Obstet 144:251-252, 1977.
57. Smith S, Gantt N, Rowe MI, et al. Dura versus Gore-Tex as an abdominal wall prosthesis in an open and closed infected model. J Pediatr Surg 24:519-521, 1989.
58. Brown GL, Richardson JD, Malagon MA, et al. Comparison of prosthetic materials for abdominal wall reconstruction in the presence of contamination and infection. Ann Surg 201:705-711, 1985.
59. Bauer JJ, Salky BA, Gelerent IM, et al. Repair of large abdominal wall defects with expanded polytetrafluoroethylene (PTFE). Ann Surg 206:765-769, 1987.
60. Bleichrodt RP, Simmermacher RK, Van der Lie B, et al. Expanded polytetrafluoroethylene patch vs. polypropylene mesh for the repair of contaminated defects of the abdominal wall. Surg Gynecol Obstet 176:18-24, 1993.
61. Stoppa RE, Warlaumont CR, Verhaeghe PJ. Prosthetic repair in the treatment of groin hernias. Int Surg 71:154-158, 1986.
62. Stoppa RE. The treatment of complicated groin and incisional hernias. World J Surg 13: 545-554, 1989.
63. Nyhus LM. The recurrent groin hernia: Therapeutic solutions. World J Surg 13:541-544, 1989.
64. Ijzermans JN, de Wilt H, Hop WC, et al. Recurrent inguinal hernia treated by classical herniaplasty. Arch Surg 126:1097-1100, 1991.
65. Nyhus LM, Pollak R, Bombeck CT, et al. The pre-peritoneal approach and prosthetic buttress for recurrent hernia: The evolution of the technique. Ann Surg 208:733, 1988.
66. Ger R. The laparoscopic management of groin hernias. Contemp Surg 39(4):15-19, 1991.
67. Glassow F. Short stay surgery (Shouldice technique) for repair of vaginal hernia. Ann R Coll Surg Engl 58:133, 1976.
68. Ger R, Ravo B, Deysire M. The management of recurrent inguinal hernias by muscle transposition—A preliminary communication. Surgery 95:712, 1984.
69. Gels WP, Salatta JD. Lumbar hernia. In Nyhus LM, Condon RE, eds. Hernia, 3rd ed. Philadelphia: JB Lippincott, 1989, pp 401-415.
70. Robinson DW. Surgical problems in the excision and repair of radiated tissue. Plast Reconstr Surg 155:41-49, 1976.
71. Granick MS, Larson DL, Solomon MP. Radiation-related wounds of the chest wall. Clin Plast Surg 20:559-571, 1993.
72. Houston GC, Drew GS, Vazquez B, et al. The extended latissimus dorsi flap in repair of anterior abdominal wall defects. Plast Reconstr Surg 81:917-924, 1988.
73. Given K. Personal communication. Medical College of Georgia: July 1993.
74. Ohtsuka H, Ochi K, Seike H. Reconstruction of the large lateral abdominal wall defect with an ileolumbar bipedicle flap. Br J Plast Surg 37:327-329, 1984.
75. Bostwick J, Hill HL, Nahai F. Repairs in the lower abdomen, groin, or perineum with myocutaneous or omental flaps. Plast Reconstr Surg 63:186-194, 1979.
76. Hershy FB, Butcher HP. Repair of defects after partial resection of the abdominal wall. Am J Surg 107:586, 1964.
77. Ger R, Duboys E. The prevention and repair of large abdominal wall defects by muscle transection: A preliminary communication. Plast Reconstr Surg 72:170-175, 1983.
78. Sensoz O, Ustuner TE, Taner OF. Use of a sartorius myocutaneous flap for reconstruction of a large full-thickness abdominal wall defect. Ann Plast Surg 25:193, 1990.
79. Core G, Kline R, Finan M. The turbo gracilis flap for perineal reconstruction. Presented at the American Society of Reconstructive Microsurgery. Kansas City, Mo.: September 1993.
80. Caffee H. Reconstruction of the abdominal wall by variations of tensor fascia lata flap. Plast Reconstr Surg 71:348-351, 1983.

81. Hill HL, Nahai F, Vasconez LO. Tensor fascia lata myocutaneous free flap. Plast Reconstr Surg 61:517, 1978.
82. Clement R, Young LV, Marsh JL. Use of greater omentum as a vascular supply for free flap transfer. Plast Reconstr Surg 74:131, 1984.
83. Earle AS, Feng LJ, Jordan RB. Long saphenous vein grafts as an aid to microsurgical reconstruction of the trunk. J Reconstr Microsurg 62:165-169, 1990.
84. Arnold PG. Personal communication. Mayo Clinic: September 1989.
85. Byrd HS, Hobar TC. Abdominal wall expansion and congenital defects. Plast Reconstr Surg 84:347-352, 1989.
86. Khouri R, Khoudsi B. Tissue regeneration. Presented at The American Society of Reconstructive Microsurgery. Orlando, Fla.: September 1991.
87. Grotting JC. The abdomen. In Jurkiewicz MJ, Mathes SJ, Krizek TJ, Ariyan S, eds. Plastic Surgery. St. Louis: Mosby, 1990.

37

Secondary Operations Following Genitourinary Reconstruction

Charles E. Horton, Jr., M.D., and Charles E. Horton, M.D.

Reoperative Problems

Fistula	Scrotal encroachment
Stricture	Inadequate skin on penile shaft
Diverticulum	Skin tags
Meatal stenosis	Recurrent chordee
Hairy urethra	Urethra of inadequate length
Spraying meatus	Tethering bands of tissue
Retrusive meatus	

The problems posed by congenital deformities of the genitalia are formidable. Over 350 different surgical techniques have been developed to repair hypospadias. Epispadias operations were considered even more challenging. Because of the difficulty in achieving successful results, these techniques commonly had complication rates of up to 50%. Recent innovations in surgical techniques have made complications much less common than in the past, although there are still many previously operated patients with complications requiring sophisticated surgery for salvage.

The following factors make reconstruction in this area a significant challenge:

1. After the initial surgery, the best tissue for repair has usually been used or discarded, leaving little ideal tissue available for secondary reconstruction.
2. The skin in the genital area is thin and becomes edematous and swollen following surgery.
3. Erections postoperatively stress delicate suture lines.
4. Urinary drainage must be accommodated within the surgical repair.
5. The potential for contamination from fecal material and clothing is a constant threat.

HYPOSPADIAS

The following complications may be seen in patients who have undergone hypospadias repair; it is not unusual for a patient to present with more than one of these conditions.

Fistula

Urethrocutaneous fistulae occur in approximately 10% of all cases of hypospadias repair. They may range in size from a minor pinhole to a major disruption of the entire urethral reconstruction. A fistula is usually diagnosed by observing the patient drip urine from an abnormal opening while voiding.

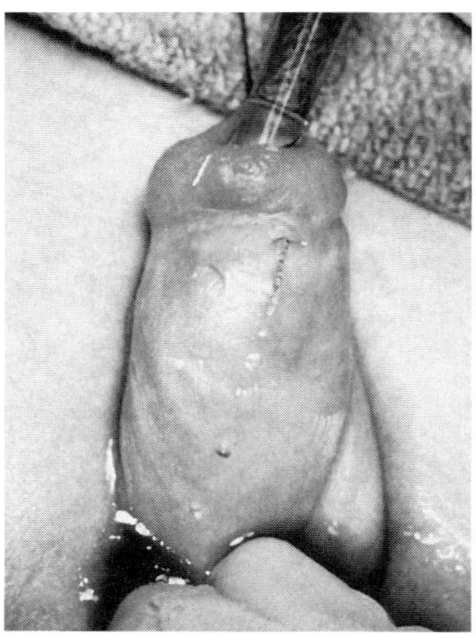

A urethral fistula that is difficult to locate may be detected by retrograde injection of saline solution tinted with methylene blue into the urethra. The saline solution will distend the urethra, and the fluid will leak out at the site of the fistula. Multiple fistulae may be present, and unless all are corrected, the repair is doomed to failure. After a fistula develops, it is best to wait at least 6 months before attempting repair; this allows the inflammatory reaction in the delicate penile tissue to subside.

The cause of the fistula must be determined. The urethra should have an adequate lumen from beginning to end. Any distal obstruction or stenosis can put undue pressure on the proximal urethra and disrupt the hypospadias repair, resulting in the formation of a fistula. ***Thus the first step in the repair of a urethral fistula is to rule out distal urethral narrowing.***

Techniques for urethral fistula repair can be divided into those applicable for small fistulae (<2 mm) and those used to close large fistulae (>2 mm). The diameter of the urethral lumen must never be compromised in an attempt to achieve uroepithelial coaptation. If a large defect is mistakenly closed primarily, the lumen will be smaller in the area of repair and the fistula can recur or a stricture or a diverticulum can develop.

For a small fistula, an incision is made directly over the area of the fistula and the track to the urethra is dissected. The fistula is closed by inverting the uroepithelial tissue and using 6-0 or 7-0 polydioxanone sutures to ensure a watertight union. The integrity of the closure can be tested with retrograde instillation of saline solution under pressure into the urethra. Multiple subcutaneous layers should be used to approximate adjacent tissue in depth over the fistula repair.

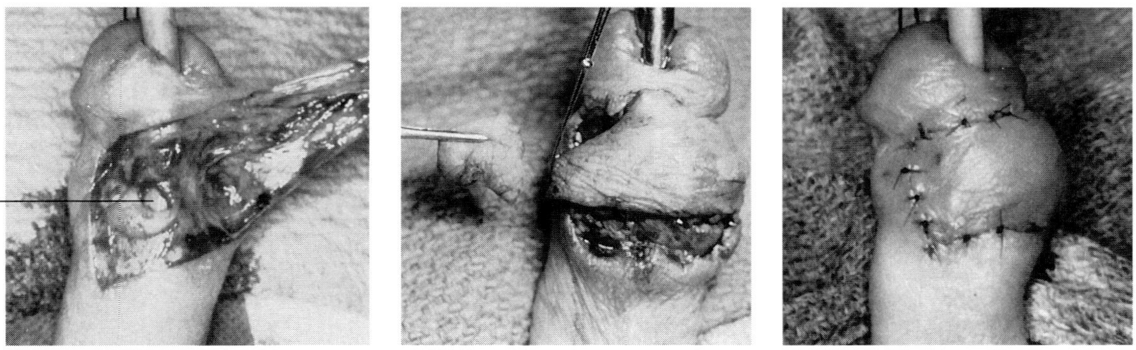

The skin can be closed directly, or a lateral skin flap can be elevated and advanced to cover the fistula, thus placing the suture lines away from the underlying fistula repair.

Large fistulae require the transfer of new epithelium into the urethra. A hinge flap or an adjacent skin flap can be used for this type of fistula closure. Extremely large defects of the urethra require either a free full-thickness graft or a tube graft using skin or vascularized skin flaps elevated on a subcutaneous dartos fascial pedicle for more extensive urethral reconstruction.

Strictures

A stricture should be suspected when the patient complains of a weak, narrow, dribbling urinary stream. Occasionally a patient with stricture will present with a urinary tract infection. The diagnosis can be made by performing a retrograde urethrogram or by calibrating the urethra with a bougie à boule to determine the extent and the length of the stricture. A stricture should not be repaired immediately after dilation because dilation can obscure the extent of involved urethra.

Depending on the severity of the stricture and quality of the epithelium of the existing urethra and surrounding skin, repair techniques will vary. Once the stricture has been opened longitudinally and healthy urethral epithelium has been identified proximally and distally, the quality of the tissue within the stricture must be assessed. If it is worthwhile to retain, a hairless full-thickness skin graft can be used to patch a small area of stricture and the original epithelium of the involved urethra can be preserved. If the adjacent skin is hairless and of good quality, skin lateral and parallel to the involved urethra can be elevated and turned into the lumen. If the urethral wall is scarred, irregular, and of poor quality, the strictured area should be resected and a new urethral segment constructed with extragenital skin, bladder mucosa, or buccal mucosa grafts.

Diverticulum

A urethral diverticulum may be diagnosed by observing a bulge in the urethra during voiding or by noting that the patient dribbles urine after micturition is otherwise complete. ***The presence of a diverticulum should immediately raise suspicion of a distal obstruction of some type.*** Diverticula form as a result of excess pressure and turbulence proximal to the obstruction. Retrograde urethrography and calibration of the entire urethra are recommended to investigate the possible cause of the diverticulum.

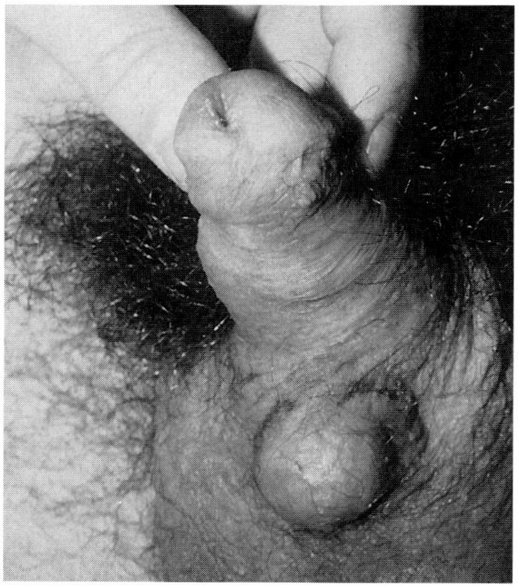

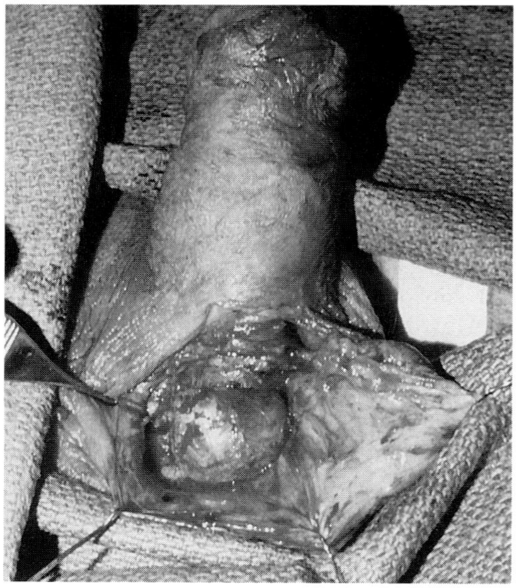

If no distal obstruction or other complication is identified, the diverticulum can be corrected by dissecting the dilated urethral wall and trimming the excess uroepithelium to a normal-sized lumen. The site should be closed with a watertight technique and tested with retrograde installation of saline solution into the urethra. In-depth subcutaneous approximation and skin closure are not difficult to accomplish in these cases because there is usually an abundance of available tissue.

If another complication is noted distal to the diverticulum (e.g., meatal stenosis), it should be corrected at the same time the diverticulum is repaired.

Meatal Stenosis

Early techniques in hypospadias repair made taking the urethra to the tip of the glans impossible and often resulted in meatal stenosis. In these older techniques the meatus was often left at the level of the coronal sulcus. A stenotic meatus results when a circular anastomosis contracts end to end, thus decreasing the diameter of the circle. This is a normal occurrence in wound healing; a circular anastomosis is simply a straight-line scar joined end to end and it is well known that a straight-line incision will contract longitudinally.

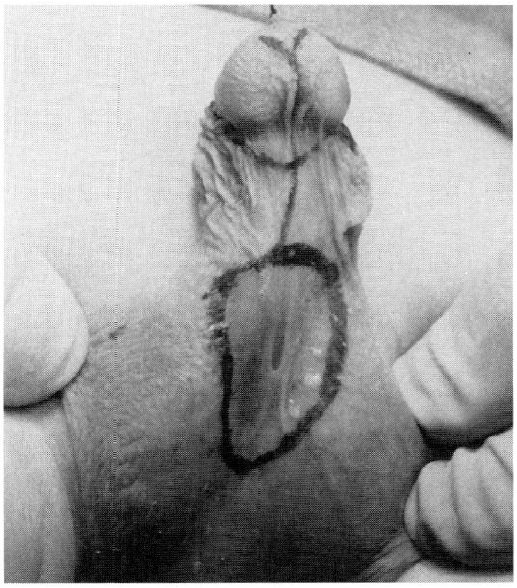

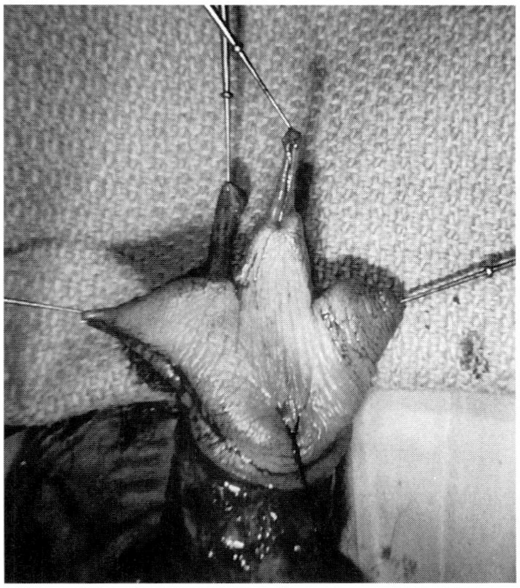

Techniques that interpose a flap into the circular anastomosis can greatly reduce the problem of meatal stenosis. We routinely employ a triangular glans flap. The midline glans flap and the lateral glans "wings" are mobilized, and the triangular glans flap is then advanced into the spatulated end of the distal neourethra.

Some patients with meatal stenosis may be treated with a simple meatotomy, but a patient with extensive meatal stenosis will need additional uroepithelium transferred to the tip of the penis. In certain cases a free full-thickness graft may be used for distal urethral enlargement. We prefer to form a flip-flap of the penile skin on the shaft just proximal to the distal stenosis. We then open the urethral segment distal to the flip-flap and insert the flip-flap into a dorsal incision that extends to the end of the urethra at the glans. The flip-flap is sutured proximally and distally as far as possible, but the flap tissue cannot be approximated in the midsurface of the glans. A stent is used to bolster the flap into the appropriate position. The skin of the flip-flap turned into the lumen provides the additional uroepithelium needed to correct the meatal stenosis.

Hairy Urethra

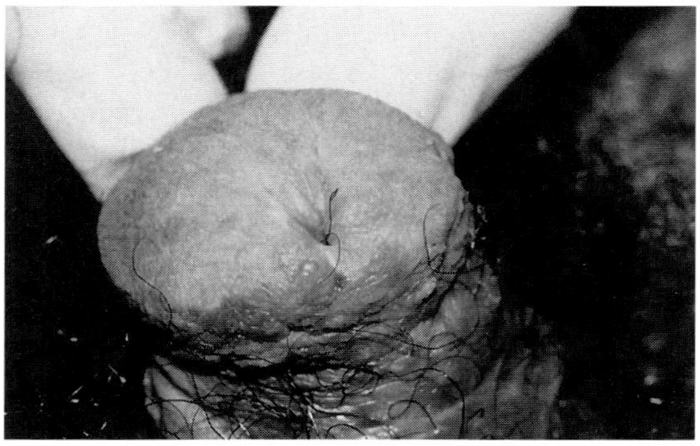

Hair grows in the urethra when scrotal tissue or hairy extragenital skin has been used in a prior repair. Hair in the urethra may not always cause problems, but when a hairy urethra is associated with infection, calcific concretions, and irritation, it must be treated. Very small, discrete areas of hair growth can be treated by excision of individual hair follicles or by transurethral electrofulguration of the hair follicle base. Large areas of hair-bearing uroepithelial tissue must be surgically approached, accurately identified, and totally excised. The urethra is then reconstructed with non–hair-bearing tissue in the form of a graft or flap. ■ ***Bladder mucosa offers an abundant source of hairless tissue.*** Our experience using free grafts of bladder mucosa for urethral reconstruction has been favorable.

Spraying Meatus

Patients who have had hypospadias repair may complain of a urinary stream that is not easily directed and that splashes and sprays in an irregular fashion. Spraying meatus is usually caused by skin tags or ridges in the urethral meatus or on the glans ridges surrounding the urethra. The pattern of the urinary stream can be demonstrated intraoperatively by antegrade instillation of saline solution injected through a needle placed percutaneously into the proximal urethra. Any irregular and uneven tissue resulting in spraying should be removed. Urethroscopy should be performed at the time of repair to look for folds or synechiae within the fossa navicularis. Graft or flap procedures for meatal stenosis can be used if necessary to resurface the irregular area.

Retrusive Meatus

Retrusive urethral meatus was more common when earlier techniques such as the Dennis Browne procedure were used to correct hypospadias. With these techniques the meatus was not brought to the tip of the penis but positioned at or below the coronal sulcus. Many patients found the result objectionable aesthetically. Meatal retrusion occasionally occurs with modern techniques if disruption of the glans wings occurs or when a MAGPI (meatal advancement and glanduloplasty) technique is used inappropriately to repair hypospadias that is too proximal.

A retrusive meatus can be treated by extensively mobilizing the urethra and advancing it distally to a new site in the glans or by creating a small flip-flap, elevating lateral glans wings, and closing the wings over the distal urethral reconstruction.

Scrotal Encroachment

In certain repairs scrotal tissue may be brought distally onto the shaft of the penis. Scrotal engulfment results in a loss of functional penile length and can cause a web of skin to form between the penis and the scrotum.

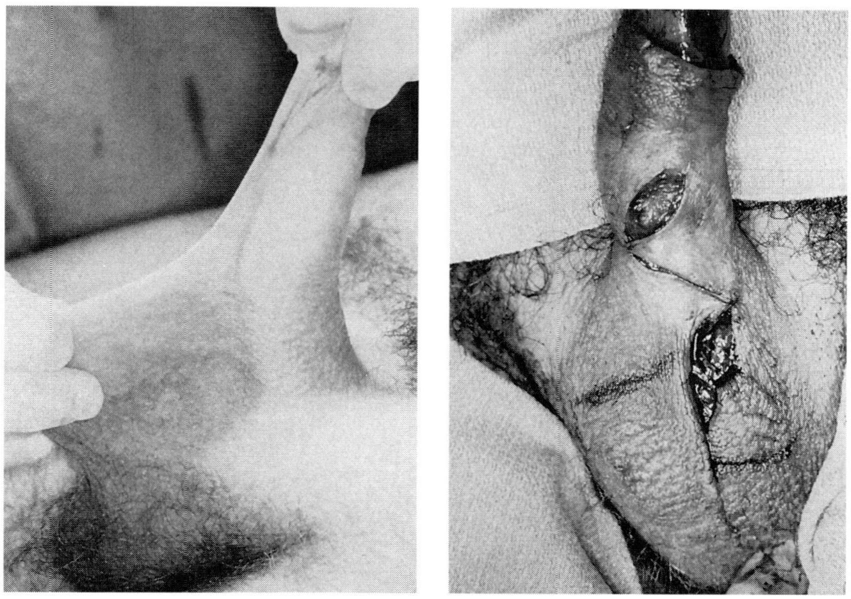

The tethering band of skin (contracture) may cause pain and bleeding during erections and sexual intercourse. Scrotal encroachment can be corrected by resecting wedges of scrotal skin (if ample skin is present) or by performing a Z-plasty at the penoscrotal junction.

Inadequate Skin on Penile Shaft

A patient who has undergone multiple prior operations to repair hypospadias or persistent fistulae may have a shortage of penile skin available for reconstruction. In these cases a full-thickness extragenital skin graft can be applied to the penile shaft. If the skin of the ventral surface of the penis is inadequate in quantity or quality, better quality dorsal penile shaft skin should be transferred to the ventrum; a hairless full-thickness skin graft harvested from the groin can then be applied to the dorsal penile shaft for skin coverage.

In extreme cases when the skin of the entire penile shaft is inadequate, a staged approach must be used. The penile shaft is initially resurfaced with full-thickness skin grafts, and 6 months later a urethroplasty is performed with a free skin graft or a bladder mucosa graft tunneled under the penile shaft skin.

Skin Tags

Skin tags and suture sinuses may occur after penile surgery. The excess skin can usually be resected with minimal difficulty, and the skin sinus tracts are opened and corrected. Subcuticular skin approximation helps to avoid these problems.

Recurrent Chordee

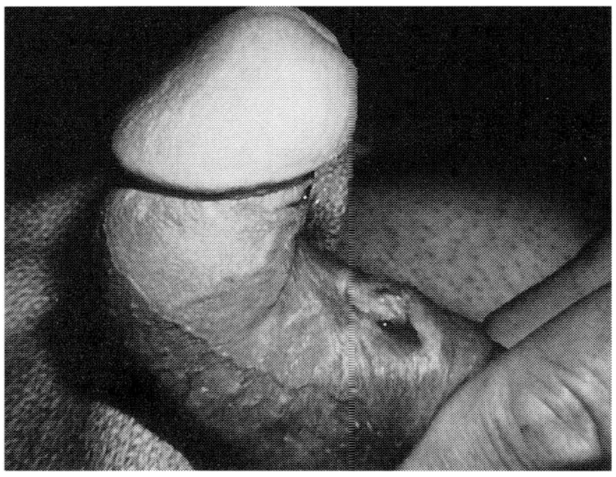

After a urethroplasty has been completed, a penile bend may persist. It may be caused by postoperative scarring, but it usually results when the tissues that cause chordee are inadequately resected at the time of the original surgery. Significant recurrent chordee may be treated by (1) shortening the long dorsal side of the penis (i.e., plicating the dorsum) or (2) lengthening the short ventral side of the penis (i.e., revising the urethroplasty). The curvature can be demonstrated intraoperatively by creating an artificial erection. If the penis is long enough, the tunica albuginea of the dorsum can be resected. Otherwise, further urethral reconstruction and release of the tissues causing persistent chordee are necessary.

If dorsal excision of tunica albuginea is chosen, the exposure is usually made through a circumcising incision, the skin is retracted proximally, and the dorsal neurovascular bundle is identified, mobilized, and carefully retracted to one side. An appropriately sized wedge of tunica albuginea is excised from the dorsal aspect of the corporal bodies, and the tunica is closed primarily with absorbable sutures.

If elongation of the urethra is preferred, an incision is made through the urethra, the tissue causing the curvature is removed, and a urethral tube is reconstructed with either a flap of hairless extragenital skin or a graft of bladder or buccal mucosa. This revision can be done as a primary one-stage procedure.

Case Presentation

B.C., a 30-year-old construction worker, was born with penoscrotal hypospadias and chordee. As a child he underwent two unsuccessful attempts at repair. Within the past year he had undergone a major procedure that included correction of chordee and an attempt at urethroplasty using a graft of bladder mucosa. Unfortunately a postoperative wound infection developed and the repair failed. The patient was highly motivated because he was engaged to be married.

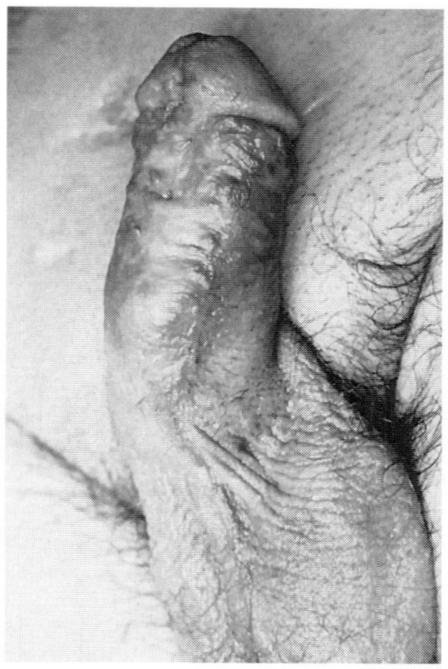

The patient's urethral meatus was positioned in the proximal penile shaft. There was persistent ventral chordee. The skin of the ventral penile shaft was quite scarred and of poor quality. Overall there was a paucity of penile skin, but the dorsal shaft skin was of good quality.

The patient underwent single-stage repair of hypospadias and correction of chordee. Cystoscopy revealed that the distal 2 cm of the existing urethra was scarred and strictured. The penile shaft was degloved of skin, and the fibrotic ventral skin was discarded. The urethra was mobilized back to the scrotum and the distal 2 cm segment was removed. An artificial erection was induced, and the dysgenetic tissue and scarred epithelium that caused the ventral curvature were excised.

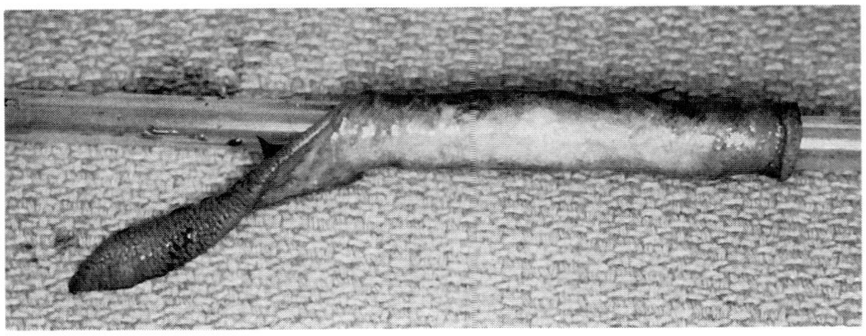

A full-thickness skin graft was harvested from a hairless area over the right anterior superior iliac spine; the tissue was tubularized over a 24 Fr catheter and used for the neourethra.

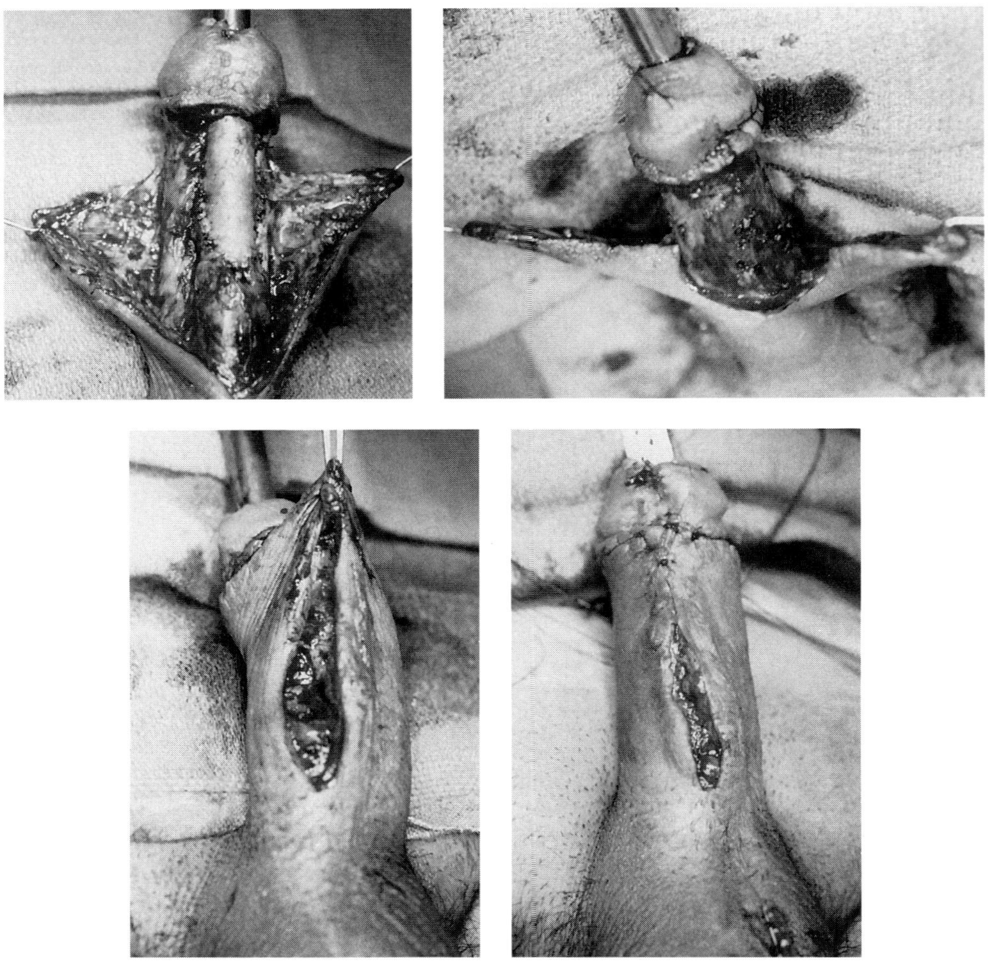

The neourethra was sutured into place after being tunneled through the glans. Because a urethra constructed with a skin graft requires healthy, well-vascularized tissue to cover it, dorsal shaft skin was divided in the midline and both flaps were rotated ventrally to close over the new urethral segment.

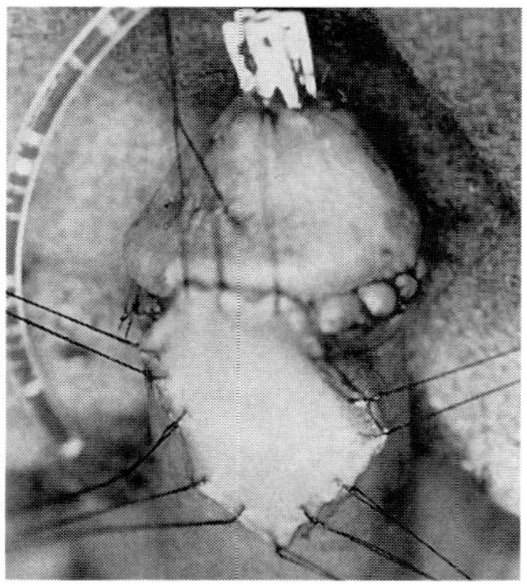

This left a bare area of penile shaft dorsally, which was covered by placing a second full-thickness skin graft in this area for shaft skin coverage.

A suprapubic drain was used for temporary urinary diversion, and a urethral stent was placed through the repair. These devices were removed after 10 days. The patient's postoperative course was uneventful, and at 1-year follow-up he is married, experiencing straight erections, and voiding from the tip of the penis.

EPISPADIAS

Fortunately epispadias is much less common than hypospadias. Isolated (simple) epispadias is quite rare (1:200,000 births). The complications of simple epispadias repair are the same as those of hypospadias and can be corrected with the techniques previously discussed.

Epispadias is more commonly seen in association with bladder exstrophy (1:30,000 births). Repair of this defect is much more complicated than simple epispadias and requires intricate reconstruction. In the patient with epispadias/exstrophy there is a general diastasis of the abdominal and pelvic musculoskeletal structures, including the pubic bones and the attachment of the corporal bodies. Also, in the adult patient the pubic hair distribution is abnormal. Pubic hair will be found growing in two separate patches lateral to the base of the penis, with a bald patch of skin in the suprapubic area. A central scar and depression may be present in the lower abdomen where bladder surgery has been performed. Many of these patients do not have an umbilicus. Because epispadias repair is usually done in childhood, any inadequacy in the repair may not become apparent until the patient has gone through adolescence. When the patient desires to begin sexual activity, the flat phallus with inadequate length and severe dorsal curvature becomes a devastating problem.

The secondary repair of epispadias deformities must be individualized on the basis of prior management of the urinary tract. If the exstrophic bladder has been closed, then the patient should void through the urethra, and urethroplasty will be a necessary part of the reconstruction. In many cases a urinary diversion with an ileal or colonic conduit will have been performed during childhood and the epispadias repair will not require a micturating urethroplasty, although a urethroplasty to enable ejaculation may be desirable. It is difficult to reconstruct a nonmicturating urethra because the urethra is not cleaned and dilated frequently with urination and so is more prone to stenosis and infection. However, if the patient understands and accepts these problems, a standard urethroplasty can be performed. Beginning 3 weeks after surgery the urethra should be irrigated and dilated frequently until the tissue matures.

The following problems are associated with secondary epispadias repair; they must be dealt with systematically, proceeding from the most superficial structures to the deeper involved tissues:

- Shortage of dorsal skin
- Skin scarring
- Tethering dysgenetic bands of tissue that cause dorsal chordee (similar to chordee in patients with hypospadias)
- Abnormal lateral displacement and attachment of the crura of the corporal bodies to the pubic bones, resulting in shortening and flattening of the phallus
- Urethra of inadequate length as a result of previous construction
- Intrinsic disproportion of the tunica albuginea of the corporal bodies (normal length on the ventral surface and shortness and lack of growth on the dorsal side)

Our approach to epispadias repair employs a W-shaped groin flap based superiorly with the apex below the base of the penis on each side. The purpose of the W flap is to provide excellent exposure of the corporal bodies where they insert on the pubic bones, to transfer good-quality skin to the base of the penile shaft, and to rotate the laterally displaced hair-bearing skin into the midline to produce a normal-looking escutcheon.

After the groin flaps are elevated, the spermatic cords must be carefully identified and preserved. The penile shaft is degloved of skin to the base, and any obvious dysgenetic tissue that would cause chordee is resected. The attachments of the corporal bodies to the underside of the pubic bones are mobilized as far proximally as seems practical. This elongates the phallus and allows the penis to dangle in a more dependent position. In some cases these maneuvers alone will provide sufficient correction.

An artificial erection is performed to detect chordee, which is often present at this stage. If the urethra is present, the adequacy of its length should be evaluated; if the urethra is short and seems to cause chordee, it is transected. Another artificial erection is performed to verify correction of chordee. If chordee persists, a dermal graft can be used to augment the deficient dorsal tunica albuginea. A transverse corporotomy incision is made through the dorsal tunica into the erectile space of each corporal body. The separate corporal bodies are then joined in the midline and an elliptically shaped dermal graft is contoured appropriately and placed into the resulting defect. A final artificial erection should confirm that the penis is straight. If the penis remains bent, then additional dermal grafting will be required.

If the existing urethra has been divided, a urethroplasty will be necessary. It is best not to place a free urethral graft over a dermal graft; therefore the new urethra should be rerouted along the ventral aspect of the corporal bodies to emerge at the tip of the glans.

The final challenge in secondary epispadias repair is resurfacing the dorsal penile shaft. In some cases the existing skin is adequate for closure. If extra skin is required and no urethroplasty or dermal graft has been utilized, then a full-thickness skin graft can be used to resurface the shaft. Occasionally the defect can be closed with adjacent skin tissue, but it is more likely that a vascularized prepucial island flap will need to be transferred from the ventral side to the dorsal surface for coverage. The ventral prepucial skin is elevated on a vascularized dartos fascial pedicle and then rotated to the dorsum of the penis.

This technique should correct any skin shortage, revise pubic hair distribution, elongate the penis and the urethra (if necessary), and augment the dorsal tunica albuginea (if necessary). The penis should now be straight when tumescent and dangle dependently in the flaccid state.

Case Presentation

A.R., a 16-year-old boy from Mexico, was born with the exstrophy-epispadias complex. As a child he underwent cystectomy and urinary diversion with an ileal conduit. He also had two previous operations on the penis for correction of epispadias. He desired revision of the epispadias repair.

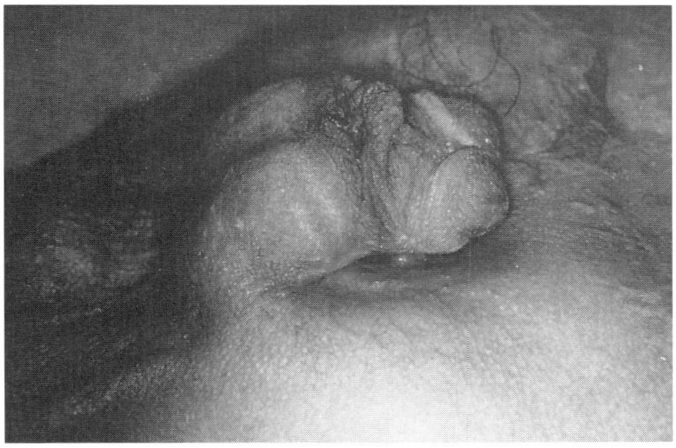

Physical examination showed a urostomy stoma present in the left lower quadrant. There was an unsightly scar and a concave depression of the skin in the suprapubic area. Pubic hair was present in two divergent patches lateral to the base of the penis. The penis was short and flat, and there was profound dorsal chordee so that the penis was tightly bound up against the lower abdomen.

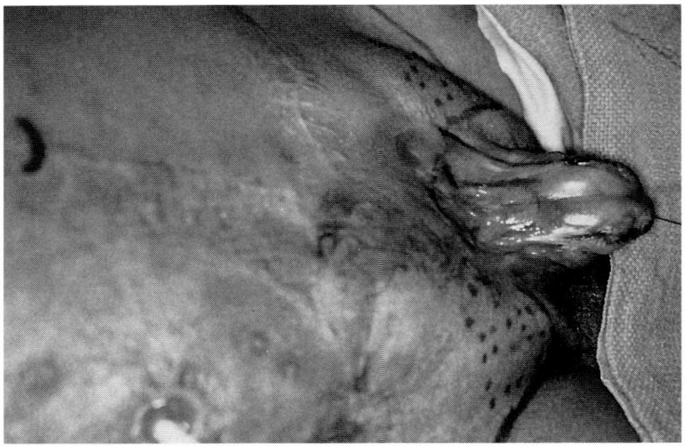

The patient was prepared for surgery, and the abdomen was marked to indicate the position of hair-bearing skin (stippled area) and the placement of the incisions for a W flap.

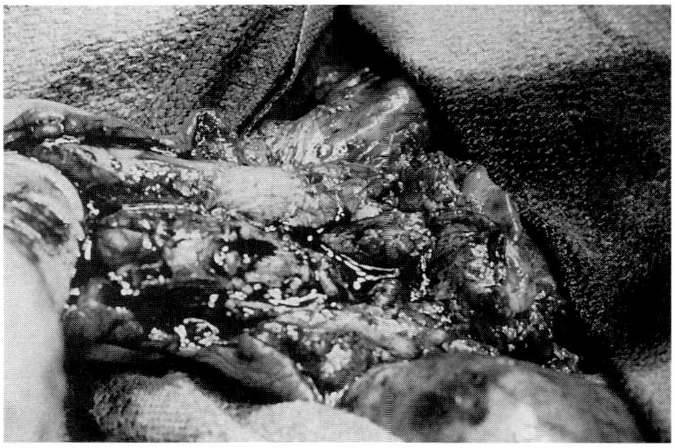

The W flap exposure provided an excellent view of the corporal bodies' attachment to the laterally displaced pubic bones. Penile lengthening was accomplished by partially detaching each corpus from the inferior pubic rami and dividing the suspensory ligament. The penile shaft was completely degloved of skin, and dysgenetic tissue and scarred epithelium were resected from the dorsal aspect of the corporal bodies.

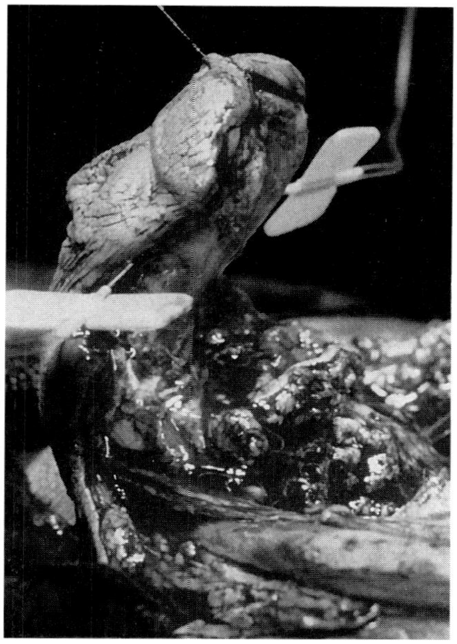

An artificial erection at this point revealed persistent chordee. A decision was made to augment the dorsal tunica with a dermal graft. The graft was harvested from hairless skin in the groin. A corporotomy was made in each corporal body at the site of maximum curvature, and the edges of the corporal defects were sutured together in the midline. This resulted in a single elliptic gap in the tunica albuginea into which a dermal graft was sutured.

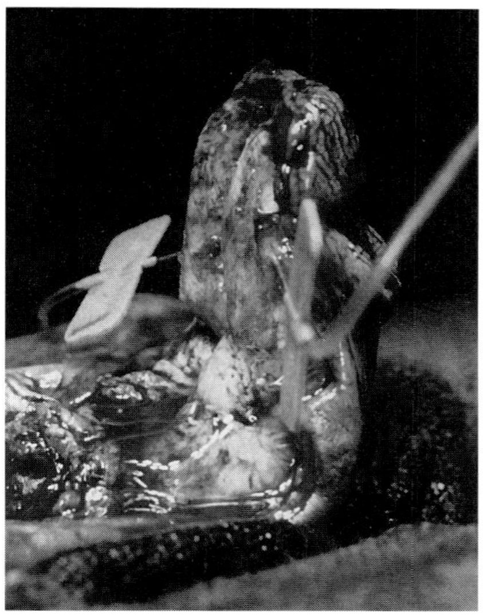

A repeat artificial erection confirmed that the penis was now completely straight. Penile shaft skin coverage was accomplished by elevating the redundant ventral prepuce on a dartos fascial pedicle and rotating the skin dorsally. Rectus abdominis muscle flaps were rotated into the midline inferiorly to provide bulk in the suprapubic area. Closure of the W flaps brought the pubic hair–bearing skin into its normal position in suprapubic area.

The repair was simplified because the patient had an ileal conduit, so there was no need for a micturating urethroplasty. A simple urethrocutaneous fistula was fashioned from the prostate at the base of the penis to accommodate ejaculation.

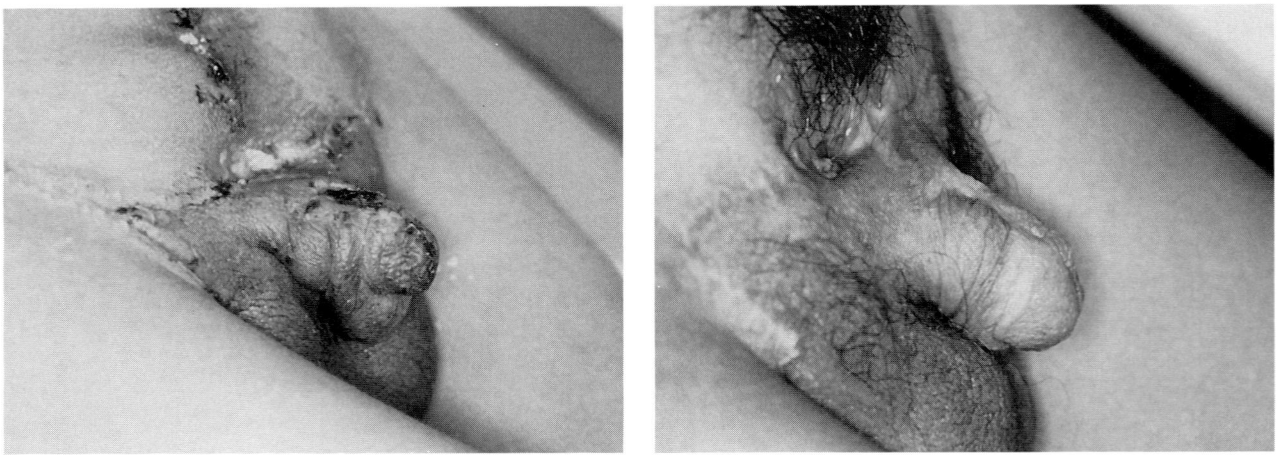

At follow-up 2 weeks postoperatively, the incisions were healing well. At follow-up 1 year postoperatively, the patient has a reasonably sized penis that dangles dependently when flaccid and is straight with erections.

Bibliography

Hendren WH, Reda EF. Bladder mucosa graft for construction of male urethra. J Pediatr Surg 21:189-192, 1986.

Horton CE Jr, Horton CE. Complications of hypospadias repair. Clin Plast Surg 15:3, 1988.

Jordan GH, Devine CJ. Surgery following the failed urethral reconstruction. In McDougal WS, ed. Difficult Problems in Urologic Surgery. Chicago: Year Book, 1989, p 289.

McCraw JB, Horton CE, Horton CE Jr. Basic techniques in genital reconstructive surgery. In McCarthy JG, ed. Plastic Surgery, vol. 6. Philadelphia: WB Saunders, 1990, p 4121.

Retik AB, Keating M, Mandell J. Complications of hypospadias repair. Urol Clin North Am 15:2, 1988.

Scherz HC, Kaplan GW, Packer MG, et al. Post-hypospadias repair of urethral strictures: A review of 30 cases. J Urol 140:1253-1255, 1988.

Stecker JF, Horton CE, Devine CJ. Hypospadias cripples. Urol Clin North Am 8:539, 1981.

Vorstman B, Horton CE, Winslow B. Repair of secondary genital deformities of epispadias/exstrophy. Urol Clin North Am 15:2, 1988.

38

Treatment of Recurrent Pressure Sores

R. Jobe Fix, M.D.

Reoperative Problems

- Recurrence
- Dehiscence
- Occurrence at other sites
- Heterotopic ossification
- Recurrence secondary to bony imbalance
- Hematoma
- Flap necrosis
- Infected retained recurrent bursa
- Residual osteomyelitis

Severe pressure sores occur in 4% or more of spinal cord–injured patients and have a significant impact on the life expectancy and lifestyle of this group of patients.[12] The recurrence rate of pressure sores that have been surgically repaired is between 10% and 50%. Hentz[4] reported an 11% recurrence in a group of 126 pressure sores. Relander and Palmer[10] noted a 48% recurrence rate in 39 patients. Although the operated pressure sore recurs in less than half, there is a subset of patients who undergo most of the operations for recurrent sores. Some of these patients may have eight to ten operations for recurrent pressure sores. However, for the vast majority, the risk of a repeat recurrence is no greater than the initial primary recurrence rate (4%). The most common problems requiring reoperation are recurrence at the same site; wound dehiscence; occurrence of pressure sores at other sites; recurrence or occurrence of a pressure sore secondary to bony imbalance, flap necrosis, hematoma, and infection; and heterotopic ossification.

PATIENT EVALUATION

To ensure success of reoperation, it is important to evaluate and correct factors that contribute to recurrence. Simply repeating the same procedure that was performed the first time is likely doomed to failure the second time. Factors that contribute to recurrence, such as debilitation of the patient, poor nutrition, psychosocial complications, poor wound bed with recalcitrant deep infection, and paucity of surrounding healthy tissue for flaps, must be recognized. Psychologic evaluation may be helpful. Preoperative planning for postoperative support services and family support at home is important. Studies that may be beneficial in the evaluation of the reoperative patient are nutritional assessment, including measurement of albumin and transferrin levels, and, if necessary, determination of nitrogen balance. A complete blood cell count may indicate an elevated white blood cell count, ongoing infection or anemia, and other nutritional disturbances. Hyperglycemia should be detected and controlled. In the quadriplegic patient it may be necessary to obtain a set of pulmonary function test results to predict the need for perioperative intubation and ventilatory assistance. A chest x-ray film may identify unsuspected pneumonia. With respect to evaluation of the affected area, a CT scan can be helpful to examine the pelvis. It may indicate soft tissue inflammation or bone erosion caused by osteomyelitis or heterotopic ossification. In addition, associated intrapelvic or ischiorectal abscesses may be identified; these defects must be addressed at the time of pressure sore treatment. Three-phase bone scans may be helpful in evaluating osteomyelitis.[2] MRI is gaining increasing acceptance as a means to diagnose osteomyelitis; however, the bone biopsy is still the most accurate standard.[6]

Urologic evaluation may be necessary. Many ischial and perineal pressure sores develop urethrocutaneous fistulae. Patients with such defects may require urinary diversion. In addition, incontinence, which is frequently present in spinal cord–injured patients, has been shown to increase the propensity toward skin excoriation and ultimate pressure sore damage. Skeletal alignment needs to be evaluated preoperatively. Some patients who have had a radical ischiectomy are off balance and have increased pressure on the side contralateral to the ischiectomy. Differential pressure–measuring devices are used for detection of this condition. Some spinal cord–injured patients may have spastic scoliosis or lordosis as demonstrated by plain radiographs. The patient who has been quadriplegic since childhood is particularly prone to lordosis because of the shifting of weight to abnormal pressure points. Skeletal realignment may be desirable. Often this treatment is deferred until soft tissue wound coverage is obtained.

In the preoperative evaluation, it is important that the surgeon understand when to operate and when to delay or recommend against surgery. In the elderly patient who is demented or very debilitated with severe contractures, it is unlikely that the conditions that caused the pressure sore can be improved and for this reason surgery is rarely recommended. It is appropriate to delay surgical repair until the patient has an improved state of mind and a willingness to participate in his care perioperatively. Depression should be treated preoperatively. In patients who have multiple recurrent pressure sores, we often find that they are not willing or are unable to comply with preventive measures against recurrence of pressure sores. Patient motivation to avoid recurrence is extremely important. It is clinically evident that psychologic counseling, social setting adjustment, and reeducation about self-care may decrease the incidence of recurrence. No amount of surgical perfection can prevent pressure sore recurrence if the patient reverts to previous behavioral patterns and repeats the pattern of injury.

With the refractory patient it is helpful to estimate how willing or able the patient is to cooperate. An outpatient test of compliance can be performed preoperatively. Initial debridement and wound care are administered. The patient is asked to remain at bed rest long enough for the wound to improve, and he is instructed that bed rest will need to be maintained for a significant period postoperatively. If the patient is not able to maintain the preoperative bed rest necessary for the wound to improve, it is unlikely that he will be able to maintain the postoperative bed rest required for the wound to heal. If the patient is unable to comply, a delay and reassessment are in the best interest of the patient and the health care system.

COMPLICATIONS

Problems that require reoperation in the pressure sore patient can be categorized as early or late problems. The most common problems requiring reoperation are recurrence of the wound, dehiscence of the wound, development of pressure sores in other locations, heterotopic ossification, flap loss, and infected recurrent bursa.

Recurrence

Recurrence of the pressure sore is the most disappointing problem for the pressure sore patient and the physician. A deep sense of loss and waste are felt by the patient who has invested weeks of bed rest and curtailment of activities and time away from friends, family, and familiar surroundings. The major causes of recurrent pressure sores are dehiscence of the wound postoperatively, residual osteomyelitis, inadequate coverage over the prominence, and poor patient compliance with resultant repeated reinjury. Contributing causes are obesity, malnutrition, smoking, urinary incontinence, diabetes mellitus, poor bedding or wheelchair support and cushioning, spasticity, scoliosis, rigidity, heterotopic ossification, and irritation by garment seams. Some recurrent sores may not be pressure sores such as ischemic gluteal slough or factitious ulcers. Recurrence of a pressure sore years later may indicate Marjolin's ulcer.[8] Recurrence can occur through a flap or through the scar at the edge of a flap. Uneven bony prominences, poor posture in a wheelchair, return to a behavioral pattern that causes damaging pressure, contractures, and scoliosis contribute to recurrence through a flap. Contributing factors in recurrence through the scar at the edge of a flap are insufficient excision of scar tissue, tension that causes local ischemia in the cicatrices, and inappropriate placement of the scar over a bony prominence.

Initial care includes resolving sepsis or infection, debriding necrotic tissue, and improving the wound hygiene. Much of this process can be accomplished on an outpatient basis. A thorough evaluation with an examination for all of the potential contributing factors must be performed. With the recognition and treatment of as many of these factors as possible, the odds of success are greater. A well-conceived plan of flap coverage is essential. A good plan requires (1) patient positioning with adequate exposure and visualization of the wounds, flaps, and changes brought on by debridement such as communication of ischial and trochanteric defects or compromise of blood supply to potential flaps; (2) for each sore at least one reliable flap and an alternative one of adequate dimensions for stable, lax coverage when the hips are fully flexed; (3) recognition of the importance of not uncovering bony prominences in flap donor sites; and (4) an understanding of how, in multiple-sore coverage, each flap closure affects other related flap closures. Intraoperatively a thorough debridement of the wound and complete excision of osteomyelitis must be obtained. However, the surgeon must keep in mind the need to maintain as much skeletal stability as possible.

Dehiscence

Dehiscence of a wound generally occurs before 3 weeks postoperatively. Dehiscence at 3 to 6 weeks is usually a result of burrowing infection from a deep plane or extreme traction across wound edges. Most cases of dehiscence tend to re-create a wound similar to the original pressure sore. Although the recurrent wound may be smaller and the tissue fresher, the wound may take just as long to close by secondary intention as any other pressure sore. The causes of dehiscence are serous fluid or hematoma accumulation, infection, flap edge necrosis, motion or movement across the lines of tension secondary to spasticity or noncompliance, and, most important, tension on closure. Fluid accumulation causing dehiscence is generally a technical problem attributed to inadequate hemostasis, inadequate drainage ports, or too early removal of the drains. The drainage from the operative site of pressure sores can be quite heavy because of the large surface areas and the potential dead space and leakage from synovial spaces. It is best to leave drains in place until egress is minimal or the wounds are securely sealed. Infection is an early cause of dehiscence and is evident by breakdown of the wound edges and purulent exudate. Infection is usually secondary to incomplete excision of the contaminated granulation tissue in the bursa, residual osteomyelitis, or primary coverage of an infected wound that would have been better treated by staged procedures. When purulence and extensive necrosis are present, the pressure sore is drained and aggressively debrided of all infected and necrotic tissue. Then in a second-stage procedure, when no further purulent drainage exists, excision and flap coverage are performed. Some lesser infections may be treated by debridement and healing by secondary intention. Tension across the operative site may pull the wound apart. Tension may be caused by spasms, too early sitting, and inappropriate positioning or moving of the patient. The single greatest contributor to dehiscence is tension across the wound. ■ ***The closure of pressure sores demands the strictest application of the principle of closure without tension.*** Adequate flap coverage must offset a negative balance of soft tissue around the sore. This negative balance exists for three reasons: (1) tissue loss in *all planes* due to pressure necrosis that is frequently wider at deeper levels, (2) tissue loss secondary to one or multiple debridements, and (3) closure performed with the trunk in an extended position so that even the slightest trunk flexion causes tension across the wound.

Dehiscence of a flap donor site is another matter. Donor sites are generally planned so that they do not cross or uncover other bony prominences or pressure points. If the donor site wounds open, they generally heal by secondary intention. Donor site dehiscence can usually be prevented by skin grafting potential areas of tension instead of attempting closure.

Occurrence at Other Sites

Another problem encountered is the occurrence of pressure sores at other sites during convalescence from the original pressure sore surgery. Often trochanteric sores develop while the patient is trying to avoid the supine position to take pressure off sacral sores, or trochanteric and sacral sores develop while the patient is at bed rest to heal ischial sores. Frequent turning and prone positioning on a good bed with a water bed or air-cushioning device can prevent this complication. Air-fluidized beds have provided a major breakthrough in the immediate postoperative period when the patient's mobility is severely restricted. Such beds are recommended for the first 3 weeks after surgery to prevent the occurrence of new sores while ensuring optimal pressure relief for the operative site. If occurrence at a different site is noted early, pressure relief measures can be taken, allowing the wound to reepithelialize and heal. However, if the damage goes unnoticed for a sufficient period of time, a new deep pressure sore may occur.

Postoperative Heterotopic Ossification

Heterotopic ossification occurs in 75% of spinal cord–injured patients.[11] Occasionally the very difficult situation arises in which heterotopic ossification develops around a pressure point that has been subjected to repeated trauma or to surgery. The result is joint immobility. When ankylosis of the hip joints occurs, the patient may be unable to sit in a wheelchair or lie flat in bed. Heterotopic ossification has also been shown to extend from the pressure sore areas up along the spine, exacerbating spine inflexibility and thus increasing the problems with positioning of the patient. As it extends into the soft tissue, heterotopic ossification also decreases tissue pliability and padding over prominent points. In addition, it creates a susceptible nidus for infection. If there is a break in the skin, infection can develop in the area of heterotopic ossification. Heterotopic ossification typically increases when there is further trauma or surgery.

Treatment may include resection of the heterotopic ossification or coverage of the affected site with a soft tissue flap. Protocols have been developed to prevent extension or recurrence. The administration of low-dose radiation immediately after surgery has been shown to decrease the incidence of heterotopic ossification.[1] Etidronate disodium (Didronel) at 20 mg/kg/day for the first 2 weeks, with the dosage decreased to 10 mg/kg/day for the next 10 weeks, and indomethacin (Indocin) at 25 mg three times a day for at least 3 weeks have also been shown to decrease the occurrence and severity of heterotopic ossification.[5] These regimens should be used in the patient with known heterotopic ossification who is prone to increased ossification, particularly in pressure sore areas.

Recurrence Secondary to Bony Imbalance

When a prominent pressure point is removed, increased pressure may be shifted to other areas that were previously without injury. Skeletal imbalance is most notably a result of radical ischiectomy, which causes pressure shifts to the pubic symphysis with consequent urethral cutaneous fistula. A Girdlestone resection of the proximal femur shifts pressure to the ipsilateral ischium. Although it is clearly necessary to remove osteomyelitic bone, it has become evident that it is necessary to retain as much healthy bone as possible for skeletal balance. If imbalance is present, seating devices such as specialized molded cushions or pressure-differentiated cushions can be provided.

Hematoma

Hematoma may be present underneath the flap, requiring reoperation in the early postoperative period. Hematoma may lead to flap necrosis, wound dehiscence, or infection. When recognized, prompt evacuation, hemostasis, and reclosure of the wound is the appropriate treatment. If hematoma is noted late, debridement of the flap may be necessary and recoverage with another flap is often required.

Flap Necrosis

Flap necrosis, when minor, may be treated conservatively and may not pose a risk of wound breakdown. However, because of the tension across the prominent areas of pressure sores and the subsequent shearing forces, even minor flap necrosis may be significant and cause wound dehiscence, leading to sinus tract formation or recurrent pressure sore. A large area of necrosis may progress to immediate wound breakdown and infection. Flap necrosis is most often caused by undue tension across the wound. It may be secondary to an inappropriate attempt to close the donor site completely when a skin graft would have sufficed and created less tension across the wound.

As mentioned previously, hematoma may cause necrosis of the flap. Venous congestion of the flap from torsion of the pedicle or compression of the pedicle is the most likely vascular cause of flap compromise. Vascular compromise may also result from injury to the pedicle. Some of the anatomic pitfalls in common flaps of the trunk may be avoided by attention to detail. For the sliding gluteus maximus flap, the superior and inferior gluteal vessels must be identified. These vessels are most easily and safely found by dissecting in the lateral avascular plane between the gluteus medius and the gluteus maximus muscles. It is easier to identify the vessels by this technique than with a medial approach. In the posterior thigh flap the pedicle is maintained with the flap by identifying the descending branch of the inferior gluteal artery in the popliteal fossa at the distal tip of the flap and dissecting from distal to proximal. In one study the descending inferior gluteal artery was found to be patent for the full length of the posterior thigh in only 25% of the anatomic dissections.[7] The tensor fascia lata pedicle may have been divided by anterior hip surgery or by pressure sore injury in that region. The V-Y biceps femoris myocutaneous advancement may be compromised by inadequate segmental perforators into the biceps femoris muscle caused by division of too many perforators. Other problems with flap necrosis are incorrect territory over the pedicle such as a tensor fascia lata flap extended more than two thirds of the length of the thigh, a flap designed off the central axis, and failure to maintain the fasciocutaneous plexus, as in the posterior thigh flap when the pedicle is separated from the flap.

Infected Retained Recurrent Bursa

Deep-seated infection or fluid accumulation caused by retained synovial fluid may result in a recurrent sore. Painting the interior of the bursa sac with methylene blue and then excising all of the blue-painted tissue helps to ensure total bursal removal. However, because of difficult exposure, portions of the bursa may be retained and may cause a recurrent sore.

TREATMENT OF SPECIFIC DEFORMITIES

Chronic Wound

The pressure sore is treated as a chronic wound. Treatment requires complete excision of scar, reduction of dead space, transfer of vascularized tissue into the space, and protection of that vascularized tissue. Improved wound perfusion, oxygenation, nutrition, and reduced contamination create a milieu of wound healing. Sclerotic or necrotic bone is excised if it is in proximity to the base of the wound.

Recurrent Sacral Pressure Sores

Recurrent sacral pressure sores most commonly occur in the quadriplegic patient. The recumbent position predisposes the patient to the sacral pressure sore. It may also be found in situations involving multiple recurrent pressure sores and may in fact result when tissue is borrowed from the gluteal areas to repair ischial or trochanteric regions. This tissue transfer causes increased tension across the sacral region in an area that is already scarred. Common causative factors of recurrent sacral sores are predisposition to osteomyelitis, poor bedding with the absence of appropriate pressure relief measures, spinal deformity that causes slumping in the chair, kyphosis, and recurrent osteomyelitis. If the quadriplegic patient remains in the recumbent position on inadequate bedding for long periods of time, the sacrum is under great pressure. This situation is aggravated by hip contractures, which increase the weight on the pelvis. The semireclining position that causes shear forces adds to the tissue damage in this area. Recurrent osteomyelitis in this area is a difficult problem. Extensive debridement of sacral bone may cause instability of the pelvis, exposure of the spinal cord, and significant bleeding.

Assessment of patients with this type of recurrent sore includes evaluation of their bedding, their seated position in the wheelchair, and their daily habits. Evaluation of the pelvic bones may be necessary with plain films, CT scan, MRI, or bone biopsy. It is important to recognize the flaps that were previously used, the scars that exist on the posterior region, and the potential areas of tension on the skin. It is also important to have an understanding of the surgical technique of the rotation flap, the previous elevation of which may have divided some of the perforators from the gluteus maximus muscle to the overlying fasciocutaneous flap or overlying skin flap. It is important to understand the technique of the gluteus maximus V-Y musculocutaneous advancement flap since this flap frequently maintains all of the perforator supply of the muscle into the fasciocutaneous flap. When flaps are planned, the design of flaps over the posterior iliac crest, superior iliac spine, posterior trochanter, or ischium is avoided. Other flaps that may be necessary to close possible recurrent ischial or trochanteric sores in the future should be taken into account.

Options for closure are as follows:

1. Readvancement of a skin or a fasciocutaneous rotation flap
2. Readvancement of a skin or fasciocutaneous rotation flap and creation of a contralateral rotation flap
3. Readvancement of a V-Y gluteus maximus musculocutaneous flap or division of one pedicle of this flap to allow advancement and rotation of the flap
4. Contralateral V-Y musculocutaneous flap
5. Transverse back fasciocutaneous flap based on its ipsilateral paraspinal perforators
6. Long posterior thigh flap based on the descending branch of the inferior gluteal artery
7. Free tissue transfer

Experience with these flaps dictates specific indications and disadvantages of each. Readvancement of the rotation flap is indicated if the perforators from the muscle are still intact. Inclusion of fascia in the flap improves the vascularity; however, some extensibility is lost. Skin grafting of the donor site from which the rotation flap is moved is nearly always necessary with a readvancement of this flap. If the first operation was a V-Y musculocutaneous gluteus maximus flap, a readvancement of this flap can be considered. In fact, the gluteus maximus musculocutaneous flap can be made to cover a greater area by dividing either the superior or the inferior pedicle, which allows a 90- to 120-degree rotation of the flap into the area. This maneuver can be helpful when covering extensive recurrent sores. Again it is necessary to recognize the potential need for a skin graft in the donor area once this flap is readvanced. If previous rotation fasciocutaneous flaps have been harvested from the gluteus maximus muscle, the musculocutaneous perforators may be disrupted in the normal territory of the V-Y advancement flap. Obviously, before either of the pedicles is divided, good pulsatile blood flow should be verified in both pedicles. Exposure of both pedicles is easily obtained by dissecting from the lateral superior edge of the gluteus maximus muscle medially and inferiorly to the superior and inferior gluteal vessels.

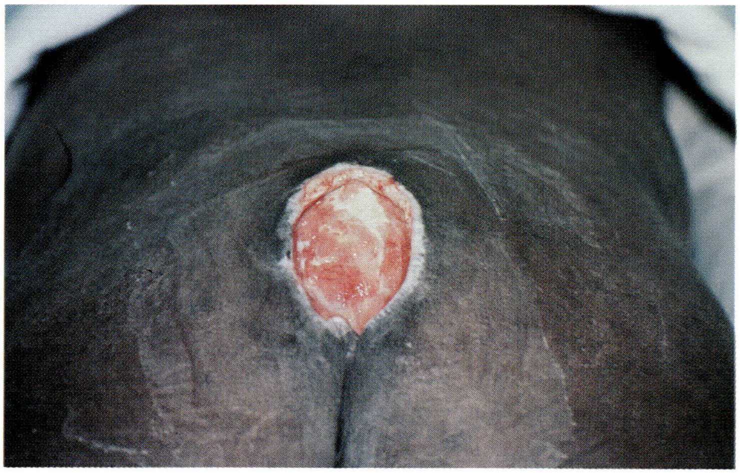

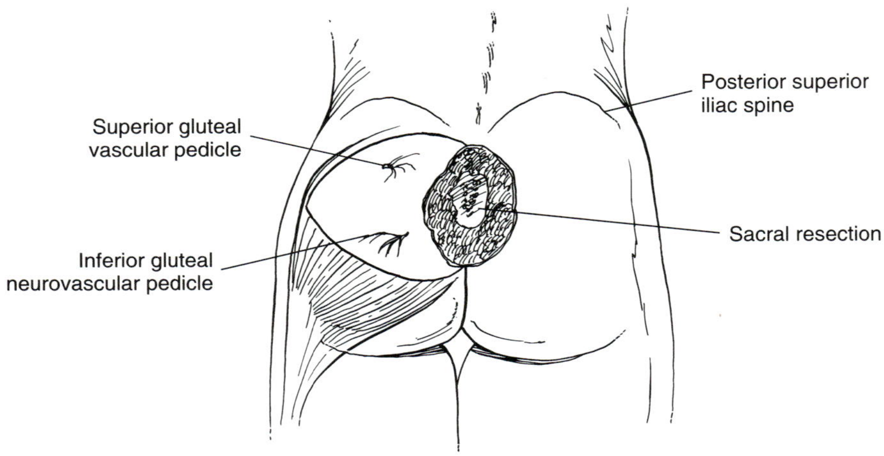

It is important to realize that a single gluteus maximus flap can cover a large defect of 8 to 12 cm. The prominences are marked so that the design of the flap will avoid uncovering the posterior iliac crest, posterior iliac spine, trochanter, and superior lateral sacrum. The V point of the flap should not lie over the trochanter.

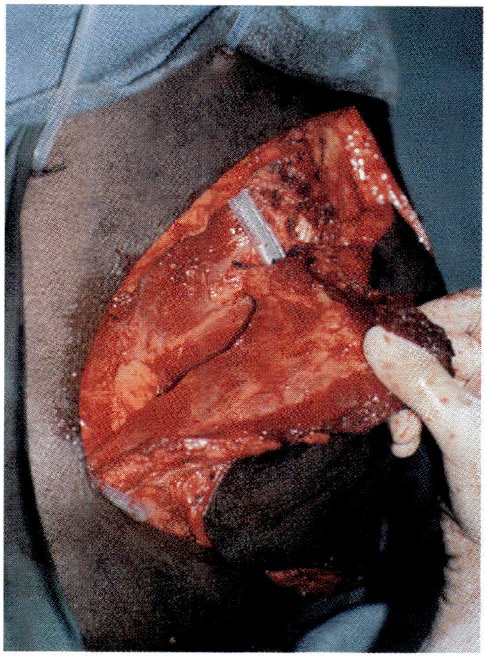

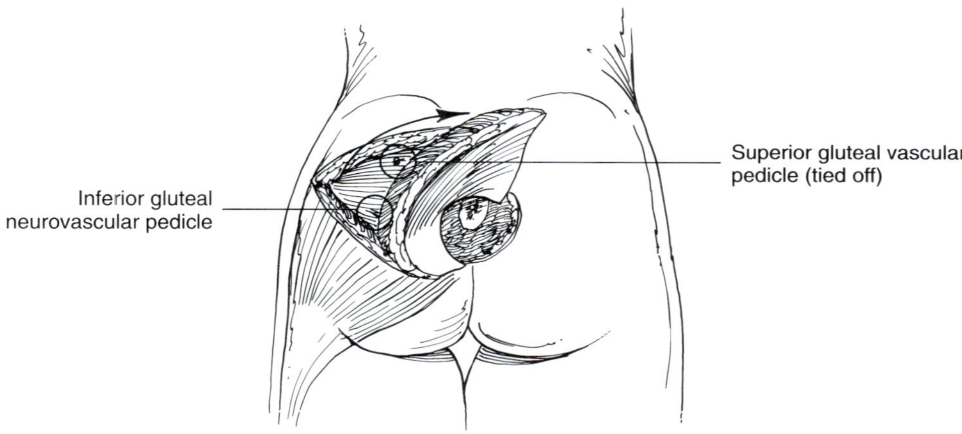

Maximal transposition is obtained by creating an island pedicle flap. This involves wide exposure and elevation of the flap from the sacrotuberous ligament, division of one of the pedicles (inferior or superior), and complete lateral and medial elevation of the flap on either side of the pedicles. In the ambulatory patient the inferior pedicle should not be ligated because it contains the inferior gluteal nerve to the gluteus maximus muscle.

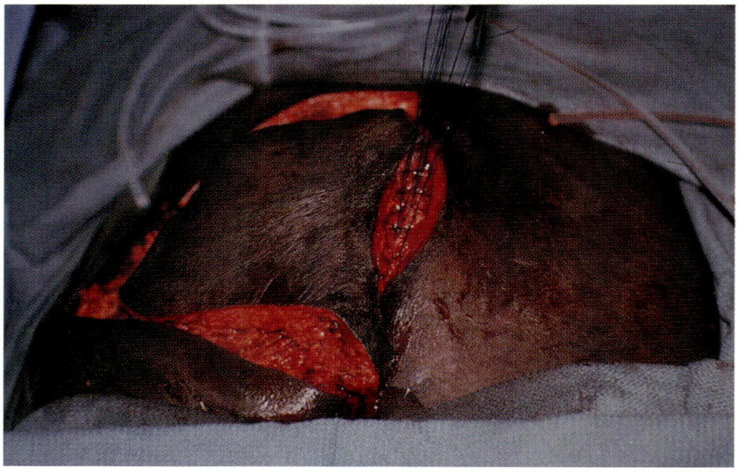

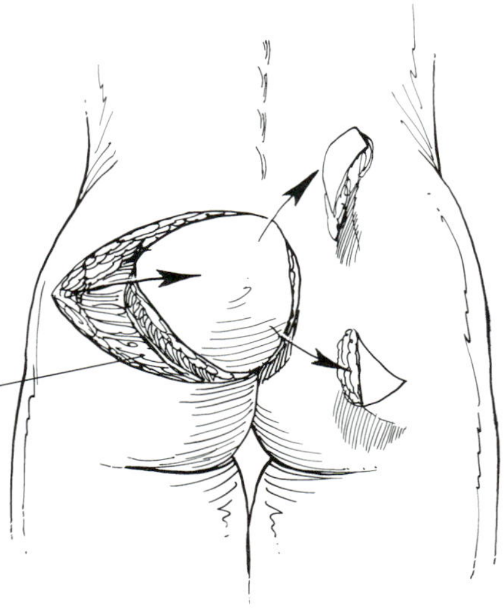

With full mobilization of the flap, the gluteus maximus muscle and fascia are approximated to the contralateral muscle and fascia, and the flap is tailored to fit the defect.

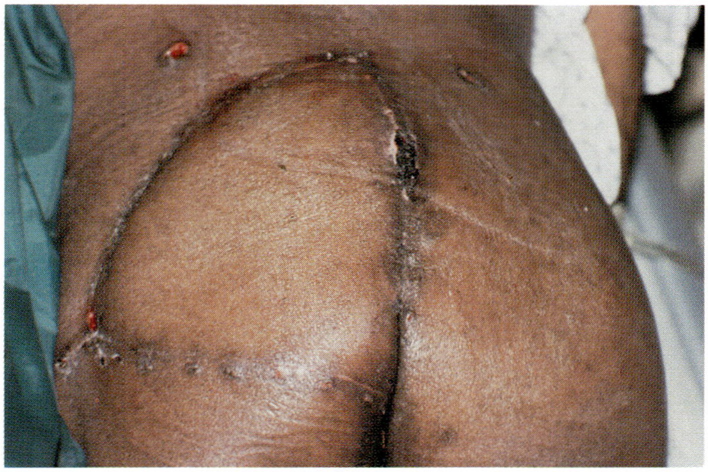

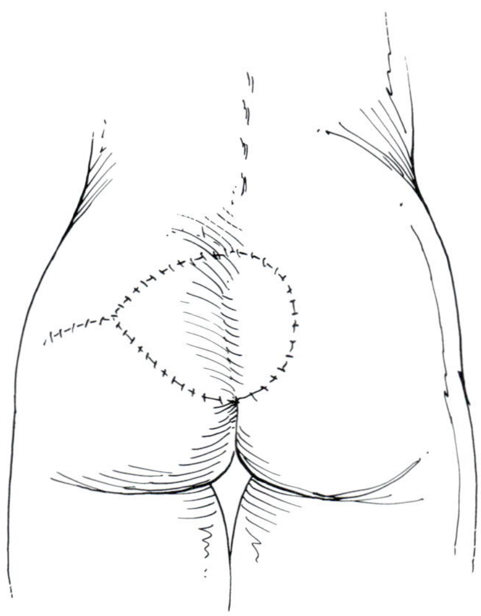

The donor site is closed as a V-Y flap or skin grafted as necessary to avoid tension.

The transverse back flap is an often forgotten but useful flap for the upper portion of the sacrum. This fasciocutaneous flap is based on paraspinal perforators on the ipsilateral side of the midline. A back cut at the midline or on the contralateral side of the midline can be made as long as the ipsilateral paraspinal perforators are maintained intact. The length of this flap can be extended to the midlateral line, and its width can vary from 8 to 15 cm as long as one recognizes that the wider the flap, the more likely that a skin graft will be necessary for donor site coverage. It is important to design these flaps so as not to uncover bony prominences. After the safe area of the transverse back flap is outlined and the perforators are marked 4 cm from the midline, the flap is incised through the fat to the fascial layer. The fascial layer can be more easily found superomedially on the flap, and dissection proceeds laterally. A thick area of subcutaneous fat is often found in the flank area; all of this fat need not be elevated with the flap. The flap is elevated more at the level of Scarpa's fascia. The appropriate dissection plane is developed laterally. The dissection then proceeds from the lateral edge of the flap and around inferiorly up to where the perforators are located at a point approximately 4 cm from the midline. A back cut can be made along the midline of the flap medial to the perforators to allow full inferior rotation of the flap down to the central sacrum. The back cut is made in much the same way as the back cut is performed for the deltopectoral flap but the perforators are still preserved. Depending on the width of the flap and evidence of previous scarring, the donor site may be closed primarily or a skin graft may be required. It is important to obtain coverage of the posterior iliac crest.

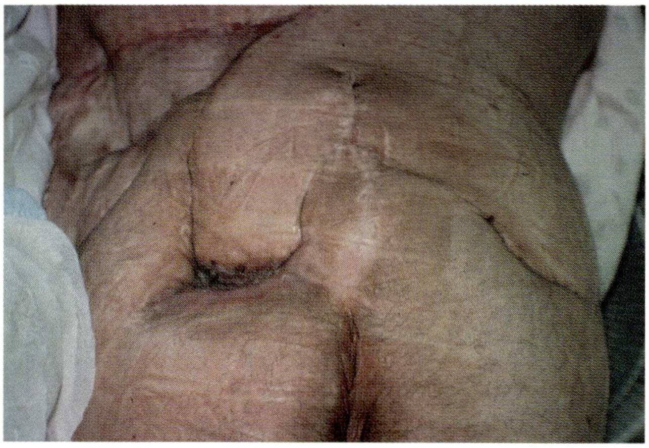

An example of the use of this flap is shown in a patient who had an L-5 to S-1 fracture and nonunion with osteomyelitis. Treatment of the recurrent sacral sore required extensive wide bony debridement, rerotation of a gluteus maximus musculocutaneous flap, and transfer of bilateral transverse back flaps to cover this extensive area. Because of the inability to obtain complete margins of all potential osteomyelitic bone, the patient was continued on long-term intravenous antibiotics for 6 weeks. At 18 months postoperatively, the patient had no recurrent signs of infection or wound breakdown in this area.

The extended posterior thigh flap based on the descending branch of the inferior gluteal artery has been described as an elegant way to cover both the ischial and sacral pressure sores simultaneously. The tip of the flap that is needed to cover the sacral area may be compromised by the extended length necessary for the flap to reach the sacrum and because the relay system of vessels that extend down the midline of the posterior thigh fasciocutaneous area has been found to be incomplete in 50% to 75% of anatomic specimens.[7]

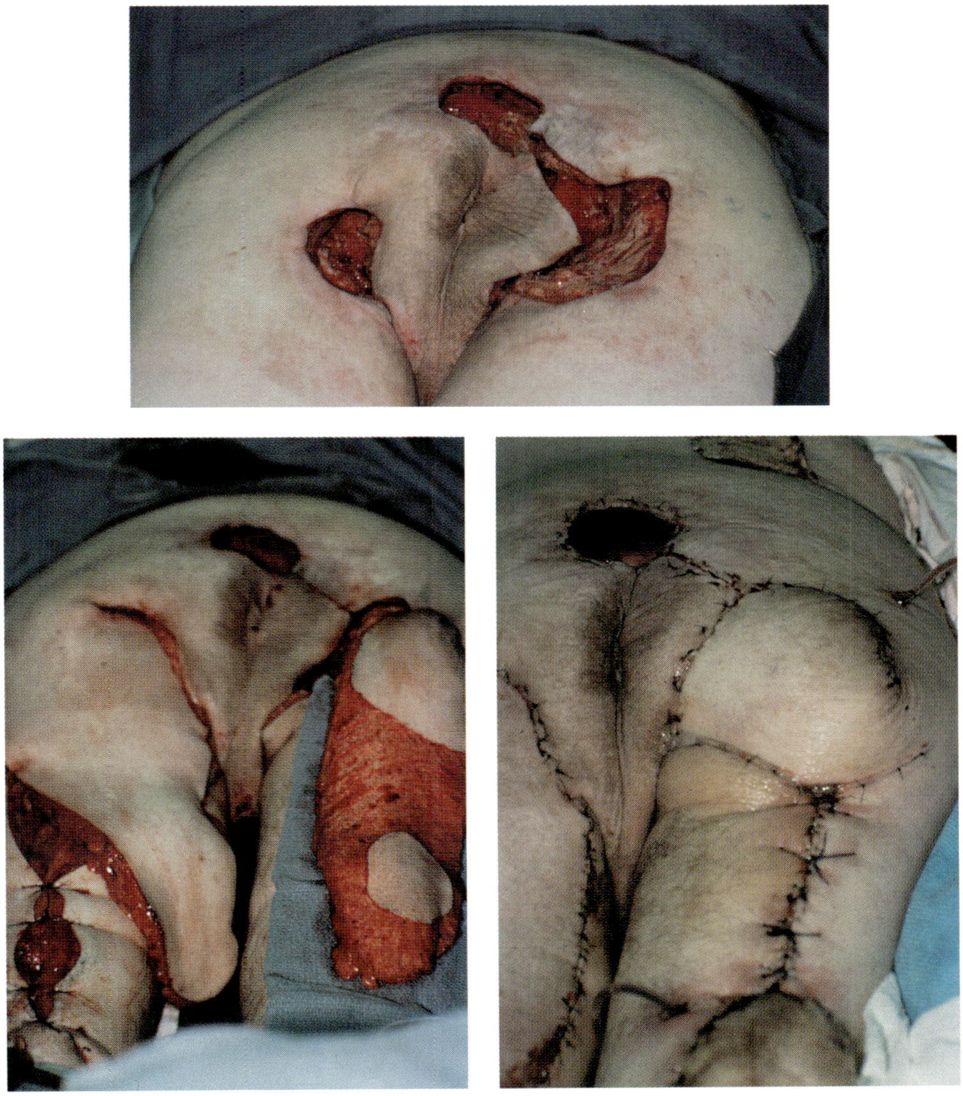

This patient had a recurrent sacral sore and new bilateral ischial sores. A left posterior thigh flap was designed for the left ischium; a right posterior thigh flap was designed for the right ischial and sacral sores. The skin paddle covering the sacrum necrosed. A subsequent gluteal rotation flap was performed for closure.

In the sacral area when there is extensive scarring or loss of flap donor tissue, it may be necessary to cover the sacral area with a free tissue transfer from the upper trunk or the lower extremities. In paraplegic patients normally it is not advisable to borrow any muscle free flaps from the upper trunk; it is desirable to maintain as much upper body function as possible. In designing a free flap, one should simultaneously consider reinnervation of the sacral area, a long nerve flap to the intercostal nerves, or a long nerve graft to the intercostal nerves.

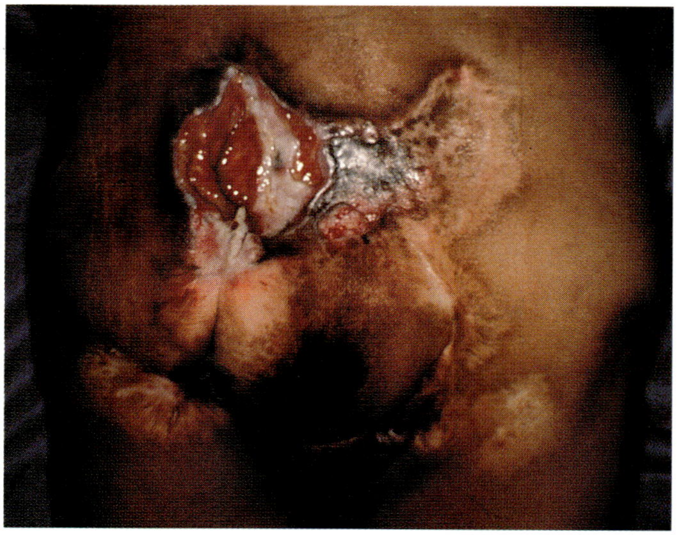

A 62-year-old T-9 paraplegic patient had a large recurrent sacral pressure sore and had previously undergone multiple attempts at reconstruction with local flaps and gluteus maximus musculocutaneous flaps. His remaining buttock area was markedly scarred from the previous surgical procedures.

Photograph from Yamamoto Y, Kunihiko N, Yoshihisa S, Igawa H, Ohura T. Reconstruction of recurrent pressure sores using free flaps. J Reconstr Microsurg 8:433-436, 1992.

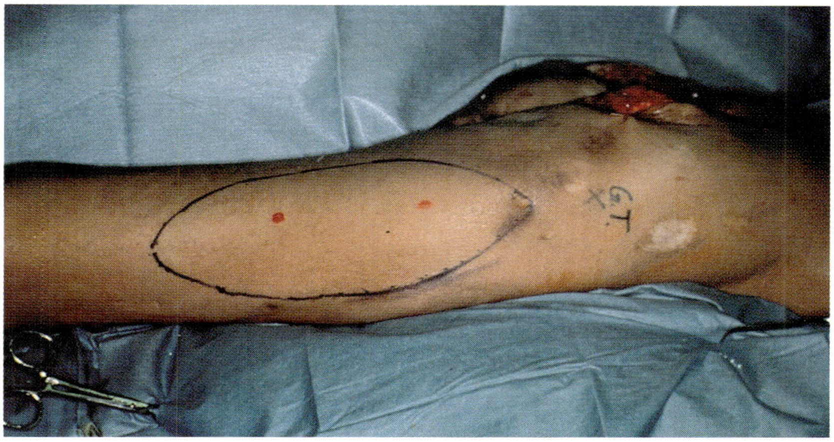

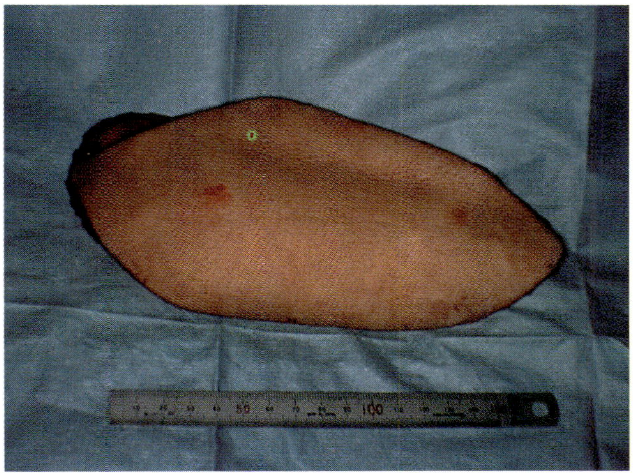

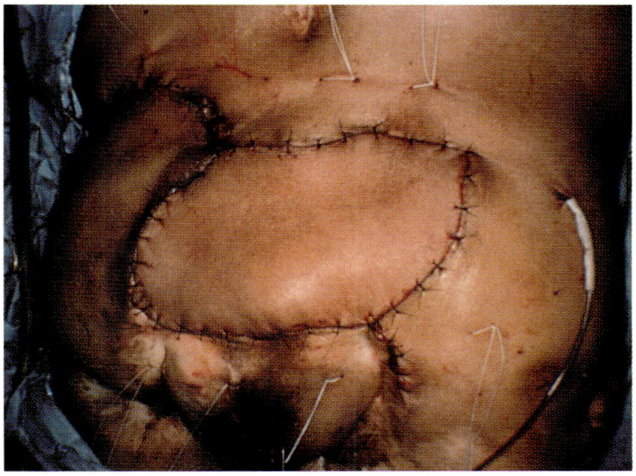

To provide tension-free and extensive coverage, free flap reconstruction was chosen. A two-stage procedure was necessary. In the first stage, infected soft tissue and bone were debrided and the right inferior gluteal artery and vein were identified as recipient vessels. Two days later, with the patient in the prone position, a lateral thigh flap 9 cm wide × 20 cm long was dissected from the right thigh based on the first and third cutaneous branches of the deep femoral vessels. The flap was transferred to cover the ulcer, and standard end-to-end arterial and venous vascular anastomoses were performed to the right inferior gluteal artery.

Postoperatively the flap became infected and the distal 5 cm became partially necrotic. Correction was obtained with the advancement of the remaining gluteus maximus musculocutaneous flap. Subsequent healing was uneventful.

Photographs from Yamamoto Y, Kunihiko N, Yoshihisa S, Igawa H, Ohura T. Reconstruction of recurrent pressure sores using free flaps. J Reconstr Microsurg 8:433-436, 1992.

Specific considerations for the postoperative care of the patient with a recurrent sacral sore are reassessment and reeducation on the prevention of the recurrent sore and pressure relief beds—in particular, the air-fluidized bed. The patient with the singular sacral pressure sore repair may begin sitting 2 to 3 weeks postoperatively because when the patient is in the upright sitting position, the direct pressure of sitting is not on the sacrum. As previously mentioned, long-term antibiotic therapy is indicated if there is a positive bone culture or bone biopsy or if there is potential osteomyelitis that could not be resected in the sacral bone.

Recurrent Trochanteric Pressure Sores

Factors associated with recurrent trochanteric sores can be divided into two categories: early postoperative problems and delayed problems. Examples of early postoperative problems are flap necrosis, flap tension, hematoma, and infection. The delayed factors specific to recurrent trochanteric pressure sores are retained trochanteric bursa with subsequent infection, osteomyelitis of the trochanter or the femoral head, pyarthrosis of the hip secondary to sinuses tracking down from the open wound to the hip joint, and protruding femoral hardware. Malalignment of the sitting posture in the wheelchair may cause the side bars to press against the trochanter.

When this wound is excised, there is usually extensive undermining in the bursal plane that can be 15 cm from the edge of the pressure sore down along the femur and superior posterolaterally along the hip. Sometimes undermining can reach all the way over to the ischial pressure sore with continuity of the ischial pressure sore cavity or a small skin bridge between the sores. Osteomyelitis of the trochanter requires wide debridement, including excision of the entire bursal cavity. Unfortunately, osteomyelitis may communicate by means of the sinus tracts to the hip joint and may extend through the femoral head. Infection of the femoral head with pyarthrosis in the trochanteric pressure sore patient generally requires a Girdlestone procedure and flap closure of the large acetabular defect and proximal femur stump. This large cavity is difficult to close because the femur tends to ride up and down during spasms in a pistonlike motion, increasing the chance of wound breakdown and recurrence.[3]

Preoperative assessment of the trochanteric pressure sore patient involves evaluation of the cause of the sore; correction of external factors such as wheelchair posture, cushion, and bedding; and education of the patient about preventive methods. Plain x-ray films of the hip joint and trochanter may identify potential bony problems, which may indicate the need for orthopedic consultation regarding the status of the hip joint. The excision of the sore is facilitated by the use of methylene blue to paint the extensive bursa. Exposure may be obtained by incising the extensive undermined area in a planned line of incision for flap coverage.

The choice of the flap used to cover the trochanteric pressure sore depends on the size of the defect after excision. The defect shape may range from a superficial flat defect to an extensive one if resection of the femoral head is necessary. Again, the flap design should avoid bony prominences such as the posterior iliac crest, posterosuperior iliac spine, ischium, and anterosuperior iliac spine.

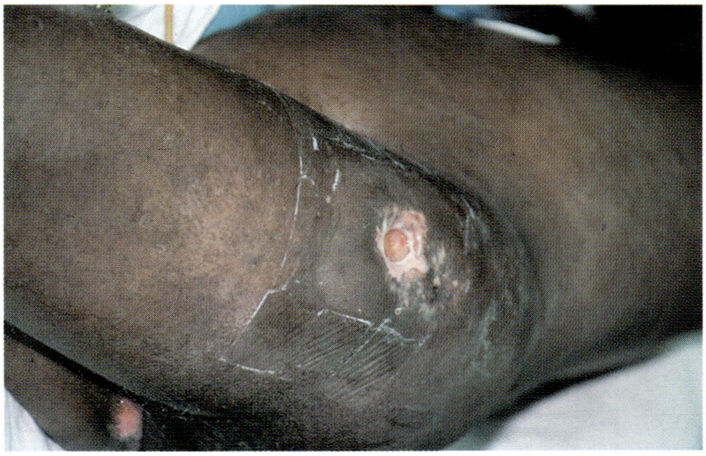

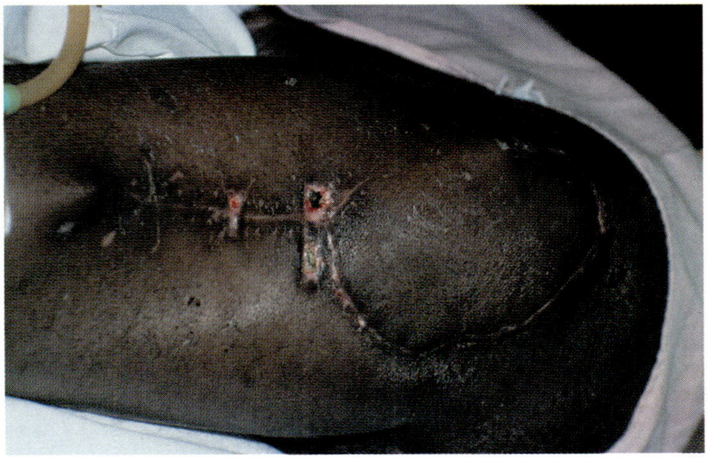

For small superficial defects a rerotation of the tensor fascia lata flap may suffice. To fill the undermined defect, deepithelialization of the distal portion of the tensor fascia lata flap is helpful. In this patient an extensive area of undermining was necessary; the defect was then covered with a tensor fascia lata flap. The rerotation of the tensor fascia lata flap often requires a split-thickness skin graft for donor site coverage on the more distal lateral thigh. The posterior thigh flap or the lateral posterior thigh flap may be used on the more distally based trochanteric defects provided the ischium is not placed at risk by thin donor site coverage.

The rectus femoris flap is especially suited for coverage of a trochanteric defect with a point of rotation in proximity but anterior to the trochanter. The donor defect is relatively remote from the posterior weight-bearing surfaces, thus posing little risk of exposing other bony prominences or pressure points. The rectus femoris flap can be used as a muscle flap to fill a deep defect with a lateral or anterior thigh random skin flap used to close the skin, or it may be transferred as a musculocutaneous flap. The rectus femoris musculocutaneous flap offers a great deal of versatility. It can be elevated en bloc and transferred, or the rectus femoris fasciocutaneous flap can be elevated from the muscle and the fasciocutaneous flap and muscle can be transposed individually to fill separate parts of the defect. The blood supply to the rectus femoris muscle is the transverse and descending branch of the lateral femoral cutaneous artery and its veins. The point of rotation is just lateral to the edge of the sartorius muscle approximately 8 to 10 cm below the anterior iliac spine. An 8 cm width of the skin flap can be harvested and still allow for primary closure. Future skin flaps may require a graft in the donor site. The flap is designed to reach all the way down to the distal three fourths of the thigh. The muscle is divided at the musculotendinous junction and elevated from distal to proximal and from lateral to medial. Once the descending branch of lateral femoral cutaneous artery is identified on the deep surface of the rectus femoris muscle, this artery can be traced up to the pedicle at its point of rotation. The muscle flap is sutured with heavy absorbable monofilament suture to the depth of the excised wound. The skin flap may be deepithelialized at its tip to allow further bulk to be inset into the undermined area. Closed suction drains are placed in the donor site of the anterior thigh and below the flaps across the surface of the debrided bone.

Occasionally an additional muscle flap may be necessary to fill an extensive deep defect. The vastus lateralis muscle is situated in proximity to the defect with its origin on the greater trochanter and linea aspera and insertion on the patellar complex. The blood supply to the vastus lateralis muscle is the lateral femoral circumflex vessels. This muscle provides adequate bulk at the point of rotation in proximity to the trochanteric defect with an easily closed donor site. Numerous vessels encountered along the linea aspera and indistinct plane between the vastus intermedius and vastus lateralis muscles cause the dissection to be somewhat bloody. Other flaps available for closure of the trochanteric pressure sore are the distal end of the gluteus maximus, which requires taking the insertion off the linea aspera and the trochanter, and random rotation flaps of the lateral thigh and hip. When feasible, innervation of the tensor fascia lata by nerve grafts or other innervated free flaps may be considered.

If a trochanteric sore is one of many sores that need to be resurfaced at the same operative setting, consideration should be given to the donor sites available with the patient in the prone position. These donor sites include the posterior thigh flap based on the descending branch of the inferior gluteal artery, inferior portion of the gluteus maximus flap as a musculocutaneous unit, lateral posterior thigh flap, and extended gluteus maximus flap combined with the posterior thigh flap as described by Ramirez, Orlando, and Hurwitz.[9]

Recurrent Ischial Pressure Sores

As with the other pressure sores, the recurrent ischial sore may be caused by early postoperative factors or delayed factors. It is important to recognize the early postoperative factors that may have caused the recurrence so as to avoid repeating the same mistakes and problems with the second operation. Factors that may cause delayed recurrence of the ischial pressure sore are insufficient soft tissue coverage with the first operation, which is aggravated by trunk and hip flexion that causes tension across the ischial coverage; rectal or urethral fistulae; residual osteomyelitis, which may extend anteriorly to the pubis; and skeletal imbalance caused by overaggressive resection of the contralateral ischium or by scoliosis or kyphosis. It is most important to reevaluate the wheelchair padding and seating position. Ankylosis of the hip from heterotopic ossification may cause relative immobility in the seated position, with pressure always occurring in the same spot. Occasionally cushions have deflated or become worn out. A serious complication of the ischial pressure sore is the ischiorectal abscess. This problem may be due to direct extension of the ischial osteomyelitis or infected bursa into the ischiorectal space, or it may be caused by a rectal fistula. A CT scan is helpful in defining the extent of the abscess and other possible bony involvement.

When a flap for ischial coverage is designed, the scars and areas of previous flap elevation are marked. Bony prominences are marked, and the remaining blood supply to potential flaps is analyzed. Options for flap coverage are readvancement of the V-Y biceps femoris musculocutaneous flap as indicated by Tobin et al.,[13] lateral posterior thigh flap based on the cutaneous perforators from the first branch of the deep femoral artery, inferior gluteal rotation flap based on multiple muscular perforators and broad-based skin blood supply, distal gluteus maximus muscle flap with a separate random skin rotation flap, tensor fascia lata fasciocutaneous flap, and readvancement of the posterior thigh flap based on the descending branch of the inferior gluteal artery.

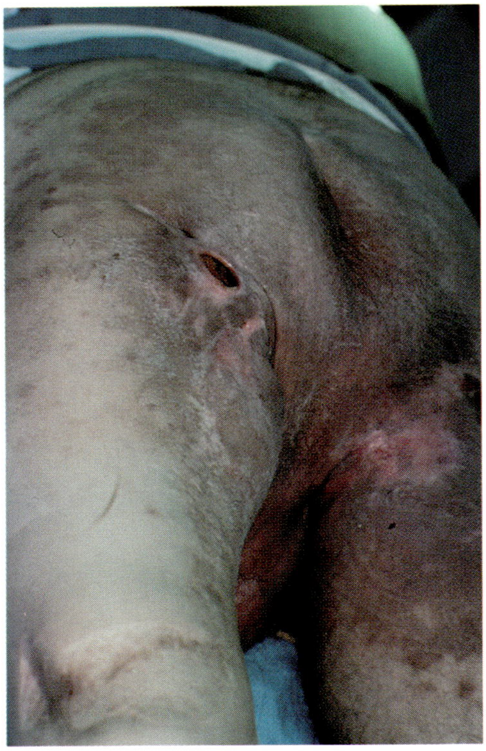

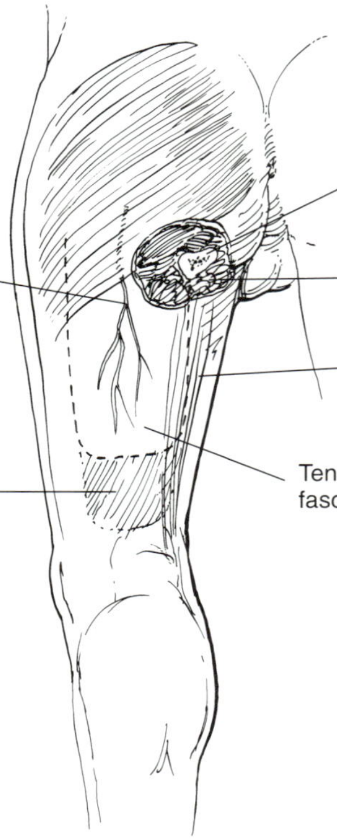

In this patient a recurrent ischial pressure sore was initially covered by a large rotation flap of the posterior thigh with the flap incised on the medial and distal aspects with a superior rotation of the flap into the defect.

The borders of the flap are outlined using lines of the previous incisions. The flap is incised medially and distally in a plane superficial to the biceps femoris muscles but deep to the descending artery branch. Once the vessels are identified, the flap is incised on its lateral edge and elevated from distal to proximal. The septal perforating vessels that connect into the system of the descending gluteal vessel must be ligated and divided. The point of rotation of the descending gluteal vessel is at the inferior edge of the gluteus maximus muscle in the midline posterior thigh. This point is one half of the distance between the trochanter and the ischial tuberosity.

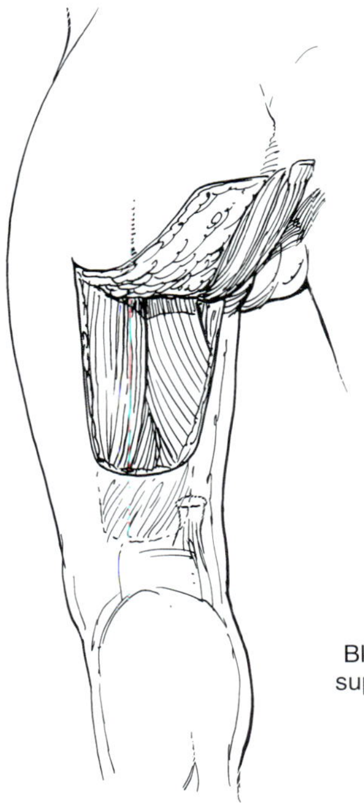

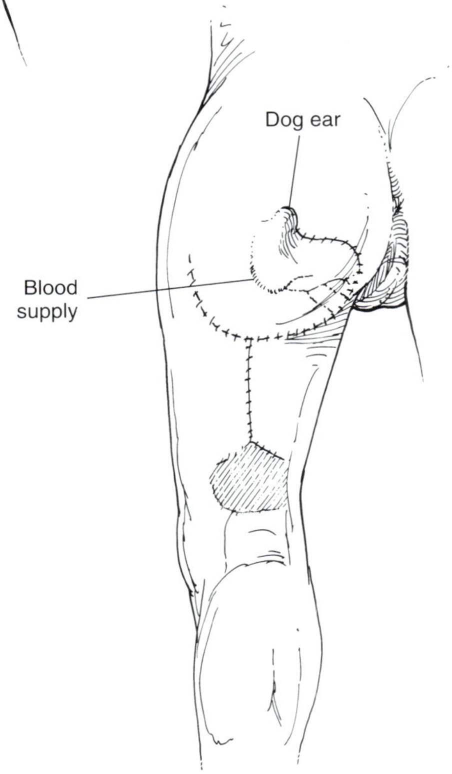

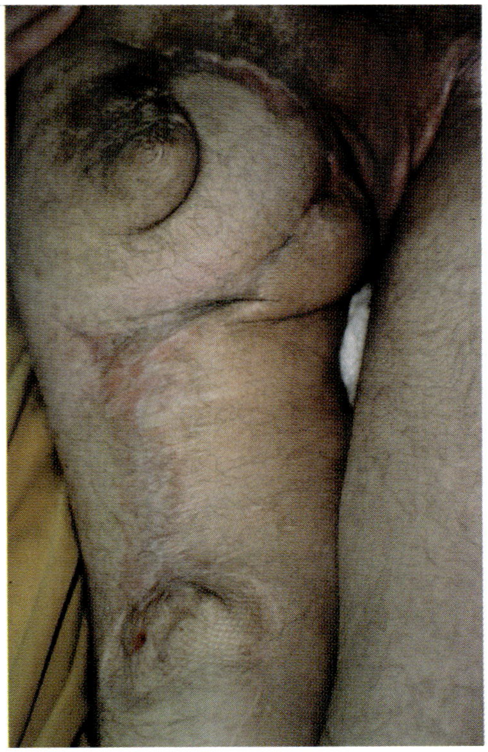

The flap is completely elevated on its medial, distal, and lateral aspects on the pedicle of the descending branch of the inferior gluteal artery. The gracilis muscle is elevated and draped across the ischium. The posterior thigh flap is inset with the distal tip deepithelialized to fill the undermined deep space. Drains are placed in the donor site and deep to the flap over the surface of the ischial bone, and 2-0 absorbable monofilament sutures are placed to secure the flap down to the periosteum and fibrous tissue around the ischium to ensure that the flap is into the deep space of the defect. The donor defect of the thigh is generally closed by primary approximation of the edges, but sometimes a skin graft is necessary.

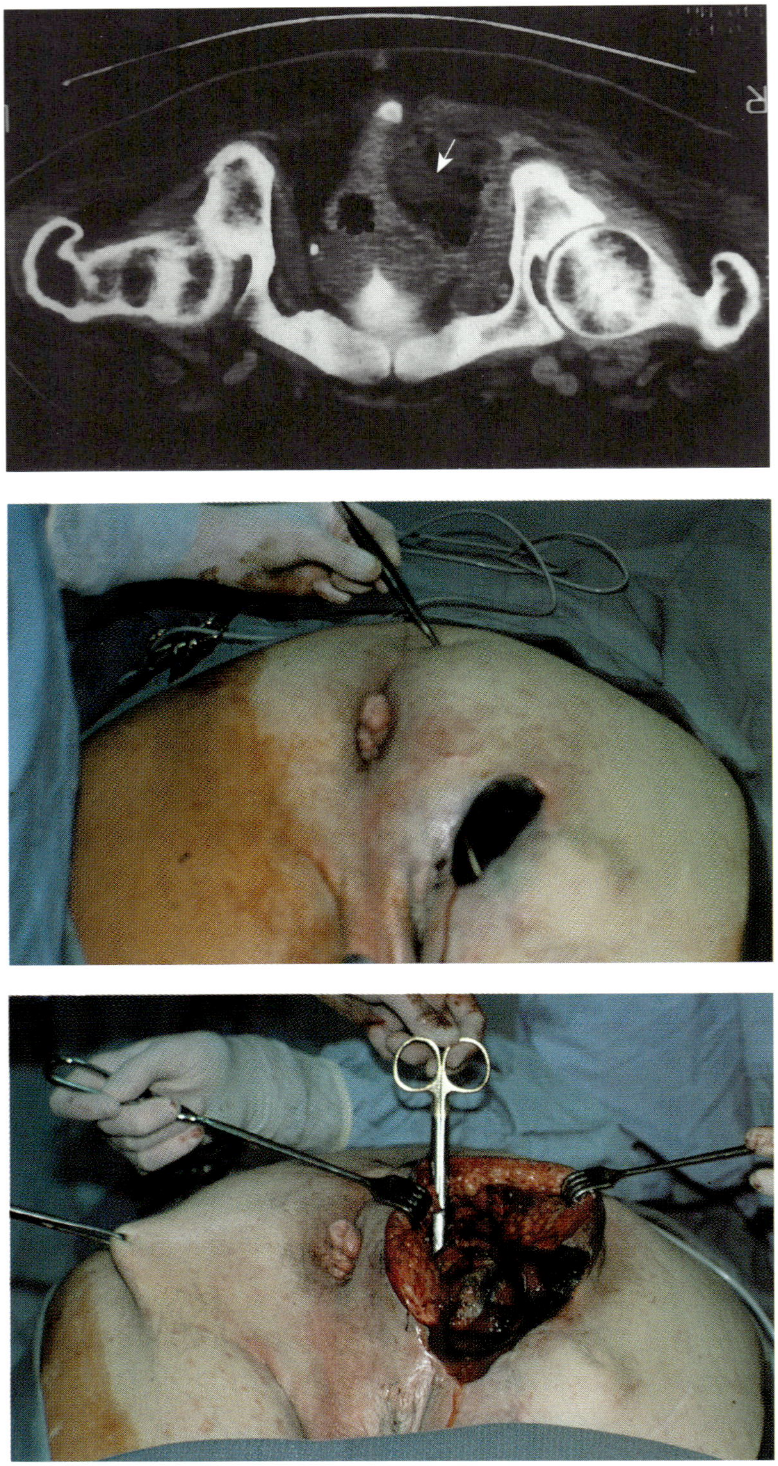

This patient presented with a right ischiorectal abscess contiguous with a right ischial sore. The wound was cavernous.

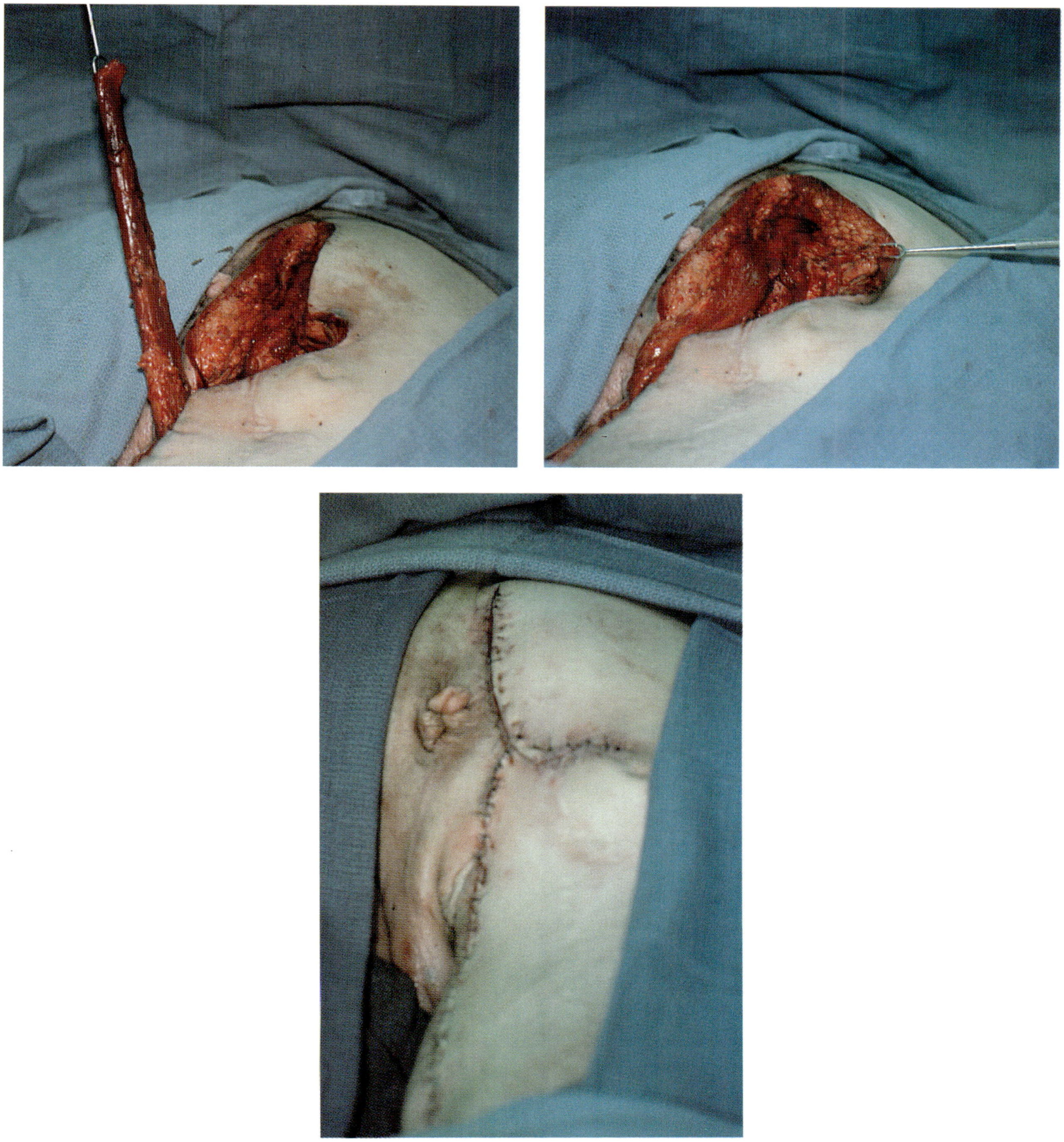

A gracilis muscle was harvested to fill the ischiorectal space, and a posterior thigh flap was rerotated into the defect.

For ischial coverage the tensor fascia lata flap should be considered. This flap taken down to the distal two thirds of the thigh can easily be rotated to cover the ischial defect. However, this approach is recommended only if there is already a scar or defect between the trochanter and ischium that also needs to be covered.

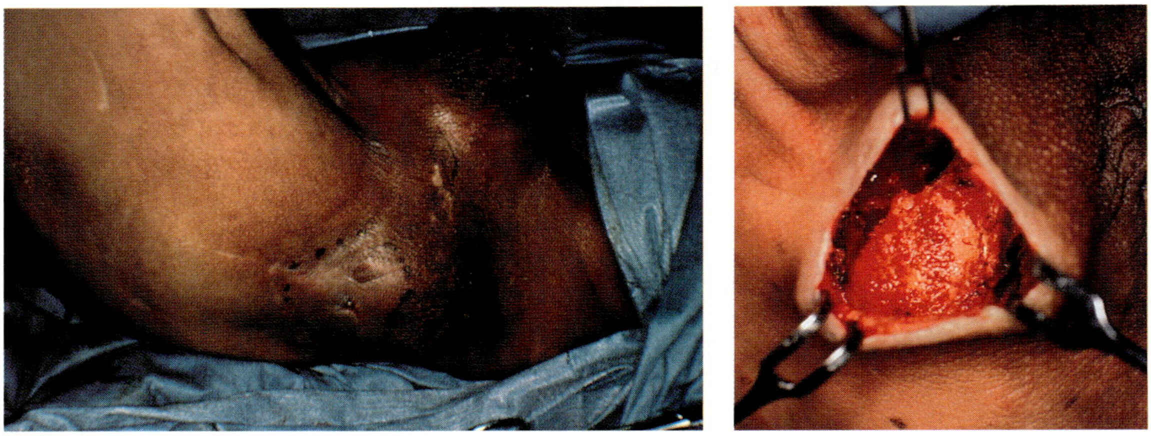

A free medial plantar flap can be used for ischial coverage.[14] The patient, with a recurrent right ischial pressure sore, was placed in a supine lithotomy position.

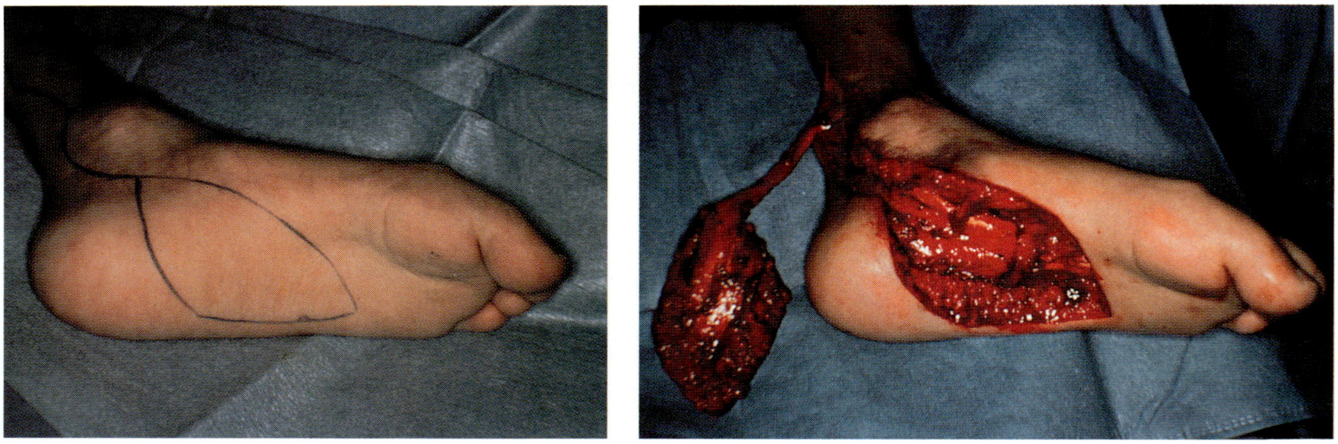

After excision, the right superficial femoral vessel was prepared as a recipient vessel. The medial plantar flap, including the flexor digitorum brevis muscle, was harvested with a long posterior tibial artery and vein pedicle.

Photographs from Yamamoto Y, Kunihiko N, Yoshihisa S, Igawa H, Ohura T. Reconstruction of recurrent pressure sores using free flaps. J Reconstr Microsurg 8:433-436, 1992.

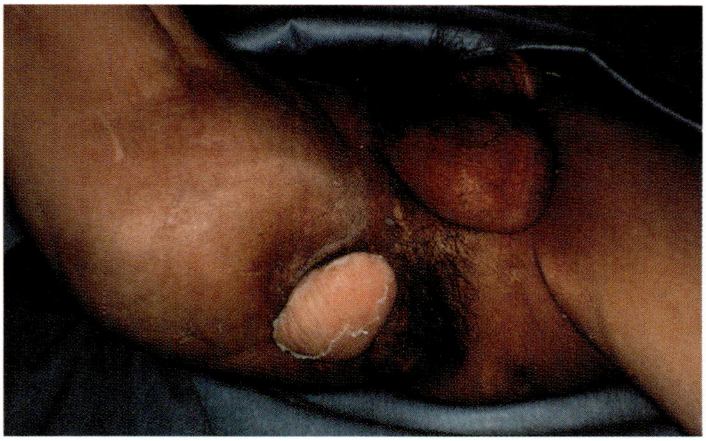

The flap was inset and shown to be well healed at 2 months. The advantage of this flap is the long pedicle of the posterior tibial artery and vena comitans.

Postoperative care includes complete pressure relief precluding any sitting for a period of 6 weeks. At the end of 6 weeks, if all wounds over the areas of pressure prominences are healed, a graduated sitting schedule is given to the patient. This regimen generally begins with 20 minutes three times a day and is doubled every 2 to 3 days until the patient is able to sit for 3 to 4 hours at the end of a 2-week period. The patient is instructed to perform pressure relief while in the sitting position and to carefully examine the pressure prominences every evening with direct visual scrutiny using a mirror. It is at this time that the appropriate wheelchair cushions need to be provided. Cushion design can be simplified by computerized pressure point evaluation. Computerized evaluation facilitates the fine-tuning of the seating cushion to help to correct areas of increased pressure caused by skeletal imbalance in the sitting posture.

Photograph from Yamamoto Y, Kunihiko N, Yoshihisa S, Igawa H, Ohura T. Reconstruction of recurrent pressure sores using free flaps. J Reconstr Microsurg 8:433-436, 1992.

Ischial Trochanteric Defects After Girdlestone Resection of the Proximal Femur

Recurrent ischial trochanteric pressure sores may result in osteomyelitis of the proximal femur with pyarthrosis. This condition necessitates a resection of the femoral head and proximal femur, leaving the acetabular defect and stump of the proximal femur in the wound. Specific problems that occur with closing these defects are related to the mechanics of the pseudoarthrosis and the extent of the osteomyelitis that necessitated the resection. Infected sinus tracts may run from the hip joint anteriorly around the anterior lip of the iliac rim and in front of the pubis and then extend posteriorly across the superior and inferior rami of the pubis. Osteomyelitis of the acetabular cup may be present. The most effective treatment involves excision of all sinus tracts and all osteomyelitic bone. The wound is unstable and difficult to cover because the proximal edge of the resected femur tends to ride up and down within the acetabular space. Optimal management of this problem is extensive coverage of the defect with well-vascularized bulky tissue, which usually requires more than one muscle flap and a skin or fasciocutaneous flap.

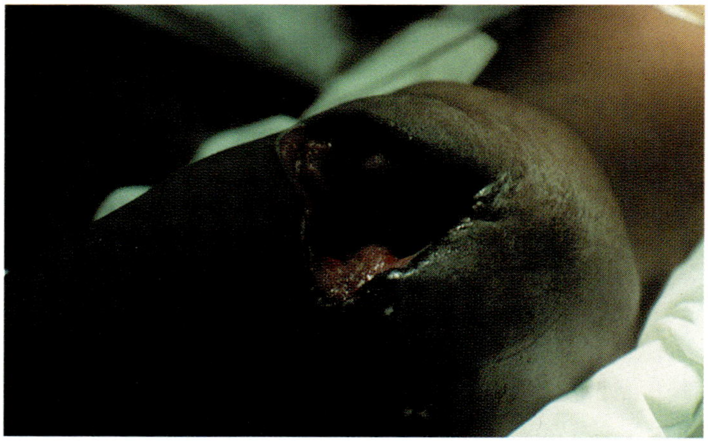

One of the most effective surgical treatments for this type of defect involves reconstruction with the vastus lateralis muscle flap and an overlying fasciocutaneous flap from the anterior lateral thigh. This technique is demonstrated in a patient with a Girdlestone wound.

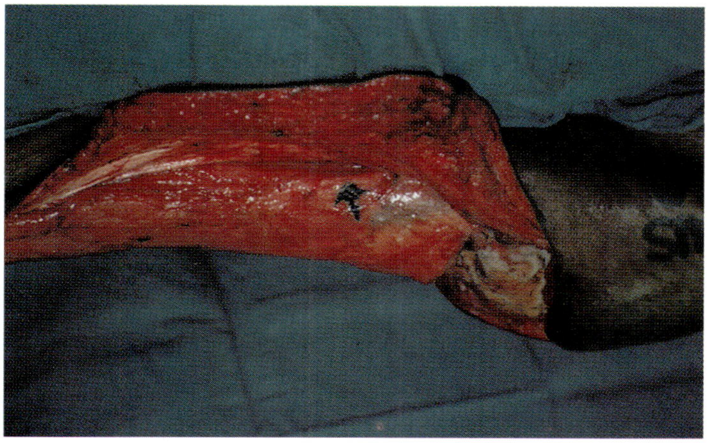

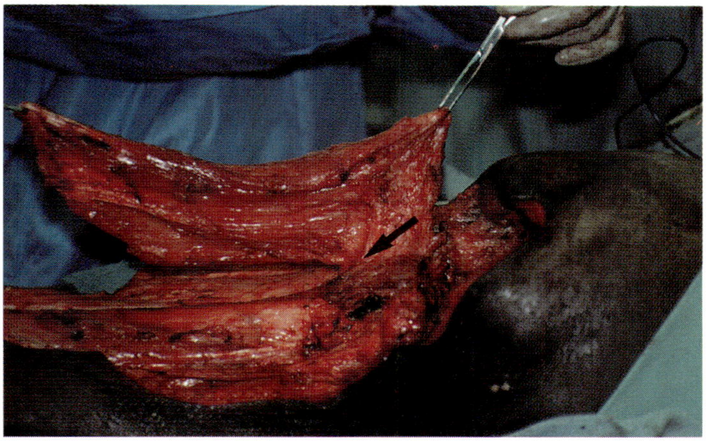

The vastus lateralis vascular pedicle is in proximity to the defect just anterior to the acetabulum and 8 to 10 cm below the anterior spine. It is mobilized from the femur and carefully separated from the vastus intermedius and rectus femoris muscles and posteriorly from the biceps femoris muscle. It is important to identify the pedicle (arrow) as it comes into the deep surface of the muscle 8 to 10 cm inferior to the anterior iliac spine. The pedicle is best located by reflecting the rectus femoris muscle away from the vastus lateralis muscle and visualizing the pedicle as it enters into the medial edge of the deep surface of the vastus lateralis muscle. Usually a portion of the origin of the vastus lateralis muscle has been previously elevated when the Girdlestone procedure was performed.

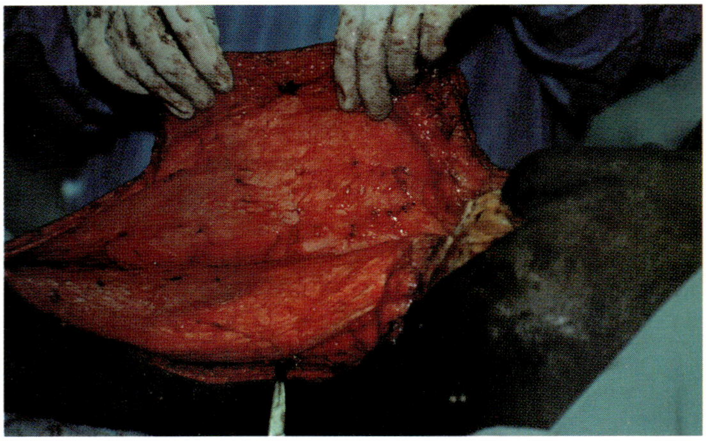

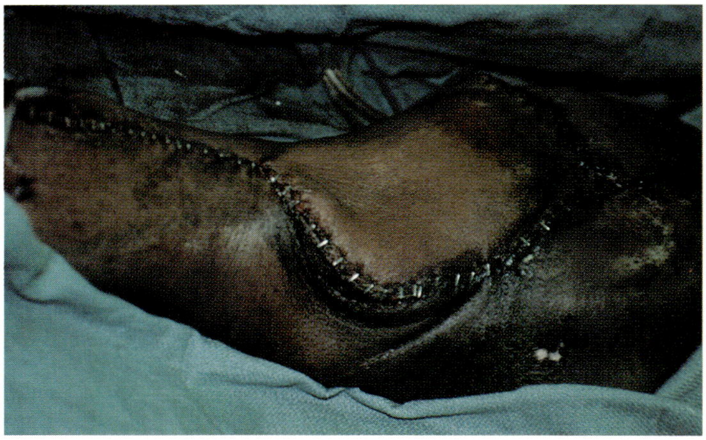

After the muscle is elevated, it is carefully and securely sutured into the acetabular defect and draped over the stump of the femur. Outer coverage is provided by a rotation fasciocutaneous flap from the anterior lateral thigh. An extremely large defect may require the transfer of a second muscle. The rectus femoris muscle is available on the same pedicle for rotation into the defect.

A recurrence of the pressure sore after a Girdlestone procedure or a dehiscence of the wound after a Girdlestone procedure commonly necessitates a disarticulation amputation of that extremity with a total thigh flap then used to cover the area. An alternative to amputation is a free flap transfer.

Extensive Recurrent Puborectal Ischial Pressure Sores

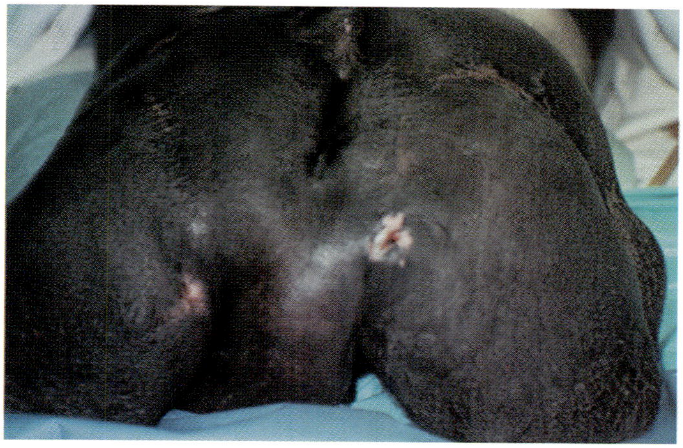

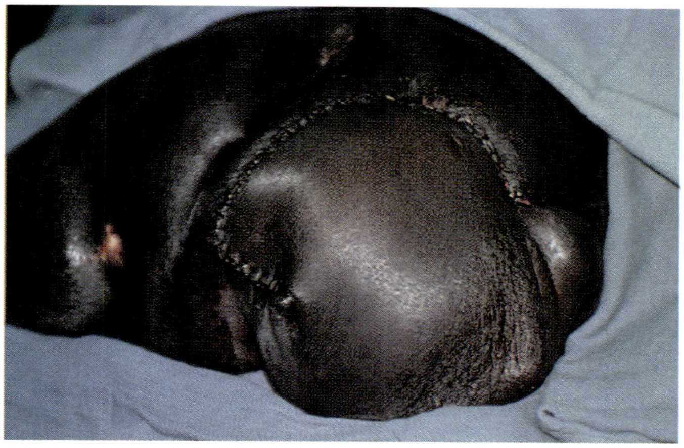

A frequent sequela of bilateral disarticulation amputation is extensive puborecto-ischial sores that develop because of direct pressure on the pubic rami, rectal tissue, and ischial bones. Generally patients with this problem have already undergone disarticulation amputations, and consideration can be given to re-advancing the total thigh flap over the area. A significant amount of redundant tissue is usually available after disarticulation amputation. For example, in this patient a recurrent ischial sore was covered by advancement of the right total thigh flap.

Consideration is given to the rectus abdominis myocutaneous flap brought down on its pedicle of the inferior deep epigastric vessels. This flap provides a large area of skin with abundant bulk to cover these extensive defects. Frequently patients who have reached this stage of recurrent pressure sore reconstruction will already have had urinary diversion and/or colostomies, which preclude a rectus abdominis flap. Consideration can be given to a free tissue transfer from the upper torso. In these advanced cases in which all other alternatives have been exhausted, consideration should be given to a total fecal and urinary diversion with colostomy and suprapubic catheter.

Recurrent Olecranon Bursa Pressure Sores

The elbow bursa pressure sore has the greatest potential to cause loss of function for the quadriplegic patient. These sores frequently occur because patients are propping the upper body on their elbows to eat, read, or watch TV. Although they have enough motor function to prop themselves up on their elbows, they may not have enough sensation to provide for protection of the skin over the olecranon bursa, and a pressure sore subsequently develops. It is necessary to rule out a pyarthrosis of the elbow, which can be done by careful physical examination and radiologic evaluation with consideration of injection of the joint to see whether any extravasation occurs.

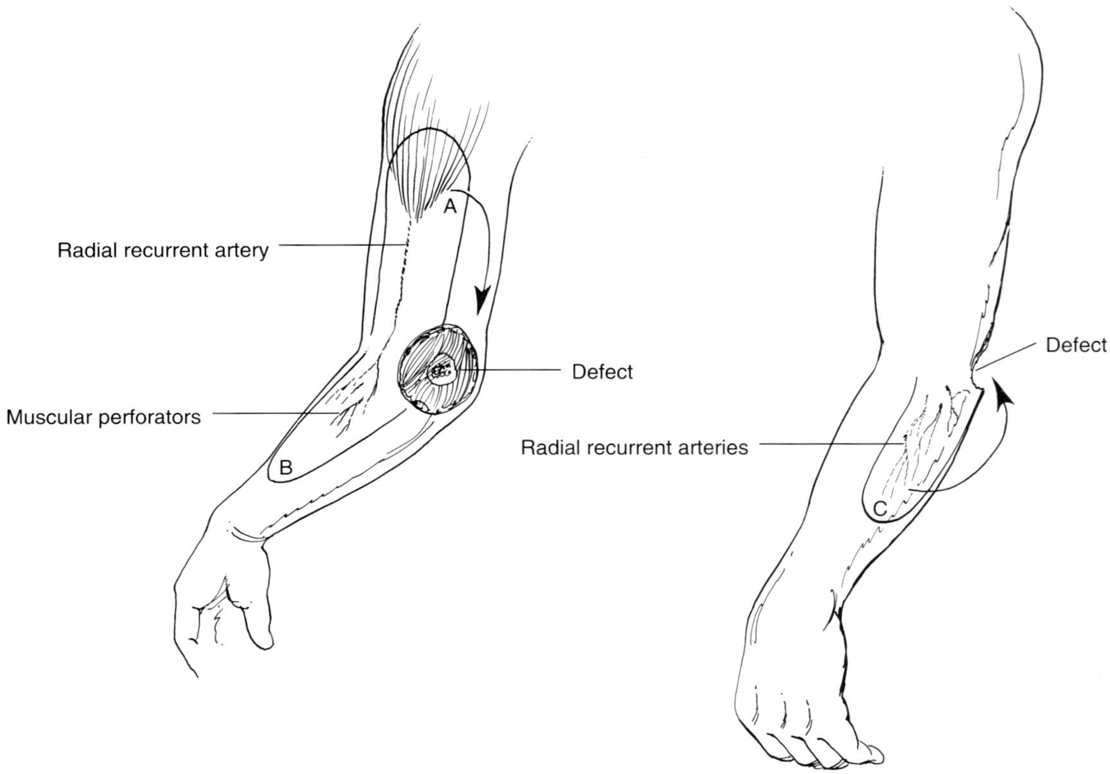

Options for coverage include the lateral arm flap distally based on the radial recurrent artery *(A),* fasciocutaneous flap based on muscle perforators from the mobile wad muscles *(B),* and an antebrachial fasciocutaneous flap based on the radial recurrent artery *(C).* The donor sites can be closed primarily.

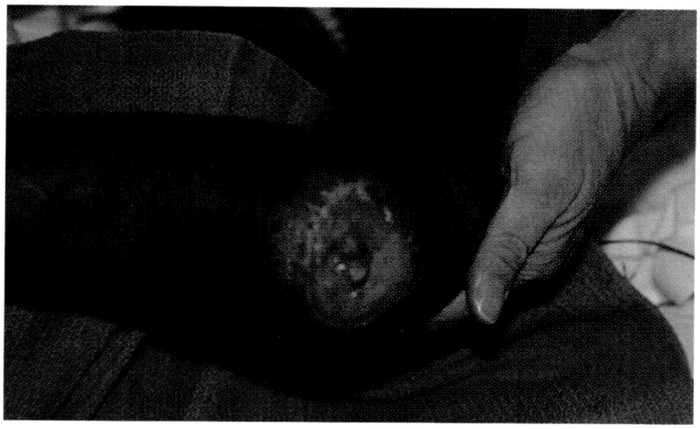

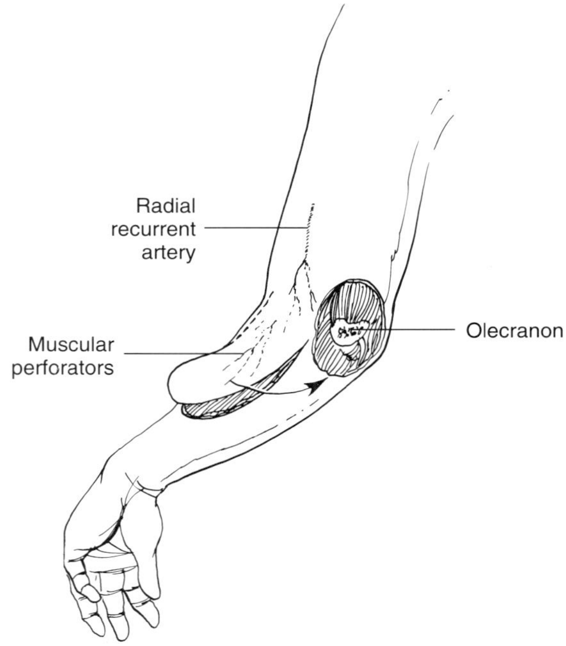

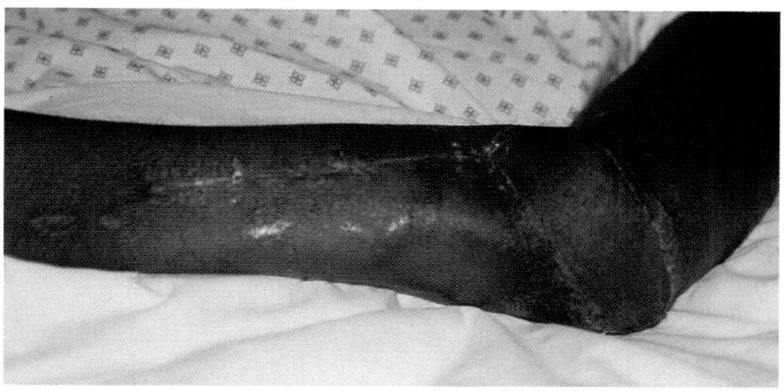

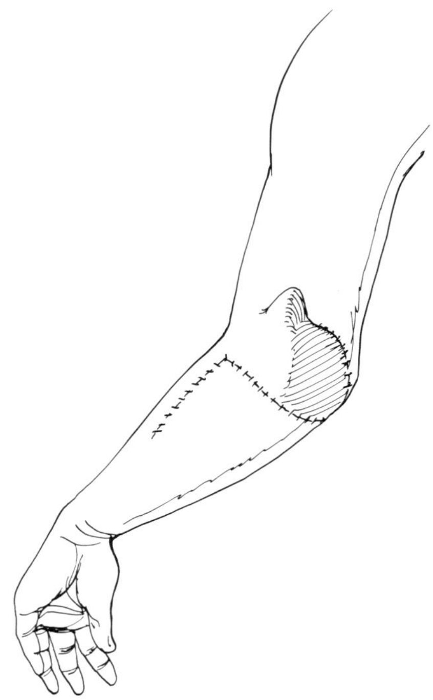

One flap that works well is the antebrachial fasciocutaneous flap elevated in the same line of axis as the lateral arm flap rotated posteriorly, with the back cut made as necessary. The donor site is closed by primary closure, and closed suction drains are placed in the donor site and beneath the flap. Postoperatively it is important to provide immobilization with the use of a well-padded plaster splint, compression, and suction drains to allow closure. Nonsteroidal anti-inflammatory drugs are helpful in reducing bursitis in the area; if not treated, bursitis and development of a bursal space may recur.

Concomitant Recurrent Sores

Ipsilateral Ischial and Trochanteric Pressure Sores

When ischial and trochanteric pressure sores exist on the same side, the descending branch of the inferior gluteal vessel may have been eroded by either one or both of the pressure sores. The sores may interconnect beneath a skin bridge. Depending on the existing scars and previous flap elevations, flaps are designed to cover both sores at the same operative setting. Options that can be considered are (1) a tensor fascia lata flap designed long enough to cover both sores, (2) a gluteus maximus rotation flap to cover both sores as an extended flap, and (3) a tensor fascia lata flap with a posterior thigh flap.

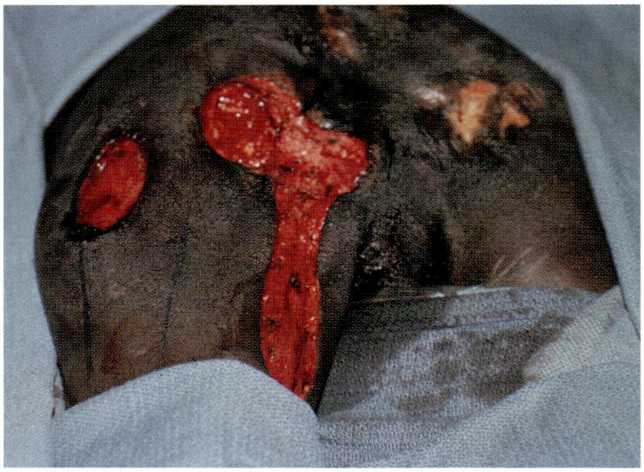

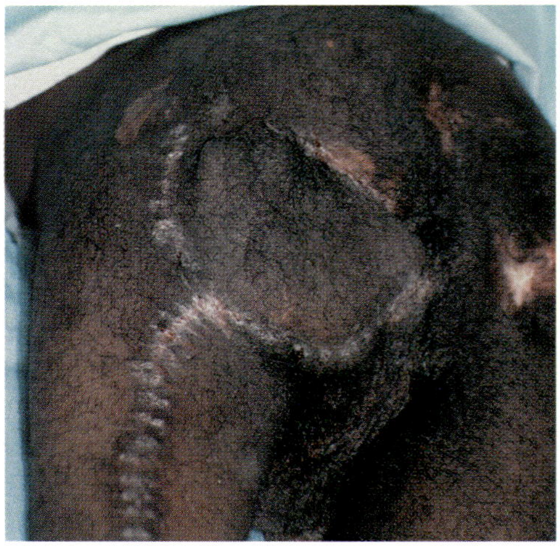

In this patient with ipsilateral trochanteric and ischial sores, the base of each sore was 10 cm in diameter. A posterior thigh flap based on the descending branch of the gluteal artery was elevated and used to cover the ischial and trochanteric sores. In this case a good skin bridge was present between the trochanter and the ischium with a robust descending branch of the inferior gluteal artery to supply the posterior thigh flap. An island pedicled flap based on the descending branch was inset into both defects. In this situation it would not have been advantageous to divide this skin bridge in order to bring a long tensor fascia lata flap across to cover both sores.

Ischial and Sacral Pressure Sores

An ischial sore coexisting with a sacral sore can be covered with an extended gluteus maximus flap as described by Ramirez, Orlando, and Hurwitz.[9] If necessary, an added transverse back fasciocutaneous flap can be used to fill and cover the upper portion of the sacral defect. This type of flap is useful if the defects tend to be flat and superficial although broad.

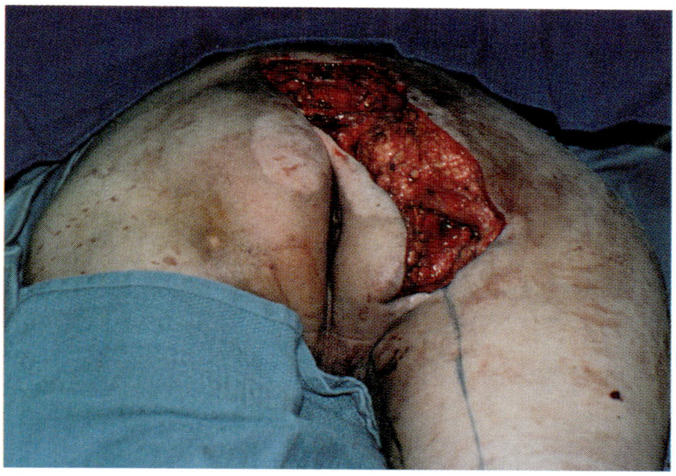

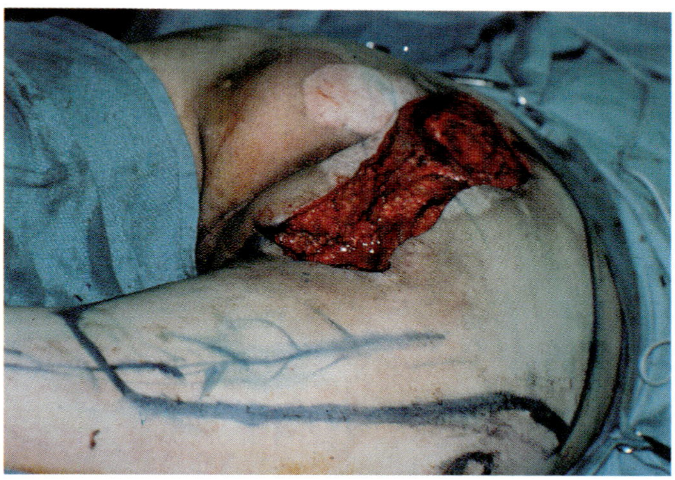

This patient had communicating sacral and ischial sores. An extended gluteus maximus musculocutaneous flap was designed based on the right inferior gluteal artery, including its descending branch.

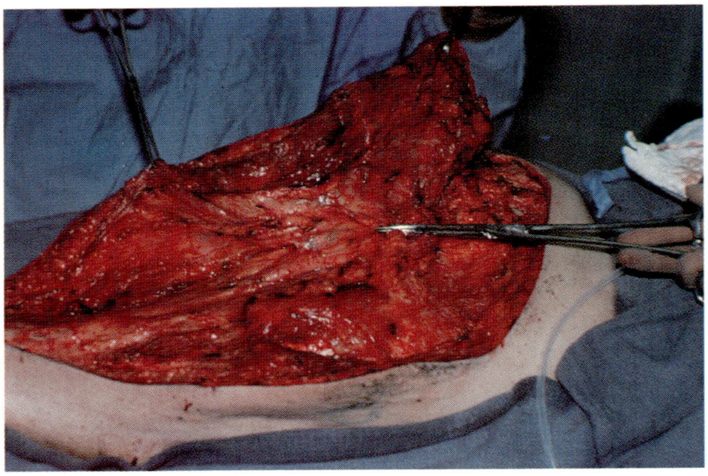

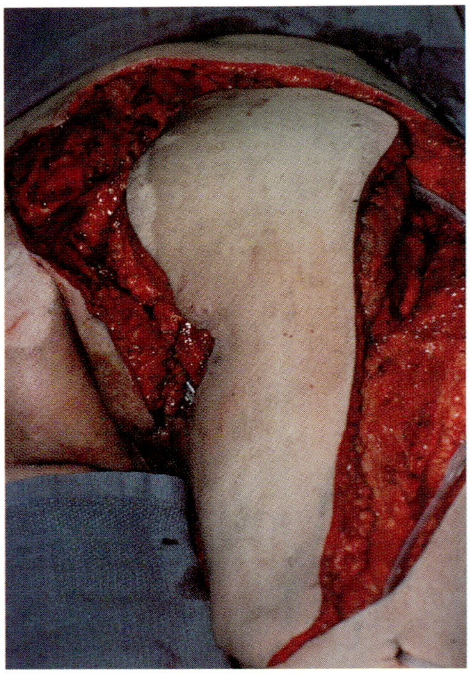

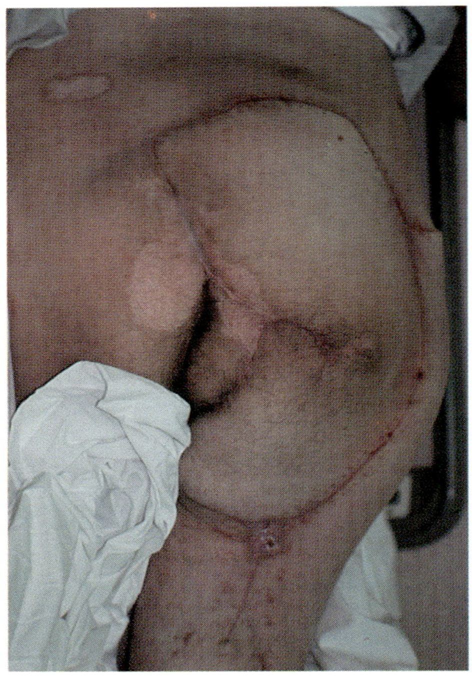

The flap was elevated by identifying the gluteal pedicle in the same way as for a V-Y gluteal flap. The flap was inset and the donor sites were closed in a V-Y fashion and skin grafted. The area is healed 12 weeks postoperatively.

Sacral, Bilateral Ischial, and Bilateral Trochanteric Pressure Sores

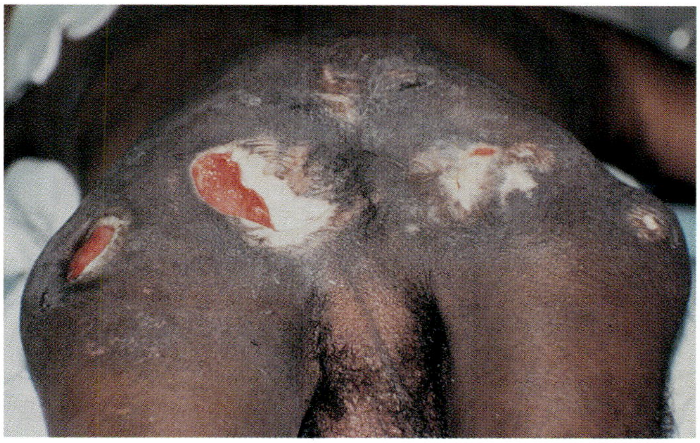

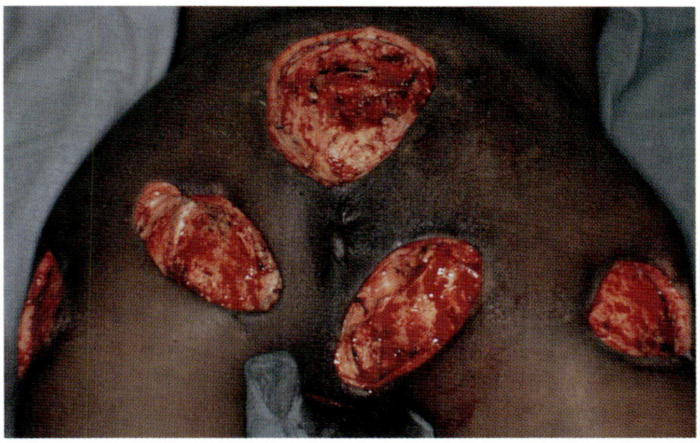

Occasionally desperate situations may arise in these unfortunate patients who have multiple sores that require closure. Preoperative evaluation includes the same examination for each pressure sore as if it were an individual pressure sore to rule out possible factors causing recurrence, osteomyelitis, and sinus tracts. Multiple pressure sores can be treated at one operative setting, which is usually completely performed with the patient in the prone position.

The patient is positioned in a slightly jack-knifed fashion. Inflatable beanbag support is helpful in that it allows support of the thoracic cage and also can be built up under the pelvis to allow exposure of the trochanteric areas and the tensor fascia lata flaps. An alternative method of positioning is the use of thick chest rolls, which again lift the pelvis off the table to allow adequate lateral exposure of the tensor fascia lata regions. The patient is prepared from the midback down to the popliteal fossa and nearly circumferential on each thigh, including all of the perineal region. All existing scars are marked, and an estimation of scarring caused by the elevation of previous flaps is made. A two-team approach is helpful in reducing operative time. Both teams work simultaneously to excise the sores, irrigate the wounds, obtain hemostasis, and develop flap coverage. Donor sites should be designed to avoid any bony prominence, and they should have a good soft tissue base. The surgeon must maintain a high index of suspicion of osteomyelitis because patients in this type of predicament frequently have had a long chronic course with exposed bone for a number of months. Therefore adequate bony debridement is most important. This requires excising down to healthy bleeding bone that is nonsclerotic. In addition, bone biopsy specimens are taken from all excised areas for examination to help to determine the need for postoperative long-term antibiotic therapy, which may be helpful. When the flaps are designed, the goal should be tension-free coverage of all sites with viable flaps while avoiding potential compromise of previously unexposed bony prominences or other pressure points. In addition, it is important to realize that borrowing tissue from one region compromises another region.

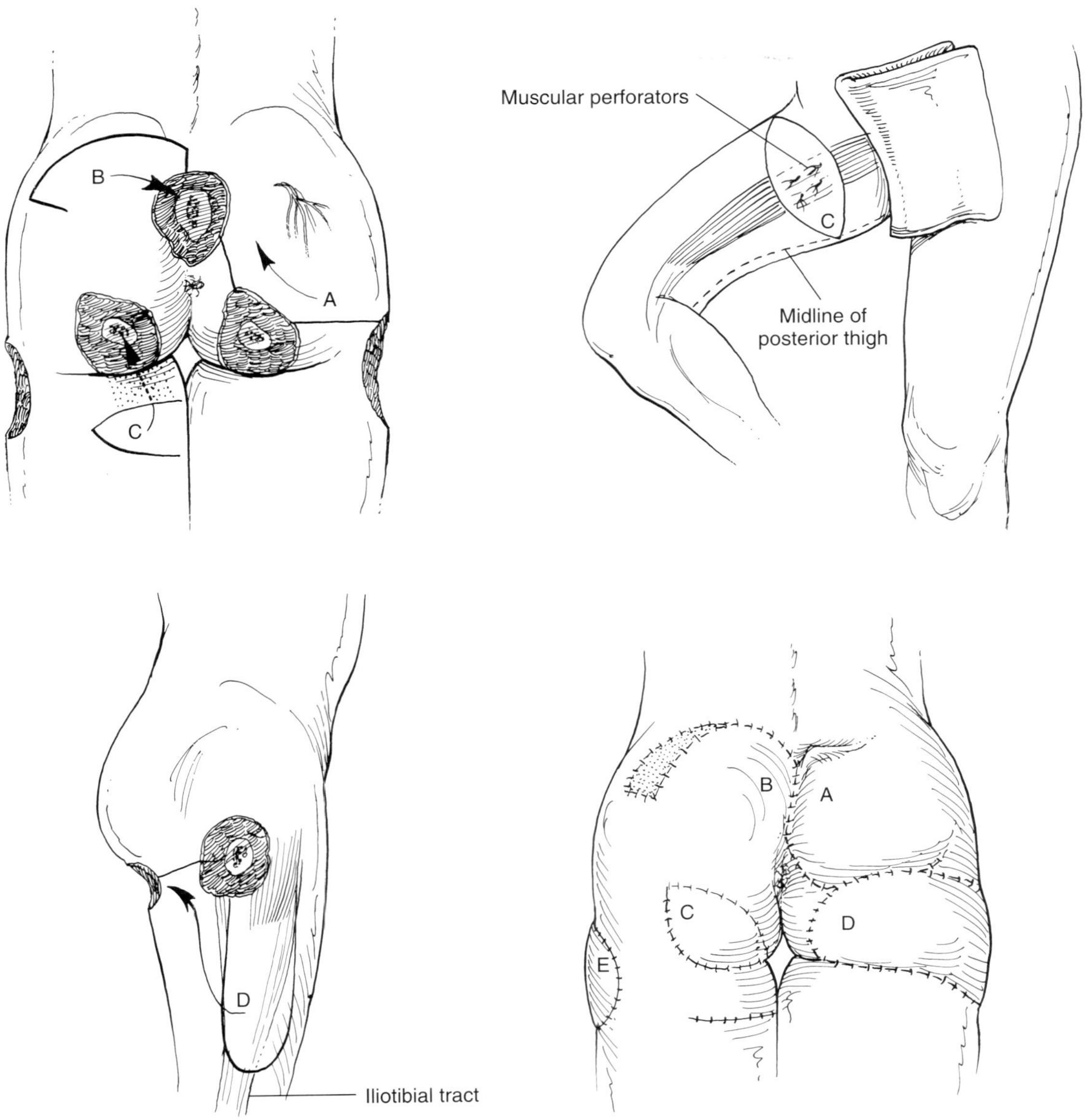

Guidelines used for flap coverage for this patient were as follows: (1) all scars and areas of potential scar resulting from flap elevation were mapped, (2) the extent of undermining of the excised pressure sores was mapped, and (3) the flaps for sacral coverage were designed and elevated first. The supermedial rotation of the gluteus maximus fasciocutaneous flap *(A)* and inferomedial rotation of the gluteus maximus fasciocutaneous flap *(B)* covered the sacrum. The right ischial and trochanteric areas were covered with an extended tensor fascia lata flap *(D)*, which was taken down to two thirds of the lateral thigh. On the left side a tensor fascia lata flap *(E)* was used to cover the trochanteric sore and a transverse gracilis flap *(C)* based on the main pedicle of the gracilis muscle 10 cm below the pubis was designed for the left ischial sore. As each flap was designed, its effect on the tension and donor sites of the other flaps was considered.

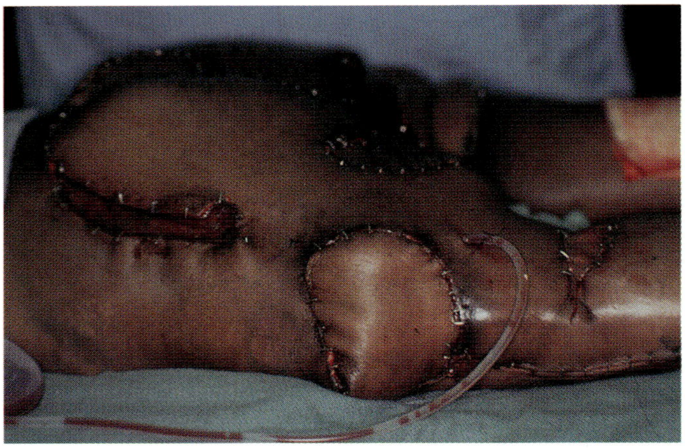

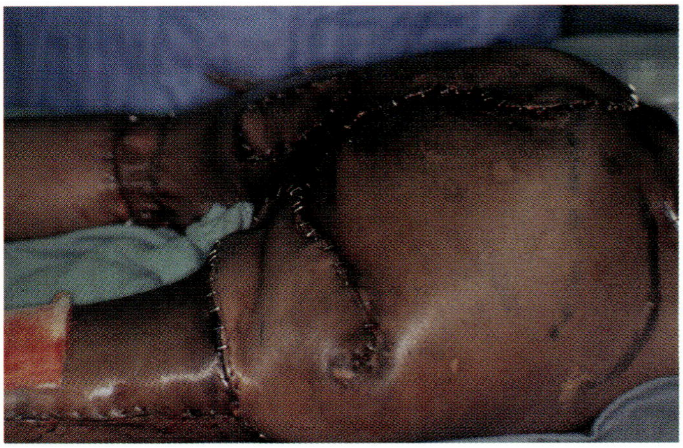

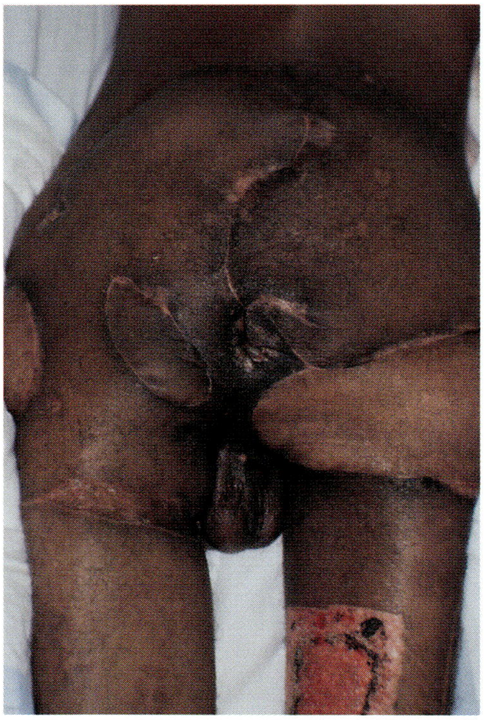

The step-by-step approach provided a tension-free closure of all areas. The patient achieved complete healing of all of these extensive pressure sores without difficulty.

CONCLUSION

Successful reoperative surgery in the pressure sore patient requires evaluation and correction of factors that contribute to reoperative problems. Factors that should be examined are debilitation of the patient, poor nutrition, psychosocial complications, poor wound bed with recalcitrant deep infection, and surrounding damage from previous surgery or pressure injury. Appropriate studies should be performed to evaluate the condition of the underlying bone. A careful plan should be developed to treat reoperative problems. This plan should include analysis of the failure of the first operation, a plan for operative positioning, selection of alternate flaps, and postoperative care. With careful evaluation, correction of contributing factors to reoperative problems, and planning of intraoperative and postoperative care, success can be obtained.

References

1. Ayers DC, Rellegrini VD, Evarts CM. Prevention of heterotopic ossification in high-risk patients by radiation therapy. Clin Orthop Rel Res 263:87-93, 1991.
2. Deloach ED, Check WE, Long R. Diagnosing osteomyelitis underlying pressure sores. Contemp Orthop 27:240-246, 1993.
3. Evans GRD, Lewis VL Jr, Manson PN, et al. Hip joint communication with pressure sore: The refractory wound and the role of Girdlestone arthroplasty. Plast Reconstr Surg 91:288-294, 1993.
4. Hentz UR. Management of pressure sores in a specialty center. Plast Reconstr Surg 64: 683-691, 1979.
5. Kjaersgaard-Andersen P, Schmidt SA. Total hip arthroplasty: The role of anti-inflammatory medication in the prevention of heterotopic ossification. Clin Orthop Rel Res 263:78-86, 1991.
6. Lewis VL Jr, Bailey MH, Pulawski G, et al. The diagnosis of osteomyelitis in patients with pressure sores. Plast Reconstr Surg 81:229-232, 1988.
7. Maruyama Y, Iwahir Y. Popliteo-posterior thigh fasciocutaneous island flap for closure around the knee. Br J Plast Surg 42:140-143, 1989.
8. Mustoe T, Upton J, Marcellino V, et al. Carcinoma in chronic pressure sores: A fulminant disease process. Plast Reconstr Surg 77:116-121, 1986.
9. Ramirez OM, Orlando JC, Hurwitz DJ. The sliding gluteus maximus myocutaneous flap: Its relevance in ambulatory patients. Plast Reconstr Surg 74:68-75, 1984.
10. Relander M, Palmer B. Recurrence of surgically treated pressure sores. Scand J Plast Reconstr Surg 22:89-92, 1988.
11. Stover SL. Heterotopic ossification after spinal cord injuries. In Management of Spinal Cord Injuries. Baltimore: Williams & Wilkins, 1986, pp 284-301.
12. Stover SL, ed. Spinal Cord Injury: The Facts and Figures. Birmingham, Ala.: The University of Alabama at Birmingham, 1986.
13. Tobin GR, Brown GL, Derr JW, et al. V-Y advancement flaps: Reusable flaps for pressure ulcer repair. Clin Plast Surg 17:727-732, 1990.
14. Yamamoto Y, Kunihiko N, Yoshihisa S, et al. Reconstruction of recurrent pressure sores using free flaps. J Reconstr Miscrosurg 8:433-436, 1992.

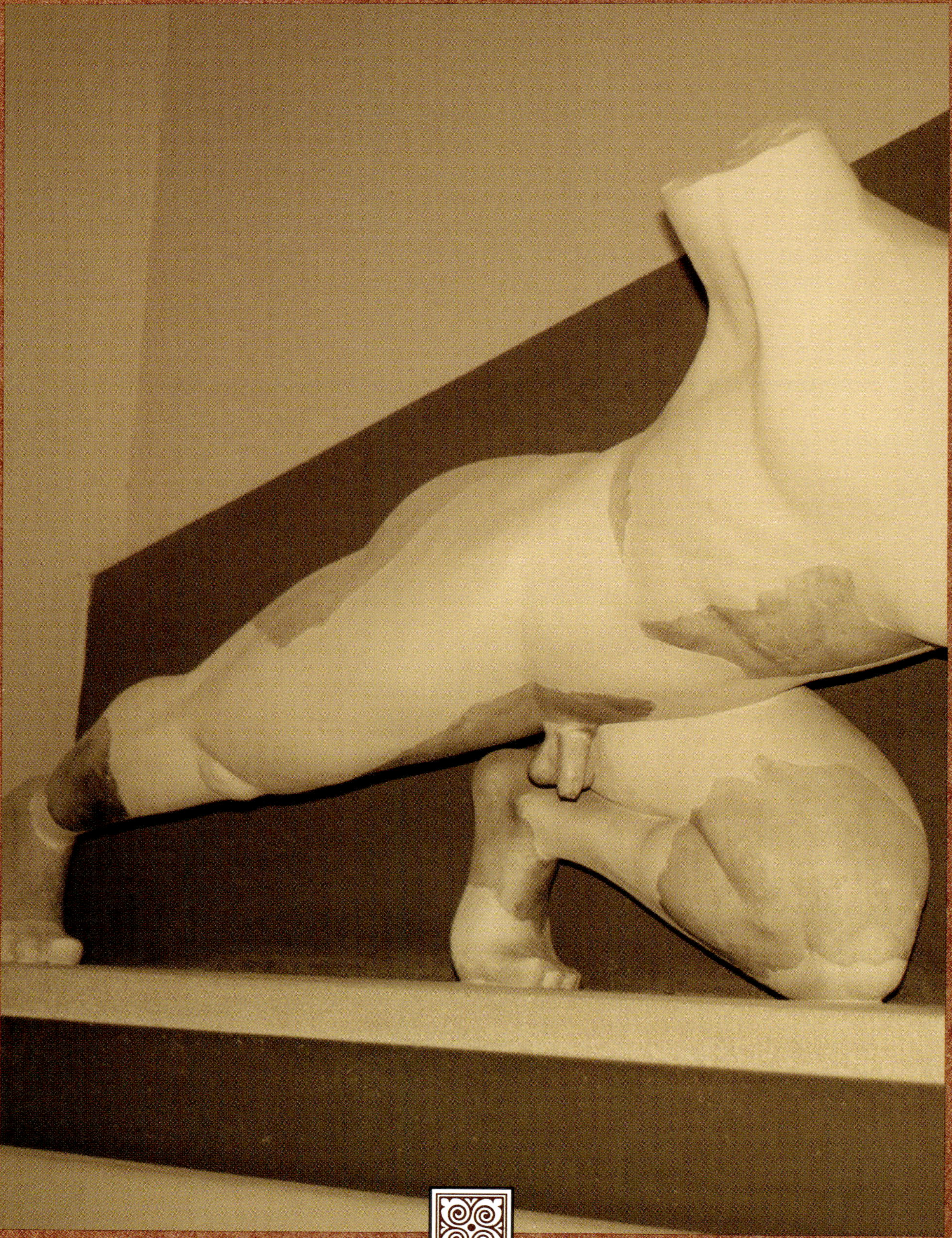

VI

Reoperative Surgery of the Extremities

39

Reoperative Hand Surgery

Victoria R. Masear, M.D.

Reoperative Problems

Dupuytren's fasciitis	Poor range of motion
Recurrent ganglion cysts	Recurrent ulnar drift
Prosthetic failure	Adhesions
Infection	Arthroplasty
Bone resorption	Flexor tendon reconstruction
Unstable fixation	

The nature of hand surgery often makes reoperation necessary, particularly in cases involving joint replacement, partial palmar fasciectomies for Dupuytren's fasciitis, staged tendon reconstructions, and recurrent ganglion cysts. Simply repeating the same procedure probably will not produce optimal results. Certain details need attention during reoperative surgery, not only the technical aspects of the procedure, but also the details related to ultimate function, potential complications, cosmesis, and pain control. ***The most important factor in attaining a good reoperative result is the postoperative supervision by a hand therapist who is familiar with both the procedure and its inherent problems.***

ARTHROPLASTY

Both interpositional and cemented total joint arthroplasties are often used to treat hand deformities caused by rheumatoid arthritis. An interpositional arthroplasty with silicone rubber is commonly used because it is dependable and predictable.[1-3] The Swanson Silastic arthroplasty probably produces the best results.[4] ***Recently, titanium grommets have been added to silicone rubber prostheses to stabilize and protect the bone-prosthesis interface. The grommets also buffer the shear stresses and thus shield the spacer from breakage.***[4,5] No distinct advantage has been seen when Niebauer silicone Dacron mesh is used for ingrowth, although the inherent stability provided by the ingrowth makes collateral ligament reconstruction unnecessary. However, the complications and outcome are similar for the two groups. The Tupper volar plate arthroplasty is an interpositional technique that may also be used as a salvage procedure.[6]

Long-term follow-up after a resection arthroplasty will show eventual resorption and shortening of the metacarpal, which ultimately leads to progressive instability, recurrence of palmar subluxation and ulnar drift, and shortening of the finger.[7] Cemented total joint prostheses provide more inherent stability, but they also carry a greater risk of loosening, prosthetic failure, infection, and stress shielding with resultant bone resorption.

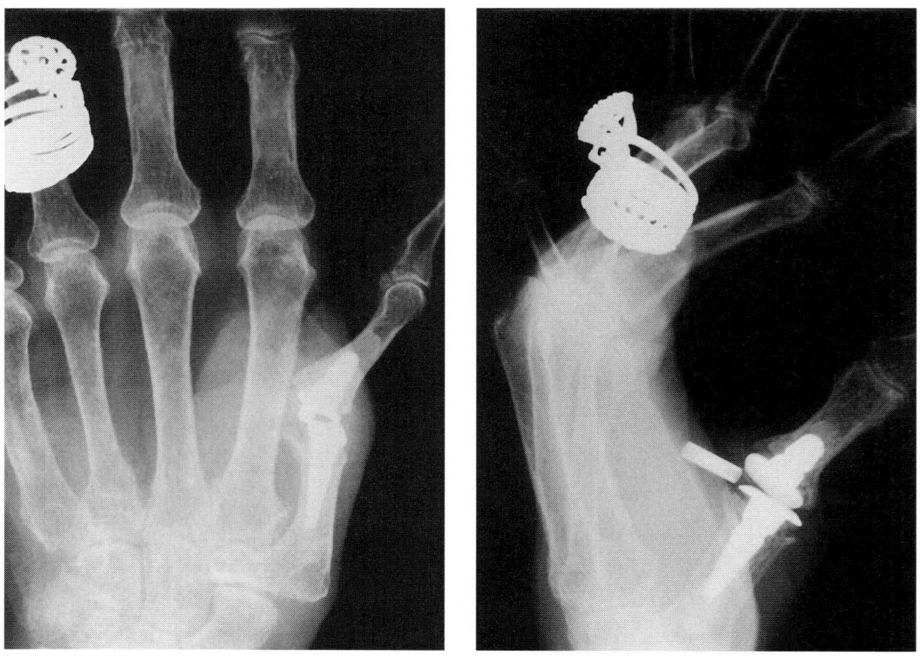

X-ray films of a failed biomeric cemented arthroplasty of the thumb show the broken hinge of the prosthesis and dislocation of the joint.

In a 10.9-year follow-up study, Adams et al.[8] noted a progressive decrease in range of motion and strength with recurrence of ulnar deviation in patients with the Schultz semiconstrained, cemented metacarpophalangeal (MP) joint replacement. The proximal phalanx component fractured at the neck level in 39% of the cases, and 22% showed extensive periarticular heterotopic bone formation.[8] However, there was no evidence of progressive loosening at the cement-bone or prosthesis-cement interface.

Metacarpophalangeal (MP) Joint Arthroplasty

Studies by Vahvanen and Viljakka[9] and by Blair et al.[10] have shown that within 4 years after silicone rubber interpositional arthroplasty patients had range of motion in the MP joint that varied from 34 to 43 degrees (average 40 degrees). Vahvanen and Viljakka[9] found that 27 of 32 patients had significant pain relief following Swanson Silastic replacement arthroplasty in the MP joints, and 28 of the 32 had cosmetic improvement as well. Kleinert and Lister[11] reported that only 50% of the Swanson silicone rubber MP arthroplasties functioned satisfactorily. According to Wilson and Carlblom,[12] the best range of motion (averaging 40 degrees) is attained in the first 2 years after replacement surgery with either a silicone spacer or a silicone Dacron prosthesis.

Most studies showed no significant improvement in grip or pinching strength following replacement arthroplasty, although pain relief and patient satisfaction were high. Derkash et al.[13] found that the Niebauer silicone Dacron mesh prosthesis provides satisfactory pain relief and correction of ulnar drift; however, as with the Swanson silicone rubber prosthesis, the range of motion was poor and both range of motion and stability decreased over time.

Recurrence of subluxation and ulnar drift and subsequent loss of function occur after breakage of the silicone Dacron prosthesis. In contrast, satisfactory function usually remains following fracture of a silicone rubber spacer, since the encapsulating scar tissue provides stability.

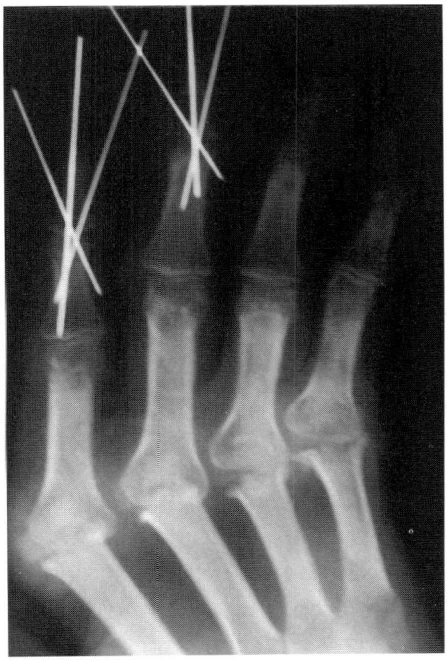

The x-ray film illustrates problems associated with silicone arthroplasty of MP joints, including implant fractures, failure to fully correct or prevent recurrence of ulnar drift, bone resorption, and a gradual loss of range of motion.

The degree of recurrent ulnar deviation following Swanson arthroplasty has been variously reported as ranging from 11% to 43%.[9,10,14,15] Ulnar deviation of a milder degree (less than 10 degrees) occurs even more frequently. Patients with rheumatoid arthritis are particularly susceptible to a gradual ulnar deviation following a Swanson arthroplasty if the wrist is unbalanced with a radial deviation deformity of the carpus and metacarpals in relation to the radius.[16-22]

The rate of fracture of a Swanson Silastic spacer has been reported to range from 1% to 26%.[2,9,10,15,22-24] The rate of fracture increases with the length of time since implantation. Following Swanson arthroplasty, infection and dislocation occur in <1% of cases; however, bone resorption recurs in 24% to 48% of implants and bone production or overgrowth in another 9% to 34%.[9,10] Hyperpronation of the index finger at the level of the MP joint is a rather infrequent complication following Silastic implant arthroplasty. Normally this should be recognized at the time of surgery and can be corrected by attaching the radial collateral ligament more dorsally on the metacarpal, thus providing a supination force. Also, by flexing the proximal interphalangeal (PIP) joint and placing a radial deviation force on the middle phalanx with therapeutic strapping postoperatively, the hyperpronation deformity can be corrected gradually over a period of several weeks.[25]

The Niebauer silicone Dacron mesh prosthesis has problems similar to those of the Swanson arthroplasty. The frequency of recurrence of ulnar drift in the MP joint increases with time with the Niebauer prosthesis. Other causes of prosthesis failure reported by Derkash et al.[13] include palmar subluxation, fracture or buckling of the prosthesis, and bone resorption. Niebauer[26] reports the infection rate at 2% and the rate of subluxation at 1%.The fracture rate of the Niebauer prosthesis has been reported at about 38%.[9,15] With the silicone Dacron prosthesis, fracture of the prosthesis seems to contribute to recurrence of the deformity, especially ulnar deviation. Beckenbaugh et al.[15] found the ulnar deviation recurrence rate for the Niebauer prosthesis to be about 44%, which is comparable to that of the Swanson arthroplasty. In a 30-month follow-up, they reported that the Niebauer prosthesis had a higher mechanical failure rate than the Swanson Silastic prosthesis and thus a higher recurrence of clinical deformity.

Surgical Techniques

Swanson Arthroplasty. A transverse dorsal incision is made over the metacarpal heads. Then the subcutaneous tissues are dissected from the underlying extensor mechanism for 2 cm proximal and distal to the joints to expose the heads of the metacarpals. Each joint is entered through a longitudinal incision in the extensor hood and the ulnar sagittal band is released longitudinally for approximately 3 cm. The ulnarly subluxed central tendon is repositioned on the radial side of the joint, then the tendon is freed from the underlying joint capsule. The capsule is incised longitudinally and the subperiosteal tissue over the metacarpal head on both the radial and the ulnar sides is resected. The metacarpal is transected with a microsagittal saw at the level of the metaphyseal flair. The cut is made perpendicular to the longitudinal axis of the metacarpal, and the metacarpal head is removed. The proximal phalangeal base is flattened by removing osteophytes if the base is cup shaped or has protruding bone edges, but the subchondral bone is left intact. A hole is drilled into the intramedullary canal at the base of the proximal phalanx to allow room for the stem of the prosthesis; a dental burr can be used to remove cancellous bone from the metacarpal shaft. Only the cortical rim of the metacarpal is left unreamed. The largest silicone rubber prosthesis that will fit into the intramedullary canal of the metacarpal when sitting flush with the hinge is selected. If too small a prosthesis is used, it may rotate within the shaft of the metacarpal. After the appropriate size is chosen, the base of the proximal phalanx is reamed to fit the stem of the corresponding trial prosthesis. A cross-section of the prosthesis stem reveals that it is rectangular, so the radial-to-ulnar reaming must be wider than the dorsal-to-palmar. The proximal phalanx must align with the dorsum of its respective metacarpal. If necessary, a No. 69 Beaver blade can be used to circumferentially dissect the subperiosteum around the base of the proximal phalanx until the palmar aspect of the proximal phalangeal base can be stacked onto the dorsum of its respective metacarpal. A .045 Kirschner wire or correspondingly small drill bit is used to drill two holes in the dorsoradial aspect of the distal metacarpal and a 4-0 nonabsorbable suture is placed through this and the proximal edge of the radial collateral ligament, which was detached previously from the head and neck of the metacarpal.

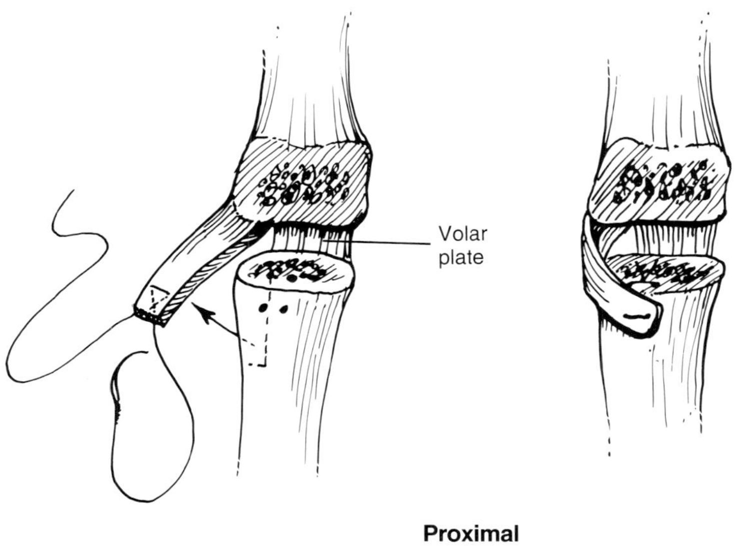

If the radial collateral ligament is unavailable, then the Swanson technique for ligament reconstruction can be employed. The radial one third of the volar plate can be split off longitudinally, leaving it attached to the base of the proximal phalanx, and the proximal end is brought dorsoradially and sutured to the drill holes in the metacarpal.

The wound is irrigated and any excess bone debris is removed. Smooth forceps are used to insert the appropriate-sized Swanson prosthesis; care should be taken to avoid making any cuts or tears in the prosthesis since this can increase the risk of particulate silicone and thus cause synovitis. After the prosthesis is inserted, the MP joint is held in extension, radial deviation, and supination while tying the sutures through the dorsoradial metacarpal and radial collateral ligaments. After soft-tissue release and insertion of the prosthesis, the extensor tendons usually become centralized and further reconstruction becomes unnecessary. The joint should be checked for alignment and range of motion. The radial sagittal bands should be imbricated if the tendons are still subluxed ulnarward when the MP joint is flexed. The skin is closed with 4-0 nylon sutures. A plaster splint is applied with the wrist in neutral position and the MP joints in full extension.

Revision Arthroplasty. The approach for revision MP arthroplasty is the same as that used for the primary procedure, except that the prosthesis is usually fractured. All fragments must be carefully searched for and removed. Dental burrs can be used to remove the pseudocapsular lining present in the intramedullary canal. If the metacarpal head has eroded and there is more bone missing on the ulnar side, the bone should be shortened slightly to get a cut perpendicular to the metacarpal shaft. The base of the proximal phalanx may need to be revised to get a smooth transverse surface, and again the proximal phalanx must be capable of being stacked onto the dorsum of its metacarpal. The same technique used in primary arthroplasty can be employed to seat the prosthesis and repair or reconstruct the radial collateral ligament.

Recurrent ulnar drift usually present at the time of revision MP arthroplasty can be repaired with a crossed intrinsic transfer procedure. On the ulnar side of the little finger the abductor digiti quinti tendon is released from its insertion on the base of the proximal phalanx and the tendon is reinserted more palmarward to give more power to MP flexion of the little finger. Other repair options include Z-plasty to lengthen the tendon and tenotomy. The ulnar-sided intrinsic muscles on the index through ring fingers are released from their insertions into the extensor hood and repositioned on the radial side of their adjacent digits. Nonabsorbable 4-0 monofilament suture is used to attach the intrinsic muscles to the bases of the proximal phalanges. The insertion is made over the original attachment of the radial collateral ligament to the base of the proximal phalanx. These are dynamic transfers and therefore under anesthesia the MP joints may still show some tendency toward ulnar deviation. However, if adequate soft tissue releases and perpendicular bone cuts have been made, when the patient awakens the intrinsic transfers will dynamically correct the tendency toward ulnar deviation. Again, the radial sagittal band is imbricated only if the extensor tendon is still subluxed ulnarward following a soft tissue correction and replacement of the implants. The closure and splinting are the same as that for primary arthroplasty.

The titanium grommets added to the Swanson silicone rubber protheses stabilize and protect the bone-prosthesis interface and thus diminish bone resorption. These prostheses are press fit devices and have a corresponding presized reamer used to prepare the canal. After reaming, choose the prosthesis size that is the same size as the reamer or one size smaller. If too large a prosthesis is inserted, it will not sit flush with the bone and rotation or pistoning of the prosthesis will occur. ***Since progressive bone resorption is a major problem with revision arthroplasty, it is probably advisable to use the grommets for revision arthroplasty.***

Postoperative Care

The bulky dressing is removed and a light dressing is applied 1 to 2 days following MP arthroplasty. If there is swelling in the fingers, Coban wraps can be applied to control the edema. A dorsal splint is fabricated with the wrist in zero or up to 20 degrees of dorsiflexion.

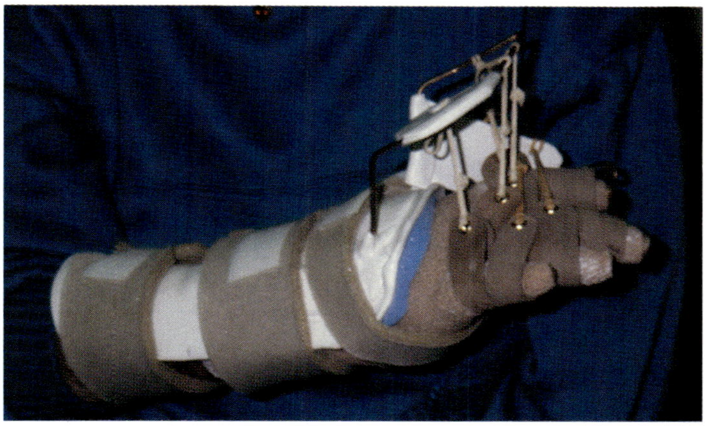

A dynamic outrigger attachment is made with elastic loops around the proximal phalanges to pull the MP joints into extension and slight radial deviation. This splint is worn at all times. The tension should be set so as to allow up to 60 to 70 degrees of active flexion. If pronation of the index or long finger is needed, a force couple can be added for those digits. The patient should actively flex the MP joints ten times each hour during the day. If PIP flexion is being substituted for MP flexion, then static PIP splints can be applied during exercise periods. The patient should be seen by the therapist one to two times weekly. If the patient has not achieved at least 45 degrees of active flexion within 3 weeks after surgery, then dynamic flexion is begun and alternated with dynamic extension during the daytime. At night the patient must continue sleeping in the dynamic outrigger for extension. Dynamic extension splinting may be needed during the day for up to 6 weeks after surgery. At that point splinting is changed to nighttime only and light active motion is allowed during the day. Continued use of the dynamic outrigger for MP extension and radial deviation at night on an indefinite basis seems to help prevent recurrence of ulnar deviation and flexion contractures at the MP joint.

Complications

The most common complication following MP arthroplasty is recurrent ulnar drift, which can be minimized in the following ways:

1. Fully release the contracted synovial capsule.
2. Make the bone cuts perpendicular to the shaft so that the titanium grommets will fit flush with the cortical rim of bone. To ensure that the metacarpal osteotomies are perpendicular to the shaft, it is best to err by taking off more bone on the radial side rather than the ulnar.[14]
3. Perform soft tissue reconstruction, especially of the radial collateral ligament.
4. Imbricate the radial sagittal band if the central tendon does not become centralized following soft tissue releases and insertion of the prosthesis. If the central tendon still tends to sublux ulnarward, ulnar drift will be accentuated.
5. Perform intrinsic muscle transfers with attachment into the adjacent digit's radial collateral insertion on the base of the proximal phalanx.
6. If the wrist is in radial deviation, stabilize it with either a tendon transfer, a joint replacement, or by arthrodesis; otherwise, a return to ulnar deviation is inevitable.

Another major complication involves insufficient release of soft tissue contractures around the base of the proximal phalanx. If the proximal phalanx cannot be stacked onto the dorsum of its respective metacarpal, then the patient will not be able to fully extend at the MP joint. Fracture of the prosthesis is also a major problem in MP arthroplasty. With the introduction of the high-performance silicone elastomer, the time to fracture has been prolonged.[11,14] Also, the rate of prosthesis fracture can be decreased by avoiding sharp edges of bone or osteophytes abutting on the prosthesis and by correcting any angular deforming forces.[14] Bone resorption is also a problem, especially in revision MP arthroplasty. The addition of titanium grommets to the silicone rubber prosthesis is probably the best method available for avoiding this complication.[4]

Proximal Interphalangeal (PIP) Joint Arthroplasty

Arthrodesis is often the procedure of choice for treating arthritis involving the PIP joint, since it provides more stability for pinch in the index finger and helps ■ facilitate motion in the MP joints following arthroplasty. ***When multiple joints of a finger have arthritic changes, arthrodesis of the PIP joint may be more advantageous than arthroplasty.*** However, when more motion is needed, such as in the more ulnar digits for gripping, then arthroplasty would be recommended.

There are several types of PIP arthroplasties, including resection, silicone interposition, and total joint replacement. Resection arthroplasty is rarely performed because it often results in instability and poor motion. Total joint replacement arthroplasty has a high rate of loosening, periosteal bone formation, recurrence of deformity, and prosthetic fracture even in the early follow-up period.[4] The Swanson silicone elastomer arthroplasty is the most commonly used procedure to treat the painful degenerative or post-traumatic PIP joint. Because of the high incidence of recurrent deformity and bone resorption, PIP arthroplasty is rarely used for multiple joint or digit involvement as in rheumatoid arthritis.

Surgical Technique

A straight longitudinal incision is made over the dorsum of the PIP joint and the subcutaneous tissues are reflected to reveal the underlying extensor mechanism. The extensor mechanism is split longitudinally over the proximal phalanx, beginning at midshaft and extending to the base of the middle phalanx at the central slip insertion. Usually the central slip attachment can be preserved to the base of the middle phalanx, but if it is disrupted or needs to be detached to provide adequate exposure, the central slip attachment can be reinserted later through drill holes in the base of the middle phalanx. After the neck of the proximal phalanx is transected with a microsagittal saw, the head of the phalanx is removed. The collateral ligaments should be preserved, but if they are detached, they can be reinserted through drill holes in the bone after the prosthesis has been inserted. The middle phalanx base is flattened and any spurs are removed. The intramedullary canal of the proximal phalanx is reamed with a dental burr to clear it of all cancellous bone, and the appropriate-sized silicone rubber implant is chosen. A hole is drilled in the base of the middle phalanx into the intramedullary canal. The canal is reamed to fit the trial silicone rubber implant. Excess bone debris is removed and the wound is irrigated. Smooth forceps are used to insert the silicone rubber prosthesis to avoid tearing or puncturing the prosthesis. The collateral ligaments can then be repaired or they can be imbricated with a 4-0 dermalon suture if the joint tends to drift into ulnar deviation following insertion of the prosthesis.

Postoperatively the wrist is held in neutral position, the MP joints are placed in about 60 degrees of flexion, and the PIP joints are placed in about 30 degrees of flexion. If boutonniere deformity exists concurrently, the lateral bands will contract palmarward and the central slip is often stretched. The transverse retinacular ligaments should be released on the palmar side of the lateral bands so the lateral bands can be mobilized dorsally. The central slip is cut transversely just proximal to the level of the PIP joint. The joint is then exposed as described earlier. After the prosthesis is inserted and the collateral ligament is repaired, the central slip is either advanced distally through drill holes in the base of the middle phalanx and brought out through a pull-out button on the palmar surface, or the tendon is repaired in a vest-over-pants fashion with a nonabsorbable monofilament suture. The lateral bands, which have already been released from palmarward, are flipped over the dorsum of the finger and the original palmar edge of the lateral band from one side is attached to the palmar edge from the opposite side with a nonabsorbable suture. Thus, the lateral bands will now act as an extension force at the PIP joint.[27]

Swan-Neck Deformity. In patients with swan-neck deformity, the dorsal skin may be tight and prevent postoperative flexion. In this case, a gentle curvilinear incision will often suffice to relax the skin.

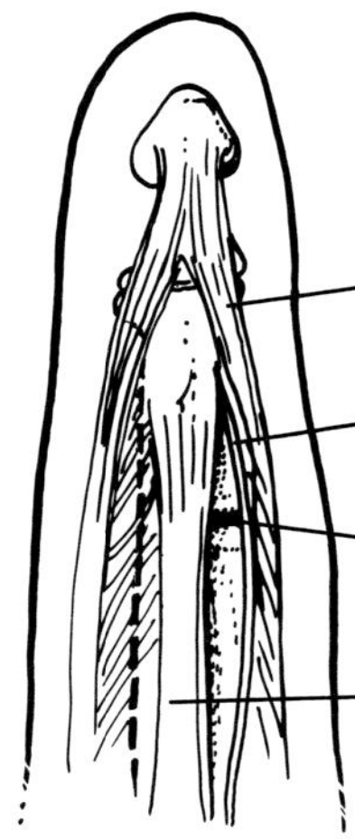

Another option would be Z-plasty of the dorsal skin. The lateral bands are mobilized from the central slip by releasing the triangular ligament over the dorsum of the base of the proximal phalanx and incising between the lateral bands and central slip on each side of the finger. The central slip is then lengthened with a Z incision in the approach to the PIP joint. After the prosthesis has been inserted and the collateral ligaments have been repaired, the central slip is snugly reattached with a 4-0 dermalon suture with the joint in 20 degrees of flexion. Following repair, the joint should be able to be brought to 90 degrees of flexion without pulling out the tendon sutures.

A flexor check must be performed with all PIP arthroplasties on patients with swan-neck deformity. An incision is made over the distal forearm and the sublimis and profundus tendons to the corresponding finger are isolated. Traction on these tendons at the level of the distal forearm should produce full flexion at the PIP joint after the prosthesis has been inserted. If not, flexor tendon adhesions are probably present and a tenolysis must accompany the procedure.[4,28] If bone resorption is a problem in the PIP joint with either severe rheumatoid arthritis or revision arthroplasty, the silicone rubber implants incorporated with titanium grommets may help prevent further resorption. However, the grommets are not made for the smaller size implants that are often needed at the PIP level.

Postoperative Care

The bulky dressing and plaster splint are removed 1 or 2 days after surgery; lighter dressings are applied to the incisional area and Coban wraps are applied to the fingers to control edema. Dorsal static splints are applied with the PIP joints in 20 to 30 degrees of flexion. For a patient with swan-neck deformity, 30 degrees of flexion is preferred, and for a patient with boutonniere deformity, 20 degrees of flexion is recommended. The splints are released distally to allow active flexion beyond that point. The patient should perform ten active flexions per hour during the day, and at night, the static splints are left in place.

Passive flexion is permitted after PIP arthroplasty that did not require a take-down or repair of the extensor mechanism. However, if the extensor tendon was lengthened or shortened, if the lateral bands were mobilized dorsally, or if the tendon had to be taken down for the approach and reattached later, passive flexion is not allowed until 6 weeks after surgery. If extensor tendon lengthening or reconstruction was not performed, dynamic flexion can be allowed 3 weeks after surgery, if needed. The extension block splints are worn continuously for 6 weeks after surgery, then they can be removed during the day and light activities of daily living allowed. Static splints in 20 or 30 degrees of flexion are continued at night until 3 months after surgery.

Complications

At 1 year postoperatively, 60 degrees of flexion can be expected following PIP arthroplasty, with a range of motion between 20 to 80 degrees or 30 to 90 degrees.[11] This range of motion will gradually diminish over the years following replacement.

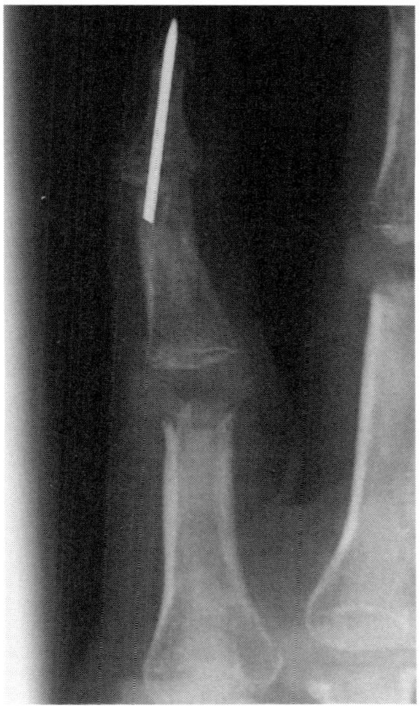

The x-ray film shows the most common problem with PIP arthroplasty, lateral instability, which is usually moderate. The lateral instability combines with settling of the prosthesis as a result of bone resorption and a gradual loss of motion.[11]

Recurrence of PIP hyperextension following arthroplasty is commonly seen in patients with swan-neck deformity,[23,29] but PIP hyperextension can also occur as a result of laxity of the volar plate, intrinsic muscle tightness, and adhesions of the flexor tendons. After the prosthesis has been inserted, an intrinsic tightness test must be performed before the incision is closed. If the intrinsic muscles are tight, a release procedure should be performed with the arthroplasty. If the joint still has a tendency to hyperextend, a sublimis tenodesis can be performed at the same time.

Pelligrini and Burton[30] reported that 35% of silicone rubber PIP arthroplasties had periarticular erosions within 2 years of surgery. Within 4 years of replacement arthroplasty extensive endosteal resorption was seen in 20% of cases.

Distal Interphalangeal (DIP) Joint Arthroplasty

Silicone rubber arthroplasty has been used occasionally in the DIP joint for patients who wish to maintain motion. Since the stability of the prosthesis depends on the collateral ligaments,[31] results have been better in patients with osteoarthritis than in patients with rheumatoid arthritis. The extensor lag normally measures about 13 degrees with 33 degrees of active motion, and the arc of motion is therefore from 13 degrees to 46 degrees of flexion.[31,32] Osteoarthritis patients with motion within this range usually have a stable result. However, arthrodesis would be the procedure of choice for DIP joint repair in patients with rheumatoid arthritis, who commonly have incompetent collateral ligaments, and in cases where DIP arthroplasties have already failed. Failure usually results from instability secondary to either incompetent collateral ligaments, fracture of the prosthesis, or bone resorption. Infection is rarely a cause for revision.

Thumb Arthroplasty Revision

Revision arthroplasties are rarely needed for the carpometacarpal (CMC) joint. Arthroplasties that have failed in either the MP or IP joints of the thumb probably should be converted to an arthrodesis. Even if both the MP and IP joints are fused, the patient will have a stronger and more stable pinch than with joint replacements. The substantial radial deviation stresses to the thumb during pinch can cause silicone rubber arthroplasties to progressively deviate with ulnar ligamentous instability and can cause cemented arthroplasties to loosen and the prosthesis to fracture. Revision arthroplasty causes progressively more bone stock to be lost. Therefore, even with failed cemented prostheses, conversion to an arthrodesis is the optimal choice.

PARTIAL PALMAR FASCIECTOMIES FOR DUPUYTREN'S FASCIITIS

The recurrence of cords and contractures of the fingers are significant problems following partial palmar fasciectomy for Dupuytren's fasciitis. ***Probably the most frequently cited reason for recurrence is inadequate or incomplete removal of all diseased tissue at the primary operation.***[33,34] The rate of recurrence ranges from 28% to 70%,[35-38] although only about 10% of patients require additional surgery after a partial palmar fasciectomy.[39] Recurrent contracture is much more common in the finger than in the palm,[31,33] and is much more likely to involve the PIP than the MP joint.

The most significant factors increasing the risk for recurrence of contracture include the following: a strong family history of Dupuytren's fasciitis, early age of onset (<40 years), fibromatosis of the feet or penis, knuckle pads, bilateral involvement of the hands, and a previous recurrence.[33,34,39,40] McFarlane[41] noted that when all of these factors were present, the recurrence or extension rate was 78%, but when all four of these factors were absent, the recurrence rate was only 17%.

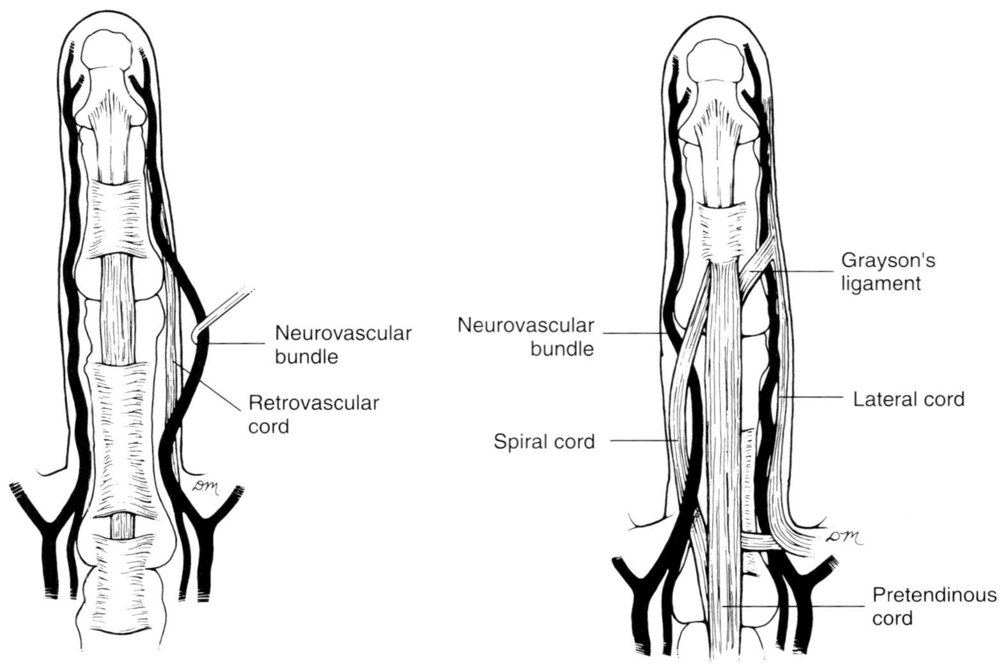

Primary PIP contracture can be caused by four types of Dupuytren's cords: central (pretendinous), spiral, lateral, and retrovascular.[42] The retrovascular cord is a longitudinally oriented fascia that lies dorsal to the neurovascular bundle.[43] The most frequent cause of recurrent contracture is probably a retrovascular cord that was not adequately excised.

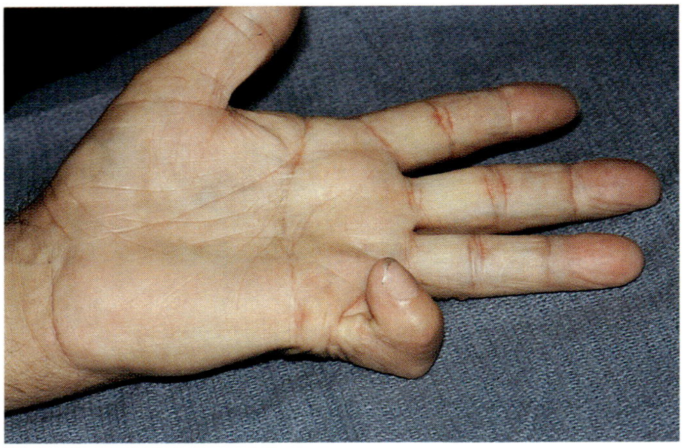

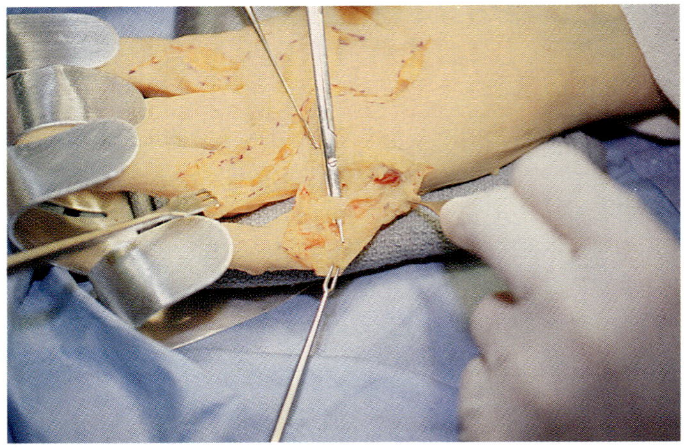

This patient has a PIP contracture secondary to a Dupuytren's cord on the ulnar side of the little finger. The intraoperative view shows a cord on the ulnar side of the finger originating from the abductor digiti quinti muscle fascia and tendon. Failure to remove a lateral or spiral cord is the most common reason for persistent or recurrent contracture involving the little finger at the MP or PIP joint. ■ ***Any operation involving the little finger should include a search for possible Dupuytren's cords.*** The least common cause of recurrent contracture involves the central cords, which usually cause MP contracture.

There are numerous reports documenting the predictability of recurrence on the basis of microscopic examination of the diseased fascia excised at the primary surgery. Rudolph and Van de Berg[44] noted an increased likelihood of recurrence when prominent myofibroblast and intracellular microtubules are found. Gelberman et al.[45] reported a correlation between clinical recurrence and electron microscopic findings of myofibroblasts in the nodules.

Rombouts et al.[39] described the following three types of Dupuytren's fasciitis: the proliferative type, which is the most active and has a 70% recurrence rate; the fibrocellular type, which has a 41% recurrence rate; and the fibrotic type, which is the least active and has an 18% recurrence rate. To reduce the rate of recurrence for high-risk patients, a more aggressive approach has been developed to excise the diseased fascia at the time of the initial surgery.[35,44,45] Hueston[46,47] advocates a dermofasciectomy (excision of both the involved fascia and the overlying skin) followed by a full-thickness skin graft because of the high recurrence rate over the PIP joint.[35,48] Tonkin et al.[36] found that recurrence almost never occurs deep to a full-thickness skin graft, although this is most likely a result of the preparation of the bed, which involves excision of the overlying skin, rather than the application of the full-thickness skin graft. They described a 33% rate of extension of the disease outside primary grafts and a 42% rate of extension outside secondary grafts. Ketchum and Hixson[49] reported that when a wider area of skin is excised and skin grafts are applied, the extension rate has been as low as 10%.

Patient Evaluation

The preoperative evaluation of a patient with recurrent Dupuytren's fasciitis should be thorough. Precise measurements must be made of the contractures involving each joint so that the postoperative rehabilitation and therapy can be tailored to the individual case. The condition of the skin overlying the diseased fascia must be carefully evaluated. Skin that is deeply pitted, extremely thin, or densely adherent to underlying cords is probably best excised. The patient should be involved in the planning and discussion before surgery concerning full-thickness skin grafting of areas where a dermofasciectomy will be performed. All cords and nodules should be documented preoperatively to give the surgeon an idea of what to expect at the time of surgery and to give a preview of the status of the neurovascular bundles. A preoperative check of both sensation and circulation to the involved finger will help determine any prior neurovascular damage. A digital Allen test should be performed on every finger with palpable cords or contracture to detect displacement of the neurovascular bundle. Almost always when there is a delay in filling of the finger on a digital Allen test, a spiral cord will be found displacing the neurovascular bundle superficially and toward the midline of the finger at the level of the proximal finger crease.

Parker[50] has described Dupuytren's nodule over the A1 pulley as a cause of triggering in the finger. However, triggering usually results from adherence and contracture of the nodule over the A1 pulley, causing the pulley itself to become contracted. Another nodule may develop secondarily in the underlying flexor tendon. Release of the A1 pulley is not always a reliable repair. The A1 pulley may thicken and scar following incision, thus causing the triggering to recur. It is best to routinely excise the A1 pulley when the patient has triggering in the fingers secondary to a Dupuytren's nodule or cord overlying the A1 pulley.

Surgical Technique

Because of the notoriously high rates of flare reactions or reflex sympathetic dystrophy following partial palmar fasciectomy for Dupuytren's contracture, it is best to follow a rigid perioperative protocol to reduce the risk of these problems.

1. Before surgery all patients should be given a long-acting supraclavicular or axillary anesthetic block for pain control and sympathetic blockade. These blocks usually keep the patient pain free for 12 to 18 hours after surgery.
2. While the anesthetic block is still in effect, early motion is begun to the involved hand; continuous passive motion is preferred.
3. All patients are kept overnight and monitored closely; the patient should still be comfortable on the following day before discharge.

With this protocol, we have not had a single flare reaction or reflex sympathetic dystrophy in more than 100 patients.

Following the administration of the long-acting anesthetic block, the patient's involved upper extremity is placed on an arm table. After exsanguination a pneumatic tourniquet is inflated on the proximal arm. The type of skin incision chosen will be determined by several factors. When multiple pretendinous nodules are involved, a transverse incision through the distal palmar crease is preferred. For either MP or PIP contractures of 30 degrees or less, a Bruner zigzag incision is normally used on the fingers. This can be extended into the palm when dealing with a single finger.

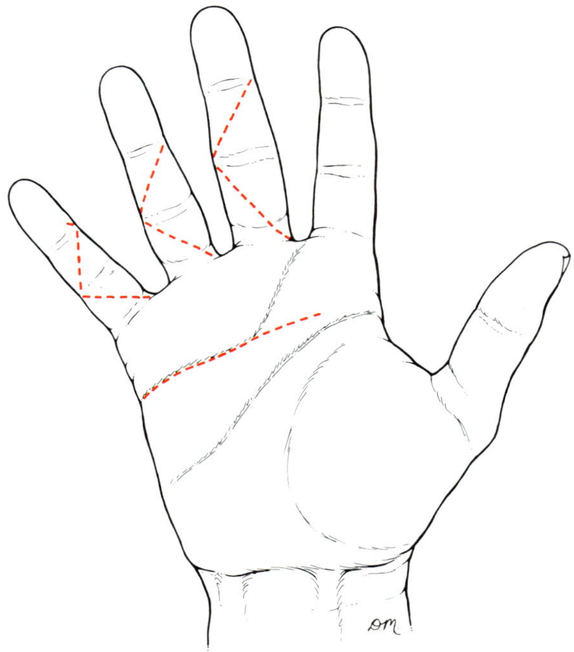

If multiple pretendinous nodules are involved in the palm, a transverse incision is made through the distal palmar crease, leaving a skin bridge between there and the proximal finger crease, and the Bruner zigzag incision is begun at the level of the proximal finger crease and extended distally. If MP or PIP contractures are 30 degrees or more, a longitudinal incision is made over the palmar aspect of the midline of the finger and extended into the palm. The longitudinal incision is converted into multiple small Z-plasties at the time of wound closure. Skin overlying the diseased fascia that is markedly thinned, deeply pitted, or densely adherent to the underlying nodules or cords should be excised and a full-thickness skin graft should be applied after the diseased fascia has been resected. ***If there is any question about whether or not to excise skin on a repeat operation in the same area for Dupuytren's fasciitis, it is safer to proceed with the excision;*** in fact, many surgeons advocate routine excision of the skin in surgery for recurrent disease in an effort to prevent further recurrence.

Controversy still exists as to the appropriate amount of fascia to remove during fasciectomy for Dupuytren's fasciitis. A simple fasciotomy carries a higher rate of recurrence, but more radical fasciectomies incur an increased rate of complications, including hematoma, skin slough, and flare reactions.[39] Hueston[33,48] advocates a dermofasciectomy for any recurrent disease. He then applies a full-thickness skin graft to the remaining defect following excision of all clinically involved fascia.

Next the neurovascular bundles are identified in the midpalmar region and are traced the full extent of the skin incision onto the involved fingers. Unless the exact location of the neurovascular bundles is known before the diseased fascia is excised, there is an excellent chance that the artery or nerve will be damaged during the excision of the involved cords. The neurovascular bundles are most susceptible to injury at the level of proximal finger crease, where the spiral cord tends to pull the neurovascular bundle superficially and toward the midline of the digit.

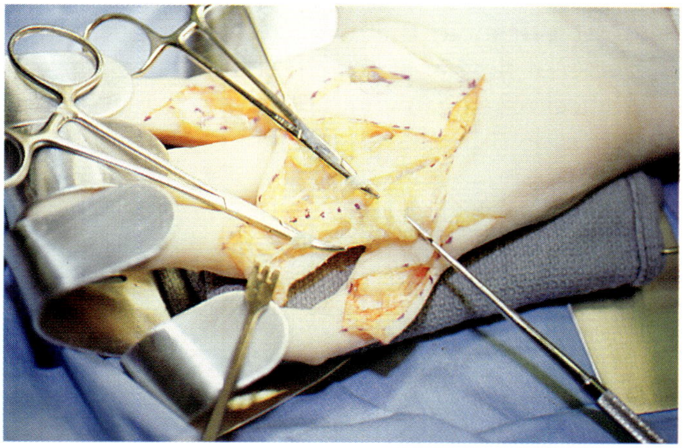

This intraoperative view shows a very tight spiral cord pulling a neurovascular bundle from one side of the digit all the way to the other side, causing it to lie over the opposite neurovascular bundle. After the neurovascular bundles have been identified throughout the length of the wound and are safely out of the way, the diseased fascia can be resected. The pretendinous cord is usually approached first since once this is released the MP and often PIP joints will extend further and the remainder of the dissection is easier. The underlying tendon sheath and fibro-osseous tunnel should be carefully avoided; if either of these are interrupted, the chances for flexor tendon adhesions become much greater. After the pretendinous cord has been excised, the retrovascular cords, spiral cords, and lateral cords can be resected.

■ ***A cord is often present in the thumb-index web when a recurrent contracture has developed elsewhere. Even if it is not yet causing a contracture of the thumb web, it is wise to remove it while operating elsewhere on that hand to prevent future contracture.*** Another area of involvement commonly seen with recurrent disease is the lateral or spiral cord originating from the tendon of the abductor digiti quinti, proceeding along the ulnar border of the little finger proximal phalanx, and usually inserting beyond the PIP joint.

If the PIP contracture is not corrected by excision of central, spiral, retrovascular, and lateral cords, it may be beneficial to make a transverse incision of the fibrous tendon sheath between the A2 and A4 pulleys. If this does not fully correct a preoperative contracture of 30 degrees or less at the PIP joint, Watson et al.[51] noted that it may be necessary to release the checkrein ligaments. Checkrein ligaments develop in long-standing flexion contractures of the PIP joint and are abnormally thick collagenous bands that extend from the proximal edge of the palmar plate to the proximal phalanx on one or both sides of the palmar plate.[51] If contracture is still present after checkrein release, Curtis[52] reported that excising the juncture between the palmar plate and accessory collateral ligament can provide further extension. Dissecting the palmar plate or opening the joint can increase stiffness in the PIP joint, thereby accentuating flexion contracture and sometimes causing loss of flexion at the PIP joint. However, since the fibrous tendon sheath and checkrein ligaments are extraarticular structures, releasing them at the level of the joint should not increase joint stiffness.

Contractures >30 degrees at the level of the PIP joint normally are not improved by fasciectomy or release of contracting structures; therefore osteotomy of the proximal phalanx, arthrodesis of the PIP joint, or joint replacement is recommended for the PIP joint contracted >40 degrees.[37,41,53-56] McFarlane[37] believes that amputation through the PIP or MP joint may be the best choice for a finger with a fixed PIP joint contracture >40 degrees or neurovascular damage after multiple operations or in the extremely debilitated elderly patient with skin maceration and hygiene problems.

Occasionally a boutonniere contracture may develop secondary to a long-standing PIP flexion contracture. Contracture that persists after removal of the cords may be attributed to a tight oblique retinacular ligament of Landsmeer, which passes palmar to the axis of the PIP joint and dorsal to the DIP joint. If the lateral bands are tight and displaced palmarward (leading to PIP flexion contracture and DIP hyperextension), the oblique retinacular ligament must either be stretched or surgically freed by transecting the transverse retinacular ligaments and allowing the lateral bands to mobilize dorsally. In cases of long-standing boutonniere deformity a Fowler tenotomy may be necessary to enable the patient to regain DIP flexion.

Microscopic visualization should be used to repair any inadvertent damage to a digital nerve or artery. Even an elderly patient with little chance of recovery of sensibility after digital surgery can benefit from nerve repair since it may prevent the development of a painful neuroma. Even if a finger has adequate circulation following interruption of one digital artery, it is important to repair the injured artery. Vascularity is already compromised to much of the skin overlying the diseased fascia and the large dissection can further compromise circulation. Repair of the digital arteries may help prevent this problem from being accentuated. The protocol for minimizing vascular trauma during fascial dissection is summarized as follows:

1. Use the bipolar cautery to maintain meticulous hemostasis.
2. Use at least 3.5× loupe magnification.
3. Coagulate all small vessels before transection.
4. Sharply dissect the dermis from underlying diseased fascia with a No. 15 knife blade; change the blade frequently to facilitate sharp dissection.

After the diseased fascia has been resected, the wound is thoroughly inspected for any small vessels that may have been transected without being cauterized. When satisfactory hemostasis is achieved, the wound can be closed or grafted with a defatted full-thickness skin graft and any necessary Z-plasties can be made. ***To minimize the risk of hematoma, the tourniquet is not deflated until after the wound is closed and a compression dressing is applied.*** Normally one 4×4 sterile gauze bandage is folded into thirds and applied over the palmar surface of each involved finger and each involved incision on the palm. A Kling bandage is wrapped around the involved fingers and palm and up above the wrist and is taped into place. Two folded ABDs are placed on the palm and two on the dorsum of the hand and the hand is wrapped snugly with a compression dressing while holding the fingers in extension. The tourniquet is then deflated.

Postoperative Care

By the time the patient arrives in the recovery room, enough time will have passed for adequate hemostasis to occur and the hand therapist can remove the compression dressing and ABDs. The Kling bandage is left in place and a wrist splint with an attached continuous passive motion unit is applied. Continuous passive motion is continued for as long as the anesthetic block is effective. Once the block wears off, the patient should begin active flexion and extension exercises of the digits. The patient should stay overnight in the hospital and if comfortable the following day can be discharged home with the continuous passive motion unit.

The continuous passive motion unit is worn at night while the patient is sleeping, and during the day the patient should perform active flexion and extension exercises. The hand therapist should check the patient's range of motion twice in the first week and give any necessary reinstruction in exercises. One week after surgery the patient should return to see the surgeon. At this time the nighttime continuous passive motion can be discontinued. If full passive extension is achieved, the patient is placed in a static splint at night holding the fingers in extension. If full passive extension cannot be obtained, then the patient is placed in a dynamic outrigger at night. During the day, the patient should continue active flexion and extension exercises. If passive extension equal to that attained on the operating room table is not gained within 2 weeks postoperatively, the patient must wear the dynamic outrigger every other hour during the day and use the alternate hours for active exercises. The patient should continue sleeping in the dynamic outrigger at night.

One week after the sutures are removed the patient can begin a regimen to aid in scar maturation and softening, including massaging the scar with vitamin E or cocoa butter lotion for 3 to 4 minutes three to four times daily and use of an elastomer mold fitted under the dynamic or static extension splint worn at night. The static night splint can usually be discontinued 4 weeks postoperatively, but the patient should continue to use the elastomer mold at night with a Coban wrap for 3 months after surgery. The dynamic outrigger splint used to attain the amount of extension gained at surgery should continue to be used for at least 6 weeks postoperatively or longer if the patient is still making gains in extension.

At 4 to 6 weeks after surgery the patient can gradually resume gripping and strengthening exercises, depending on the amount of motion gained and the amount of scar tenderness present. The patient should be seen by the hand therapist two to three times per week if swelling is present. Any edema still present by the third postoperative week should be controlled by Coban wrapping to prevent stiffness. The Coban wraps should be reapplied daily by the patient or the therapist.

Complications

Repeat surgery for Dupuytren's contracture carries a significant risk of postoperative stiffness.[33,41–43] Most MP joint contractures can be relieved by excising the problematic cords, but PIP joint contractures, even when present for only several months, may not be fully correctable. Most PIP joint contractures >30 degrees, even if fully corrected at the time of surgery, tend to have some PIP ■ flexion contracture at the final outcome. ***An even greater incidence of joint stiffness is encountered if too much joint dissection is performed in an attempt to regain motion at the time of surgery. Therefore only extraarticular release of contracting structures should be performed.***

Blood supply to the palmar skin arises from the digital arteries and reaches the skin via vertical septa piercing the palmar fascia. When a palmar fasciectomy is performed, the overlying skin is relatively devascularized. Furthermore, removal of the dermis intimately involved with the diseased fascia can lead to further devitalization of the more superficial layers of skin and increase the risk of skin slough and hematoma seen with repeat operations for Dupuytren's contracture.

The neurovascular bundles are also at more risk for injury with repeat operations than with the primary operation.[40,41,43,57] Sennwald[43] reports that only one nerve was cut in 77 primary operations and seven were cut in 26 operations for recurrent disease. The increased incidence of neurovascular bundle damage when operating for recurrent disease can be attributed to several factors. In the palm Dupuytren's cords are superficial to the neurovascular bundles, but in the fingers the cords may encircle the bundles and draw them more toward the midline of the digit and superficially. Hueston[57] found that in primary disease the neurovascular bundles are easily separated from the diseased fascia, but in recurrent disease the plane of dissection is much more difficult because of the incorporating scar tissue, and neurovascular damage is much more common.

Flexor Tendon Repair

Tendon adhesions occur whenever the surface of the tendon is violated, either from a traumatic injury or by surgical manipulation such as puncture by a forceps or needle.[58-61] Amadio[62] noted that increased fibrosis and contracture following flexor tendon surgery can also result from sacrifice of the vinculae, which results in devascularization of the tendon, and from the use of reactive suture material. Kleinert et al.[63] reported that staged flexor tendon reconstruction is needed when extensive adhesions develop as in crush injuries, nearby fracture, skin loss or damage, previous operations, healed infections, joint contractures, and destruction of critical pulleys. Excision of the flexor digitorum sublimis tendon at the PIP joint can also lead to adhesions on the flexor digitorum profundus, which diminishes tendon healing and gliding. Diminished gliding results from both loss of an important gliding surface for the profundus tendon and loss of the vinculum longus to the profundus tendon, decreasing the tendon's vascularity and therefore increasing fibrosis.

Primary flexor tendon grafting or staged grafting may be necessary when partial tendon lacerations cause diminished gliding, triggering on the pulley system, or tendon rupture. A repaired tendon is also more likely to rupture when only one of the two flexor tendons is repaired.[63] If a ruptured flexor tendon repair is identified and treated within the first 2 weeks, it can often be repaired again without grafting. However, with time, shortening of the proximal tendon and muscle unit occurs and the tendon cannot be advanced enough for primary repair. If the profundus tendon ruptures off the insertion on the base of the distal phalanx or loses tendon substance, it is sometimes possible to advance the flexor tendon to make a primary repair. The index flexor digitorum profundus is more independent than the other profundus tendons and may often be advanced as much as 1.5 cm. The remainder of the profundus tendons usually tolerate only 1 cm advancement; anything more than that causes a flexion contracture in the repaired digit and a flexor lag in the other digits.

Patient Evaluation

Supple joints and skin are prerequisites for flexor tendon grafting. The maximum range of motion must be attained preoperatively by splinting and passive exercises. If motion cannot be attained by splinting, then capsular releases may be indicated as a preliminary surgery to flexor tendon reconstruction. Capsulectomies can be performed simultaneously with the insertion of the first-stage tendon rod. The scars from previous surgery and injury must be supple and mature before grafting so that passive motion may be maintained in the first stage of the tendon grafting.

A contraindication to flexor tendon reconstruction is damage to either both digital arteries or both digital nerves in the same finger. Patients with insensate fingers make very limited gains in motion postoperatively and the results are usually dismal.[64–66] Unless nerve repair and regeneration precede the flexor tendon reconstruction, postoperative stiffness usually precludes a good result.

Wilson[65] believes the greatest prognostic indicator for flexor tendon grafting is the patient's age. The best results are obtained in patients between the ages of 10 and 30. Staged tendon grafting in children usually should not be done until the child is at least 7 years old and can cooperate with rehabilitation.[67–70] Other than that, there is no absolute contraindication to tendon grafting in children. Technically the smaller rods are more difficult to work with and to anchor. However, the main problem seems to be the patient's inability to cooperate in therapy.

Other factors that lead to a poorer prognosis with flexor tendon grafting include crush injury to the local soft tissues, adjacent fracture or joint injury, skin loss, infection, nonunited fracture, previous surgeries, and a joint contracture.[64,66] Boyes and Stark[71,72] believed that the factors that predicted the outcome after flexor tendon surgery were (in order of importance): scarring, joint involvement, age, bilateral digital nerve injury, the digit involved, scarring of the pulley system or graft bed, and joint stiffness that had not been successfully eliminated preoperatively. An associated fracture or open joint gives a poorer prognosis with subsequent tendon grafting. Wilson[65] advises that all fractures must be reduced and healed and joint motion needs to be restored before grafting.

Single nerve involvement in a digit and simultaneous pulley reconstruction seem to have no effect on results of flexor tendon reconstruction.[65] Wilson[65] felt that the location of injury was of little significance for prognosis after staged grafting. However, most others agree that the poorest results occur in zones I and II, whereas those outside the fibro-osseous tunnel do better.[64,67] Amadio et al.[67] found that the best results have been obtained in zones III and IV and when all postoperative therapy is under the direct supervision of the treating surgeon.

If a patient does not have good prognostic indicators preoperatively, then alternatives to flexor tendon grafting must be sought. Patients who have not regained passive motion, fracture stability, and sensibility preoperatively, as well as those patients who cannot cooperate with a strict therapy regimen and those who do not have supple skin coverage, should not undergo flexor tendon grafting. In these patients either arthrodesis or amputation may be a better alternative.[64]

Stage I Repair

Surgical Technique

The Bruner zigzag incision is made over the flexor surface of the involved digit, extending from the pulp of the finger to the midpalmar level but leaving the carpal tunnel region intact. A separate incision is made over the palmar aspect of the distal forearm, beginning at the wrist flexion crease and proceeding proximally approximately 4 to 5 cm. The pulley system is identified and any remaining intact pulleys are preserved, particularly the A1, A2, and A4 pulleys.

Any remnants of the flexor tendons are excised from the fibro-osseous tunnel, except for the sublimis tendon from its insertion to just proximal to the PIP flexion crease and a 0.75 cm stump of profundus tendon at its insertion site. In an adult, a size three Hunter rod is usually needed for the little finger and size four rods are used for the other digits. Kleinert et al.[63] found that a rod that is too large will stretch the pulleys and contribute to bowstringing. Also, a large rod or a pulley that is too tight will cause the rod to buckle because it cannot glide beneath the pulley system with passive flexion of the finger.[73] Beyond the remaining stump of profundus tendon, the Silastic rod is fixed distally with a wire suture or nonabsorbable monofilament suture to periosteum on either side of the base of the distal phalanx and the stump of profundus tendon is sutured over the rod. The rod is passed through the remaining pulley system and then through the carpal tunnel. The pass through the carpal tunnel is normally made deep to the profundus tendons with a large hemostat. With the finger in full extension and the rod attached distally, the remaining length of the Silastic rod is cut about 3 to 5 cm proximal to the wrist. Finger dissection is then carried proximally into the forearm deep to the profundus tendons to make a tunnel in which the rod can glide. The involved finger is then taken through a passive range of motion to ensure there is no buckling of the rod. Buckling would indicate that the proximal tunnel is not large enough in the distal forearm, or a pulley is too tight and not allowing the rod to glide, or the pulley system is insufficient. If any of these factors are present, they must be corrected. A large suture (No. 2 Mersilene or Tevdek) attached to a disrupted profundus or sublimis tendon that has good excursion in the distal forearm can serve as a marker so very little dissection will need to be done at stage II surgery. The skin is closed and the patient is placed in a bulky hand wrap. The tourniquet is then deflated. Because of the risk of infection, perioperative antibiotics are given for 48 hours.

Pulley Reconstruction. Pulley reconstruction combined either with flexor tenolysis or a one-stage tendon graft usually leads to adhesions between the pulley system and the tendon, causing dismal results. Therefore, when pulley reconstruction is necessary, it is imperative to proceed with staged tendon grafting and reconstruct the pulley system over a Silastic rod.

At least two pulleys (A2 and A4) must be retained or reconstructed,[63,74-78] and Schneider[79] recommends a minimum of three pulleys. Other investigators[67,77,80,81] have suggested that even a four- or five-pulley system is preferred because of increased efficiency. When reconstructing pulleys for the thumb, a minimum of two pulleys is required. If fewer than two or three pulleys are present, bowstringing will usually develop in the flexor tendon, displacing it more palmarward, thus increasing the flexor force at the joint level and leading to a diminished range of motion and ultimately a fixed flexion contracture.[63-65,79] Basically, any area of destroyed pulley system >1.5 cm in length should be reconstructed from the DIP joint to the level of distal palmar crease.

There are numerous methods of pulley reconstruction.[64] The most common method employs a piece of flexor tendon or palmaris longus. A sublimis or profundus tendon is quite broad but may be split in half or into thirds for a more appropriate working size.

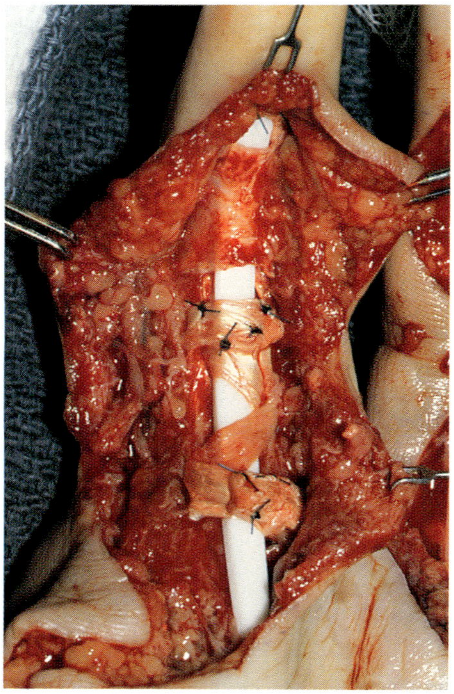

This intraoperative view shows a tendon encircled around the phalanx.[82,83]

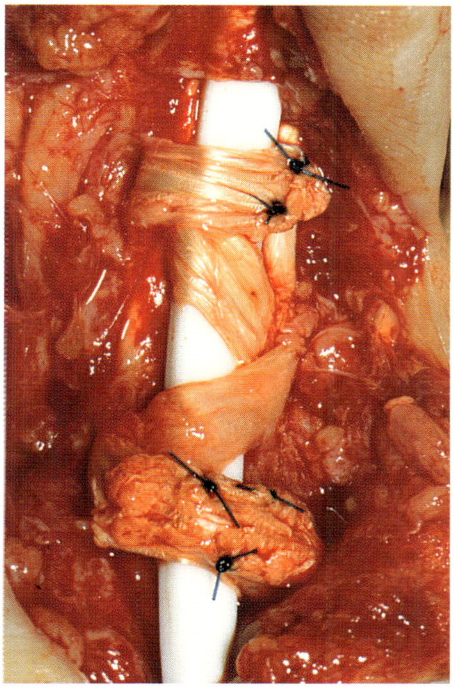

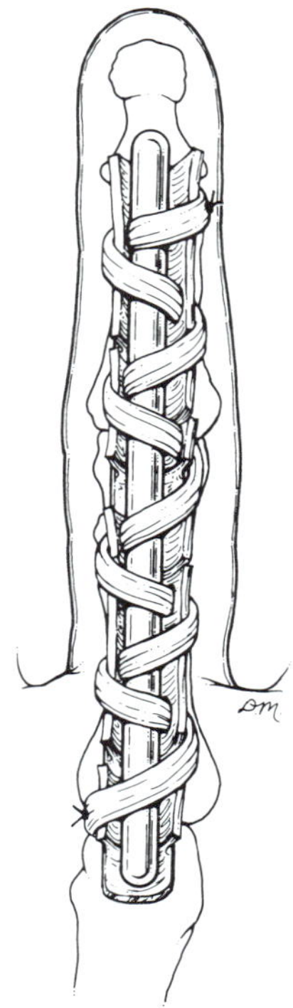

This view shows the tendon interwoven in a running shoelace fashion through remnants of the fibro-osseous tunnel.[83,84]

Postoperative Care

The bulky dressing is usually removed in the recovery room and a light dressing is applied to the involved digits and hand. The wrist is supported with a splint and a continuous passive motion unit is applied. The patient is usually more comfortable if a long-acting regional block has been given either before the surgery or before the institution of passive motion. The patient should wear the continuous passive motion unit at night during sleep for 1 week. During the day, the involved joints and fingers are periodically taken through a passive range of motion. The patient should spend 5 minutes per hour doing the exercises. If adjacent fingers have normal flexor tendons and motion, the involved finger can often be buddy taped to an adjacent digit and thereby get a more continuous passive motion pull. If the pulley system has been reconstructed, that area is protected with either a Coban wrap or thermoplastic rings. Scar massage and softening techniques are instituted after the sutures are removed, along with more intense passive range of motion exercises. At this time, dynamic splints are applied if needed for any joint contractures.

Complications

Synovitis is the most common complication of Silastic rod placement, occurring in 15% to 20% of patients.[79,85,86] The patient will present with warmth over the involved finger, crepitus with passive motion, an increase in swelling, and often fluid in the pseudosheath. There is still some debate over whether or not synovitis influences the end results of tendon grafting, but most practitioners feel that it will lead to a poorer result following stage II surgery.[64,81,87] Schneider[79] found that a thickened and less pliable sheath occurred after the stage II procedure if synovitis was present after the stage I operation.

The implant should not be handled with gloves during insertion and should be kept in a saline solution to prevent the accumulation of talc, lint, and dust, which could lead to synovitis.[63,79] Other possible causes of synovitis include breakdown of the distal juncture with detachment of the rod and buckling of the implant secondary to either inadequate or tight pulleys.[64] When synovitis occurs after stage I flexor tendon grafting, the finger needs to be placed in a resting splint and a diminished passive motion exercise program should be instituted. If the synovitis does not subside, then the stage II procedure should be performed at an earlier date than normal.

Wehbe et al.[86] found that infection occurs in 5% to 6% of implants. Initially, the patient should be placed on antibiotics and the finger is drained, irrigated, and immobilized. If no improvement is seen within several days, the rod must be removed. If the scar is maturing, the rod can be replaced with a new implant 3 months after the infection has cleared.

Erosion usually occurs over the distal juncture of a rod when it does not glide smoothly, either because of inadequate or too tight pulleys, and the rod buckles. Also, erosion over the rod can result when the skin is damaged and does not provide adequate coverage. Hunter and Salisbury[80] and Bora[88] have found skin erosion over the rod to be quite common in the insensate finger. If the distal juncture of the rod is placed deep to the stump of profundus tendon, the problem of skin erosion can be avoided. If erosion does occur, motion exercises of the finger should be delayed and the patient placed on antibiotics until skin healing occurs.

One further complication during stage I is migration of the rod. This usually occurs when an inadequate distal fixation ruptures, forming an inadequate pseudosheath. This problem can be corrected by reattaching the distal juncture of the rod. Lateral x-ray films of the distal forearm with the finger first in full extension and then in full passive flexion will usually show the tip of the rod. If the rod is moving with the finger, then it is still attached distally.

Stage II Repair
Surgical Technique

Stage II surgery should not be performed any sooner than 8 weeks after the stage I surgery. If the patient has not attained a passive range of motion equal to that present before the stage I surgery or if the scar from the stage I surgery is still thickened and indurated, then the stage II surgery should be delayed for several weeks.

A tourniquet is again used after exsanguination of the arm. A 2 cm zigzag incision is made distally through the old scar over the DIP joint. The stump of profundus tendon superficial to the rod is identified and elevated off the rod. The rod is left in place at this time, sutured to the periosteum. Passive flexion of the involved finger should enable the surgeon to feel the underlying Silastic rod in the distal forearm as it glides. The pseudosheath around the rod is then opened and the tip of the rod is identified.

At this point, a graft is harvested from either the palmaris longus, plantaris, toe extensors, or extensor indices proprius tendons. Unless the tendon graft is being used for a thumb, the palmaris longus is usually not long enough to reach from the distal phalanx to the distal forearm, replacing a profundus tendon. Strickland[89] reported no difference among the different donor tendons as far as ultimate results. However, the plantaris tendon is often absent and when present is usually quite small and technically more difficult to suture; therefore, a toe extensor tendon is preferred. The tendon graft may be harvested by making multiple small incisions and dissecting subcutaneously beneath the incisions to release the tendon, or the tendon can be removed with a tendon stripper. Controversy exists as to whether the peritenon should be left with a graft. It is unknown whether the peritenon will facilitate gliding or lead to increased adhesions.[64,82,83,90–96]

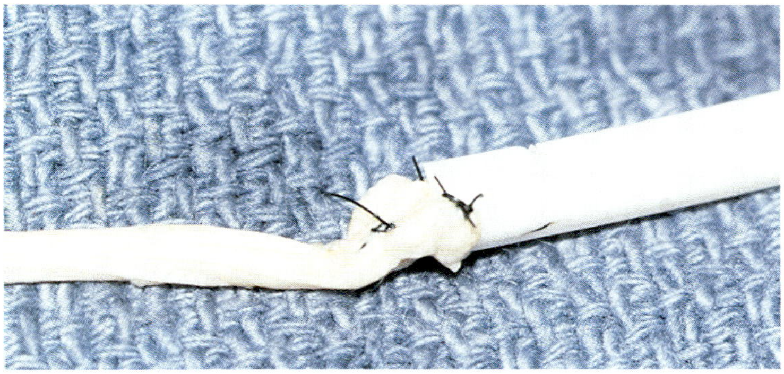

The tendon graft is sutured end-to-end to the proximal end of the Silastic rod in a fashion similar to a tendon repair.

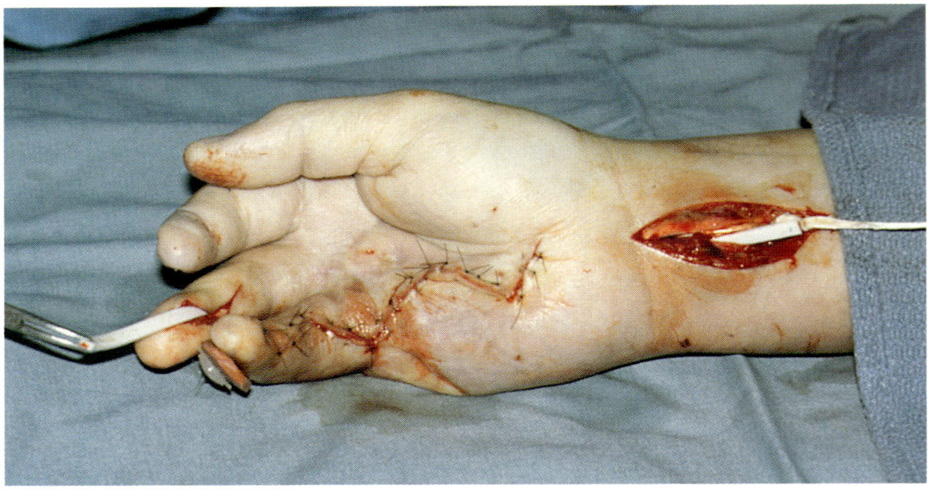

The intraoperative view shows the distal end of the Silastic rod being released from its attachment on the distal phalanx and being pulled through the sheath, bringing the tendon graft with it. The distal edge of the tendon graft is freshened and a pull-out suture is placed.[93,97,98] A 4-0 dermalon suture on a small needle works well, but wire suture or nylon may also be used; a monofilament, nonabsorbable suture facilitates removal of the suture from the tendon at a later date. The suture is either brought through drill holes in the distal phalanx or may be brought out through the pulp or dorsum of the finger by going around the distal phalanx.

Next the periosteum over the base of the distal phalanx on the palmar surface is roughened with a curette so good tendon graft–to-bone contact and early healing can be obtained. The tendon suture is pulled snug over a pull-out button, and under visualization the tendon graft is pulled up into the roughened area of the bone. The suture is tied over the button and the distal skin incision on the finger is closed. Attention is now turned back to the wrist, where traction on the tendon graft is applied to ensure that the suture has holding power and to confirm that the pulley system does not impinge on the graft. The large Tevdek or Mersilene suture previously used for marking the motor flexor tendon is then identified at the level of the wrist, and that tendon is freed from surrounding tendons and the suture is removed. The proximal edge of the tendon graft is woven through the motor tendon in a Pulvertaft weave,[70,93,97-100] which is the strongest of suturing techniques. After the first weave is performed, tension should be adjusted before suturing. Bunnell[82] felt that the tendon graft should be put in with some excessive length since the grafts tend to shrink. However, Pulvertaft[70] felt that grafts do better if put in with slightly more tension than normal since the muscle will gradually stretch somewhat with exercise. The involved digit is usually placed in slightly more flexion than normal while performing the proximal weave. Difficulty in attaining active flexion is more common than a flexion contracture after staged flexor tendon grafting. A finger with a slight flexion contracture postoperatively is much less of a functional problem than a finger that cannot attain enough active flexion.

The wrist wound is then closed and a sterile bulky dressing and plaster splint are applied. The wrist is flexed approximately 30 degrees in the dressing with the MP joints in 70 or 80 degrees flexion.

Amadio et al.[67] and Rowland[101] have found no difference between grafts that extend into the midpalmar region versus those that extend to the distal forearm region. In the rare instance in which the palm is uninjured by trauma, a shorter graft may be used and motored by the profundus tendon at the origin of the lumbrical muscle. Amadio et al.[67] report no difference in ultimate results between a flexor digitorum sublimis versus a profundus motor at the distal forearm level. If distal phalangeal motion is not obtainable or if the tendon graft ruptures and a secondary repair of the graft would be too tight to advance it distally, the distal tendon may be inserted into the middle phalanx rather than the distal phalanx, thus creating a sublimis finger.[94,102-104]

In the thumb the stage II procedure can be done with a free tendon graft, but Schneider and Wiltshire[105] report that transferring a sublimis tendon through the pseudosheath at the stage II surgery provides stronger, earlier healing because it is not necessary to await revascularization of a tendon graft. Also, simple arthrodesis of the thumb interphalangeal joint in skeletally mature patients may be preferable to staged tendon grafting for flexor pollicis longus.[64]

Postoperative Care

On the first or second postoperative day the patient is seen by the hand therapist and the bulky dressing is removed. Either a suture placed through the fingernail at the time of surgery or a hook glued to the fingernail is attached to a rubber band and the finger is pulled into flexion with a Kleinert-type traction. Lister et al.[106] recommend blocking finger extension at the MP joint level at 60 to 70 degrees and holding the wrist in 30 degrees flexion. Tension is adjusted to obtain maximum flexion of the digit.

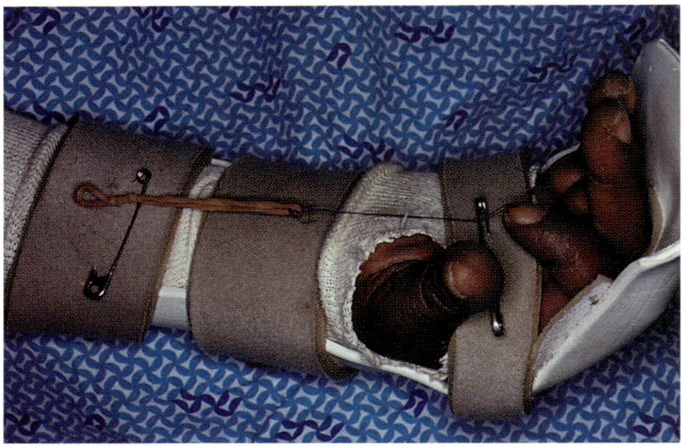

To increase PIP joint flexion, the patient can be fitted with a sling with a rubber band going beneath an artificial pulley at the distal palmar area. The artificial palmar pulley gives greater passive PIP and DIP joint flexion, better finger curl, a closer approximation of the finger pulp to the distal palmar crease, and improved total active motion.[106,107] The patient should perform active extension exercises within the splint (i.e., attempt to touch the extension block) and passive flexion exercises ten times per hour. Splinting remains unchanged until the fourth postoperative week when the wrist is brought to a neutral position; then the patient should add five to ten exercises for passive flexion with active hold to the hourly exercise regimen. Five weeks after surgery the dorsal extension block splint is removed, but the dynamic traction is continued for another week. Ten weeks after surgery dynamic extension splinting is used if needed to correct any flexion contractures, and passive exercises for extension are added. Resistive exercises are not begun until 16 weeks after surgery, when passive stretching exercises with simultaneous wrist and finger extension are added. Before that, all passive stretching exercises were done one joint at a time. By 18 weeks, heavy resistive exercises and grip strengthening can be added.

Complications

Kleinert et al.[63] and Wehbe et al.[86] have found that adhesions are the most common complication following stage II flexor tendon grafting. Adhesions lead to both limited passive extension of the fingers and flexor lag. A graft that is traumatized by surgical manipulation or one that does not glide well beneath the pulleys will have an increased incidence of adhesions. Hunter and Salisbury[80] reported that most adhesions occurred between the graft and pseudosheath rather than at the proximal tendon juncture. The most common problem is adhesions between the graft and flexor digitorum sublimis,[63,108–111] resulting in flexion contracture of the finger and flexor lag. Fewer adhesions occur if the graft is passed around the sublimis tendon rather than through the chiasm. Artificial membranes such as cellophane, silicone rubber sheeting, polyethylene film, gelatin sponge, amniotic membrane, fascia, peritenon, and tunica vaginalis have been used to prevent recurrence of adhesions.[112–117]

Amadio et al.[67] and Strickland[89] have found that graft rupture occurs in 4% to 7% of cases, usually within the first 2 months after surgery. The incidence of rupture is related to the strength of the repair before active flexion and passive extension exercises are begun. The graft is more likely to rupture if these exercises are begun before the graft has adequately revascularized and healed. The strength of the repair also depends on the repair technique, suture material, and the duration of immobilization; grafts attain strength more quickly with controlled motion than when immobilized. Kleinert et al.[63] have found that low-grade infections and uneven, protruding bone surfaces can also result in graft rupture. Wilson[65] notes that disruption occurs more commonly at the proximal juncture rather than at the insertion site or in midsubstance. When distal ruptures do occur, they are usually about a centimeter proximal to the point of bony attachment. Early reoperation can often salvage the distal rupture.

Flexion contractures are common after staged tendon grafting[64,65,79,86] especially when the finger is immobilized in a position that allows flexion contracture to occur at the PIP joint. Schneider[79] reports that late flexion deformity can be aggravated either by an inadequate pulley system or by poor nutritional status of the tendon graft. Kleinert et al.[63] state that mallet finger deformity following staged tendon grafting results from several factors: the tendon graft may be too short, the A4 pulley may be inadequate, postoperative splinting may have been suboptimal, or adhesions may be present. Swan-neck deformity may also develop and be related to one of the following: a mallet deformity, excision of the flexor digitorum sublimis distal to the PIP joint, an inadequate PIP joint volar plate, adhesions, or from the tendon graft being too long.

Improper length of the tendon graft can lead to diminished motion. A graft that is too short will prevent full extension of the fingers. A graft that is too long will lead to a flexor lag; also, the profundus tendon may retract into the palm, putting increased tension on the lumbrical muscle and thereby lead to a lumbrical plus deformity.[63,118-121] When flexion is attempted, the profundus tendon will glide proximally, thus putting more tension on the lumbrical muscle, leading to a paradoxical extension of the IP joints with attempted flexion. Lumbrical plus deformity is most common in the middle finger. Colville and Dickie[118] note that in the ring and little fingers, the profundus tendon is limited by the bicipital lumbrical muscle origin.

If the tendon graft is put in with too much tension, a flexion contracture or even quadregia may develop. This complication occurs most commonly in the middle through little fingers. The index profundus tendon is more independent and is not as heavily involved with quadregia. If any of the long through little finger profundus tendons are attached to a graft that is too short, the common profundus tendon will be pulled distally, thus limiting proximal excursion with attempted active flexion and causing a flexor lag to occur even in the uninvolved fingers.

Pulley breakdown can occur after staged tendon grafting if the pulleys are not properly protected with blocking or external rings for 2 months after reconstruction. If too large a rod is used, stretched pulleys will result; stretched or inadequate pulleys lead to bowstringing, which may result in flexion contracture and diminished motion. If this happens, the pulleys must be reconstructed after digital range of motion has plateaued. The best time to reconstruct the pulleys is when the Silastic rods are implanted.

Several other complications can occur during stage II grafting, but they are less common. Amadio et al.[67] reported infection in as many as 15% of cases. However, most authors report a much lower incidence of infection, around 2% to 3%. Other poor results include skin slough secondary to compromised vascularity, reflex sympathetic dystrophy in about 1% of cases, and ultimate amputation in 4%.[67,89]

Anticipated Outcome

The finger salvaged by staged flexor tendon grafting often has the best motion and softest scar while the Silastic implant is in place. LaSalle and Strickland[122] report that stiffness and joint contracture commonly return after the stage II operation. Virtually all patients will have some flexion contracture at the PIP or DIP joint. In 43 tendon reconstructions, LaSalle and Strickland[122] found a flexion contracture in all digits. Only 20% to 40% of patients will have a final total active motion of greater than 180 degrees;[67,79] 30% do not regain any useful motion. The preoperative passive range of motion is a good indicator of final total active motion following staged grafting. Strickland[89] reports that about 40% of digits will gain 60% or better of the passive range of motion that was present before the stage I operation. Compared with the passive range of motion before the stage II procedure, half of the patients will regain an active range of motion that is at least 80% of the pre-stage II passive range of motion.

Schneider[123] found that 90% of the ultimate active range of motion was regained within 22 weeks after the stage II procedure. An optimal interval has not yet been found between the stage I and stage II procedures[89]; however, most people recommend 6 to 8 weeks between the two stages. Normally it is best to wait until the scar begins to mature and soften and to allow the passive range of motion to return to what it was before the stage I operation. Strickland[89] tested different types of rod materials and designs and did not find any effect on the final outcome; this author also showed that early mobilization did not significantly influence the final performance. However, most practitioners feel that early motion aids in preventing adhesions and ultimately gives a better total active motion and that motion is regained more quickly.

Secondary Operations

The most common secondary operations following staged tendon grafting are repair of graft rupture and tenolysis.

Graft Rupture Repair

Graft ruptures usually occur around the tenth postoperative day but can occur as late as 7 weeks after stage II surgery. The preferred treatment for graft rupture is early exploration and repair[63,64,89]; early reattachment can often salvage the situation. If the tendon graft ruptures distally and is not long enough to reach the distal phalanx for reattachment, a sublimis finger may be made by reattaching the graft to the base of the middle phalanx and performing tenodesis or arthrodesis of the DIP joint. If the graft ruptures proximally, a new tendon graft can be inserted if the pseudosheath is still open and in good condition. If the fibro-osseous tunnel has collapsed or adhesions have formed due to either late rupture or late identification of a rupture, then either a stage I Silastic rod implant procedure should be repeated or the digit should be amputated or fused.

Tenolysis

Various sources[67,69,89,121] have reported the rate of tenolysis following staged flexor tendon grafting as ranging between 7% and 47%. Tenolysis should not be performed until at least 3 months after tendon repair or 6 months after grafting. Stripping the soft tissue connections to the tendon graft endangers the circulation of the tendon and increases the risk of rupture, but if tenolysis is delayed long enough for revascularization and tendon healing to occur in the graft, the risk of rupture is decreased. Other preoperative criteria for tenolysis include no further improvement in the range of motion, an intact flexor tendon, supple joints, a softened scar, healthy skin, and a well-motivated patient.[64,124–126] When all of these factors are present, 50% to 60% of patients will show improvement following tenolysis. Tenolysis is contraindicated with concomitant tendon repair or graft, skin grafting, osteotomy, capsulotomy, patient age >40 years, nerve repair, tenolysis >1 year previously, tenolysis requiring a long operative time, associated pulley reconstruction, and any procedure that may require immobilization in the postoperative period.[127]

■ ***Patients scheduled for tenolysis must be prepared preoperatively for a staged tendon graft procedure since it is difficult to tell the difference between tendon rupture and tendon adhesions.*** Even if the tendon itself is intact, there may be such massive scarring that tenolysis will not be of benefit. Although use of a long-acting regional anesthetic is standard, some practitioners use a local anesthetic so the patient can cooperate during the surgery. However, tenolysis surgery is often prolonged, so it is difficult to keep a tourniquet inflated on the arm during the entire case under local anesthesia.

An incision is initially made over the volar aspect of the distal forearm and a flexor check is made of the involved tendons. Pulling on the involved flexor tendon at the level of distal forearm will show an adequate release of the tendon adhesions when the finger comes to the full range of flexion possible passively. The finger is approached through the previous Bruner zigzag incision, keeping in mind that all pulleys or pulley reconstructions need to be maintained. The tendon is gradually freed from the underlying bone as well as the overlying pulleys and may also need to be freed from adjacent tendons in the distal forearm. The carpal tunnel region usually does not need to be opened. Many practitioners add steroid preparations to the tendon bed following tenolysis.[128-133] After the wound is closed, the patient is placed in a bulky dressing for hemostasis. In the recovery room the bulky dressing is removed and a continuous passive motion unit is applied while the anesthetic block is still effective. The continuous passive motion unit is worn at night for 1 to 2 weeks. During the day the patient practices individual joint blocking and individual finger flexion as well as active flexion and extension of all fingers together. For the first 48 hours an 18-gauge angiocath is left in the carpal tunnel region and a 5 ml dose of 0.05% plain Marcaine (bupivacaine) is administered every 6 hours. By keeping the median nerve anesthetized, the fingers can be moved without discomfort, thus providing more effective immediate mobilization. Coban wraps are used to control edema. Dynamic extension splinting is used if needed during the day and alternated with active range of motion exercises. At 2 weeks postoperatively, when the sutures are removed, scar remodeling techniques are used with massage and ultrasound. Graduated resistance exercises are begun 4 to 6 weeks postoperatively.

Active Tendon Implants

The primary advantage of an active tendon implant is that it is performed in one operation. Pseudosheath formation does occur; the results of the active and passive implants are comparable. The difference in the exercise program is that with the active implant the patient's own muscles provide the necessary motion of the rod rather than having to perform passive motion. The rod is made of silicone rubber with a Dacron core. It has a proximal loop for flexor tendon attachment in the distal forearm and a metal plate distally. The metal end of the active implant is usually fixed with a screw or the Dacron cords can be used for distal attachment through drill holes in the distal phalanx.[64] The active implant can be used with pulley reconstruction and if so, the pulleys are protected with rings or with direct digital pressure blocking exercises for 2 months afterward. Results are similar to the two-stage grafting procedure, with total active motion improving an average of 72 degrees after insertion of the active rod.[134] Complication rates are also similar to staged grafting with a passive rod. There are problems in creating a permanent attachment both proximally and distally. Either of the junctures may rupture, although the proximal juncture is more likely to rupture. If this occurs, stage II grafting should be performed within 3 weeks. Most active implants are replaced by a tendon graft within 2 years. The search for a long-term or permanent tendon prosthesis continues.[135]

Ganglion Excision

Although primary excision of dorsal or volar wrist ganglions has a recurrence rate of 5% to 10%, excision of recurrent ganglions has a recurrence rate of 30% to 40%. The most common dorsal wrist ganglions are at the level of the scapholunate ligament. Although a transverse incision is commonly used, a longitudinal incision is much easier to extend if needed. Also, the cutaneous nerves are much more easily dissected and mobilized since they lie parallel to the incision rather than perpendicular. Longitudinal scars normally do not cause any difficulty over the dorsal aspect of the wrist.

Surgical Technique

Dorsal Wrist Ganglion Cyst. The longitudinal incision is carried down to the cyst, which lies usually beneath the fourth dorsal compartment. The distal third of the extensor retinaculum through second, third, and fourth compartments is released so the second and third compartment tendons can be retracted radially and the fourth compartment tendons ulnarward. The stalk of the cyst is traced to the level of the joint, which is normally the scapholunate joint for dorsal wrist ganglia. In surgery for recurrent ganglions, the scar tissue often makes it difficult to be sure exactly where the stalk extends. If the stalk is lost, it is best to take out a small section of dorsal capsule directly over the scapholunate interval. Dissection between the scaphoid and lunate bones must be avoided, since this would disrupt the interosseous membrane and lead to potential wrist instability.

Volar Wrist Ganglion Cyst. Volar ganglia usually lie between the flexor carpi radialis and first dorsal compartment tendons. Again, a longitudinal incision is made directly over the cyst. After opening the volar antebrachial fascia, the radial artery adhering to the cyst must be dissected free throughout the length of the incision and preserved. The ganglion cyst is then traced to the level of the joint capsule. The stalk for the volar ganglion normally extends either to the radioscaphoid joint or scaphotrapezial joint. Since the most common location is the radioscaphoid joint, if the stalk cannot be absolutely identified at surgery, a small section of capsule over the radioscaphoid joint should be removed. Great care must be taken when removing any of the palmar capsule and only a small section can be safely removed. The most substantial wrist ligaments are on the palmar side; these ligaments can be disrupted easily and thus lead to a wrist instability if too much capsule is excised.

Postoperative Care

The wrist is splinted for 2 weeks. Normally the patient has full range of motion by 4 weeks postoperatively. If not, an Oppenheimer splint alternating wrist flexion and extension may be added and full range of motion should be attained within 2 months after surgery.

Complications

Recurrent ganglia are common because of the difficulty in tracing the stalk to the appropriate joint level; if the entire stalk is not excised, a recurrence may develop. Because of the proximity of the radial artery to volar ganglia, it is too risky to aspirate or inject volar ganglia. However, it is reasonable to repeatedly aspirate dorsal ganglia even if they are recurrent. Often after repeated aspirations, the cyst will scar enough that it becomes smaller or nonpalpable.

Pain is a frequent complication of ganglionectomy. Pain usually occurs after resection of a dorsal wrist ganglion and is associated with a neuroma in the posterior interosseous nerve. The terminal branch of the posterior interosseous nerve, which innervates the dorsal wrist capsule, is invariably in the area of capsular resection for dorsal ganglia and is commonly injured. If the patient has point tenderness at the level of the radial carpal joint dorsally after a ganglionectomy, whether or not a ganglion has recurred, a posterior interosseous neuroma must be suspected of causing the pain. The treatment for this is to simply resect the posterior interosseous nerve about 2.5 cm proximal to the level of radial carpal joint. The nerve is thus in an area where no traction is placed on it with wrist motion.

References

1. Millender LH, Nalebuff EA. Metacarpophalangeal joint arthroplasty utilizing the silicone rubber prosthesis. Orthop Clin North Am 4:349-371, 1973.
2. Swanson AB. Flexible implant arthroplasty for arthritic finger joints. J Bone Joint Surg 54A:435-455, 1972.
3. Swanson AB. Surgical Techniques for Flexible Implant Arthroplasty in the MP, PIP, DIP Joints of the Hand. Grand Rapids, Mich., 1980.
4. Beckenbaugh RD, Linscheid RL. Arthroplasty in the hand and wrist. In Green DP, ed. Operative Hand Surgery, 3rd ed. New York: Churchill Livingstone, 1993, pp 143-187.
5. Swanson AB, Swanson G. Flexible implant arthroplasty of the digits: Indications, methods, and results. Acta Orthop Belg 51:679-699, 1985.
6. Weilby A. Resection arthroplasty of the metacarpophalangeal joint a.m. Tupper using interposition of the volar plate. Scand J Plast Reconstr Surg Hand Surg 11:239-242, 1977.
7. Riordan DC, Fowler SB. Arthroplasty of the metacarpophalangeal joints: Review of resection-type arthroplasty. J Hand Surg 14A:368-371, 1989.
8. Adams BD, Blair WF, Shurr DG. Schultz metacarpophalangeal arthroplasty: A long-term follow-up study. J Hand Surg 15A:641-645, 1990.
9. Vahvanen V, Viljakka T. Silicone rubber implant arthroplasty of the metacarpophalangeal joint in rheumatoid arthritis: A follow-up study of 32 patients. J Hand Surg 11A:333-339, 1986.
10. Blair WF, Shurr DG, Buckwalter JA. Metacarpophalangeal joint implant arthroplasty with a Silastic spacer. J Bone Joint Surg 66A:365-370, 1984.
11. Kleinert JM, Lister GD. Silicone implants. Hand Clin 2:271-290, 1986.

12. Wilson RL, Carlblom ER. The rheumatoid metacarpophalangeal joint. Hand Clin 5:223-237, 1989.
13. Derkash RS, Niebauer JJ, Lane CS. Long-term follow-up of metacarpal phalangeal arthroplasty with silicone Dacron protheses. J Hand Surg 11A:553-558, 1986.
14. Ferlic DC, Clayton ML. Complications following surgery for rheumatoid and arthritic conditions. In Boswick JA, ed. Complications in Hand Surgery. Philadelphia: WB Saunders, 1986.
15. Beckenbaugh RD, Dobyns JH, Linscheid RL, et al. Review and analysis of silicone-rubber metacarpophalangeal implants. J Bone Joint Surg 58A:483-487, 1976.
16. Backhouse KM. The mechanics of normal digital control in the hand and an analysis of the ulnar drift in rheumatoid arthritis. Ann R Coll Surg Engl 43:154-173, 1968.
17. Flatt AE. The Care of the Rheumatoid Hand, 3rd ed. St. Louis: CV Mosby, 1974.
18. Hakstian RW, Tubiana R. Ulnar deviation of the fingers: The role of joint structure and function. J Bone Joint Surg 49A:299-316, 1967.
19. Harrison SH. Rheumatoid arthritis of the hand. Conn Med 41:199-204, 1977.
20. Pagowski S, Piekarski K. Biomechanics of the metacarpophalangeal joint. J Biomech 10:205-209, 1977.
21. Shapiro JS. The etiology of ulnar drift: A new factor [abstr]. J Bone Joint Surg 50A:634, 1968.
22. Smith RJ, Kaplan EB. Rheumatoid deformities at the metacarpophalangeal joints of the fingers: A correlative study of anatomy and pathology. J Bone Joint Surg 49A:31-47, 1967.
23. Ferlic DC, Clayton ML, Holloway M. Complications of silicone implant surgery in the metacarpophalangeal joint. J Bone Joint Surg 57A:991, 1975.
24. Madden JW, Devore GL, Arem AJ. A rational postoperative management program for metacarpophalangeal joint implant arthroplasty. J Hand Surg 2:358-366, 1977.
25. Devore GL, Muhleman CA, Sasarita SG. Management of pronation deformity in metacarpophalangeal joint implant arthroplasty. J Hand Surg 11A:859-861, 1986.
26. Niebauer JJ. Dacron-silicone prostheses for the metacarpophalangeal and interphalangeal joints. In Cramer LM, Chase RA, eds. Symposium on the Hand. St. Louis: CV Mosby, 1971, pp 96-105.
27. Ferlic DC. Boutonniere deformities in rheumatoid arthritis. Hand Clin 5:215-222, 1989.
28. Nalebuff EA. The rheumatoid swan-neck deformity. Hand Clin 5:203-214, 1989.
29. Swanson AB. Silicone rubber implants for replacement of arthritic or destroyed joints in the hand. Surg Clin North Am 48:1113-1127, 1968.
30. Pellegrini VD, Burton RI. Osteoarthritis of the proximal interphalangeal joint of the hand: Arthroplasty or fusion? J Hand Surg 15A:194-209, 1990.
31. Zimmerman NB, Suhey PV, Clark GL, Wilgis EFS. Silicone interpositional arthroplasty of the distal interphalangeal joint. J Hand Surg 14A:882-887, 1989.
32. Brown LG. Distal interphalangeal joint flexible implant arthroplasty. J Hand Surg 14A: 653-656, 1989.
33. Hueston JT. Dupuytren's contracture: The trend to conservatism. Ann R Coll Surg Engl 36:134-151, 1965.
34. Hakstian RW. Long-term results of extensive fasciectomy. Br J Plast Surg 19:140-149, 1966.
35. Millesi H. Dupuytren-Kontraktur. In Nigst H, Buck-Gramko D, Millesi H, eds. Handchirurgie, Band 1, New York: Thieme, 1981, pp 15.1-15.57.
36. Tonkin MA, Burke FD, Varian JPW. Dupuytren's contracture: A comparative study of fasciectomy and dermofasciectomy in one hundred patients. J Hand Surg 9B:156-162, 1984.
37. McFarlane RM. Dupuytren's contracture. In Green DP, ed. Operative Hand Surgery, 3rd ed. New York: Churchill Livingstone, 1993, pp 563-591.
38. Watson HK, Fong D. Dystrophy, recurrence and salvage procedures in Dupuytren's contracture. Hand Clin 7:745-755, 1991.
39. Rombouts JJ, Noel H, Legrain Y, et al. Prediction of recurrence in the treatment of Dupuytren's disease: Evaluation of a histologic classification. J Hand Surg 14A:644-652, 1989.

40. Ketchum LD. The use of full thickness skin graft in Dupuytren's contracture. Hand Clin 7:731-741, 1991.
41. McFarlane RM. Complications of Dupuytren's disease. In Boswick JA, ed. Complications in Hand Surgery. Philadelphia: WB Saunders, 1986, pp 294-299.
42. McFarlane RM. Patterns on the diseased fascia in the fingers in Dupuytren's contracture. Plast Reconstr Surg 54:31, 1974.
43. Sennwald GR. Fasciectomy for treatment of Dupuytren's disease and early complications. J Hand Surg 15A:755-761, 1990.
44. Rudolph R, Van de Berg J. The myofibroblast in Dupuytren's contracture. Hand Clin 7:683-692, 1991.
45. Gelberman RH, Amiel D, Rudolph R, et al. Dupuytren's contracture: An electron microscopic, biochemical, and clinical correlative study. J Bone Joint Surg 62A:425-432, 1980.
46. Hueston JT. Digital wolf grafts in recurrent Dupuytren's contracture. Plast Reconstr Surg 29:342-344, 1962.
47. Hueston JT. The control of recurrent Dupuytren's contracture by skin replacement. Br J Plast Surg 22:152-156, 1969.
48. Hueston JT. Dermofasciectomy for Dupuytren's disease. Bull Hosp Joint Dis 44:224-231, 1984.
49. Ketchum LD, Hixson FP. Dermofasciectomy and full-thickness grafts in the treatment of Dupuytren's contracture. J Hand Surg 12A:559-563, 1987.
50. Parker HG. Dupuytren's contracture as a cause of stenosing tenosynovitis. J Maine Med Assoc 70:147-148, 1979.
51. Watson HK, Light TR, Johnson TR. Checkrein resection for flexion contracture of the middle joint. J Hand Surg 4:67-71, 1979.
52. Curtis RM. Capsulectomy of the interphalangeal joints of fingers. J Bone Joint Surg 36A:1219-1231, 1954.
53. Moberg E. Three useful ways to avoid amputation in advanced Dupuytren's contracture. Orthop Clin North Am 4:1001-1005, 1973.
54. Watson HK, Lovallo JF. Salvage of severe recurrent Dupuytren's contracture of the ring and small fingers. J Hand Surg 12A:287-289, 1987.
55. Watson HK, Schaffer SR. Concentric arthrodesis in joints of the hand. J Plast Reconstr Surg 46:368-371, 1970.
56. Haimovici N. Die Alloarthroplastik-Therapie Alternative bei der arthrogenen Beugekontraktur der Finger bei Dupuytren's cher Krankheit. Hand Chir 10:135-148, 1978.
57. Hueston JT. Unsatisfactory results in Dupuytren's contracture. Hand Clin 7:759-763, 1991.
58. Lindsay WK, Thomson HG. Digital flexor tendons: An experimental study. I. The significance of each component of the flexor mechanism in tendon healing. Br J Plast Surg 12:289-316, 1960.
59. Peacock EE. Biological principles in the healing of long tendons. Surg Clin North Am 45:461-476, 1965.
60. Potenza AD. Tendon healing within the flexor digital sheath in the dog. J Bone Joint Surg 44A:49-64, 1962.
61. Potenza AD. Prevention of adhesions to healing digital flexor tendons. JAMA 187:187-191, 1964.
62. Amadio P. Effect of vincular injury on the results of flexor tendon surgery in "no man's land." Presented at the American Academy of Orthopaedic Surgeons Meeting. Atlanta: 1984.
63. Kleinert HE, Steyers CM, Kalisman M. Complications from flexor tendon surgery. In Boswick JA Jr, ed. Complications in Hand Surgery. Philadelphia: WB Saunders, 1986, pp 19-28.
64. Schneider LH, Hunter JM. Flexor tendons—Late reconstruction. In Green DP, ed. Operative Hand Surgery, 3rd ed. New York: Churchill Livingstone, 1993, pp 1853-1924.
65. Wilson RL. Flexor tendon grafting. Hand Clin 1:97-107, 1985.

66. Lister G. Pitfalls and complications of flexor tendon surgery. Hand Clin 1:133-146, 1985.
67. Amadio PC, Wood MB, Cooney WP III, et al. Staged flexor tendon reconstruction in the fingers and hand. J Hand Surg 13A:559-562, 1988.
68. Schneider LH. Injuries to tendons in children. In Bora FW, ed. The Pediatric Upper Extremity. Philadelphia: WB Saunders, 1986, pp 91-119.
69. Hunter JM, Salisbury RE. Use of gliding artificial implants to produce tendon sheaths: Techniques and results in children. Plast Reconstr Surg 45:564-572, 1970.
70. Pulvertaft RG. Tendon grafts for flexor tendon injuries in the fingers and thumb: A study of technique and results. J Bone Joint Surg 38B:175-194, 1956.
71. Boyes JH. Evaluation of results of digital flexor tendon grafts. Am J Surg 89:1116-1119, 1955.
72. Boyes JH, Stark HH. Flexor tendon grafts in the fingers and thumb. J Bone Joint Surg 53A:1332-1342, 1971.
73. Urbaniak JR, Bright DS, Gill LH, et al. Vascularization and the gliding mechanism of free flexor tendon grafts inserted by the silicone rod method. J Bone Joint Surg 56A:473-482, 1974.
74. Doyle JR, Blythe WF. The finger flexor tendon sheaths and pulleys: Anatomy and reconstruction. In American Academy of Orthopaedic Surgeons: Symposium on Tendon Surgery in the Hand. St. Louis: CV Mosby, 1975.
75. Doyle JR, Blythe WF. Anatomy of the flexor tendon sheath and pulleys of the thumb. J Hand Surg 2:149-151, 1977.
76. Brand PW, Cranor KC, Ellis JC. Tendon pulleys at the metacarpophalangeal joint of a finger. J Bone Joint Surg 57A:779-784, 1975.
77. Hunter JM, Cook JF. The pulley system: Rationale for reconstruction. In Strickland JW, Steichen JB, eds. Difficult Problems in Hand Surgery. St. Louis: CV Mosby, 1982.
78. Solonen KA, Hoyer P. Positioning of the pulley mechanism when reconstructing deep flexor tendons of the finger. Acta Orthop Scand 38:321-328, 1967.
79. Schneider LH. Staged tendon reconstruction. Hand Clin 1:109-120, 1985.
80. Hunter JM, Salisbury RE. Flexor tendon reconstruction in severely damaged hands: A two-stage procedure using a silicone-Dacron reinforced gliding prosthesis prior to tendon grafting. J Bone Joint Surg 53A:829-858, 1971.
81. Schneider LH. Staged tendon reconstruction using the method of Hunter. Clin Orthop 171:164-171, 1982.
82. Bunnell S. Surgery of the Hand. Philadelphia: JB Lippincott, 1944.
83. Koch SL. Complicated contractures of the hand: Their treatment by freeing fibrosed tendons and replacing destroyed tendons with grafts. Ann Surg 98:546-580, 1933.
84. Kleinert HE, Bennett JB. Digital pulley reconstruction employing the always present rim of the previous pulley. J Hand Surg 3:297-298, 1978.
85. Schneider LH. Complications in tendon injury and surgery. Hand Clin 2:361-371, 1986.
86. Wehbe MA, Hunter JM, Schneider LH, et al. Staged tendon reconstruction. Presented at the American Academy of Orthopaedic Surgeons Meeting. Las Vegas: January 1985.
87. Hunter JM. Staged flexor tendon reconstruction. J Hand Surg 8:789-793, 1983.
88. Bora FW. Profundus tendon grafting with unimpaired sublimus function in children. Clin Orthop 71:118-123, 1970.
89. Strickland JW. Results of flexor tendon surgery in zone II. Hand Clin 1:167-179, 1985.
90. Boyes JH, Stark HH. Flexor tendon grafts in the fingers and thumb. In Verdan C, ed. Tendon Surgery of the Hand. Edinburgh: Churchill Livingstone, 1979, p 85.
91. Littler JW. Free tendon grafts in secondary flexor tendon repair. Am J Surg 74:315-321, 1947.
92. Peacock EE. Some technical aspects and results of flexor tendon repair. Surgery 58:330-342, 1965.
93. Boyes JH. Operative technique of digital flexor tendon grafts. In American Academy of Orthopaedic Surgeons: Instructional Course Lectures, vol 10. Ann Arbor: JW Edwards, 1953.

94. Tubiana R. Technique of flexor tendon grafts. Hand 1:108-114, 1969.
95. Weiner LJ, Peacock EE. Biologic principles affecting repair of flexor tendons. Adv Surg 5:145-188, 1971.
96. White WL. Tendon grafts: A consideration of their source, procurement, and suitability. Surg Clin North Am 40:402-413, 1960.
97. Pulvertaft RG. Suture materials and tendon junctures. Am J Surg 109:346-352, 1965.
98. Littler JW. The digital flexor-extensor system. In Converse JM, ed. Reconstructive Plastic Surgery, 2nd ed. Philadelphia: WB Saunders, 1977, p 366.
99. Bruner JM. The zigzag volar-digital incision for flexor tendon surgery. Plast Reconstr Surg 40:571-574, 1967.
100. Urbaniak JR, Cahill JD, Mortenson RA. Tendon suturing methods: Analysis of muscle strengths. In American Academy of Orthopaedic Surgeons: Symposium on Tendon Surgery in the Hand. St. Louis: CV Mosby, 1975, p 70.
101. Rowland SA. Palmar fingertip use of silicone rubber followed by free tendon graft. In American Academy of Orthopaedic Surgeons: Symposium on Tendon Surgery in the Hand. St. Louis: CV Mosby, 1975, p 145.
102. Osborne GV. The sublimus tendon replacement technique in tendon injuries. J Bone Joint Surg 42B:647, 1960.
103. Schneider LH, Hunter JM, Fietti VG. The flexor superficialis finger: A salvage procedure. In Hunter JM, Schneider LH, Mackin EJ, eds. Flexor Tendon Surgery in the Hand. St. Louis: CV Mosby, 1987, pp 528-532.
104. Chuinard RG, Dabezies EJ, Mathews RE. Two stage superficialis reconstruction in severely damaged fingers. J Hand Surg 5:135-143, 1980.
105. Schneider LH, Wiltshire D. Restoration of flexor pollicis longus function by flexor digitorum superficialis transfer. J Hand Surg 8:98-101, 1983.
106. Lister GD, Kleinert HE, Kutz JE, et al. Primary flexor tendon repair followed by immediate controlled mobilization. J Hand Surg 2:441-451, 1977.
107. Edinburg M, Widgerow AD, Biddulph SL. Early postoperative mobilization of flexor tendon injuries using a modification of the Kleinert technique. J Hand Surg 12A:34-38, 1987.
108. Jaffe S, Weckesser E. Profundus tendon grafting with the sublimus intact: The end result of thirty patients. J Bone Joint Surg 49A:1298-1308, 1967.
109. McClinton MA, Curtis RM, Wilgis EFS. 100 tendon grafts for isolated flexor digitorum profundus injuries. J Hand Surg 7:224-229, 1982.
110. Pulvertaft RG. The treatment of profundus division by the free tendon graft. J Bone Joint Surg 42A:1363-1371, 1960.
111. Parker A. The "lumbrical plus" finger. J Bone Joint Surg 53B:236-239, 1971.
112. Wheeldon T. The use of cellophane as a permanent tendon sheath. J Bone Joint Surg 21:393-396, 1939.
113. Wilmouth CL. Tendoplasty of flexor tendons of the hand: Use of tunica vaginalis in reconstructing tendon sheaths. J Bone Joint Surg 19:152-156, 1937.
114. Williams CW, Dickie WR, Colville J. Silastic sheeting in hand surgery. Hand 4:273-276, 1972.
115. Suzuki K. Delayed flexor tendon repair in the digital sheath with end to end suture and fascial graft. Hand 8:141-144, 1976.
116. Stark HH, Boyes JH, Johnson L, et al. The use of paratenon, polyethylene film or Silastic sheeting to prevent restricting adhesions to tendons in the hand. J Bone Joint Surg 59A: 908-913, 1977.
117. Nichols HM. Discussion of tendon repair with clinical and experimental data on the use of gelatin sponge. Ann Surg 129:223-234, 1949.
118. Colville J, Dickie WR. Tendon graft length. Br J Plast Surg 22:37-40, 1969.
119. Mayou BJ, Harrison SH. The length of flexor tendon grafts. Hand 10:48-51, 1978.
120. Parkes A. "Lumbrical plus" finger. Hand 2:164-165, 1970.

121. Chamay A, Verdan C, Simonetta C. The two-stage graft: A salvage operation for the flexor apparatus (a clinical study of 28 cases). In Verdan C, ed. Tendon Surgery of the Hand. Edinburgh: Churchill Livingstone, 1979.
122. LaSalle WB, Strickland JW. An evaluation of the two-stage flexor tendon reconstruction technique. J Hand Surg 8:263-267, 1983.
123. Schneider LH. Staged flexor tendon reconstruction using the method of Hunter. Clin Orthop Rel Res 171:164-171, 1983.
124. Weeks PM, Wray RC. Rate and extent of functional recovery after flexor tendon grafting with and without silicone rod preparation. J Hand Surg 1:174-180, 1976.
125. Fetrow KO. Tenolysis in the hand and wrist: A clinical evaluation of two hundred twenty flexor and extensor tenolyses. J Bone Joint Surg 49A:667-685, 1967.
126. Rank BK, Wakefield AR, Hueston JJ. Surgery of Repair as Applied to Hand Injuries, 4th ed. Baltimore: Williams & Wilkins, 1973.
127. Verdan C. Tenolysis. In Verdan C, ed. Tendon Surgery of the Hand. Edinburgh: Churchill Livingstone, 1979, p 137.
128. Carstram N. Prevention of experimental tendon adhesions by cortisone. Acta Orthop Scand 22:15-24, 1953.
129. Gonzalez RI. Experimental tendon repair within the flexor tunnels: The use of hydrocortisone without improvement of function of the dog. J Bone Joint Surg 35A:991-993, 1953.
130. James JIP. The value of tenolysis. Hand 1:118-119, 1969.
131. Ketchum LD. Effects of triamcinolone on tendon healing and function: A laboratory study. Plast Reconstr Surg 47:471-484, 1971.
132. Whitaker JH, Strickland JW, Ellis KK. The role of flexor tenolysis in the palm and digits. J Hand Surg 2:462-470, 1977.
133. Wrenn RN, Goldner JL, Markee JL. An experimental study of the effect of cortisone on the healing process and tensile strength of tendons. J Bone Joint Surg 36A:588-601, 1954.
134. Hunter JM, Singer DI, Jaeger SH, et al. Active tendon implants in flexor tendon reconstruction. J Hand Surg 13A:849-859, 1988.
135. Jaeger SH, Hunter JM, Schneider LH, et al. Development of a long-term flexor tendon prosthesis. In Hunter JM, Schneider LH, Mackin EJ, eds. Flexor Tendon Surgery in the Hand. St. Louis: CV Mosby, 1986, pp 491-500.

Bibliography

Bassett CAL, Carroll RE. Formation of tendon sheaths by silicone rod implants. J Bone Joint Surg 45A:884-885, 1963.

Hunter JM. Artificial tendons: Early development and application. Am J Surg 109:325-338, 1965.

Hunter JM, et al. Study of early sheath development using static nongliding implants. J Biomed Mater Res 5:155-161, 1974.

Hunter JM, et al. Sheath formation in response to limited active gliding implants (animals). J Biomed Mater Res 5:155-161, 1974.

Hunter JM. Staged flexor tendon reconstruction. J Hand Surg 8:789-793, 1983.

Malerich MM, Baird RA, McMaster W, et al. Permissible limits of flexor digitorum profundus tendon advancement: An anatomic study. J Hand Surg 12A:30-33, 1987.

Salisbury RE, et al. Tendon sheath reconstruction with artificial implants: A study of ultrastructure. In American Academy of Orthopaedic Surgeons: Symposium on Flexor Tendon Surgery in the Hand. St. Louis: CV Mosby, 1975, pp 59-65.

Urbaniak JR, Goldner JL. Laceration of the flexor pollicis longus tendon: Delayed repair by advancement, free graft or direct suture. J Bone Joint Surg 55A:1123-1148, 1973.

Wagner CJ. Delayed advancement in the repair of lacerated flexor profundus tendons. J Bone Joint Surg 40:1241-1244, 1958.

40

Secondary Surgery Following Digit Replantation

William C. Lineaweaver, M.D.

Reoperative Problems

Soft tissue loss	Poor sensation
Skeletal nonunion or deformity	Joint contracture
Soft tissue contraction	Tendon adhesion and rupture

Replantation of amputated digits is probably the single most common clinical application of microsurgery.[1,2] The rate of successful replantation has steadily improved from <50% in early reports to >90% in more recent reviews.[3,4] By the 1980s clinicians realized that a digit that survived following replantation was not necessarily functional, and the reported incidence of secondary surgery to improve replanted digit function increased[5-11] (Table 40-1). Reports of finger replantation yield widely varying statistics regarding postreplantation surgery. In a series from Scott et al.[7] that included all levels of finger amputation, up to 80% of patients underwent a secondary operation. ***However, fingers replanted distal to the superficialis tendon insertion rarely require further reconstruction.***[8-12] Table 40-1 summarizes data collected on 482 replantation patients, 30% of whom underwent secondary surgery. A total of 283 reconstructive operations were performed, an average of nearly two operations per reoperated patient.

Table 40-1 Incidence of Secondary Surgery Following Successful Digit Replantation

Author	*No. of Patients*	*No. of Secondary Procedures*	*No. of Patients Having Secondary Surgery*
Morrison et al.[5] (1977)	100	22	14 (14%)
Schlenker et al.[6] (1980)	64	20	12 (19%)
Scott et al.[7] (1981)	38	53	30 (80%)
May et al.[8] (1982)	18	1	1 (6%)
Pitzler et al.[9] (1982)	106	104	49 (46%)
Meyer[10] (1985)	105	57	24 (23%)
Urbaniak et al.[11] (1985)	51	26	15 (27%)
TOTAL	482	283*	145 (30%)

*1.95 procedures per patient undergoing secondary surgery.

Table 40-2 Incidence of Various Types of Postreplantation Surgery

Author	*No. of Procedures*	*Skin*	*Skeleton*	*Nerve*	*Joint*	*Tendon*	*Amputation*
Schlenker et al.[6] (1980)	20	3	2	3	2	9	1
Scott et al.[7] (1981)	53	7	1	5	13	25	0
May et al.[8] (1982)	1	1	0	0	0	0	0
Pitzler et al.[9] (1982)	104	27	9	20	18	30	0
Meyer[10] (1985)	57	13	7	11	6	20	0
Urbaniak et al.[11] (1985)	26	0	4	2	9	9	2
Tamai[13] (1982)	98	24	18	13	20	23	0
Steichen[14] (1987)	55	0	0	0	19	36	0
TOTAL	414	75 (18%)	41 (10%)	54 (13%)	87 (21%)	152 (37%)	3 (1%)
Davies Medical Center (1990)	140	24 (18%)	7 (15%)	15 (11%)	42 (30%)	48 (34%)	3 (2%)

The types of secondary operations itemized in Table 40-2 include tendon surgery (which accounts for 37% of the total); reconstruction of skin, bone, nerve, and joint (each accounts for 10% to 20% of the total); and amputation (rare).[6-11,13] These cases include only procedures done on successfully replanted digits and do not include debridements and acute revascularizations.[14] At the Davies Medical Center (DMC) secondary reconstructive operations on replanted digits constitute over 10% of the annual surgical case load, and over 100 such cases have been performed each year since 1985.[15] Although some useful progress has been made in establishing a complex data base of elective transplant patients,[16] the many variables of replantation surgery and its consequences make specific calculation of the incidence of secondary surgery an elusive task. For example, the DMC unit performs approximately 110 primary replantation operations per year,[17] but the incidence of patients having secondary surgery cannot be determined until the clinical data are sufficiently organized to sort out patients who underwent multiple secondary procedures.

The literature contains only a few reports of studies describing results of post-replantation surgery. Steichen[14] and Jupiter et al.[18] have documented significant improvement in total range of motion in replanted fingers following tenolysis, and our unit at DMC has reported successful secondary skeletal stabilization following nonunion or malrotation of the replanted fingers.[19]

Digit replantation is creating a large population of patients who undergo secondary reconstructive surgery. The detailed work of clearly defining the incidence and results of such surgery remains to be done.

Relationship Between Primary Replantation Surgery and Secondary Surgery

As the incidence of secondary surgery of replanted digits increases, it becomes imperative that the surgeon discuss this probability as part of the initial presentation of replantation to patients referred for emergency treatment of amputation. Most of these patients (except those with distal replantation[8-12]) face an approximately 30% to 50% chance of needing one or more later operations to achieve useful function in their replanted fingers. Some patients, especially those with single finger amputations, may decide to go on to complete amputation. Patients who decide to undergo replantation will enter their recuperation and therapy with some realistic expectations about their future. They will be able to discuss with surgeons, therapists, and fellow patients the details of possible future surgery and its consequent recovery time. When these patients come to secondary surgery, they are generally well informed, realistic, and motivated.

When postreplantation surgery is being planned, it is necessary to have clear, detailed records of the original replantation procedure. I generally perform digit replantation with Kirschner wire skeletal fixation, repair of a single flexor tendon, single arterial and venous anastomoses, and primary repair of the digital nerves and extensor tendon.[20,21] Unusual components, such as a vein graft crossing over a flexor tendon, must be clearly recorded to prevent their damage during reoperation, and knowledge of the location of arterial repairs can influence incision placement. ***Before secondary surgery is performed on a replanted digit, the details of the replant surgery and any subsequent procedures should be outlined and the summary used to plan the later procedure*** (see box).

I usually do not attempt to accomplish or initiate secondary procedures at the time of replantation. The risk of infection is such that I believe it is unwise to place silicone joints or tendon rods in severed digits at the time of replantation. However, Scott et al.[7] have reported anecdotal success with immediate prosthetic placements. As more experience is reported, the feasibility of these maneuvers may become more established. ***Nerve grafting should not be performed at the time of replantation since the true extent of nerve injury and the viability of the replanted digit are usually too uncertain to justify the expense of donor nerve.[22] However, vein conduits may be used to bridge short nerve gaps in digital nerves,[23,24] particularly when vein grafts were already harvested to repair vascular defects.*** Measurable sensation may develop in some cases, but even if no sensation develops, the vein graft could help to mobilize the margin of the nerve defect for later grafting.

SELECTION OF PATIENTS AND TIMING OF SECONDARY SURGERY

Postreplantation reconstruction is an excellent example of surgery as "an interpretive activity," a concept used by K.M. Hunter to describe the integration of medical technology into the verbalized goals of the patient.

> Medicine is an interpretive activity, a learned inquiry that begins with the understanding of the patient and ends in therapeutic action on the patient's behalf. Far from being objective . . . medicine is grounded in subjective knowledge . . . [of] the physician's understanding of the particular patient. Physicians need not only an encyclopedic, Sherlock Holmes–like knowledge of clinical cases but also a sense of the life stories in which illness and medical care take place.[25]

When planning postreplantation surgery, the patient and the surgeon need to have a clear understanding of each other's anticipated outcome of the procedure. The patient proceeds from a general desire "to have my finger back to normal" to statements of functional goals, such as "I need a better grip on the steering wheel"; "My hand needs to be flatter to work in close spaces"; "I have to find a way to keep from cutting my finger at work" and specific structural proposals, such as, "I need more flexion in the last joint of my thumb"; "The middle joints of my fingers should straighten out more"; "I need better sensation on the outside of my little finger." Responding to the patient, the surgeon can then move from general technical planning to specific connections between the patient's detailed goals and possible surgical procedures; for example, "Breaking up scar around

Surgical Summary

Injury

Amputation of index, middle, and ring fingers of right hand

Replantation Surgery

Index
- Kirschner wire, proximal phalanx
- Repair, UDA
- Repair, UDN
- Tag, RDN (2 cm gap)
- Repair, FDP
- Resection, FDS
- Repair, extensor
- Repair, two dorsal veins

Middle
- Kirschner wire fusion, PIPJ
- Vein graft, UDA to distal RDA
- Repair UDN
- Vein graft interposition, RDN (1 cm)
- Repair FDP
- Resection FDS
- Debridement, extensor

Ring
- Fusion DIPJ with Kirschner wires
- Repair RDN
- Repair UDN, RDN
- Repair FDP and extensor

Secondary Surgery (5 Months Postoperative)

Sural nerve grafts to RDN, index finger and to RDN, middle finger

Current Defects (Proposed Surgery)

Index
- Deficit: Flexion contracture, PIPJ, flexion deficit
- Planned operation: PIPJ capsulotomy, tenolysis of flexor, possible tendon rod
- Comment: Note position of previous arterial repair and nerve grafts during dissection.

Middle
- Deficit: Fused PIPJ
- Planned operation: Silicone PIPJ arthroplasty, extensor tendon reconstruction
- Comment: If extensor tendon remnants are unfavorable, consider delayed reconstruction with rod placement. If flexor tenolysis is necessary later, note cross-over vein graft.

DIPJ: distal interphalangeal joint; FDP: flexor digitorum profundis; FDS: flexor digitorum superficialis; PIPJ: proximal interphalangeal joints; RDA: radial digital artery; RDN: radial digital nerve; UDA: ulnar digital artery; UDN: ulnar digital nerve.

the flexor tendon could improve your thumb function"; "Scar releases of the skin and joint capsule should help straighten your finger, but scar releases of your flexor tendon may be also necessary later"; "A nerve graft could really improve the sensation in your little finger." The patient should also make realistic plans for convalescence and therapy based on information given by the surgeon, the therapist, and fellow patients, and the patient's postoperative demands should be coordinated with occupational and vocational rehabilitation requirements. This level of precise communication and planning must be established before proceeding with complicated postreplantation surgery.

At each stable stage of the reconstruction process the patient and surgeon should reevaluate the patient's level of function. Further pursuit of finer function should be performed only if the patient's expectations and the surgeon's confidence in an improved result remain realistic. These decisions should be made with the realization that there is a small but real chance of loss of the replanted finger following repeated surgery. Rarely, postreplantation procedures may be complicated by substantial necrosis of the replanted finger and amputation. This possibility should be discussed frankly with each patient considering such surgery.

The timing of reconstructive surgery is primarily determined by the course of the finger in therapy. For initial secondary surgery it is best to wait until returning nerve, joint, and tendon function are stable and the skin of the finger is supple. Generally this plateau occurs 4 to 6 months following replantation. However, skeletal nonunion or angulation that interferes with therapy and function should be corrected as soon as it is recognized.[19]

PRIORITIES AND PLANNING FOR SECONDARY SURGERY

The different categories of secondary surgery have definite relationships to each other. These relationships determine the order in which the procedures should be performed. These relationships can be defined by the preoperative and postoperative conditions necessary to promote the success of the planned procedure (Table 40-3). After replantation, stable skin coverage is necessary before any further reconstruction can take place. Skeletal stabilization and alignment are the next priorities, and these procedures can sometimes be performed at the same time that the skin is reconstructed. The postoperative immobilization necessary after major skin and skeletal procedures makes it unwise to perform tenolysis at the same time. Nerve grafting and secondary nerve repairs can be performed at the same time as skin and skeletal reconstruction as long as the dissection for exposure is not too extensive, but the immobilization necessary following nerve repairs again makes tenolysis inappropriate at this time. Joint reconstruction,

Table 40-3 Preconditions and Postoperative Requirements for Postreplantation Reconstruction

Secondary Reconstruction	*Necessary Preconditions*	*Postoperative Requirements*
Skin	Viable replanted finger	Immobilization, edema control
Skeleton	Stable skin cover	Immobilization, edema control
Nerve	Stable skin and skeletal structures	Immobilization
Joint	Skin and skeletal stability, protective and proprioceptive sensation	Passive and active mobilization
Tendon	Skin and skeletal stability, protective and proprioceptive sensation, supple joints	Active and/or passive mobilization

either by capsulotomy or arthroplasty, requires skin coverage, skeletal stability, and protective and proprioceptive sensation to maximize the chance for a functional success. Finally, tendon reconstruction, including grafting, tenolysis, and transfer are best done after joint reconstruction (and its preconditions) have been completed.

Each step in the reconstructive sequence should be explained to the patient to ensure that the goals of the operation are specific and clear. It is also advisable to plan sequences of surgery to avoid operating on both sides of a replanted finger at one time. An example of a combination to avoid is placing a Silastic implant into a proximal interphalangeal joint through a dorsal approach and simultaneously performing a flexor tenolysis through a volar incision. Such extensive dissections can result in excessive swelling, marginal necrosis of the incision, and cellulitis. ***Finally, the planned operation should be discussed with the patient's hand therapist to ensure that a therapy plan is prepared and to confirm that no postoperative therapy requirements of a multicomponent operation are mutually incompatible.***

SECONDARY SURGICAL PROCEDURES

Most of the aspects of reconstructive surgery unique to replanted digits concern patient selection and the timing of procedures. The operations themselves generally do not vary greatly from descriptions available in current hand surgery texts.[26,27] The following discussion reviews the most frequently performed operations and points out special considerations relevant to replanted fingers.

Skin Reconstruction

Skin Grafting to Repair Small Defects

Most replanted digits develop small areas of marginal suture line necrosis that heal spontaneously with local care. If the patient develops an eschar or an open, granulating wound >1 cm^2, skin grafting should be considered, especially if allowing the wound to heal secondarily might cause a contracture that could compromise a joint or web space. Small full-thickness skin grafts that are carefully defatted into the dermal layer are convenient solutions to this coverage problem, and they may undergo less contraction with time than split-thickness grafts.[28]

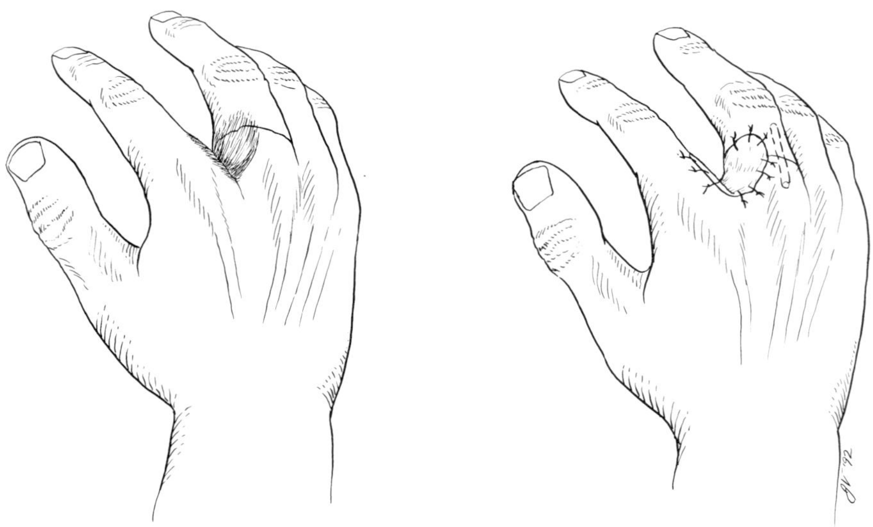

An example of acute skin loss following replantation is this eschar involving the second web space and middle finger. The damaged skin is excised and a full-thickness skin graft is taken from the wrist or groin area and carefully fixed to the contour of the defect with 5-0 or 6-0 chromic sutures. The sutures are carefully placed to avoid any underlying microvascular repair. The patient can resume digit motion according to postreplantation therapy guidelines[29] within 3 to 4 days.

Web Space Releases

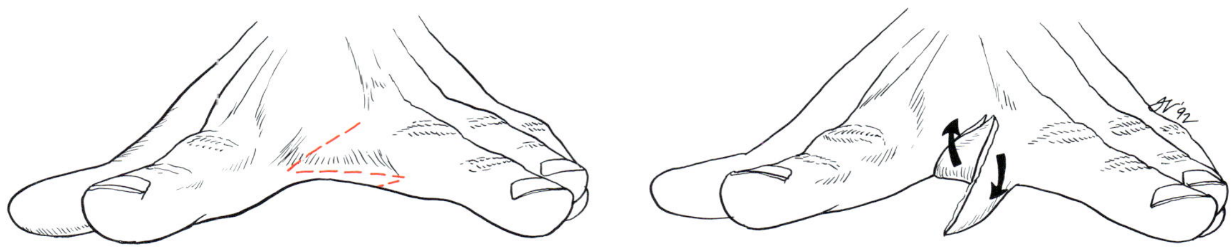

Web space scarring and contractures are common between adjacent replanted fingers with amputation levels just distal to the web space. In a patient with supple dorsal and volar skin and a small contracture, a Z-plasty is performed in the web space. Transposition of the flaps releases the contracture.

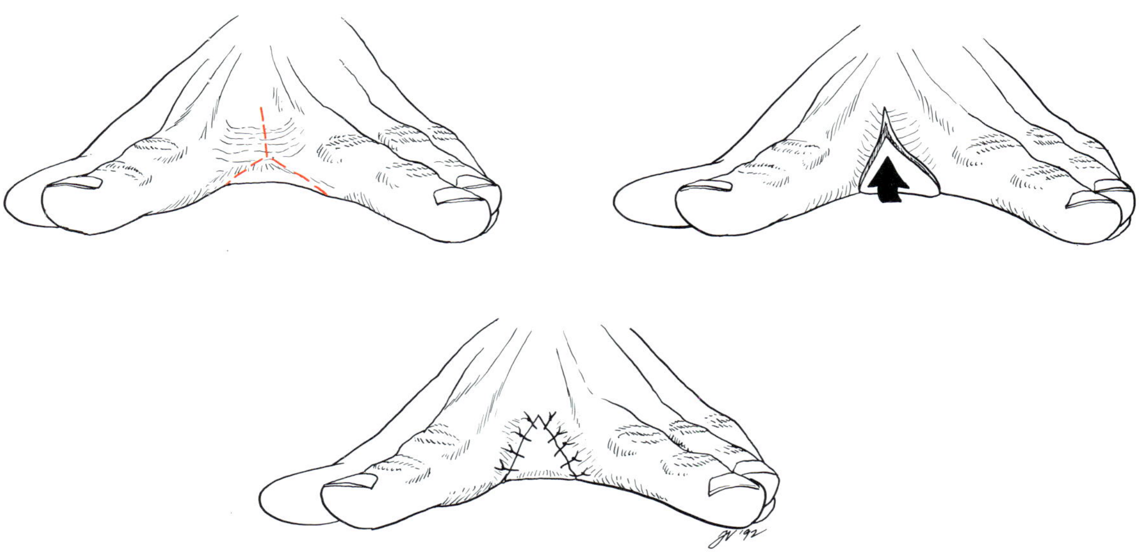

Large contractures or contractures with only one adjacent plane of supple skin are released with a Y-V advancement flap technique, using the supple skin for the flap. Small triangles excised at the base of the flap permit primary closure. However, if dense scarring is present and there is insufficient adjacent skin for local flaps, the scar tissue is excised and the web space resurfaced with a full-thickness skin graft.

Correction of Volar Joint Contractures

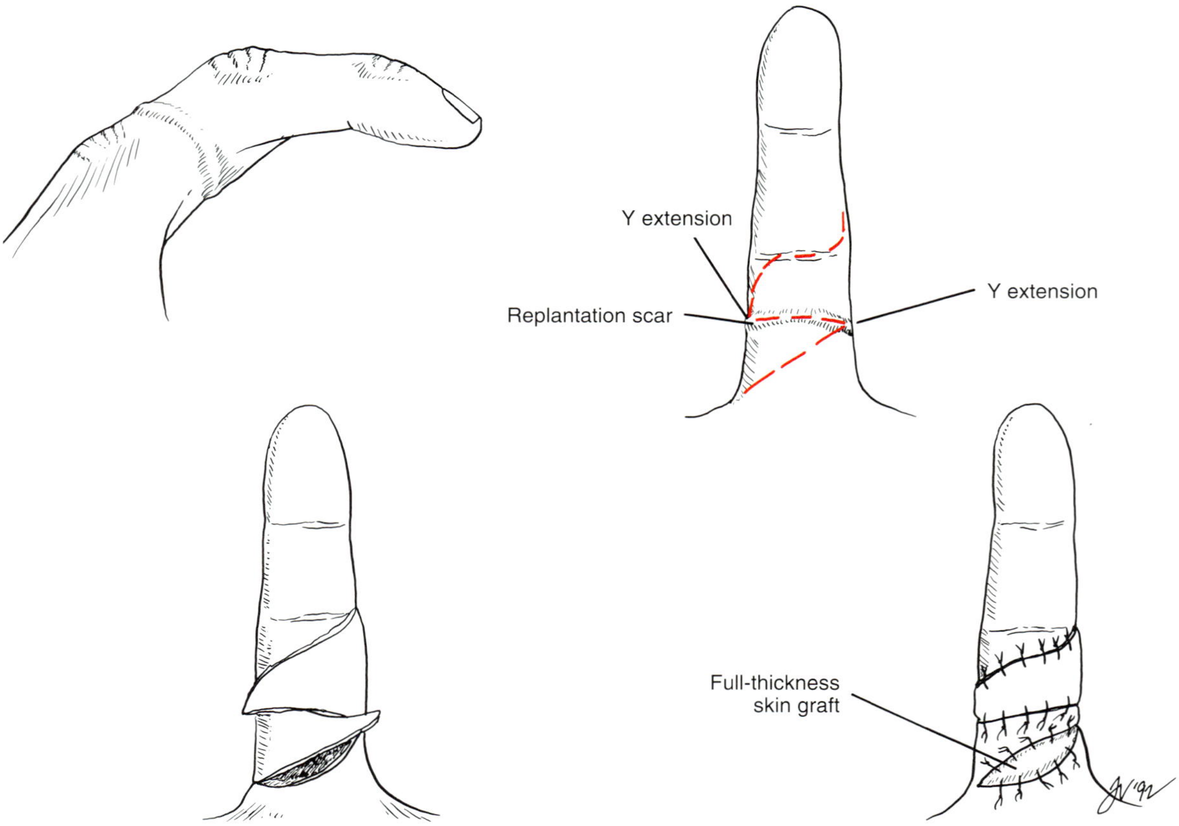

Skin contractures can complicate flexion contractures, and this deformity occurs most frequently at the proximal interphalangeal joint. In releasing such a contracture, the surgeon should incorporate the replantation scar into a Bruner-type incision as illustrated. The incision defines the flaps, which are elevated, permitting underlying capsulotomy as necessary. Y extensions are then made at each V of the skin incision, thereby releasing the skin contracture. The skin flaps are then advanced into the opened limbs of the Y extensions, covering the volar joint surface with intact skin and subcutaneous tissue. This advancement will usually leave an open area proximal to the flaps. This open area will leave sufficient subcutaneous tissue to permit coverage with a full-thickness skin graft that will not interfere significantly with postoperative mobilization.

Skeletal Reconstruction

Secondary skeletal procedures should be performed only after the establishment of stable skin coverage.

Repair of Nonunion

At DMC, skeletal fixation of most replanted fingers is accomplished with crossed Kirschner wires. As many as 11% of these fingers eventually require later skeletal surgery for nonunion or malrotation.[19] Nonunion is usually immediately evident after Kirschner wire removal 4 to 8 weeks after replantation. Sometimes the nonunion will heal with splinting, but it may be best to operate on these failures as they are recognized to reduce splinting time and facilitate therapy.

The nonunion is approached through a dorsal skin incision made over the area of the defect and the extensor tendon is split with a longitudinal incision. Dorsal vein repairs cannot always be spared by this approach, but if the dissection is not extended to the volar surface of the finger, no vascular embarrassment should occur. After the nonunion is opened, all fibrous tissue, bone irregularities, and nonviable bone are removed. Both the extensor and flexor tendons are carefully inspected to ensure that a traumatic flap of tendon tissue has not intruded between the bone margins. Any such flaps are debrided when noted. If solid, well-matched bone ends can be fashioned, another set of Kirschner wires can be used for fixation if they can be placed without crossing a joint. Otherwise, a small plate or an interosseous wire is used.

Bone Grafts

If resection of a nonunion will result in unacceptable shortening of a finger, a bone graft can be used to repair the defect caused by debridement of the nonunion. An example of bone graft reconstruction of a proximal phalangeal nonunion is illustrated.

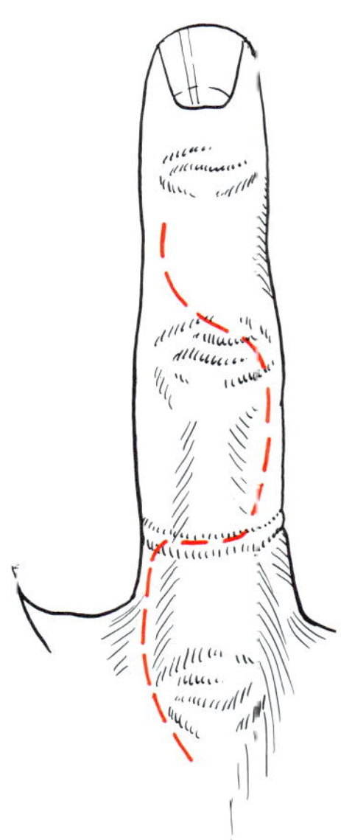

The replantation scar is incorporated into the S incision for maximum exposure.

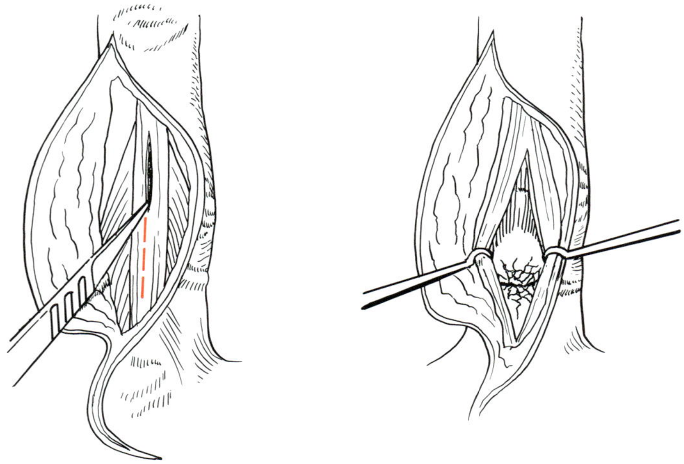

The extensor mechanism is incised longitudinally. After the phalanx is exposed, a fibrous nonunion with unstable fragmentation is revealed.

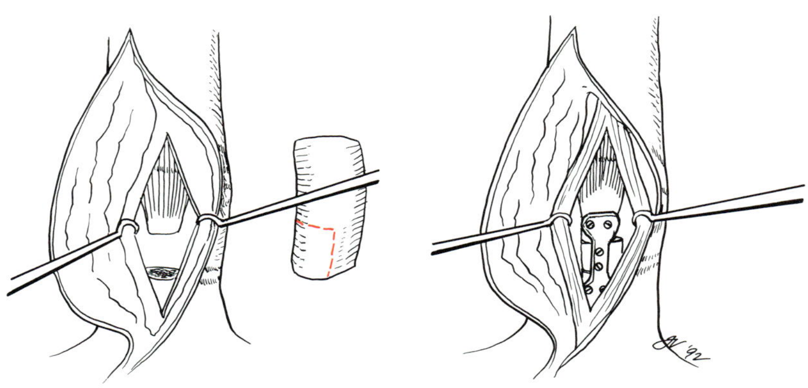

After debridement the defect is filled with bone graft material obtained from the fifth or sixth ribs. These grafts can be harvested through small incisions that heal well when closed with subcuticular sutures. Short rib segments readily lend themselves to shaping to obtain solid cortical contact in irregular defects. Fixation is obtained with a plate, Kirschner wires, or interosseous wires.

Correctional Osteotomies

Replanted fingers can develop either angular, rotational, or combination angular-rotational deformities. These defects can be corrected when the patient acquires sufficient sensation and motion to notice that the deformity interferes with the function of the digit. The unsatisfactorily healed fracture is exposed with a dorsal incision and the extensor tendon is split longitudinally as described above. The fracture is then incised with a side-cutting saw. An attempt can be made to cut out the angulation and to leave matched bone ends, but it may be best to make a simple incision and trim the bone ends until a proper fit is achieved. Rarely is so much bone lost that a graft is necessary. After the bone ends are realigned, satisfactory fixation can be obtained with either Kirschner wires or small plates; small plates seem to give a more precise realignment.

If the original fracture site appears too fragile to tolerate revision without fragmentation or if the soft tissue coverage over the fracture site is tenuous, it may be advisable to perform the correctional osteotomy proximal to the fracture on the same bone or even more proximally on an adjacent bone. For example, a rotational deformity of a proximal phalanx may be better aligned by rotating its metacarpal. However, such compensatory alignments should be observed closely, for even though complementary skeletal deformities may add up to a straight finger, angulations of tendon and joint structure may progress to mechanical defects with time.

Nerve Reconstruction

Nerve reconstruction should only be undertaken after stable skin coverage and stable skeletal structures have been established.

Positions of Neurovascular Bundles

■ ***In any reconstruction of neurovascular structures, flexor tendons, or volar joint structures in a replanted finger the surgeon must recognize that the neurovascular bundles of such fingers may be in unexpected positions.*** Bone shortening and disruption of the compartment formed by Grayson's and Cleland's ligaments can place the neurovascular bundles abnormally volar and bowstrung toward the middle of the finger. Digital nerves and arteries may develop differing degrees of dislocation. Dissection of the neurovascular bundles should begin well proximal to the level of replantation and each nerve and artery should be clearly identified. Certainly the original notes of the replantation must be reviewed to see if any unusual revascularization procedures were performed (e.g., vein grafts crossing the finger from one digital artery to another).

Vein Conduits

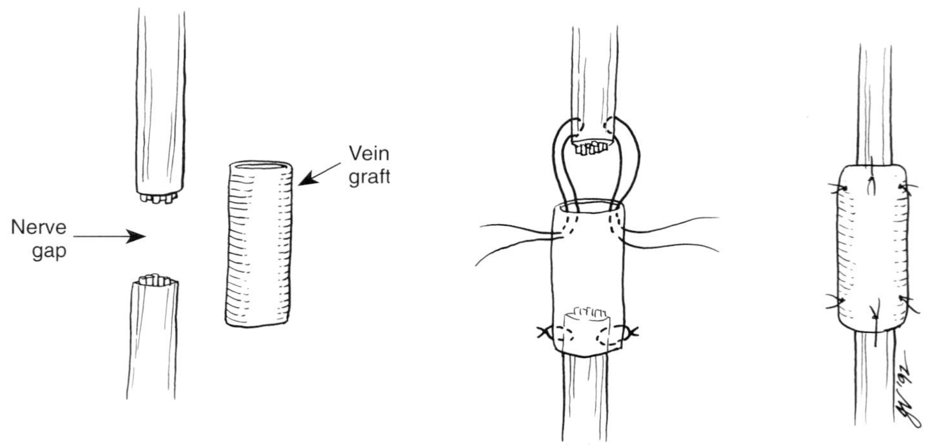

At the time of replantation, a vein graft already harvested for digital artery reconstruction can be used to bridge a small digital nerve gap of 3 cm or less. Sutures are placed, intussuscepting the nerve into the vein. Reinforcing sutures can be placed along the vein cuff.

Neurolysis

Poor but measurable sensation can be significantly improved by neurolysis of the digital nerves. This procedure can be performed simultaneously with flexor tenolysis, but the nerves should be carefully inspected to ensure that no nerve resection and reconstruction are required before the tenolysis is actually performed.

Neurectomy and Primary Repair

If the patient has very poor or no useful sensation and attempted neurolysis reveals waxy, scarred nerves with gross loss of any fascicular configuration or if neuroma in continuity is found, the grossly abnormal nerve should be resected under magnification until normal-appearing fascicles are revealed. If the nerve ends can be mobilized and primarily approximated at this point, it is reasonable to do so.

Nerve Grafts

Nerve grafts should be used when primary nerve gaps exist from the time of primary replantation or when significant lengths of damaged nerve have been resected in a secondary procedure. ***The dimension of the nerve defect should be clearly determined before the graft is harvested.***

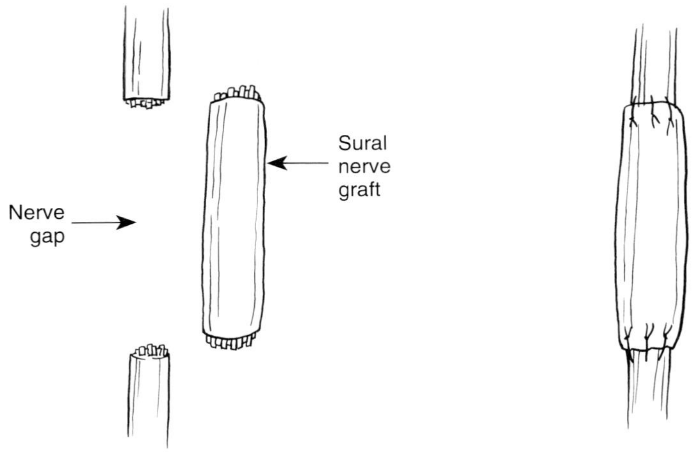

The sural nerve is a good source for nerve grafting since it is consistently larger than the digital nerves, allowing intussusception of both digital nerve ends.

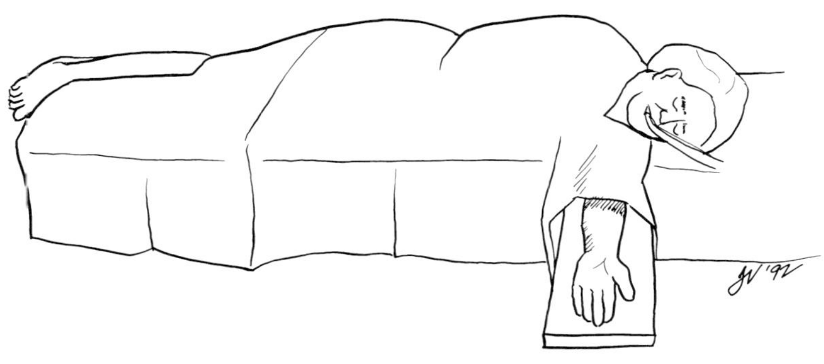

Positioning the patient on his or her side during the operation dramatically improves access to the sural nerve.

Rose et al.[30] have attempted to make a case for using vascularized nerve grafts in postreplantation surgery. Their clinical data, derived from a small and curiously designed study, do not compellingly warrant a decision to adopt this technique in the face of extensive experimental evidence indicating that vascularized nerve grafts have no long-term advantages over properly executed conventional grafting.[31]

Joint Reconstruction

Secondary reconstruction of joints in replanted fingers should be performed only after stable skin coverage, stable skeletal structures, and protective and proprioceptive sensation have been established.

Capsulotomy

After replantation, capsulotomies are performed almost exclusively on proximal interphalangeal joints. Distal interphalangeal joint stiffness is not reliably or usefully corrected by capsulotomy, and metacarpophalangeal joints rarely become stiff unless they are bound by adhesions of the extensor tendon. Direct crushing trauma to the dorsum of the metacarpophalangeal joint can cause true capsular scarring, which can be successfully released by incision.

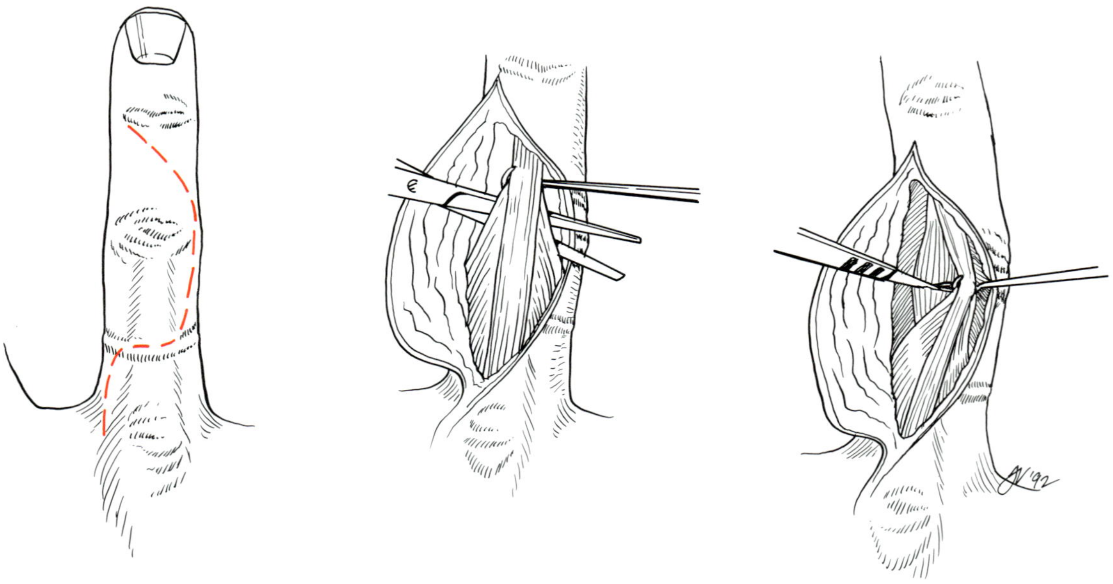

Dorsal capsulotomy requires wide exposure of the extensor mechanism and incision of the dorsal hemisphere of the joint capsule. The capsular incision should include both collateral ligaments. The extensor hood is completely mobilized. The extensor tenolysis may be extended proximally since the extensor mechanism often has adhesions involving the joint, the fracture site, the intrinsic slips, and the skin. All these sites must be inspected and any adhesions released. Intrinsic releases can be considered if scar excision does not relieve intrinsic tightness. The dorsum of the capsule is sharply incised.

In replanted fingers, I do not explore the flexor mechanism at the time of capsulotomy, as can be done in a simple finger injury.[32] If good passive flexion and active extension are not accompanied by active flexion, I reexplore the flexor mechanism after therapy has maximized the gains of the dorsal operation.

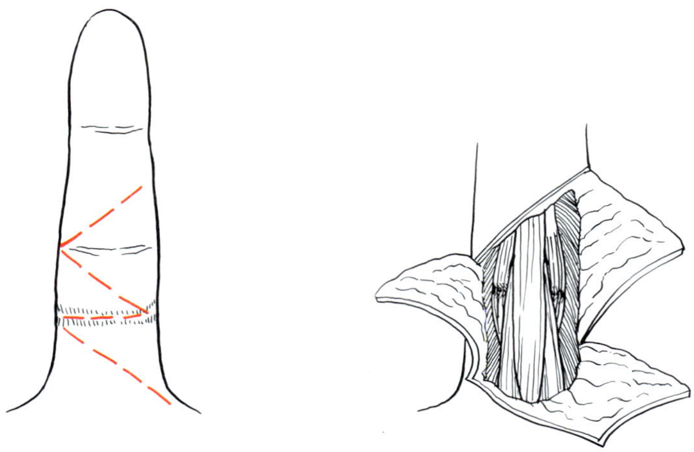

Flexion contractures are approached through a volar incision as illustrated. The replantation scar is incorporated into the zig-zag incision, which can be modified by Y-V flaps.[32] The likelihood of aberrant neurovascular structures must be considered, and wide exposure allows better identification of the digital arteries and nerves. Dissection is carried down to the flexor sheath, which is opened over the joint.

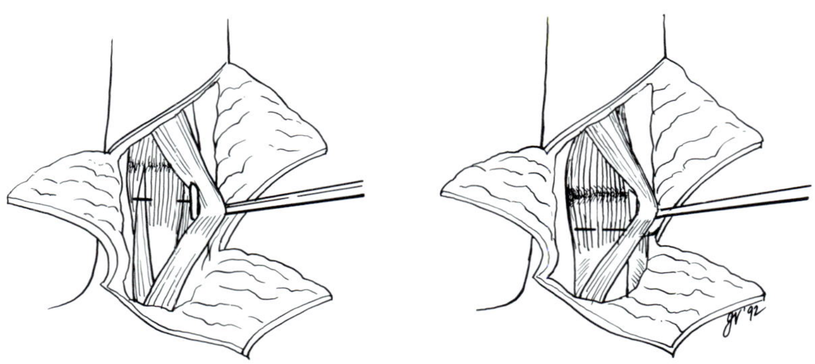

The profundus tendon is retracted, thus exposing the superficialis insertion. If the profundus tendon is contributing to the contracture or is not gliding, tenolysis is performed. If the superficialis remnant is contracted, it may be incised. The volar plate is usually diffusely thickened and the checkrein ligaments are often obscured. The volar plate should be incised at the level of the condyles of the proximal phalanx and the incision should be carried as laterally as necessary to permit joint extension. Postoperative therapy should include dorsal splinting to prevent hyperextension.

Arthrodesis

If flexion contractures of the interphalangeal joints of the thumb and the distal interphalangeal joints of the fingers cannot be corrected by tenolysis or, in the case of the thumb, after an attempt at capsulotomy, then arthrodesis should be performed. Amputation should be considered if the distal phalanx is insensate or if inadequate pulp is present. Arthrodesis is performed with a dorsal exposure, resection of the joint, and Kirschner wire fixation in about 10- to 15-degree flexion. This slight angulation seems to enhance pulp-to-pulp contact without producing any objectionably noticeable deformity.

Capsuloplasty

Individuals who have undergone replantation at the level of the proximal phalanx and have developed active extension and good passive range of motion at the proximal interphalangeal joint may have flexor tendon adhesions along with hyperextension of the proximal interphalangeal joint, possibly related to unopposed extensor tendon and intrinsic muscle action, therapy, and original injury.

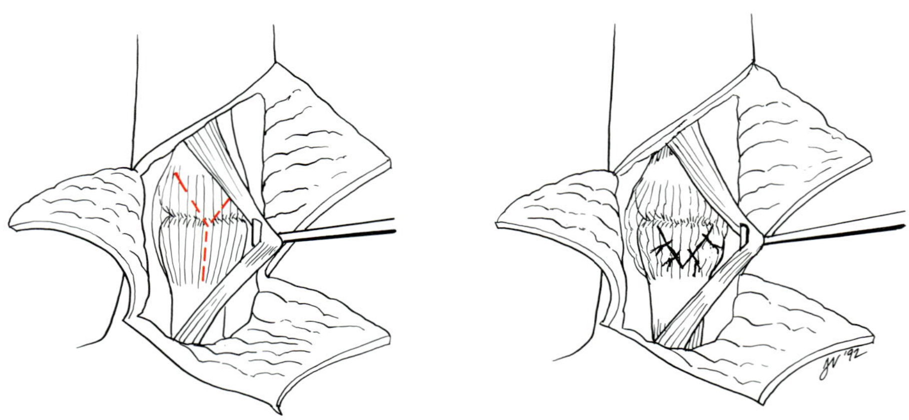

At the time of flexor tenolysis, exploration of the volar plate will show it to be stretched, allowing hyperextension. A Y flap is made on the volar plate. The Y flap is advanced to a V, thus shortening the volar plate and, in conjunction with a functioning flexor tendon and postoperative splinting, correcting the hyperextension.

Arthroplasty

Arthroplasty using silicone joint prostheses has produced functional results in metacarpophalangeal joints and proximal interphalangeal joints. The fingers treated with arthroplasties had joint injury at the time of amputation and underwent joint fusion with the replantation. Low-profile Silastic implants work well in these patients.[33] I avoid using implants that might adhere to bone and result in further bone shortening during later implant replacement. The standard Swanson implant technique can be used in these cases.[33] ***The surgeon must take special care to obtain good seating of the implant into the bone and secure recentering of the extensor mechanism since there is no dorsal capsule to close over the implant.***

Tendon Reconstruction

Tendon reconstruction should be performed only after successful and functional reconstruction of the skin, skeleton, nerves, and joints has been accomplished.

Flexor Tendons

Flexor tenolysis is probably the single most common postreplantation reconstructive operation performed at DMC (see Table 40-2) and the only one reported in any detail. Steichen[14] reported a significant improvement in total active range of motion following flexor tenolysis in 13 replanted fingers. Jupiter et al.[18] described a similar overall functional improvement following flexor tenolysis in 37 fingers, but could not document consistent improvement in four thumbs. Fingers replanted at DMC have only single flexor repairs, usually of the profundus tendon. Tenolysis is performed by incorporating the replantation scars into a Bruner zig-zag incision. Tenolysis is carried out (as necessary) from distal to the proximal interphalangeal joint to proximal to the metacarpophalangeal joint, preserving whenever possible the second annular pulley or its scarred remnant.

If the tendon is ruptured or appears hopelessly attenuated after tenolysis, then a silicone tendon rod is placed to establish a pseudosheath for later tendon grafting. Tendon rod and tendon graft procedures in replanted digits are generally the same as those for nonreplanted digits.[34-36] Generally, 2 to 4 mm diameter rods are used and the surgeon should choose the largest size that will permit secure tension-free skin closure.

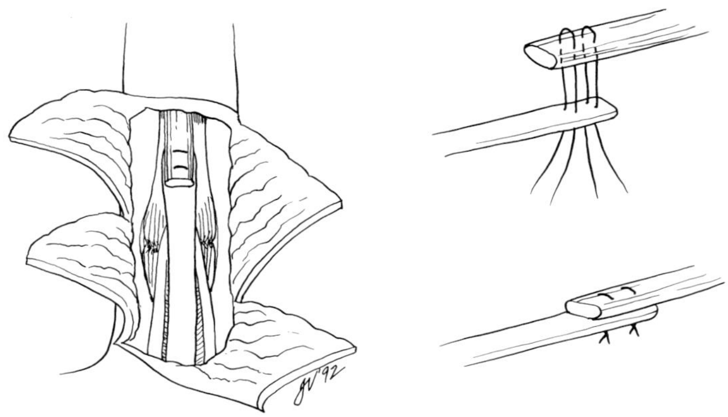

The rod is positioned beneath the flexor tendon distal to the proximal interphalangeal joint and is attached with nonabsorbable mattress sutures, taking care that the rod end is tucked beneath the tendon and the suture knots are beneath the rod. This arrangement prevents the edge of the rod or the suture knot from pushing through the sometimes thin overlying skin and initiating a disastrous infection. The proximal end of the rod is left free in the palmar space, if this area is unscarred, or in the flexor compartment of the wrist. The rods should be left in place for 10 to 12 weeks, until the overlying tissue regains suppleness, before placing the tendon grafts.

Extensor tenolysis and tendon grafting are performed with the same general approach. When placing the rod for extension reconstruction, the distal end should be sewn to the extensor hood of the proximal interphalangeal joint.

Pulley Reconstruction

The second annular pulley is often damaged by either the original amputation or later tenolysis. This defect can result in marked bowstringing of the flexor tendon and loss of flexor function.

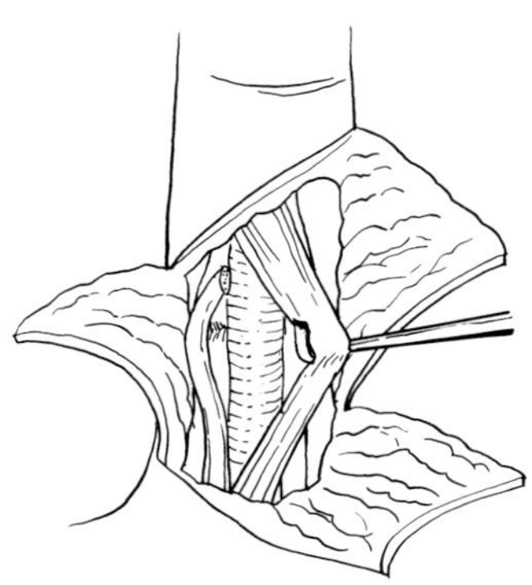

In the replanted finger, a portion of the superficialis insertion can be used to create a pulley attached to the proximal phalanx. A slip of the superficialis insertion is mobilized in the replanted finger.

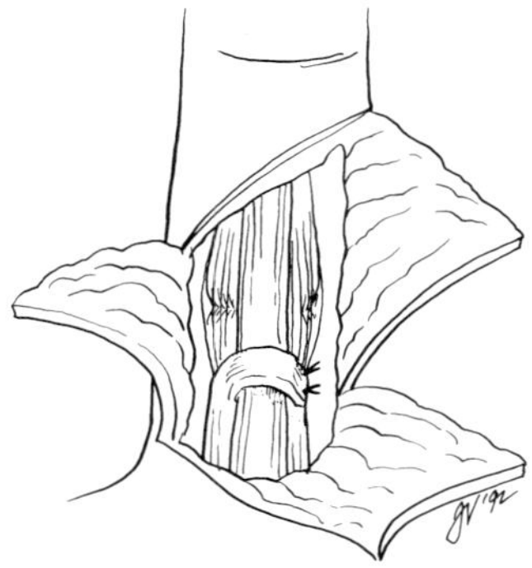

The slip is then sewn to the other border of the superficialis, creating a proximal phalangeal pulley for the profundus tendon.[34] This technique requires minimal dissection in addition to the exposure obtained for flexor tenolysis, volar capsulotomy, or rod placement.

Amputation

As noted in Table 40-2, amputation is performed on very few replanted digits. These fingers usually have a combination of sensory, joint, and tendon malfunction that renders them stiff and insensate. ***Amputation should be at least mentioned by the surgeon throughout the course of postreplantation reconstruction, and it should be seriously considered whenever the patient raises this option.*** Such amputations are performed just proximal to the most proximal stiff joint. Optimistically, I contend that the low incidence of late postreplant amputation is an indirect testimony to the functional status of most replanted fingers, although this contention has not been rigorously investigated.

HAND THERAPY

Hand therapists play a critical role in all aspects of care following digit replantation. At DMC, replantation patients are seen by our staff of hand therapists immediately after surgery and a comprehensive postoperative plan is developed, including initial splinting, injury-specific mobilization protocols, and arrangement of therapy sites convenient to the patient. After the patient is discharged, the therapist continues to monitor wound healing and functional progress.[29] This process provides the basis for identifying the need for later operations as well as the timing of future surgery.

The hand therapist also becomes immediately involved in postoperative management following subsequent reconstructive surgery. All skeletal and soft tissue reconstructions are splinted before the patient is discharged and appropriate mobilization for tendon and joint procedures is begun. After discharge the patient is followed closely in hand therapy to monitor progress and to note problems.

- ***Hand therapists implement the return to function restored by the replantation and reconstruction operations, and they generate the data by which the results of these procedures will eventually be judged.*** Innovations, such as continuous passive motion units, can only be safely introduced and evaluated within a comprehensive hand therapy program.

CASE EXAMPLES

Postreplantation reconstruction has a growing patient population and there are almost no data available for evaluating the results of these procedures. The few careful analyses of postreplantation tenolyses[4,18] need to be emulated and expanded to larger populations and other procedures. The surgical approaches described in this chapter reflect my own preference and empiric experience and should be considered a work in progress, performed in dim, emerging light. This situation is appropriately summarized by Peacock[37]: "Deductions based on lack of data are subject to sudden refutation when data become available." The following three cases, however, illustrate some details of my current approaches.

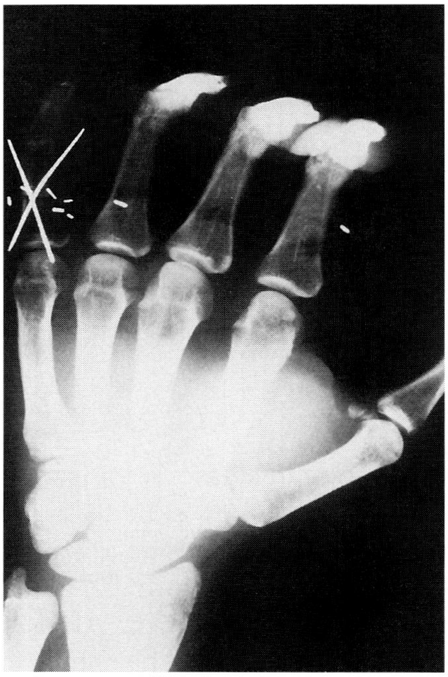

This x-ray film shows the replantation level of the little finger of a 28-year-old patient with a saw injury of his left hand. Emergency surgery consisted of full-thickness skin grafting of the thumb pulp; revascularization, flexor repair, and digital nerve repair of the index finger; ulnar digital nerve repair of the middle finger; digital nerve repair of the ring finger; and replantation of the little finger at the level of the midproximal phalanx.

Six months later, following good return of sensation and joint mobility, the patient underwent tenolysis and annular pulley reconstruction of the index and flexor tenolysis of the little finger. Local scar tissue was used to reconstruct the pulley. Two months later the flexor to the little finger ruptured and a tendon rod was inserted. A tendon graft was performed 12 weeks later.

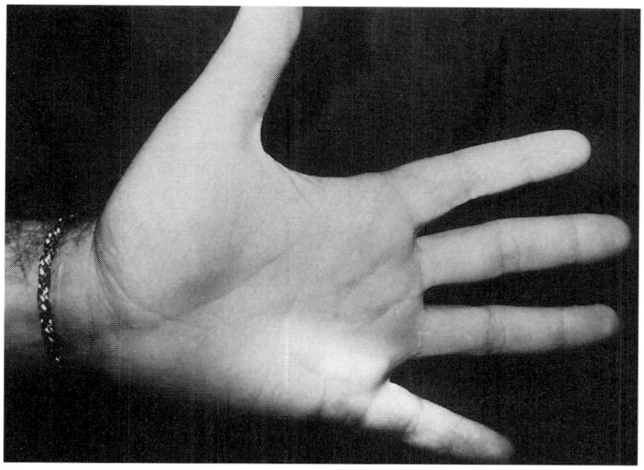

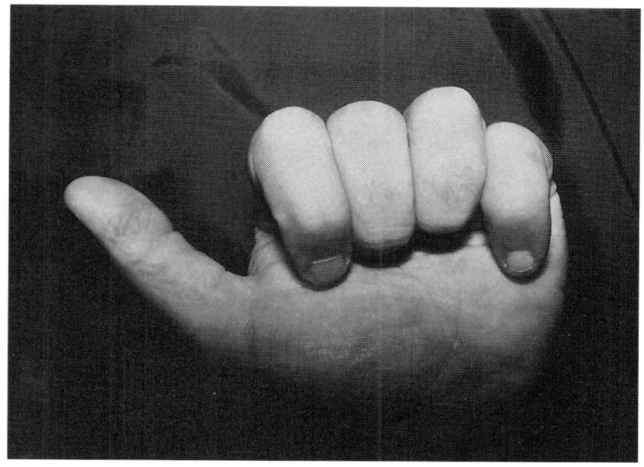

One year later the patient shows full extension and can flex all fingers to his palm. His total active range of motion is 210 degrees for the index finger and 150 degrees for the little finger.

■ ■ ■

When a 23-year-old man sustained a crush injury to his left hand, emergency surgery was performed to replant the index finger and revascularize the middle, ring, and little fingers, all at the level of the web spaces. Seven months later the patient underwent flexor tenolysis and flexion improved in all fingers except the middle finger. Fifteen months after his injury the patient complained of poor sensation of the middle and ring fingers, a contracture of his third web space, and lack of flexion of his middle finger. He underwent Z-plasty release for the web space, nerve grafting to previously unrepaired nerves to the middle and ring fingers, and placement of a flexor tendon rod from his middle finger to his palm. Postoperatively the middle finger was immobilized for 4 weeks; then passive range of motion exercises were started. Ten weeks after rod placement the patient underwent tendon grafting. A year after this procedure the distal phalanx of the index finger was fused due to persistent flexion deformity and volar capsulotomies were performed on the proximal interphalangeal joints of his middle and ring fingers. Sixteen months later, he again underwent proximal interphalangeal joint capsulotomies. One year postoperatively the patient had protective sensation in all fingers and was employed in engine rebuilding.

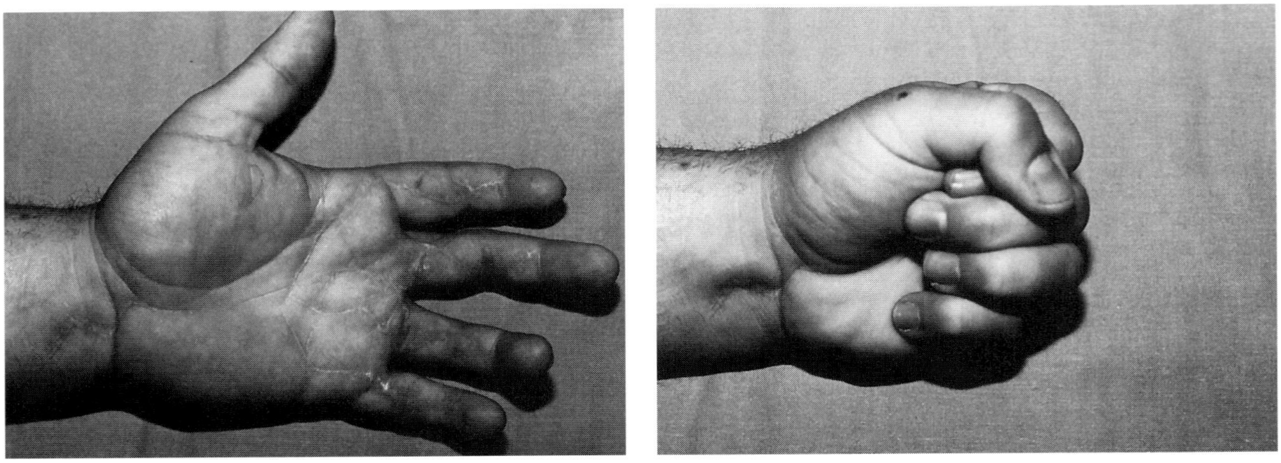

Full extension is still hampered by 20-degree flexion contractures of the proximal interphalangeal joints of the patient's middle and ring fingers. The patient's fused index finger is stable and he has active flexion to his palm.

▪ ▪ ▪

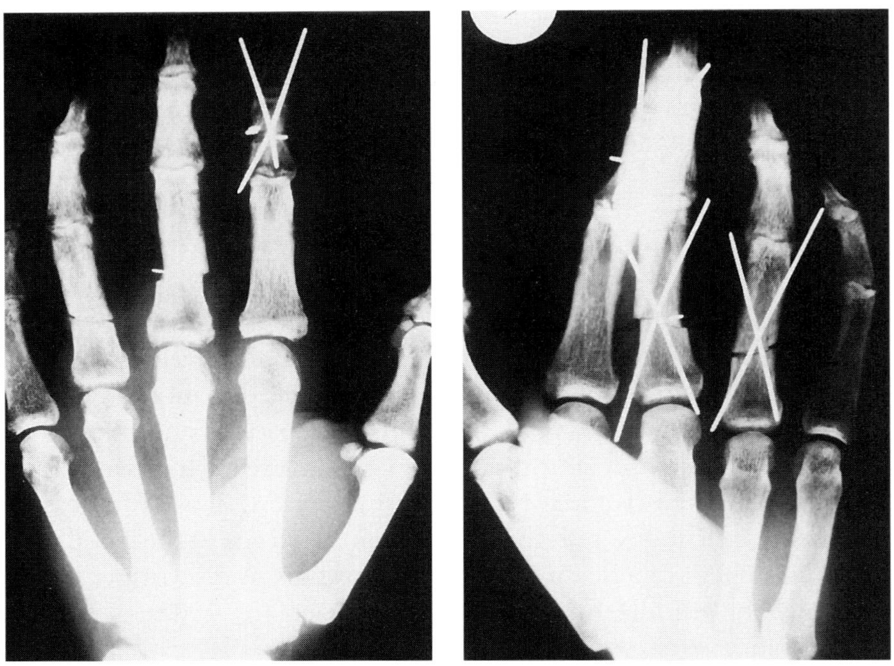

These x-ray films show the level of amputation of middle and ring fingers and the level of replantation of the index finger of a 31-year-old man. All fingers were replanted, the index finger at the level of the middle phalanx and the ring and middle fingers at the level of the midproximal phalanges. A proximal second level laceration required repair of the extensor hood and the metacarpophalangeal joint capsule of the index finger. Six months later with good return of sensation, an extensor tenolysis and metacarpophalangeal joint capsulotomy were performed on the index finger with good resultant fusion.

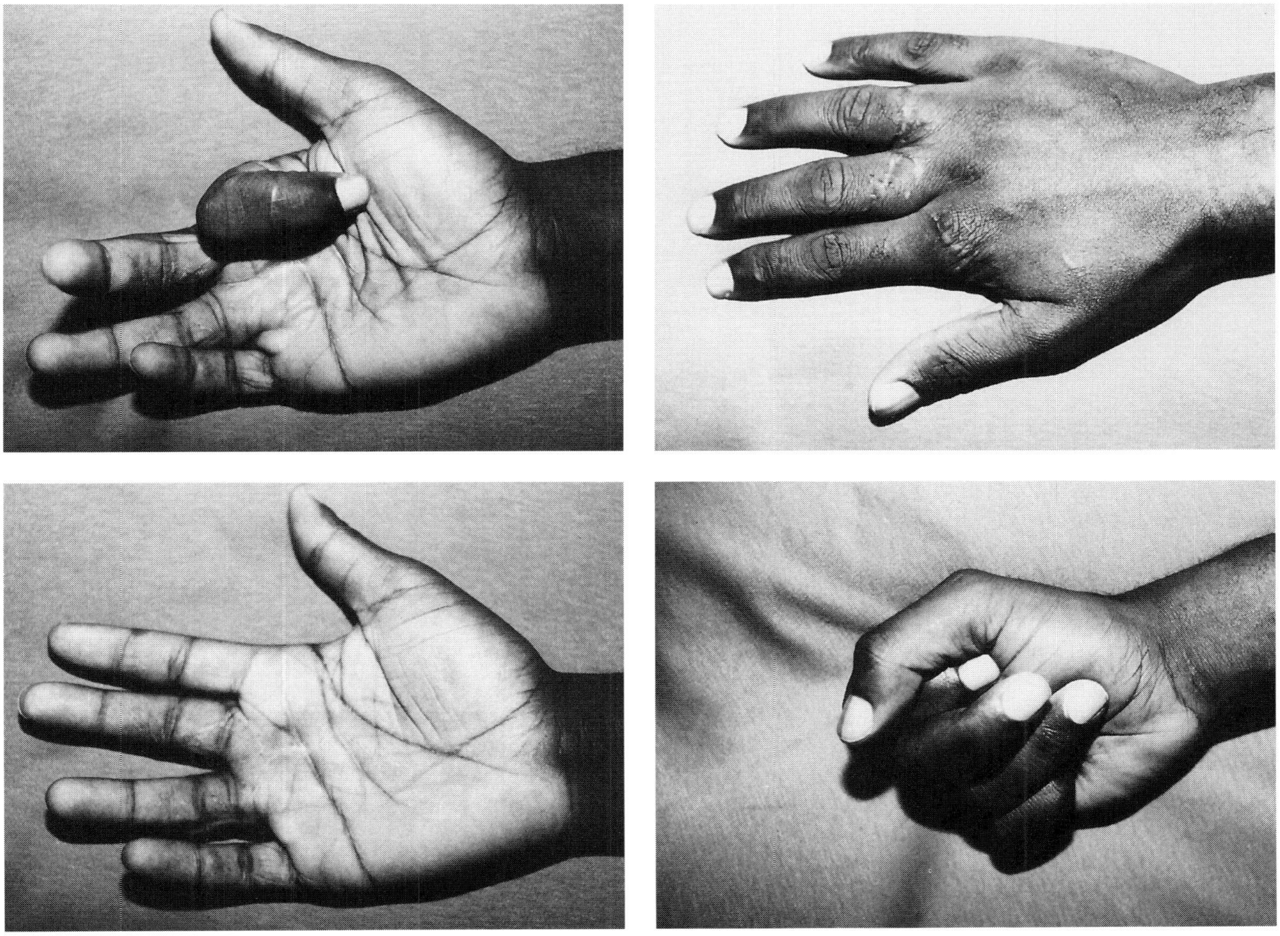

Three months later the patient underwent flexor tenolysis of the ring finger and placement of a tendon rod in his middle finger and palm. The rod was replaced with a graft 12 weeks later and a contracture of the third web space was relieved with a Y-V flap. Eighteen months later the patient has full extension, preservation of the web space, and flexion to his palm.

References

1. Biemer E, Duspiva W. Reconstructive Microvascular Surgery. Berlin: Springer-Verlag, 1982, p 97.
2. O'Hara M, Lineaweaver W. Microsurgical replantation: Development and current status. Crit Care Nurs Q 13:1, 1990.
3. Weiland AJ, Villareal-Rios A, Kleinert H, et al. Replantation of digits and hands. J Hand Surg 2:1, 1977.
4. Urbaniak JR. Digital replantation: A 12-year experience. In Urbaniak JR, ed. Microsurgery for Major Limb Reconstruction. St. Louis: Mosby, 1987, p 12.
5. Morrison WA, O'Brien B, MacLeod AM. Evaluation of digital replantation: A review of 100 cases. Orthop Clin North Am 8:295, 1977.
6. Schlenker JD, Kleinert HE, Tsai T. Methods and results of replantation following traumatic amputation of the thumb in sixty-four patients. J Hand Surg 5:63, 1980.
7. Scott FA, Howar JW, Boswick JA. Recovery of function following replantation and revascularization of amputated hand parts. J Trauma 21:204, 1981.
8. May JW, Toth BA, Gardner M. Digital replantation distal to the proximal interphalangeal joint. J Hand Surg 7:161, 1982.
9. Pitzler D, Buck-Gramcko D. Secondary operations after replantation. Ann Chir Gynaecol 71:19, 1982.
10. Meyer V. Upper Extremity Replantation. New York: Churchill Livingstone, 1985, p 96.
11. Urbaniak JR, Roth JH, Nunley JA, et al. The results of replantation after amputation of a single finger. J Bone Joint Surg 67A:611, 1985.
12. Foucher G, Henderson HR, Maneau M, et al. Distal digital replantation: One of the best indications for microsurgery. Int J Microsurg 3:253, 1981.
13. Tamai S. Twenty years' experience of limb replantation: Review of 293 upper extremity replants. J Hand Surg 7:549, 1982.
14. Steichen JB. Management of flexor tendon injury associated with digital replantation of revascularization. In Hunter JM, Schneider LH, Mackin E, eds. Tendon Surgery of the Hand. St. Louis: Mosby, 1987, p 156.
15. Buncke HJ, Whitney TM. Secondary reconstruction after replantation. In Buncke HJ, ed. Microsurgery: Transplantation-Replantation: An Atlas Text. Philadelphia: Lea and Febiger, 1991, p 651.
16. Lineaweaver W, Buncke HJ, Whitney TM, et al. Factors associated with microvascular flap failure and direction for research. Plast Surg Forum 12:252, 1989.
17. Buncke GM, O'Hara M, Siko P. Statistical evaluation of replant patients at Davies Medical Center. Crit Care Nurs Q 13:65, 1990.
18. Jupiter JB, Pess GM, Bour W. Results of flexor tendon tenolysis after replantation in the hand. J Hand Surg 14A:35, 1989.
19. Whitney TM, Lineaweaver W, Buncke HJ, et al. Clinical results of bony fixation methods in digital replantation. J Hand Surg 15A:328, 1990.
20. Buncke HJ, Whitney TM, Valauri F, et al. Replantation surgery. In Buncke HJ, ed. Microsurgery: Transplantation-Replantation: An Atlas Text. Philadelphia: Lea and Febiger, 1991, p 594.
21. Lineaweaver WC, Buncke GM, Alpert BS, et al. Pitfalls in replantation surgery. In Vistnes L, ed. Procedures in Plastic and Reconstructive Surgery. Boston: Little, Brown, 1991, p 699.
22. Mackinnon SE, Dellon AL. Surgery of the Peripheral Nerve. New York: Thieme Medical Publishers, 1988, p 108.
23. Chiu DT, Janecka I, Krizek TJ, et al. Autogenous vein graft as a conduit for nerve regeneration. Surgery 91:226, 1982.
24. Walton RL, Brown RE, Matory WE, et al. Autogenous vein repair of digital nerve defects in the finger: A retrospective clinical study. Plast Reconstr Surg 84:944, 1948.

25. Hunter KM. Doctors' Stories: The Narrative Structure of Medical Knowledge. Princeton: Princeton University Press, 1991, pp xx, xxiii.
26. Green DP. Operative Hand Surgery, vols 1 to 3, 2nd ed. New York: Churchill Livingstone, 1988.
27. Jupiter JB. Flynn's Hand Surgery, 4th ed. Baltimore: Williams & Wilkins, 1991.
28. Rudolph R, Ballantyne DL. Skin grafts. In McCarthy J, ed. Plastic Surgery. Philadelphia: WB Saunders, 1990, p 221.
29. Petrilli J, Milne E, Nugent K, et al. Hand therapy. In Buncke HJ, ed. Microsurgery: Transplantation-Replantation: An Atlas Text. Philadelphia: Lea and Febiger, 1991, p 748.
30. Rose EH, Kowalski TA, Norris MS. The reversed venous arterialized nerve graft in digital nerve reconstruction across scarred beds. Plast Reconstr Surg 83:593, 1989.
31. Millesi H. The current state of nerve microsurgery. In Reidiger D, Ehrenfeld M, eds. Microsurgical Tissue Transplantation. Chicago: Quintessence, 1989, p 159.
32. Watson HK, Turkeltaub SH. Stiff joints. In Green DP, ed. Operative Hand Surgery, vols 1 to 3, 2nd ed. New York: Churchill Livingstone, 1988, p 537.
33. Swanson AB, Swanson G. Flexible implant resection arthroplasty in the upper extremity. In Jupiter JB, ed. Flynn's Hand Surgery, 4th ed. Baltimore: Williams & Wilkins, 1991, p 342.
34. Schneider LH, Hunter JM. Flexor tendon: Late reconstruction. In Green DP, ed. Operative Hand Surgery, vols 1 to 3, 2nd ed. New York: Churchill Livingstone, 1988, p 1969.
35. Kleinert H, Smith RI, Pulvertaft RG. Flexor tendon grafting in the hand. In Jupiter JB, ed. Flynn's Hand Surgery, 4th ed. Baltimore: Williams & Wilkins, 1991, p 283.
36. Hunter JH, Aulicino PL. Salvage of scarred tendon systems using passive and active Hunter tendon implants. In Jupiter JB, ed. Flynn's Hand Surgery, 4th ed. Baltimore: Williams & Wilkins, 1991, p 300.
37. Peacock EE. Surgery of scars. In Serafin D, Georgiade NG, eds. Pediatric Plastic Surgery. St. Louis: Mosby, 1984, p 126.

41

Reoperative Surgery Following Excision and Grafting of Upper Extremity Burns

James C. Grotting, M.D., and F. Raymond Ortega, M.D.

Reoperative Problems

Unstable scars	Elbow contracture
Interdigital contracture	Axillary contracture
Wrist contracture	

The reconstruction of the burned upper extremity presents the surgeon with a difficult challenge. Reoperative surgery further intensifies this challenge. Primary excision and grafting of upper extremity burns will frequently result in acceptable function without additional correction. Yet certain deformities may develop secondarily that continue to restrict function. Although reoperative surgery is usually elective, it is often essential if maximum rehabilitation potential is to be achieved. The goals of primary and reoperative surgery of the burned upper extremity are usually the same: function restoration. Complications from primary surgery may be significant because of the functional problems that they create. Aesthetic corrections are secondary to the restoration of function.

Usually these patients are managed with a team approach by the surgeon, the patient and his family, and the occupational and physical therapists. The decision to operate on these patients is influenced by the functional requirements of the patient and the surgeon's ability to fulfill these requirements. If the patient is able to function well in his everyday life, particularly in his occupation, no surgery may be required. In older, debilitated patients with severe contractures, amputation occasionally may be the best option.

Usually by the time a patient becomes a candidate for reoperative surgery of a burned upper extremity, he has become acutely aware of the physical limitations that continue to restrict his ability to function normally. Accustomed to living with a certain amount of pain, this patient has a keen understanding of the hard work required to overcome the biologic forces that continue to work against him. In general, patients in this situation are willing partners in the planning of reoperative surgery. They will very specifically mention those functional problems that have the most significant effect on their daily lives. In this way a list of priorities can be established for the reconstructive plan.

In addition, the patient at this stage usually understands that there are no "miracle cures" to completely erase all of the scarring and persistent aesthetic deformities. Therefore an understanding of very reasonable expectations can be reached between the reoperative surgeon and the patient.

TIMING

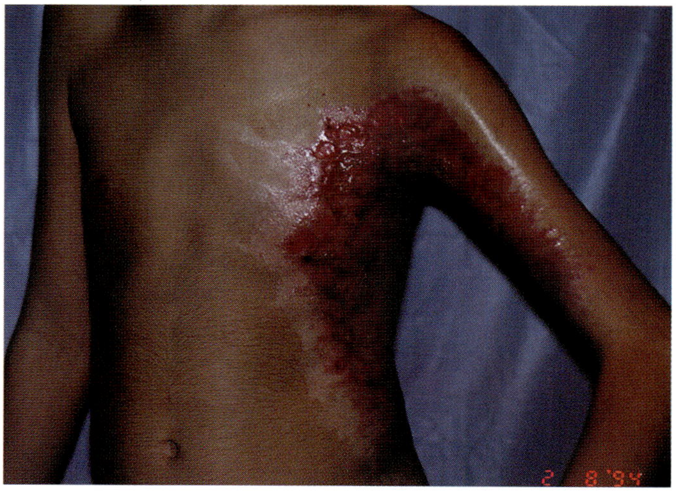

Immature scar 3 months after burn

- ***The timing of reoperative surgery for upper extremity burns is key in maximizing the functional result.*** Ideally this surgery is best performed in a mature scar. If reoperation is performed on tissue that is erythematous, hypertrophic, and edematous, such as in the patient shown above, one can anticipate that this very active scar response will limit the degree of contracture release and therefore compromise the end result. Therefore, if secondary corrections can be delayed for 6 months to 1 year, scar maturation will be much more favorable. The use of elastic garments may hasten scar maturation. The burn scars are observed at intervals until there is no further improvement and the patient is no longer gaining motion in physical therapy. ***When the skin is pale, soft, and pliable, the time for secondary surgery is ideal.***

Infrequently the reoperative surgeon will encounter a patient who would benefit from early contracture release, particularly in the neck, axilla, and elbow regions. In general, these patients received either head injuries or severe smoke inhalation injuries in association with their burns. They may have been comatose and unable to cooperate with any type of early physical therapy intervention. Donor sites may have limited the ability to excise and graft each of these areas so that healing by secondary intention has occurred, with resultant thick, hypertrophic scars. When such a patient is making no progress in therapy and is severely restricted functionally, early releases may be indicated with the understanding that it is likely that additional tertiary corrections may well be necessary even 9 months to 1 year later.

PATIENT EVALUATION

Patients referred for reoperative correction generally fall into two groups: those who have reached scar maturation with persistent burn scar contractures and those who are still gaining ground in therapy but in whom the burn scars remain immature and active. In the latter group, future corrections usually can be anticipated to some degree, but the patient is advised that it would be best if he would continue to work with the therapist until gains in motion have plateaued and scars have matured. Nevertheless, these patients can begin to develop an understanding of what possible corrections can be accomplished through secondary surgery. In the former group, several issues are important. The reoperative surgeon must know what type of employment to which the patient has either returned or intends to return following the completion of surgical treatment. It is uncommon that a patient with severely burned upper extremities is able to return to his former type of employment. Nevertheless, by this point in time the patient may well have developed an idea of the type of work that he desires or he may have been reassigned within his workplace. He may also have particular hobbies or vocations for which a particular functional range is needed. By discussing these issues, the patient and the surgeon can establish a list of priorities so as to address those problems that are most debilitating to the patient. In most cases, multiple problems exist simultaneously, so the reoperative plan must establish whether all can be addressed in a single operation or if staged procedures are necessary. If the patient has returned to work, the plan must be modified so time away from work can be minimized. For the patient who will not return to work until all surgery has been completed, it may be possible to do multiple procedures in fewer operations in the interest of speeding up the overall "downtime."

Contracture releases should be performed in a proximal to distal fashion. Unless the hand can be properly positioned in space, the hand is of little use to a patient. Therefore the release of axillary and elbow contractures may be necessary before a patient can even fully understand the limitations in the hand. When secondary deformities and contractures are present in both hands, it may be necessary to stage the procedures. The dominant or perhaps the least injured hand should be reconstructed first in order to provide a better intermediate level of function. Surgical planning should be designed so that following each operation the patient has an improved level of function. It is also essential that continued therapy to the unoperated portions of the upper extremity remains unrestricted.

The hand therapist or physical therapist should be involved in the surgical planning. Therapists may give valuable insight into how independently the patient is functioning at any given time. In addition, the ultimate goals of treatment may vary according to how the therapists can adapt the patient's environment for maximal independence.

Some patients may place limitations on the reoperative surgeon. Although surgical correction might be an option for certain deformities, these defects may be of little or no significance to the patient. On the other hand, certain deformities that might appear minimal to the reoperative surgeon could represent a major problem for patients involved in certain types of activities. Therefore, instead of developing a reconstructive plan that addresses every conceivable surgical possibility, the surgeon must carefully listen to the patient and compile a list of priorities according to what will maximally benefit that particular individual.

Certain general principles must be applied when developing a surgical plan. Even though burn scars may have maximally matured, the pliability of the ultimate coverage may vary greatly. Superficial burns may well have virtually normal skin elasticity, whereas certain thin grafted areas may be quite rigid. One can always assume that an incised graft or burn scar will retract to the point where reclosure may be difficult or impossible. Therefore additional grafts are commonly an important aspect of reoperative surgery in the burned upper extremity. Only when there is nearby unburned normal skin can one hope to divide or excise burn scar contractures and resurface using local flaps without additional grafts. One must assess how much surface area can be achieved from the mobilization or transposition of the nearby normal skin. Tissue expansion might even be a consideration. However, in most instances it will not be possible to totally excise upper extremity burns and resurface with nearby normal or expanded skin flaps. Therefore these local techniques are most valuable for covering the wrist, elbow, and axilla, particularly if release of the burn scar leaves the underlying vital structures at risk for exposure.

Certain patients may have been told at initial treatment that a plastic surgeon would be able to remove all of the burn scars later. Obviously this is only possible in very limited burned or grafted areas and cannot be accomplished without creating permanent scars. Realistic expectations by the patient will be helped by focusing on the importance of achieving maximum function of the upper extremity. Some patients may benefit by a discussion of makeup techniques and clothing, which can be used to cover permanent scars.

SURGICAL CONSIDERATIONS

Burn scar contractures are caused by the primary healing of burned tissue, improper splinting, or lack of adequate physical therapy. They result in the limitation of motion secondary to the loss of sufficient amounts of elastic skin across mobile joints.

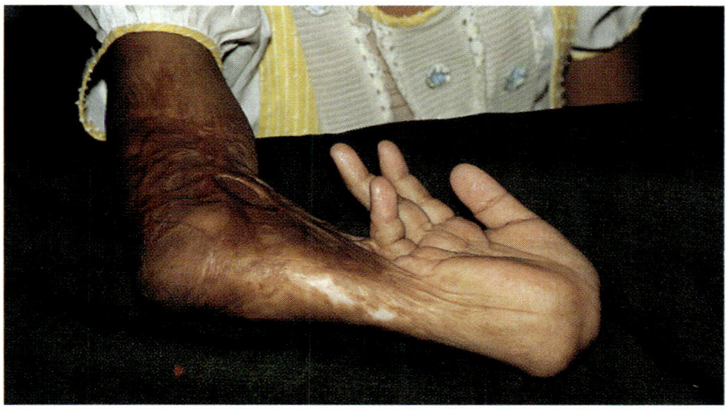

This Filipino child demonstrates the natural history of a burned wrist and hand that has not been treated. Complete dislocation of the wrist has occurred as a result of inexorable scar contracture. Wound contraction is a natural consequence of healing. Contractures of soft tissue and joints can occur even in spite of adequate excision and grafting of burn scars with proper splinting and therapy.

As in virtually all types of reconstructive plastic surgery, the simplest modality that will correct the problem is usually the best. If the contracture consists only of a tight band that is narrow and surrounded by normal skin, a simple excision of the band and Z-plasty is all that is required. However, often a contracture band will be surrounded by burned skin, in which case transposition of the flaps will yield an unclosable donor site. Therefore Z-plasties often must be supplemented with additional skin grafts.

Large Z-plasties are often helpful in designing coverage for the contracted axilla and elbow. However, only rarely can these types of Z-plasties be transposed and closed with adequate contracture release.

The anticipated recipient bed usually dictates the surgical plan. If release of the contracture will most likely result in exposed tendons or other vital structures, the transfer of a local or distant flap is indicated. Similarly, if exposed tendons are anticipated or if tendon transfers are planned, flap coverage is essential to create an environment for gliding structures.

Skin grafts virtually always play a major role in reoperative surgery in the burned upper extremity. Usually donor sites are readily available, even in the patient who had extensive excision and grafting of primary burns. We prefer to use unmeshed grafts on the dorsum of the hand and fingers in secondary releases unless mesh grafts were used primarily due to the limitations of donor skin available.

The thickness of harvested skin grafts should be in accordance to the requirements of the recipient site. For the palmar surfaces, grafts of a thickness of 0.02 to 0.024 inch are required to replace the thick dermis. Medium-thickness skin (0.016 to 0.018 inch) will suffice for the thin dorsal skin of the hands. The lateral buttocks below the belt line is a good site for this donor tissue. Estimates of graft requirements should be made after excision and release of scars. Split-thickness skin grafts provide as satisfactory a result as do full-thickness skin grafts.

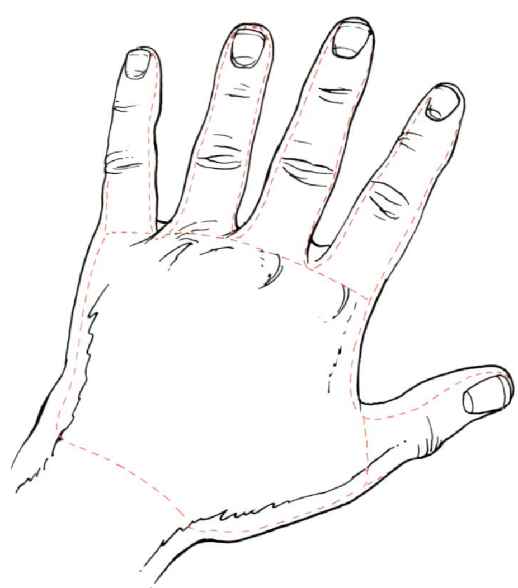

When skin grafts are placed on the dorsum of the hand, the boundaries of the aesthetic subunits must be respected. The most important aesthetic subunits are the dorsum of the hand between the distal wrist crease and the metacarpal-phalangeal joints and the dorsum of the fingers themselves.

Occasionally, local flaps are available. The more pliable and nonfibrotic these flaps are, the more easily they can be transposed. Unfortunately, scarred tissue may not survive elevation. Local flaps must be designed larger than initially estimated. Contractures must be fully released and scars must be excised before local flaps are designed. Frequently the size of the defect that requires coverage is extensive. Therefore contingency plans for the transfer of additional grafts are a requirement of the surgical planning for the correction of upper extremity contractures.

Scar excision and contracture release will result in the creation of new scars and the formation of new contractures. Therefore the placement of reoperative incisions must follow the same principles as for the placement of the primary incisions. It is advantageous to adjust scar excisions and the shape of the defect to allow a local flap to be rotated along acceptable skin tension lines.

The incisions around the scar should be beveled toward it to prevent the retraction of the subdermal plexus. These incisions should be made under tension, which will aid in separating the scar from the normal tissues. If previously skin-grafted tissue is to be excised, minimal undermining should be undertaken because the vascularity of the tissue may be considerably compromised. Hemostasis must be meticulous. Tourniquets should be lowered, the arm elevated, and the wound reexamined for hemostasis before closure with grafts and flaps.

SPECIFIC PROBLEMS

Unstable Scars

■ ***Unstable scars are the result of full-thickness burns in which most of the dermis has been destroyed.*** Loss of the dermis causes the formation of a disorganized scar that is prone to ulceration due to recurrent inflammation in the area. Chronic irritation from joint motion or mechanical shear force from clothing or opposing skin surfaces further contributes to the chronic inflammation. Unstable scars may be isolated or may occur on top of scar contracture bands. The ulceration may be surrounded by mature, pliable scar.

The treatment of unstable scar is excision, much like one would perform for the treatment of skin cancer. The excision should leave only mature pliable scar or healed skin behind. The defect is closed with either skin grafts or local flaps depending on the condition of the surrounding tissues.

In 1828, Jean Nicolas Marjolin described the classic "carcinomatous ulcer." Since that time the term "Marjolin's ulcer" has become widely used to denote a carcinoma that occurs in a chronic burn wound. Many authors have reported squamous cell carcinoma in other areas of chronic scarring such as osteomyelitis, fistulae, and posttraumatic wounds; however, most surgeons consider Marjolin's ulcers as burn scar carcinomas. A review of burn scar carcinoma by Novick et al.[1] revealed that the average age of patients with burn scar carcinoma is 58 years. The development of a carcinoma within a burn scar occurs on average 35 years following the initial burn. However, when the carcinoma does develop, it is a particularly lethal condition with a 32% mortality rate at 5 years in the series of Novick et al.[1]

When the reoperative surgeon encounters a chronic ulceration within a burn scar that occurred many years following the burn injury, he must certainly consider the diagnosis of burn scar carcinoma. A chronic ulceration that has within it an area of exophytic papillary-type growth must raise the suspicion of pseudo-epitheliomatous hyperplasia, the forerunner of burn scar carcinoma; these two conditions frequently coexist.

Although a variety of treatment regimens have been advocated for the treatment of burn scar carcinoma, none is highly effective. In general, wide local excision and flap coverage are the accepted primary means of obtaining local control and wound closure. Burn scar carcinoma tends to be radioresistant, although pre-operative topical 5-fluorouracil treatment has been promising.[2]

Axillary Contracture

The major considerations in reoperative management of axillary contracture are protection of vital structures and restoration of function. Structures that must be protected are the axillary vein and artery and the branches of the brachial plexus. Functional considerations include the range of motion of the shoulder. Aesthetic improvement is a minor factor in this region. Surgery should be considered when the range of motion is functionally disabling and the soft tissue protection of these vital structures is compromised. Scars should be allowed to mature fully for 6 months to 1 year. The patient should undergo physical and occupational therapy to achieve maximum gains in function before surgery is considered. If therapy fails to obtain superficial functional results, surgery should be contemplated.

In general, axillary contractures involve the posterior or anterior axillary fold, both folds together, or the entire axilla (including both folds and the axillary dome). The unburned axilla may be foreshortened due to adjacent trunk and upper arm scars. In addition, some contractures have been classified as edge contractures, which limit motion due to a tight axillary web or a strip contracture at the anterior or posterior axillary lines.

The reconstructive approach depends on the location and severity of the burn contracture. Rigid scar tissue that comprises the contracture and split-thickness skin grafts that may surround the scar do not provide supple tissue for reconstruction. Scarred tissue is inelastic and does not tolerate mobilization well. Therefore it is necessary to include as much subcutaneous tissue as possible when mobilizing flaps and to design flaps from the areas of undamaged or ungrafted tissue when possible.

Small axillary contractures are best treated by Z-plasty, V-Y- or Y-V-plasties. Again, rigid scar tissue should not be mobilized but either incised and allowed to retract or excised. Axillary contractures must be fully released to allow the greatest possible range of motion. Contractures and unstable scars create a net tissue loss that must be adequately compensated by skin grafting.

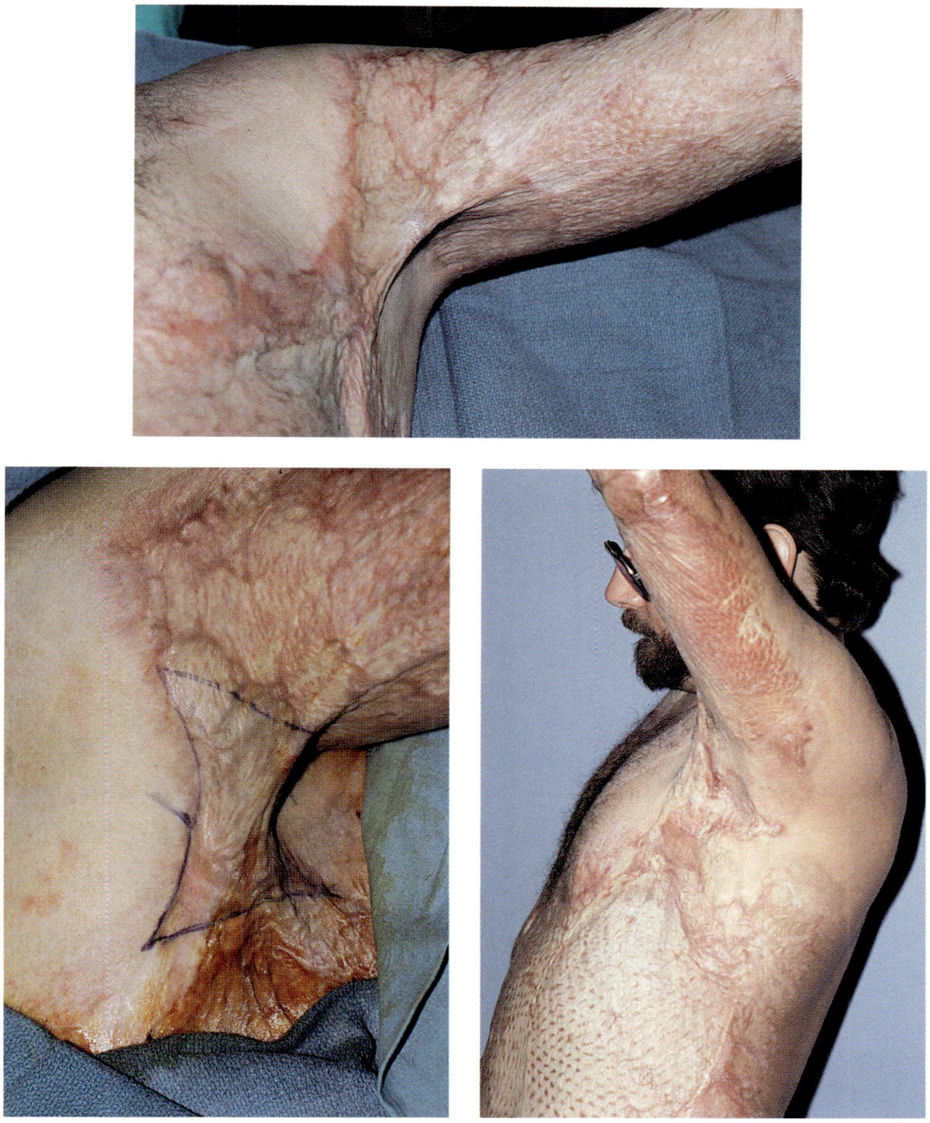

In this patient with anterior axillary contracture the scar was actually excised to allow complete release. Local flaps were insufficient to resurface the area. Therefore an additional skin graft was used to obtain the result shown.

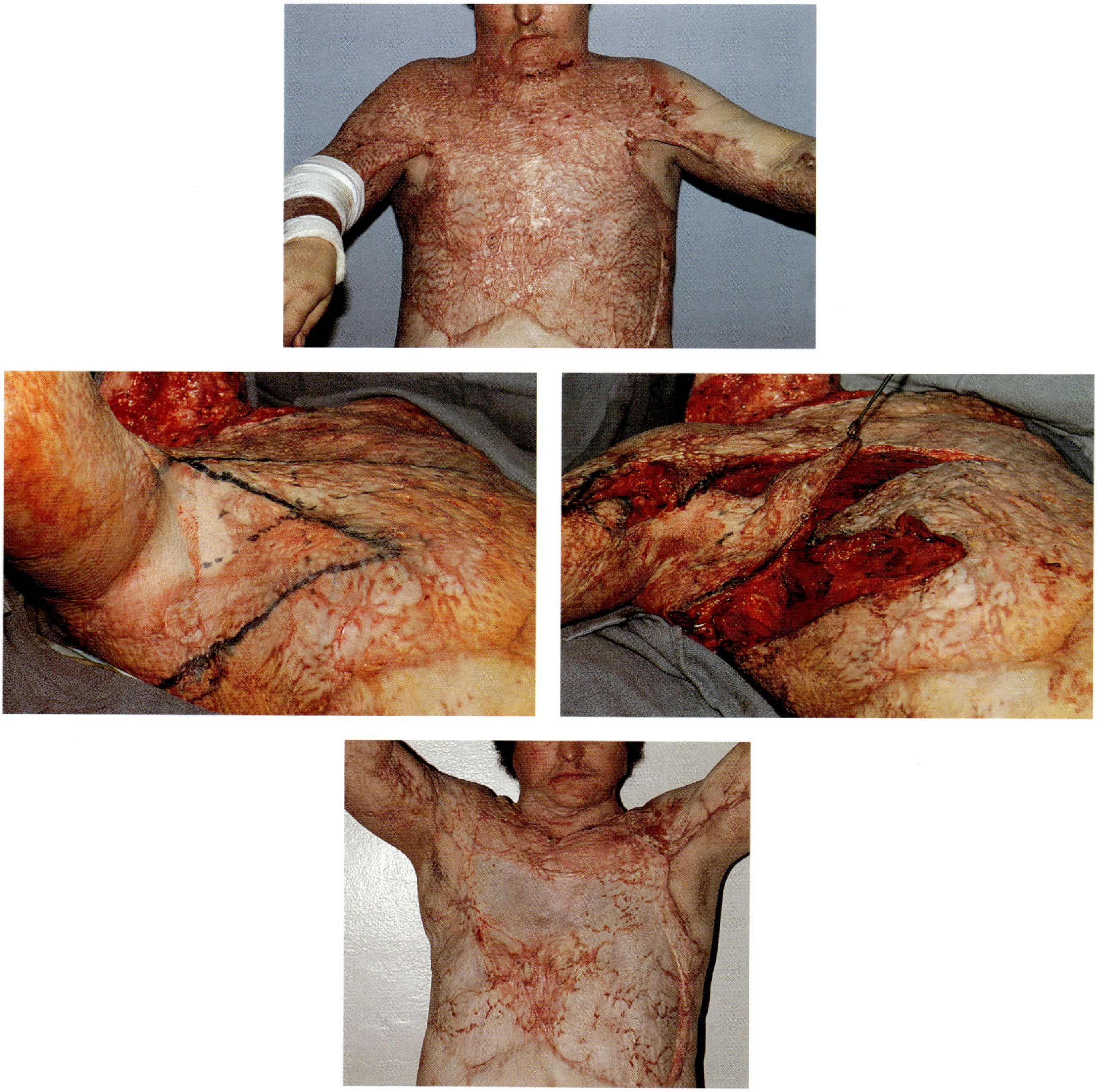

This patient had severe axillary contracture. The scar tissue was mobilized as a large Z-plasty to preserve thicker coverage in the dome of the axilla. Donor sites for skin grafts were limited. Following release and retraction of the burn scar, the mobilized flaps provided only limited coverage of the area. The remainder was covered by split-thickness skin grafts. The result is shown 1 year after surgery.

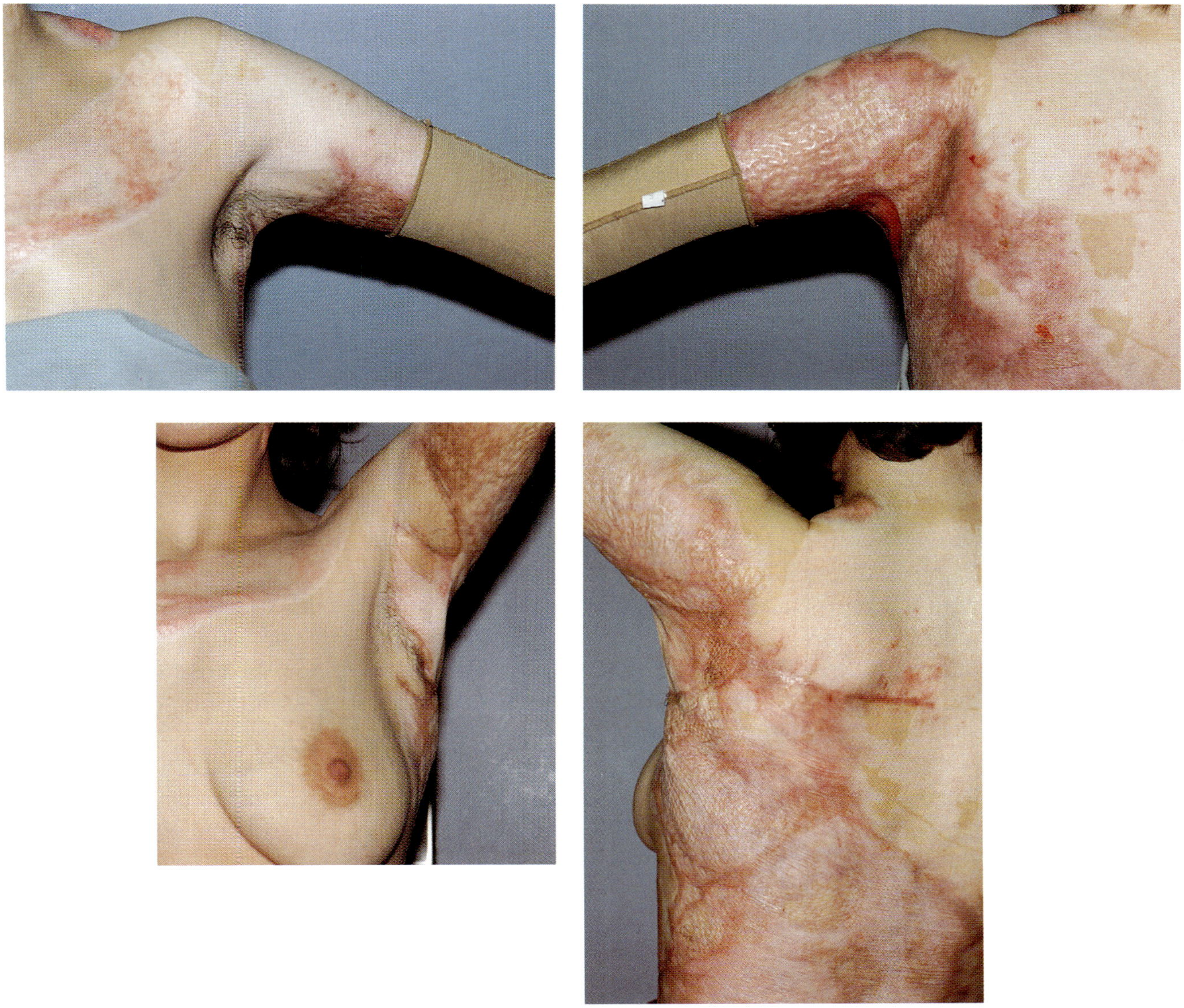

The anterior axillary contracture in this patient was surrounded by relatively mobile skin and scar. Only Z-plasty was necessary for correction. The patient is shown 6 months postoperatively.

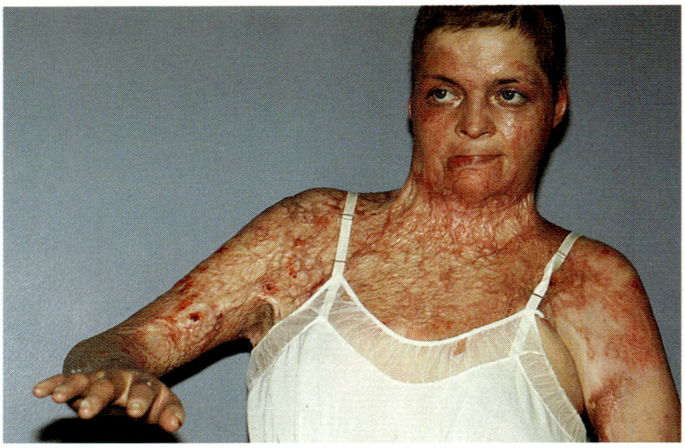

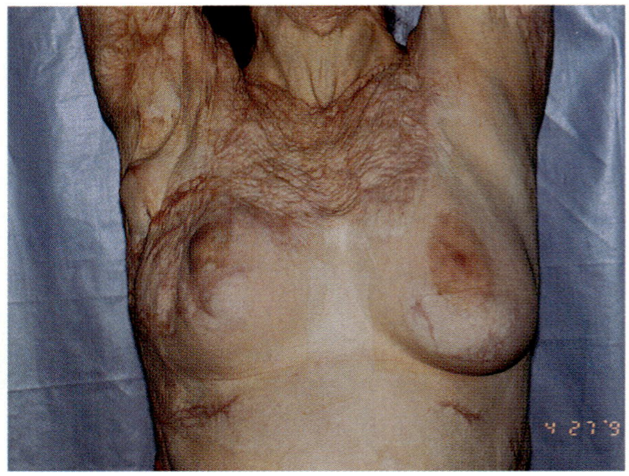

Axillary contracture in this patient was corrected by wide release and combined Z-plasty and skin grafting.

Once a well-vascularized bed is prepared, the grafts may be applied. They are secured with absorbable staples or sutures when necessary. The grafts are covered with a Xeroform dressing. Bolsters of cotton soaked with mineral oil are secured over the graft sites with nylon sutures to ensure immobilization of the grafts. Immobilization is further ensured by splinting the hand in the position of function. The grafts are then examined after 4 days, and range-of-motion exercises are begun when appropriate.

Vascularized flaps, including advancement flaps, propeller and subcutaneous pedicled flaps, and bilobed and rhomboid random flaps, are a good alternative to skin grafts if they can be designed over mobile, relatively unscarred tissue.

Fasciocutaneous flaps and muscle flaps can provide a large area of dorsal tissue. Fasciocutaneous flaps available for anterior defects include the thoracoacromial flap, lateral arm flap, and lateral thoracic flap. For posterior axillary contractures the scapular, parascapular, dorsal thoracic, or lateral thoracic flaps can be used. Lateral defects are served by medial or posterior upper arm fasciocutaneous flaps. Total axillary resurfacing can be achieved with parascapular flaps even when the donor site is scarred, as demonstrated in the following patient.

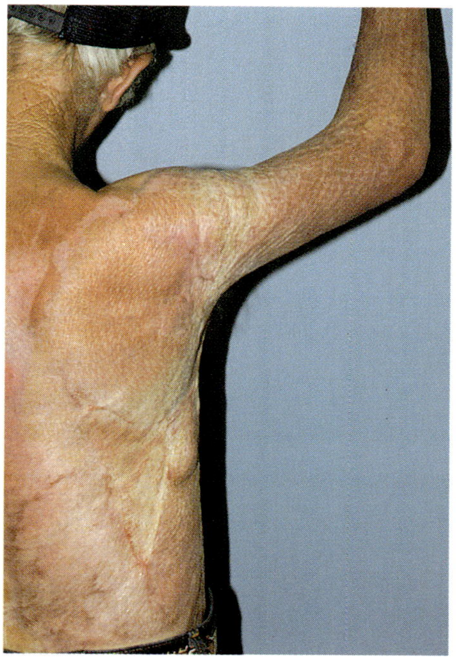

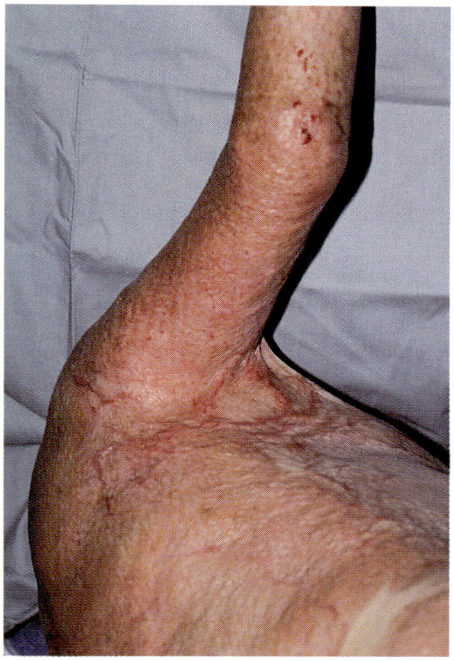

In this patient with a posterior axillary contracture, the scar was released, a scapular flap was elevated and inset in the defect, a split-thickness skin graft was transferred to the donor site, and a bolster was secured over the graft site.

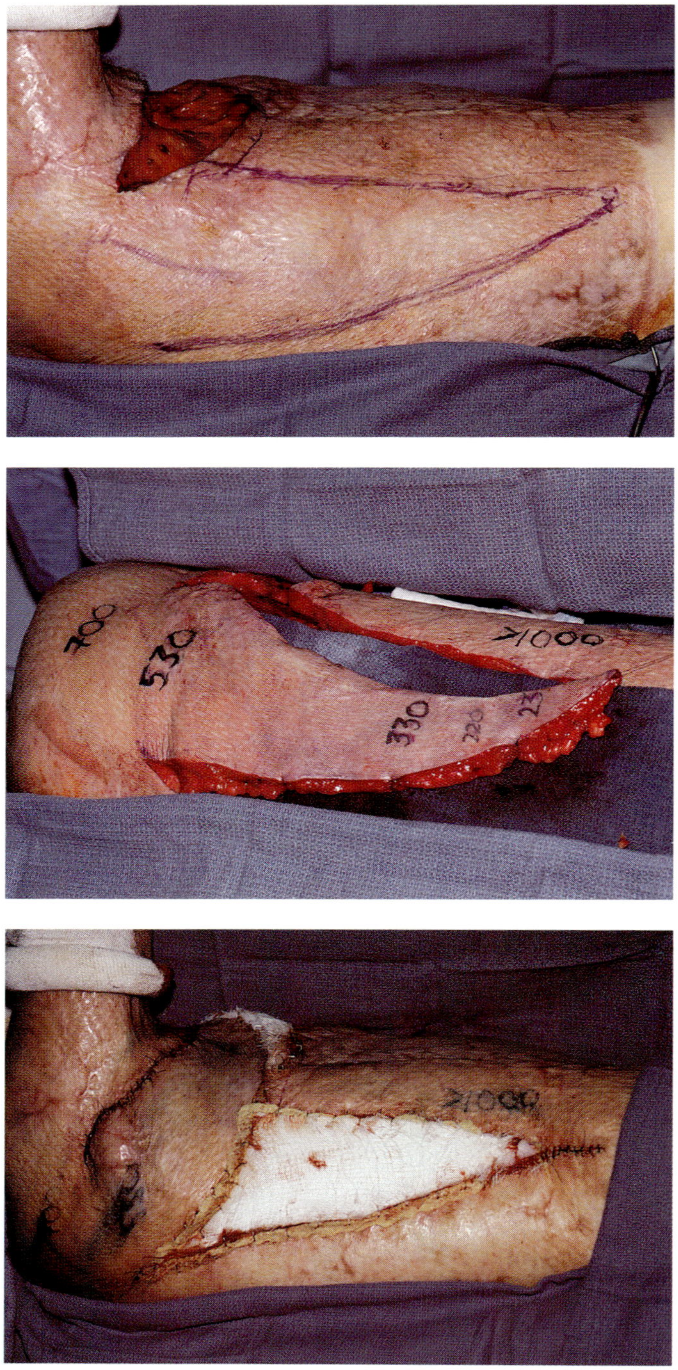

The dermal photofluorometer was used to measure vascularity of the flap with volumes recorded on the skin as shown. Any portion of the flap that measures below 15% of control (or 105 in this example) will not survive. The tip of this flap was debrided.

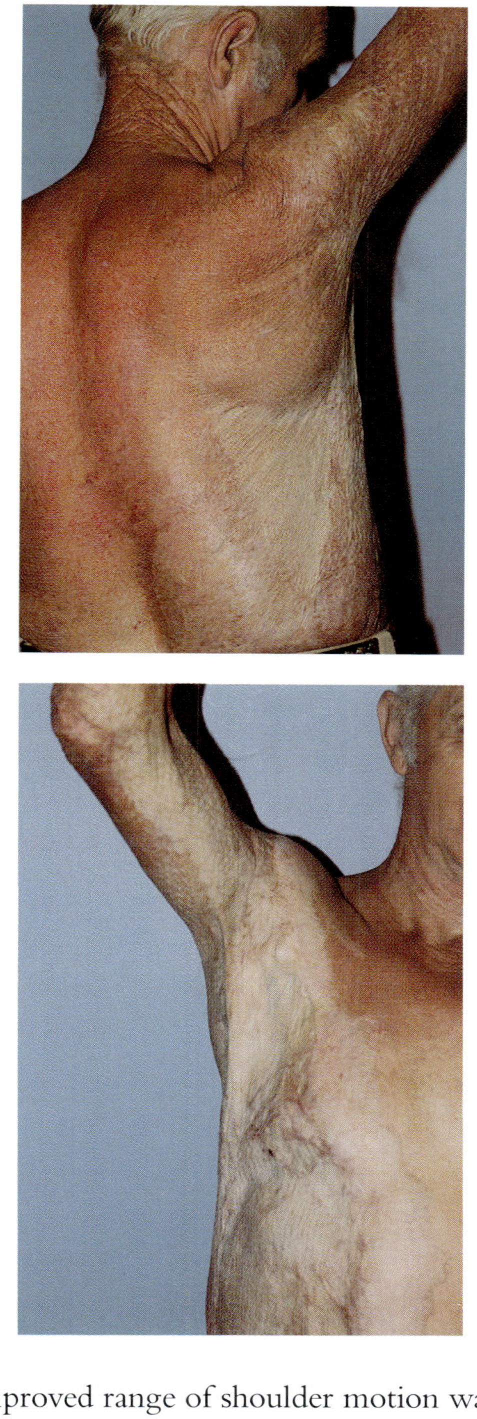

Postoperatively an improved range of shoulder motion was achieved.

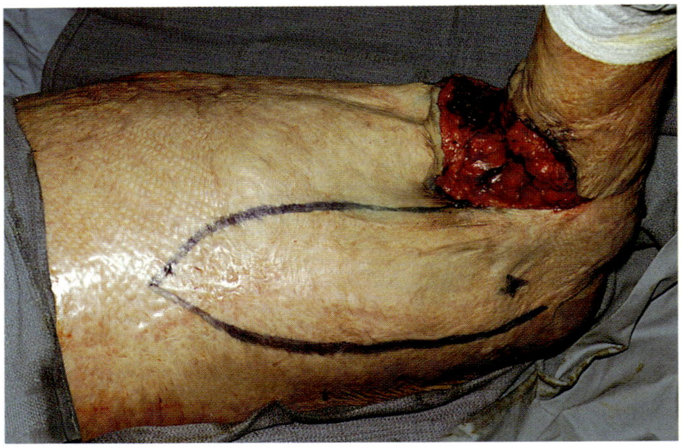

In this patient the axillary contracture was released and a parascapular flap was designed for rotation into the defect. The donor site was skin grafted.

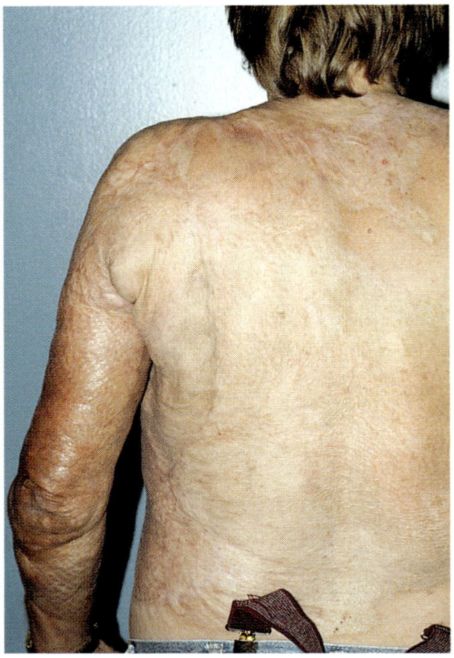

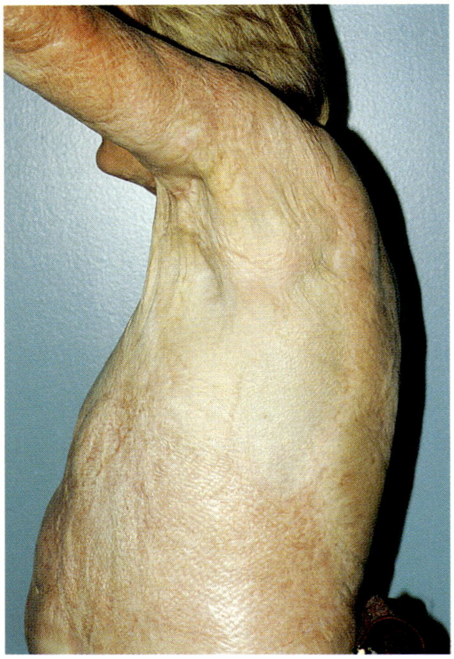

Postoperatively the range of motion is considerably improved.

The distal portion of fasciocutaneous flaps may not be as reliable due to burn damage to the subdermal plexus. It is important that the flap be designed to ensure adequate coverage of vital structures. The donor site as well as those portions of the recipient site that do not need flap coverage often require skin graft closure.

For anterior defects the pectoralis major and pectoralis minor muscle flaps are available. Posterior defects are served by latissimus dorsi, teres major, and lower trapezius muscle flaps. Muscle flaps for axillary contractures are usually considered second to fasciocutaneous or local flaps and grafts.

Elbow Contracture

Functional problems of the elbow are usually the result of skin contractures. Contractures less than 35 degrees do not require correction. As previously discussed, these contractures are usually amenable to Z-plasties or by Z-plasty supplemented with skin grafts. If no Z-plasty can be designed to adequately release the contracture and cover the resulting defect, the transfer of a fasciocutaneous flap may be required. Fasciocutaneous flaps to repair elbow contractures are designed to be either laterally or medially based to cover the defect created by scar excision and contracture release.

Wrist Contracture

A common complication of dermal burns is flexion contractures of the wrist. These contractures, like most contractures of the joints involving dermal injuries, are usually the result of improper or inadequate splinting, insufficient tissue replacement, and normal wound contraction. The ability to correct these problems is a function of the length of time the contracture has been present and the severity of the contraction.

Tenotomies of the flexor carpi radialis, flexor carpi ulnaris, and palmaris longus muscles may relieve small flexion contractures of the wrist. These tenotomies will heal with scars that resemble normal tendon within a year. Physical therapy and prolonged splinting must follow. Great care must be taken to avoid injury to the major arterial and nerve structures in the area such as the ulnar artery and nerve and the median nerve when performing tenotomies. For moderate contractures, skin grafts may be sufficient. However, more severe contractures may require tissue replacement in addition to tenotomy. When the median nerve or flexor tendons are exposed, a flap is mandatory for coverage with preservation of gliding function and a reduced recurrence of contractures.

Metacarpophalangeal Finger Joint Contracture

Contractures of the metacarpophalangeal finger joints following thermal injury may be in either extension or flexion. Extension contractures are more common. Given that the intrinsic muscle system is intact and functioning, these deformities are corrected by capsulectomy and collateral ligament division. The intrinsic muscles will provide the necessary secondary lateral support. The extensor tendon may need to be divided or actually excised to release the contracture.

Release of extension contractures of the metacarpophalangeal joints virtually always requires either skin grafting or flap resurfacing, especially if the fingers are fully flexed and the extent of the tissue deficit is revealed. First, a longitudinal incision is made over the proximal phalanx to the metacarpophalangeal joint. The skin is left intact at the point of maximum tension over the metacarpophalangeal joint after it is brought into flexion. This incision splits the extensor tendon longitudinally without cutting into the periosteum and lifts it to expose the joint directly. If the extensor tendon restricts metacarpophalangeal flexion and is not amenable to Z-plasty lengthening, it must be divided or excised. The thickened dorsal joint capsule is then excised. If this maneuver does not give adequate release, the second step is to excise the collateral ligament on the ulnar side of the joint by grasping it with a thin hemostat and cutting on each side. Passive flexion is tested again. If more release is required, the third step is to excise the dorsal half of the origin of the collateral ligament on the radial side of the joint. A part of the radial collateral ligament is saved whenever possible because finger drift is usually ulnar. With severe ankylosis a complete excision of the radial collateral ligament may be necessary, which is the final possibility for release. After all necessary ligament excision is completed, a smooth probe is passed around the head of the metacarpal bone to break any adhesions that are limiting flexion. Any soft tissue deficit must be dealt with using skin grafts or, if a gliding surface is required, distant pedicle flaps or free flaps. A cast is placed postoperatively to maintain the flexion gained by the surgery. Skin sutures are removed after 10 days, the cast is immediately replaced with an elastic splint, and the patient begins therapy with active extension exercises. Any delay in splinting will result in a considerable loss of the function gained operatively.

Displacement of the lateral bands of the intrinsic muscle dorsal to the axis of rotation of the metacarpophalangeal joints may cause extreme metacarpophalangeal hyperextension and dorsal displacement of the proximal phalanges. The lateral bands can become extremely shortened. Severing the bands around the joint along with the joint ligaments to allow the joint to be brought again into flexion may result in instability with ulnar drift. In this case resection arthroplasty, which preserves and repositions the lateral band, is preferable. It is difficult to restore satisfactory flexion to these joints. Flexion contractures of the metacarpophalangeal joints that limit extension are common with neglected deep palmar burns. When they occur, there may be extensive cutaneous or soft tissue damage and therefore grafts or resurfacing should be part of the reconstructive plan. In this case the palm is explored and the volar plate and any other restricting scar bands are severed. The neurovascular bundles must be dissected free using continuous slow finger extension to avoid ischemia and spasm. The metacarpophalangeal joints are then stabilized with Kirschner wires in extension until vigorous therapy can be initiated.

Interdigital Contracture

Restricting web contractures are a common sequela of hand burns. These contractures frequently occur between the fingers dorsally and distal to the normal webs. Tissue loss is the cause of the syndactyly.

Z-plasty is a possible treatment option. However, this correction usually suffices only for small contractures. Moderate webbing is better repaired with excision and skin grafting.

Correction also can be accomplished similar to the repair of congenital syndactyly. A proximally based flap can be developed from the side of one of the involved digits. The volar margin should be oblique to avoid creating a longitudinal scar. This flap is then rotated so that the apex can be placed into the dorsal aspect of the web space. A length-to-width ratio of 2:1 can be used. The residual defects can then be skin grafted.

Adduction contractures of the thumb, or thumb space webbing, are also a common sequela of thermal hand injuries. This is due to the pull of the extensor pollicis longus muscle, which pulls the thumb toward the second metacarpal bone. In addition, burns of the dorsum of the hand frequently involve the thumb-finger web space. The repair of small contractures of the thumb-finger web space may be accomplished by Z-plasties and local flap transfer.

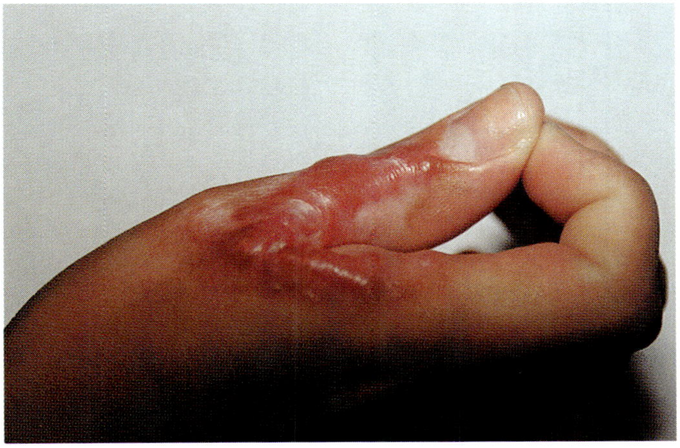

This female patient presented with an adduction contracture of the left thumb–index web space and an extension contracture of the interphalangeal joint.

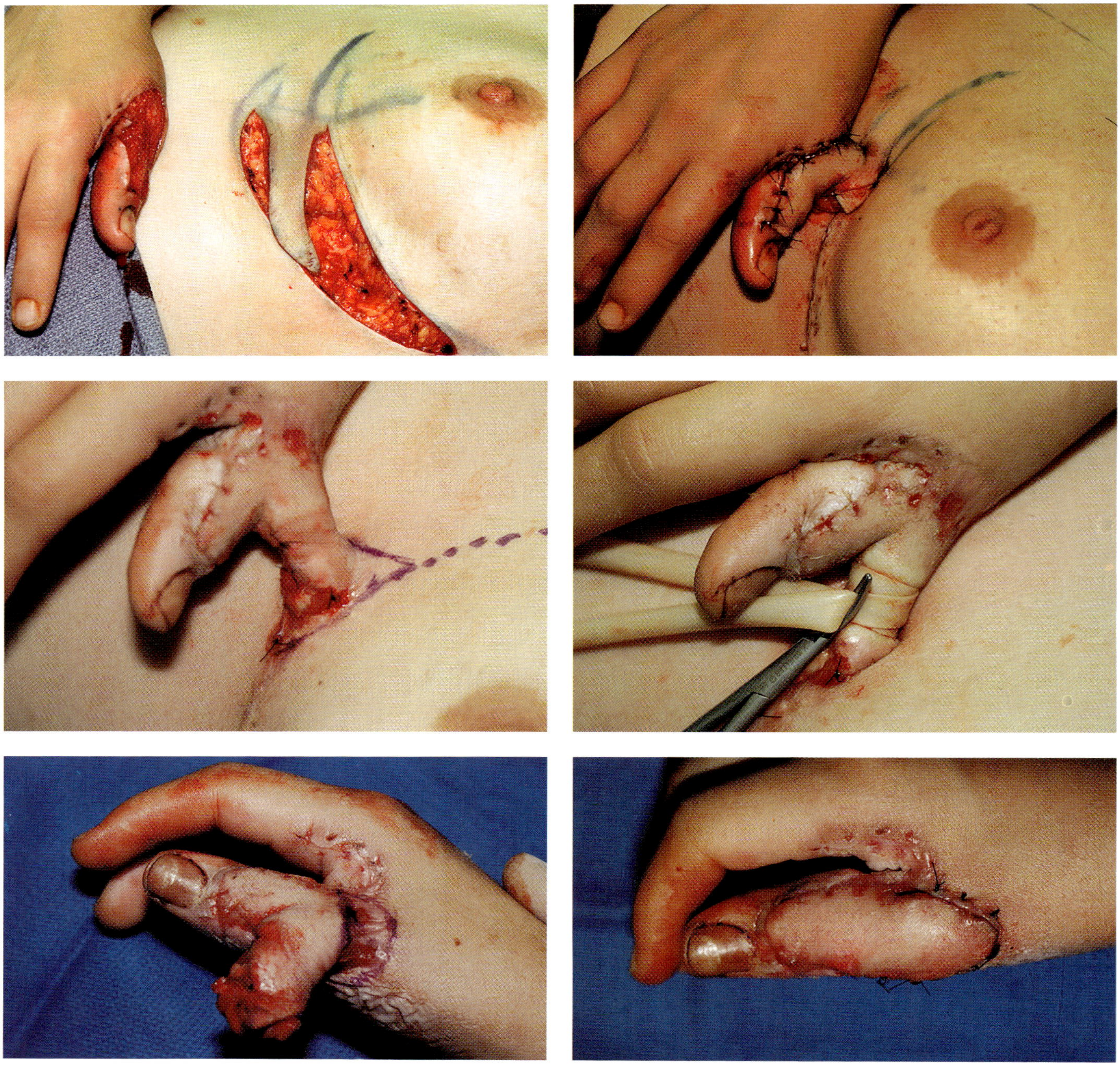

Following release of all contractures and burn scar excision, a chest wall flap developed from the inframammary fold was used to provide tissue coverage.

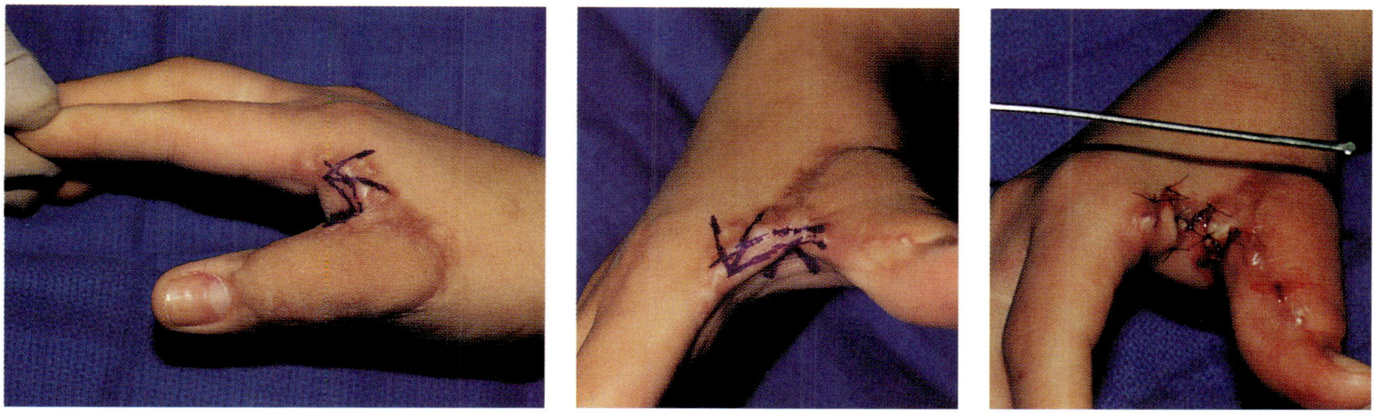

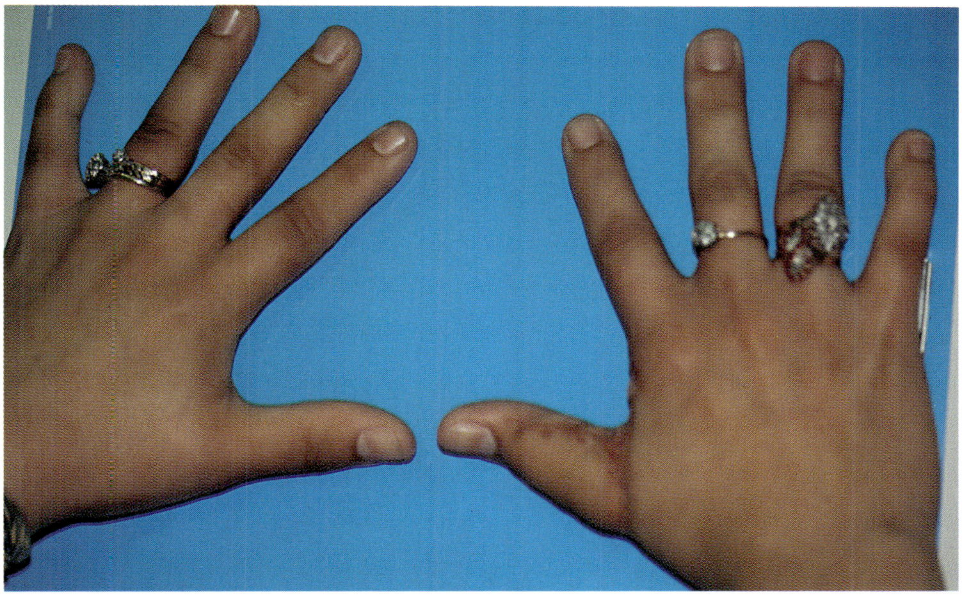

In a second procedure four-flap Z-plasty was performed to release the first web space contracture.

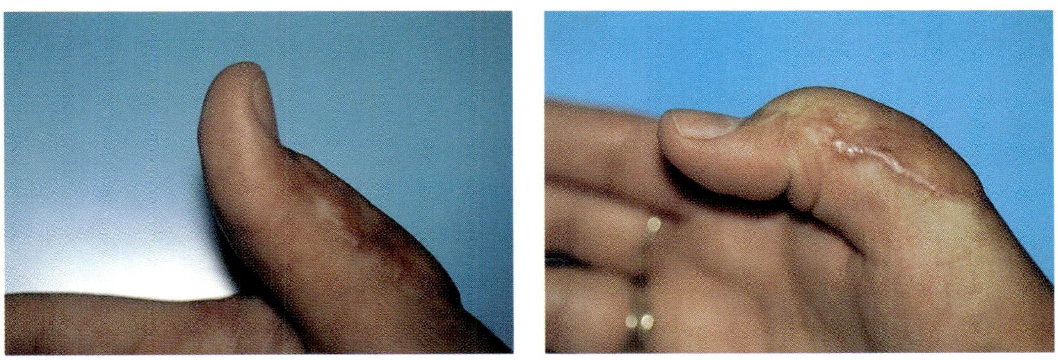

The final result is shown following flap thinning.

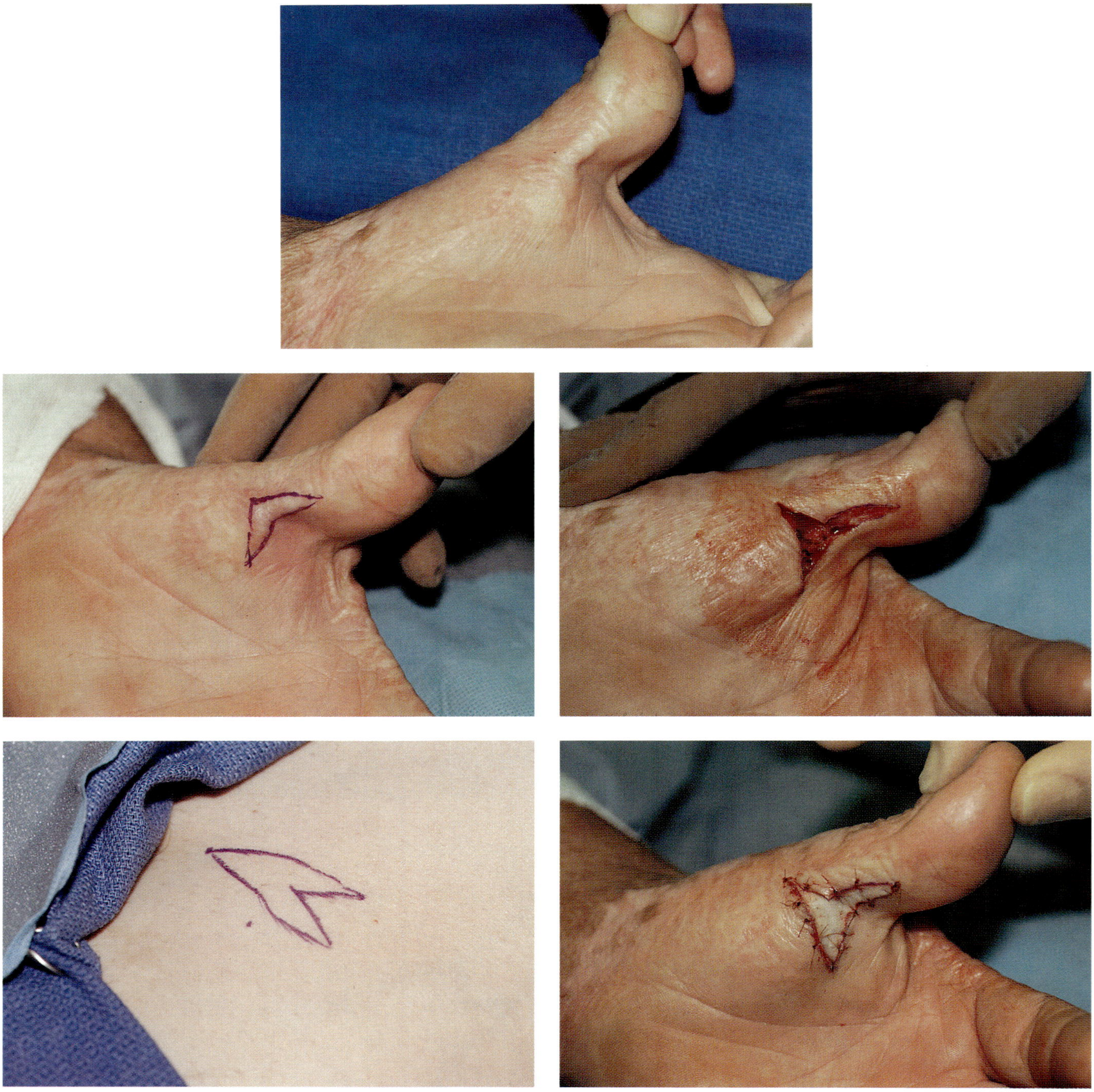

In this case of thumb contracture, the scar was excised and a full-thickness skin graft harvested from the abdominal wall was inset into the defect.

Proximal Interphalangeal Joint Contracture

Frequent exposure of the thin skin over the dorsal surface of the proximal interphalangeal joints often results in damage. Although this injury may be caused by direct exposure of the joint, it is usually the result of secondary contractures to the structures in the joint. If implant arthroplasty is considered for treatment, good tissue coverage and intact tendon systems are required. However, with burn injuries, these tendon systems are frequently not present and thus preclude this type of repair. Given this situation, arthrodesis in the position of function is the usual recourse for either proximal or distal interphalangeal joints that have been destroyed by heat injury. Contractures can fix these joints in either extension or flexion.

With normal proximal interphalangeal joint flexion, the lateral band of intrinsic muscles slides anteriorly, volar to the axis of rotation in the joint. When scarring occurs secondary to a dermal injury, this shift in the lateral band cannot occur and the joint therefore cannot be fixed. This problem may occur despite the presence of intact, serviceable skin over the joint. When the skin is destroyed, the extensor system underneath suffers more damage than just adhesion. Relief may be obtained by a bilateral resection of the bands, leaving an intact central slip for extension of the joint. It may be necessary to resect the dorsal portion of the collateral ligaments; great care must be taken not to make the joint unstable. The prognosis for restoring flexion is favorable.

In flexion contractures there is a disruption of the flexor arch of the finger, which impairs function. Surgical release is difficult since there is no secondary system for lateral joint stability. Despite the presence of collateral ligaments in the proximal interphalangeal joint, other support tissues—flexor tendon sheath, volar plate, and all of the deep transverse fascia complex—are folded with joint flexion and cannot provide stability.

Deep dorsal burns destroy the central strip of the extensor mechanism. The lateral bands shift volarly, becoming a proximal interphalangeal flexor rather than extensor. The loss of the restraint of the extensor system permits the whole extensor system to move more proximally and results in excessive pull through the lateral bands and hyperextension of the distal interphalangeal joint. This is the classic boutonnière deformity: proximal interphalangeal joint flexion and distal interphalangeal joint hyperextension. Disruption of the central slip by burn injury will not allow direct repair of the central slip mainly because of tissue loss; lack of coverage would result.

Several attempts to repair this deformity have been described, but no satisfactory treatment exists. We recommend the repair outlined by Littler. Beasley[3] described this repair as follows:

> The lateral bands are severed transversely over the middle phalanx just distal to the normal level of the central slip insertion at the base of the middle phalanx. This releases the abnormal extension pull on the distal joint. The distal joint is thereafter extended by tenodesis as the oblique retinacular ligaments of Landsmeer lie deep and remain intact. Next, the anteriorly displaced lateral bands are dissected free on each side of the proximal interphalangeal joint but with great care not to detach them from the remnant of central slip attachment at the base of the middle phalanx. The freed volar margins of the lateral bands are turned upwards and sutured together directly over the proximal interphalangeal joint. This accomplishes two things. First, the lateral bands can no longer displace anteriorly to become flexors. Second, it restores continuity of the central slip, but the entire extension system now acts only on the proximal interphalangeal joint. . . . The extensor system repairs can, with careful planning, be done in conjunction with dorsal tissue replacement with appropriate flaps.
>
> . . . [implant arthroplasty] may occasionally be used to restore some range of motion in a damaged joint with central slip disruption. The joint and distal end of a proximal phalanx are resected until the end of the disrupted central slip reaches the area of normal attachment at the base of the middle phalanx with the proximal interphalangeal joint implant in place. The collateral ligaments of the joint are carefully preserved and subsequently reattached to give lateral joint stability while the end of the advanced central slip is fixed to bone at its normal insertion. In this manner, a restricted but useful active range of motion may be recovered and a severe flexion contracture simultaneously relieved in selected cases.
>
> With extreme damage, arthrodesis of the proximal interphalangeal joints in a functional position may be the only solution, especially if they are rigidly fixed in more than 90 degrees of flexion. When poor skin coverage is also present, arthrodesis must be accomplished without undermining the skin. This can be done by a carefully planned wedge resection of both scarred skin and bone without any undermining. Obviously, with arthrodesis of the proximal interphalangeal joints every effort should be made to restore maximum range of motion to the metacarpophalangeal joints.

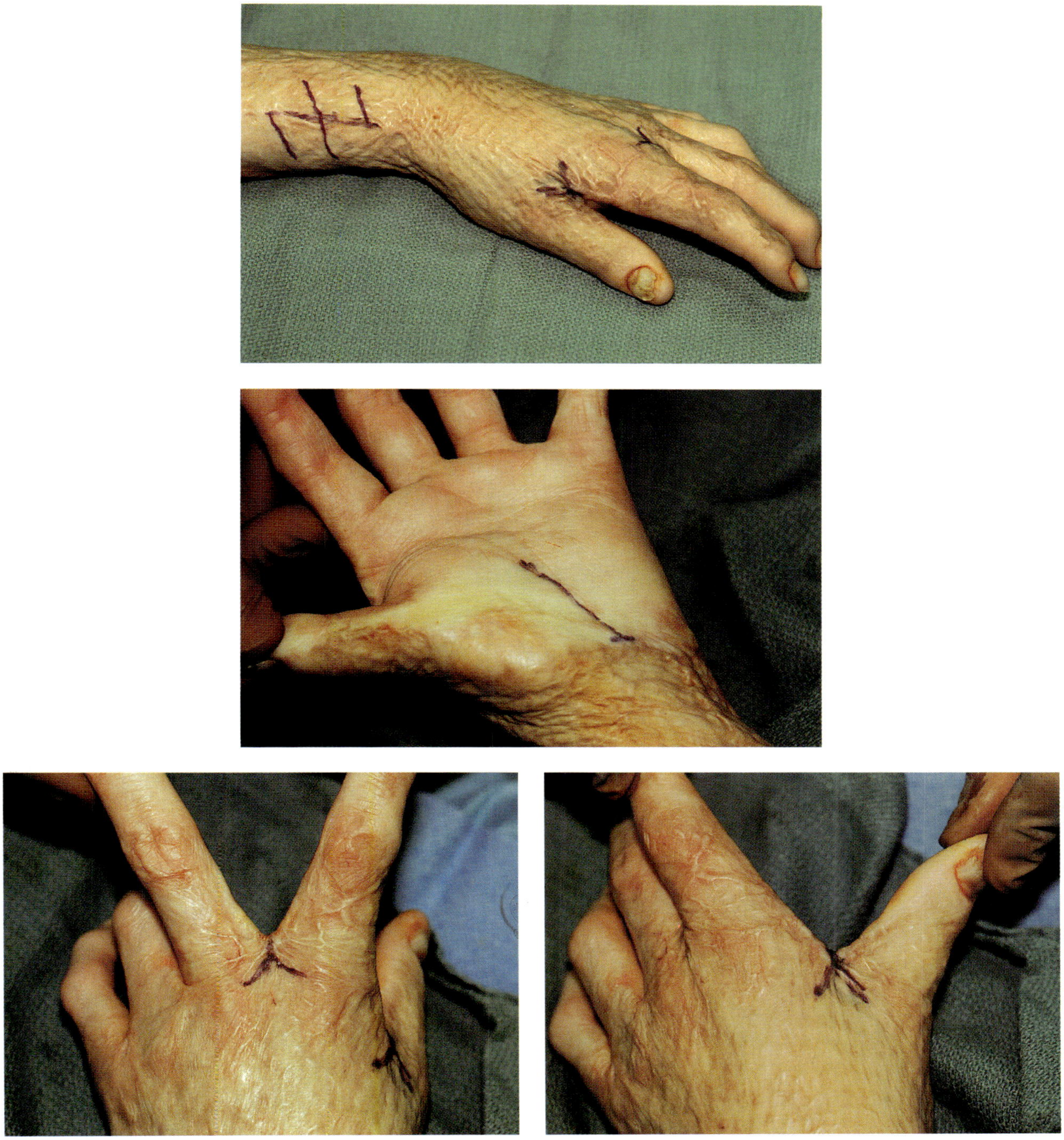

It is often advisable to release multiple joint contracture in a single operation. Double opposing Z-plasty and split-thickness grafts were performed in this 43-year-old woman with dorsal, ventral palm, and web space contractures of the left hand.

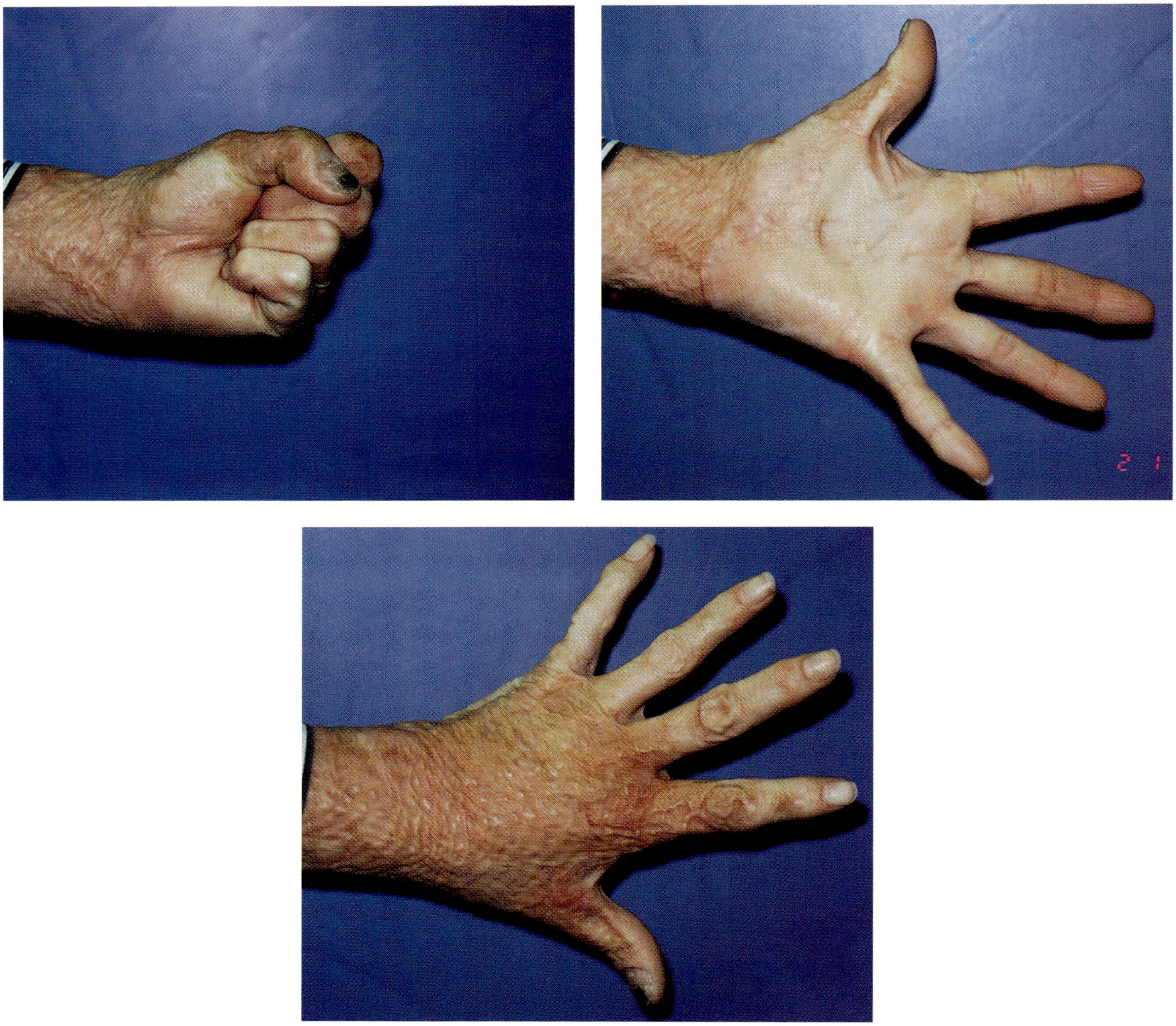

Postoperative results at 3 months demonstrate good return of function.

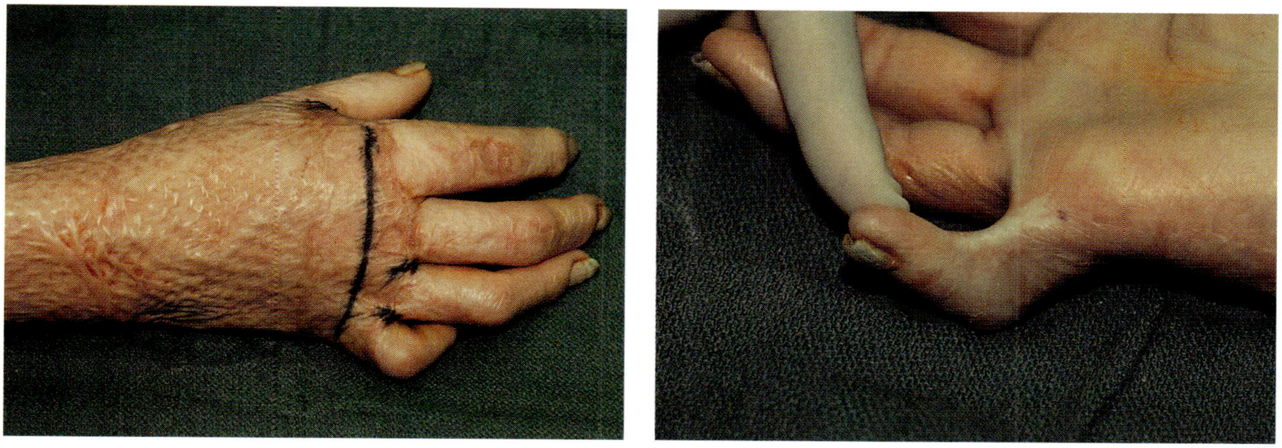

Dorsal metacarpophalangeal release with split-thickness grafts was performed in the same woman's right hand. Temporary Kirschner wire fixation of the metacarpophalangeal joints maintains the release and facilitates immobilization until the grafts are adherent.

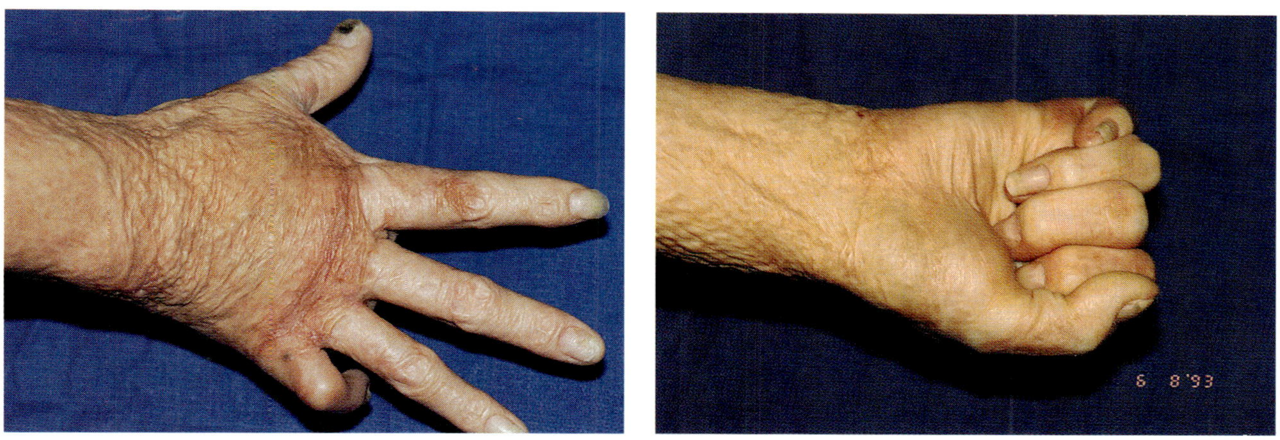

Arthrodesis is planned for the correction of the little finger proximal interphalangeal contracture.

Distal Interphalangeal Joint Contracture

Arthrodesis is usually the method of choice for treatment of distal interphalangeal joint contractures because the stabilizing elements of the joint are often unrepairable. The best approach is arthrodesis of the joint in extension in women or in slight flexion in manual laborers.

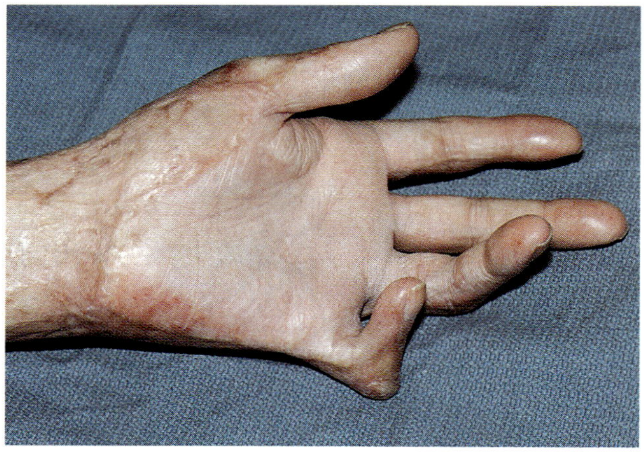

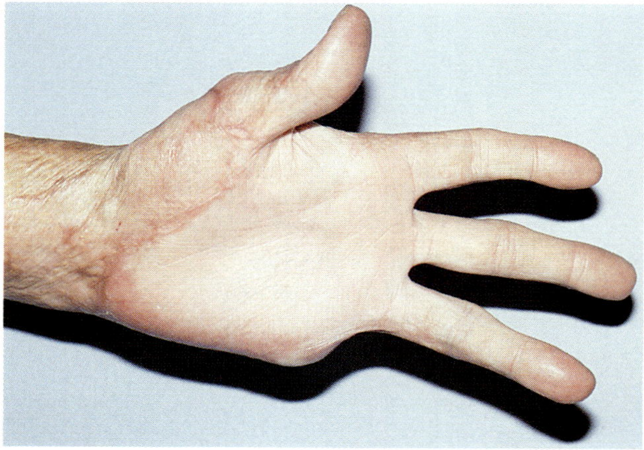

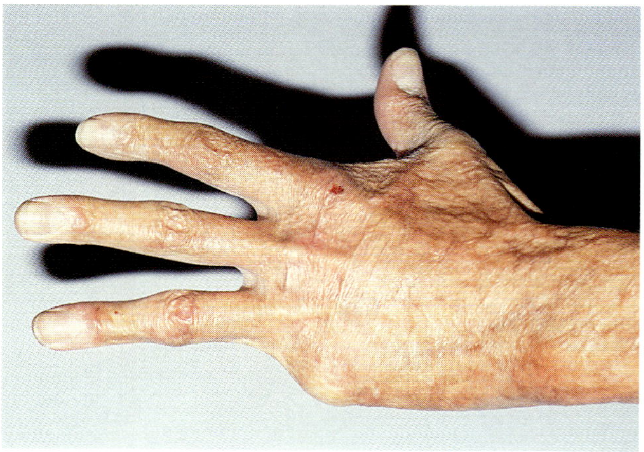

At times when flexor contractures are severe and tissue coverage is not adequate, amputation is the best option, as was the case for this patient.

ROLE OF THE THERAPIST

The therapist plays a crucial role in reoperative surgery of the burned upper extremity. First, through active therapy, many of the poor outcomes of primary surgery can be avoided. Second, with effective therapy good function of the affected areas can be achieved, and the need for reoperative surgery may be obviated. Third, the therapist can determine the limits of therapy. He will establish when the maximum gains that can be expected from therapy have been attained and when surgery is necessary. Fourth, the therapist can provide advice as to the optimal staging of operations to achieve a reasonable level of functioning between procedures. Fifth, the therapist can maximize postoperative gains with effective rehabilitation.

UNSOLVED PROBLEMS

Resurfacing of the forearm following burn injury requires large amounts of tissue. Tissue expansion has been used for this purpose, but this approach is limited by the problems associated with the expansion of burn scar skin. Cosmetic goals are often limited by the lack of available normal skin and the inability of any procedure to completely eliminate scarring.

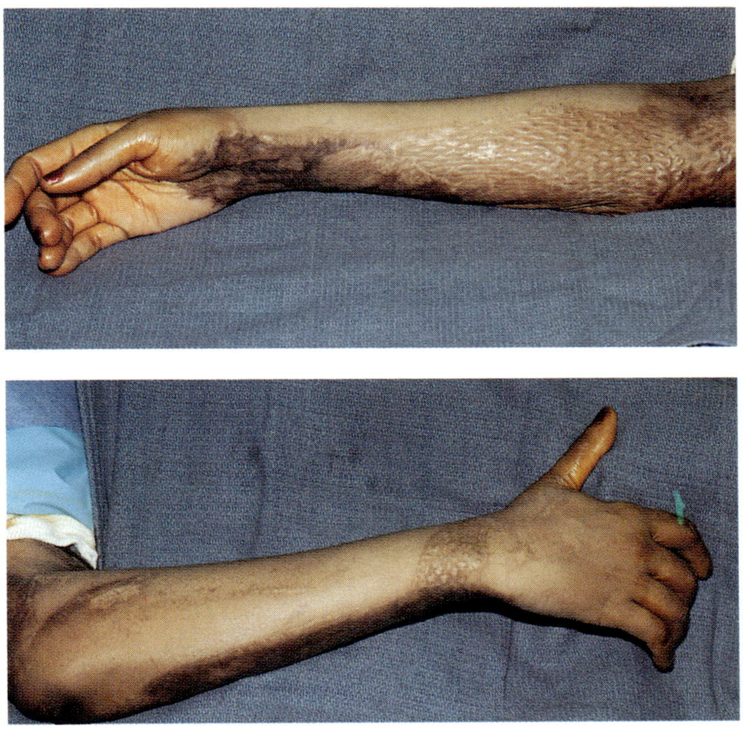

This patient is shown before an attempt was made to resurface the forearm with local tissue after two episodes of tissue expansion.

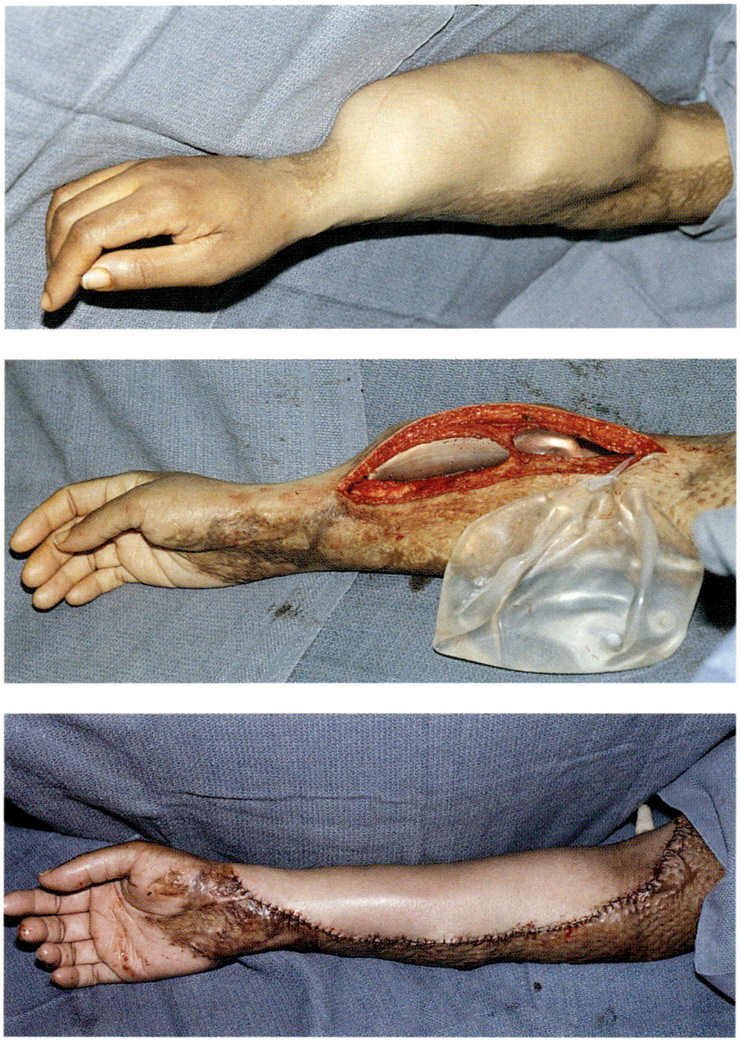

Although expansion yielded good-quality skin for near circumferential resurfacing, as shown, too much burn scar was resected at the second procedure, resulting in postoperative compartment syndrome.

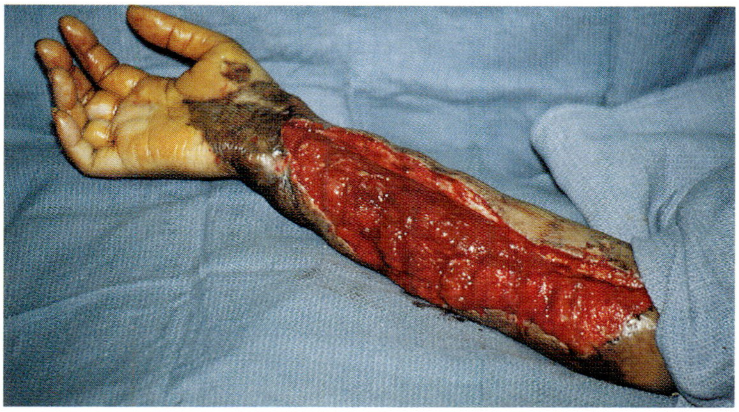

The sutures were released following development of a median nerve sensory deficit.

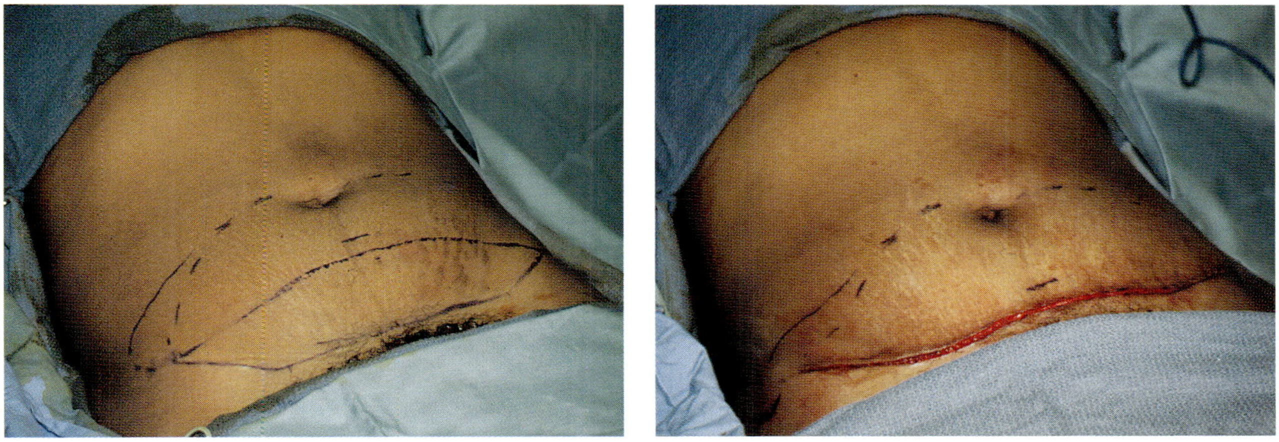

After compression symptoms resolved, wound closure was accomplished using a full-thickness skin graft from the suprapubic area.

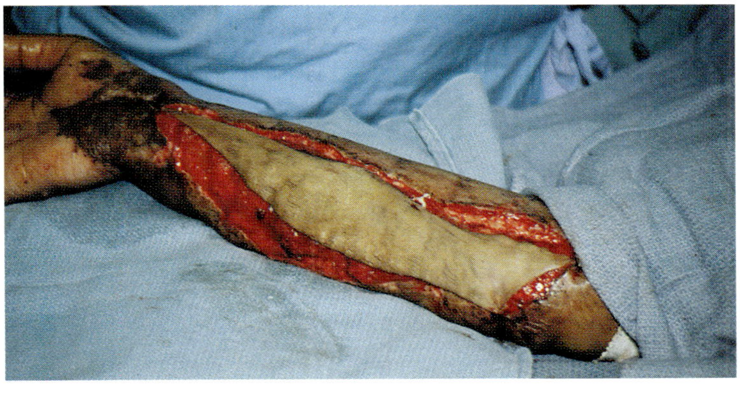

The immediate postoperative view is shown.

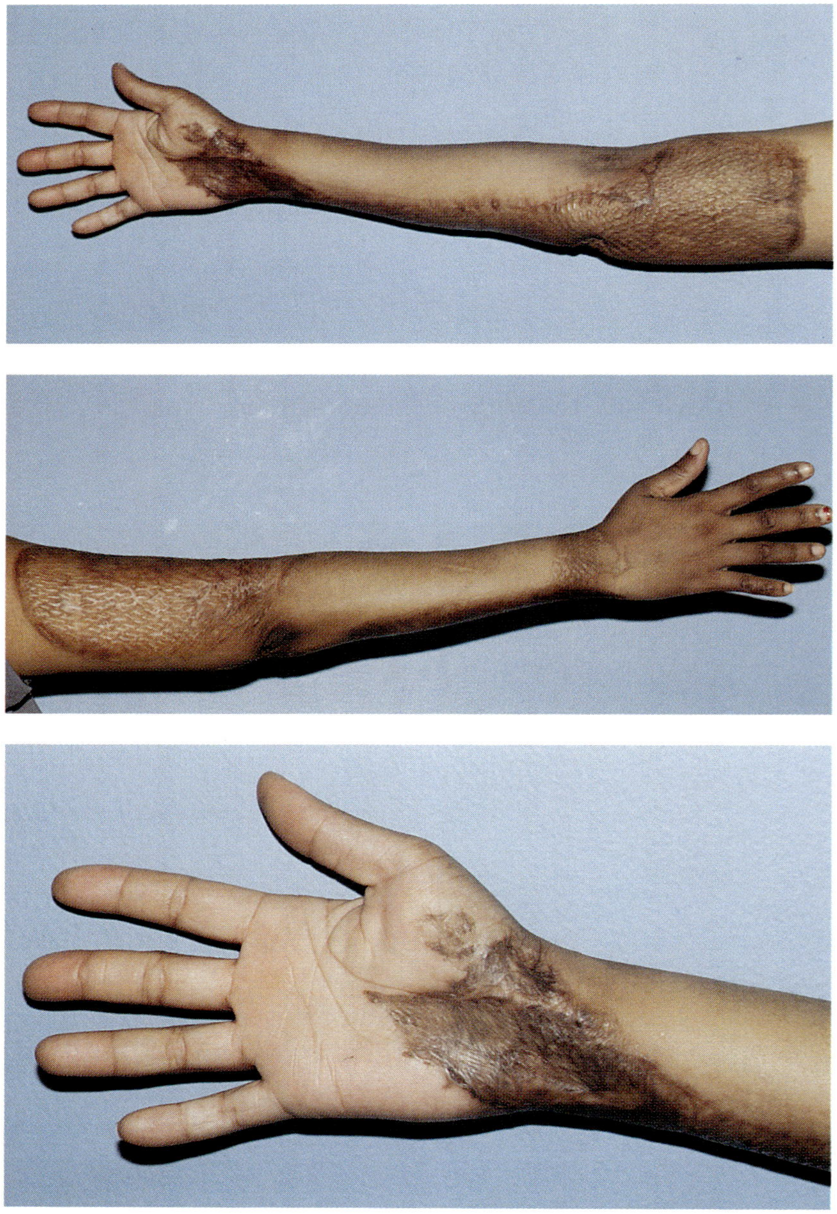

The final result shows an improvement in appearance but not to the degree that might have been possible had the use of the expanded flap been more conservative.

PREVENTION

The prevention of the need for reoperative surgery following burns of the upper extremity involves proper primary therapy, adequate debridement, and burn wound coverage. Splinting and rehabilitative therapy are the essentials of gaining optimal function. Still, despite proper therapy, burn scar and joint contractures may occur.

References

1. Novick M, Gard DA, Hardy SB, Spira M. Burn scar carcinoma: A review and analysis of 46 cases. J Trauma 17:809, 1977.
2. Ryan RF, Litwin MS, Krementa ET. A new concept in the management of Marjolin's ulcers. Ann Surg 193:598, 1981.
3. Beasley RW. Secondary repair of burned hands. Hand Clin 6:319, 1990.

42

Secondary Lymphedema

A. Esteban Reyes, M.D., and Gabriela Guzman-Stein, M.D.

Reoperative Problems

Severe functional impairment	Recurrent lymphangitis
Increased tissue turgor	Lymphangiosarcoma

The management of lymphedema, whether primary or secondary, is a challenge for surgeons. Lymphedema in the upper and lower extremities and the genitals presents major problems. The disfigurement and chronic changes caused by primary lymphedema have led to multiple proposals for medical treatment and corrective surgery.

No form of treatment offers a complete cure, and most operative procedures are followed by deformity of the affected extremity and partial recurrence of the edema. Since the disease is chronic and unremitting and because there is no single effective operation, afflicted patients may consult with many physicians in the course of their care. A basic understanding of the problem involves a frank discussion with the patient of the treatment options and consequences.

Lymphedema is usually divided into primary and secondary types based on Allen's classification table. In this chapter we limit our discussion to the analysis of secondary lymphedema and its management.

INCIDENCE AND ETIOPATHOGENESIS

An estimated 150 million people worldwide suffer from lymphedema, an ancient medical problem that remains unsolved. The most common cause of secondary lymphedema is infection. Approximately 45 million people suffer from filarial lymphedema, elephantiasis, and hydrocele. Other infectious causes of lymphedema are *Streptococcus* organisms, lymphogranulomas, tuberculosis, syphilis, and leprosy. Secondary lymphedema also results from iatrogenic (surgical trauma) or obstructive problems after lymphatic dissection for cancer, tumor obstruction of lymphatic vessels, and sequelae of irradiation.

PHYSIOLOGY AND PATHOPHYSIOLOGY

The lymphatic vessels are formed by the budding of the venous epithelium from the jugular and iliac regions. These vessels form a network of three recognized layers: a superficial plexus and an intermediate plexus in the dermis, both of which are devoid of valves, and a deep dermal plexus furnished with valves at the junction of the dermis and subcutaneous tissue. Lymphatic vessels have not been found in muscle, bone, or tendons, but they are present in the intermuscular fascial planes.[1]

Lymphatic vessels ascend alongside superficial veins in the subcutaneous layer where they are connected by horizontal arcades; they then continue along the main lymphatic trunks close to the deep fascia and end in the regional (axillary, iliac, and inguinal) lymph nodes.

The propulsive force of lymph flow is furnished (1) by the pulsation of the lymphangions (segments of lymphatic vessel bordered by distal and proximal valves), (2) by propulsion against gravity through intermittent compression caused by muscular activity, and (3) in the deep lymphatic vessel by the pulsation of adjacent arteries.[2]

The primary function of the lymphatic system is the removal of excess water and solutes from the interstitial space to maintain protein balance. It is believed that almost 50% of the total circulatory plasma protein is filtered and returned daily to the venous system through the thoracic duct.

Under normal circumstances the amount of capillary filtrate that becomes lymph varies from tissue to tissue with the state of physical activity, amount of capillary pressure, and permeability of the capillaries. Physiologically the major lymphatic channel pressure is intermittent, either below or equal to venous pressure.

The lymphatic system normally can accommodate a sizable increase in lymphatic protein overload by what is called the "lymphatic *safety* factor." It is for this reason that a generalized system increase in lymph filtration with normal transport capacity (highest possible lymph flow per unit of time) does not invariably lead to lymphedema.

In disease states, when lymph formation (load) exceeds "transport capacity," lymphatic resorption of extra plasma protein is inadequate, intralymphatic pressure then becomes positive, and lymphedema results. To understand secondary lymphedema, the concept of insufficiency of the lymph vascular system has to be defined as the insufficiency of transport capacity.

With respect to lymphatic load, there are two basic forms of lymph vascular insufficiency. One form occurs when the lymphatic transport capacity is reduced to a level unable to process the normal lymphatic load, which results in a state of low lymph flow by what is called "mechanical insufficiency." The result of this state is lymphedema—a protein-rich edema. A second form occurs when an already reduced transport capacity is overwhelmed by an increase in lymphatic load; in this instance even a dynamic insufficiency of the healthy lymphatics would terminate in what has been called by Foldi and Clodius "safety valve insufficiency."

Edema substantially changes the biophysical parameters of the tissue. Oxygenation is impaired, tissue scavengers and macrophages are less functional, and the balance of the injury remodeling process is inhibited. In the extreme case protein-rich edema with necrotic cells results. The balance between deposition and lysis of collagen is shifted toward fibrosclerosis, and induration of the perilymphatic interstitial tissue gradually progresses. Whether lymphedema is congenital or acquired, progressive pressure and perfusion impairment produce skin changes and thickening.

Because of the accumulation of lymph, which is an ideal culture medium, the affected tissues are extremely prone to frequent episodes of lymphangitis and cellulitis. Increased fibrosclerotic changes occur in the affected extremity.

SECONDARY LYMPHEDEMA

Acquired lymphedema develops after obstruction of the proximal lymphatic vessel because of infection, chronic disease, or interruption of the lymphatics after surgical resection, lymphadenectomy, or trauma.

We do not believe that cardiac and renal failure, venous thrombosis, and hypoproteinemia are causes of lymphedema. Experimental and clinical data have demonstrated that chronic edema does not arise as a consequence of the ligature of a large vein. However, if the lymphatics are blocked and regeneration is prevented, chronic irreversible lymphedema can result.

Confusing lymphedema (localized high-protein edema) with generalized (low-protein) edema secondary to cardiac or renal failure shows a poor understanding of the pathophysiology of lymphedema. Lymphedema results from a quantitative deficit between the lymphatic transport capacity and lymphatic load, resulting in accumulation of macromolecules and protein.

The primary disorder in secondary lymphedema is attributable to an acquired lymphatic obstruction in the proximal extremity. The distal normal lymph trunk undergoes secondary dilation and tortuosity that make the valves incompetent. The increased hydrostatic pressure with the consequent decreases in backflow of lymph produces a protein-rich edema.

The microfilaria *Wuchereria bancrofti* (Bancroft's filaria) is responsible for tropical lymphangitis.[3,4] The most common infecting organism in lymphedema is microfilaria; it has a particular predilection for the lymphatic trunks and nodes, which become obstructed by the adult worm. Local infection can obliterate lymphatic vessels and produce additional fibrosclerosis with increased severity in edema formation. Acute infectious lymphangitis may progress to chronic recurrent lymphangitis if not adequately treated. After recurrent episodes of infection, progressive blockage of the lymphatics can occur. Historically the most common organisms encountered in recurrent lymphangitis are *Streptococcus* organisms. *Staphylococcus* organisms are occasionally present; other organisms are encountered depending on the geographic region.

Blockage of the lymphatic channels by malignancy is not common; however, in the late phase of disease such blockage can result from surgical extirpation of the tumor and regional lymphatic vessels. The incidence of lymphedema after lymphadenectomy varies widely among reported series, despite the fact that most of the axillary iliac and inguinal node dissections are performed in essentially the same fashion.

Postoperative irradiation greater than 5000 cGy will produce definitive vascular and lymphatic sclerosis. Other forms of lymphatic obstruction occur with ligation of the thoracic duct at the cervical level, in the thorax, at the cisterna chyli, and at the iliac level.

Clinical Presentation

The edema is slowly progressive, taking a period of months or years to become fully established. Initially in the first stage lymphedema is a soft, pitting edema, usually more noticeable in the distal extremity. In the second stage nonpitting, brownish edema develops. The edema is maximal toward evening or after prolonged periods of standing or walking. It is rare for durable spontaneous regression to occur. The edema may fluctuate with fluid loading or dependent position.

The patient complains about the weight of the limb and that it impairs physical activity and produces fatigue, especially at the end of the day when swelling is maximal. Pain is rare, but when maximal swelling occurs, discomfort may result from the sensation of distention of the skin.[5]

The diseased skin is thickened, coarse, and hairless. The subcutaneous tissue is also thickened. Slight trauma to the skin can induce weeping of lymph because of lymph stasis and impaired circulation. Ulcers are frequent. Pigmentation of the skin is seen at the sites of recurrent ulceration. The nails have a yellowish tinge and nail growth is delayed.

The area involved varies according to etiology. Primary lymphedema usually affects the entire lower extremity; in 50% of patients it may affect to some degree the contralateral extremity, lower abdomen, scrotum, or genitals. Secondary lymphedema resulting from ablative surgery of the breast involves the entire upper extremity. Lymphedema caused by filariasis or bacterial infection is often limited to the lower leg or foot, seldom rising above the knee to affect the thigh.[6,7]

The possibility of lymphedema should be considered in any individual (child or adult) with a persistent increase in the volume of a limb. Interrogation of a family member facilitates recognition of the hereditary forms.

Textbooks often state the need to differentiate lymphedema from hemangioma and neurofibroma; making this distinction is usually not difficult. Lymphedema is frequently clearly discernible by a typical history and characteristic symptoms and physical findings. Hemangioma can be readily compressed; neurofibroma is much firmer and has fibromatous strands that can be detected. Both have specific clinical characteristics quite different from those of lymphedema.

Diagnostic Studies

The diagnosis of lymphedema can be made in the majority of patients by clinical evaluations on the basis of the characteristic historic and physical findings. In the case of follow-up the most reliable method of diagnosing lymphedema of an extremity is water displacement volume determinations. The use of lymphography must be avoided in these patients because of the high morbidity and increased edema after the procedure.[8]

When microsurgical reconstruction is being considered, preoperative diagnostic evaluation, including lymphatic and venous isotopic scintigraphy, Doppler flowmetrics, and pressure manometry, plays an essential role in assessing the status of both the lymphatic and venous systems and in determining which procedure, if any, is indicated.

The practice of performing routine venography to diagnose lymphedema should be condemned. Venography is not without hazards and in certain cases may aggravate lymphedema. Venous disease is assessed by inspection and noninvasive methods. The presence of symptoms and signs of venostasis should provide evidence of associated blockage of the venous system.

Lymphedema of the Upper Extremities

Lymphedema of the upper extremity is rare except after treatment of the axillary lymphatic bed for breast carcinoma. Standard measurements of the upper extremity show that slight swelling of the arm is invariably present after mastectomy with axillary lymphadenectomy. Significant swelling is delayed for at least 6 months. Varying degrees of lymphedema occur in approximately 50% of patients. Approximately 10% will have pronounced to severe edema with the consequent functional and cosmetic impairment of the extremity.[9,10] Lymphedema may not develop in some patients until 15 or more years postoperatively.

The reported incidence of lymphedema of the upper extremity varies from 3% to 42%. In a review of the literature consisting of 2330 cases collected from 14 series of patients who had been treated by mastectomy for breast cancer from 1937 to 1966, 13% were reported to suffer from lymphedema as a complication of surgical or combined treatment of axillary lymphatics.[11]

Using premastectomy and postmastectomy lymphangiography, Bower et al.[12] have postulated that the extent of surgical excision may be less important in the etiology of secondary lymphedema than primary failure of lymphatic proliferation, which means effective collateral lymphatic circulation cannot be restored. The lymphatic obstruction has been demonstrated by various researchers. The contribution of the venous system to arm edema is usually nonexistent.[12,13]

Some patients may follow a cycle wherein the primary defect in the lymphatics results in chronic edema and secondary fibrosis of the subcutaneous tissue, which may on occasion lead to venous obstruction and venous stasis.

The incidence of lymphedema is increased when radiotherapy is used to treat the axillary area. This treatment modality also results in interstitial fibrosis and consequent sclerosis of the lymphatics.[13]

The most serious long-term complication of lymphedema is lymphangiosarcoma. In a series of 894 patients surviving 5 years after mastectomy, the incidence of lymphangiosarcoma was 0.45%. Most reported cases have occurred in lymphedematous extremities of patients after axillary node dissection. Few cases have been reported after primary lymphedema.[10,14]

Lymphedema of the Lower Extremities

The course of the lymphatic outflow tract of the lower extremities follows the division of the venous system, superficial lymphatic system (greater saphenous and lesser saphenous lymphatics), and deep lymphatic system.

Lymphedema resulting from blockage of the lymphatic channels by tumor is an uncommon early presentation. In the late phases of malignancy, there may be extensive tumor encasement. One of the major objections to elective inguinal and deep inguinal lymphadenectomy is the predictable development of lymphedema. Lymphedema often occurs after iliac node dissection or extensive radiation of the pelvis for malignant gynecologic tumors. Edema is worse in the lower extremity than the upper extremity because the lymphatics are channeled through the inguinal-iliac region, collateral routes are distant, and the dependent position of the leg makes gravity an adversary rather than an ally. Postoperative radiation or local infection increases the incidence and severity of edema formation.

Genital Lymphedema

The testes drain directly to the lymphatic nodes of the pelvis and upper region. Lymphatic vessels descend along the course of the spermatic cord and bypass the male nodes. The penis, vulva, and scrotum drain to the medial superficial inguinal nodes.

The most common cause of secondary lymphedema of the genitals is obstruction, most frequently secondary to infection. The most accepted management of genital lymphedema is surgery; conservative medical management (diuretics, elevation, scrotal support) is of little value. The use of benzopyrones in the treatment of genital lymphedema has been unsatisfactory.

In male lymphedema the penis becomes crooked and thickens, and the enlarged scrotal mass may cause problems during walking and sex. Shusutrua (600 BC) was the first to perform excisional surgery for genital lymphedema. Different techniques have been described in the reconstruction of the scrotum to create a new lymphatic bed for preservation of testicular function. During initial attempts the genital area was excised and left to spontaneously heal. Later, coverage was achieved with a free skin graft and/or pedicle flap. Because of altered testicular thermoregulation, testicular function was inhibited when skin grafts were used.

Delpech (1820) described reconstruction of penis and scrotum with local flaps. Subcutaneous pouches prepared bilaterally at the medial thigh also failed to prevent thermoregulation.[15,16] Other authors have advocated reconstruction using posterior scrotal flaps after excision of lymphoid tissue.

Yormuk et al.[15] proposed the creation of U-shaped flaps from the suprapubic region and posterior scrotal skin with anterior repositioning of the penis and split-thickness skin graft as the best method of reconstruction. This approach basically offers an acceptable outcome in testicular function with normal sexual activity.

With respect to lymphangioplasty procedures (autogenous or prosthetic materials), they have been beneficial in certain patients. Gillies proposed the use of a skin bridge for treatment of genital lymphedema. Modifications were described by McDonald and Huggins (scrotal and thigh anastomoses)[15a] and Chitale (tensor fascia lata musculocutaneous transposition).[16] However, these procedures do not augment lymphatic drainage significantly.

Lymph drainage prosthetic materials have been used for a long time. Initially long silk sutures were used to form fibrotic bridges; silicone tubes that acted as wicks to absorb lymph fluid by capillary action have also been employed. Limited success has been achieved with these materials.

We believe that for lymphedema of the penis and scrotum, regardless of etiology, the best approach is the excision technique in which the superficial lymphatics, subcutaneous tissue, and skin at the level of Buck's fascia of the penis are excised and direct dissection of the spermatic cord and testicle from the scrotal mass is performed.

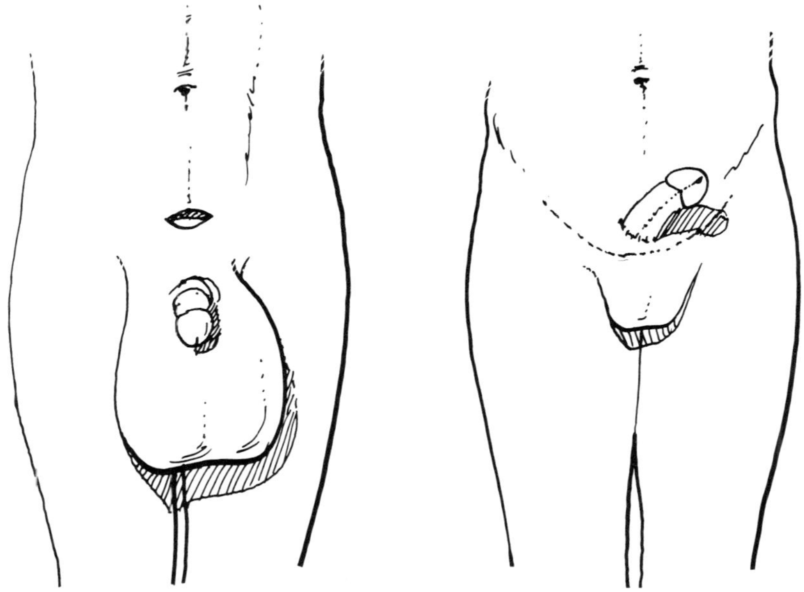

Reconstruction techniques vary according to the degree or severity of lymphedema and the type of excision.[17] The nonaffected skin of the scrotum should be used to cover the testis. If not, both testes can be sewn together and covered with a split-thickness skin graft.

For the penis we have found that a combination of local flaps and split-thickness skin graft (0.018 to 0.23 μm) spiraled around the penis or a split-thickness skin graft applied as a Z-plasty is effective and decreases the possibility of contracture. Postoperatively painful erection should be avoided by hormonal manipulation or aromatic ammonia.

MANAGEMENT

The treatment of lymphedema attempts to restore equilibrium between tissue lymph protein load and lymphatic vascular capacity. Medical management includes multicompartment pneumatic pumps and massage, limb elevation, weight control, and meticulous hygiene in order to avoid secondary problems such as cellulitis and lymphangitis.[8]

The treatment of lymphedema with intermittent pressure devices and compression stockings is associated with long-term maintenance of reduced limb girth in 90% of patients.[18]

Although many surgical techniques for the treatment of lymphedema have been described in the literature, none has evolved as the ideal operation; therefore surgical intervention is reserved for extreme situations in which there is recurrent infection or severe disability.

When the surgical procedure is being selected, particular consideration should be given to the surgeon's experience with different techniques, clinical stage of the lymphedema, and realistic expectations about functional recovery and aesthetic appearance. During the early postoperative period reduction in size or volume of an extremity is frequently achieved only to be followed by relapse.

Objective improvement with any type of surgical treatment should be evaluated by the following criteria:

1. Decrease in the circumferential standardized measurements at fixed anatomic points on the lymphedematous extremity at different periods after treatment
2. Increased function of the affected limb
3. Marked decrease in tissue turgor of the lymphedematous extremity
4. Complete resolution or a significant decrease in the frequency of episodes of cellulitis or lymphangitis of the lymphedematous limb

A great number of operations have been described for the treatment of lymphedema, but basically they can be divided into two categories: (1) physiologic procedures (attempts to reconstruct lymphatic flow) and (2) excisional or resectional procedures (removal of varying amounts of skin and subcutaneous tissue by surgery or liposuction).

Encouraging results with the use of lymphatic grafts and microlymphaticovenous anastomoses have recently been reported; although improvement is seen, cure is still not possible.[19-22] Other physiologic procedures attempt to restore lymphatic flow by introducing a pedicle of omentum as skin flap, prosthetic material, or buried dermis, thus creating a bridge to drain the involved edematous area into normal tissue. Various reports appear in the literature supporting the described techniques.[23,24] Generally the above-mentioned techniques are supplemented by operations that remove subcutaneous tissue by liposuction and/or by the use of compressive devices, thus raising serious doubts as to which aspects of the treatment were responsible for the clinical improvement.

Suction lipectomy in selected lymphedema patients is offered now as a procedure that has a low infection risk with minimal scarring and rapid healing. Sando and Nahai[25] suggest that patients with good skin elasticity and limited fibrosis would benefit from liposuction of the upper extremity. The procedure would be especially useful in patients with breast carcinoma following brachial radioneuritis. In these patients, because of restricted limb movement, the muscle pump mechanism to propel the lymph is lost.[26] Liposuction has been used as an initial procedure in patients with primary lymphedema and in patients with obstructive lymphedema when no lymphatic vessels were available for lymphogenous anastomoses. For the lower extremity a combined approach of liposuction with a conventional debulking technique is recommended (Table 42-1).

Pharmacologic management has been attempted, including use of anti-inflammatories, diuretics (low-dose, short-lived), emollients (antiliposclerotics), connective tissue enzymes (e.g., mucinolytic derivatives), and lymphotropes such as benzopyrones and rutosides. Although these agents can be used at any stage, their beneficial value is more noticeable during the early stages of lymphedema.

Special consideration should be given to the benzopyrones, which exert their moderate therapeutic effect by stimulating macrophages to scavenger the stagnating plasma proteins. Clinical trials show a 20% reduction in volume after 6 months of treatment. Still under study are the possible long-term effects of protein catabolism, a consequence of the continuous degradation of protein molecules that escape to the microcirculation.[8]

In chronic lymphedema the presence of fibrosis makes any reconstitution of lymphatic conduits less likely. In this late stage operations are directed at attempts to reduce the size of the limb by excision of subcutaneous tissue and skin. The three well-known excisional procedures were proposed by Charles,[27] Kondoleon, and Sistrunk.[29,30] The Charles procedure is the most frequently used (see p. 1553). The other two have been practically abandoned. Two procedures that attempt to reduce the size of the extremity and improve lymph drainage are Thompson's buried dermal flap[11] and Miller's staged subcutaneous and dermal excision[31-33] (see p. 1555).

Table 42-1 Treatment Comparison

Treatment Type	*Decrease in Circumferential Measurements*	*Functional Improvement*	*Decrease in Tissue Turgor*	*Decrease in Episodes of Cellulitis and Lymphangitis*
Clinical massage	Beneficial in early stages	Improvement	N/A	N/A
Intermittent pressure devices	3-5 cm	Variable	50%	Variable
Pharmacologic benzopyzones	1-2 cm	Variable	20% during 6 months' treatment	Not available
Surgical debulking procedures	Depends on the amount of tissue excised; 3-4 cm recommended	Variable	40%-50%	Variable improvement
Microsurgery	3-4 cm	Improvement	48%-80%	Clear improvement
Liposuction	2-3 cm	Improvement	2.3%-8%	Difficult to assess, requires multiple procedures

In the case of reoperation for lymphedematous extremities, the same principles of conservative management and prophylactic measures are applied. Reoperation for lymphedema is indicated only for patients who after relapse fail to respond to appropriate medical management and suffer severe functional impairment.

Choosing the most appropriate surgical approach for a reoperation depends on the severity of the case (mild, moderate, or severe) and the type of lymphedema (primary or secondary). The approach is limited by the initial surgical procedure that was performed on the extremity. In the case of recurrent incapacitating lymphedema, a more radical surgical approach is recommended (Table 42-2).

The excisional type of surgical procedure is indicated (i.e., the Charles procedure, Thompson's buried dermal flap, or Miller's staged excision) once medical management or a lesser operation fails. At the far extreme of radical treatment, ligation of the superficial femoral artery immediately below the takeoff of the deep femoral artery has been suggested as a last resort before amputation. We have no experience with this procedure.

Table 42-2 Lymphatic Microsurgical Procedures

Technique	*Follow-up*	*Volume Reduction*	*Functional Improvement*	*Infection Control*	*Lymphatic Visualization (Flow Control)*
Lymphatic venous anastomosis—O'Brien (upper limb)	5 years	42%	Yes	Yes	Lymphatic scintigram
Lymphatic venous anastomosis—Degni	2 months-6 years	76%	Yes	Yes	N/A
Segmental lymphatic anastomosis—Baumasteir and Siuda	Upper limb, 3 years average; lower limb, 2 years average	Upper limb, 80%; lower limb, 60%	Yes	Yes	Lymphatic scintigram, good flow
Lymphatic-venous lymphatic anastomoses—Campisi	3-5 years	75%	Yes	Yes	Isotopic lymphography, good flow

After preoperative investigation, if the examining physician has no previous experience in the surgical treatment of lymphedema and is uncertain about the best operative procedure, he should refer the patient to a surgeon who is experienced in these techniques instead of subjecting the patient to an inadequate procedure.

The Charles Procedure

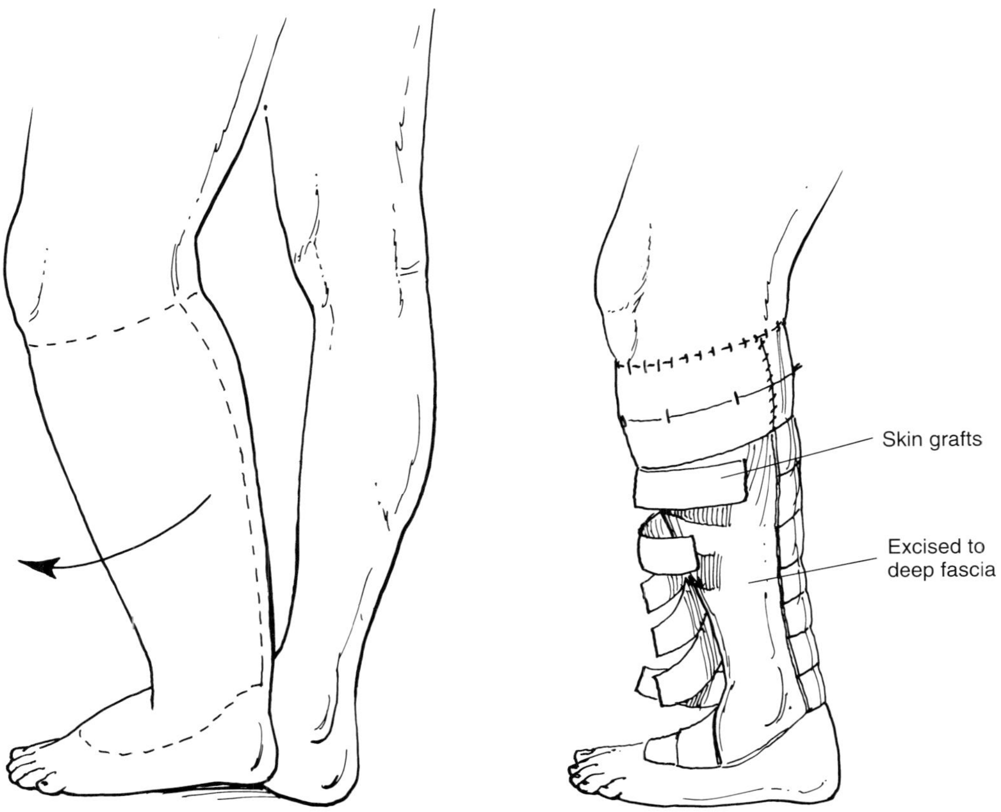

The Charles procedure consists of radical excision of all involved skin, subcutaneous tissue, and fascia with subsequent partial-thickness skin graft coverage.[27,28] The donor skin should be taken from anatomic sites other than the affected limb.

The postoperative appearance is grotesque, with hypertrophic scar formation, exophytic keratosis, contracture, graft loss, sensory deficit, ulceration, and aggravated distal edema. This procedure should be reserved for extreme cases in which other surgical methods of treatment have failed.

Miller's Staged Subcutaneous and Dermal Excision

The staged excision of skin and subcutaneous tissue represents the more reasonable alternative for most patients with recurrent lymphedema. Miller[31-33] describes the procedure as a two-stage approach that allows the relatively safe removal of large amounts of lymphedematous tissue.

The first stage is usually performed in the medial aspect of the extremity. To limit blood loss, a high pneumatic tourniquet is placed proximally. A longitudinal incision is made along the medial malleolus. Skin flaps, approximately 1.5 to 2 cm in thickness, are raised anteriorly and posteriorly to the midsagittal plane. Conservative undermining is advised about the malleolus. All underlying fat, fibrotic tissue, and fascia are then excised except for a strip of fascia underlying the posterior tibial artery at the ankle. (In Servelle's method, muscle fascia and subcutaneous tissue are removed.[34]) The saphenous vein is usually sacrificed, but it is desirable to preserve it. The sural nerve should be positively identified and preserved. Equal amounts of the anterior and posterior soft tissues under the skin flaps are removed, allowing for closure under minimal tension. After hemostasis has been obtained, the flaps are closed over suction drains. Closure in two layers allows for early suture removal at about 2 weeks. If the viability of the skin flap is in question, the use of intravenous fluorescein (15 mg/kg) is helpful for diagnostic purposes. Approximately 2 to 4 months later the second stage is performed in the lateral aspect of the extremity if it is necessary. In some cases a single procedure has proved effective. Special attention should be paid to the preservation of the sural and peroneal nerves when performing the lateral approach. With proper attention to atraumatic technique, hemostasis, and avoidance of excessive tension, complications are minimal.

The most common problems have been small areas of skin flap necrosis, dehiscence, and hematoma. Any sizable hematoma should be drained. Minor flap dehiscence or loss is treated conservatively. Occasionally skin grafting may be required.

The extremity is elevated to facilitate lymph drainage, and appropriate antibiotics are administered to prevent infection. An indwelling catheter is placed to protect the thigh from contamination from urine. Dressings are not removed until the sutures are removed unless wound infection is suspected. After suture removal dressings and elastic bandages must still be used to prevent formation of blisters under the graft or flap. The patient can be partially ambulatory but must remain in bed most of the time. At 3 months the patient is allowed to resume activities with the following precautions: (1) fitted compressive stockings must be worn for the rest of the patient's life to protect the grafted limb, (2) the limb must be elevated at regular intervals during the day for 20 to 30 minutes, (3) careful hygiene must be maintained, and (4) early treatment of infection is mandatory.

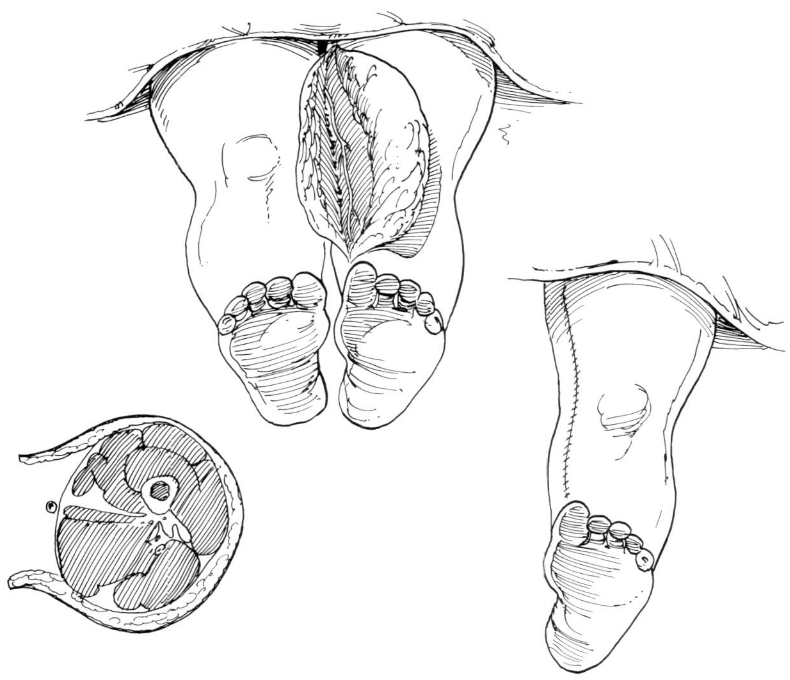

First stage: Excision via medial incision

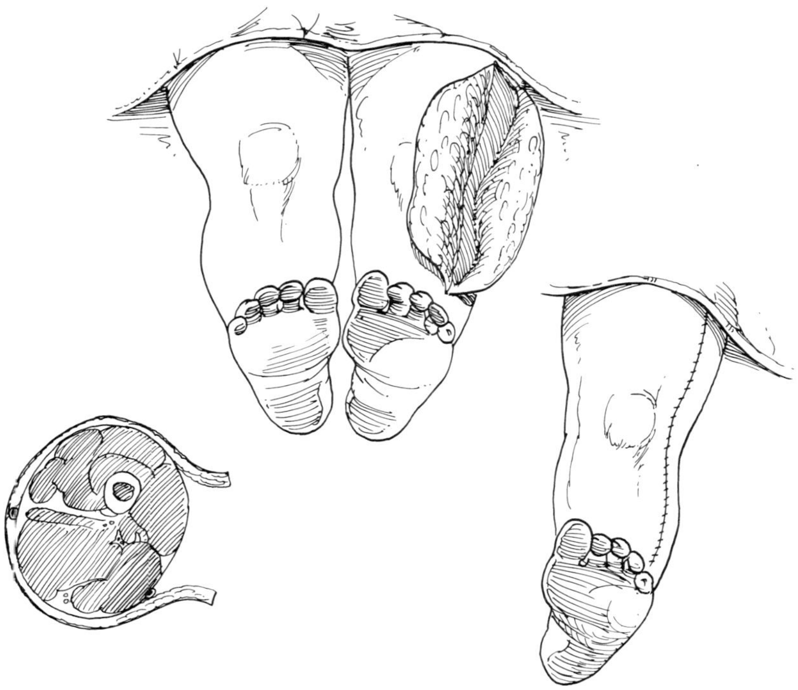

Second stage: Excision via lateral incision

Lymphatic Microsurgical Procedures

Promising results have been documented in the literature with different microsurgical techniques in the treatment of patients with long-standing secondary lymphedema in whom nonoperative treatment has failed.[21]

The described techniques are indicated in all cases of benign pathologic or iatrogenic blocked lymphatic vessels when lymph scintigraphic controls show blockage at a definite level and demonstrate normal valves and permeability of lymphatic vessels.

The only absolute contraindications to microlymphaticovenous anastomosis and autogenous transplantation of lymph nodes are (1) primary lymphedema because of the presence of hypoplastic lymphatic vessels unsuitable for anastomosis and (2) venous hypertension in cases of obstructive lymphedema due to the reverse flow from vein to the lymphatic vessel.[20]

Lymphatic microsurgical procedures basically are physiologic surgeries that are designed to create a bypass around an obstructed area via lymphaticovenous anastomoses, lymphatic-lymphatic anastomoses, or lymphatic graft interposition. These operations do not solve the problem of quantitative relation between the lymphatic load and lymphatic transport capacity. Lymphscintigraphic controls have shown improvement but not necessarily normalization of lymph flow.[20,21]

Microlymphatic anastomosis as the main method of treatment either alone or in combination with other procedures has been used since 1974.[35-37] Many techniques have been described. A review of the literature indicates improvement in technique as evidenced by 40% to 80% volume reduction.[20,21] Especially good results have been seen in the upper limb (Table 42-2).

We believe the results are convincing, particularly with lymphatic and venous graft interposition. Such techniques apparently have high anastomotic patency rates because of the lower coagulability of the lymph compared with that of blood and the lower lymphatic pressure at the anastomotic site compared with that at the lymphaticovenous anastomosis.[21,38]

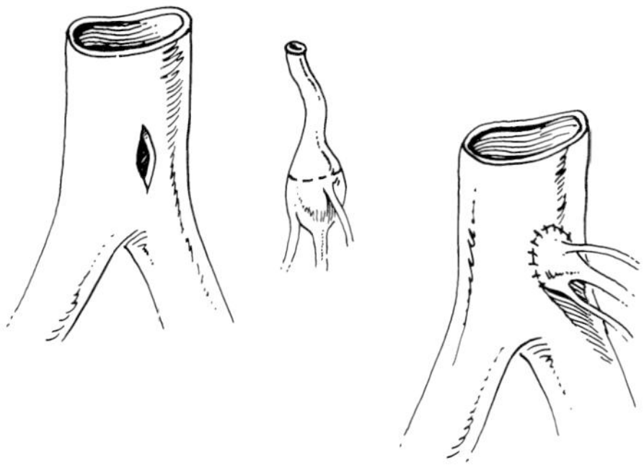

Lymph nodal–venous anastomosis

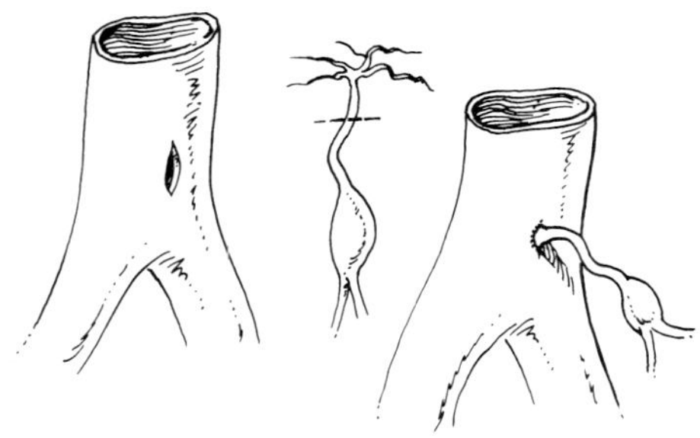

Lymphaticovenous anastomosis

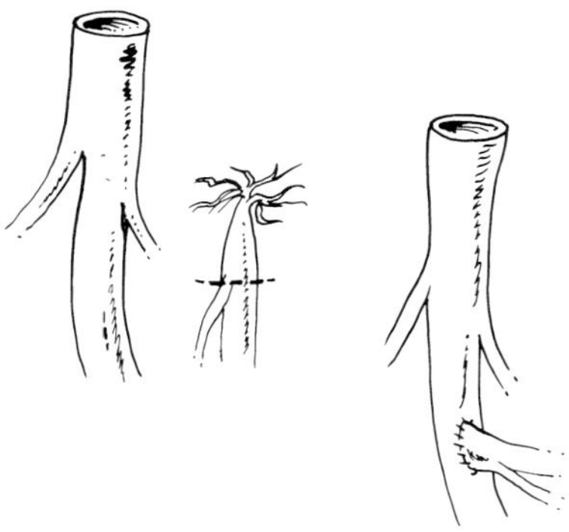

Lymphaticovenous capsular anastomosis

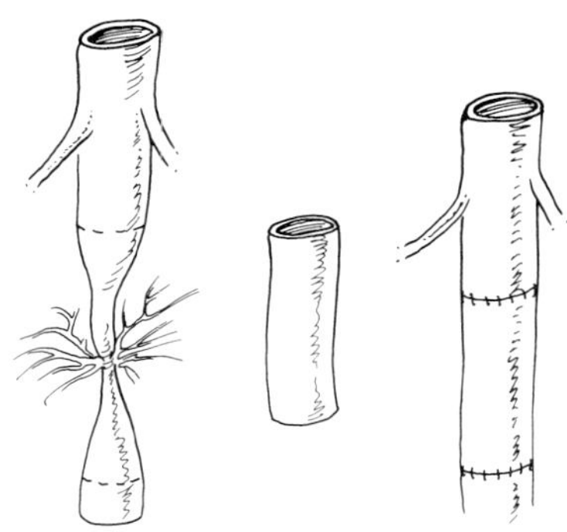

Segmental lymphatic autotransplant
Segmental lymphatic allotransplant

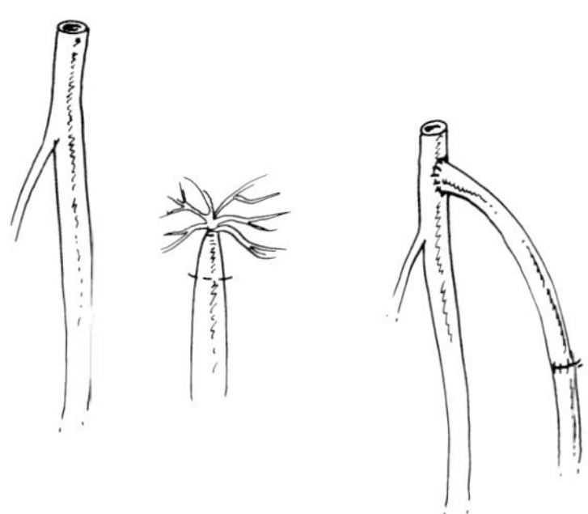

Lymphaticovenous-lymphatic anastomosis

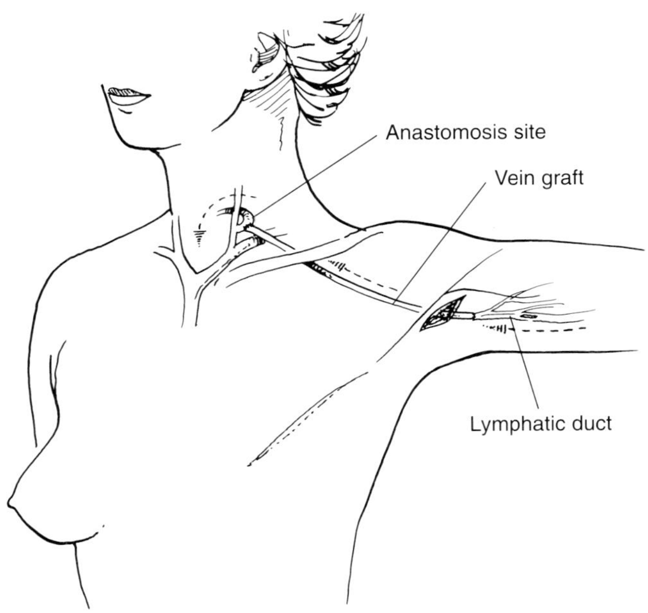

Lymphatic bypass

References

1. Crockett DJ. Lymphatic anatomy and lymphoedema. Br J Plast Surg 18:12, 1965.
2. Starling EH. On the absorption of fluids from the connective tissue spaces. J Physiol 19:312, 1896.
3. Dandapat MC, Nohapatro SK, Mohanty SS. Filarial lymphoedema and elephantiasis of lower limb: A review of 44 cases. Br J Surg 73:451-453, 1986.
4. Jamal S. Lymphogenous anastomosis in filarial lymphedema. Lymphology 13:64-68, 1981.
5. Song R, Gao X, Li S, et al. Surgical treatment of lymphedema of the lower extremity. Clin Plast Surg 9:113-114, 1982.
6. Jamal S. Lymphogenous anastomosis in filarial lymphedema. Lymphology 14:64-68, 1981.
7. Schirger A, Harrison EG, Janes JM. Idiopathic lymphedema. JAMA 182:14-22, 1962.
8. Foldi E, Foldi M, Clodius L. The lymphedema chaos: A lancet. Ann Plast Surg 22:505-515, 1989.
9. Tracy GD, Reeve TS, Fitzsimmons E, et al. On the swollen arm after mastectomy. Aust N Z J Surg 30:204, 1960.
10. Schirger A, Harrison EG, Janes JM. Idiopathic lymphedema. JAMA 182:14, 1962.
11. Thompson N. The surgical treatment of chronic lymphoedema. Surg Clin North Am 47:445-503, 1967.
12. Bower R, Danese C, Debbas J, et al. Advances in diagnosis of diseases of the lymphatic. JAMA 181:687, 1962.
13. Treves N. An evaluation of the etiological factors of lymphedema following radical mastectomy. An analysis of 1007 cases. Cancer 10:444, 1957.
14. Peterson LF. Surgical treatment of lymphedema and treatment of lymphangiosarcoma. Mod Treat 6:413-421, 1969.
15. Yormuk E, Sevin K, Emiroglu M, et al. A new surgical approach in genital lymphedema. Plast Reconstr Surg 86:1194-1197, 1990.

15a. McDonald DF, Huggins C. Surgical treatment of elephantiasis. J Urol 63:187, 1950.

16. Chitale VR. Role of tensor fascia lata musculocutaneous flap in lymphedema of the lower extremity and external genitalia. Ann Plast Surg 23:297, 1989.
17. Sauer P, Bueschen A, Vasconez L. Lymphedema of the penis and scrotum. Clin Plast Surg 15:507-511, 1988.
18. Pappas CJ, O'Donnell TF Jr. Long-term results of compression treatment for lymphedema. J Vasc Surg 16:555-564, 1992.
19. Campisi C. A rational approach to the management of lymphedema. Lymphology 24:48-53, 1991.
20. O'Brien BMcC, Mellow CG, Khazanchi RK, et al. Long-term results after microlymphaticovenous anastomoses for the treatment of obstructive lymphedema. Plast Reconstr Surg 85:562-572, 1990.
21. Baumeister RG, Siuda S. Treatment of lymphedema by microsurgical lymphatic grafting. What is proved? Plast Reconstr Surg 85:64-74, 1990.
22. Degni M. New technique of lymphatic-venous anastomosis for the treatment of lymphedema. J Cardiovasc Surg 19:577-580, 1978.
23. Hen HC, O'Brien BMcC, Rogers IW, et al. Lymph node transfer for the treatment of obstructive lymphoedema in the canine model. Br J Plast Surg 43:578-586, 1990.
24. O'Brien BMcC, Hickey MJ, Hurly JV, et al. Microsurgical transfer of the greater omentum in the treatment of canine obstructive lymphoedema. Br J Plast Surg 43:440-446, 1990.
25. Sando WC, Nahai F. Suction lipectomy in the management of limb lymphedema. Clin Plast Surg 16:369-373, 1989.
26. O'Brien BMcC, Khazanchi RK, Kumar PAV, et al. A preliminary report. Br J Plast Surg 42:530-533, 1989.

27. Charles RH. Surgical treatment of lymphedema. In Latham A, English TC, eds. A System of Treatment, vol 3. London: Churchill Livingstone, 1912, p 504.
28. Dellon AL, Hoopes JE. The Charles procedures for primary lymphedema. Plast Reconstr Surg 60:589, 1977.
29. Sistrunk WE. Contribution to plastic surgery. Ann Surg 85:185-193, 1927.
30. Sistrunk WE. Further experiences with the Kondoleon operation for elephantiasis. JAMA 71:800-806, 1918.
31. Miller TA. Lymphedema. In Grabb WC, Smith JW, eds. Plastic Surgery. Boston: Little, Brown, 1979, pp 826-837.
32. Miller TA. Surgical management of lymphedema of the extremity. Plast Reconstr Surg 56:633-641, 1975.
33. Miller TA, Harper JD, Longmire WP Jr. The management of lymphedema by staged subcutaneous excision. Surg Gynecol Obstet 136:558-592, 1973.
34. Servelle M. Surgical treatment of lymphedema: A report on 652 cases. Surgery 101:485-495, 1987.
35. O'Brien BMcC, Sikes P. Microlymphatic anastomosis for obstructive lymphedema. Plast Reconstr Surg 60:197-211, 1977.
36. O'Brien BMcC, Shofizoff B. Microlymphaticovenous and resectional surgery in obstructive lymphedema. World J Surg 3:3, 1979.
37. Campisi C. Use of autologous interposition vein graft in the management of lymphedema: Preliminary experimental and clinical observations. Lymphology 24:71-76, 1984.
38. Yoffery JH, Courtice FE. Lymphatics Lymph and the Lymphomyeloid Complex, 2nd ed. New York: Academic Press, 1970.

43

Reoperative Peripheral Nerve Surgery

A. Lee Dellon, M.D.

Reoperative Problems

Scarring	Adhesions
Neuroma	Recurrent nerve entrapment
Anomalous anatomic structures	Persistent numbness
Pain	Sensory loss

Operations on the peripheral nerve are performed for three general reasons: (1) to restore function by decompression of the nerve (e.g., carpal tunnel syndrome), (2) to restore function by reestablishing continuity by either a nerve repair or a graft, and (3) to interrupt function by division of the nerve (e.g., neuroma of the radial sensory nerve). Reoperation on the peripheral nerve presupposes that one of these three indications has not had the desired outcome: (1) the nerve remains compressed (e.g., recurrent carpal tunnel syndrome), (2) the nerve repair or graft has not sufficiently restored function (e.g., incontinuity neuroma), or (3) neural function persists or has recurred in the form of a disturbing, recurrent neuroma. This chapter discusses each of these conditions as they relate to problems in the upper and lower extremity.

At the outset it must be recognized that many surgical disciplines view surgery of the peripheral nerve as their province: neurosurgeons, hand surgeons, plastic surgeons, orthopedic surgeons. It is common practice for these surgeons to wear operating loupes and to use intraoperative (disposable) nerve stimulators when they encounter critical problems. Certainly even the most experienced surgeon has patients in whom despite the best preoperative planning, intraoperative care, and postoperative rehabilitation, the surgical outcome does not meet the expectations of the patient or the surgeon or both. Such an outcome is unfortunate, but it does not constitute medical malpractice. The reoperative techniques discussed in this chapter may correct many of these problems.

The surgeon who operates on patients with complex peripheral nerve problems will often encounter extensive scarring about the nerve intraoperatively. Such scarring significantly increases the possibility of iatrogenic injury to the nerve by either direct transection of a fascicle or nerve or infarction due to disruption of remaining critical circulation. Preoperative discussion of the inherent risks of such reoperation and documentation of that discussion in the patient's chart should indemnify the surgeon reoperating on the peripheral nerve from successful medical malpractice litigation. Unfortunately, such discussion cannot guarantee that a claim will not be brought, and this is a risk that must be assumed by those who perform difficult reoperative surgery.

Any time an incision is made in the skin, minute sensory nerves will very likely be cut. Most of the time this does not result in a situation that requires treatment. It is perhaps only a matter of semantics as to whether surgery to treat an iatrogenic injury to a peripheral nerve constitutes a reoperation on that nerve. If an injury to a critical peripheral nerve is recognized at the time it occurs, one must decide whether to repair it or resect it at a more proximal level. If the nerve is a less critical cutaneous nerve, no treatment is necessary. If the injury is not recognized and either critical sensory or motor function is lost or the cutaneous nerve forms a painful neuroma, then reoperation is required. Unfortunately, division or stretch injuries to cutaneous nerves are common because these small nerves lie between the skin and the anatomic structures that are often the focus of primary surgery (e.g., gallbladder, abdominal wall, uterus). In these circumstances anatomic variations are usually to blame, not the surgeon. However, appropriate postoperative care should include recognition of the fact that the resulting postoperative pain is possibly due to a nerve injury, and consultation should be obtained from a colleague who is adept at reoperative or secondary surgery on the peripheral nerve.

An additional set of problems often accompanies the patient being evaluated for reoperation on the peripheral nerve: psychosocial adjustment. Frequently the patient has been unemployed for more than 2 years, has pending litigation for a motor vehicle or workmen's compensation claim, is hostile to physicians because of previous outcomes, and may be drug dependent. None of the discussion in the rest of the chapter will be of help in managing these problems! Close cooperation is encouraged between you and at least one psychiatrist experienced in chronic pain management. You must derive your own plan for narcotic management and you must determine if the patient should be detoxified preoperatively. Often this narcotic dependence will be detected only postoperatively. You will want to consult with another physician who is knowledgeable about psychotropic drugs or neuropharmacology. You do not want to be the one prescribing drugs to raise cortical serotonin levels and to restore sleep patterns. Another colleague with whom to combine services is an anesthesiologist knowledgeable about chronic pain management who can provide diagnostic nerve blocks, steroid Bier blocks, and sympathetic blocks.

Patient Evaluation

In contrast to most peripheral nerve entrapments for which careful physical examination plus quantitative sensibility testing suffice to make the diagnosis[1,2] and for which there are often false negative nerve conduction and electromyography results,[3] the preoperative evaluation of the patient being considered for reoperation on the peripheral nerve usually should include electrodiagnostic testing. The inherent limitation of nerve conduction testing is that it indicates only what is happening to the fastest-conducting and largest myelinated fibers. Thus problems within individual fascicles or with the smaller myelinated or unmyelinated fibers are not detected. When you write your referral, you must be specific: for example, "Rx: evaluate cervical disc disease at C5-6, C6-7 vs. median nerve entrapment in the forearm vs. recurrent median nerve compression at the wrist." It must be remembered that a previously decompressed peripheral nerve, even if clinically it is not a source of symptoms, may have slowed conduction time or prolonged latency because it never completely remyelinated. An abnormal electrodiagnostic finding, other than denervation potentials on the electromyogram, does not mean that the involved area is necessarily the source of the patient's problems nor that you must surgically intervene. The electrodiagnostic report must be correlated with clinical impressions and used to support and guide the findings based on careful physical examination and common sense.

Reoperative Technical Considerations

Role of Internal Neurolysis

My introduction to internal neurolysis was through the teaching of Raymond M. Curtis for whom the indications were persistent sensory change, muscle wasting, abnormal two-point discrimination, and recurrence of nerve compression.[4] It was his experience that patients with these clinical findings did not do well without internal neurolysis. With the development of a model for chronic nerve compression of the monkey median nerve,[5] it was possible to test different treatment strategies. Whereas it was demonstrated that with microsurgical training internal neurolysis could be performed in the plane of interfascicular fibrosis without injuring the nerve fibers, internal neurolysis was not shown to improve morphometric or electrodiagnostic results in this model.[6]

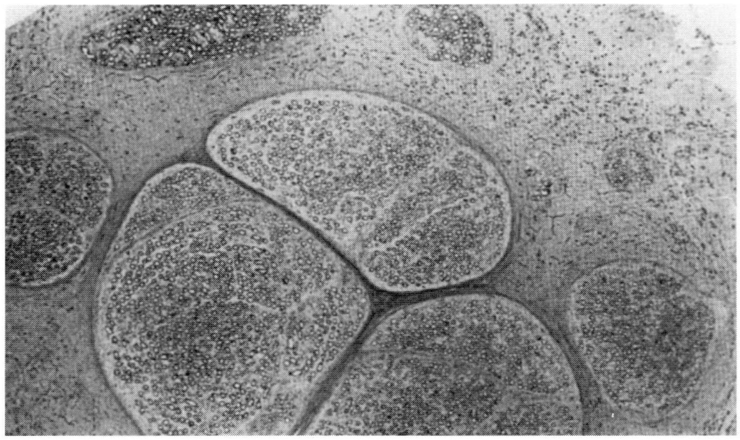

The surgical plane for internal neurolysis is between the fascicles. The perineurium, which provides a special environment for the nerve fibers including an increased endoneurial pressure,[6] must not be violated.

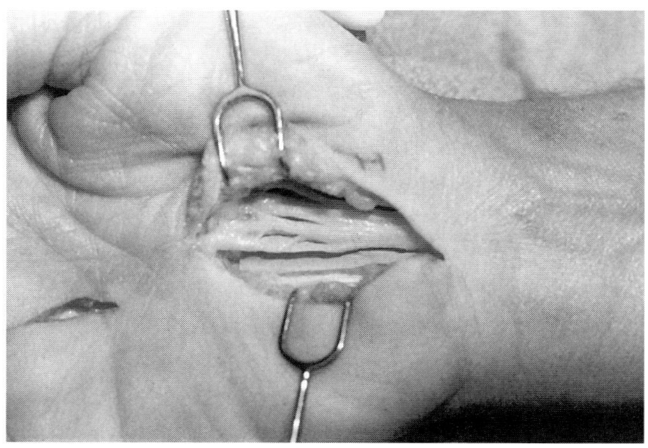

Plexus formation between fascicles can occur even in the distal portions of the peripheral nerve, such as shown here within the median nerve in the carpal tunnel.

In a prospective clinical randomized trial, it was demonstrated that adding internal neurolysis as an adjunctive procedure to carpal decompression for the routine patient with carpal tunnel syndrome did not significantly improve postoperative results.[7] That study did not stage the patient intraoperatively nor did it include patients with recurrent carpal tunnel syndrome. My personal approach is to open the epineurium, and if there is firmness within the nerve and the perineurial markings are not clearly visible, then I perform internal neurolysis.[8] If the fascicles are translucent consistent with axonal degeneration, then intraneural fibrosis is not present, the fascicles have decompressed themselves during the process of wallerian degeneration, and there is no need for internal neurolysis. Internal neurolysis is frequently required during reoperative surgery of the peripheral nerve.

Blood Supply to the Nerve

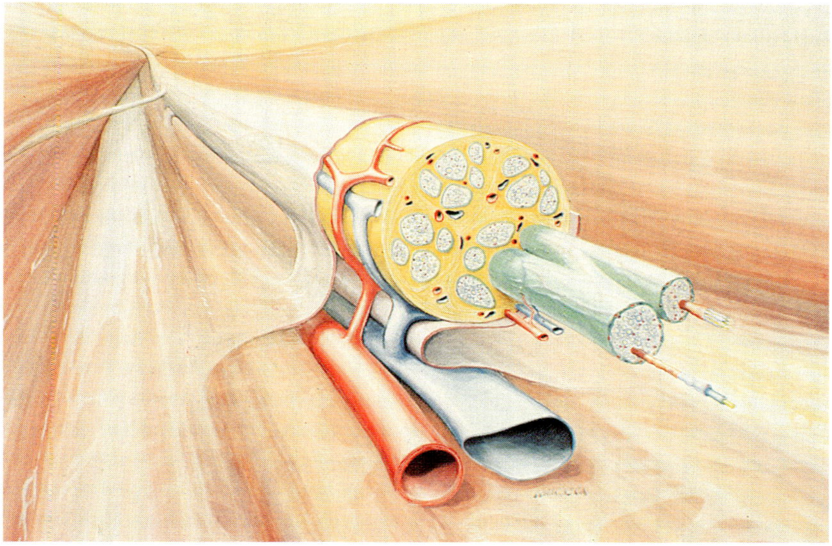

Lundborg[9] has extensively studied the anatomy of the blood supply to the peripheral nerve. The critical aspect for reoperative surgery is that there is a significant intrinsic blood supply to the peripheral nerve that permits the surgeon to lift the nerve from its anatomic bed, open the epineurium, and operate between the fascicles. The endoneurial and perineurial microvessels maintain an excellent vascularity to the peripheral nerve. Segmental blood vessels enter the peripheral nerve through the mesoneurium. In addition, an extensive number of longitudinal vessels in the epineurium, perineurium, and endoneurium supply the nerve.[1] However, pressures above 20 mm Hg will decrease blood flow. Recently, Breidenbach et al.[10] demonstrated that the "safe" length a nerve can be elevated from its bed (i.e., its segmental vascular supply) is a distance that is 63 times the diameter of the nerve. Therefore the surgeon should consider primarily the need to move the nerve into an area that is free from forces that might externally compress the nerve rather than be concerned about the length to which the nerve has been neurolysed. Breidenbach's observations were made on a normal rabbit tibial nerve. It has been my sad experience to cause infarction in two ulnar nerves. These patients were both above the age of 60, and in one patient the neurolysis was the second and in the other the neurolysis was the third procedure that the patient had. I therefore recommend extreme caution when performing neurolysis, even if the nerve is hard and fibrotic, the patient is over the age of 60 years, and the nerve has undergone neurolysis previously.

Illustration from Mackinnon SE, Dellon AL. Surgery of the Peripheral Nerve. New York: Thieme, 1988.

RECURRENT NERVE ENTRAPMENT IN THE UPPER EXTREMITY

Recurrent Carpal Tunnel Syndrome

An extensive review of the results of carpal tunnel decompression for carpal tunnel syndrome has been reported[11] and suggests that at least 10% to 20% of patients do not achieve an excellent result. Thus there are many patients who could potentially present for reoperation. Furthermore, perhaps 2% of patients who undergo carpal tunnel decompression will experience a complication other than failure before a good result is achieved. The general subject of secondary carpal tunnel surgery has also been reviewed recently.[12]

The indications for reoperation in the patient who has already undergone carpal tunnel decompression are (1) the patient has not obtained relief of numbness and tingling and (2) there is pain in and/or about the scar. Rarely the patient who had severe thenar atrophy may have a functional problem with thumb apposition; in this case tendon transfer may be considered. I have not ever found this procedure necessary in this situation, not so much because the results of the peripheral nerve surgery have been so good but because there is usually sufficient ulnar nerve innervation to ensure thenar muscle function.

The differential diagnosis for the patient with persistent numbness after carpal tunnel decompression is critical to the success of reoperative surgery. You must be sure there is not a proximal source of compression such as in the forearm (beneath a fibrous sublimus arch, the deep head of the pronator teres muscle) or at the elbow (the laceratus fibrosus or a ligament of Struthers). You must be sure that a coexisting brachial plexus compression in the thoracic inlet (not "outlet") or cervical disc disease at C5-6 and C6-7 is not present. Clearly if the symptoms are originating at another site, then "reoperative surgery" should be directed at this region rather than the carpal tunnel. The patient who complains of numbness in the index finger and thumb after carpal tunnel decompression must be asked if the numbness is present on the dorsum of those fingers. Radial sensory nerve compression[13] can present as failed carpal tunnel syndrome, and the radial nerve can innervate a significant portion of the thumb pulp.[14]

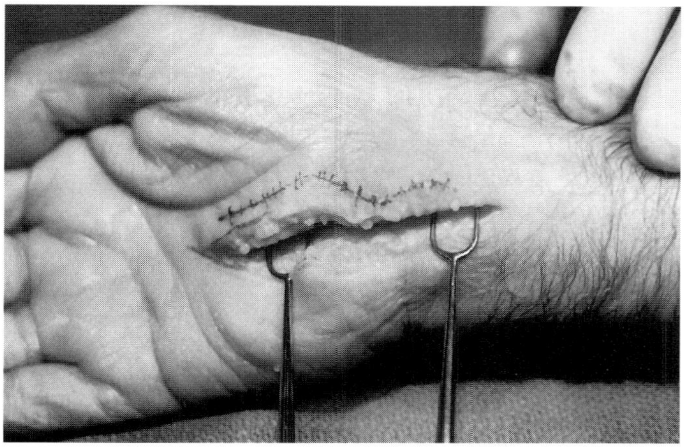

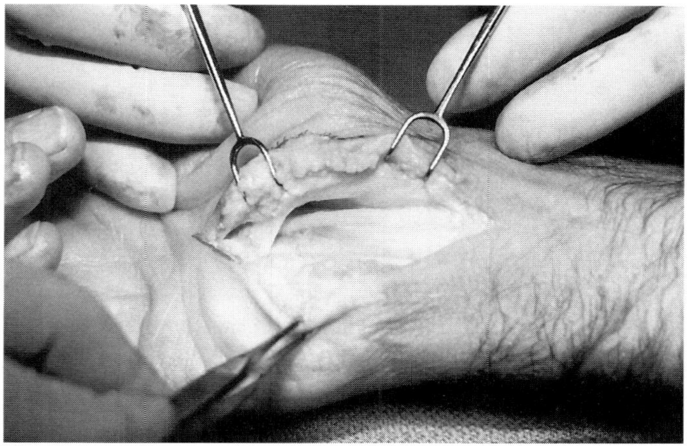

My personal approach to reoperation on the median nerve in the carpal tunnel after previous carpal tunnel decompression has been reported.[15,16] A new incision is made to the ulnar side of the first incision. This access avoids the risk of the scalpel incising the median nerve itself since the nerve is usually densely adherent to the undersurface of the palmar skin and is encased between the divided edges of the deep transverse carpal ligament. From the vantage of Guyon's canal, neurolysis of the median nerve can begin distal to the adherent site and the incision can be extended into the forearm to begin dissection distally from another unscarred area. If needed, use of a nerve stimulator can help to identify the motor branch. You must determine if there is a separate tunnel for this branch as it courses between layers of transverse carpal ligament instead of directly entering thenar muscles, which occurs in about 25% of the patients.[17]

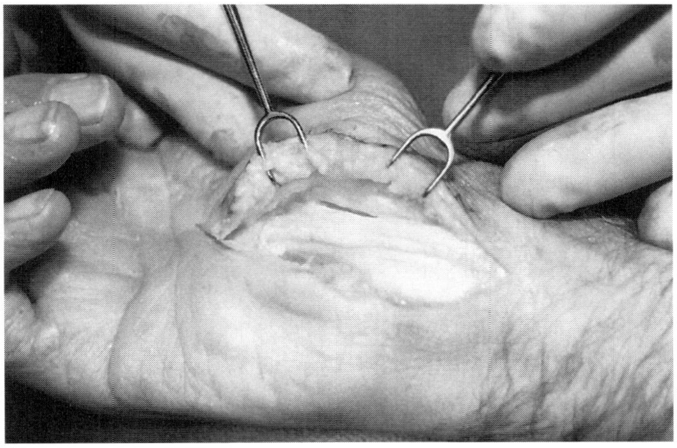

Microsurgical intraneural neurolysis to the median nerve is then performed. A flexor synovectomy is always performed as well, and the specimen is sent for pathologic examination; findings consistent with rheumatoid arthritis or another collagen vascular disease may be present. A small rim of the transverse carpal ligament should also be sent with a request for amyloid staining if this diagnosis is being considered or if the patient has some chronic disease, for which secondary amyloidosis is a possibility (e.g., renal disease).

The wrist is splinted in the neutral position for 7 to 8 days; the patient is then allowed to move the wrist in the full range of motion. Finger movement begins on the first postoperative day. In 30 patients with 35 reoperated hands treated with this approach, improvement was achieved in 32 patients (91.4%).[16] In that report a new numerical grading system was reported for the median nerve that permits statistical analysis of these complicated patients with varying degrees of sensory and motor deficits. In that system 0 is normal and 10 is severe intrinsic atrophy. The mean preoperative numerical score of the 35 hands was 6.7, and the mean postoperative score was 1.8 at a mean follow-up of 23.5 months; this improvement was statistically significant ($p < .001$). It has been helpful for us to use this grading system in the evaluation of peripheral nerve function.

At reexploration one of several congenital anomalies may be noted such as the presence of lumbricales manus muscles within the carpal canal, a high division of the median nerve so that it occupies a greater than expected volume within the tunnel, or a persistent median artery, which is often found in conjunction with a high division of the median nerve. If present, the persistent median artery should be preserved, but it should be separated from the median nerve via microsurgical dissection to prevent any vascular compression of the nerve. Its blood supply may be needed for an incomplete vascular arch. If there has been a history of a wrist fracture, especially a distal radius fracture, it is critical to extend the incision proximally and release the distal antebrachial fascia to well above the fracture site. The median neurolysis also may need to extend to this level.

When pain is one of the indications for surgery, you must determine if the source is adherence of the median nerve to the incision, so-called adhesive neuritis, neuroma of the palmar cutaneous branch of the median nerve (PCBM nerve), or both. If palpating or touching the incision causes sensations into the index or middle finger, then you must plan to provide some interface between the median nerve and the incision; my personal preference is to rotate an abductor digiti minimi manus muscle flap into this position.[18] This is a salvage procedure and probably should be reserved for the patient undergoing a third operation on the median nerve at the wrist. Most often neurolysis performed from the ulnar side provides sufficient soft tissue coverage. However, if the median nerve is very close to the surface, an interposition of vascularized muscle bulk is indicated.

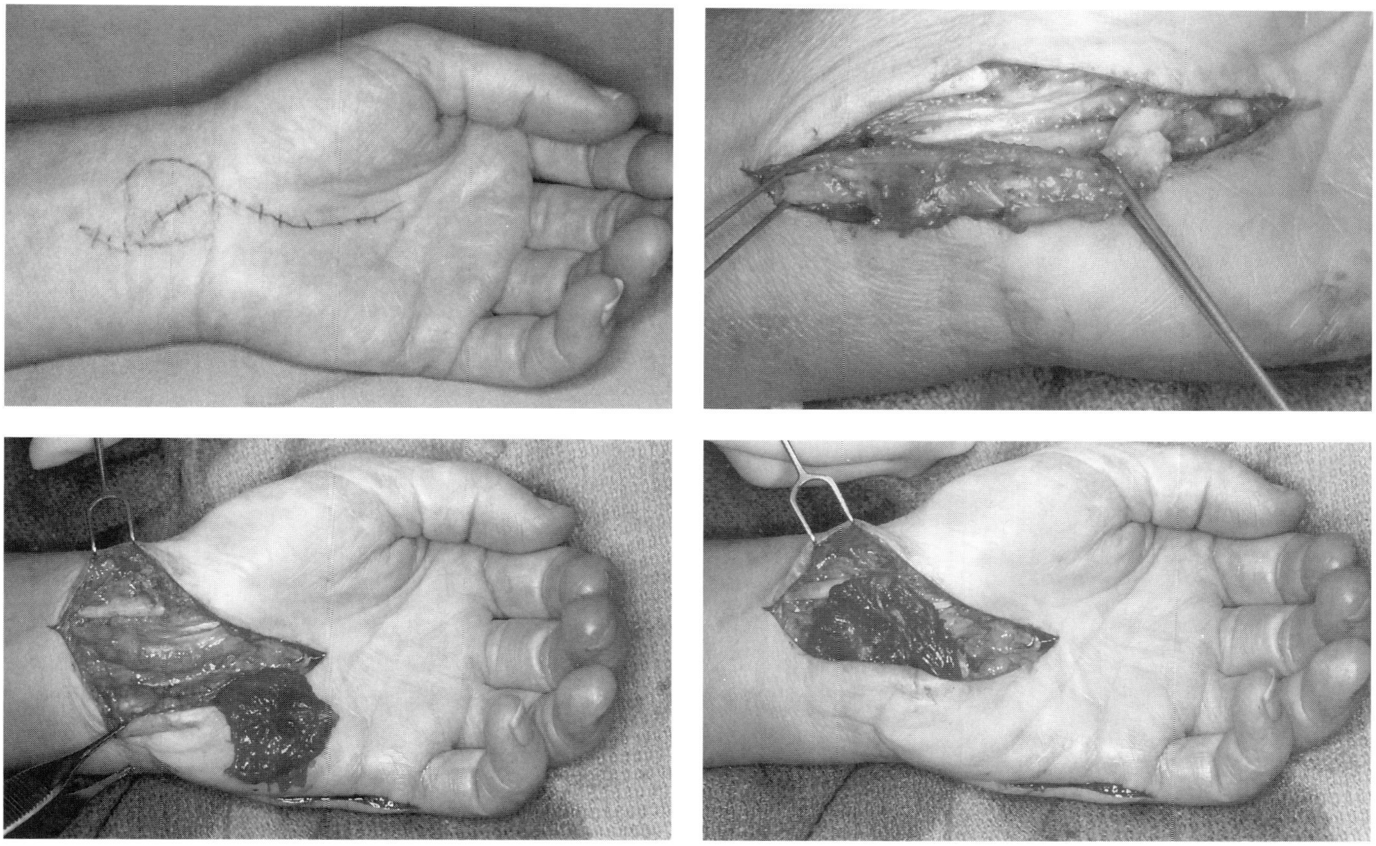

In this patient with an incontinuity neuroma of the median nerve, the interposition of the abductor digiti minimi manus muscle flap provided vascularized bulky tissue between the neurolysed median nerve and overlying thin cutaneous tissue and scar.[18]

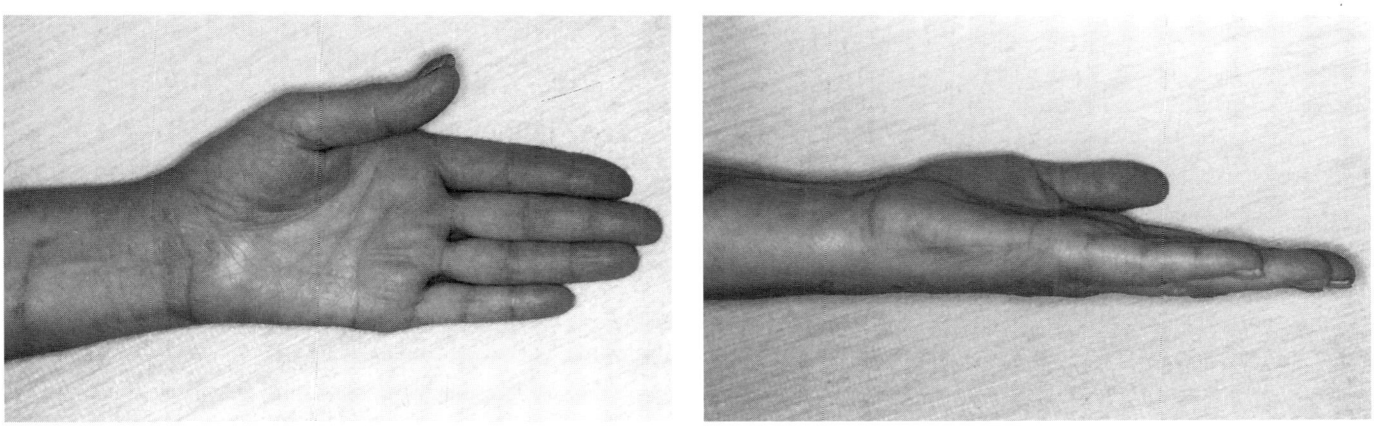

The postoperative appearance of the hand is cosmetically acceptable.

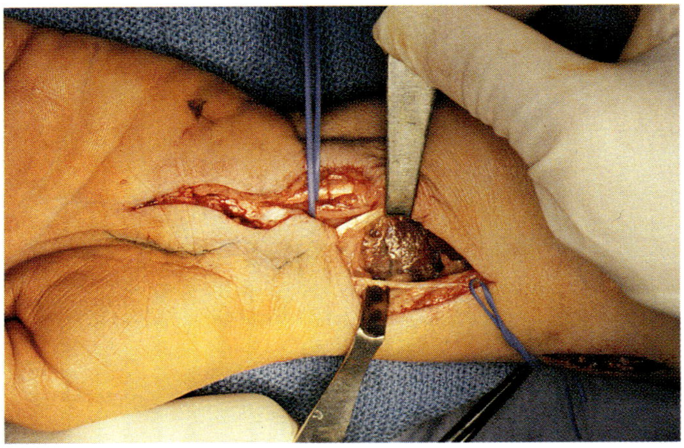

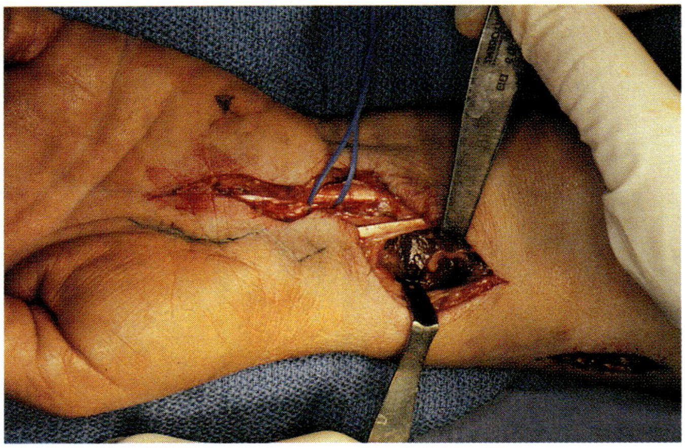

When a neuroma of the PCBM nerve has been demonstrated by nerve block, then interruption of the PCBM nerve function must be included in the operative plan. My preference is to divide the PCBM nerve at the tubercle of the trapezoid and implant the PCBM nerve into the pronator quadratus muscle.[19] This strategy prevents the nerve from regenerating into palmar or wrist skin, protects the transected end of the nerve for wrist and tendon range of motion, and places the "live" end of the nerve away from cutaneous stimulation or traction. Results with this approach to neuroma of the PCBM nerve have been good to excellent in 12 of 13 patients in whom this treatment was performed with a mean follow-up of 13.3 months (range, 6 to 22 months).

Photographs from Evans GRD, Dellon AL. Implantation of the palmar cutaneous branch of the median nerve into the pronator quadratus for treatment of painful neuroma (submitted for publication).

Recurrent Ulnar Nerve Entrapment at the Elbow

Cubital tunnel syndrome refers to entrapment of the ulnar nerve in the postcondylar groove, which implies that at least the roof of the tunnel and the band described by Osborne between the two heads of the flexor carpi ulnaris muscle have been released at the first operation. Reoperation then is indicated for ulnar nerve entrapment at the elbow regardless of where the ulnar nerve is located; it may be in situ or it may be transposed anteriorly and lie subcutaneously, intramuscularly, or submuscularly. If the first operation was a medial epicondylectomy, the ulnar nerve may be adherent to the medial humeral epicondyle. In one patient in whom the flexor-pronator muscle mass had been elevated to include a portion of the medial humeral epicondyle that was then reattached by a corticocancellous screw, the ulnar nerve was found compressed between bone! Reoperation for ulnar nerve entrapment must therefore be a true exploration of the ulnar nerve because unfortunately the previous surgeons' operative notes are not always an accurate guide as to the present location of the nerve.

The subject of successful ulnar nerve surgery at the elbow has been reviewed recently.[20] A modified list of the anatomic structures that may be responsible for recurrent compression or persistence of symptoms is provided in the accompanying box. This list is of perhaps more importance to the surgeon performing the primary procedure to the ulnar nerve because attention to each of these structures will go a long way toward obtaining a successful result initially.

Anatomic Structures Related to Recurrent or Persistent Ulnar Nerve Entrapment at the Elbow

Medial intermuscular septum
Fascia from medial head of triceps brachii muscle to medial intermuscular septum
Thickened brachialis fascia
High origin of pronator teres muscle, superficial head
Common flexor tendon
Periosteal origin of ulnar head of flexor carpi ulnaris muscle
Tethering by motor branch of flexor carpi ulnaris muscle
Unreleased Osborne's band or roof of tunnel
Overgrowth of medial humeral epicondyle after medial epicondylectomy
Adherence of ulnar nerve in acceptable location due to prolonged splinting

From Dellon AL. Techniques for successful management of ulnar nerve entrapment at the elbow. Neurosurg Clin North Am 2:57-73, 1991.

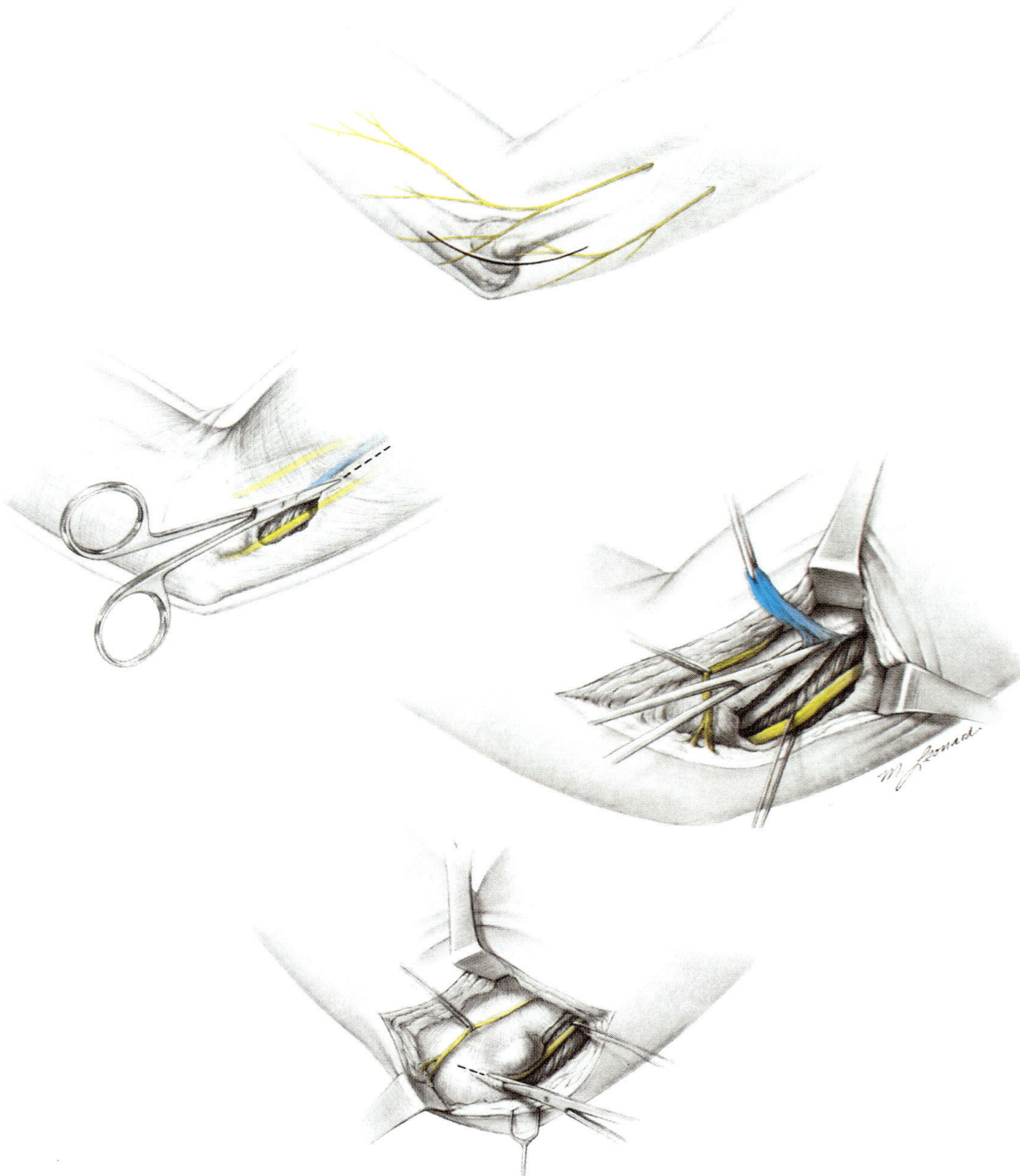

The procedure that I have developed creates a musculofascial step-type lengthening of the flexor-pronator muscle mass.[21] When this elongated muscle mass is used to cover the ulnar nerve, enough slack should be allowed so that the surgeon's finger can fit between the muscle above and the nerve below; in this way postoperative pressure from the reattached muscle mass is minimized.

Illustrations from Dellon AL. Submuscular transposition of the ulnar nerve at the elbow: Musculofascial lengthening technique. Neurosurg Oper Atlas 3:459-466, 1993.

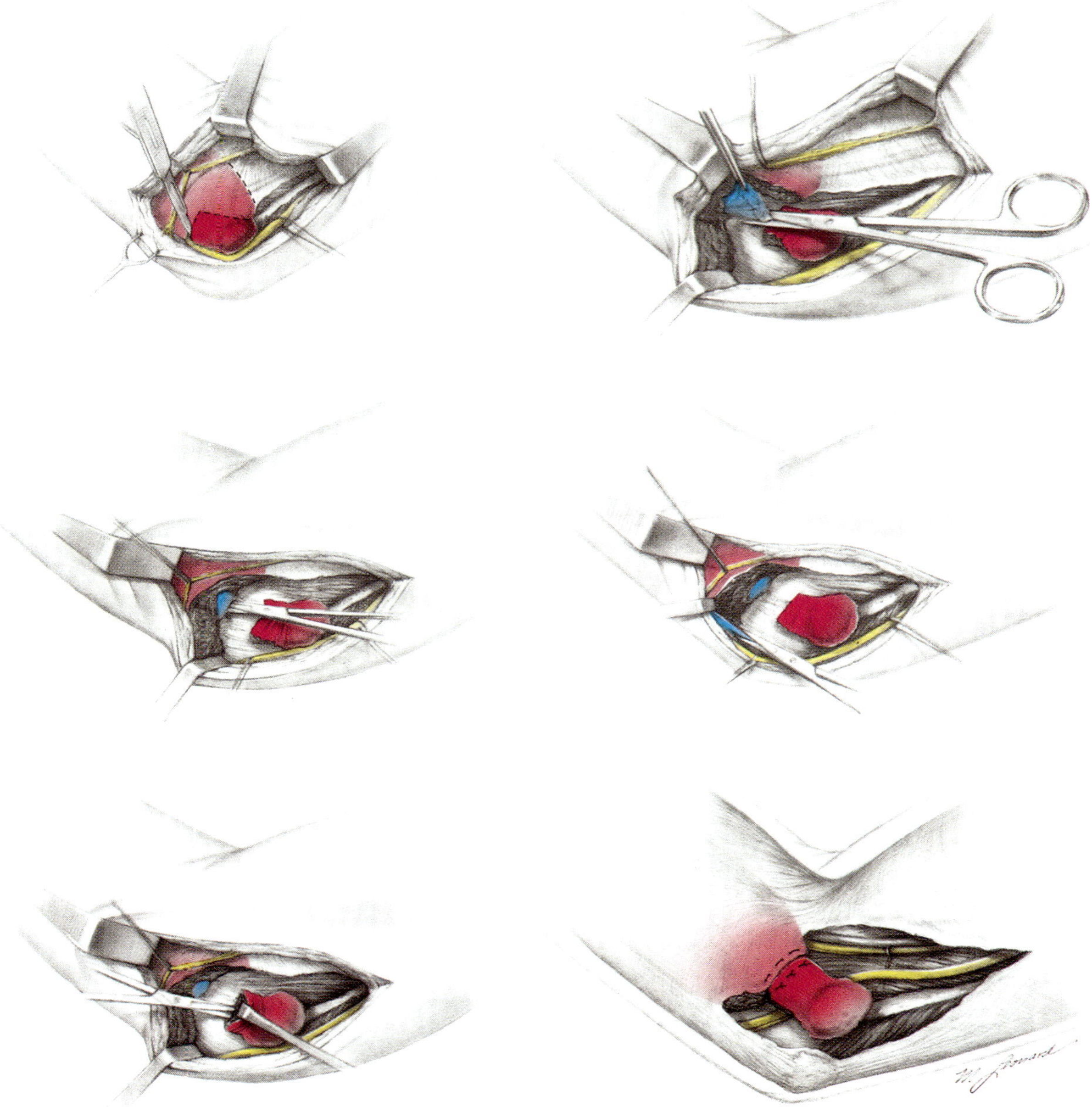

The periosteal origin of the ulnar head of the flexor carpi ulnaris muscle must also be considered. This structure forms a sharp edge at the point where the transposed ulnar nerve will cross and thus must be divided or excised as was done to the medial intermuscular septum proximally.

Illustrations from Dellon AL. Submuscular transposition of the ulnar nerve at the elbow: Musculofascial lengthening technique. Neurosurg Oper Atlas 3:459-466, 1993.

The need for reoperation for recurrent or persistent ulnar nerve entrapment at the elbow is significant as suggested by the review of worldwide results for ulnar nerve surgery at the elbow.[22] Although the results following the initial procedure to decompress the ulnar nerve are excellent in most cases if the degree of compression is minimal, if the degree of compression is moderate or severe, regardless of which decompression technique is used, most techniques are associated with an approximately 33% failure or recurrence rate.

Of more than theoretical interest is the technique used by almost all surgeons if their initial "less complicated" technique is not successful: submuscular transposition. My experience with musculofascial lengthening as the initial procedure for cubital tunnel syndrome has been quite satisfactory. Of more than 800 patients I have reoperated on, only two of my own patients required reoperation for recurrence or persistence of symptoms. One patient had postoperative bleeding and severe fibrosis developed; the second patient suffered recurrence after return to work in a "cumulative-trauma," assembly line job. For this reason I prefer the musculofascial lengthening approach to submuscular transposition.[23]

The differential diagnosis for the patient who has persistent or recurrent numbness in the little finger associated with weakness must include determining if there is an additional compression site of the ulnar nerve distally in Guyon's canal, or if the not so uncommon double-crush situation of brachial compression in the thoracic inlet, the so-called thoracic outlet syndrome, is present. In the setting of automobile trauma this double-crush injury is common, and I have found that it is often bilateral. Furthermore, automobile accident patients, who usually present about 2 years after their injury, often have associated carpal tunnel syndrome. In this circumstance, when the patient presents with multiple bilateral peripheral nerve entrapments, you must investigate for not only the presence of cervical disc disease, but also for any medically treatable disease such as diabetes, hyperthyroidism or hypothyroidism, collagen vascular disease, and alcoholism. Outside the United States the possibility of leprosy must also be considered. Referral to a neurologist or rheumatologist for workup is appropriate.

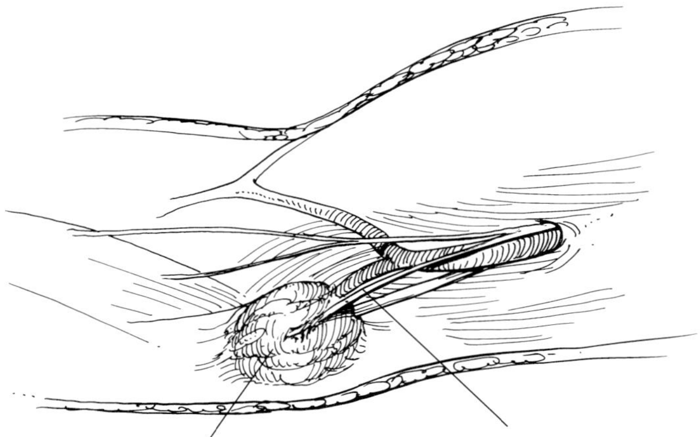

Medial aspect of elbow

Recurrent chronic ulnar nerve entrapment at the elbow does not cause elbow pain. Acute degeneration of the ulnar nerve might cause this type of referred pain, but I have not encountered this situation. Associated elbow pain must be considered as caused by a neuroma of the medial antebrachial cutaneous nerve.[24] There will be an area in the scar, usually anterior and distal, from which pain radiates not to the little finger but to the elbow or just distal and anterior or posterior to the scar. This pattern represents the distribution of the medial antebrachial cutaneous nerve, usually its posterior branch. This diagnosis can be confirmed by a diagnostic nerve block proximal to the antecubital crease that relieves this pain while preserving sensibility in the little finger. My preferred treatment is to resect the neuroma and implant the proximal end of usually just the posterior branch into the triceps brachii muscle lateral to (deep to) the ulnar nerve.[23]

Recently three patients on whom I had reoperated for recurrent ulnar nerve entrapment at the elbow had incisional pain for which I resected the neuroma of the medial antebrachial cutaneous nerve; unfortunately these patients had some residual pain. Their pain was present in the proximal scar and posterior and inferior to the scar. Nerve block of the medial brachial cutaneous nerve relieved the pain. This nerve arises from the medial cord of the brachial plexus just proximal to the origin of the medial antebrachial cutaneous nerve. Treatment by neuroma resection and implantation of the nerve into the triceps brachii muscle deep to the ulnar nerve has been successful in all three cases.[25]

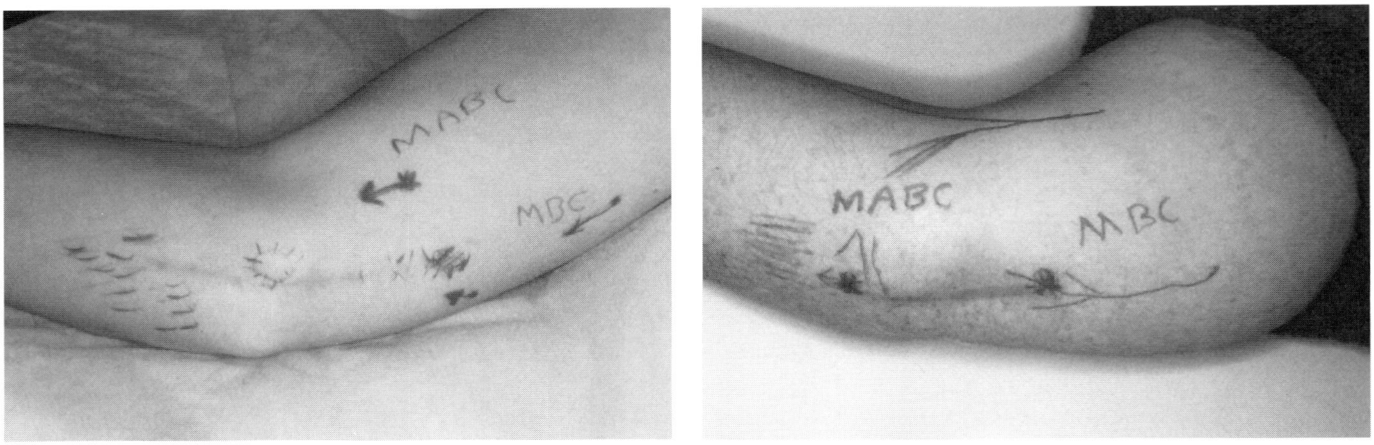

As shown in these two patients, the medial brachial cutaneous (MBC) nerve and associated neuroma are distinct from the medial antebrachial cutaneous (MABC) nerve and its neuroma.

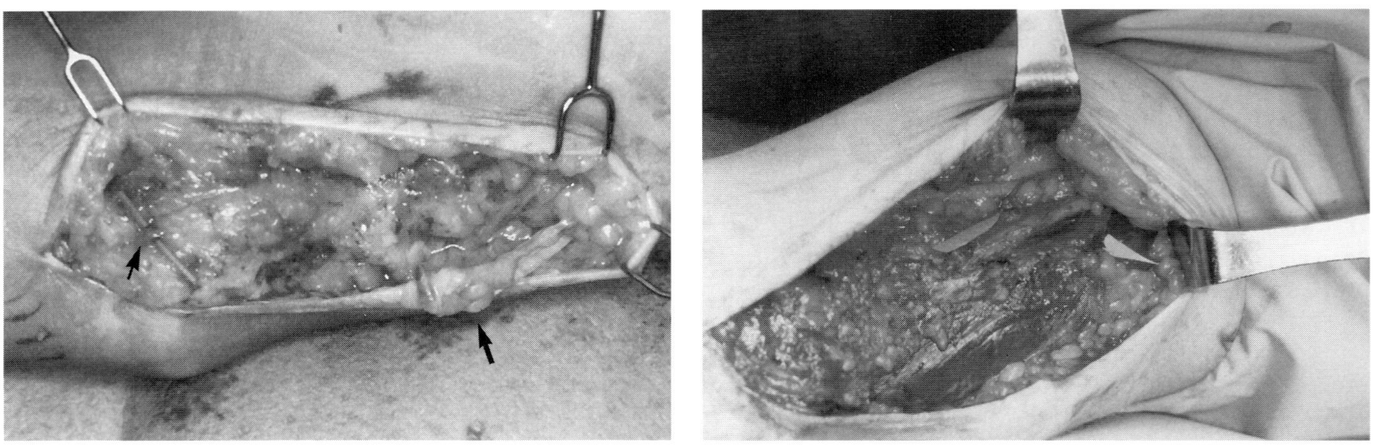

Note the vessel loop, medial antebrachial cutaneous nerve (small arrow), and the medial brachial cutaneous nerve (large arrow).

Successful management may be achieved by neuroma resection and implantation of each nerve (at paper arrows) into the triceps brachii muscle.

At surgery the medial brachial cutaneous nerve was found to be scarred not only in the incision but also in the fascia from the medial head of the triceps brachii muscle on which it travels; this fascia is incised from its connection to the medial intermuscular septum. Clearly, for reoperation when pain is a component of the patient's complaint, the possibility of these two painful cutaneous neuromas must each be explored by physical examination and by nerve blocks.

Recurrent Radial Nerve Entrapment

Once radial sensory nerve entrapment in the forearm has been released,[13] reoperation is rarely necessary. The more common situation is that the patient has had de Quervain's disease treated by the release of the first dorsal extensor compartment and has not recovered. The differential diagnosis must include consideration of the second compartment for the extensor pollicis brevis muscle, radial sensory nerve entrapment in the forearm, and injury to a branch of the radial sensory nerve during the first operation.[26] In this scenario the surgeon reoperating on this patient must consider the need to resect the radial sensory nerve and possibly the lateral antebrachial cutaneous nerve (see the section on neuromas of the dorsoradial wrist area). In the differential diagnosis of recurrent or persistent numbness in the distribution of the radial sensory nerve, one must also consider compression of the radial nerve in the radial tunnel and a C6 radiculopathy. The physical examination and electrodiagnostic evaluation are both necessary for a correct diagnosis.

Reoperation for radial nerve compression in the proximal forearm and the elbow region suggests that one or more structures in that region may not have been released at the first operation. The operative technique for this complicated area has been described in detail.[27] The concept underlying reoperation is that the radial nerve from the spiral groove of the humerus to the midforearm must be considered as coursing through a "multiple crush" region like the median nerve in the forearm does. The structures that must be considered during the surgical exploration are listed in the box on p. 1578. The differential diagnosis must include entrapment at the more distal site for the radial sensory nerve in the forearm and C6 radiculopathy. When the patient with a failed posterior interosseous nerve release has had denervation for a significant period of time (greater than 1 year), tendon transfers should be considered. When the patient has coexisting lateral humeral epicondylitis, this condition should be thoroughly treated before reoperation on the radial nerve is considered.

Anatomic Structures Related to Recurrent or Persistent Radial Nerve Compression

Scarring in the spiral groove (s/p humeral fracture)
Fibrotic bands from humerus to lateral humeral epicondyle
Anomalous muscular origins of brachioradialis muscle
Pathologic condition affecting radial head (rheumatoid arthritis, fracture callus)
Fibrous edge of extensor carpi radialis brevis muscle
Fibrous edge of supinator muscle (arcade of Frohse)
Fibrous surface of entire superficial head of supinator muscle
Vascular leashes crossing posterior interosseous nerve
Thickened fascia between brachioradialis tendon and extensor carpi radialis brevis muscle distally
Radial sensory nerve exiting between slips of brachioradialis tendon

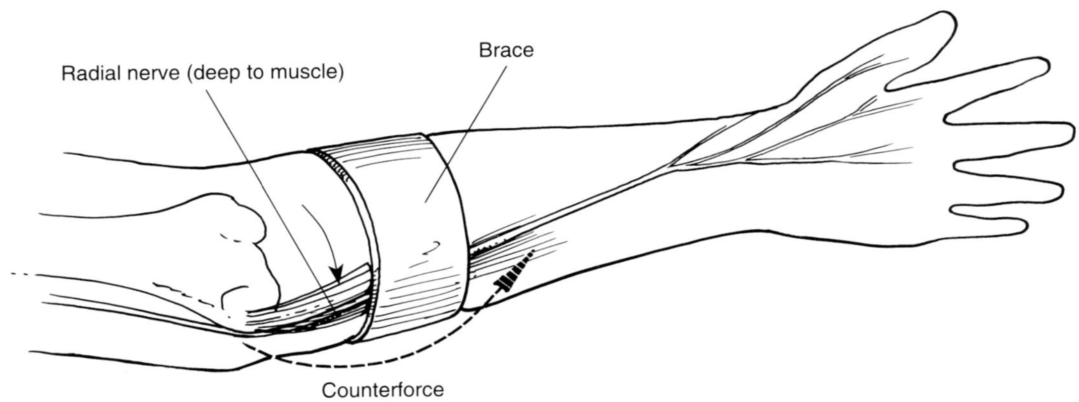

The surgeon must make sure that the patient is not wearing any type of counterforce brace, which causes compression of the radial nerve in the radial tunnel (short arrow) as it attempts to transfer the force of the musculotendinous unit from the lateral humeral epicondyle to the brace (long arrow).

Recurrent Median Nerve Entrapment in the Forearm

Reoperation for recurrent or persistent median nerve compression in the forearm is not common. By far the more common situation is median nerve entrapment in the forearm following carpal decompression. When reoperation is necessary for recurrent median nerve compression in the forearm, the situation is analogous to that of the radial nerve in this same region: there is a potential for multiple-crush injury of many anatomic structures in a short length of the arm (see accompanying box).

Anatomic Structures Related to Recurrent or Persistent Median Nerve Entrapment in the Forearm

Ligament of Struthers
Lacertus fibrosus
High origin of superficial head of pronator teres muscle[33]
Deep (fibrous) head of pronator teres muscle
Deep (fibrous) head of flexor sublimus muscle
Vascular leash crossing nerve

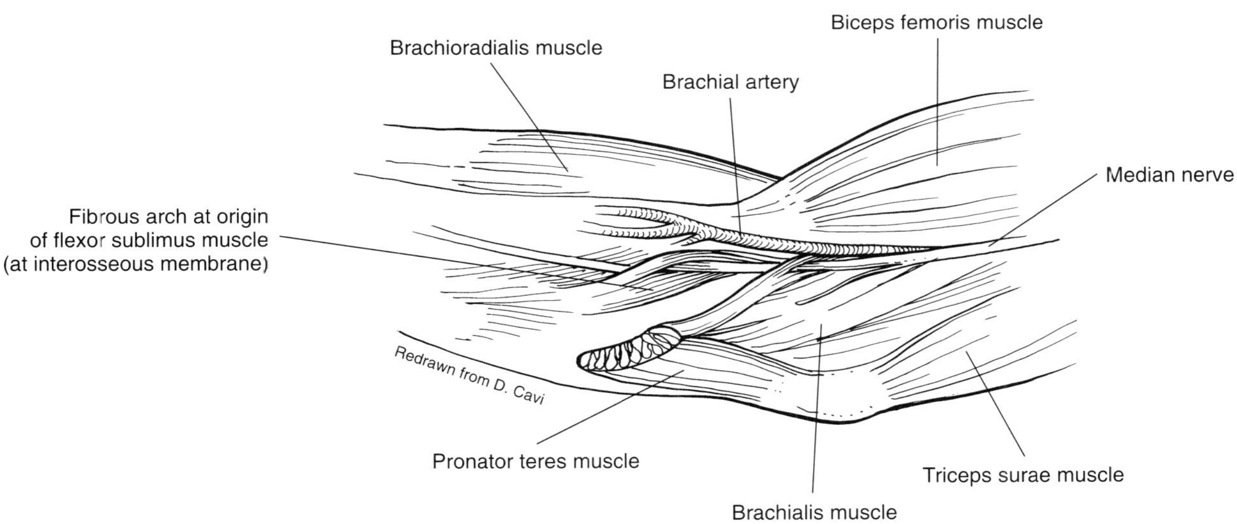

Perhaps the structure most commonly requiring release at reoperation is a second fibrous arch due to the flexor digitorum sublimus muscle originating from the interosseous membrane.[27,28] The surgical technique for this difficult anatomic area has been described in detail.[29]

A structure not described extensively is the high origin of the superficial head of the pronator teres muscle, which has been found in 20% of cadaver dissections.[30] This muscle origin can compress the median nerve against the trochlear process of the humerus.

Recurrent Ulnar Nerve Entrapment at the Wrist

This problem is rare. The differential diagnosis should include thrombosis of the ulnar artery and pisio-triquetrial arthritis, both of which can cause symptoms similar to those of ulnar nerve compression in Guyon's canal. Of course, wrist ganglia and lipomas should also be considered. Appropriate vascular testing and imaging studies are required.

RECURRENT PAINFUL NEUROMA IN THE UPPER EXTREMITY

Basic research has facilitated some of the decision making with regard to the surgical treatment of the painful neuroma. The relevant conclusions of this research and the appropriate references follow.

1. The mature end-bulb neuroma is the source of the pain-generating mechanisms due to spontaneous activity in A-delta and C fibers. Furthermore, the neuroma is very sensitive to mechanical and chemical stimuli. Rather than simply move this mature end-bulb to a new quiet place, it is critical to resect it and permit neural regeneration to begin anew.[31]
2. The classic painful neuroma forms in an environment in which tension and neurotrophic stimuli from denervated skin are present. If the microenvironment of neural regeneration is altered, a classic neuroma will not form histologically. This has been demonstrated by the implantation of the transected sensory nerve into innervated muscle.[32]
3. The failure of neuroma treatment is often due to either resecting the wrong nerve or not recognizing that more than one cutaneous nerve has been injured. Diagnostic nerve blocks are critical to the successful planning of neuroma resection. For instance, in 75% of the population the lateral antebrachial cutaneous nerve overlaps the radial sensory nerve.[33] Another example of two nerves causing pain in one region is the possibility of both the medial antebrachial and the medial brachial cutaneous nerves being the source of the painful scar following ulnar nerve transposition.

Recurrent Neuroma: Dorsoradial Aspect of the Forearm

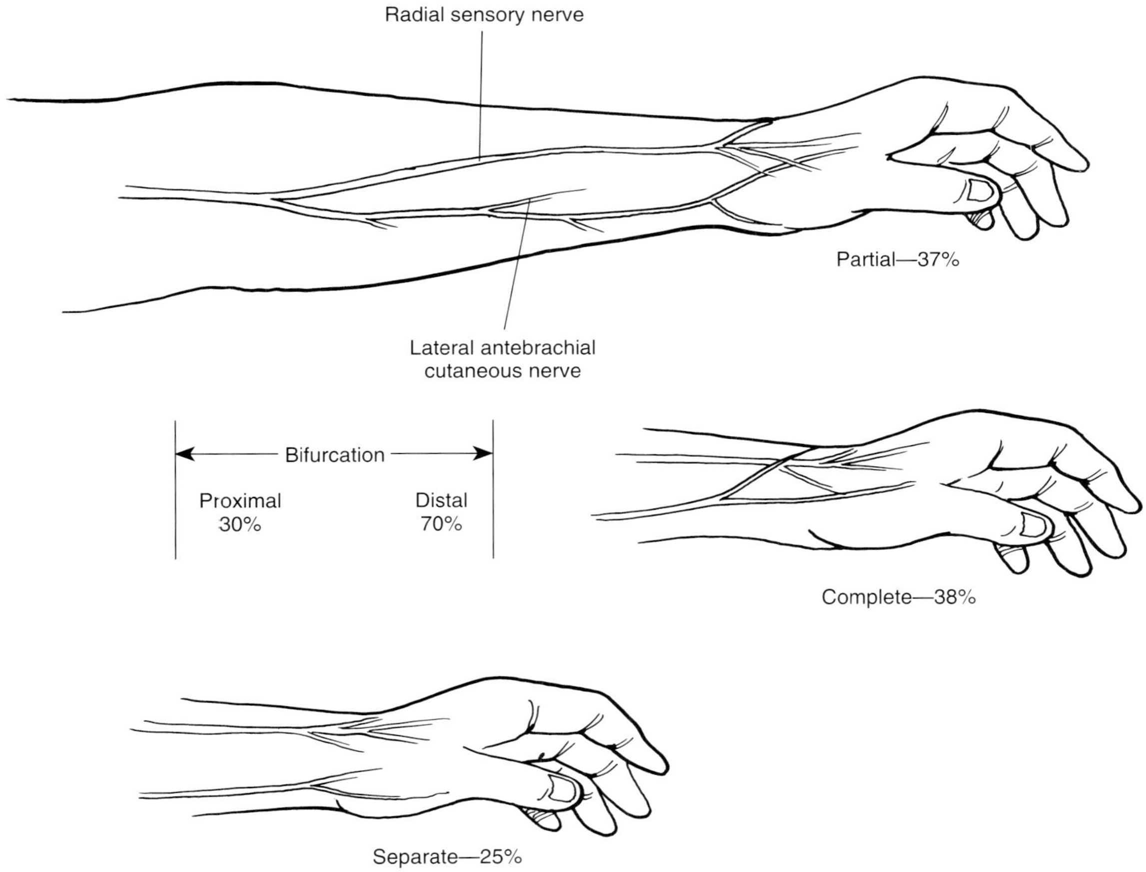

Reoperation for painful neuroma is most commonly performed for problems over the dorsoradial aspect of the forearm and wrist. The most common situation, as mentioned earlier in terms of radial sensory nerve entrapment, is that the patient will have had dorsal ganglion excision or first dorsal extensor tendon release for de Quervain's disease with iatrogenic injury to a branch believed to be a branch of the radial sensory nerve. Thus in the first operation for the painful neuroma of the radial sensory nerve (RSN), the nerve is usually resected to a more proximal level. Typically the pain is either not improved, worse, or recurs within a few weeks, and sensation is lost in the painful area. As mentioned earlier, the most common cause for reoperation is because the lateral antebrachial cutaneous (LABC) nerve overlaps the RSN to some degree in 75% of patients.[33]

The approach to this problem begins with searching for a positive Tinel sign over the proximal course of cutaneous nerves that may be contributing to the pain other than the RSN. Most common is the LABC nerve. In the few patients I have had who have had some residual pain following resection of the RSN and the LABC nerve the involved nerves with anomalous distributions have been the palmar cutaneous branch of the median (PCBM) nerve and the posterior cutaneous nerve of the forearm. Therefore diagnostic nerve blocks are performed first to the LABC nerve at the antecubital crease and then 15 minutes later to the RSN over the dorsoradial forearm. If the pain remains, then nerve blocks are performed to the PCBM nerve and the posterior cutaneous nerve of the forearm just anterior to the radial head to search for a possible anomalous overlap of these nerves. The dorsal cutaneous branch of the ulnar nerve rarely enters this area.

Although there have been reports of the occasional inclusion of a PCBM nerve extending into the dorsoradial wrist area among series of anatomic dissections of this nerve,[34,35] there has not been a case report of a neuroma of this nerve being involved in this type of pain syndrome. I have encountered this condition twice; the first case was a man in whom a saw injury to the dorsoradial aspect of the wrist led to RSN and LABC resections.

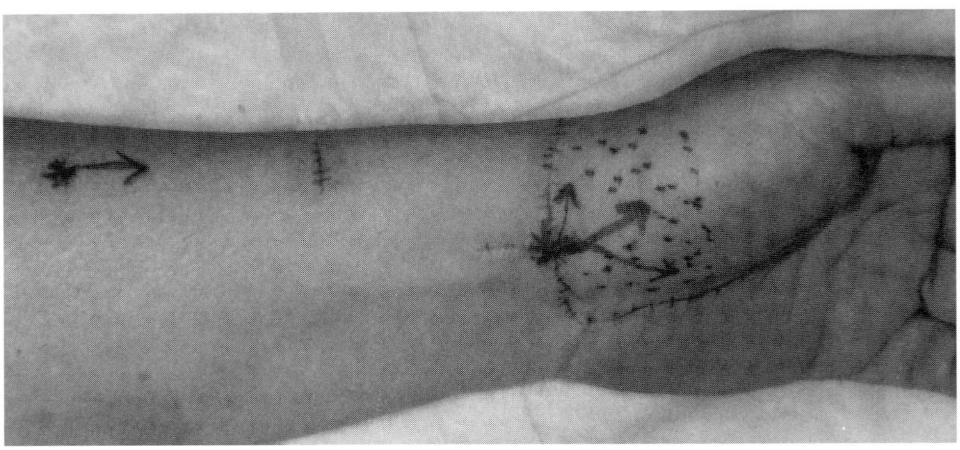

In the second case, which is documented here, a woman sustained a crush injury to this area and the blocks of the LABC nerve and then the RSN did not relieve the pain. At a second session the blocks were first instituted with the PCBM nerve, which successfully relieved the pain.

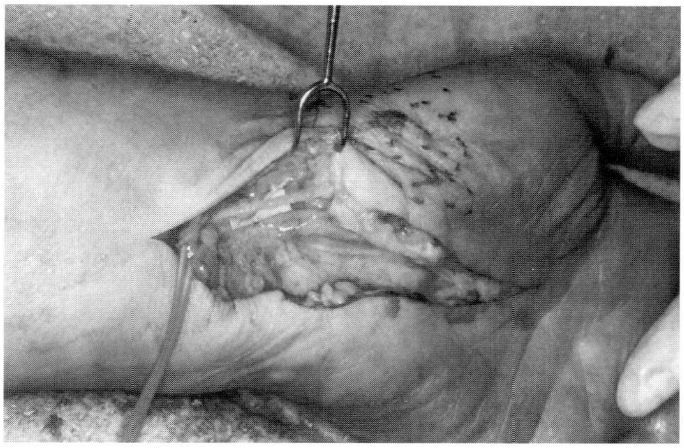

Note the small branch of the PCBM nerve coursing toward the dorsoradial area (nerve is above marker).

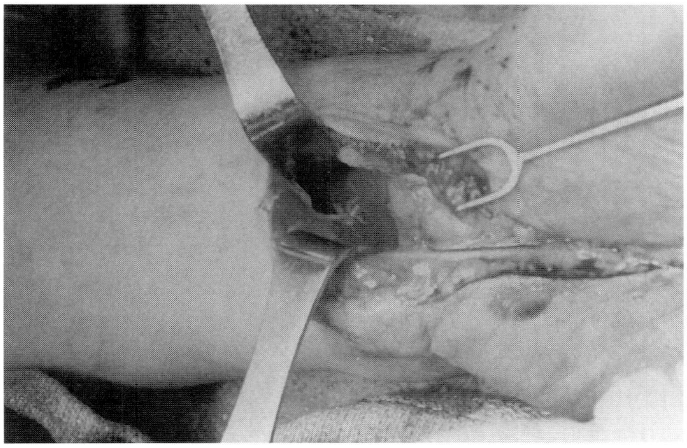

The treatment for this unusual situation is the same as that described for treatment when the PCBM nerve complicates carpal tunnel decompression: resect the nerve and implant the PCBM nerve into the pronator quadratus muscle.

If performed as a primary operation for pain relief, this treatment regimen involving diagnostic nerve blocks, resection of both the RSN and the LABC nerve, and implantation of the nerves into the proximal thick portion of the brachioradialis muscle has a success rate for pain relief and return to work approaching 90%. The success rate still approaches 50% even if the patient has had more than three previous operations.[36,37]

Painful Neuroma: Posterior and Anterior Interosseous Nerves

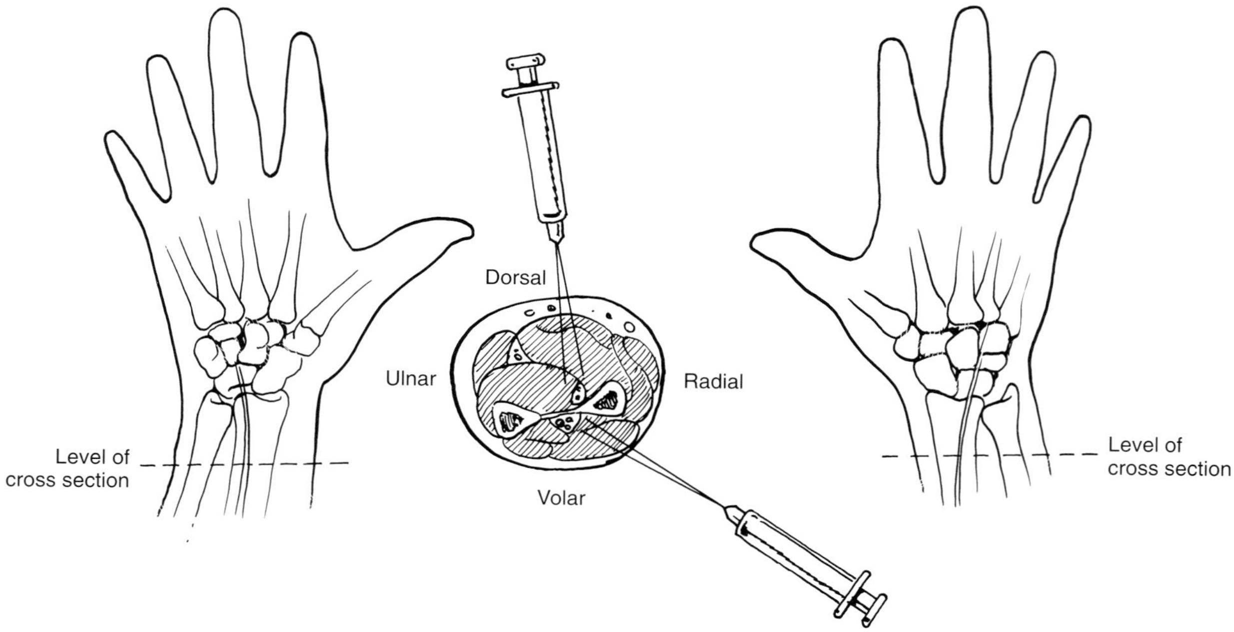

Partial wrist denervation block for posterior interosseous nerve and terminal branch of anterior interosseous nerve

With the description of the terminal branch of the posterior interosseous nerve,[38,39] it became clear that reoperation to treat pain that arises from the dorsal wrist capsule was possible. It followed logically that the anterior interosseous nerve could be related distally to volar wrist pain.[40] Interruption of the function of these nerves is indicated for (1) wrist pain after sprain that is not relieved by appropriate splinting and anti-inflammatory medication, (2) wrist pain after distal radius fracture when radiographically the radius is in the best position and the pain is not radiating from the distal radial-ulnar joint or due to a positive ulnar variance, and (3) pain due to a triangular fibrocartilaginous tear for which arthroscopy has not relieved pain and a more extensive surgical intervention is not acceptable to the patient or the surgeon. Partial wrist denervations are generally contraindicated in patients with carpal instabilities because even though the pain may be relieved, progressive collapse patterns occur and fusion of some type will most certainly be required anyway.

Illustration modified from Dellon AL. Partial wrist denervation. In Horner G, Levin S, eds. Problems in Plastic and Reconstructive Surgery: The Wrist. Philadelphia: JB Lippincott, 1993.

I am not aware of a cutaneous distribution to the posterior interosseous nerve, and none of the patients for whom I have performed a dorsal wrist denervation has experienced a postoperative sensory loss. Therefore I know of no basis to suggest that this nerve should be divided in patients with dorsoradial (cutaneous) wrist or forearm pain. Of course, it is true that the posterior interosseous nerve originates more proximally from the radial nerve and ultimately from the C6 dermatome, so some referred pain pathways may exist.

REOPERATION FOR NERVE RECONSTRUCTION IN THE UPPER EXTREMITY

Neurotization During Reoperation

Neurotization is a technique that supplies nerve fibers to a target end-organ for which normal innervation is no longer available. If normal innervation is still available, the reoperation technique would be a nerve repair or nerve graft. The need for neurotization is unusual. There are two types of situations in which neurotization is needed: sensory and motor.

An example of neurotization for sensory function would be a patient with an irreparable median nerve injury or a failed median nerve graft for whom the goal of reoperation is to provide sensation for a critical pinch area such as the radial side of the index finger. In this case the transfer of the digital nerve to the ulnar side of the ring finger to the digital nerve to the index finger would neurotize the median territory by the ulnar nerve.[41] This past year I have had the opportunity to try this type of neurotization in reverse for patients with an irreparable ulnar nerve injury who, because of lack of sensation, have repeatedly burned or injured the ulnar side of the little finger. In three patients I have transferred a median nerve–innervated digital nerve (e.g., ulnar digital nerve to the middle finger) to the little finger and sutured it to the ulnar digital nerve in that finger. Within 3 months sensibility began to recover in the little finger. To this approach I have added the transfer of the radial sensory nerve to the dorsal cutaneous branch of the ulnar nerve. This maneuver has been successful in neurotizing the hypothenar eminence in two patients. In a third patient who did not wish the radial sensory nerve to be transferred, the palmar cutaneous nerve was used for the neurotization.[42]

In neurotization for motor function the first operation has to result in a muscle, critical for function, that does not have a distal portion of nerve into which a nerve graft can be placed. This situation has been most unusual in my experience. Areas in which nerve traction injuries may cause avulsion of the motor branches from the muscles are the musculocutaneous nerve as it innervates the coracobrachialis and the biceps brachii muscles, the deep peroneal nerve as it innervates the anterior tibialis, and the posterior interosseous nerve at the level of the supinator muscle.

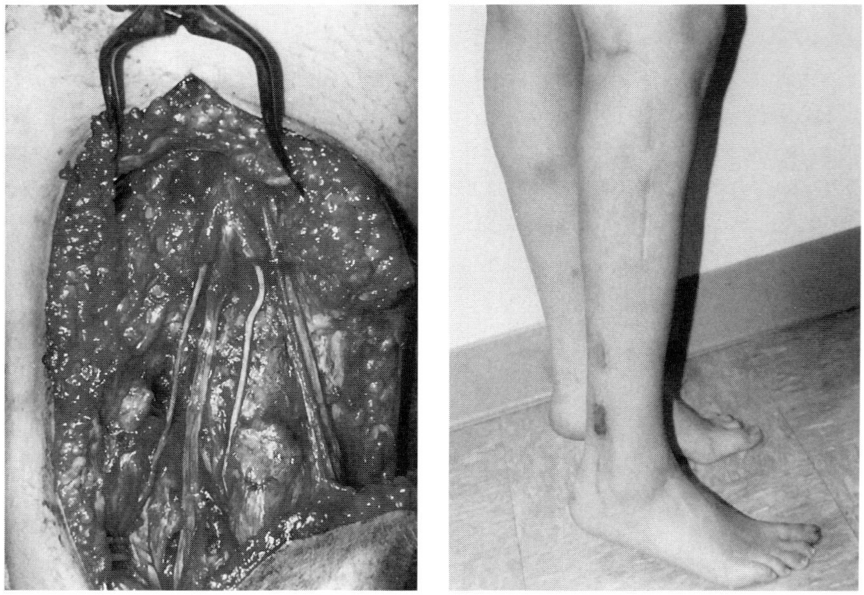

This patient sustained an injury to the posterior tibial nerve in the popliteal fossa during arthroscopy. At subsequent exploration she was found to have a large nerve defect and was referred for reoperation and nerve grafting. Although the sensory portion of the posterior tibial nerve was available for interfascicular nerve grafting, distal motor nerve branches to the gastrocnemius muscle were not present.[43] Direct neurotization of the gastrocnemius muscles was performed with 15 cm sural nerve grafts from the proximal posterior tibial nerve. Postoperative muscle contraction was present at 18 months.

Motor neurotization is possible but the result is not as successful as muscle reinnervation with either nerve repair or by a nerve graft.

Nerve Repair or Grafting During Reoperation

During reoperation to restore nerve function when the nerve has been either divided inadvertently at the first operation or left for secondary repair because of some unfavorable condition present during the first operation, the surgeon must be prepared to perform a nerve graft instead of a nerve repair.

The main concern of the surgeon at reoperation is to restore function and relieve pain. If the mechanism of injury was anything but a glass or knife laceration, then at reoperation, when the scarred proximal and distal ends of the nerve are resected, there will be a gap that in most instances cannot be closed by secondary sutures without placing an unacceptable degree of tension on the repair site. Tension on the repair without grafting is likely in the case of digital nerve and common volar digital nerve injuries. In the forearm, where nerves can be mobilized more easily, a nerve defect of 1 or 2 cm *may* be overcome without grafting. ■ *However, when in doubt, nerve graft.*

Preferred Nerve Graft Donor Sites

Medial antebrachial cutaneous nerve
Lateral antebrachial cutaneous nerve
Sural nerve (lateral sural nerve from common peroneal nerve can provide an extra 20 to 30 cm of donor graft when present)
Terminal posterior interosseous nerve (suitable for distal digital nerve grafts only)
Radial sensory nerve (suitable when grafting radial nerve for motor function)
Superficial peroneal nerve (suitable when grafting deep peroneal nerve for tibialis anterior muscle function)

Preferred nerve donor site areas are listed in the accompanying box. It is my belief that in the future reoperation for reconstruction of nerve gaps of less than 3 cm will employ bioabsorbable nerve guides such as the Neurotube. It has already been demonstrated that excellent functional sensory recovery can be achieved in humans with repair employing these polyglycolic acid tubes.[44] With the availability of these tubes, surgeons will be less reticent to reconstruct a nerve defect at reoperation, and they will be less likely to attempt a secondary nerve repair under tension. These tubes will probably be used extensively at initial operations when the mechanism of injury is a saw or avulsion and it is clear that some amount of peripheral nerve must be debrided. The placement of a primary nerve graft in this situation would be incorrect because the exact degree of nerve tissue to debride cannot be ascertained at the time of injury.[45]

Tendon Transfer for Reoperation on Nerve

The penultimate reoperation for nerve repair, at least motor nerve repair, is tendon transfer. This approach is taken when there is no possibility of reinnervation of the muscle. If a muscle has not had neurotrophic stimuli for more than 2 years, its receptivity for motor axon sprouts to form a successful motor endplate is rare. Although the muscle cell is still alive, it has become greatly reduced in size, its sarcolemma has thickened, and there is fibrosis between muscle fibers. In this situation the options at reoperation are free muscle transfer or tendon transfer.

Recurrent Nerve Entrapment in the Lower Extremity

The nerves in the lower extremity have the same neurophysiology and pathophysiology as the nerves in the upper extremity. The principles that apply to the diagnosis and treatment of upper extremity peripheral nerve problems apply to the nerves of the lower extremity as well.

Recurrent Tarsal Tunnel Syndrome

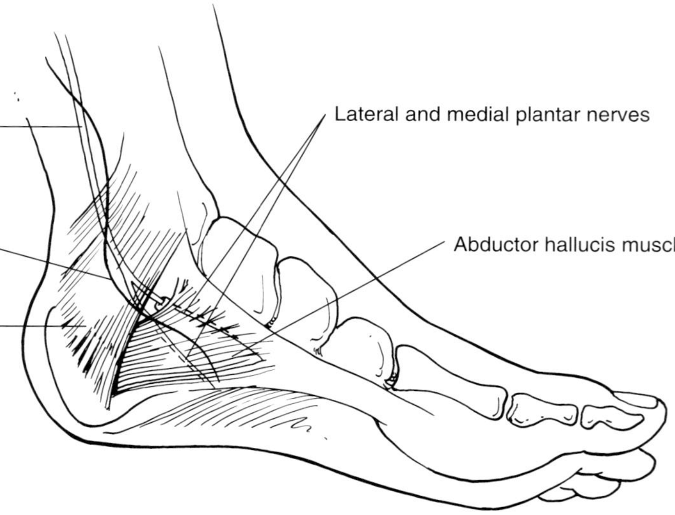

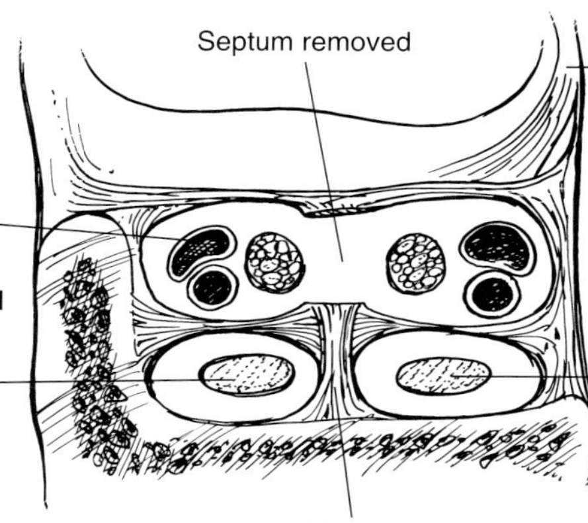

Tarsal tunnel syndrome, recognized in 1962 as the compression of the posterior tibial nerve in the tarsal tunnel, is the most common chronic peripheral nerve compression syndrome of the lower extremity. Its history, diagnosis, treatment, and results have been described extensively.[46] Unfortunately, reoperation is not rare. The original descriptions of tarsal tunnel syndrome gave the impression that the area of compression was limited to the region of the nerve beneath the flexor retinaculum. However, it is clear based on anatomic dissections that there is also a separate medial plantar tunnel and a separate lateral plantar tunnel. When correlated to the anatomic structures of the upper extremity, the tarsal tunnel represents the distal forearm, the medial plantar tunnel is analogous to the carpal tunnel, and the lateral plantar tunnel represents Guyon's canal.[47]

Reoperation for recurrent or persistent complaints of numbness in the toes or burning beneath the metatarsal head is most often required because these distal two tunnels were not released at the first operation. Signs of this condition on

Illustrations redrawn from Mackinnon SE, Dellon AL. Surgery of the Peripheral Nerve. New York: Thieme, 1988.

physical examination are (1) the incision will not extend much distal to the medial malleolus and (2) there may be a Tinel sign over the medial plantar nerve just beneath the tubercle of the navicular bone or over the lateral plantar tunnel with appropriate radiation of sensation into the big or the little toe. Heel numbness or pain may be due to compression of the calcaneal nerve in its own separate tunnel beneath the fascia from the calcaneus to the abductor hallucis brevis muscle.

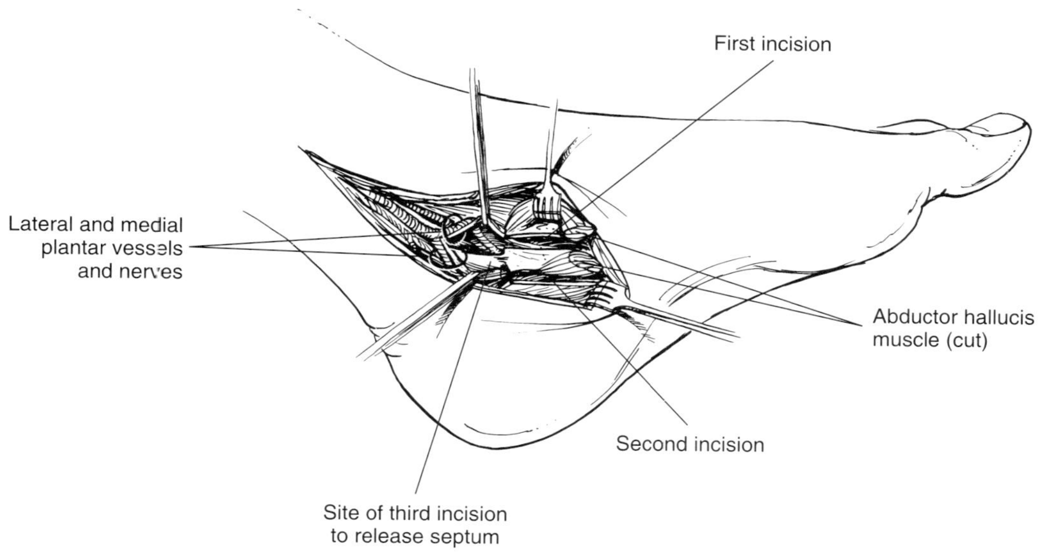

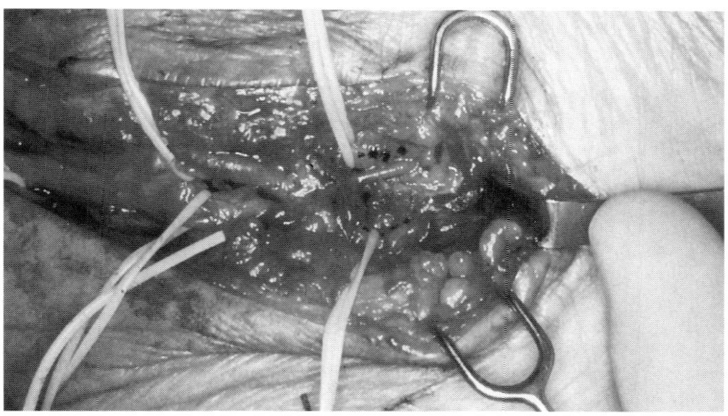

The indicated surgical treatment is to reexplore the entire posterior tibial nerve, identify the calcaneal branch or branches, retract the abductor hallucis brevis muscle, and release each of the distal tunnels separately. I recommend excision of the interfascicular septum that separates the two tunnels, thereby creating one large tunnel for both nerves. This maneuver is similar to excision of the hook of the hamate in the hand. The surgeon's finger should pass easily to the plantar aspect of the foot. The epineurium should be opened; internal neurolysis for intraneural fibrosis is especially required at the junction of the medial and lateral plantar nerves and the posterior tibial nerve.

Illustration redrawn from Mackinnon SE, Dellon AL. Surgery of the Peripheral Nerve. New York: Thieme, 1988.

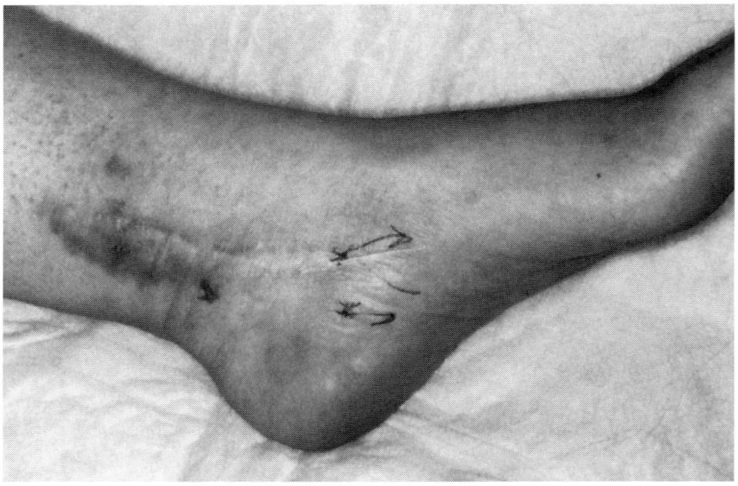

When pain is one of the indications for reoperation in the patient with previous tarsal tunnel release, the surgeon must check for the presence of the neuromas. One potential site is the saphenous distal branch, which lies close to the medial malleolus; if the original incision was near this site, then it is likely that the saphenous nerve is part of the problem. (Note the asterisk and the arrow anterior to the distal scar pointing to the top of the big toe.) Once a neuroma at this location is confirmed with a diagnostic nerve block, the saphenous nerve is resected proximal to the ankle and the nerve is implanted into muscle in the distal anterolateral compartment. The nerve can be found adjacent to the saphenous vein lying on top of the fascia.

Another potential neuroma site is the calcaneal nerve. This nerve may be a branch arising from the posterior tibial nerve and/or the lateral plantar nerve. A small branch arising from the medial plantar nerve and crossing anterior to the posterior tibial vessels has also been noted; at this location the nerve is vulnerable to transection during the initial division of the flexor retinaculum. Neuromas of the calcaneal nerve often develop after surgery for plantar fasciitis or a calcaneal bone spur. Treatment involves resection of the neuroma and then implantation of the nerve into a muscle. The choice of muscle depends on the origin of the calcaneal nerve: soleus muscle or flexor hallucis longus muscle for a calcaneal branch arising from the posterior tibial nerve or abductor hallucis brevis muscle for a branch arising from the medial or lateral plantar nerve.

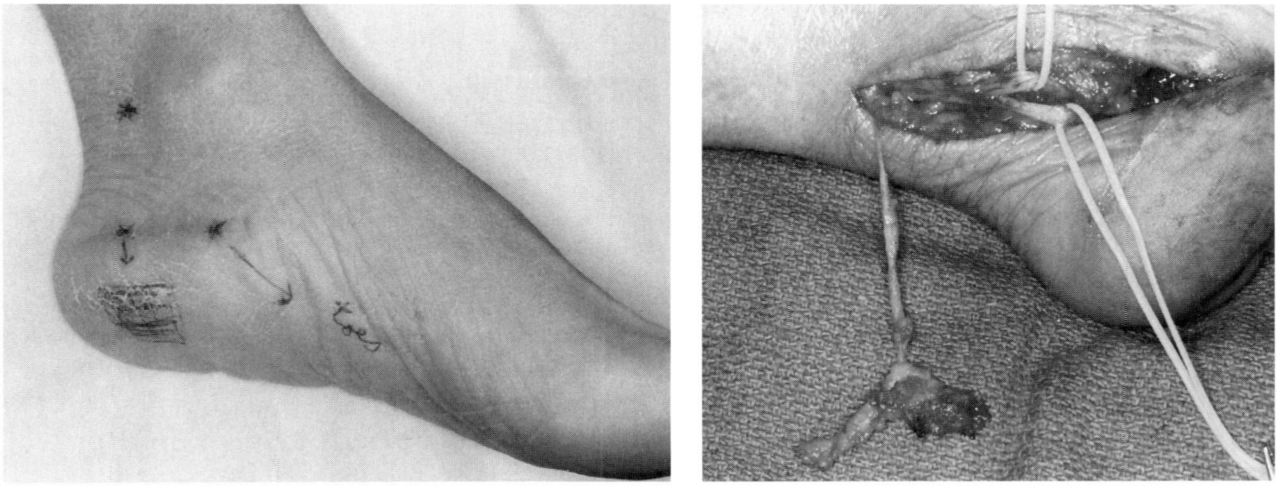

In this patient the asterisks mark the sites of pain. The calcaneal nerve arose from the posterior tibial nerve; the neuroma was implanted into a muscle proximally, away from the ankle.

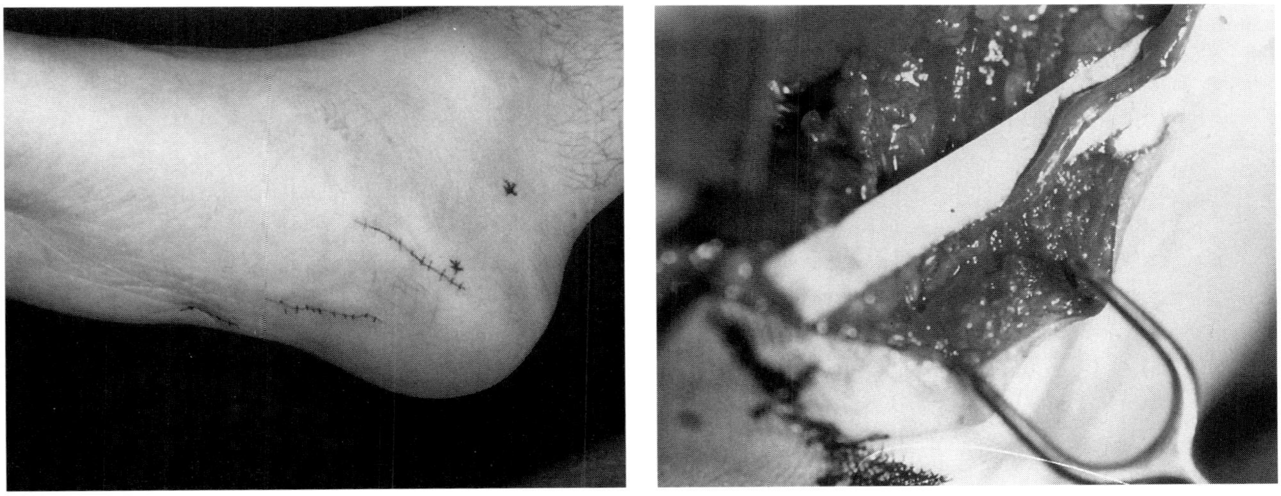

In another patient the calcaneal branch arose from the lateral plantar nerve and resection could not be performed without the risk of losing intrinsic muscle function or sensation to the little toe. In this case the neuroma was implanted into the abductor hallucis brevis muscle.

Recurrent Compression of the Common Peroneal Nerve

Although the common peroneal nerve at the knee may be compressed related to various knee injuries, surgical positioning, or ganglia, its release is usually successful. Failure of the initial attempt at release is usually due to long-term denervation of the muscles preoperatively rather than failure of the initial decompression. I have not personally reoperated on this nerve for this problem.

Recurrent Compression of the Deep Peroneal Nerve

The deep peroneal nerve may be compressed beneath the inferior extensor retinaculum at the ankle (i.e., anterior tarsal tunnel syndrome) or over the dorsum of the foot.[48] Failure of operations to decompress this nerve is usually not due to recurrent compression but to injury to the deep peroneal nerve, which requires neuroma resection, or to the superficial peroneal nerve during the primary surgery. I have not personally operated on this nerve for recurrent entrapment.

RECURRENT PAINFUL NEUROMA IN THE LOWER EXTREMITY

Neuroma of the Posterior Tibial Nerve

Ankle trauma sufficient to require ankle fusion may result in compression of the posterior tibial nerve. Attempts at neurolysis of this nerve may lead to severe pain relieved only by anesthetic block of this nerve. Amputation is frequently suggested to these patients. Because an anesthetic plantar aspect to the foot is likely to cause future problems related to infection and soft tissue ulceration, resection of the posterior tibial nerve and muscle implantation is *not* recommended. Rather I have had excellent results with the excision of the damaged nerve and interfascicular nerve grafting of the posterior tibial nerve.[49] This difficult procedure will be rewarded by relief of pain and recovery of better than protective sensation in the plantar aspect of the foot. The patient must be informed before surgery that during neural regeneration postoperatively there may be 3 to 6 months of dysesthesias. If there is severe scarring posterior to the medial malleolus, an extra-anatomic route (i.e., anterior to the medial malleolus) may be chosen for the nerve grafting.

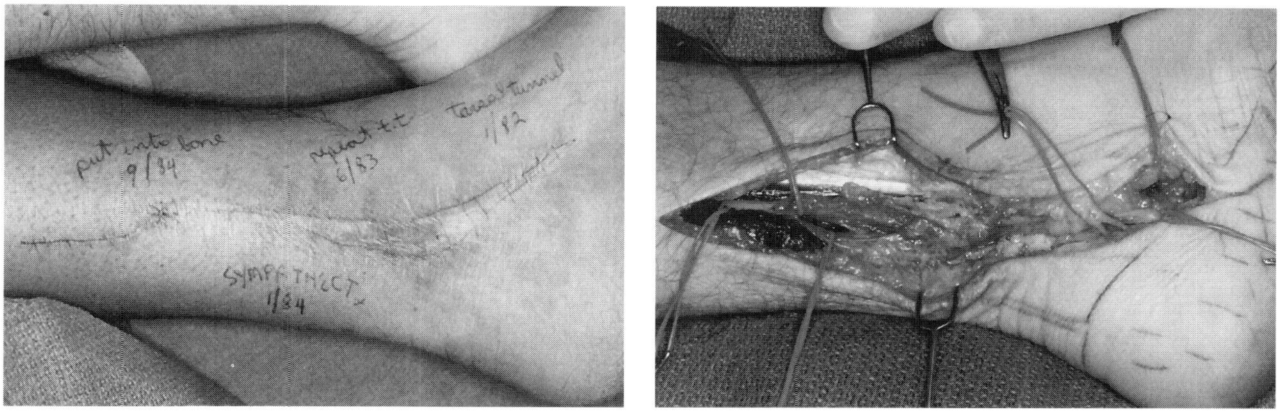

In this patient nerve grafting of the posterior tibial nerve was indicated because of pain. Note the scarring around the posterior tibial nerve.

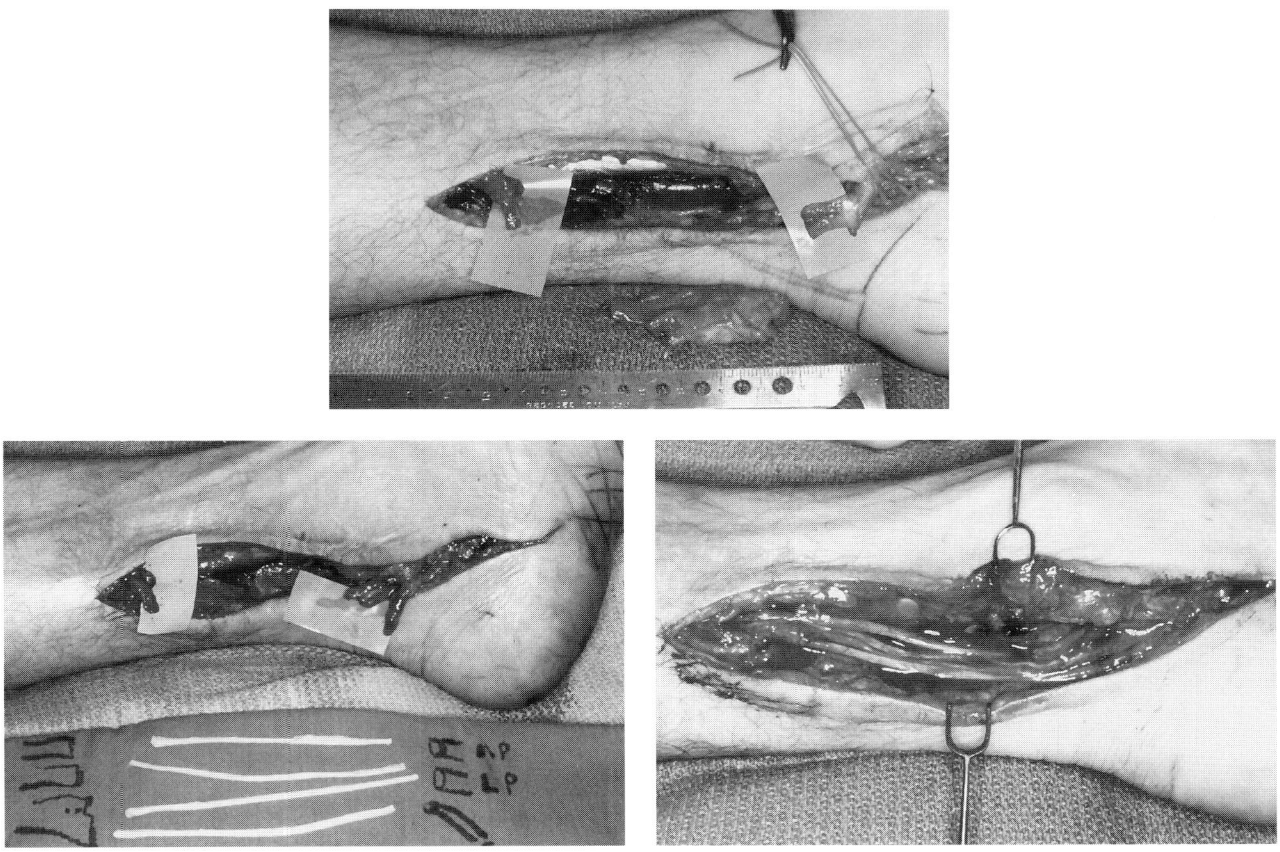

The scar tissue around the posterior tibial nerve was excised, and multiple interfascicular sural nerve grafts were used to reconstruct the posterior tibial nerve.

Photographs reprinted with permission from Dellon AL, Mackinnon SE. Results of posterior tibial nerve grafting at the ankle. J Reconstr Microsurg 7:81-83, 1991.

Recurrent Neuroma of the Deep and Superficial Peroneal Nerves

Many surgeons have recognized that pain after surgery for Morton's "neuroma," metatarsal fracture, and ganglia is the result of injury to the small cutaneous nerves over the dorsum of the foot. Unfortunately, often treatment has been to resect the neuroma to a more proximal level (i.e., to the ankle) or to implant the nerve into a metatarsal bone. With plantar flexion and extensor tendon activation, recurrent pain is predictable.

Based on the considerations for the management of the painful neuroma, I have developed the following approach to this difficult and disabling problem.[50] Diagnostic nerve blocks are necessary to determine if both the deep peroneal nerve and the superficial peroneal nerve need to be resected. Most often both nerves must be resected; the patient must fully understand that with this surgery the dorsum of the foot will then be completely and permanently anesthetic. The surgeon must ensure by appropriate blocks that neither the sural nerve nor the saphenous nerve is related to the pain syndrome. Confirmation of the involved structures will require repeat blocks and more than one office visit.

The peroneal nerves marked for resection must be divided over the anterior ankle to be properly identified. Then an incision is made over the anterolateral compartment, and the peroneal nerves are pulled up into the leg from the ankle. The deep and superficial peroneal nerves are individually implanted into different muscles of the anterolateral compartment. Although this procedure will successfully relieve pain, it does not guarantee that when the patient resumes extensive ambulation, the disuse atrophy sustained by these muscles will not cause compartment syndrome–like symptoms in 6 months. To avoid this problem, a fasciotomy of the anterolateral compartment must be performed.

In two patients in whom I have transferred these nerves into the anterolateral compartment, each patient successfully returned to work only to present to me about 6 months later complaining of aching in the anterolateral compartment toward the end of each day. This sensation was not recurrent neuroma pain but was caused by muscle ischemia due to the anterolateral compartment muscles bulking up with use and attempting to function within the restricted compartment.

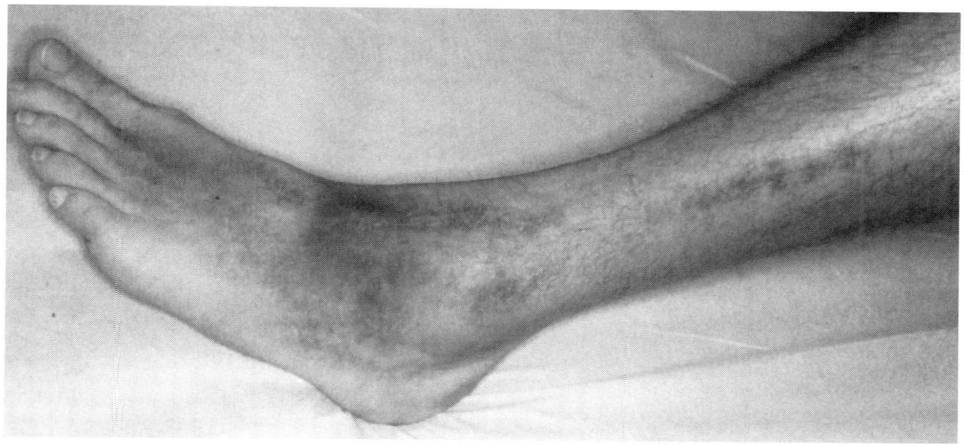

In this patient neuromas of the deep and superficial peroneal nerves were resected at the ankle and the nerves were transferred to the anterolateral compartment. Pain relief was excellent. However, subsequent activity caused an aching sensation consistent with anterolateral compartment symptoms. Fasciotomy was performed.

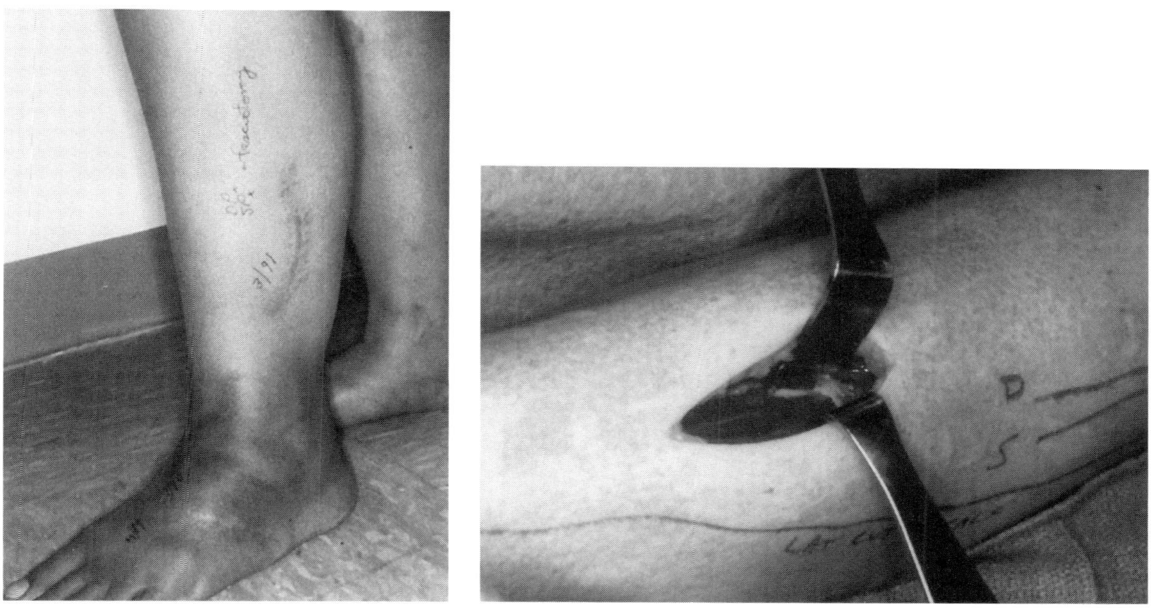

In this patient fasciotomy was performed concomitantly with neuroma resection and implantation of the peroneal nerves into the extensor digitorum communis and peroneus longus muscles.

REOPERATION FOR NERVE RECONSTRUCTION IN THE LOWER EXTREMITY

Nerve Repair or Grafting

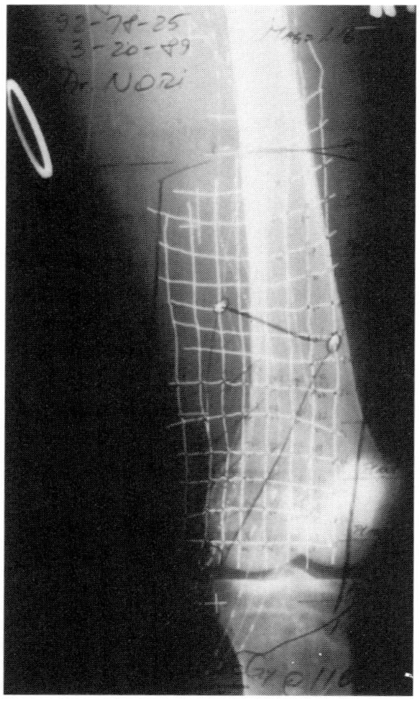

Reoperation in the lower extremity for nerve repair or grafting is unusual. I personally have reoperated on only one patient for nerve grafting in the lower extremity. This patient had a soft tissue sarcoma resected from the posterior thigh and was treated postoperatively with implantation of radioactive material, which lay in close proximity to the sciatic nerve. He experienced a slowly progressive loss of function of the sciatic nerve.

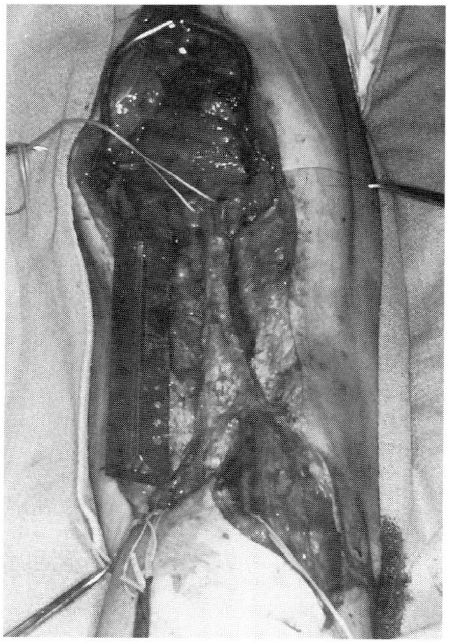

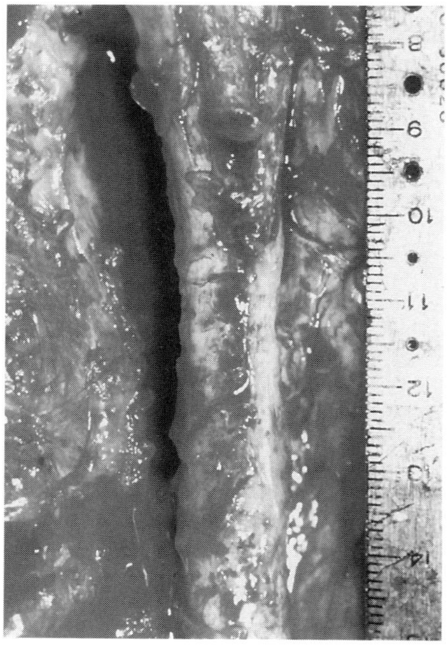

Six months following the onset of functional loss, vascularized muscle flaps from the biceps femoris muscle were placed over the sciatic nerve. The dense, white, functionless sciatic nerve was noted.

At 1 year following the onset of the paresis, he presented for consultation because it was clear that revascularization had not altered the radiation fibrosis of the sciatic nerve, and he had lost function in both the posterior tibial and common peroneal components of the sciatic nerve.

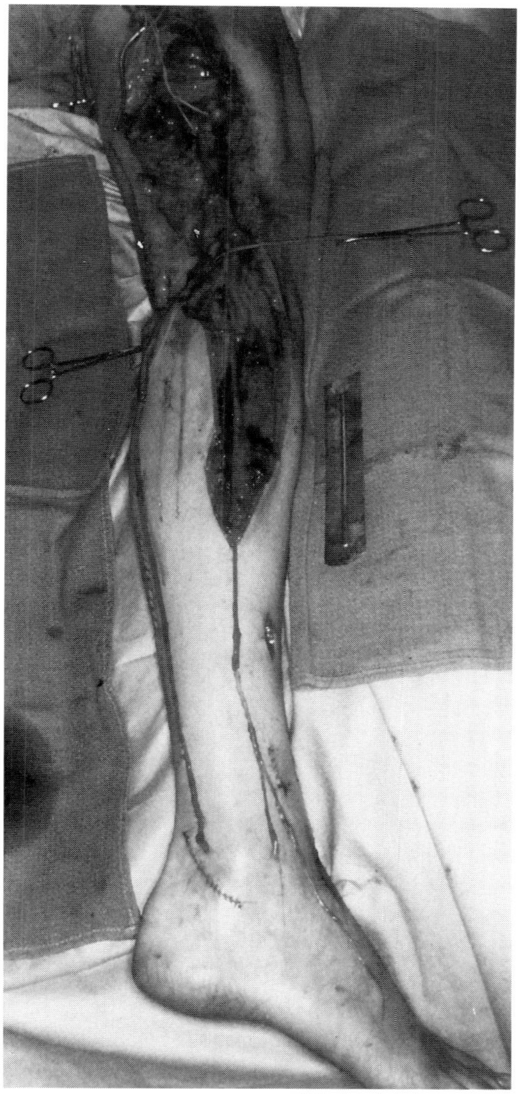

Donor nerve grafts were harvested from the ipsilateral sural nerve, including its lateral sural component, and from the superficial peroneal nerve.

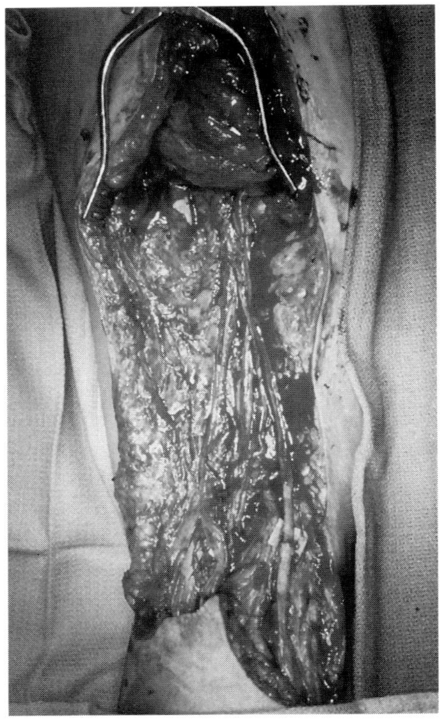

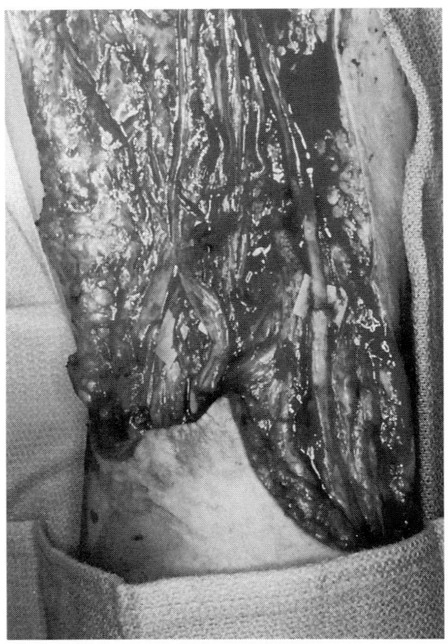

The plan was to recover sensation to the plantar aspect of the foot through nerve grafts to the distal posterior tibial nerve, to recover foot dorsiflexion by nerve grafting to the deep peroneal nerve, and to recover gastrocnemius muscle function for plantar flexion by nerve grafting the tibial branches to each of these two muscle bellies. There is an advancing Tinel sign, but it remains too early to report ultimate recovery in this difficult situation.

POSTOPERATIVE CARE

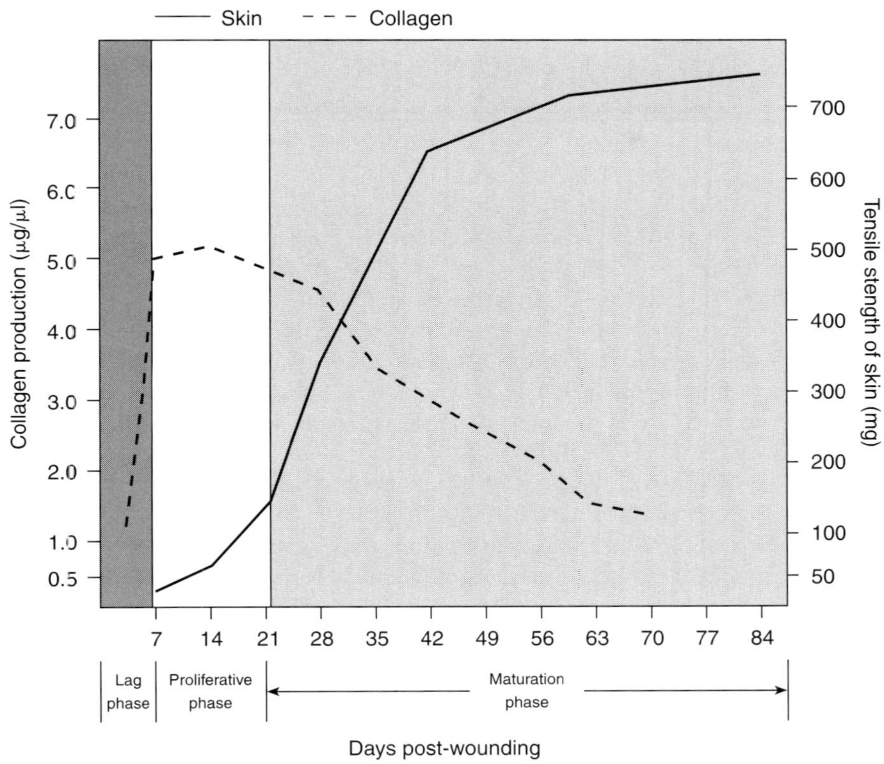

Wound healing concepts can and should be applied to the peripheral nerve.[50] Among the concepts derived from such an analysis is the fact that during the first week after surgery, the nerve will lie in an environment that is mostly inflammatory cells, with collagen not deposited into the wound until the second week and cross-linking of the collagen not occurring until the third week. If the nerve is kept immobile during the second and third postoperative week, then the nerve will become adherent to the surrounding tissues. Conversely, in order for the nerve to be loose and able to slide through its surrounding tissues, you must permit movement of the nerve with respect to its bed after the first 7 or 8 days of splinting. The fact that a nerve will not adhere to a bed of cut muscle and fibrous tissue if it is allowed to glide early in the postoperative period was demonstrated for the ulnar nerve at the elbow in the baboon model.[51] An intramuscular transposition performed on one arm and a submuscular transposition (without musculofascial lengthening) was performed on the other. There was no splinting. At 3 months, evaluation demonstrated no adherence of the nerve to the muscle, with a good neuromysial plane having developed histologically. ***Therefore in reoperation on the peripheral nerve it is essential that the postoperative regimen include some movement of the joints during the first week and the removal of all splints at 8 days.*** If a nerve graft has been performed, you may wish to continue protective splinting to prevent extension into the second or third postoperative week but have the patient begin active flexion during the second week.

Another adjunct, which I use in almost every patient, is to have them apply a steroid-containing cream such as 0.1% dexamethasone to the scar twice a day beginning the third postoperative week.

References

1. Mackinnon SE, Dellon AL. Physical examination. In Surgery of the Peripheral Nerve. New York: Thieme, 1988.
2. Dellon AL. Physical examination in nerve compression. In Gelberman R, ed. Operative Management of Peripheral Nerve Injury. Philadelphia: JB Lippincott, 1991.
3. Dellon AL. Pitfalls in electrodiagnosis. In Gelberman R, ed. Operative Management of Peripheral Nerve Injury. Philadelphia: JB Lippincott, 1991.
4. Curtis RM, Eversmann WW Jr. Internal neurolysis as an adjunct to carpal tunnel surgery. J Bone Joint Surg 55A:733-740, 1973.
5. Mackinnon SE, Dellon AL, Hudson AR, Hunter DA. A primate model for chronic nerve compression. J Reconstr Microsurg 1:185-194, 1985.
6. Mackinnon SE, Dellon AL. Evaluation of microsurgical internal neurolysis in a primate median nerve model of chronic nerve compression. J Hand Surg 13A:54-61, 1988.
7. Mackinnon SE, McCabe S, Murray JF, Szalai JP, Kelly L, Novack C, Burke GM. Internal neurolysis fails to improve the results of primary carpal tunnel decompression. J Hand Surg 16A:211-216, 1991.
8. Mackinnon SE, Dellon AL. Internal neurolysis. In Surgery of the Peripheral Nerve. New York: Thieme, 1988.
9. Lundborg G. Nerve Injury and Repair. Edinburgh: Churchill Livingstone, 1988.
10. Breidenbach W, et al. Blood flow in the rabbit tibial nerve after neurolysis. Presented at the Plastic Surgery Research Council meeting. Washington, D.C.: April 1990.
11. Mackinnon SE, Dellon AL. Carpal tunnel syndrome. In Surgery of the Peripheral Nerve. New York: Thieme, 1988.
12. Mackinnon SE. Secondary carpal tunnel surgery. Neurosurg Clin North Am 2:75-91, 1991.
13. Dellon AL, Mackinnon SE. Radial sensory nerve entrapment in the forearm. J Hand Surg 11A:196-198, 1986.
14. Dellon AL. Radial sensory nerve entrapment. Arch Neurol 43:833-835, 1986.
15. Chang B, Dellon AL. An alternate incision for approaching recurrent median nerve compression at the wrist. Plast Reconstr Surg 89:576-577, 1992.
16. Chang B, Dellon AL. Surgical treatment for recurrent carpal tunnel syndrome. J Hand Surg 18B:467-470, 1993.
17. Dellon AL, Mackinnon SE. Anatomic dissection about the median nerve in the wrist. I. Orientation of the motor fascicle of the median nerve in the carpal tunnel. Ann Plast Surg 21:32-35, 1988.
18. Reisman NR, Dellon AL. The abductor digiti minimi muscle flap: A salvage technique for wrist pain. Plast Reconstr Surg 72:859-863, 1983.
19. Evans GRD, Dellon AL. Implantation of the palmar cutaneous branch of the median nerve into the pronator quadratus for treatment of painful neuroma (submitted for publication).
20. Dellon AL. Techniques for successful management of ulnar nerve entrapment at the elbow. Neurosurg Clin North Am 2:57-73, 1991.
21. Dellon AL. Operative technique for submuscular transposition of the ulnar nerve at the elbow. Contemp Orthop 16:17-24, 1988.
22. Dellon AL. Review of treatment results for ulnar nerve entrapment at the elbow. J Hand Surg 14A:688-699, 1989.

23. Dellon AL. Musculofascial lengthening technique for the treatment of recurrent ulnar nerve entrapment at the elbow. Presented at the American Society of Surgery of the Hand. Vancouver: October 1992.
24. Dellon AL, Mackinnon SE. Injury to the medial antebrachial cutaneous nerve during cubital tunnel surgery. J Hand Surg 10B:33-36, 1985.
25. Dellon AL. Unpublished observations, 1992.
26. Saplys R, Mackinnon SE, Dellon AL. The relationship between nerve entrapment versus neuroma complications and the misdiagnosis of de Quervain's disease. Contemp Orthop 15:51-57, 1987.
27. Mackinnon SE, Dellon AL. Radial nerve entrapment at the proximal forearm and brachium. In Surgery of the Peripheral Nerve. New York: Thieme, 1988.
28. Dellon AL, Mackinnon SE. Musculoaponeurotic variation about the course of the median nerve in the proximal forearm. J Hand Surg 12B:359-363, 1987.
29. Mackinnon SE, Dellon AL. Median nerve entrapment in the proximal forearm and brachium. In Surgery of the Peripheral Nerve. New York: Thieme, 1988.
30. Dellon AL. Musculotendinous variations about the elbow. J Hand Surg 11B:175-181, 1986.
31. Meyer RA, Raja SN, Campbell JN, Mackinnon SE, Dellon AL. Neural activity originating from a neuroma in the baboon. Brain Res 325:255-260, 1985.
32. Mackinnon SE, Dellon AL, Hudson RA, Hunter DA. Alteration of neuroma formation by manipulation of its microenvironment. Plast Reconstr Surg 76:345-352, 1985.
33. Mackinnon SE, Dellon AL. Overlap of the lateral antebrachial cutaneous nerve and the superficial sensory branch of the radial nerve. J Hand Surg 10A:522-526, 1985.
34. Carroll RE, Green DP. The significance of the palmar cutaneous nerve at the wrist. Clin Orthop Rel Res 83:24-28, 1972.
35. Taleisnick J. The palmar cutaneous branch of the median nerve and the approach to the carpal tunnel. J Bone Joint Dis 55A:1212-1217, 1973.
36. Dellon AL, Mackinnon SE. Treatment of the painful neuroma by neuroma resection and muscle implantation. Plast Reconstr Surg 77:427-438, 1986.
37. Mackinnon SE, Dellon AL. Results of treatment of recurrent dorsoradial wrist neuromas. Ann Plast Surg 19:54-61, 1987.
38. Dellon AL, Seif SS. Neuroma of the posterior interosseous nerve simulating recurrent ganglion: Case report and anatomical dissection relating the posterior interosseous nerve to the carpus and etiology of dorsal ganglion pain. J Hand Surg 3:326-332, 1978.
39. Dellon AL. Partial dorsal wrist denervation: Resection of posterior interosseous nerve. J Hand Surg 10A:527-533, 1985.
40. Dellon AL, Mackinnon SE. Terminal branch of anterior interosseous nerve as source of volar wrist pain. J Hand Surg 9B:316-322, 1984.
41. Stocks GW, Cobb T, Lewis RC Jr. Transfer of sensibility in the hand: A new method to restore sensibility in ulnar nerve palsy with use of microsurgical digital nerve translocation. J Hand Surg 16A:219-226, 1991.
42. Dellon AL. Restoration of sensibility to the ulnar-deprived hand (submitted for publication).
43. Francel T, Dellon AL. Functional limb salvage combining gastrocnemius neurotization and posterior tibial nerve grafting: A case report. J Reconstr Microsurg [in press].
44. Mackinnon SE, Dellon AL. Clinical nerve reconstruction with a bioabsorbable polyglycolic acid tube. Plast Reconstr Surg 85:419-424, 1990.
45. Zacchary L, Dellon AL, Seiler WA IV. Relationship of intraneural damage in the rat sciatic nerve to the mechanism of injury. J Reconstr Microsurg 5:137-140, 1989.
46. Mackinnon SE, Dellon AL. Tarsal tunnel syndrome. In Surgery of the Peripheral Nerve. New York: Thieme, 1988.
47. Dellon AL, Mackinnon SE. Homologies between the tarsal and carpal tunnels: Implications for surgical treatment in the tarsal tunnel syndrome. Contemp Orthop 14:75-78, 1987.

48. Dellon AL. Deep peroneal nerve compression over the dorsum of the foot. Foot Ankle 11:73–80, 1990.
49. Dellon AL, Mackinnon SE. Results of posterior tibial nerve grafting at the ankle. J Reconstr Microsurg 7:81–83, 1991.
50. Dellon AL, Aszman O. Treatment of dorsal foot neuromas. Foot Ankle (submitted for publication).
51. Dellon AL. Wound healing in nerve. Clin Plast Surg 17:545–570, 1990.
52. Dellon AL, Mackinnon SE, Hudson AR, Hunter DA. Effect of submuscular versus intra-muscular placement of ulnar nerve: Experimental model in the primate. J Hand Surg 11B:117–119, 1986.

44

Reoperative Surgery Following Tissue Transplantation in Extremity Reconstruction

Randy Sherman, M.D.

Reoperative Problems

Persistent infection	Inability to wear preinjury footwear
Contour deformity	Flap failure
Difficult ambulation	Refracture or bone grafting
Hypertrophic nonunion	Tendon adhesions
Nerve reconstruction	Tendon reconstruction or transfer

Extraordinary progress has been made in reconstructive extremity surgery since the advent of vascularized tissue transfer for either wound coverage or functional restoration.[1,2] Whether a particular problem is addressed by local flap rotation or microsurgical free tissue transfer, tissue transplantation has allowed a whole spectrum of successive reoperative procedures to be performed in grievously wounded, previously unsalvageable extremities. Whereas a blast injury to the hand previously meant entire loss of function of that extremity, composite tissue transfer can restore essentially all missing structures, leading to potentially significant functional rehabilitation. Whereas a malignant fibrous histiocytoma of the proximal tibia previously meant amputation and prosthesis, wide en bloc excision with simultaneous flap reconstruction results in limb salvage in a majority of cases. Whereas before a chronic nonunion of the distal tibia with subsequent infection and sinus tract formation led to chronic osteomyelitis, radical pseudotumor excision of the infected tissue followed by obliteration of dead space with free tissue transfer can arrest the infection and result in subsequent long bone healing in most affected patients.[3] The frequency with which new and more comprehensive reconstructive procedures are being described mandates a close review and assessment of how and when subsequent surgical procedures should be performed in these previously injured but initially reconstructed regions.

Oftentimes a local muscle flap will be turned or a free muscle flap transferred with the intention of returning to the operative site within 2 to 6 months to perform further reconstructive surgery. Prime examples include elevating a previously placed muscle flap after coverage of a type IIIB tibial fracture for the placement of a cancellous bone graft, elevating a local muscle flap or free tissue transfer about the knee to replace a previously removed artificial joint complex, or performing a tendon transfer under a recently placed flap for the restoration of finger flexion, extension, and/or pinch. Given the initial strategies for multistaged reconstructive procedures using the augmented tissue bed provided by the primary flap transfer, secondary procedures should proceed in concert with originally planned goals. Conversely, transfers should be chosen, designed, and transplanted with full consideration given to possible subsequent elevation, reorientation, or revision.

Due to the nature of most complex extremity injuries, there often may be more than one practitioner involved in the patient's reconstruction and rehabilitation. It is crucial for the plastic surgeon to develop an active and harmonious relationship with his colleagues involved in resolving these difficult problems. The quality of this relationship can be directly proportional to the timing and success of the patient's outcome. The value of a team approach is most noticeable when dealing with patients who have sustained complex open fractures of the lower extremity. Nearly all patients who undergo muscle or musculocutaneous transfer for the reconstruction of compound lower extremity fractures will eventually require bone grafting. The timing of the bone grafting will be affected by reliable and complete wound closure, which in turn will depend on timely stabilization and debridement of the initial fracture site. In type III fractures about the ankle or foot, the above problems might be compounded by a need to further revise the soft tissue envelope in order to achieve comfortable shoe fit. Prolonged intervals between these numerous surgeries can be minimized by developing and maintaining constant communication with orthopedic and rehabilitation medicine colleagues. It is crucial that the plastic surgeon responsible for initial wound coverage be present for all subsequent procedures involving the local flap or free tissue transfer. Elevation, transposition, or other revisional procedures involving the tissue transfer should not be left to persons unfamiliar with the original operative procedure. Consideration should be given to pedicle orientation, probable sources of collateral revascularization, and flap configuration before any decisions can be made regarding flap elevation.

In reoperative surgery of the hand and upper extremity, the same principles apply but must be directed toward an open and honest relationship with the hand therapist. Inevitably, after major tissue transfers for reconstruction of the hand or phalanges, occupational therapy will be central to restoration of function. Reoperation for tenolysis, tendon transfer, web space deepening, or flap debulking must be undertaken as soon as the patient plateaus in the rehabilitation progress. The timing of these procedures depends entirely on a clear understanding of the therapist's perception of presence or absence of progress in the rehabilitation environment and his subsequent recommendations.

One of the greatest challenges presented to the reconstructive plastic surgeon in these cases involves patient understanding, acceptance, and compliance. In most cases it is not inherently obvious to an individual who has sustained a complex extremity injury as to why tissue transfer is required and, more important, why reoperative surgery—sometimes in multiple stages—may be the safest and most reliable option for an ultimately successful outcome. Extra time spent educating and empathizing with the patient and his family is key to ensuring their support in achieving ultimate rehabilitative goals. Surprisingly, patient acceptance is quite high when basic wound healing principles are explained and illustrated. This approach applies as well to the description and discussion of plans for subsequent reoperative surgical procedures. A clear outline given to the patient as to the expected number and timing of secondary procedures will help him to gain a clear perspective of the length and complexity of the healing process. Frustration and disappointment can be replaced by acceptance and even enthusiasm, with the patient actually looking forward to the reoperative surgical procedure as a milestone in the restorative process.

TIMING

Subsequent elective reoperative surgery can be performed anywhere from several days to several years after flap transfer in the upper and lower extremity. The ultimate functional and aesthetic goals of the particular reconstruction will influence the timeliness of any subsequent intervention. There are very few hard and fast rules regarding how long after a successful transfer a subsequent reconstructive or reoperative procedure may be undertaken. Surgical preferences vary widely on any number of reoperative issues including elevation for nerve grafting, tendon transfer, iliac crest bone grafting, flap reorientation, and debulking. There are those who would argue that accomplishing as much as possible at the time of transfer has the advantage of earlier incorporation and quicker return of function. Others, however, believe that successful wound closure, as evidenced by the healed musculocutaneous flap or completed epithelialization of the skin graft over a muscle flap, is an important physiologic marker for successful wound closure and a prerequisite for any subsequent attempts to reconstruct other component structures such as bone, tendon, or nerve. Teleologically, there should be no strict contraindication to reelevating a transferred flap, whether it be pedicled or free, shortly after a successful transfer. Conversely, there are no apparent disadvantages to lifting a flap years after its initial application. So much is dependent on the particular goals of the restorative strategy.

PLANNING

Initial Considerations

Consideration of possible secondary surgery of a particular flap, once transferred, should be part of the initial planning process. Muscle flaps are the preferred choice for the obliteration of dead space in osteomyelitic defects but may present problems for debulking at a later date. Fasciocutaneous flaps often provide a superior cosmetic result initially but over time may require debulking when used in the hand or ankle and foot regions because of their tendency to swell or develop segmental trapdoor deformities. Pedicle length and position in relationship to the flap inset must be considered at initial tissue transfer when there is any possibility of subsequent flap elevation. In an overwhelming majority of lower extremity compound fractures, the open wounds are anteriorly oriented. Most high-energy impact fractures of the tibia are sustained by a direct, oncoming blow to the patient as exemplified by the automobile bumper vs. pedestrian injury. Because of the lack of cushioning soft tissue along the anterior crest of the tibia, those forces that result in highly comminuted fractures of the diaphysis of the tibia can decimate overlying skin, subcutaneous tissue, and anterior compartment musculature. With this predominant pattern of injury, the anterior tibial vessels are rarely, if ever, chosen for recipient anasto-

Considerations in Reoperative Surgery of the Extremities

- Maintenance of vascular supply
- Limited elevation of flaps to meet the specific needs of the reoperative problem
- Liberal use of tourniquet control for flap reelevation and resuture
- Early and prolonged use of compressive garments in reoperated lower extremities
- Development of comprehensive surgical strategy including possible reoperative events before choosing initial flap

moses. Vascular anastomoses in free tissue transfer should be consistently performed outside the zone of injury whenever possible. This not only ensures the highest rate of anastomotic patency at the time of inset but also helps to separate the vascular supply of the flap from the target area of the initial injury and subsequent reconstructive site. We preferentially choose muscle flaps with long pedicles that can be anastomosed well proximal to the zone of injury. When available, the posterior circulation is preferential because of its ease of exposure and relative lack of side branches in the mid and distal thirds of the leg. Release of the soleus muscle fibers from the medial tibial diaphysis is all that is required to gain clear exposure to the posterior tibial artery and concomitant veins in this area. Godina[4] has suggested a posterior approach to the trifurcation. Anastomosis of the donor vessels is performed with the patient in a prone position after initial tacking of the tissue transfer anteriorly. This is one alternative with which we have not had much experience but that clearly has the distinct advantage of ultimate separation of the injury site from the vascular pedicle.

At the time of initial flap transfer, subdivision or partial reorientation of flap subunits can positively affect reoperative surgical outcomes. Muscle flaps can be partially divided along lines of vascular axes for simultaneous wound coverage and deep space obliteration. We favor using the rectus abdominis muscle with a longitudinal split for simultaneous osseous defect obliteration and cutaneous coverage. Buncke and colleagues[5] have had favorable experience with the serratus anterior muscle: they subdivide this transplant into its multiple slips, which in turn can be reoriented in several planes. The latissimus dorsi muscle, with its two predominant subunits, can be used in a similar fashion. Another option is to take the entire latissimus dorsi muscle with the contiguous serratus anterior muscle on a common subscapular pedicle. Although some orthopedists still use antibiotic beads, silicone block, or methylmethacrylate spacers, subdivided vascularized muscle units have predominantly replaced these previously popular alloplastic implants because they provide more physiologic dead space obliteration. At the time of revisional surgery, elevation of the muscle transfer can then be confined to excision of the deep dead space subunit with replacement using cancellous bone, vascularized cortical bone, or endoprosthesis implantation or replacement.

When a flap is chosen for the reconstruction of composite defects of the hand, muscle transplants are less favorable for those injuries requiring subsequent tendon transfers or nerve grafting procedures. Thin fasciocutaneous flaps such as the lateral arm or radial forearm flaps tend to provide the ideal bed for secondary procedures in this area. Parascapular flaps have the advantage of being able to cover large defects but may bring with them an excess of fatty tissue and require secondary debulking. Temporoparietal fascia transferred as a bilaminar flap is advantageous for subsequent tendon transfer because of its exquisite vascularity and lack of bulk.

Flap Debulking

Primary inset of muscle flaps, either pedicled or freely transferred, often results in objectionable contour deformity. However, muscle atrophy will usually occur beginning as early as 8 to 12 weeks after surgery and stabilize at roughly 1 year. With thorough preoperative counseling and periodic patient reeducation, our experience has shown that if a complete progression of muscle atrophy is allowed to occur, patients rarely request further debulking of the muscle flap. In those cases in which reduction of muscle volume is requested because of a persistent aesthetic contour deformity, two methods may be used.[6] Elevation of the entire muscle on its pedicle with advancement and partial excision can be undertaken in limited situations. This approach is oftentimes difficult because of the progressive lack of pliability of the muscle as it becomes increasingly fibrotic. Once the flap has conformed to the wound size and shape, it may be more difficult to reorient or reduce the flap in a segmental fashion. Another method is the tangential excision of the muscle flap's most superficial layers. This approach requires first removing a previously placed skin graft followed by planar excision of the protruding parts of the muscle flap itself. Other authors have described harvesting the mature, previously placed skin graft and reapplying it as a mesh graft. In our experience this leads to a markedly inferior aesthetic result and negates any advantage of improvement of contour deformity. In such cases we have applied a new sheet graft to further improve the desired aesthetic appearance. Because the transferred pedicle and vascular anastomoses are usually deep and proximal to the main body of the muscle flap, this planing technique is quite safe in terms of maintaining vascularity throughout the muscle transfer.

Fasciocutaneous flaps on the other hand may be inset at the time of primary transfer with greater attention toward contour considerations. However, more often than not these flaps will eventually require debulking or defatting because of subsequent enlargement. Fasciocutaneous flaps applied in the lower extremity, particularly about the lower third of the tibia, ankle, or foot, tend to become increasingly bulky with time, dependency, and ambulation. Most likely this condition is the result of a less than efficient outflow system for lymphatic and other extracellular fluid within the most superficial elements of the flap. Patients should be educated as to the probability that one and sometimes up to three subsequent flap debulking and defatting procedures in the distally placed fasciocutaneous flap will be necessary to achieve maximal aesthetic restoration. When the fasciocutaneous flap is elevated for the removal of skin and wedge excision of fat, the primary vascular pedicle should be maintained if at all possible. In addition, as much of the cutaneous marginal scar as possible should be left undisturbed.[7] Closure under moderate tension with subsequent compression wrapping is usually very well tolerated.

Another option for volume removal in the fasciocutaneous flap is liposuction. Just as for use in free tissue transfer, the application of liposuction in this setting should not vary significantly from other, more classic applications.

Direct Flap Manipulation

Besides debulking, segmental reelevation, and flap reorientation, direct limited manipulation may be required in certain circumstances. Procedures include tunneling for the placement of tendon grafts or tendon transfers, placement of fine-wire stabilizing devices for Ilizarov distraction or compression, and placement of osteointegrated implants for prosthetic mounting. In addition, staged separation of previously inset flaps can be performed.

In those patients requiring tendon transfer or tendon grafting through the bed of a previously transferred flap, we have performed classic tunneling techniques using a blunt-nosed tendon passer with excellent results. If a tendon suture is required under the region of the transferred flap, small, albeit adequate, incisions can be made directly in the flap to avoid large-plane disruption, which occurs with flap elevation. As is the case with classically described principles of tendon transfers and tendon grafting, tissue equilibrium and maximal passive range of motion of the involved joints must be obtained. These goals should be obtained in those tissues affected by the free flap transfer as well as in the surrounding soft tissues and joints.

Fine-wire pin fixation of the fractured and comminuted tibia in conjunction with the application of the Ilizarov device can be performed within the substance of a free flap.[8,9] Several authors have described successful outcomes with the application of an Ilizarov device simultaneously with (or sometime after) flap transfer for wound coverage in the extremities. Once initial take of the muscle transfer is achieved, distraction or compression osteosynthesis using the Ilizarov device presents no significant problem to transplant viability. Buncke and colleagues[5] believe that certain muscles including the latissimus dorsi, rectus abdominis, and gracilis allow for easier fine-wire movement than other muscles because of the parallel nature of the muscle fibers. In certain circumstances in which the muscle flap is initially applied for both cutaneous wound coverage and obliteration of deep osseous dead space, secondary limited elevation and removal of that interposed muscle segment may be required to successfully allow for final bony docking.

When AO-type half-frame external fixators are used, primary pin fixation in or around the flap is discouraged. Conversely, wrapping a flap around an external pin that is not placed through intact, nontraumatized skin also can lead to sinus tract formation and subsequent problematic wound closure. Once the defect is closed with the flap well healed, placement of external pin fixation through the substance of the flap, while rarely indicated, can be safely performed.

Osteointegrated implant insertion is more germane to free flaps used in the head and neck and oromandibular region than those placed in the extremities. In those infrequent circumstances in which a partial prosthesis might be mounted in the extremity, placement of osteointegrated implants can be performed once primary wound coverage is complete and tissue equilibrium is achieved.

In certain cases in which the geometry of the wound prevents a tailored inset of the transferred flap, an umbrella-type transplant may be performed with secondary flap subdivision. This problem is usually encountered in patients who sustain composite degloving injuries to the dorsum of the hand and phalanges. A planned syndactylization of the digits may be performed with subsequent separation after 4 to 6 weeks depending on the condition of the recipient wound beds. Just as in congenital syndactyly release, additional skin grafting in the web spaces is required. If there is concern about the underlying vascularity, releases can be performed in a staged fashion.

Vascular Considerations

When reoperative surgery is considered in the field of a previously transferred flap, it is wise to elevate the flap via its previously inset margins. This approach allows the maintenance of blood flow through the natural axes of the specific flap as it was designed and transferred. Although there are anecdotal reports of pedicle division as soon as 2 weeks after transfer without complication, there are also occasional reports of delayed flap loss up to 12 months postoperatively secondary to acute division at the anastomotic site.[10,11] It is only logical that maintenance of the pedicle, if possible, is the most advantageous option when reelevating a transferred flap. The larger the surface area that can be left undivided at any reoperative event, the more reliable the blood supply to the flap. In most cases underlying blood supply need not be deemed critical in that an overwhelming majority of transfers is performed initially due to lack of recipient site vascularity at the base of the wound. Examples include osseous dead space caused by comminuted fracture, exposure of total knee or total hip arthroplasty, and exposure of Achilles tendon with loss of paratenon.

GOALS OF TREATMENT

As the problems that require flap transfer in the upper and lower extremities are multiple and varied, the goals and strategies of reoperative surgery for these various conditions are numerous. Clearly each procedure has a common end point: the restoration of function or form to the previously traumatized, congenitally deformed, or iatrogenically ablated extremity. Principal procedures performed for these purposes include tendon transfers, tendon grafting, nerve grafting, bone grafting, flap reorientation or division, flap debulking, recontouring, defatting, and simple elevation for revisions on underlying devices such as endoprostheses. In all of the above circumstances, the goal of the initial surgery is to provide an anatomic and physiologic environment in which reoperative procedures have the best chance of success in transforming the diseased extremity into a useful one.

Reoperative Procedures

As previously outlined, an overwhelming majority of reoperative surgery procedures in the extremities after flap transfer is the result of a continuing need for functional restoration. A representative spectrum of clinical examples illustrating the specific secondary reconstructive problems and their solution after successful flap transfer is presented.

Staged Tendon Reconstruction and Release of Flap Syndactylization

With complex composite injuries of the dorsum of the hand and finger in which both soft tissues and extensor tendons have been lost, multicomponent reconstruction using the temporoparietal fascial flap in a bilaminar fashion can be accompanied by staged extensor tendon reconstruction using temporary Silastic implants.

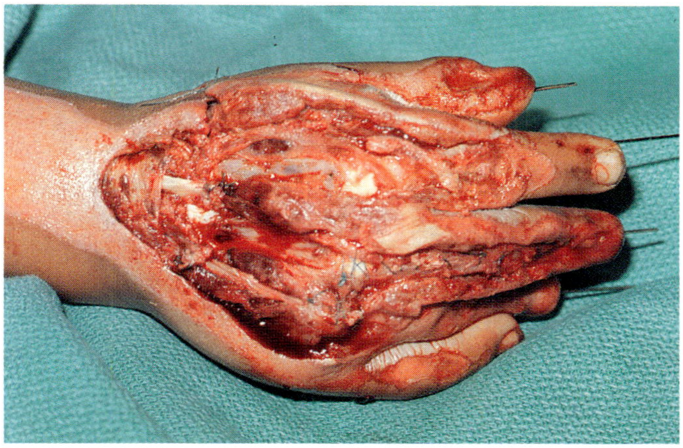

A 7-year-old child sustained an avulsive injury to the dorsum of the hand and digits in a lawn mower accident. There was a loss of skin, subcutaneous tissue, and extrinsic extensor tendons on all four fingers to the level of the middle phalanx. Stripping of the periosteum and cortices of the metacarpal bones and phalanges was also noted, with some loss of the dorsal hood complex over the metacarpophalangeal joints.

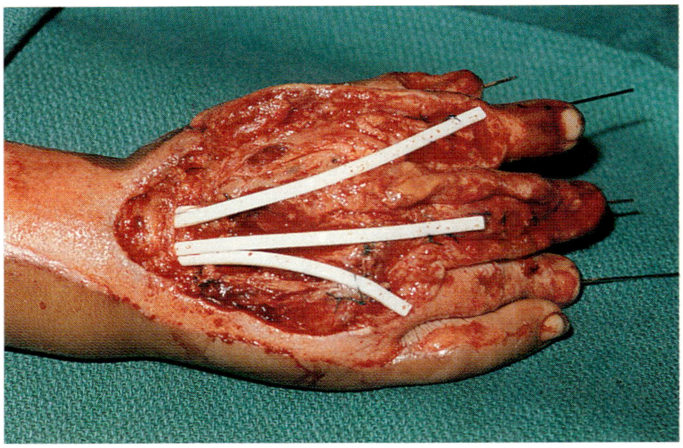

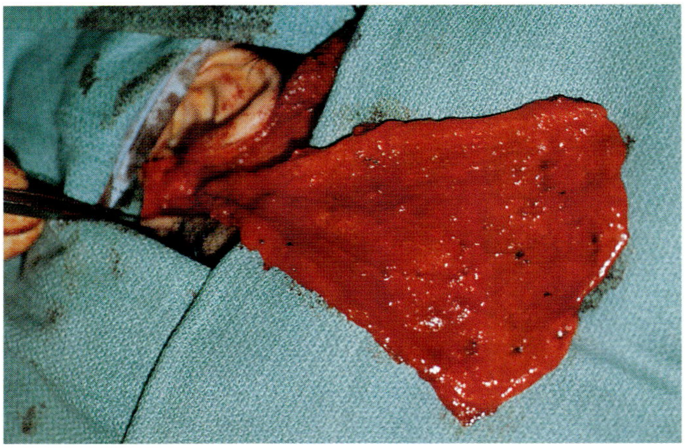

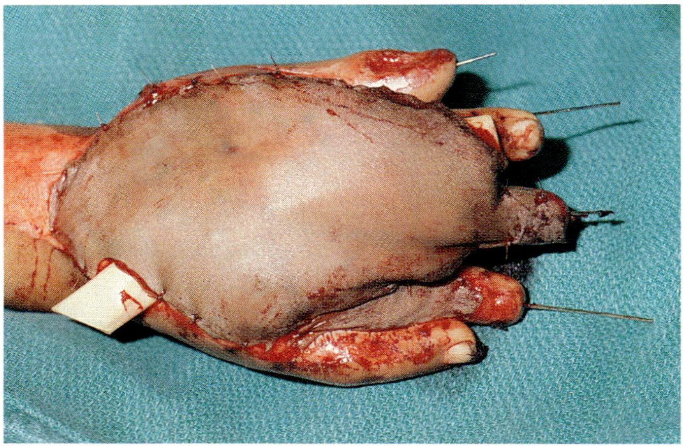

Soft tissue reconstruction was accomplished using a bilaminar temporoparietal fascial flap with simultaneous placement of Hunter rod Silastic implants. The digits were purposely syndactylized to allow simultaneous coverage of both the dorsum of the hand and phalanges with one flap. After initial flap healing the child received progressive occupational therapy for joint mobilization. During the postoperative course one of the Silastic implants became exposed on the distal surface and required removal.

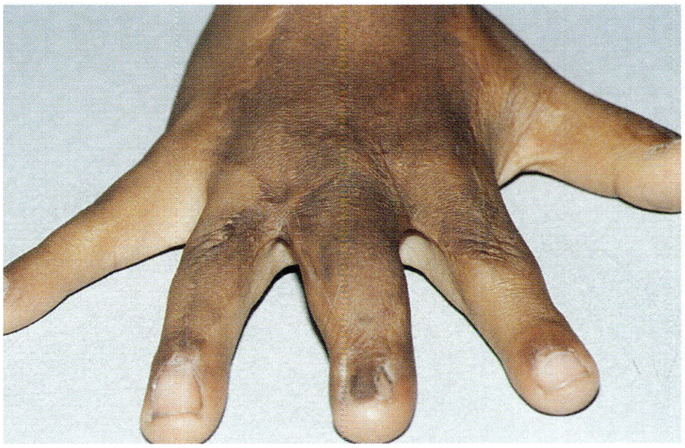

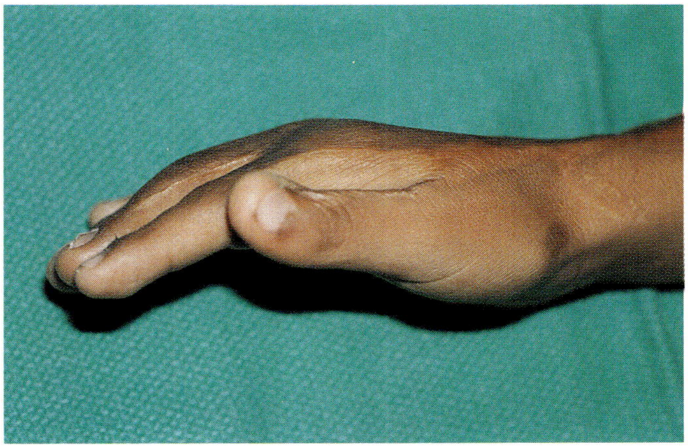

At 3 months postoperatively the remainder of the fingers underwent secondary tendon reconstruction with interpositional tendon grafts applied to the extensor digitorum communis muscle proximally and inserted into the middle phalanx distally. Simultaneous syndactyly release with additional split-thickness skin grafting in the web spaces was accomplished. The hand was held in an extension splint for 4 weeks after which controlled passive range-of-motion and then active assisted range-of-motion therapy was undertaken. The postoperative result is shown.

Secondary Tendon Reconstruction

In composite injuries that disrupt tendon function with substantive loss of tendon structure, stabilization of the underlying bony architecture, anatomic reduction of the joint surfaces, and wound closure with vascularized tissue are clearly a priority. Once these goals have been achieved, planning may proceed for the restoration of active joint function using either tendon grafts or tendon transfers. Classic principles of tendon transfer cannot be short-circuited and must be followed in order to achieve maximal possible functional return. Solid union of bony fractures must be achieved both clinically and radiographically. Passive joint motion must be maintained and preferably maximized using frequent and often daily occupational therapy for stretching, passive range-of-motion exercises, and modality therapy. Tissue equilibrium as first described by Bunnell must be achieved to provide for the most favorable recipient bed. Classic transfers for particular nerve or musculotendinous unit deficits may then be safely carried out. In those cases in which a soft tissue flap makes up a majority of the interposing tissue between originating muscle and end affector joint, subcutaneous tunnels are developed within the flap using tendon passers just as one might perform this procedure on native, uninjured tissues. As is classically described, the reorientation of the transferred musculocutaneous unit must achieve a straight-line pull to the transferred joint complex. Ultimate success of the functional restorative surgery demands that the flap transfer address these ultimate needs at the initial inset.

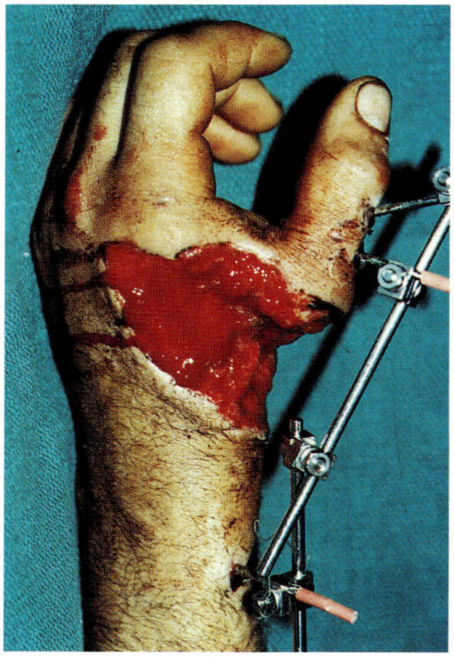

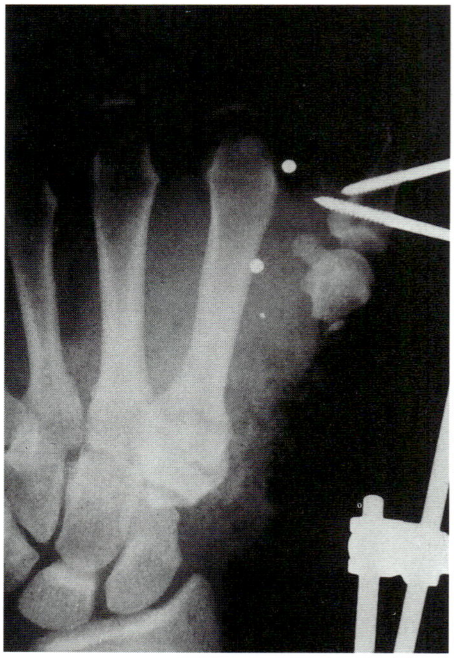

This 27-year-old, right hand–dominant man sustained a close-range shotgun injury to the radial side of the left hand. Tissues lost included the first metacarpal, trapezium, and trapezoid bones; extensor pollicis longus, extensor pollicis brevis, and abductor pollicis longus muscles; portions of the first interosseus dorsalis manus muscle; superficial branch of the radial nerve; and overlying skin and subcutaneous tissue on the radial dorsum of the hand extending around the palmar surface to include portions of the thenar eminence. Amazingly enough the distal aspect of the thumb from metacarpophalangeal joint onward remained viable, with a vascularized base including the digital vessels, both digital nerves, and a bridging soft tissue base within the palmar web space. Fortunately the flexor pollicis longus muscle was uninjured. After initial debridement, stabilization was achieved with external minifixation.

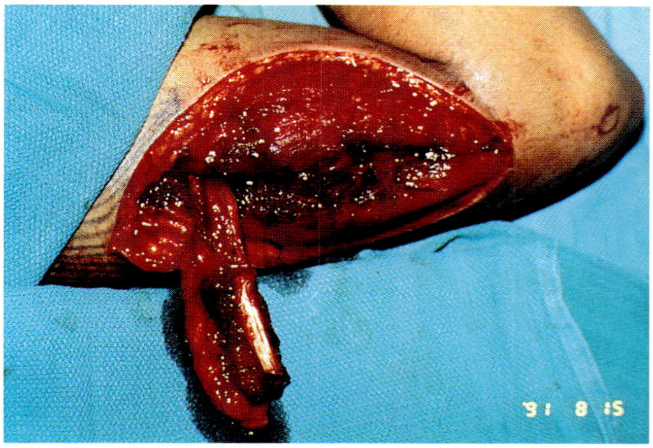

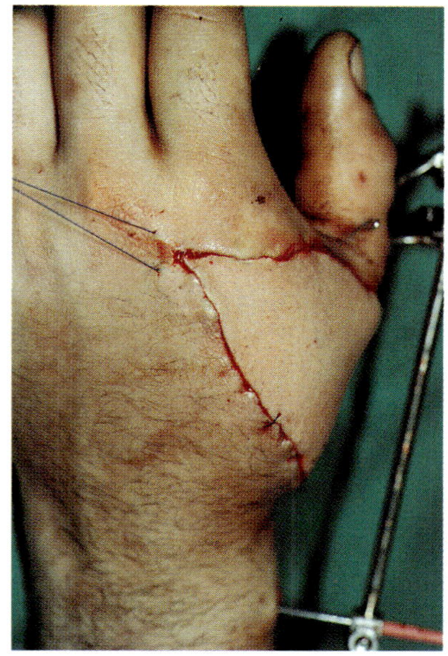

The first stage of reconstruction addressed the issue of bony stability and soft tissue coverage with the transfer of a lateral arm osteocutaneous flap. The cutaneous nerve to the forearm was carried with the osteocutaneous flap and used as a flow-through vascularized nerve graft to repair the superficial branch of the radial nerve defect. The external fixation was maintained and the humeral bone was further stabilized with internal pin fixation to allow thumb-interphalangeal range-of-motion exercises during osseous healing.

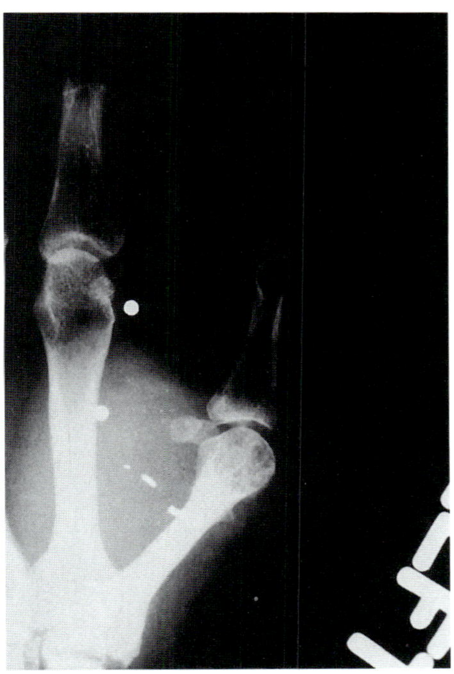

Once bony stabilization had been achieved at 4 months postoperatively, the residual inability to extend the thumb-interphalangeal joint was addressed with a tendon transfer using the extensor indicis proprius muscle to reconstruct the lost extensor pollicis longus muscle.

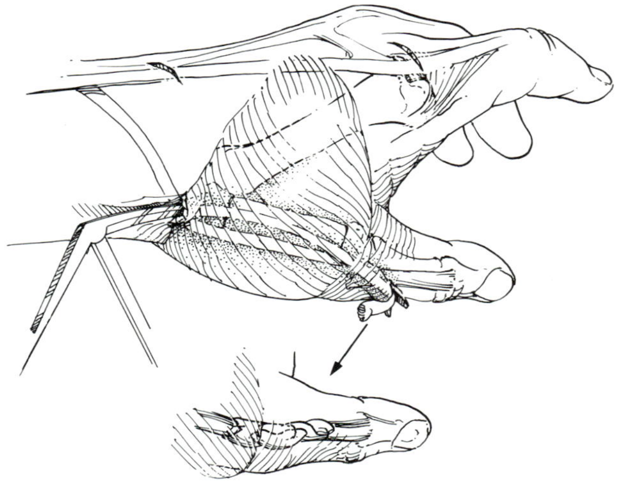

As classically described, the extensor indicis proprius muscle was harvested through a small longitudinal incision over the index finger metacarpophalangeal bone and proximal phalanx and further freed proximally using a small incision over the distal forearm dorsally. After the tendon was rerouted out of its compartment, it was passed through a tunnel made in the cutaneous portion of the lateral arm osteocutaneous flap. The tunnel was developed from distal to proximal, retrieving the extensor indicis proprius tendon for subsequent tendon juncture over the thumb–proximal phalangeal area. Although classic extensor indicis proprius–extensor pollicis longus muscle transfers are coapted more proximally than in this situation, no option was available for a more proximal juncture because of the nature of the segmental defect over the dorsum of the metacarpal bone. A modified Kessler tendon juncture was accomplished, and the thumb was held in extension with a spica splint for 4 weeks. A spica-type brace replaced the initial immobilizer and controlled motion exercises were initiated.

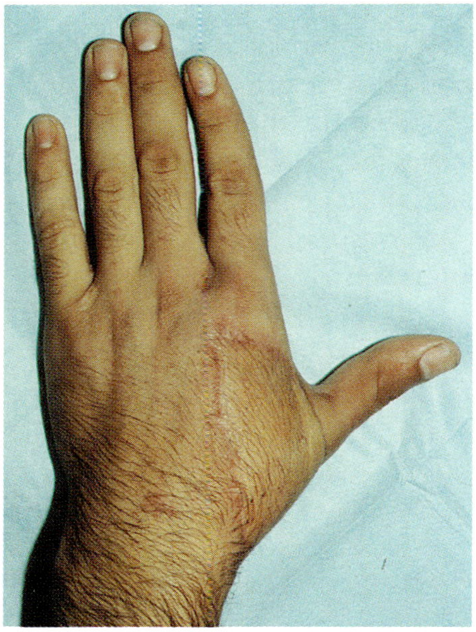

After a complete course of therapy, virtually complete thumb interphalangeal extension was restored.

Periodic reports in the literature have described simultaneous tendon transfers or tendon grafts placed under or accompanying free flaps. We have used this technique with limited success in cases in which osseous stability or joint destruction was not in question (see pp. 1620-1622). In those situations, however, in which bony union must be achieved, simultaneous tendon transfer or tendon grafting has not led to a more rapid return to functional restoration and has required tenolysis or revisional tendon surgery.

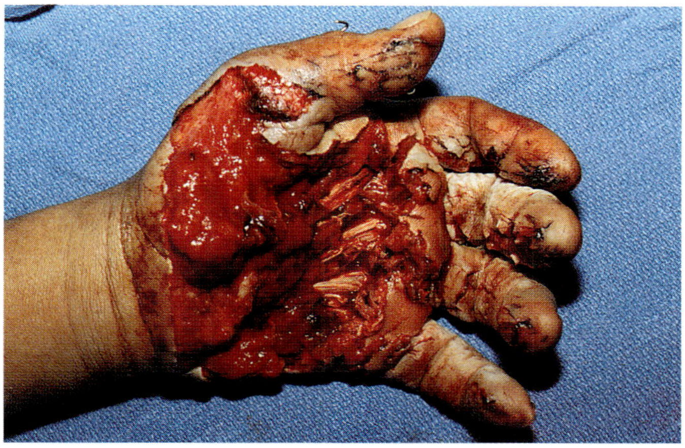

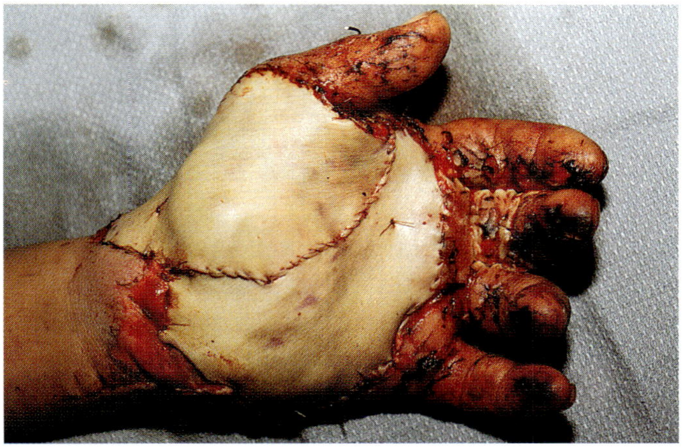

This patient, a right hand–dominant man in his mid-30s, sustained a crushing degloving injury of the left palm. This trauma resulted in the destruction of the thenar intrinsics and the motor branch of the median nerve, as well as the exposure and denuding of the entire flexor tendon apparatus and zone III. The patient was initially treated with debridement and the wound was covered using temporoparietal fascia supplemented with a full-thickness skin graft.

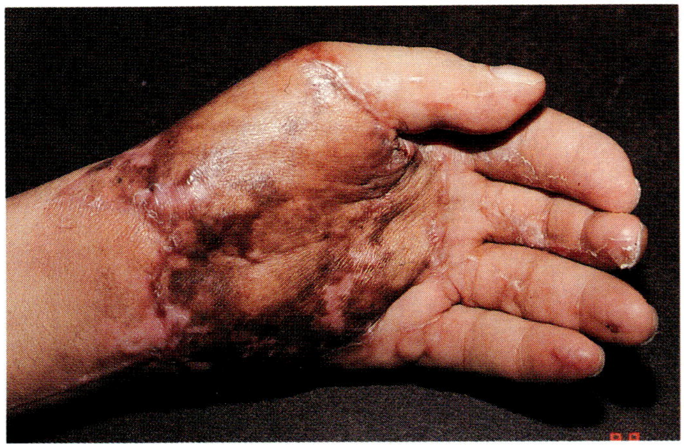

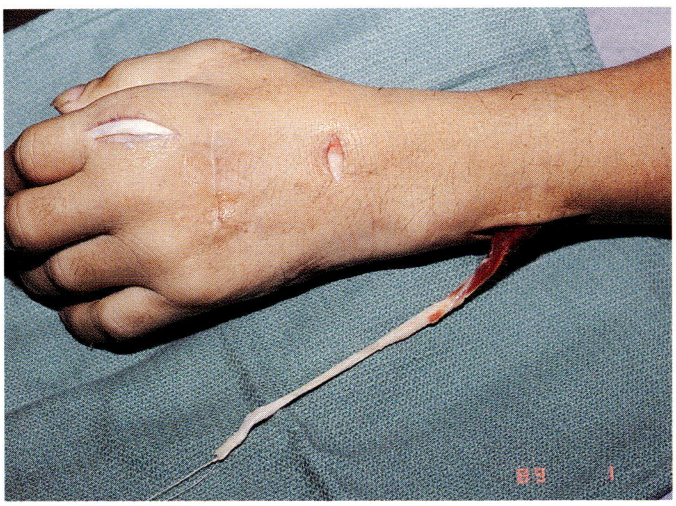

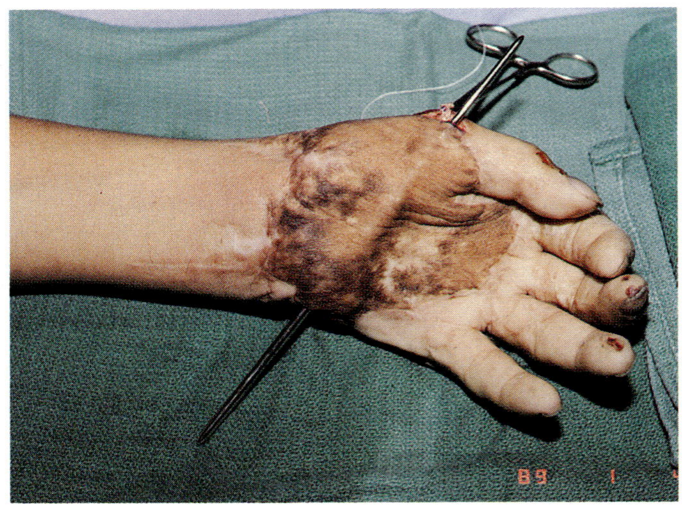

Despite the achievement of wound closure and tissue equilibrium, the patient had no residual opposition of the thumb and fingers. Thus an extensor indicis proprius muscle–opponensplasty (Zancolli-Burkhalter) was performed. The extensor indicis proprius muscle was harvested through an incision over the index metacarpophalangeal joint and a more proximal incision dorsally over the wrist and ulnarly at the origin of the muscle. A tendon passer was then used to create a tunnel beneath the reconstructed palmar soft tissues, and the extensor indicis proprius muscle was threaded without difficulty. The tendon was secured to the first metacarpal bone, with tendon juncture to the insertion of the adductor pollicis muscle and implantation into the metacarpal bone.

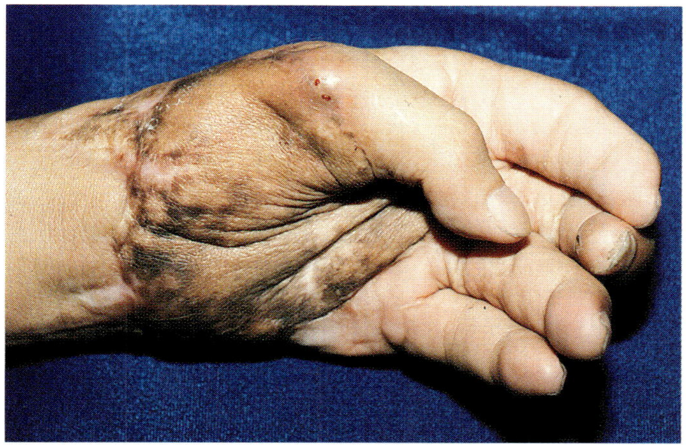

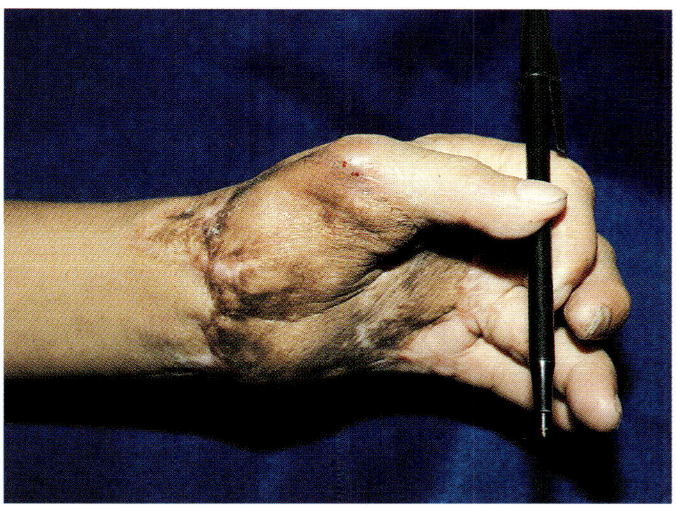

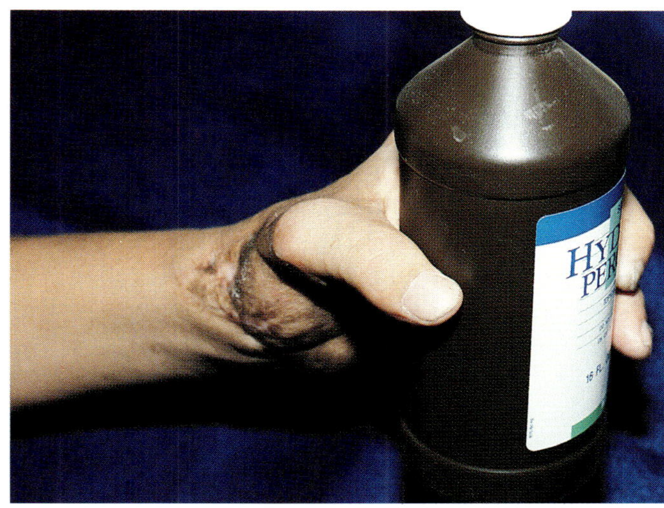

The thumb was held in opposition using a specially molded thermoplastic splint, and active-assist controlled range-of-motion therapy was instituted at 4 weeks. The splint was worn continually for an additional 3 weeks after which functional opposition was achieved as demonstrated by fine pinch and power grasp.

Once again, after successful wound closure was obtained with restoration of soft tissue mass, the secondary tendon transfer proceeded as it might have for an isolated nerve injury alone. All principles of tendon transfer were heeded, with the interposed free flap serving to normalize the initial soft tissue deficit.

Tenolysis

In specific circumstances in which tendon reconstruction was accomplished primarily under free tissue transfers, limited elevation or direct incision of the flap for release of underlying tendon adhesions may be safely accomplished. Again, in keeping with the established principles of secondary tendon surgery, this procedure should not be attempted until passive range of motion of all joints and maturation of all scar tissue have occurred. Because of localized anesthesia in the flap bed, tenolysis oftentimes can be carried out with the patient under minimal anesthesia, which allows the patient to test the tenolysis in real time on request by the surgeon.

This 43-year-old right hand–dominant man sustained an avulsion injury to the dorsum of the left hand, which destroyed the skin and subcutaneous tissues, caused untidy lacerations of the entire extensor digitorum communis muscle complex, and stripped the underlying periosteum and cortices of the index through the ring metacarpal bones.

Composite reconstruction was obtained in a single stage by the transfer of a bilaminar temporoparietal fascial flap with primary suture of the partially debrided and revised tendon ends. A skin graft was applied over the superficial layer of the temporoparietal fascia and the wound was splinted. Once wound closure was ensured and the skin graft had completed its epithelialization, the patient began an extended course of joint mobilization.

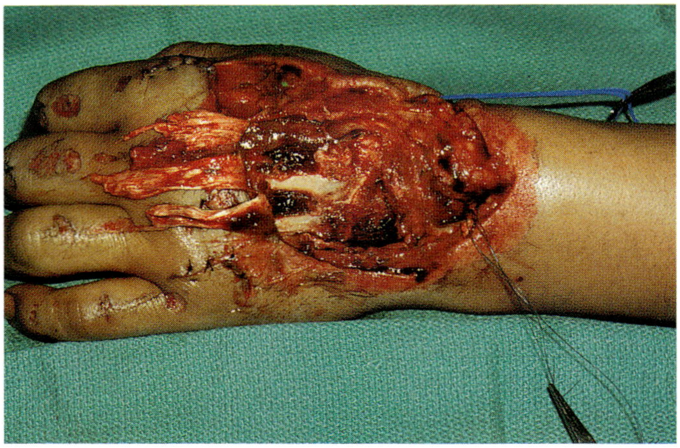

Avulsion injury

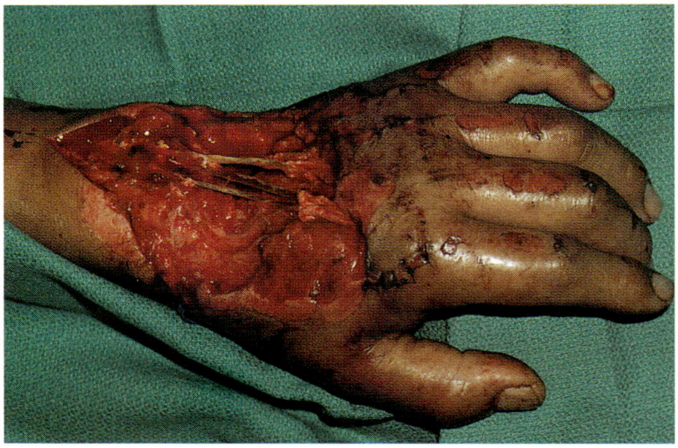

Primary debridement and resutured tendon ends

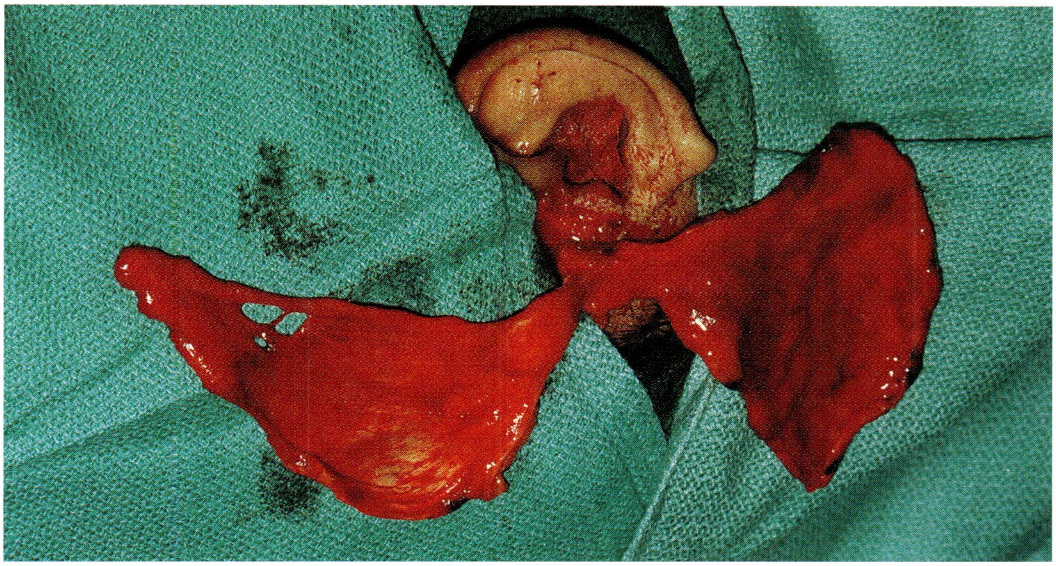

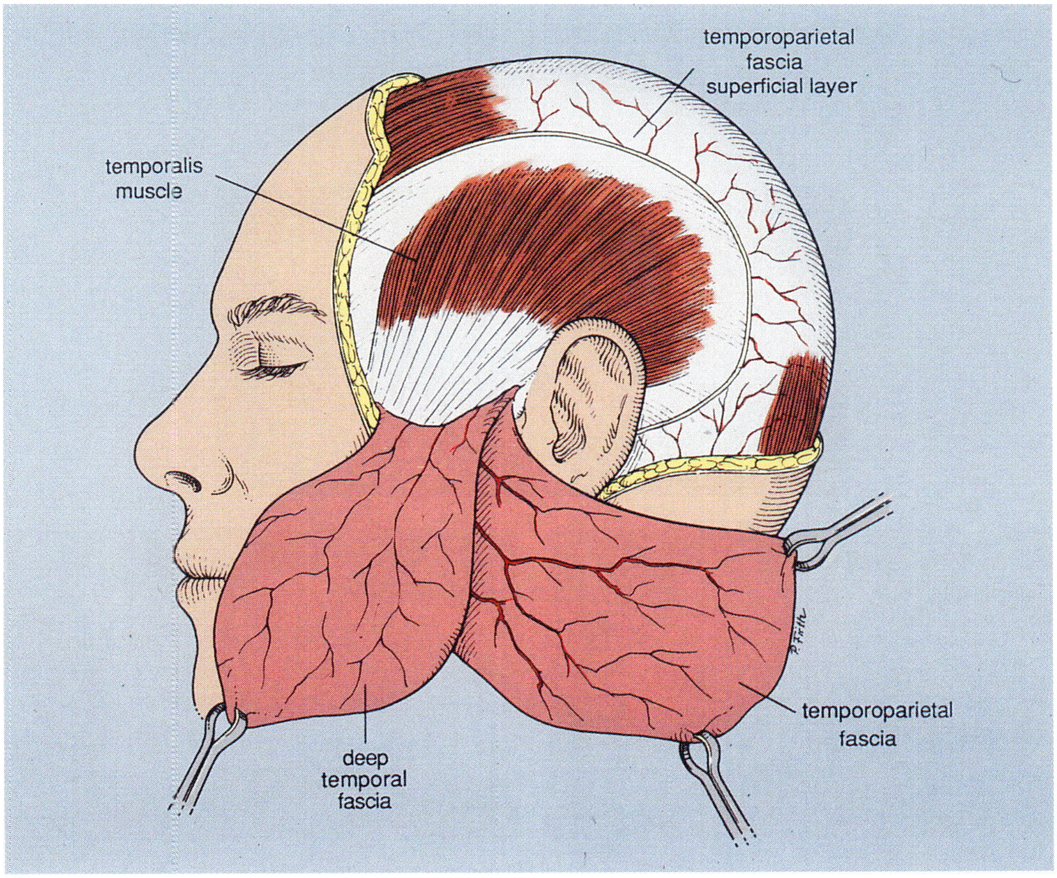

Elevation of bilaminar temporoparietal flap

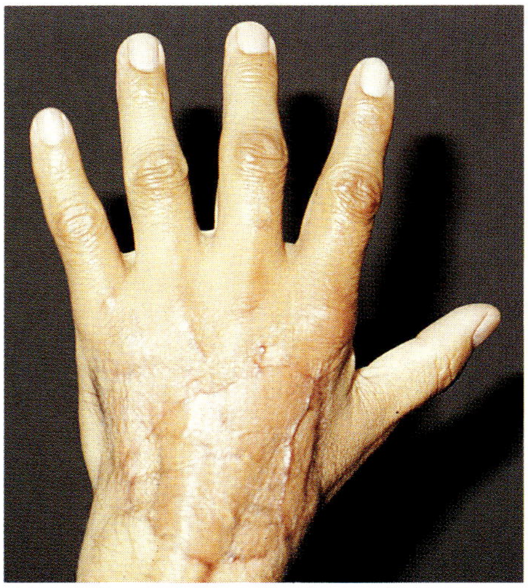

At 4 months, passive range of motion of the wrist and finger joints had returned to a near normal level. However, active range of motion was impeded by tendon scarring at the site of tendon juncture.

With the patient under local anesthesia and tourniquet control, a small longitudinal incision was made in the midbody of the temporoparietal flap. Tenolysis was undertaken and the patient then asked to pull through on the extensor tendon reconstruction. Once the patient demonstrated restoration of active motion, the tourniquet was let down. Hemostasis was achieved and the wound was closed.

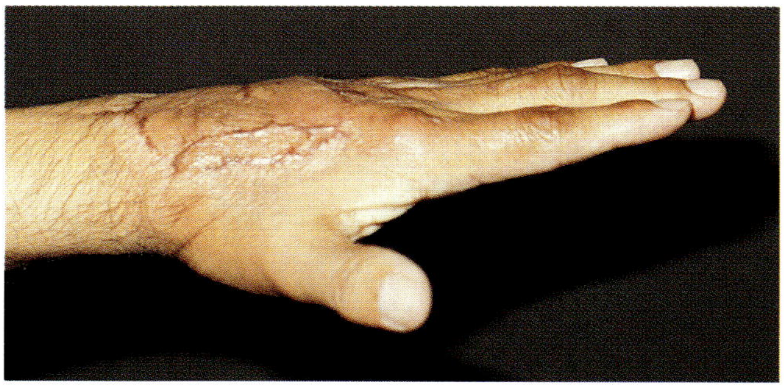

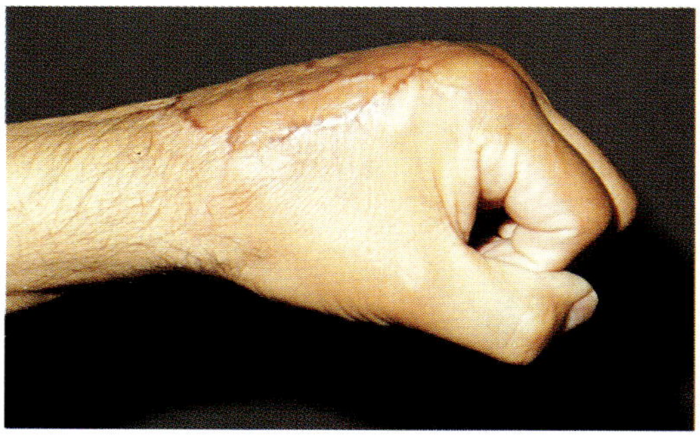

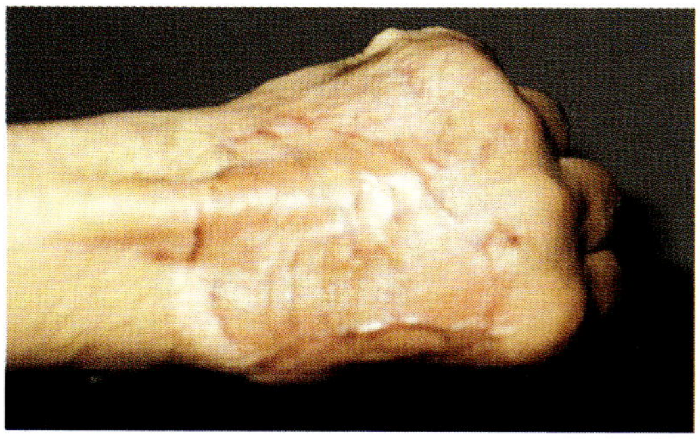

The patient returned to the therapist shortly after surgery for continued postoperative rehabilitation including maintenance of the newly achieved range of motion and active resistance exercises designed to strengthen the extensor digitorum communis musculotendinous units.

Secondary Nerve Grafting

In composite injuries to the upper extremity that disrupt major peripheral nerves, distal and proximal mobilization for advancement and primary suture of nerve ends is limited to the repair of small segmental defects measuring not more than 2 to 3 cm. It has been well proven by Millesi that nerves repaired primarily under tension have a poorer functional return than those treated with interpositional nerve grafting. Long segmental defects associated with overlying soft tissue loss presage a poor prognosis regardless of the surgical option used for reconstruction. Bridenback and Terzis underscore the importance of improving the vascular bed of the nerve graft for optimal axonal regeneration. They have performed and reported on a series of interpositional nerve grafts for this purpose. An alternative method for nerve repair is the primary reconstruction of the soft tissue defect with a vascularized flap followed by re-elevation of the flap for interpositional nerve grafting using nonvascularized autogenous sural nerve.

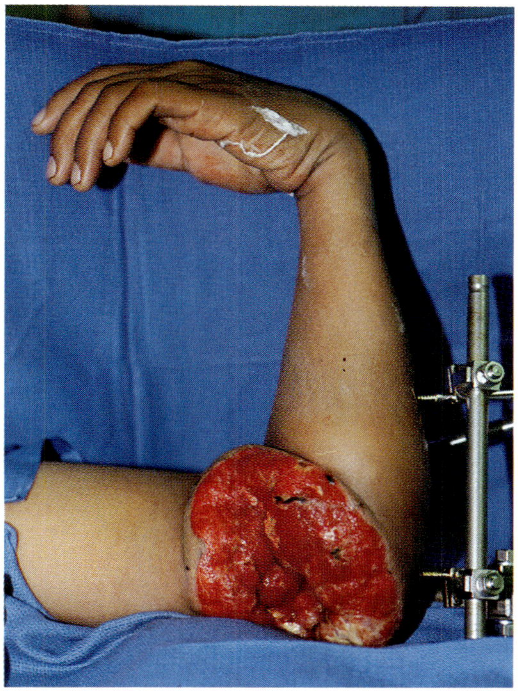

This 37-year-old Oriental man sustained a gunshot blast to the left antecubital fossa with resultant loss of medial and posterior skin, a 9 cm loss of ulnar nerve, and destruction of both the medial epicondyle of the olecranon and distal humerus (type IIIB fracture). Initial stabilization was accomplished with an AO external fixation device, and debridement was performed to remove all nonviable soft tissue and bone.

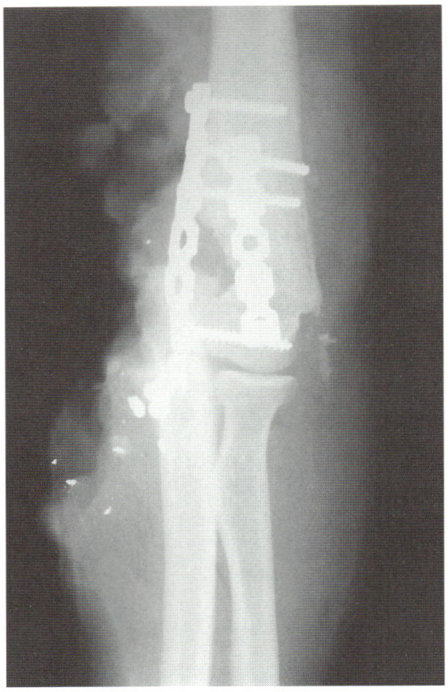

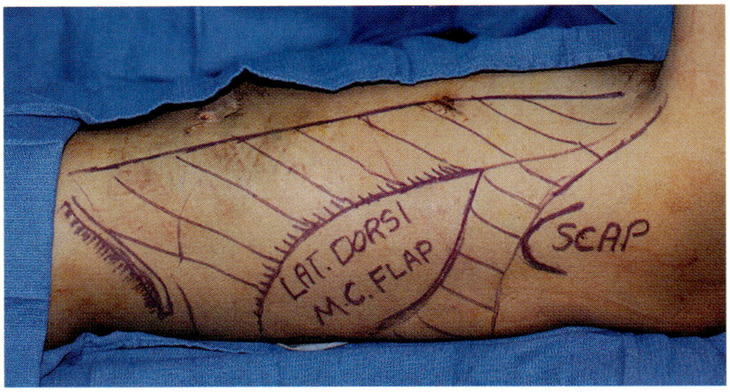

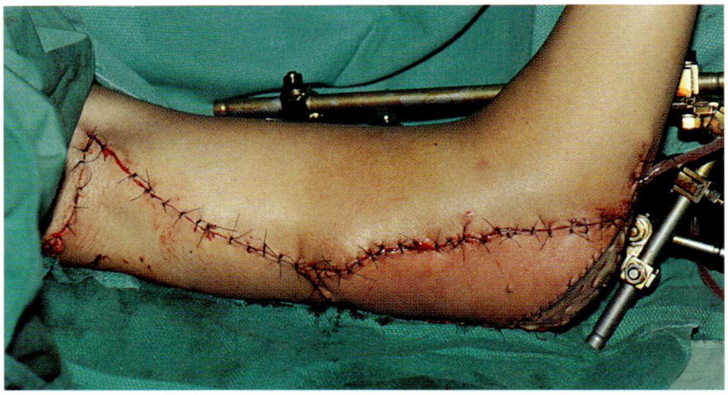

Fracture reduction was subsequently completed with conversion of the external fixation to a combination of posteriorly placed reconstruction plates on the humeral condyles. Simultaneously a pedicled latissimus dorsi musculocutaneous flap was transferred for coverage of the defect.

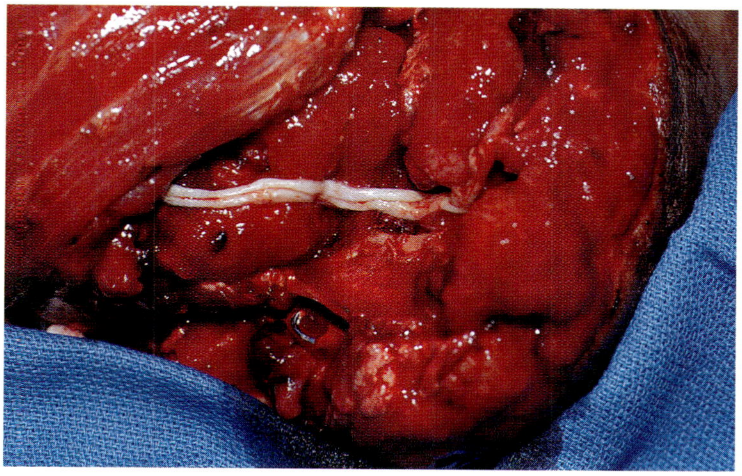

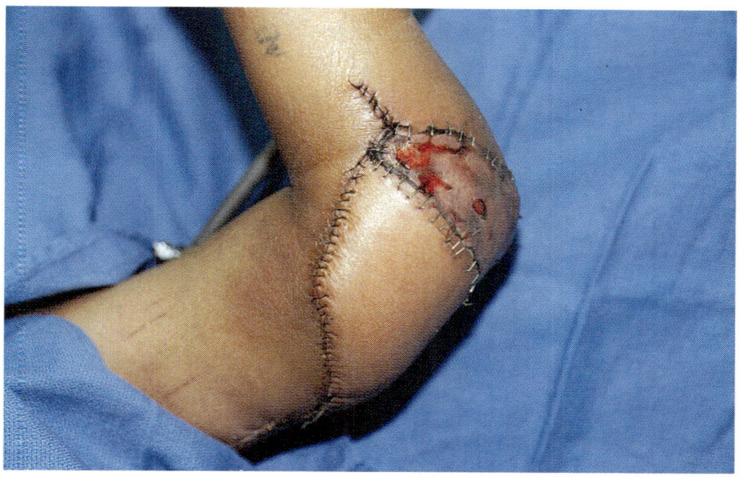

Shortly thereafter nerve reconstruction using multiple sural nerve grafts facilitated by limited flap elevation was performed. At the time of nerve grafting the soft tissues appeared clean and well vascularized.

Flap Elevation for Secondary Iliac Crest Bone Grafting

One of the most common secondary procedures after flap transfer in the extremities is limited but direct reexposure of a comminuted fracture site for subsequent iliac crest bone grafting.[12,13] The orthopedic literature has clearly documented the need for secondary, augmentational bone grafting for eventual union of type IIIB fractures in both the upper and lower extremities.[14] Although early coverage of these complex fractures with vascularized soft tissue has significantly decreased the untoward sequelae of infection,[15-17] there are no data to support the idea that soft tissue coverage alone imparts increased potential for decreased time to bony union. The restoration of a vascularized soft tissue envelope, however, has allowed the orthopedic traumatologist to bone graft directly at the fracture site in a timely fashion. Before the advent of flap coverage of these types of injuries, the standard practice was to indirectly bone graft through a separate posterior approach. Posterior lateral bone grafting for the treatment of type IIIB tibial fractures was hampered by the long delay in attempting to achieve closure of the primary wound by secondary intention and biomechanically by application of the bone graft in an area other than the direct diaphyseal shaft defect.

Although simultaneous iliac crest bone grafting and vascularized wound closure have been reported with favorable results, the accepted standard of treatment at this time is early secondary iliac crest bone grafting 4 to 6 weeks after successful wound closure. The procedure is performed with both the orthopedist and plastic surgeon's participation. With the extremity under tourniquet control, the previously transferred flap can be elevated with care taken to maintain the vascular pedicle. Any muscle component that is used for the obliteration of the osseous dead space can then be directly excised. The iliac crest bone graft is then packed into the osseous defect directly, obliterating the diaphyseal defect completely. Wound cultures are taken to determine if any persistent deep space infection is present; if so, this finding might then alter the postoperative antibiotic strategy. The flap is resutured under tourniquet control after the placement of drains. Tourniquet release before wound closure after iliac crest bone grafting is not recommended because the rapid onset of flap swelling would impair wound closure and compromise the primary objective. Appropriate bulb suction drainage allows for the evacuation of any residual bleeding under the flap.

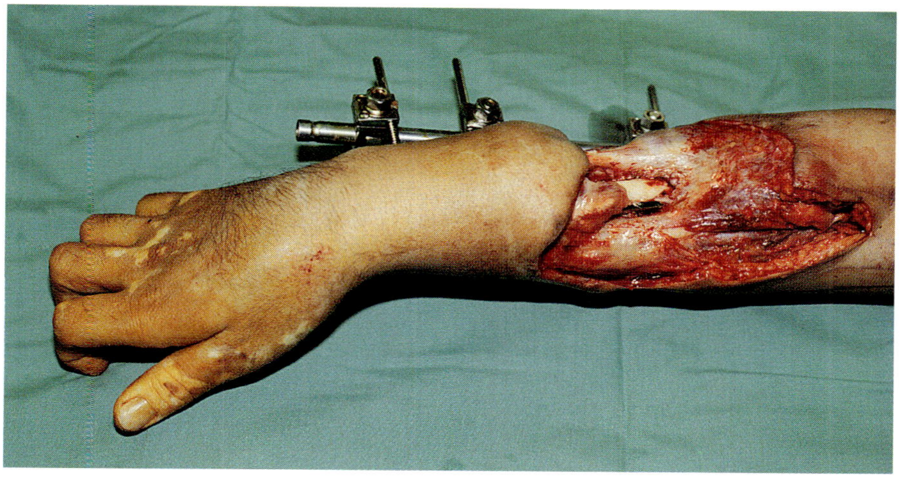

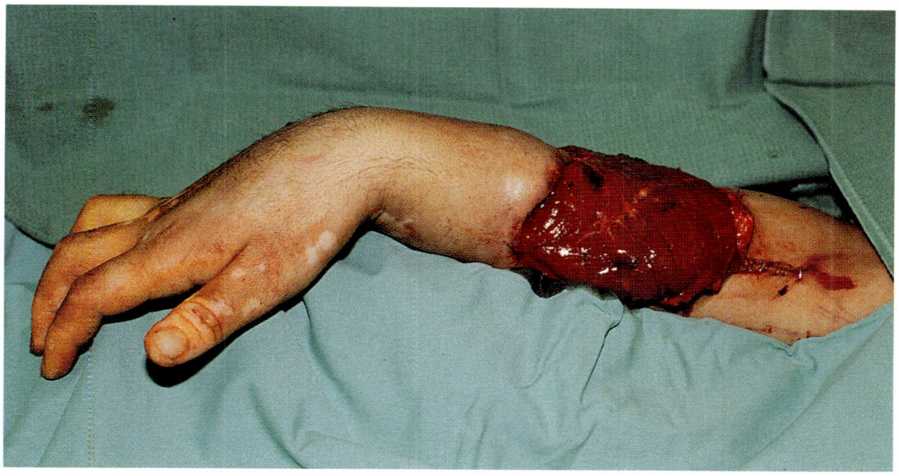

This 41-year-old right hand–dominant construction worker sustained a type IIIB fracture of the radius and ulna in the right upper extremity after a crane boom fell on his dominant arm. Injuries included a comminuted fracture of the mid-body of the ulna, a 6 cm loss of the mid and distal radius, and the loss of nearly the entire extrinsic extensor compartment and the majority of the overlying skin and subcutaneous tissue. Initial stabilization was accomplished using an AO external fixation device accompanied by radical debridement of all nonviable structures. Initial wound coverage was achieved 72 hours after injury using a rectus abdominis muscle flap covered with split-thickness skin grafts. A frame extension was applied to the distal pins for the application of an outrigger splinting device. This allowed therapists to begin the process of early joint mobilization and maintenance of flexor function.

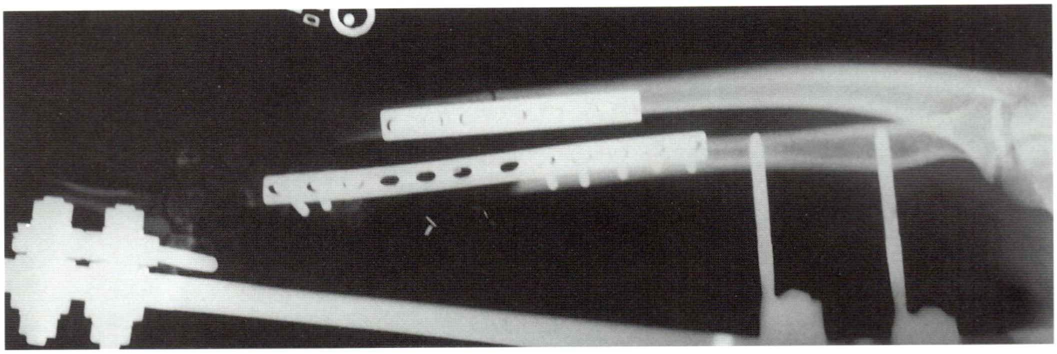

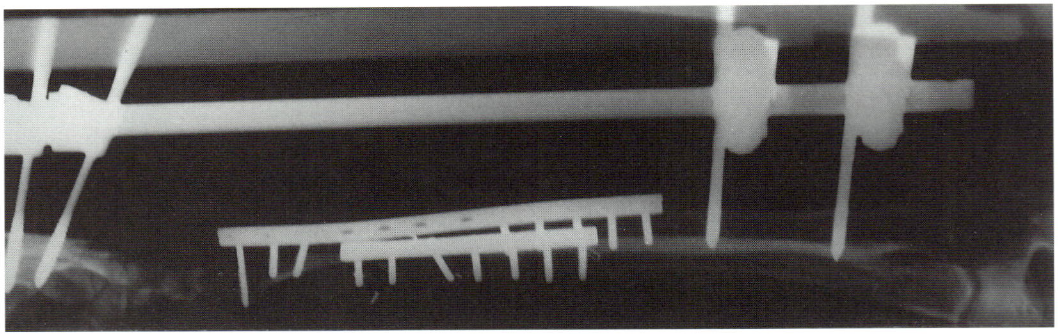

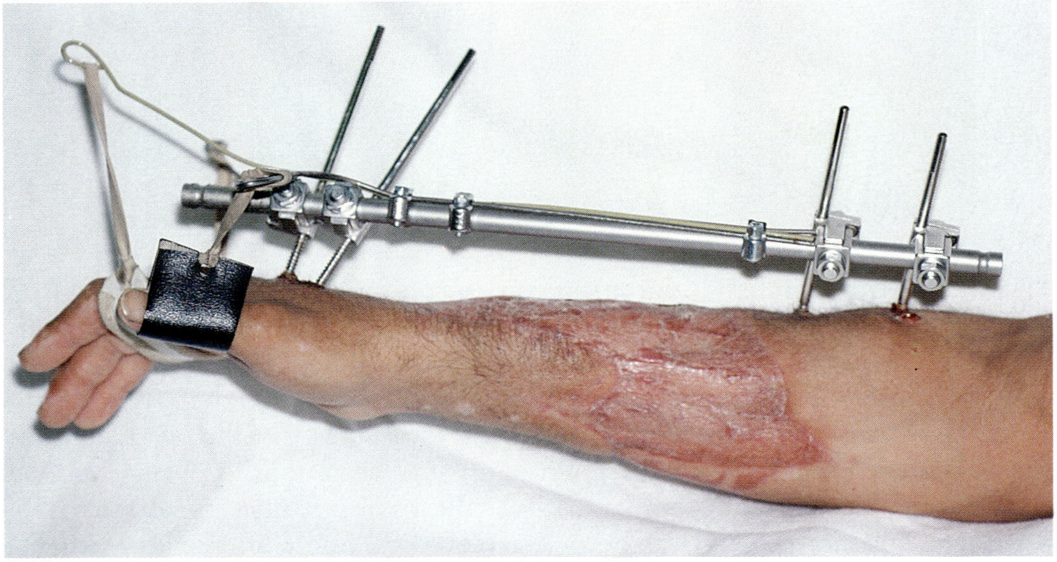

Eight weeks after injury the patient was returned to the operating room for massive iliac cancellous bone grafting and reconstruction plating of both the radius and ulna. Flap elevation was accomplished without incident. The external fixator was maintained for an additional 4 weeks to maximize the passive range of motion of the wrist and finger joints. The device was then removed in the office with the patient under local anesthesia.

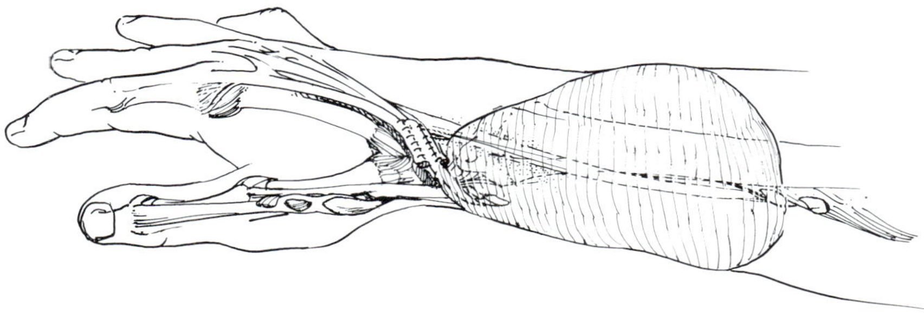

Six months following the bone grafting, the patient was returned to the operating room once again for a modified Brand, Starr, Tsuge tendon transfer for the restoration of wrist, finger, and thumb extension.

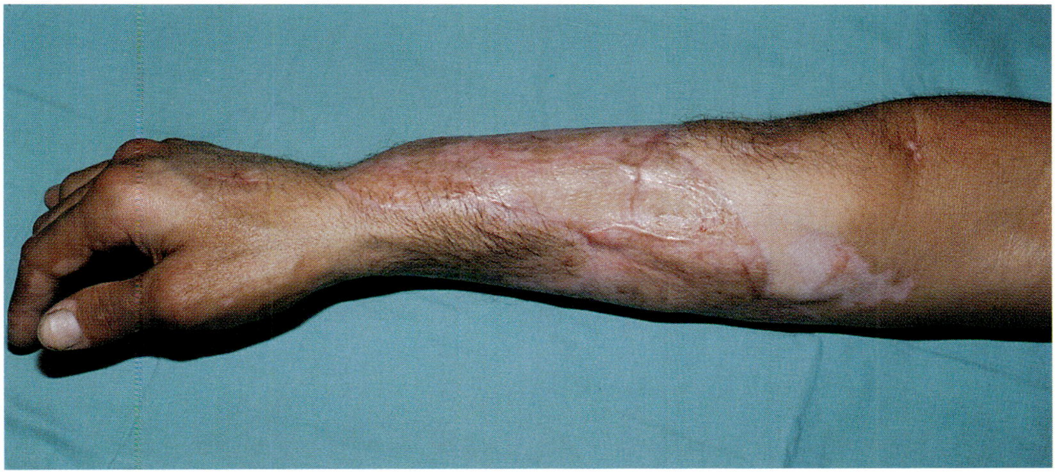

Therapy continued for several months with resultant fracture healing, wound closure, and good restoration of wrist and finger extension using the pronator teres and flexor carpi radialis muscles, respectively. The patient returned to light modified work 16 months after initial injury.

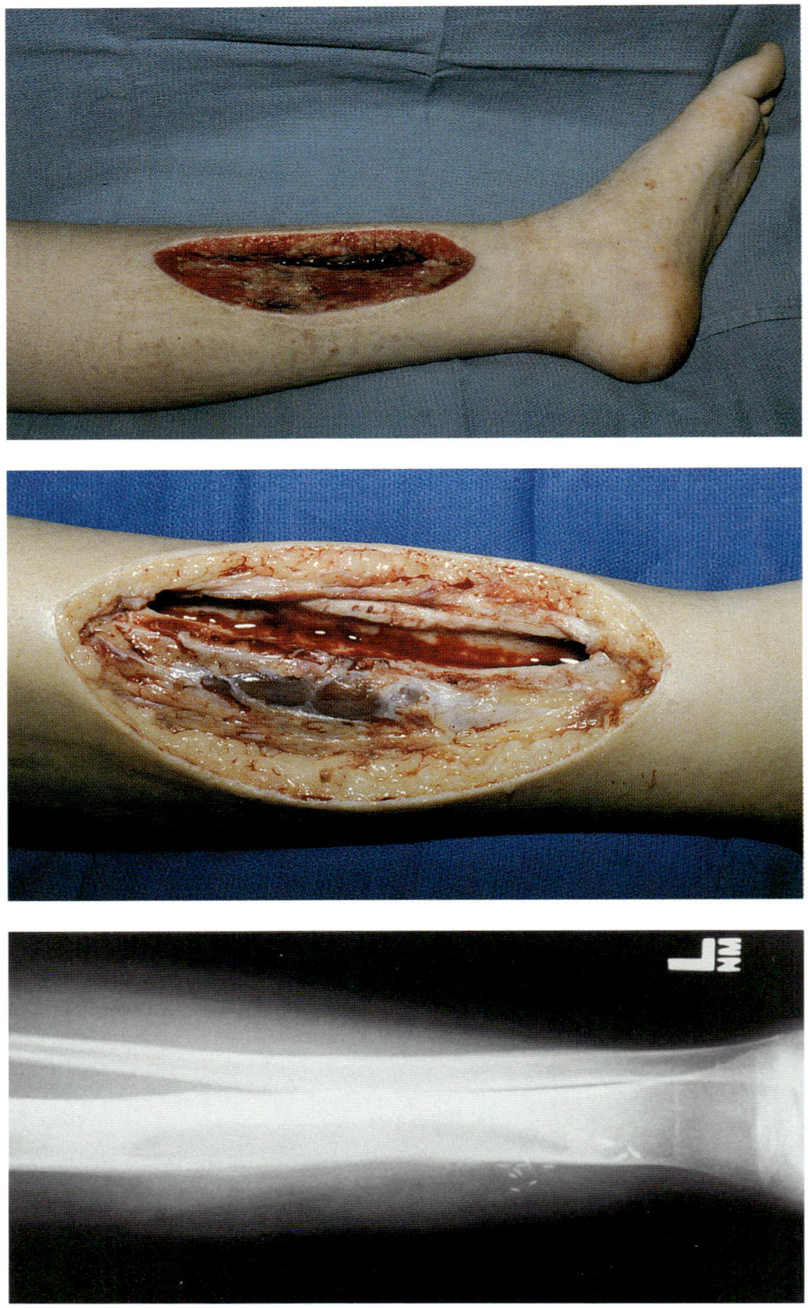

This 31-year-old woman was treated for a type IIIA tibial fracture with primary plating and wound closure. Several weeks after the initial surgery, the wound broke down, with drainage of purulent material. Debridement with removal of the internal fixation device resulted in an open wound with bony nonunion.

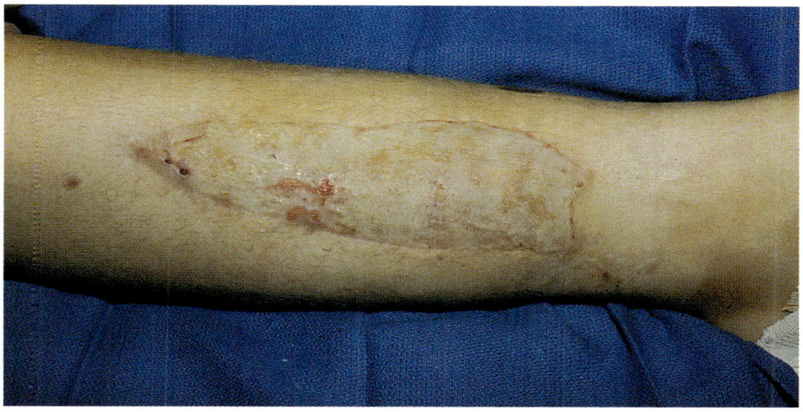

After transfer to our facility several months later, a radical en bloc excisional debridement was undertaken followed by free flap transfer using the rectus abdominis muscle and split-thickness skin graft.

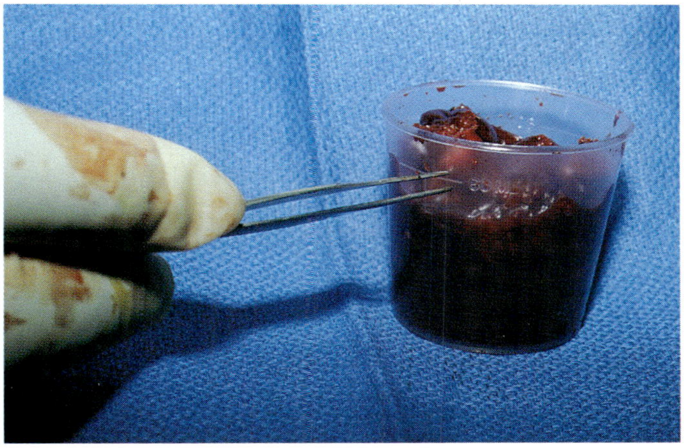

Harvested iliac crest cancellous bone graft

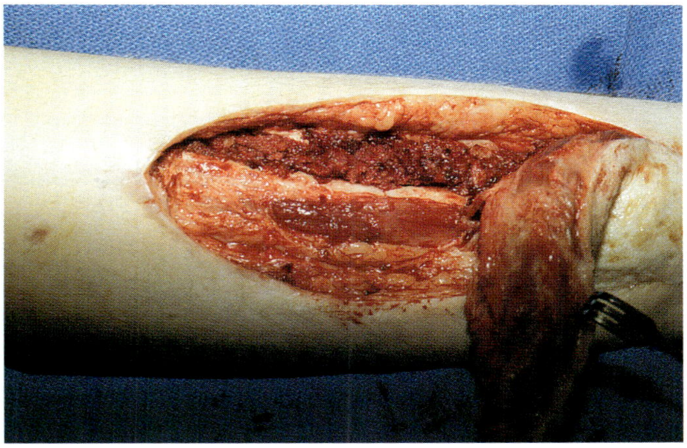

Flap elevation on vascular pedicle with placement of bone graft in osseous defect

Six weeks after wound closure the patient was returned to the operating room where the rectus abdominis flap was raised under tourniquet control to allow for the placement of simultaneously harvested bone graft. Close attention was paid to the maintenance of the vascular anastomoses. That component of the flap that had been used to obliterate the diaphyseal dead space was excised in order to accommodate the cancellous bone graft. Drains were placed and the flap resutured before the release of the tourniquet. The overlying skin graft on the rectus abdominis muscle remained undisturbed throughout the reelevation procedure.

Bony union was achieved with complete wound closure and no subsequent evidence of drainage. She is now fully ambulatory without bracing or assistive devices.

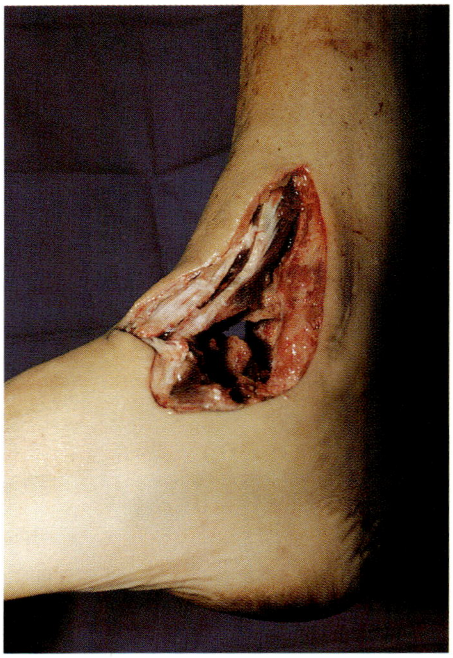

This 53-year-old psychotherapist sustained a devastating type IIIB plafond fracture to the ankle. Initial attempts at internal fixation and wound closure resulted in infection and further soft tissue loss. Because of the complex nature of the fracture with an extensive intra-articular component, internal fixation was left in place despite continued drainage. The patient underwent a prolonged course of antibiotic therapy, which resulted in a superinfection with *Aspergillus* organisms.

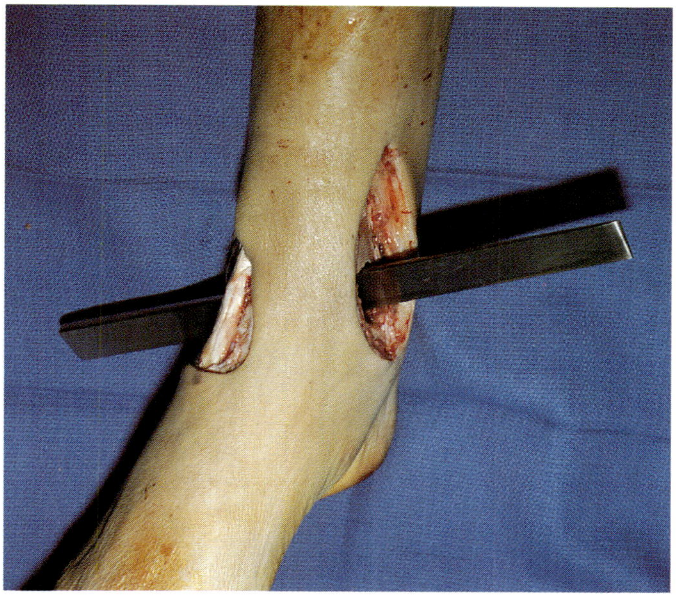

On transfer to our facility the patient was switched to antifungal medications and taken to surgery for a wide en bloc radical debridement of all involved structures. Two subsequent debridements were required to arrest the continued, ongoing necrotizing process.

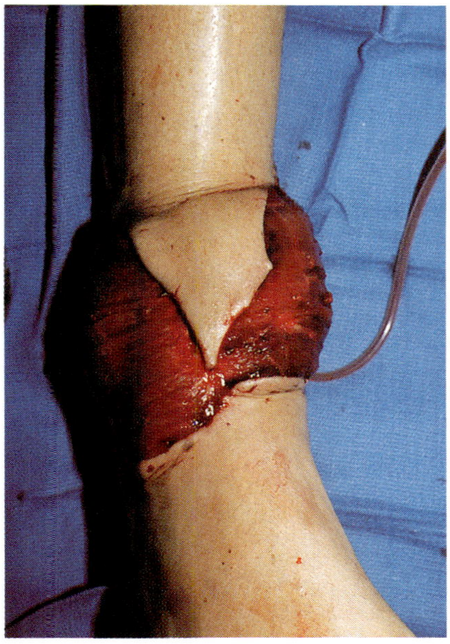

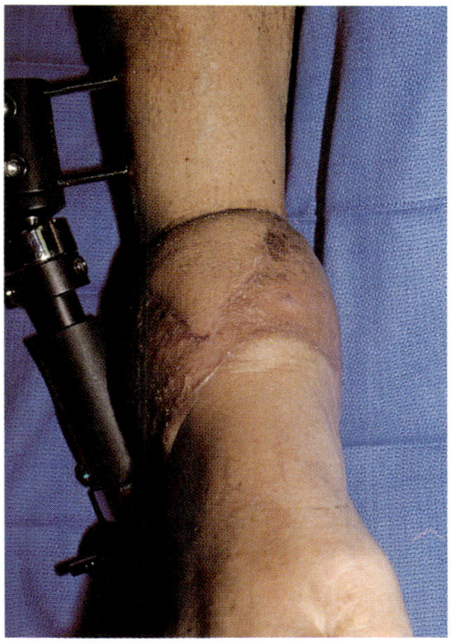

Once the wound was stabilized, a rectus abdominis flap was transferred for wound coverage and complete obliteration of dead space. The wound was simultaneously split-thickness skin grafted. Antifungal agent therapy was continued for an additional 6 weeks.

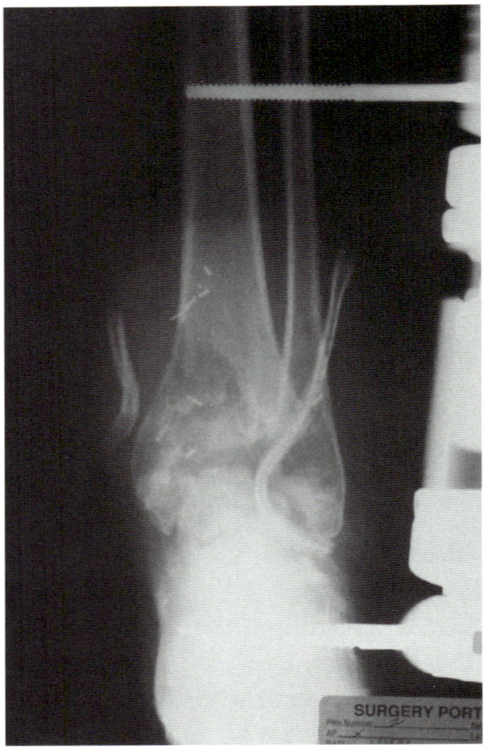

Residual osseous defect

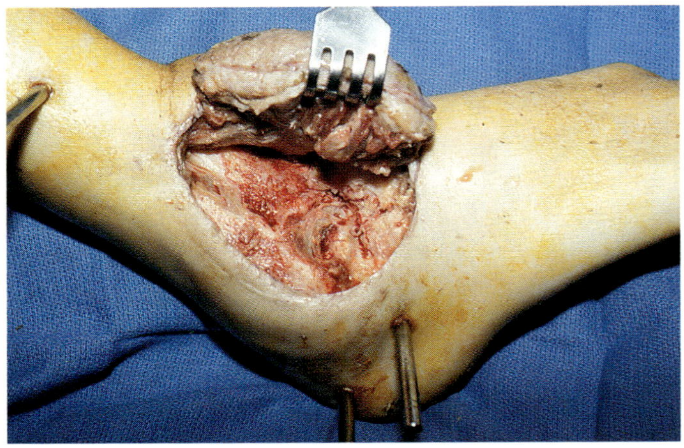

Reelevation of flap for bone grafting and ankle fusion

Three months postoperatively the patient was returned to the operating room for extensive cancellous bone grafting and ankle fusion. The flap was elevated away from the site of the anastomoses and a deep portion of the flap was removed to accommodate the bone graft. Drains were placed and the flap was resutured before tourniquet release. Marked shrinkage of the flap had occurred in the 3 months between initial transfer and reelevation.

The patient has achieved solid ankle fusion with no recurrence of drainage or other signs of infection. Continued atrophy of the flap has occurred, and the patient is now able to wear a tennis shoe.

Vascularized Bone Transfer After Soft Tissue Coverage

Occasionally a type IIIB fracture of the upper or lower extremity results in not only massive skin and soft tissue loss but also long segmental cortical defects in the diaphysis that are not amenable to repair by iliac crest bone grafting alone. According to classic reconstructive principles, 6 cm is the limit for bone grafting; beyond this point cancellous bone grafting alone is considered insufficient for successful bony union and preservation of extremity length. Although isolated reports have documented successful fracture healing under free tissue transfers of defects up to 12 cm with nonvascularized cancellous bone graft, most surgeons favor either vascularized long bone transfer using the fibula or more recently use of the Ilizarov device for compression osteosynthesis with subsequent, or in some cases simultaneous, distraction via distant corticotomy. Vascularized fibula transfer has been popularized by Weiland and Daniel[18] and has since been reported by multiple centers for numerous applications.[19] Modification of the fibula transfer has allowed the addition of soleus muscle and/or overlying skin panels for soft tissue augmentation. In our hands wound closure with muscle or musculocutaneous flap transfer provides the most favorable environment for the subsequent microvascular transfer of the fibula. Before osteosynthesis using the interpositional fibula, it is important to ascertain the correct length of the defect, with the injured extremity being held out to its normal length using external fixation devices.

In the upper extremity the latissimus dorsi flap has served nicely to quickly and completely cover complex humeral defects without requiring microvascular anastomoses. Injuries to the forearm that require significant soft tissue coverage with the expectation of future long bone interpositional fibula transfer usually require early free muscle or fasciocutaneous flap transfer for wound coverage. Similarly in the lower extremity those diaphyseal defects that are more proximally located can be initially covered with rotational flaps of either gastrocnemius or soleus muscles. Those injuries of the distal third of the tibia first require wound coverage using muscle or musculocutaneous flaps as free tissue transfers. Muscle or fasciocutaneous flap elevation must be extensive to allow for complete visualization of the osseous defect with adequate distal and proximal exposure to allow for various combinations of plate and screw fixation across each fracture site. An additional sleeve of fibular periosteum is harvested from the distal and proximal ends at the transection site to allow for wrapping of the osteosynthetic site at the recipient defect.

Various options for osteosynthesis include long reconstruction plating incorporating both the proximal and distal native humerus as well as the fibula, dual short reconstructive plating of each osteosynthetic site separately, and screw fixation with augmented external fixation performed with either a tongue and groove technique or a step-cut technique. Finally cross Kirschner wire fixation along with supplemented external fixation can be used but is discouraged because it does not provide enough strength and stability.

Problems with fibular fracture have been late refracture at one of the two osteosynthetic sites or osteoplastic deformation, both requiring an additional revisional surgery for bone graft augmentation and plating at the failed osteosynthetic site. Despite these occasional late complications, all fibular transfers we have performed later achieve complete healing.

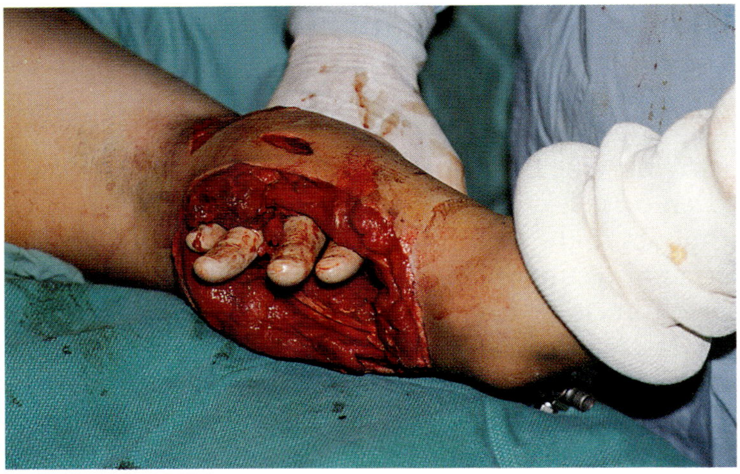

This 17-year-old Hispanic man sustained a gunshot wound to the left mid and proximal humerus. Through-and-through soft tissue loss and segmental loss of the mid and proximal humerus occurred. Overlying skin was destroyed as well as significant distances of the radial and median nerves.

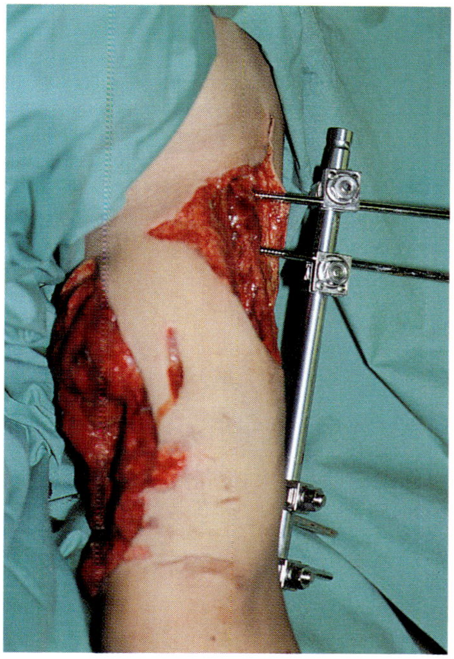

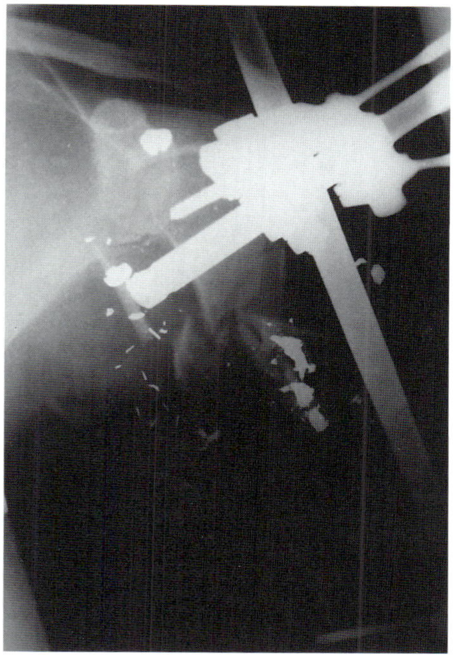

The distal upper extremity remained vascularized. Initial stabilization was achieved by AO external fixation with debridement of nearly 11 cm of diaphyseal humerus. The x-ray film demonstrates the extensive osseous loss of the humerus.

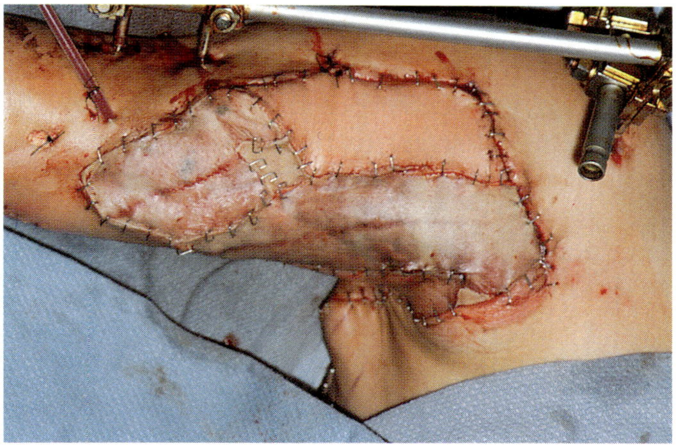

The ipsilateral latissimus dorsi muscle was transferred as a pedicled musculocutaneous flap, allowing early wound closure.

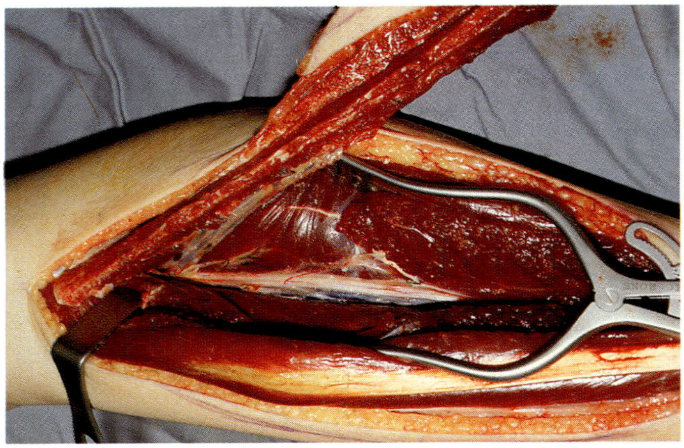

Harvest of fibular osteocutaneous flap

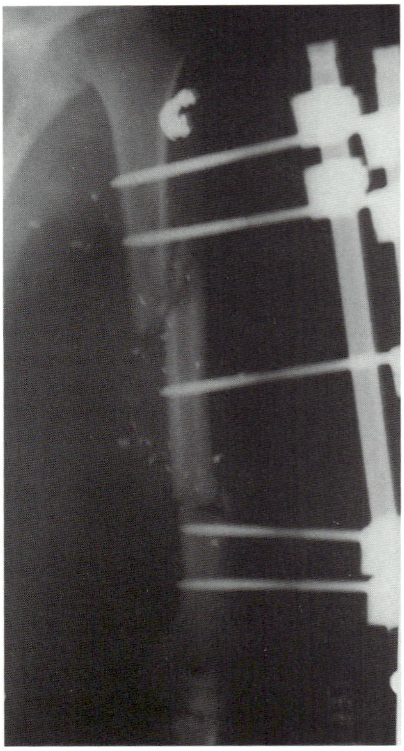

Fibular osteocutaneous flap interposed for humeral reconstruction

The patient was returned to surgery 2 months postoperatively for the transfer of an interpositional fibular osteocutaneous flap. This flap was fixed with both external fixation and internal screw fixation. Fracture healing occurred at the proximal and distal osteosynthetic sites.

After increased use, however, a refracture occurred at the proximal site, requiring subsequent reelevation of the latissimus dorsi musculocutaneous flap, plate fixation, and augmentation with an iliac crest bone graft. With healing complete bony union of the humerus was achieved. Continued occupational therapy revealed a persistent radial nerve deficit for which he received radial nerve transfers.

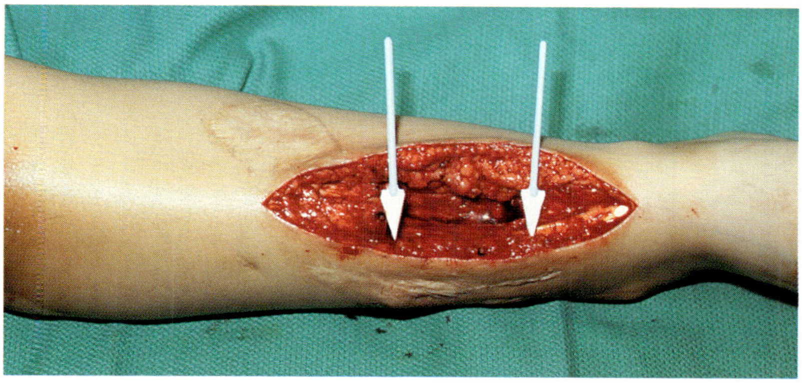

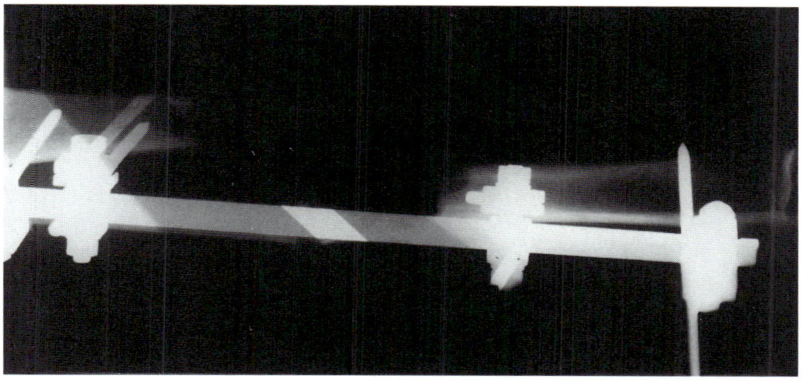

This patient, a 27-year-old man, sustained a type IIIB midthird tibial fracture of the right lower extremity with loss of 10 cm of the tibial shaft.

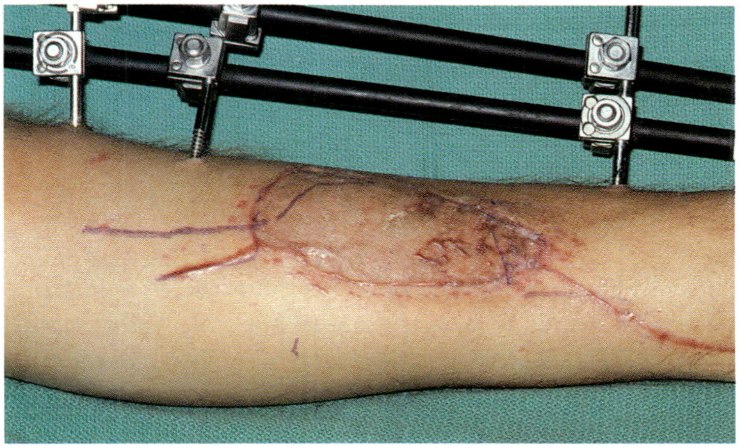

Initial wound closure was achieved with a soleus muscle transposition flap (because surprisingly the soft tissue defect was much smaller than the osseous one) and a split-thickness skin graft. Length and alignment were obtained with an AO half-frame external fixator.

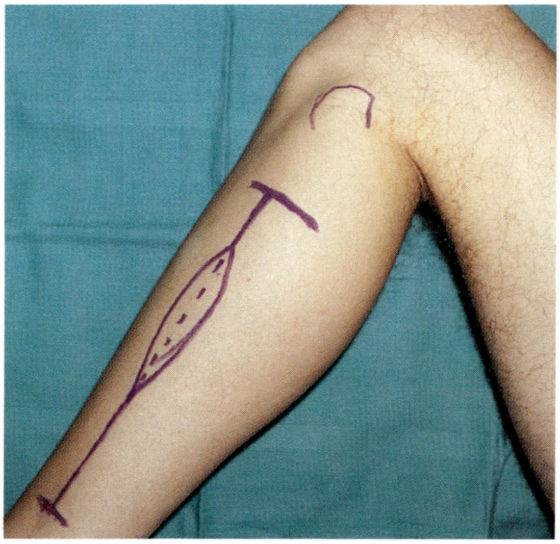

Outline of fibular osteocutaneous flap

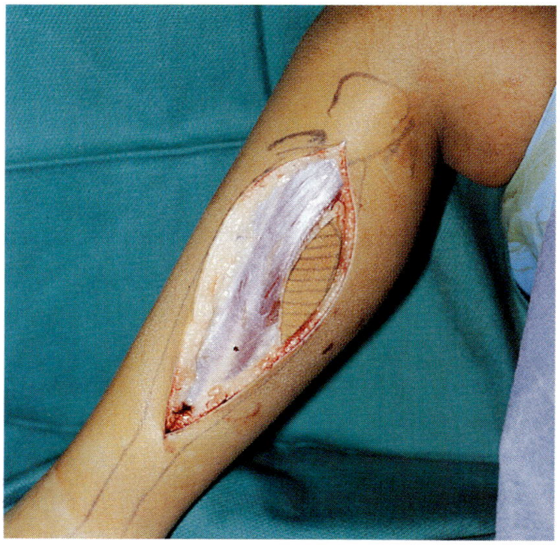

Initial incision revealing posterior intercrural septum

Eight weeks after wound coverage, with no evidence of infection, the contralateral fibula was transferred as a vascularized flap. Note the septal vessels supplying the skin paddle. A combination of maintained external fixation and internal screw fixation was used to stabilize the transfer. Successful union occurred at both osteosynthetic sites, with progressive ambulation being undertaken.

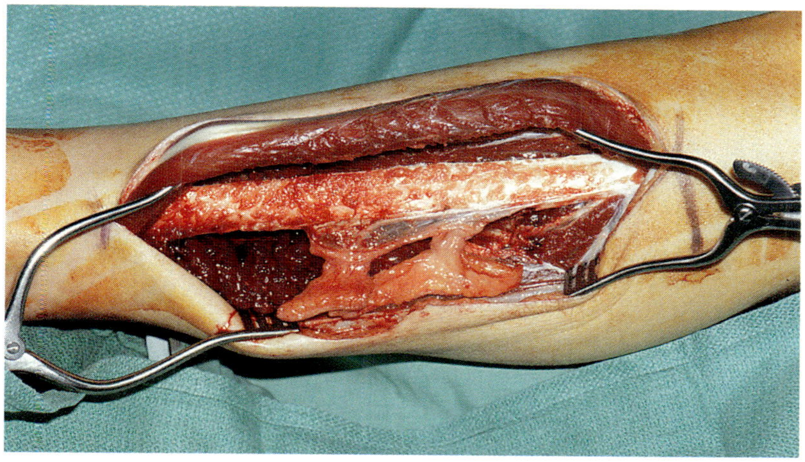

Fibular osteocutaneous flap isolated in situ

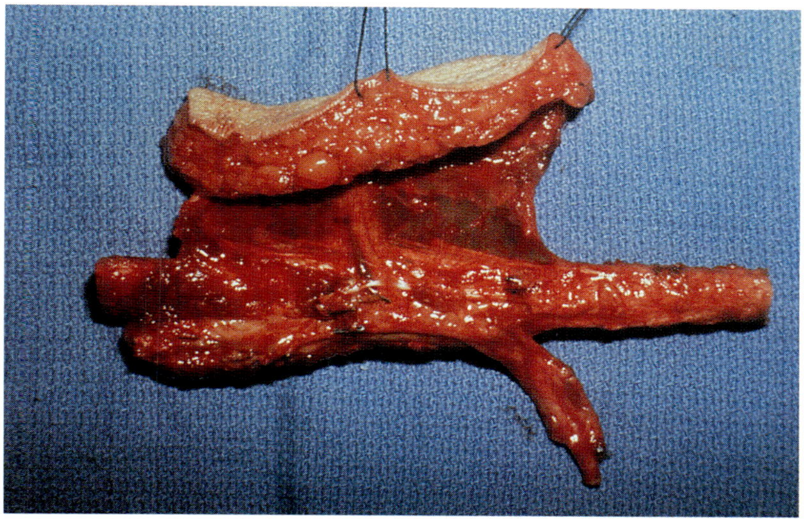

Flap ready for transfer

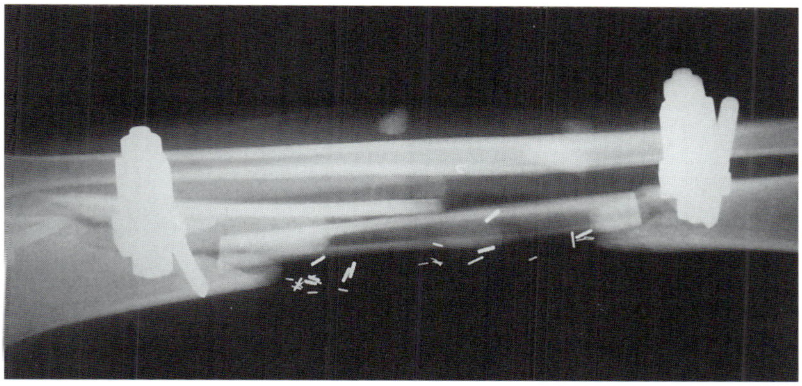

Fibular osteocutaneous flap interposed for tibial reconstruction

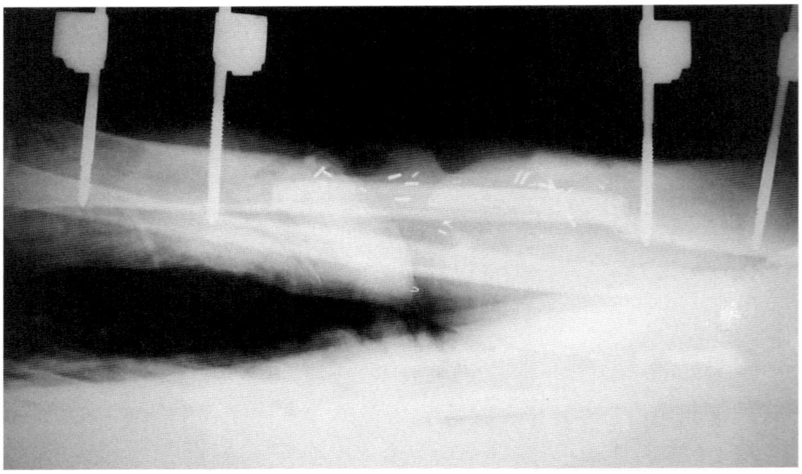

Three months after the flap transfer before the external fixation was removed, some fibular hypertrophy was noted.

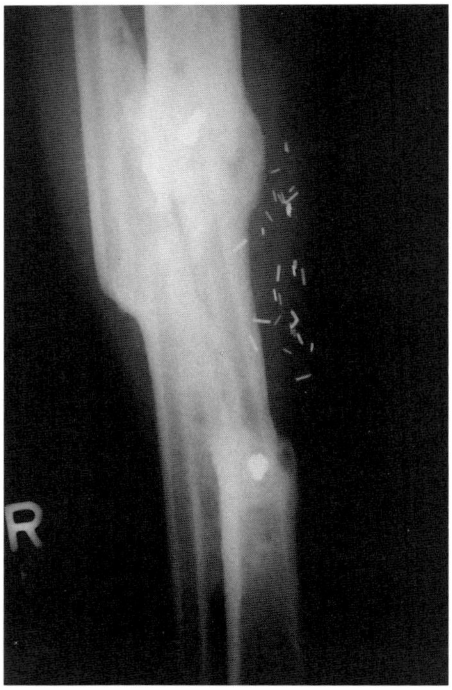

Six months following the fibular transfer, the proximal osteosynthetic site was noted to have undergone osteoplastic deformation with valgus angulation.

This defect was corrected by a second reelevation of the soleus muscle and osteotomy with plating of the proximal healed osteosynthetic site. The patient eventually achieved full weight-bearing, nonassisted ambulation with complete bony union.

Ilizarov Application After Free Tissue Transfer

As orthopedists have gained experience with the Ilizarov device, distraction and compression osteosynthesis using bony transport has allowed the correction of large segmental diaphyseal long bone defects without the need for distantly harvested bone graft. Osseous defects of considerable length can be obliterated by slow but steady bone transport using a series of ring guides and fine-wire fixators. A distant corticotomy is performed in the proximal uninjured tibia or humerus, allowing distraction of the cortex toward the bony portion of the deficit. Once the defect is obliterated, compression osteosynthesis can be performed. Most complex open fractures that result in segmental bone defects are accompanied by significant overlying skin and subcutaneous tissue loss. Early wound closure allows more rapid undertaking of Ilizarov distraction, culminating in a shorter time to bony union. Both pedicled and free tissue transfers have been liberally used in association with the Ilizarov frame.[9] Fine-wire fixation devices can be placed directly into the flap substance without fear of flap compromise. Problems with the progressive transport of the device through the flap have not been reported. If muscle flaps are used initially to obliterate deep osseous dead space, that part of the flap might interfere with the ultimate docking of the two bone ends. A small revision requiring elevation of that section of the flap might be required and should be performed as close to final bony contact as can be afforded. If the Ilizarov device is to be used before or simultaneous with the placement of a muscle flap, consideration should be given to the location of the vascular pedicle for access for the initial anastomoses and in the case of potential revision.

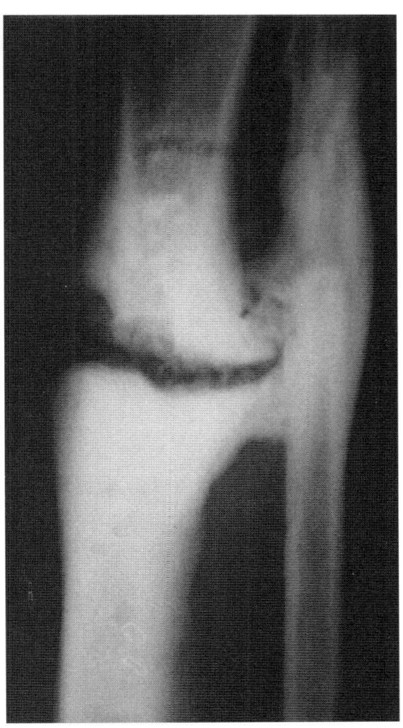

This 32-year-old Hispanic man sustained a type IIIB midthird tibial fibular fracture and was initially treated with internal fixation using plates and screws. This site became infected, so the internal hardware was removed and an external fixation device was placed. A series of incisions and debridements led to the eventual formation of a sinus tract and hypertrophic nonunion at 2½ years following injury.

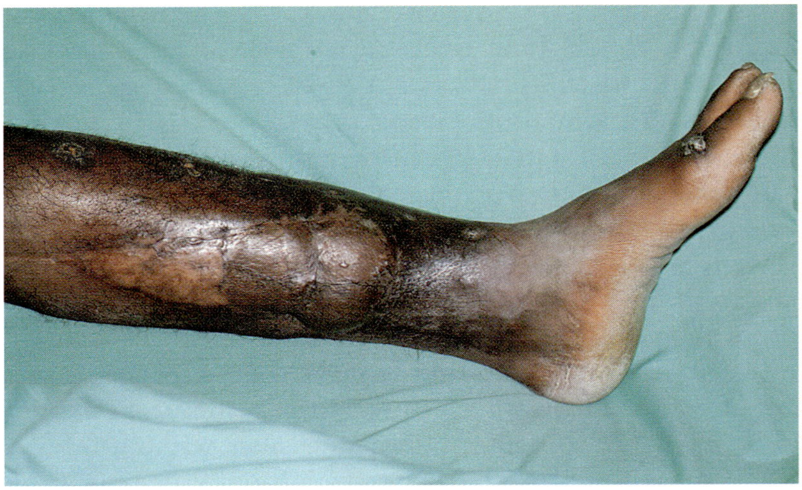

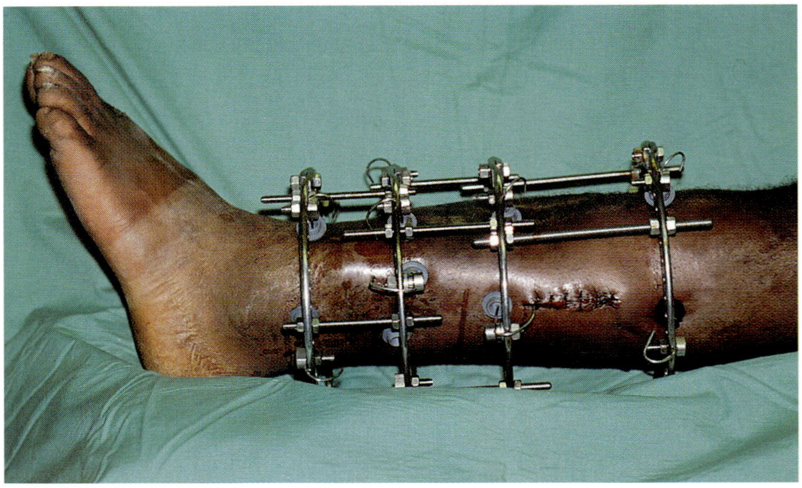

At this point the patient underwent radical debridement with subsequent transfer of the rectus abdominis muscle with overlying split-thickness skin graft for obliteration of dead space. The external fixator was converted to an Ilizarov device, and the resected hypertrophic nonunion was then obliterated and compressed to gain bony union. Fine-wire fixation pins were placed through the substance of the flap and transport occurred without any deleterious effect to the soft tissues.

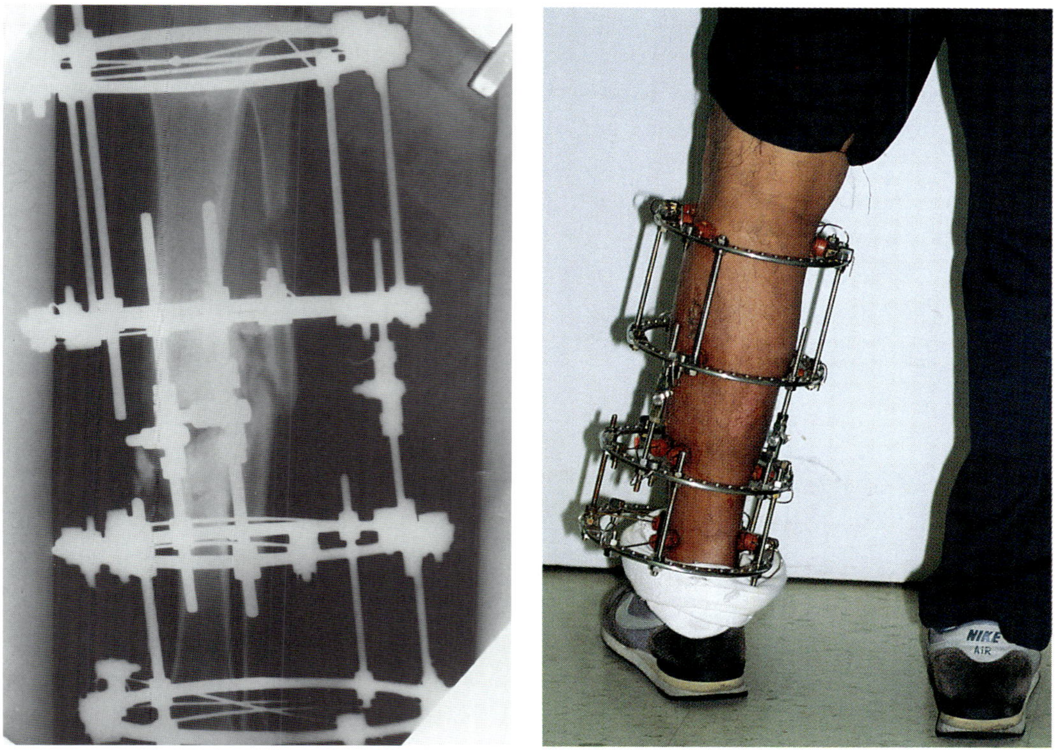

Union was achieved both clinically and radiologically 3 months after application of the device. The x-ray film demonstrates the successful docking of the tibial fragments.

Flap Debulking, Reorientation, and Recontouring

Both fasciocutaneous and muscle flaps are now commonly used in lower extremity reconstruction with great success.[19] Of the two, fasciocutaneous flaps tend to give an initial superior cosmetic result. With time, however, dependency, edema, and lack of anchoring to the normal underlying structures may result in bulky, redundant skin paddles. Residual contour deformities become more pronounced and focused on by the patient as the other, more serious problems are resolved. These deformities can be minimized somewhat by the application of compression devices such as Jobe stockings or elastic wrap bandages. Despite these adjunctive measures, however, most contour deformities of the lower leg do not improve and tend to worsen. Functional problems about the ankle or foot can occur because of difficulty with ambulation and shoe fit. Fortunately skin paddle elevation for debulking, recontouring, or flap reorientation is quite safe. If skin excess is not a problem, liposuction can be used to remove unwanted fatty tissue. Few extra precautions are necessary when performing this procedure. Cannulation in and around the pedicle should be avoided if possible.

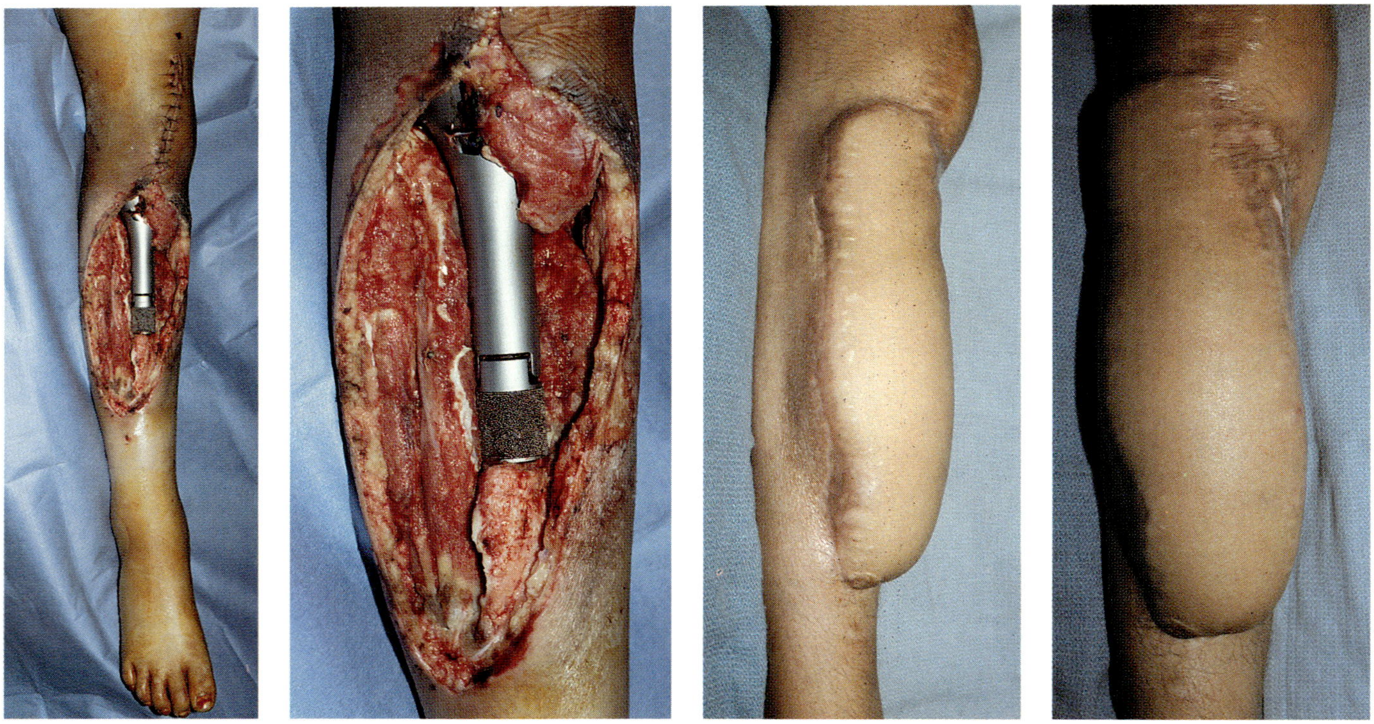

This 10-year-old girl required en bloc excision of the proximal tibia and all overlying skin and soft tissues secondary to a high-grade sarcoma. A custom endoprosthesis was implanted to replace the tibia and knee joint. Wound closure was achieved with a rectus abdominis musculocutaneous flap. Due to some truncal obesity, the musculocutaneous transfer brought with it unwanted subcutaneous tissue.

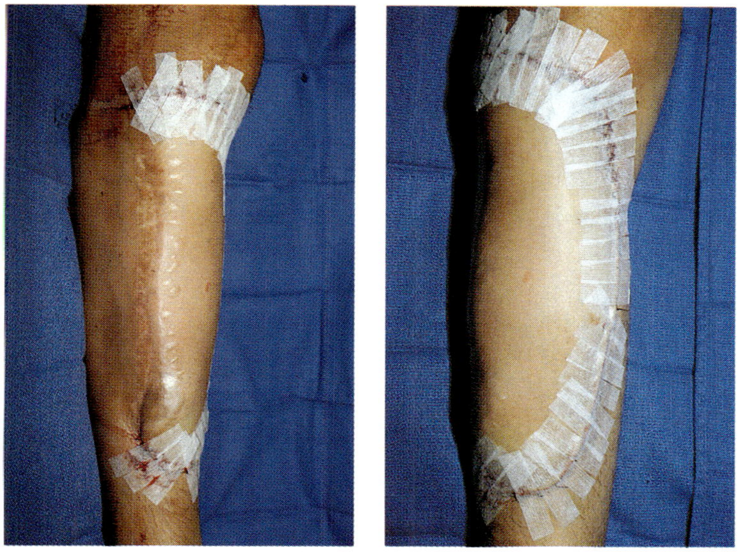

Once the patient was well past the 6-month course of chemotherapy with no evidence of local or systemic recurrence, she underwent two successive debulking procedures of the previously placed transfer. The second debulking was performed 6 months after the first. Each procedure was confined to the skin and subcutaneous tissue without any reexploration of the vascular pedicle region. Elevation was confined to no more than half of the circumference of the marginal wound, and wedge excision of the underlying fat was performed. The second elevation was oriented toward the opposite side, thus completing the defatting circumferentially.

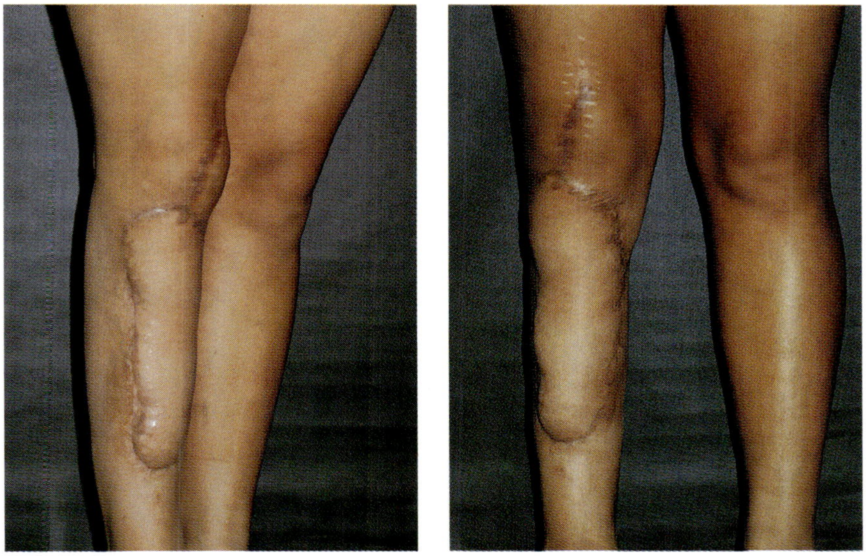

A significant improvement of the aesthetic and contour deformities resulted as shown 2 years following flap transfer.

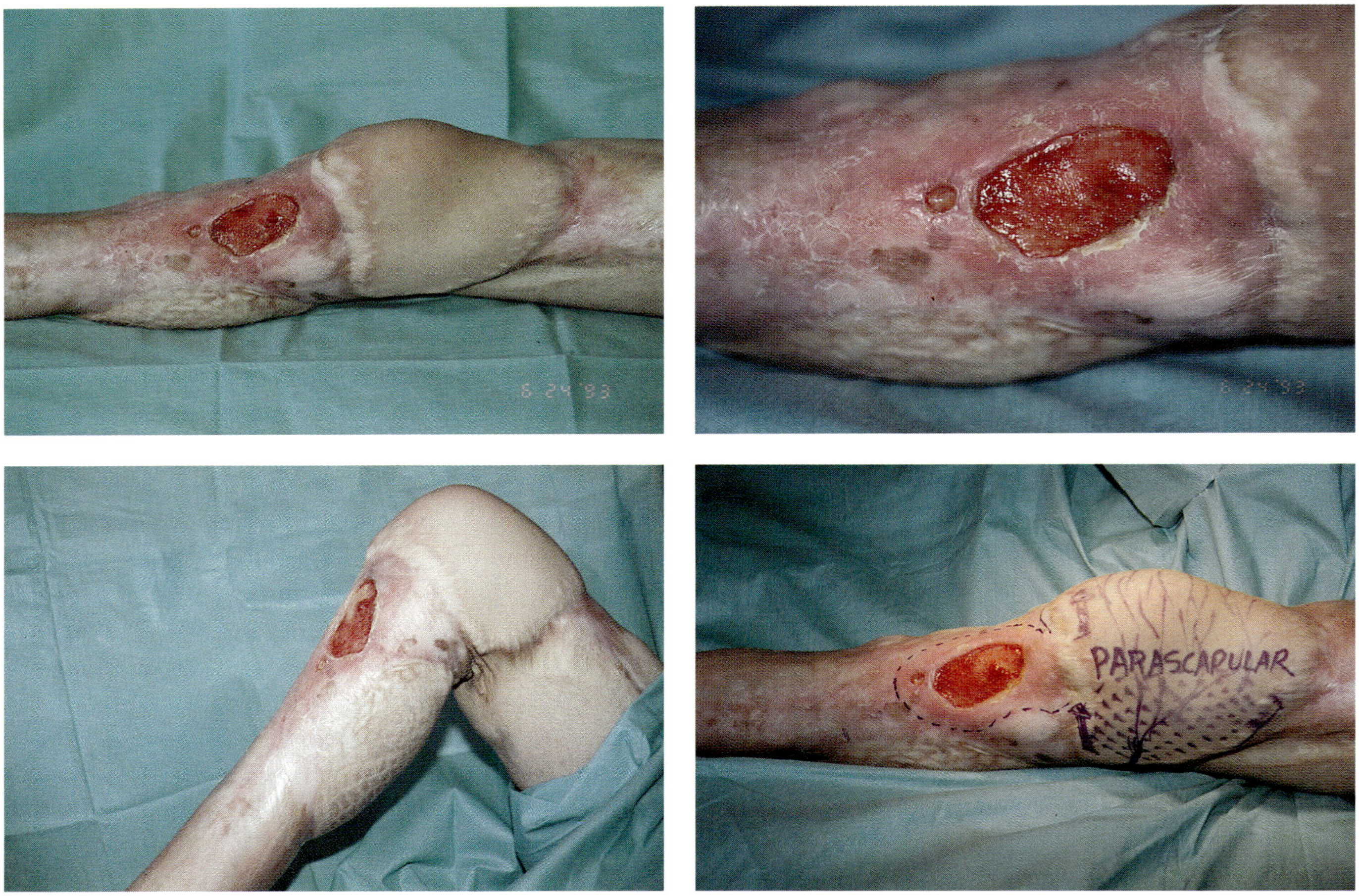

Courtesy Vysevelod Rybchonok, M.D.

This 11-year-old girl sustained a third-degree burn injury of the left distal thigh, knee, and proximal tibia anteriorly. These wounds were treated by serial debridements and secondary wound contracture and closure. Unstable scars throughout the burn injury led to secondary breakdown with reinfection along the distal thigh and knee. Composite excision of the burn wound superiorly was then followed by transfer of the parascapular fasciocutaneous flap with anastomoses to the lateral superior genicular artery and vein. One year after transfer although the flap remained in place, there was subsequent breakdown of the inferior wounds over the proximal tibia (top). Full range of motion was retained (bottom left). Doppler examination verified the patency of the lateral anastomosis of the subscapular vessels (bottom right).

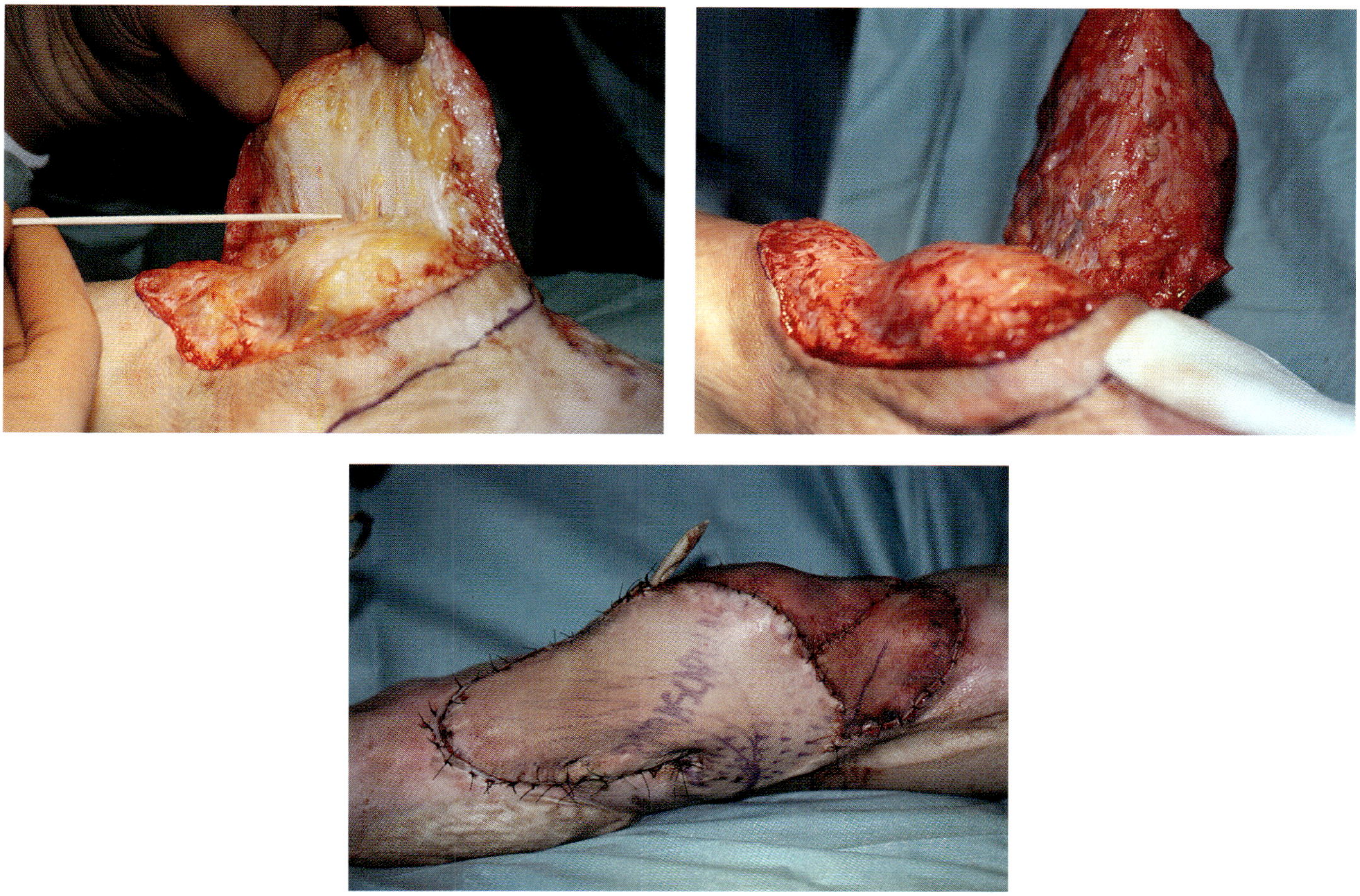

This problem was addressed by inferior wound excision and re-elevation of the parascapular flap, with close attention paid to its subtending vascular pedicle. The pointer indicates the patent vascular pedicle (top left). A layer of well-vascularized subcutaneous tissue was left superiorly as the flap was transposed to cover the inferior wound. Based on the Crane principle, an excellent bed remained superiorly for the placement of a split-thickness skin graft while the flap was used to close the recalcitrant inferior wound without problem. The patient healed without incident. The wound has remained closed and a full range of knee motion has been retained.

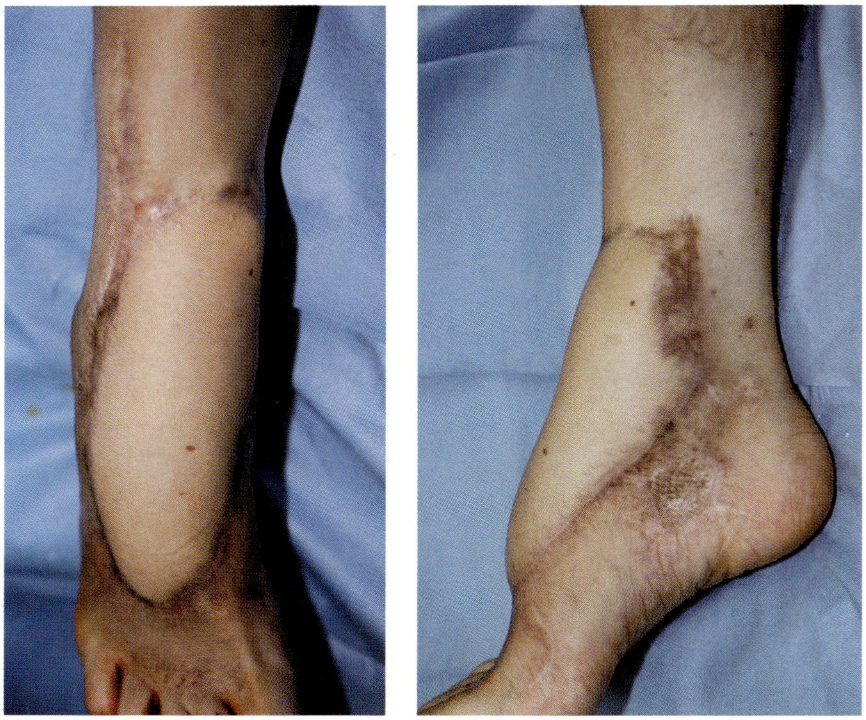

This 27-year-old warehouse worker sustained an avulsion injury of the dorsum of the foot, losing skin, subcutaneous tissue, and some toe extensors. The dorsal metatarsal joints were exposed and initially treated with debridement and temporoparietal fascia flap with overlying skin graft. Unfortunately, the flap failed to survive, leaving a chronic open wound. This wound was repeatedly skin grafted without success. Six months after the initial injury we addressed the problem with aggressive debridement of the entire wound and transfer of the parascapular fasciocutaneous flap vascularized by the anterior tibial artery and vein. Wound closure was achieved with excellent initial inset and contour. However, over the course of the next 4 months, progressive swelling and fullness of the fasciocutaneous flap were noted. This swollen state was made worse with progressive ambulation despite the consistent use of compressive wraps.

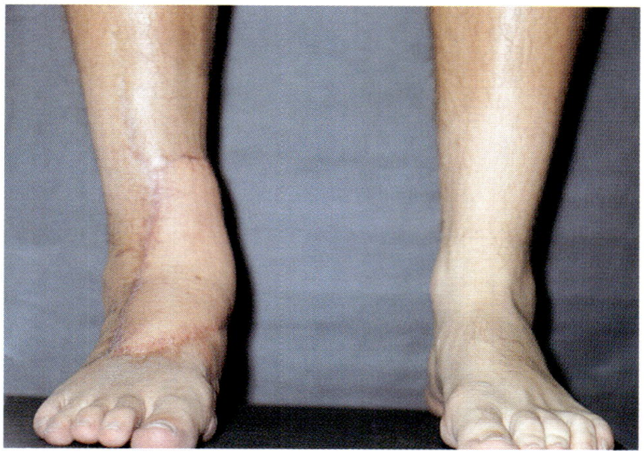

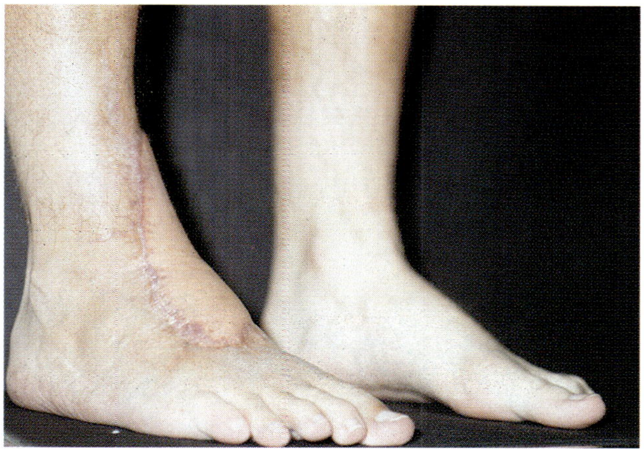

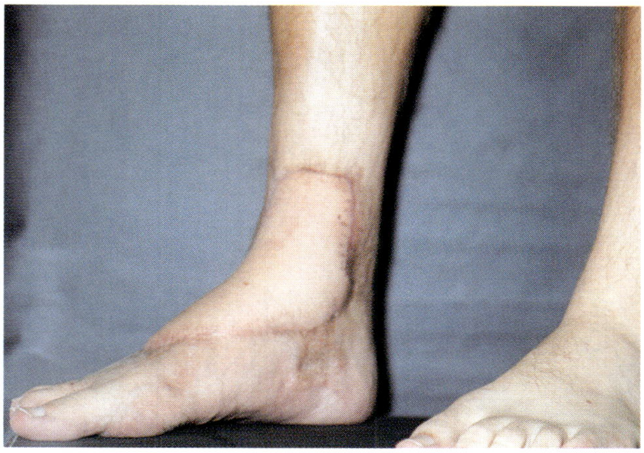

At the patient's request 6 months following flap transfer he underwent elevation and excision of the redundant skin and subcutaneous tissue. The vascular pedicle was maintained as was the 50% of the marginal incision between the flap and native tissues. The flap was reclosed under a moderate degree of tension and compressive hose was applied at the time of surgery. This support was worn for 6 weeks postoperatively and then changed to a light support hose, which was worn for the ensuing 6 months. The patient is now able to wear his preinjury shoes and stockings.

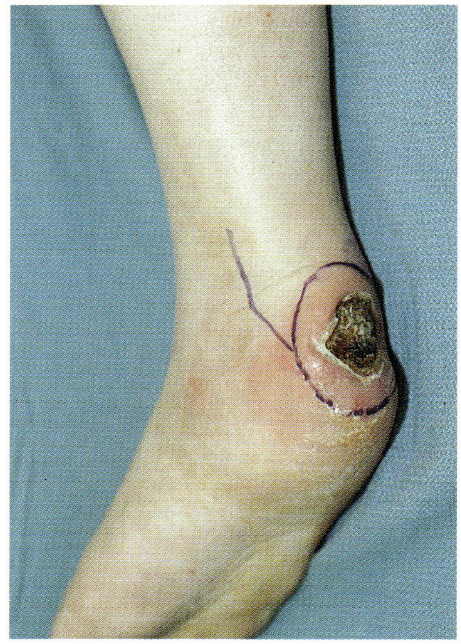

This 33-year-old woman sustained a type IIIB calcaneal fracture with necrosis of overlying posterior skin. This injury was initially casted for 3 weeks. At the time of the second cast change, an eschar over the posterior calcaneus was noted. X-ray films demonstrated persistent malalignment at the fracture site.

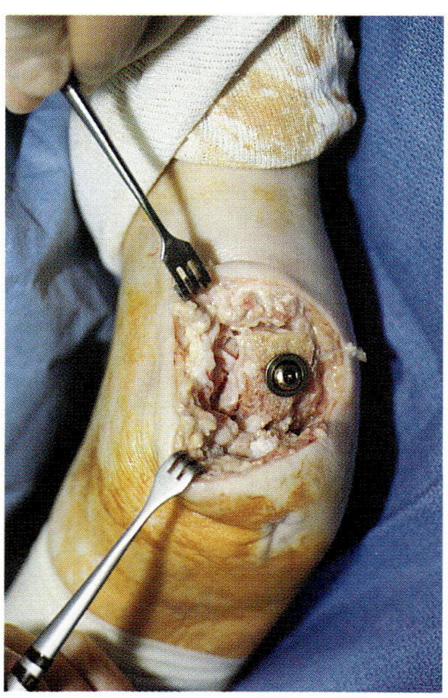

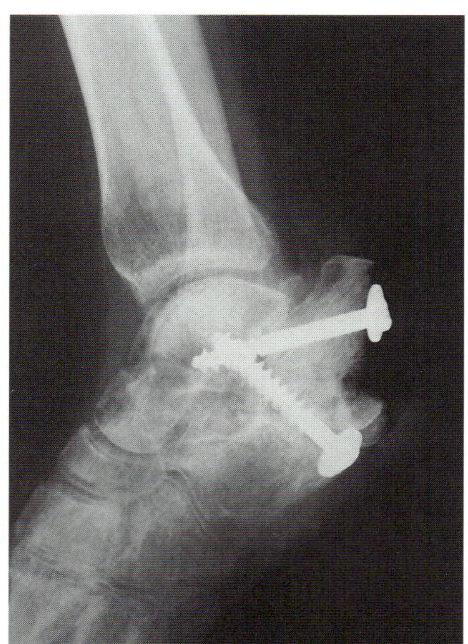

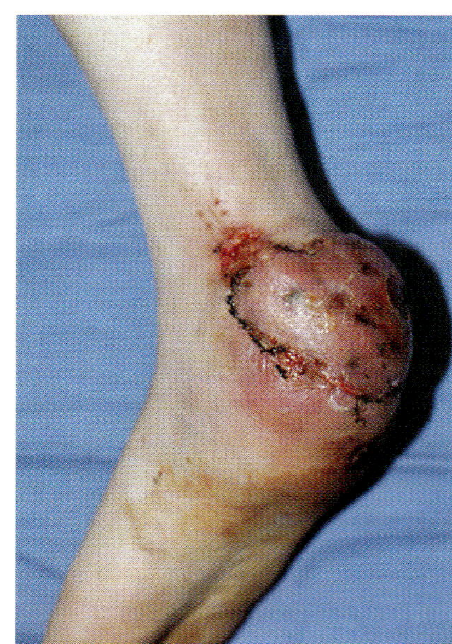

Consequently the patient was taken to the operating room where excision of all involved skin and soft tissue was performed and the calcaneus was reduced and rigidly fixated with screws. Wound closure was obtained with gracilis muscle transfer and split-thickness skin graft. Healing occurred with some initial loss of the skin graft.

Eight months after flap transfer some shrinkage was noted. The patient continued to complain of a sheering sensation over the calcaneus and the contour deformity that prevented her from wearing most of her preinjury footwear. Again the vascular pedicle was left undisturbed. The patient was returned to surgery for wedge excision and reclosure of the muscle flap. A marginal wedge of muscle was removed without difficulty after raising it intact from the posterior defect. The patient was treated postoperatively with a compressive device for several weeks followed by the application of a compressive elastic bandage for the next 4 months.

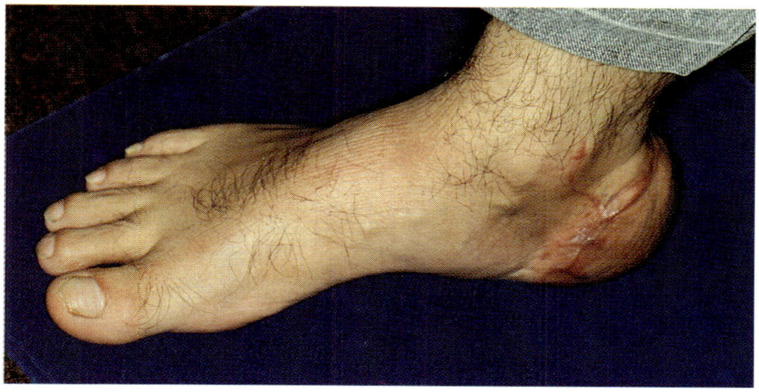

Normal contour and shoe fit with successful debulking was achieved with minimal flap reelevation and reorientation.

CONCLUSION

Ideally there may come a day when refinements in reconstructive surgery allow us to address functional and aesthetic problems in a single operative procedure with one composite tissue transfer. Isolated but encouraging reports that describe single-stage comprehensive reconstruction of multiorgan defects are surfacing.[21] Presently, however, most injuries that involve multiple structures, including significant loss of overlying skin and soft tissue, require at least one additional and often multiple staged secondary procedures to achieve maximal restoration of function and cosmesis. Most important in our considerations during the planning of reoperative procedures in the previously wounded extremities are those regarding vascularity.[22] Although it is generally accepted that delayed transection of a vascular pedicle and a transferred flap may be safely performed after some arbitrary period, it should be remembered that in most circumstances initial flap transfer was required for a relative lack of vascularity to the wound space. In this regard maintenance of vascular pedicles in secondarily operated tissue transfers should be maintained whenever possible. Elevation of flaps for subsequent revision or for further operation to subtending structures should be limited to only that amount deemed necessary for the completion of the objective for two reasons: (1) it helps to maintain maximal blood flow to the revised flap and (2) it minimizes the operative trauma to the surgically disrupted tissue planes. Timing of reoperative flap surgery varies widely with the intended goals of the procedure. Flaps have been reelevated electively as soon as 2 days after initial placement and as long as several years after transfer. Reoperation for the restoration of tendon function can be maximized by allowing tissue equilibrium to be achieved as is classically taught for all tendon transfers. Compression garments are well tolerated in revised flaps and should be used liberally to minimize postoperative swelling.

As it is in the quest for a universal cancer cure, the best way to avoid the problems of secondary or reoperative surgery after flap transfer in the extremities is to prevent occurrence initially. As previously stated, given the further maturation and refinement of free tissue transfer and extremity reconstructive surgery, the more that can be achieved at the primary operative setting, the less the need for secondary surgery at the outset.

References

1. Acland RD. Refinements in lower extremity free flap surgery. Clin Plast Surg 17:733-744, 1990.
2. Melissinos EG, Parks H. Post-trauma reconstruction with free tissue transfer: Analysis of 442 consecutive cases. J Trauma 29:1095-1103, 1989.
3. Anthony JP, Mathes S, Alpert BS. The muscle flap in the treatment of chronic lower extremity osteomyelitis: Results in patients over five years after treatment. Plast Reconstr Surg 88:311, 1991.
4. Godina M. Selection of recipient vessels in the lower leg for microvascular flap transfer. Thesis on the Management of Injuries to the Lower Extremity. Ljublijana: Presernova Irbzba, 1991.
5. Feibel RJ, Oliva A, Buncke GM, et al. Soft tissue reconstruction in orthopedic surgery: Secondary procedures. Orthop Clin North Am 24:537-548, 1993.
6. Chowdary RP, Murphy RX. Delayed debulking of free muscle flaps for aesthetic contouring. Br J Plast Surg 45:38-41, 1992.
7. Tsur H, Daniller A, Strauch B. Neovascularization of skin flaps: Route and timing. Plast Reconstr Surg 66:85, 1980.
8. Brandt KE, Howell RL, DeLozier JB, et al. Management of traumatic soft tissue injuries during Ilizarov external fixation. Plast Surg Forum 14:388-391, 1991.
9. Jupiter JB, Kour AK, Palumbo MD, et al. Limb reconstruction by free-tissue transfer combined with the Ilizarov method. Plast Reconstr Surg 88:943-951, 1991.
10. Black MJ, Chait L, Sykes P, et al. How soon may the axial vessels of a surviving free flap be safely ligated: A study in pigs. Br J Plast Surg 31:295, 1978.
11. Khoo CTK, Bailey BN. The behavior of free muscle and musculocutaneous flaps after early loss of axial blood supply. Br J Plast Surg 35:43-46, 1982.
12. Khouri RK, Shaw WW. Reconstruction of the lower extremity with microvascular free flaps: A 10-year experience with 304 consecutive cases. J Trauma 29:1086, 1989.
13. Gordon L, Chiu EJ. Treatment of infected nonunions and segmental defects of the tibia with staged microvascular muscle transplantation and bone grafting. J Bone Joint Surg 70(A):377, 1988.

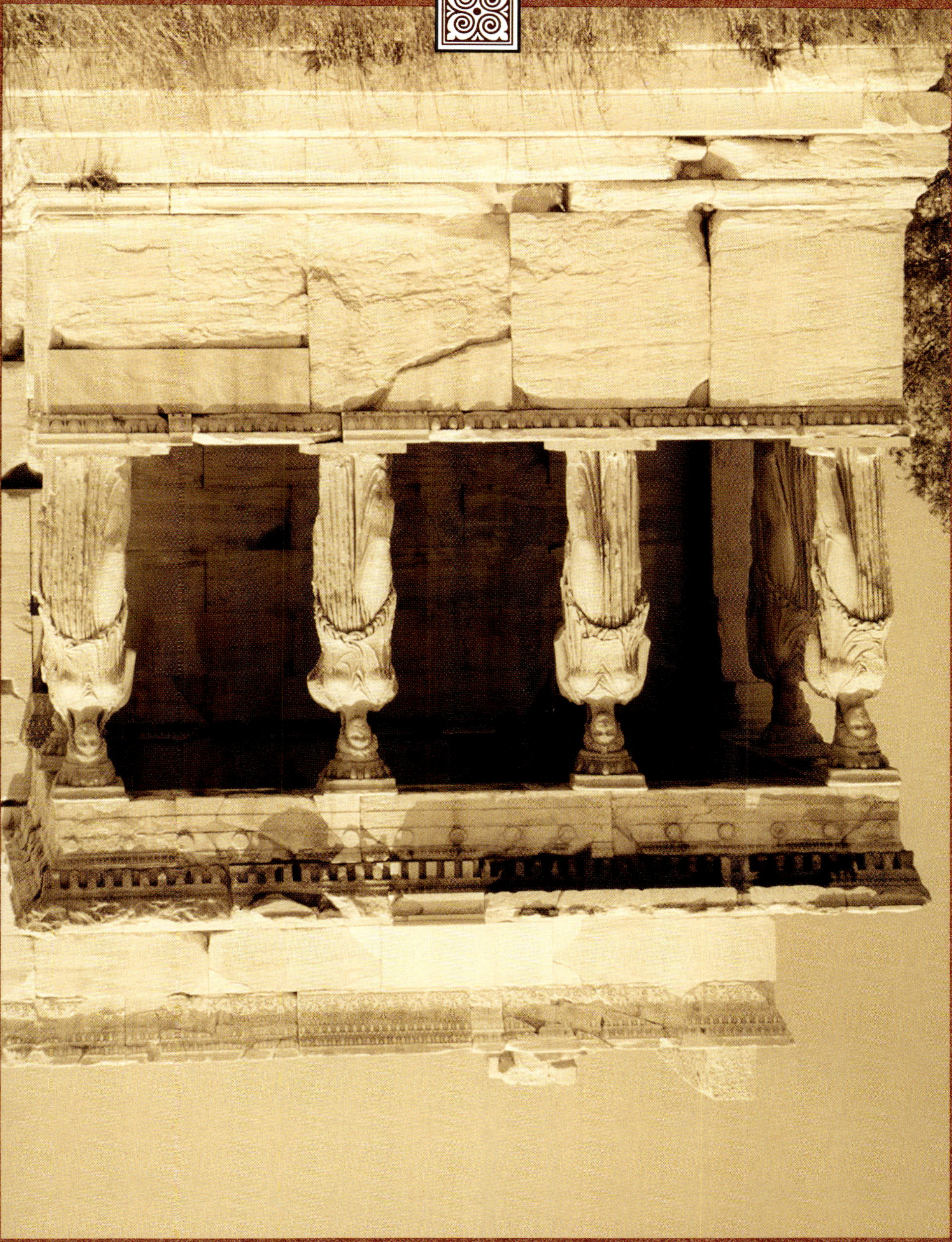

14. Blick SS, Brumback RJ, Lakatos R, et al. Early prophylactic bone grafting of high-energy tibial fractures. Clin Orthop 240:21-41, 1989.
15. Ger R. Muscle transposition for treatment and prevention of chronic posttraumatic osteomyelitis of the tibia. J Bone Joint Surg 59(A):784, 1977.
16. Chang N, Mathes JS. Comparison of the effect of bacterial inoculation in musculocutaneous and random-pattern flaps. Plast Reconstr Surg 70:1, 1982.
17. Francel TJ, Vander Kolk CA, Hopper JE, et al. Microvascular soft tissue transplantation for reconstruction of acute open tibial fractures: Timing of coverage and long-term functional results. Plast Reconstr Surg 89:478-487, 1992.
18. Weiland AJ, Daniel RK. Microvascular anastomosis for bone grafts in the treatment of massive defects in bone. J Bone Joint Surg 61(A):98, 1979.
19. Minami A, Kimura T, Matsumoto O, et al. Fracture through united vascularized bone grafts. J Reconstr Microsurg 9:227-232, 1993.
20. Coleman JJ III. Long-term evaluation of muscle and musculocutaneous flaps. In Mathes SJ, Nahai F, eds. Clinical Applications for Muscle and Musculocutaneous Flaps, 1st ed. St. Louis: Mosby, 1982.
21. Godina M. Early microsurgical reconstruction of complex trauma to the extremities. Plast Reconstr Surg 78:285, 1986.
22. Millican PG, Poole MD. Peripheral neovascularization of muscle and musculocutaneous flaps. Br J Plast Surg 38:369-374, 1985.

VII

In Closing

45

In Closing

James C. Grotting, M.D.

The ancient Greeks built the Acropolis with the intention that it would endure for eternity. A similar optimism motivates most plastic surgeons in their operative attempts to preserve and restore the human form. Just as monuments are subject to natural and man-made assaults, however, so is our surgical artistry susceptible to the ravages of time, disease, and biologic processes. Thus reoperative plastic surgery becomes a practical necessity as we use the newest technology and most advanced surgical techniques in our efforts to correct complications, refine results, and reverse the stigmata of aging.

The ongoing challenge for the reoperative surgeon is defining the end point for surgical intervention. When is the result considered final and unimprovable? Can we be satisfied with an exceptionally well-contoured breast reconstruction that remains insensate or will nerve grafts performed at the time of reconstruction or in a secondary procedure achieve a more perfect reconstruction? In the case of mandibular reconstruction, is restored contour sufficient or is dental restoration needed to enable normal mastication? Reoperative plastic surgery continues to evolve. Each time one operates, something new is learned. Each secondary procedure offers the potential for devising new solutions to old problems and enhancing one's appreciation of how scarred tissue planes respond to traction and tension. Innovation and technology further influence this learning process and contribute to redefining our expectations for the final result.

Technologic improvements and new ideas have simplified certain secondary procedures and have made others possible. Tissue expansion, endoscopy, and liposuction have proved to be viable solutions for a number of reoperative reconstructive problems. With tissue expansion, scar-damaged skin or grafts can now be replaced with nearby expanded flaps of similar color and texture. Endoscopy also offers tremendous potential for reoperative surgery, making it possible to approach operative sites through distant ports with minimal incisions. Now implant malposition after transaxillary augmentation mammaplasty can be corrected via endoscopic visualization without the need for an additional inframammary incision. Similarly the recurrence of glabellar creases following coronal browlift can be addressed secondarily through an endoscopic approach.

The tumescent technique for liposuction and the use of small cannulas for fat contouring in the superficial plane both have helped to prevent secondary deformities and to treat them when they do occur. For example, persistent malar bags following blepharoplasty may be effectively treated with a 2 mm suction cannula. Other difficult reoperative problems as well as formerly untreatable areas such as dorsal back folds are now amenable to treatment with superficial suction using the tumescent technique. With the advent of better fat removal techniques has also come improved methods of autologous fat grafting. Fat injection can now be used to treat secondary contour deformities and dermal adhesions to underlying fascial planes. As our understanding and appreciation of these new technologies deepen, the applications continue to evolve and we are challenged as to how to best use these new tools. In light of the changes that are affecting health care today, sound clinical judgment is a skill as essential as technical expertise.

Health care reform has significant implications for reconstructive and aesthetic plastic surgery. Global fee policies by insurance carriers will place an added burden on patients and surgeons as we try to accomplish as much as possible in one operation since a subsequent procedure may not be reimbursed, regardless of whether the surgeon and patient believe the surgery is necessary. Thus the final result for the patient may be determined by the policies instituted by managed care groups or insurance companies rather than by the limits of the reoperative plastic surgeon's creativity.

This book represents a collection of thoughts and techniques in evolution. Often the person who learns the most from writing scientific material is the author himself; one of the benefits of having edited this book is what I have learned from each of the contributors. My patients have been the benefactors of the information and techniques garnered from the contributors of this book. It is my hope that *Reoperative Aesthetic and Reconstructive Plastic Surgery* will stimulate readers to reflect on the ways they have solved particular operative problems, to develop means of minimizing the need for reoperations and increasing the safety and predictability of primary procedures, and to communicate their innovations through the literature. With carefully documented outcome studies, we can influence managed care decisions regarding the quality of treatment for our patients. By educating one another, we can vitalize and elevate the discussion of solutions to our common problems.

INDEX

A

C

G

M

N

O

R

S

T

U

V